MODERN SURGICAL CARE

Third Edition
Volume 2

MODERN SURGICAL CARE

Physiologic Foundations and Clinical Applications

Third Edition
Volume 2

editor-in-chief

Thomas A. Miller, M.D.

Ammons Professor of Surgery
Division of General Surgery
Department of Surgery
Virginia Commonwealth University School of Medicine and Medical Center
Chief of Surgery
Hunter Holmes McGuire Veterans Affairs Medical Center
Richmond, Virginia, USA

informa

healthcare

New York   London

Informa Healthcare USA, Inc.
270 Madison Avenue
New York, NY 10016

© 2006 by Informa Healthcare USA, Inc.
Informa Healthcare is an Informa business

No claim to original U.S. Government works
Printed in the United States of America on acid-free paper
10 9 8 7 6 5 4 3 2 1

International Standard Book Number-10: 0-8247-2869-6 (Hardcover)
International Standard Book Number-13: 978-0-8247-2869-4 (Hardcover)

Visit the Informa Web site at
www.informa.com

and the Informa Healthcare Web site at
www.informahealthcare.com

DEDICATION

To all trainees in surgery,
medical students rotating on surgical services,
and surgeons in practice
who recognize the importance of
understanding the physiologic underpinnings of
treating surgical disease
in order to ensure optimal patient care.

Preface

When the first edition of this book was published in 1988 under the title *Physiologic Basis of Modern Surgical Care*, its goal was to bridge the gap that commonly exists between basic science information regarding human disease and the ability to apply this knowledge to everyday clinical care. In teaching medical students rotating on surgery, as well as residents embarking on surgical careers, many of my colleagues and I, serving on medical school faculties across the country, were all too acutely aware that management of surgical disorders by these trainees was frequently based on memorized schemes or protocols rather than a thorough understanding of the pathophysiology underlying a particular disease. To address this issue, we published the initial edition with the intent to approach surgical disease as a derangement in normal physiology and that the best way to diagnose and treat it was to understand thoroughly this deviation from normal. We were very gratified with the acceptance of the book by the surgical community and its adoption by many program directors as essential reading to prepare residents for various examinations, such as the annual in-service training examination in surgery and the board certification examination following completion of surgical training. We also received many positive comments from established surgeons regarding its usefulness in preparing for recertification exams.

Because of the wide acceptance of the first edition as an important vehicle to train house officers in the physiologic underpinnings of surgical disease, a second edition was published in 1998 under the title *Modern Surgical Care: Physiologic Foundations and Clinical Applications*. The title change was made to more adequately reflect the linkage between physiology and clinical care. We have been especially pleased with the continuing acceptance of the second edition as an important educational tool and were extremely grateful when Informa Healthcare (formerly Marcel Dekker, Inc.) asked us to produce a third edition.

In addition to being thoroughly updated, the third edition reflects the capable assistance and counsel of a group of associate editors who have contributed greatly in streamlining chapters, minimizing repetitive material, adding new chapters to include cutting-edge material, and selecting a more diverse and mainstream authorship who are the current leaders in their fields. Their recommendations were responsible for the inclusion of 91 new authors not involved in the previous editions. These associate editors include Drs. Barbara Bass, Jeff Fabri, Carl Haisch, Dave Mercer, Ron Merrell, and Stuart Myers. To each of them, I offer my utmost thanks and gratitude.

As reflected in the previous editions, the needs of the general surgeon continue to be emphasized in the present edition. Further, the goal of this third edition remains the same, namely to approach surgical disease as a derangement in normal physiology, which needs to be corrected to as near normal as possible to effectively manage and treat the underlying disorder. This book is divided into nine parts, with the first part devoted to information pertinent to the body as a whole, and the eight remaining sections focused on specific organ systems or themes. Diseases affecting the reproductive organs, disorders of the head and neck (other than the thyroid and parathyroid glands), and disorders of the musculoskeletal system are not specifically dealt with because the current practice of surgery only rarely involves these disciplines. Finally, this book is not meant to replace standard textbooks of surgery and, accordingly, is not a comprehensive discussion of all surgical diseases. For less common types of surgical problems or those not regularly encountered in the practice of general surgery, such books should be consulted.

I would personally like to offer my sincere appreciation to the folks at Informa Healthcare who have worked with us during the production of the book. I have found everyone with whom I have collaborated to be extremely professional, cordial, and helpful in making sure that this third edition meets the goals that we have set. I would especially like to recognize two people with whom I have had a very close working relationship. The first is Joe Stubenrauch who has been the project editor. He has more than met my expectations and has demonstrated unusual adaptability when I thought something should be done for which initially he and I had differing viewpoints. The second individual is Joanne Jay who was responsible for the final editing of each chapter and preparing the galley proofs. Her attention to detail has been exemplary. I have been very pleased with the outstanding quality of her editorial review. To both of these individuals I say "Thank you!" They made the process of finalizing this book most pleasurable.

Thomas A. Miller, M.D.

Contents

VOLUME 2

PART THREE: THE CARDIOTHORACIC SYSTEM

■ **Lung**

Contributors

Ramzi Alami, MD Fellow in Advanced Laparoscopic Surgery, Department of Surgery, Stanford University Medical Center, Palo Alto, California, U.S.A.

Joseph F. Amaral, MD President and CEO, Rhode Island Hospital, Professor of Surgery, Brown University Medical School, Providence, Rhode Island, U.S.A.

Paul A. Armstrong, DO Clinical Assistant Professor of Surgery, Department of Surgery, University of South Florida College of Medicine, Tampa, Florida, U.S.A.

Dennis F. Bandyk, MD Professor of Surgery, Director, Division of Vascular Surgery, University of South Florida College of Medicine, Tampa, Florida, U.S.A.

Ronald M. Barton, MD Associate Professor of Surgery Emeritus, Director of the Burn Center Emeritus, Division of Plastic Surgery, Department of Surgery, Virginia Commonwealth University School of Medicine and Medical Center, Richmond, Virginia, U.S.A.

Giacomo P. Basadonna, MD Professor of Surgery, Department of Surgery, University of Massachusetts Medical School, Worcester, Massachusetts, U.S.A.

Barbara L. Bass, MD Professor of Surgery, Department of Surgery, Weill Medical College of Cornell University, New York, New York; Carolyn and John F. Bookout Chair, Department of Surgery, The Methodist Hospital, Houston, Texas, U.S.A.

David J. Bentrem, MD Assistant Professor of Surgery, Department of Surgery, Surgical Oncology, Northwestern University Feinberg School of Medicine, Chicago, Illinois, U.S.A.

Timothy R. Billiar, MD The George Vance Foster Professor and Chair, Department of Surgery, Presbyterian University Hospital, University of Pittsburgh Medical Center, Pittsburgh, Pennsylvania, U.S.A.

Karen Bitzer, OTR/L, CHT Musculoskeletal Division Coordinator, Department of Rehabilitation Services, University Hospitals of Cleveland, Cleveland, Ohio, U.S.A.

Mark Bloomston, MD Fellow in Surgical Oncology, Ohio State University Medical Center, Columbus, Ohio, U.S.A.

Edward L. Bove, MD Helen and Marvin Kirsh Professor of Surgery, Professor and Section Head, Cardiac Surgery, Director, Pediatric Cardiac Surgery, University of Michigan, C. S. Mott Children's Hospital, Ann Arbor, Michigan, U.S.A.

William C. Broaddus, MD, PhD Hord Professor, Department of Neurosurgery, Virginia Commonwealth University Health System; Chief of Neurosurgery, Hunter Holmes McGuire Veterans Affairs Medical Center, Richmond, Virginia, U.S.A.

Robert E. Brolin, MD Adjunct Professor of Surgery, University of Pittsburgh Medical Center, Pittsburgh, Pennsylvania, Director

of Bariatric Surgery, University Medical Center at Princeton, Princeton, New Jersey, U.S.A.

Kevin Bruen, MD Resident in Surgery, Department of Surgery, University of Utah School of Medicine, Salt Lake City, Utah, U.S.A.

M. Ross Bullock, MD, PhD Reynolds Professor, Department of Neurosurgery, Virginia Commonwealth University Health System, Richmond, Virginia, U.S.A.

Michael D. Caldwell, MD, PhD Director of Marshfield Medical Research and Education Foundation, Director of the Wound Healing Clinic, Marshfield, Wisconsin, U.S.A.

Thomas C. Chelimsky, MD Associate Professor of Neurology, Department of Neurology, Case Western Reserve University School of Medicine, Cleveland, Ohio, U.S.A.

G. Patrick Clagett, MD Professor and Chairman, Division of Vascular and Endovascular Surgery, Department of Surgery; Ian and Bob Pickens Distinguished Professorship in Medical Science; Director, Center for Vascular Disease, University of Texas Southwestern Medical Center, Dallas, Texas, U.S.A.

Neri M. Cohen, MD, PhD Chief, Division of Thoracic Surgery, Greater Baltimore Medical Center Health Care, Baltimore, Maryland, U.S.A.

Sheila M. Coogan, MD Assistant Professor of Surgery, Vascular Surgery Service, Palo Alto Veterans Affairs Hospital, Stanford University School of Medicine, Palo Alto, California, U.S.A.

Peter F. Crookes, MD Associate Professor of Surgery, Director of Bariatric Surgery Program, Department of Surgery, University of Southern California Keck School of Medicine, Los Angeles, California, U.S.A.

Eric J. DeMaria, MD Professor and Chief, Endoscopy and Bariatric Surgery, Vice Chair, Network General Surgery, Chief, Duke General Surgery at Durham Regional Hospital, Duke University Medical Center, Durham, North Carolina, U.S.A.

Daniel T. Dempsey, MD Professor and Chairman, Department of Surgery, Temple University School of Medicine, Philadelphia, Pennsylvania, U.S.A.

Gerard M. Doherty, MD Norman W. Thompson Professor of Surgery, Head, Section of General Surgery; Chief, Division of Endocrine Surgery, University of Michigan, Ann Arbor, Michigan, U.S.A.

Philip E. Donahue, MD Professor of Surgery, Department of Surgery, University of Illinois Medical Center at Chicago; Chairman, Division of General Surgery, John H. Stroger, Jr. Hospital of Cook County, Chicago, Illinois, U.S.A.

Egon M. R. Doppenberg, MD Former Chief Resident, Department of Neurosurgery, Virginia Commonwealth University

Health System, Richmond, Virginia; presently in neurosurgery private practice in Chicago, Illinois, U.S.A.

Akinsan Dosekun, MD   Associate Professor of Internal Medicine, Department of Internal Medicine, The University of Texas Medical School at Houston, Houston, Texas, U.S.A.

Ashley E. Ducale, MPT, PhD   Post-Doctoral Fellow, Department of Surgery, Wound Healing Laboratory, Virginia Commonwealth University School of Medicine, Richmond, Virginia, U.S.A.

Rodney Durham, MD   Professor of Surgery, Department of Surgery, Division of Trauma and Critical Care, University of South Florida College of Medicine, Tampa General Hospital, Tampa, Florida, U.S.A.

Douglas B. Evans, MD   Professor of Surgery, The University of Texas M.D. Anderson Cancer Center, Houston, Texas, U.S.A.

B. Mark Evers, MD   Professor and Robertson-Poth Distinguished Chair in General Surgery, Department of Surgery, The University of Texas Medical Branch, Galveston, Texas, U.S.A.

Peter J. Fabri, MD   Professor of Surgery, Associate Dean for Graduate Medical Education, University of South Florida College of Medicine, Tampa, Florida, U.S.A.

Andrew C. Fiore, MD   Professor of Surgery, Division of Cardiothoracic Surgery, Department of Surgery, St. Louis University School of Medicine; Chief of Cardiothoracic Surgery, Cardinal Glennon Children's Hospital, St. Louis, Missouri, U.S.A.

John R. Foringer, MD   Assistant Professor of Internal Medicine, Department of Internal Medicine, The University of Texas Medical School at Houston, Houston, Texas, U.S.A.

O. Howard Frazier, MD   Professor of Surgery, University of Texas Health Science Center at Houston; Professor of Surgery, Baylor College of Medicine; Chief of Cardiopulmonary Transplantation; Director of Cardiovascular Surgery Research, Texas Heart Institute, Houston, Texas, U.S.A.

Julie A. Freischlag, MD   William Stewart Halstead Professor of Surgery, Chair, Department of Surgery; Surgeon-in-Chief, Johns Hopkins Medical Center, Baltimore, Maryland, U.S.A.

Janette Gaw, MD   Former Chief Resident, Department of Surgery, Yale University School of Medicine, New Haven, Connecticut; presently in colorectal surgery private practice, Fort Myers, Florida, U.S.A.

Bruce L. Gewertz, MD   Dallas B. Phemister Professor and Chair, Department of Surgery, The University of Chicago, Chicago, Illinois, U.S.A.

Rafik M. Ghobrial, MD, PhD   Professor of Surgery, Director, Liver, Pancreas and Small Bowel Transplantation, The Dumont-UCLA Transplant Center, David Geffen School of Medicine of the University of California at Los Angeles, Los Angeles, California, U.S.A.

George K. Gittes, MD   Surgeon-in-Chief, Children's Hospital of Pittsburgh, Professor of Surgery, Division Chief, Pediatric Surgery, Department of Surgery, University of Pittsburgh Medical Center, Pittsburgh, Pennsylvania, U.S.A.

Deborah T. Glassman, MD   Clinical Assistant Professor, Department of Urology, Thomas Jefferson University, Philadelphia, Pennsylvania, U.S.A.

Bobby S. Glickman, MD   Instructor of Surgery, Department of Surgery, University of Nebraska Medical Center, Omaha, Nebraska, U.S.A.

R. Scott Graham, MD   Associate Professor of Neurosurgery, Department of Neurosurgery, Virginia Commonwealth University School of Medicine and Medical Center, Richmond, Virginia, U.S.A.

Bartley P. Griffith, MD   Professor of Surgery, Chief, Division of Cardiac Surgery, Director, Heart and Lung Transplantation, Maryland Heart Center, University of Maryland Medical Center, Baltimore, Maryland, U.S.A.

Dipin Gupta, MD   Fellow, Cardiovascular Surgery, New York University School of Medicine, New York, New York, U.S.A.

Carl E. Haisch, MD   Professor of Surgery, Department of Surgery, East Carolina University Brody School of Medicine, Director of Surgical Immunology and Transplantation; Attending Surgeon, Pitt County Memorial Hospital, Greenville, North Carolina, U.S.A.

Nahid Hamoui, MD   Assistant Professor of Surgery, Department of Surgery, University of Southern California Keck School of Medicine, Los Angeles, California, U.S.A.

Sean P. Harbison, MD   Associate Professor of Surgery, Department of Surgery, Temple University School of Medicine, Philadelphia, Pennsylvania, U.S.A.

Kenneth S. Helmer, MD   Assistant Professor of Surgery, Department of Surgery, University of Texas Medical School at Houston, Houston, Texas, U.S.A.

Ana O. Hoff, MD   Assistant Professor of Endocrinology, The University of Texas M.D. Anderson Cancer Center, Houston, Texas, U.S.A.

Kathryn Holloway, MD   Professor of Neurosurgery, Department of Neurosurgery, Virginia Commonwealth University Health System; Neurosurgical Director of the Southeast Parkinson's Disease Research, Education and Clinical Care Center of Excellence (PADRECC) at Hunter Holmes McGuire Veterans Affairs Medical Center, Richmond, Virginia, U.S.A.

Kamal M. F. Itani, MD   Professor of Surgery, Boston University Medical Center, Chief of Surgery, VA Boston Health Care System, Boston, Massachusetts, U.S.A.

Lindsey N. Jackson, MD   Resident in General Surgery, Department of Surgery, The University of Texas Medical Branch, Galveston, Texas, U.S.A.

Mark R. Jackson, MD   Former Associate Professor of Surgery, Division of Vascular Surgery, University of Texas Southwestern Medical School, Dallas, Texas; presently in vascular surgery private practice, St. Francis Hospital, Greenville, South Carolina, U.S.A.

Raymond J. Joehl, MD   Professor of Surgery, Program Director General Surgery Residency, Department of Surgery, Loyola University Medical Center, Maywood; Chief, Surgical Service and Manager, Surgery Service Line, The Charles B. Puestow Surgical Service, Edward Hines, Jr VA Hospital, Hines, Illinois, U.S.A.

Haytham M. A. Kaafarani, MD   Resident in Surgery, Department of Surgery, University of South Florida Medical School, Tampa, Florida, U.S.A.

Lillian S. Kao, MD   Assistant Professor of Surgery, Department of Surgery, University of Texas Medical School at Houston, Houston, Texas, U.S.A.

Gregory Kennedy, MD   Chief Resident in Surgery, Department of Surgery, University of Wisconsin Medical School, Madison, Wisconsin, U.S.A.

Jonathan Kiev, MD   Assistant Professor of Surgery, Division of Cardiothoracic Surgery, Department of Surgery, Virginia Commonwealth University School of Medicine and Medical Center, Richmond, Virginia, U.S.A.

V. Suzanne Klimberg, MD   Professor of Surgery, Department of Surgery, Director, Breast Surgical Oncology, University of Arkansas for Medical Services and the Arkansas Cancer Research Center, Little Rock, Arkansas, U.S.A.

Evan R. Kokoska, MD   Assistant Professor of Surgery, Department of Surgery–Pediatric Surgery Service, University of Arkansas for Medical Sciences, Little Rock, Arkansas, U.S.A.

Bruce C. Kone, MD   The James T. and Nancy B. Willerson Chair, Chairman, Department of Medicine, Professor of Internal Medicine and of Integrative Biology and Pharmacology, The University of Texas Medical School at Houston, Houston, Texas, U.S.A.

Kara C. Kort, MD   Assistant Professor of Surgery, Department of Surgery, State University of New York–Upstate Medical University, Syracuse, New York, U.S.A.

Maria A. Kouvaraki, MD, PhD   Fellow in Endocrine Surgery, The University of Texas M.D. Anderson Cancer Center, Houston, Texas, U.S.A.

Rosemary A. Kozar, MD, PhD   Associate Professor of Surgery, Department of Surgery, University of Texas Medical School at Houston, Houston, Texas, U.S.A.

Rakhshanda Layeeque, MD   Assistant Professor of Surgery, Department of Surgery, Surgical Oncology Section, University of Massachusetts Memorial Medical Center, Worcester, Massachusetts, U.S.A.

Jeffrey E. Lee, MD   Professor of Surgery, The University of Texas M.D. Anderson Cancer Center, Houston, Texas, U.S.A.

Kangmin Lee, MD   Resident in Neurosurgery, Department of Neurosurgery, Virginia Commonwealth University Health System, Richmond, Virginia, U.S.A.

Denise Lester, MD   Assistant Professor, Department of Anesthesiology, Virginia Commonwealth University School of Medicine and Medical Center; Director, Chronic Pain Clinic, Anesthesiology Service, McGuire Veterans Affairs Medical Center, Richmond, Virginia, U.S.A.

Terrence H. Liu, MD   Associate Clinical Professor of Surgery, Residency Program Director, UCSF–East Bay Surgery Program, University of California San Francisco School of Medicine, East Bay Campus, Oakland, California, U.S.A.

Walter E. Longo, MD   Professor and Vice Chairman, Chief, Division of General Surgery, Department of Surgery, Yale University School of Medicine, New Haven, Connecticut, U.S.A.

Patricia A. Lowry, MD   Associate Professor of Radiology, Department of Radiology, Virginia Commonwealth University School of Medicine and Medical Center, Richmond, Virginia, U.S.A.

Michael P. Macris, MD   Medical Director, Cardiovascular Surgery, Memorial Hermann Northwest Hospital, Houston, Texas, U.S.A.

Ajai K. Malhotra, MD   Assistant Professor of Surgery, Division of Trauma and Critical Care, Department of Surgery, Virginia Commonwealth University School of Medicine and Medical Center, Richmond, Virginia, U.S.A.

James F. McKinsey, MD   Associate Professor of Clinical Surgery and Site Chief of Vascular Surgery, Columbia University of New York Presbyterian Hospital System, New York, New York, U.S.A.

Irvine G. McQuarrie, MD, PhD   Associate Professor of Neurosurgery and Neuroscience, Department of Surgery, School of Medicine, Case Western Reserve University; Cleveland VA Medical Center, Cleveland, Ohio, U.S.A.

Margaret M. McQuiggan MS, RD, CNSD   Clinical Instructor, Department of Surgery, University of Texas Medical School at Houston, Houston, Texas, U.S.A.

Sheilendra S. Mehta, MD   Former Research Fellow in Pediatric Surgery, Division of Pediatric Surgery, Children's Mercy Hospital, Department of Surgery, University of Missouri School of Medicine at Kansas City, Kansas City, Missouri, U.S.A.

David W. Mercer, MD   Professor of Surgery and Vice Chairman, Department of Surgery, The University of Texas Health Science Center–Houston; Chief of Surgery, Lyndon Baines Johnson General Hospital, Houston, Texas, U.S.A.

Ronald C. Merrell, MD   Professor of Surgery, Department of Surgery, Virginia Commonwealth University School of Medicine and Medical Center, Richmond, Virginia, U.S.A.

Thomas A. Miller, MD   Ammons Professor of Surgery, Division of General Surgery, Department of Surgery, Virginia Commonwealth University School of Medicine and Medical Center; Chief of Surgery, Hunter Holmes McGuire Veterans Affairs Medical Center, Richmond, Virginia, U.S.A.

Sina L. Moainie, MD   Resident in Cardiothoracic Surgery, Maryland Heart Center, University of Maryland Medical Center, Baltimore, Maryland, U.S.A.

Jeffrey F. Moley, MD   Professor of Surgery and Chief, Endocrine and Oncologic Surgery, Washington University School of Medicine; Associate Director, Alvin J. Siteman Cancer Center; Attending Surgeon, Barnes-Jewish Hospital, St. Louis, Missouri, U.S.A.

Frederick A. Moore, MD   Professor of Surgery and Vice Chairman, Department of Surgery, Medical Director, Trauma Services, University of Texas Medical School at Houston, Houston, Texas, U.S.A.

Ralph S. Mosca, MD   Associate Professor of Surgery, Columbia University College of Physicians and Surgeons; Associate Attending Surgeon, New York Presbyterian Hospital/Columbia University Medical Center, New York, New York, U.S.A.

Carlos A. Murillo, MD   Resident Instructor, Department of Surgery, Texas Tech University Health Sciences Center, El Paso School of Medicine, El Paso, Texas, U.S.A.

Stuart I. Myers, MD   Professor of Surgery, Division of Vascular Surgery, Department of Surgery, Virginia Commonwealth University School of Medicine and Medical Center; Attending Surgeon, Hunter Holmes McGuire Veterans Affairs Medical Center, Richmond, Virginia, U.S.A.

Attila Nakeeb, MD   Associate Professor of Surgery, Department of Surgery, Indiana University School of Medicine, Indianapolis, Indiana, U.S.A.

Lena M. Napolitano, MD   Professor of Surgery, Director, Surgical Critical Care; Associate Chair, Department of Surgery, University of Michigan Health System, Ann Arbor, Michigan, U.S.A.

Leigh Neumayer, MD   Professor of Surgery, Program Director, Utah Building Interdisciplinary Research Careers in Women's Health, University of Utah Medical Center, Salt Lake City, Utah, U.S.A.

John E. Niederhuber, MD   Acting Director, National Cancer Institute, Bethesda, Maryland; Former Director, University of Wisconsin Comprehensive Cancer Center, Madison, Wisconsin, U.S.A.

Unyime O. Nseyo, MD   Adjunct Professor, Department of Urology, University of Florida School of Medicine; Chief, Urology Section, Malcom Randall VA Medical Center, Gainesville, Florida, U.S.A.

Fiemu E. Nwariaku, MD   Associate Professor and Vice Chairman, Division of Gastrointestinal and Endocrine Surgery, Department of Surgery, University of Texas Southwestern Medical Center, Dallas, Texas, U.S.A.

Daniel J. Ostlie, MD   Associate Professor of Surgery, Division of Pediatric Surgery, Children's Mercy Hospital, Department of Surgery, University of Missouri School of Medicine at Kansas City, Kansas City, Missouri, U.S.A.

Lucian Panait, MD   Former Postdoctoral Research Fellow, Department of Surgery, Virginia Commonwealth University School of Medicine, Richmond, Virginia, U.S.A.

Donald H. Parks, MD   Professor and Chief, Division of Plastic and Reconstructive Surgery, Department of Surgery, University of Texas Medical School at Houston, Houston, Texas, U.S.A.

Jose R. Parra, MD   Former Assistant Professor of Surgery, Division of Vascular Surgery, Department of Surgery, Johns Hopkins Medical Center, Baltimore, Maryland, U.S.A.

Christina Paylan, MD   Former Fellow in Trauma and Critical Care, Department of Surgery, University of South Florida College of Medicine, Tampa General Hospital, Regional Trauma Center, Tampa, Florida, U.S.A; presently in plastic surgery private practice, Tampa, Florida, U.S.A.

Melissa F. Perkal, MD   Assistant Professor of Surgery, Director, Veterans Affairs Hospital Surgical Intensive Care Unit, Director, Surgical Preceptor Program, Department of Surgery, Yale University School of Medicine, New Haven, Connecticut, U.S.A.

Henry A. Pitt, MD   Professor and Vice Chairman, Department of Surgery, Indiana University School of Medicine, Indianapolis, Indiana, U.S.A.

Jose M. Prince, MD   Surgical Resident, Department of Surgery, University of Pittsburgh Medical Center, Pittsburgh, Pennsylvania, U.S.A.

Frank J. Quayle, MD   Resident in Surgery, Department of Surgery, Division of General Surgery, Washington University School of Medicine, St. Louis, Missouri, U.S.A.

J. Robert Ramey, MD   Chief Resident in Urology, Department of Urology, Thomas Jefferson University, Philadelphia, Pennsylvania, U.S.A.

Cristiana Rastellini, MD   Associate Professor, Department of Surgery, University of Massachusetts Medical School, Worcester, Massachusetts, U.S.A.

Lorita Rebellato, PhD   Associate Professor of Pathology, Department of Pathology, East Carolina University Brody School of Medicine, Greenville, North Carolina, U.S.A.

Kathryn A. Richardson, MD   Assistant Professor, Department of Surgery, Louisiana State University Health Sciences Center, Shreveport, Louisiana, U.S.A.

Alexander S. Rosemurgy, MD   Professor of Surgery and Medicine, Director, Division of General Surgery, Surgical Director, Tampa General Hospital Digestive Disorders Center, University of South Florida College of Medicine, Tampa, Florida, U.S.A.

Ronnie Ann Rosenthal, MS, MD   Associate Professor of Surgery, Yale University School of Medicine, New Haven; Chief, Surgical Service, Veterans Affairs Connecticut Healthcare System, West Haven, Connecticut, U.S.A.

Shawn D. St. Peter, MD   Assistant Professor of Surgery, Division of Pediatric Surgery, Children's Mercy Hospital, Department of Surgery, University of Missouri School of Medicine at Kansas City, Kansas City, Missouri, U.S.A.

Jeannie F. Savas, MD   Associate Professor of Surgery, Division of General Surgery, Department of Surgery, Virginia Commonwealth University School of Medicine and Medical Center; Attending Surgeon, Hunter Holmes McGuire Veterans Affairs Medical Center, Richmond, Virginia, U.S.A.

Henry J. Schiller, MD   Associate Professor of Surgery, Department of Surgery, Mayo Clinic School of Medicine, Rochester, Minnesota, U.S.A.

Lelan F. Sillin, MD, MS(Ed)   Professor of Surgery, Vice Chair for Educational Affairs, Department of Surgery, University of Rochester Medical Center, Rochester, New York, U.S.A.

Michael Sobel, MD   Professor and Vice Chairman, Department of Surgery, University of Washington; Professor and Chief, Puget Sound Veterans Affairs Health Care System, Seattle, Washington, U.S.A.

James C. Stanley, MD   Handleman Professor of Surgery, Section of Vascular Surgery, Department of Surgery, University of Michigan Medical Center, Ann Arbor, Michigan, U.S.A.

Heinrich Taegtmeyer, MD, DPhil   Professor of Medicine, Division of Cardiology, Department of Internal Medicine, University of Texas Medical School at Houston, Houston, Texas, U.S.A.

Daniel G. Tang, MD Chief Resident in General Surgery, Department of Surgery, Virginia Commonwealth University School of Medicine and Medical Center, Richmond, Virginia, U.S.A.

Jon S. Thompson, MD Professor and Vice Chairman, Department of Surgery, University of Nebraska Medical Center, Omaha, Nebraska, U.S.A.

Hari Siva Gurunadha Rao Tunuguntla, MD, MBBS, MS (Surgery), MCh Resident, Department of Urology, University of Miami, Miller School of Medicine, Miami, Florida, U.S.A.

Richard H. Turnage, MD Professor of Surgery and Chairman, Department of Surgery, Louisiana State University Health Sciences Center, Shreveport, Louisiana, U.S.A.

Douglas J. Turner, MD Assistant Professor of Surgery, Division of General Surgery, Department of Surgery, University of Maryland School of Medicine, Baltimore, Maryland, U.S.A.

Henry Ty, MD Former Chief Resident in Neurosurgery, Department of Neurosurgery, Virginia Commonwealth University Health System, Richmond, Virginia; presently in neurosurgery private practice, North Andover, Massachusetts, U.S.A.

Kathryn M. Verbanac, PhD Professor of Surgery, Division of Transplantation, Department of Surgery, East Carolina University Brody School of Medicine, Greenville, North Carolina, U.S.A.

David J. Wainwright, MD Associate Professor of Surgery, Division of Plastic and Reconstructive Surgery; Department of Surgery, University of Texas Medical School at Houston, Houston, Texas, U.S.A.

Jian-Ying Wang, MD, PhD Professor of Surgery and Pathology, Associate Chair for Basic Research, Department of Surgery, University of Maryland School of Medicine, Baltimore, Maryland, U.S.A.

Andrew S. Wechsler, MD Stanley K. Brockman Professor and Chairman, Department of Cardiovascular Medicine and Surgery, Drexel University College of Medicine, Philadelphia, Pennsylvania, U.S.A.

Glenn J. R. Whitman, MD Professor of Surgery, Division of Cardiothoracic Surgery, Temple University School of Medicine, Philadelphia, Pennsylvania, U.S.A.

Charles Williams, MD Associate Professor, Vice Chair for Veterans Affairs, Department of Anesthesiology, Virginia Commonwealth University School of Medicine and Medical Center; Chief, Anesthesiology Service, Hunter Holmes McGuire Veterans Affairs Medical Center, Richmond, Virginia, U.S.A.

Ryan M. Wolfort, MD Resident in Surgery, Department of Surgery, Louisiana State University Health Sciences Center, Shreveport, Louisiana, U.S.A.

Kenneth J. Woodside, MD Chief Resident in General Surgery, Department of Surgery, The University of Texas Medical Branch, Galveston, Texas, U.S.A.

Dorne R. Yager, PhD Associate Professor of Surgery, Physiology and Biochemistry, Director, Wound Healing Laboratory, Department of Surgery, Virginia Commonwealth University School of Medicine, Richmond, Virginia, U.S.A.

Christopher K. Zarins, MD Chidester Professor of Surgery, Chief, Division of Vascular Surgery, Stanford University Medical Center, Palo Alto, California, U.S.A.

Emmanuel E. Zervos, MD Assistant Professor of Surgery, Department of Surgery, Surgical Oncology, University of South Florida College of Medicine, Tampa General Hospital, Tampa, Florida, U.S.A.

Yuan Zhai, MD Assistant Professor of Surgery, Department of Surgery, Section of Liver and Pancreas Transplantation, David Geffen School of Medicine at University of California at Los Angeles, Los Angeles, California, U.S.A.

Huiping Zhou, PhD Assistant Professor, Department of Microbiology and Immunology, Virginia Commonwealth University School of Medicine, Richmond, Virginia, U.S.A.

31

Pathobiology of Surgically Relevant Pulmonary Disease

Daniel G. Tang, Jonathan Kiev, and Neri M. Cohen

INTRODUCTION

The pulmonary system is the body's gateway for exchange of gasses, principally oxygen and carbon dioxide. This critical function is essential to maintain the vital processes that enable the body to carry out its many functions. An understanding of the various derangements that may alter normal lung function is mandatory for the surgeon involved in the care of seriously ill patients. This chapter reviews the normal physiology of the pulmonary system and how aberrations from the norm present in surgically relevant lung disease.

ANATOMY AND PHYSIOLOGY

The airway consists of the oropharynx, trachea, bronchi, and bronchioles. The trachea extends from the cricoid cartilage of the larynx to the carina, where it branches into the left and right main bronchi. Bronchial branching is more acute on the left than the right, creating a more direct path to the right, which is therefore more frequently involved in aspirations and inadvertent bronchial main stem intubations. From the carina, the bronchi undergo approximately 25 subdivisions to the alveoli. The bronchi sequentially divide into lobar bronchi, segmental bronchi, bronchioles, and then alveoli. Anatomically, the lungs are divided into lobes and then segments based on the bronchial branching. There are three lobes on the right (upper, middle, and lower) and two lobes on the left (upper and lower; the lingula corresponds to the middle lobe) (Fig. 1).

Airway

The trachea is supported by 15 to 20 C-shaped cartilaginous rings anteriorly. The bronchi are also supported by cartilaginous plates, whereas the bronchioles and alveoli lack such support and are therefore susceptible to collapse. The trachea and the first 16 divisions of the bronchi to the terminal bronchioles constitute the conducting zone of the airways. The conducting zone has a continuous mucosal lining, which is not involved in gas exchange, creating an anatomic dead space. The mucosa is lined with pseudostratified columnar epithelium predominantly made up of ciliated cells interspersed with mucus-secreting goblet cells. Ciliated cells are estimated to contain approximately 200 cilia each, which beat approximately 1000 times/min. Goblet cells secrete mucus as well as immunologic proteins such as immunoglobulin A. The mucus and beating cilia produce a mucociliary escalator that provides the first line of defense against inhaled particles, moving these particles up to the pharynx to be swallowed or expectorated. Smoking is associated with both abnormalities in ciliary motility and mucus production, thereby compromising this protective mechanism.

Distal to the conducting zone, the next few divisions of the bronchioles leading to the most proximal alveoli consist of respiratory bronchioles or the transitional zone. The remaining subdivision lies within the lung parenchyma itself. These branches are lined with alveolar ducts and make up the respiratory zones of the airways. This efficient branching organization leads to approximately 300 million alveoli, which provide $7 \, m^2$ of surface area for gas exchange (2,3).

Alveoli

The alveoli make up the functional respiratory unit. The alveolar wall provides an alveolar epithelial and capillary endothelial interface. The alveolar epithelium has two types of cells. These cells are joined by tight junctions, forming a monolayer barrier to the diffusion of solutes. Type I alveolar

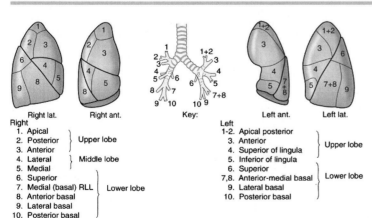

Right lat.   Right ant.   Key: Left ant.   Left lat.

Right
1. Apical ⎫
2. Posterior ⎬ Upper lobe
3. Anterior ⎭
4. Lateral ⎫ Middle lobe
5. Medial ⎭
6. Superior ⎫
7. Medial (basal) RLL ⎬ Lower lobe
8. Anterior basal ⎪
9. Lateral basal ⎪
10. Posterior basal ⎭

Left
1-2. Apical posterior ⎫
3. Anterior ⎬ Upper lobe
4. Superior of lingula ⎪
5. Inferior of lingula ⎭
6. Superior ⎫
7,8. Anterior-medial basal ⎬ Lower lobe
9. Lateral basal ⎪
10. Posterior basal ⎭

Figure 1 Segmental anatomy of the lung. *Source*: From Ref. 1.

cells are thin and make up the vast majority of the epithelial layer (>95%). These cells contain few intracellular organelles and appear to be relatively metabolically inert, allowing for maximal oxygen delivery with minimal energetic demand. These cells also function to reabsorb pathologic accumulation of alveolar fluid (4).

In contrast, type II alveolar cells are sparsely interspersed cuboidal cells with an abundance of intracellular organelles and are metabolically active. These cells produce surfactant and can regenerate the epithelium by differentiating into type I cells. Surfactant is a lipoprotein complex containing large amounts of saturated lecithins and other proteins and serves two main functions. Surfactant reduces surface tension at the air–tissue interface of the lung, reducing inhalational work. It also stabilizes the alveoli, thereby contributing to the general compliance of the lung. Surfactant also has an immunoprotective role. Two surfactant proteins, SP-A and SP-D, have been described to have a host of immune functions, including pathogen opsonization, regulation of inflammatory mediators, and even direct antimicrobial activity by increasing membrane permeability (5,6).

The capillary endothelial cell makes up the other half of the blood–air interface. The endothelial cells are water permeable, but impermeable to macromolecules. They are metabolically active and secrete prostaglandins, and can deactivate bioactive compounds such as histamine and serotonin.

The alveolar epithelium and capillary endothelium are supported by a thin interstitium, composed of a proteoglycan matrix embedded with elastin and collagen, which is produced by fibroblasts. Elastin can stretch to 130% of its length while retaining recoil properties and is the prime determinant of the mechanical properties of the lung. Its loss, as seen in patients with emphysema, leads to hyperexpansion and loss of elastic recoil. Stimulation of fibroblasts during disease processes can lead to severe pathology such as pulmonary fibrosis or acute respiratory distress syndrome (ARDS). Interspersed in the interstitium are alveolar macrophages, which provide a further layer of immunologic defense. They appear to be derived from a pluripotential cell—possibly circulating monocytes, which remain dormant until needed for differentiation. Alveolar macrophages actively engulf bacteria and inert particles and experimentally have been demonstrated to clear 95% of aerosolized bacteria within four hours of exposure (7).

The Chest Wall and Diaphragm

Bony Thorax

The chest wall is supported by the 12 thoracic vertebrae and the associated ribs. Movement of the ribs during forced respiration changes the dimension of the thorax facilitating inspiration and expiration. Movement of the upper six ribs during respiration has been likened to that of a water-pump handle, increasing the anterior–posterior dimension. Movement of the 7th through 10th ribs has been likened to that of a water bucket handle, increasing the lateral thoracic dimension.

Muscles of Respiration

The diaphragm is the chief muscle of inspiration. Concentric contraction of its muscle fibers lowers the central tendon from the level of the nipples to the costal margin, greatly increasing the thoracic vertical dimension. Between the ribs are the external, internal, and innermost intercostal muscles.

Contraction of the interchondral intercostal muscles rotates the ribs upward, while contraction of the interosseous intercostal muscles rotates the ribs downward. Contraction of the neck muscles and other chest wall muscles (scalenes, sternocleidomastoid, pectoral muscles, etc.) can also contribute to movement of the ribs and changes in thoracic dimension during active respiration. Additionally, contraction of the abdominal wall muscles compresses the abdomen, pushing the diaphragm upward and augmenting active expiration.

Pleura

The parietal pleura lines the inner chest wall, while the visceral pleura lines the lungs. The two pleurae are continuous with each other, joining at the lung hilum. The space between the parietal and visceral pleura is normally only a potential space containing a few milliliters of serous fluid. It can become abnormally enlarged in conditions such as pneumothorax, pleural effusion, hemothorax, and empyema.

Lung Volumes and Pulmonary Function Tests

The inspiratory–expiratory cycle can be divided into four lung volumes (Fig. 2). The *tidal volume* (TV) is the volume of air inspired during a normal breath. The *inspiratory reserve volume* (IRV) is the volume of air, beyond the TV, that can be inspired with maximal inspiratory effort. The *expiratory reserve volume* (ERV) is the volume of air that can be expelled with maximal effort following a normal passive exhalation. The *residual volume* (RV) is the volume that still remains in the lung following maximal expiration.

These volumes can also be grouped into four standard capacities. The *total lung capacity* is the total volume of air in the lung at maximum inhalation and is equal to the sum of all four volumes (TV + IRV + ERV + RV). The *vital capacity* (VC) is the maximal amount of air that can be moved in one breath and is equal to the sum of TV + IRV + ERV. The *functional residual capacity* (FRC) is the volume that remains in the lung after normal passive exhalation and is equal to the sum of ERV + RV. The *inspiratory capacity* is the maximal amount of air that can be inhaled after a normal passive exhalation and is equal to the sum of TV + IRV.

Although whole body plethysmography is considered the gold standard in the measurement of lung volumes and capacities, it is not clinically practical to use. Lung volumes and capacities that do not include RV are easily measured with a spirometer. Measurements with a spirometer are also performed over time. The simple and clinically useful measures of pulmonary function obtained with spirometry include the forced expiratory volume in one second (FEV$_1$) and the forced vital capacity (FVC). Normal values can vary based on sex, age, and height. A

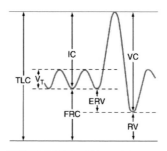

Figure 2 Spirometry. *Abbreviations*: ERV, expiratory reserve volume; FRC, functional residual capacity; IC, inspiratory capacity; RV, residual volume; TLC, total lung capacity; TV, tidal volume; VC, vital capacity. *Source*: From Ref. 8.

Table 1 FEV₁ and FVC in Normal and Diseased Lungs

Normal lung	FVC = normal
	FEV$_1$ = normal
	FEV$_1$/FVC > 75%
Obstructive lung disease	FVC = normal or decreased
	FEV$_1$ = decreased
	FEV$_1$/FVC < 75%
Restrictive lung disease	FVC = decreased
	FEV$_1$ = decreased
	FEV$_1$/FVC > 75%

Abbreviations: FEV$_1$, forced expiratory volume in 1 second; FVC, forced vital capacity.

normal 70-kg adult male will have an FEV$_1$ of about 4 L and an FVC of about 5 L. The ratio of FEV$_1$ to FVC can be used to define normal, restrictive, and obstructive patterns of lung function. Normal healthy individuals have an FEV$_1$/FVC of 80%. FEV$_1$ is determined in part by airway resistance, which is increased with various diseases such as asthma and chronic bronchitis, and pulmonary irritants such as smoke. With increased airway obstruction, FEV$_1$ will fall by a much greater level relative to the FVC and the ratio will drop. With restrictive patterns of lung disease, there will also be a reduction in FVC, but not as large a drop in FEV$_1$, and the ratio may be normal or even elevated (Table 1).

Genetics and environmental factors can also affect pulmonary function tests (PFTs). Spirometry and genomic scanning of individuals enrolled in the Original and Offspring Cohort Framingham studies demonstrated loci on chromosomes 4, 6, and 21 that strongly influence FEV$_1$ and FVC (9). Diets high in vitamin C have also been associated with a lower age–related decrease in FEV$_1$ (10).

Mechanics of Respiration

Air movement into and out of the lungs is driven by changes in thoracic pressure. Thoracic pressure is created by a balance between the elastic nature of the lungs, the respiratory muscles, and the chest wall. During quiet respiration (near FRC), inspiration is active, while expiration is passive. At the end of a normal passive exhalation, the atmospheric and alveolar air pressures are equal, and there is no pressure gradient for gas movement. The respiratory muscles are relaxed and the inward elastic contractive force of the lungs equals the outward expansive force of the chest wall. Active contraction of expiratory muscles, as described above, can further enhance expiration by compressing the thoracic cavity. Active contraction of inspiratory muscles increases the thoracic volume, lowering intrathoracic pressure and causing inward movement of air. At end-inspiration, potential energy has been stored into the tissues and elastic recoil drives expiration.

In the compression and expansion of gas, work (W) is defined by the product of pressure (P) and volume (V), where

$$W = PV$$

Pressure volume loops (Fig. 3) during respiration can be constructed, and the total area represented by TV multiplied by dP (the change in intrapleural pressure) is proportional to the work of breathing. Normally, the work of breathing represents 2% to 3% of resting oxygen consumption.

Lung compliance and airway resistance are the principal determinants of respiratory work. Compliance (C) is

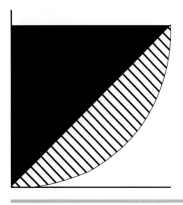

Figure 3 The mechanical work required to overcome the compliance of the respiratory system (*triangular area*) and the airway resistance (*curved loop*) during lung inspiration. The total work is the sum of the two. *Source:* From Ref. 11.

defined by the change in volume (V) produced by a change in pressure (P) where,

$$C = dV/dP$$

Using the same pressure volume loops, the compliance of the lung is equal to the slope of the line from the beginning to the end of inspiration. Total compliance is the sum of chest wall and lung compliance. Generally, chest wall compliance remains fairly constant, and clinically significant changes in compliance are due to changes in lung compliance.

Perfusion

The lungs have a dual blood supply: the pulmonary vasculature and the bronchial vasculature. Systemic venous blood returning to the heart is mixed with cardiac venous blood (via the coronary sinus and thebesian veins) with an oxygen saturation of 68% to 76% normally. The entire output of the right ventricle is then ejected into the pulmonary artery. The pulmonary artery branches into lobar, then segmental branches corresponding to the bronchopulmonary segments (Fig. 4). The pulmonary arterial vessels are thinner and less muscular than systemic vessels, resulting in a distensible, low-pressure, low-resistance circuit. Normal pulmonary blood pressure is approximately one-fifth of systemic circulation (15–30/6–12 mmHg). After passage through the pulmonary capillaries, blood is then returned by right and left, superior and inferior pulmonary veins.

In contrast, the bronchial arteries receive 1% to 2% of the cardiac output from the left ventricle, with an oxygen saturation of 100% because they arise from the aorta. Some bronchial arteries will bypass the capillary network and drain directly into the pulmonary venous system, contributing to physiologic shunting.

Distribution of blood flow within the lung is not uniform. Gravity and alveolar pressure influence regional lung perfusion. West described three zones of perfusion in an upright individual from cranial to caudal relating P_A, P_a, and P_V (Fig. 5). When moving from the lung apices to the bases, hydrostatic pressure in the blood vessels increases while the alveolar pressure remains constant. Thus the vessels in the dependent portions of the lungs are at higher pressures and receive greater blood flow. In zone 1, near the lung apices, the alveolar pressure, P_A, may exceed both P_a and P_V, preventing blood flow, and thus creating dead space (areas of ventilation but no perfusion). This does not occur normally, but can occur if the P_a pressures are abnormally low (such as in hypovolemia) or if the P_A is abnormally high

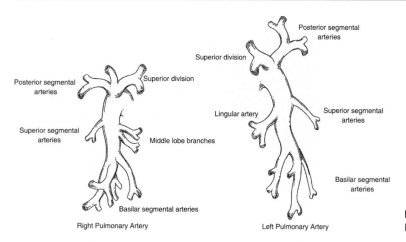

Figure 4 Pulmonary artery segmental anatomy. *Source*: From Ref. 12.

(such as in mechanical ventilation). In contrast, reduced blood flow can be seen at the base of the lung as well if pulmonary venous pressures (P_V) are abnormally high, as in left heart failure (3).

Blood flow is also affected by the local alveolar oxygen tension. Local hypoxia produces pulmonary vasoconstriction, which is further potentiated by hypercapnia and acidosis. Functionally, *hypoxic pulmonary vasoconstriction* helps match pulmonary blood flow to alveolar ventilation by shifting blood flow to alveoli with higher oxygen levels (which is locally related to the alveolar ventilation).

Ventilation

Ventilation refers to the movement of gases between the lungs and the atmosphere. Not all of the gases taken in participate in gas exchange at the alveolar capillary membrane. As described above *anatomic dead space* ventilation occurs within the conducting airways that do not participate in gas exchange. Additional *physiologic dead space* ventilation occurs in alveoli that are underperfused and thus not able to fully participate in gas exchange. The volume of gas that reaches the alveoli and is able to participate in gas exchange is referred to as alveolar ventilation.

Carbon dioxide is about 25 times more soluble than oxygen. CO_2 is then rapidly converted to bicarbonate and approximately 90% of carbon dioxide is transported as bicarbonate. The remaining fraction is transported as dissolved carbon dioxide and protein-bound carbamino compounds. Only a small gradient is required to facilitate carbon dioxide uptake from peripheral tissues and elimination at the alveolus [normal venous partial pressure of CO_2 (P_{CO_2}) of 46 mmHg; and arterial P_{CO_2} = alveolar P_{CO_2} of 40 mmHg—Fig. 6]. At steady state, CO_2 production is directly proportional to the product of alveolar ventilation (V_A) and the P_{CO_2}, where

$$V_{CO_2} \ (CO_2 \ \text{production}) \sim V_A \times P_{CO_2}$$

Therefore, if CO_2 production is relatively constant, V_A is inversely proportional to P_{CO_2}. Practically, this can be used to predict how changes in minute ventilation, V_E (assuming a relatively small effect from dead space ventilation), will affect P_{CO_2}. For example, changing a patient with a minute ventilation of 10 L/min and an arterial P_{CO_2} of 40 mmHg to a V_E 8 L/min would be expected to change the arterial P_{CO_2} to 50 mmHg ($10 \times 40/8$).

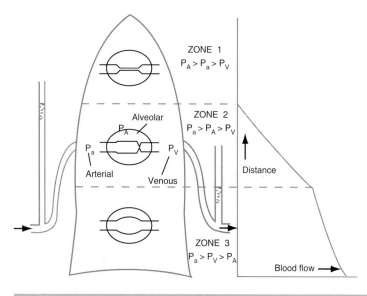

Figure 5 Differential pulmonary perfusion in an upright individual. *Note*: Three-zone model designed to account for the uneven topographic distribution of blood flow in the lung. *Abbreviations*: P_a, pulmonary arterial pressure; P_A, pulmonary alveolar pressure; P_v, pulmonary venous pressure. *Source*: From Ref. 13.

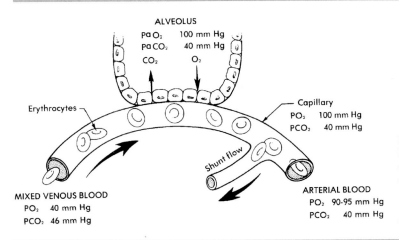

Figure 6 Gas exchange across the alveolus. Relationship between driving pressures for oxygen and carbon dioxide exchange at alveolocapillary membranes. *Abbreviations*: CO_2, carbon dioxide; O_2, oxygen; Pa_{CO_2}, partial pressure of arterial carbon dioxide; Pa_{O_2}, partial pressure of arterial oxygen; P_{CO_2}, partial pressure of carbon dioxide; P_{O_2}, partial pressure of oxygen. *Source*: From Ref. 2.

Similar to pulmonary perfusion, there are also regional differences in lung ventilation. At FRC, dependent alveoli are less distended due to increased hydrostatic pressure from gravity. Thus, dependent alveoli expand more with inspiration and receive greater ventilation. Accordingly, in an upright healthy individual, during normal respiration the lung bases receive more ventilation than the apices. However, with lower lung volumes approaching RV, intrapleural pressure can exceed intraluminal pressure, resulting in peripheral airway collapse and atelectasis. This volume is called the *closing volume* (CV). In normal individuals, the CV is about 10% of the VC. As patients age, and especially in bedridden patients, the CV can approach and exceed FRC, resulting in peripheral airway collapse during a significant portion of the respiratory cycle.

Oxygenation

The oxygen requirement for a normal healthy adult is about 200 mL/min. The normal oxygen gradient at room air is about 60 mmHg (alveolar P_{O_2} of 100 mmHg, arterial P_{O_2} of 90–95 mmHg; and venous P_{O_2} of 40 mmHg). As oxygen diffuses across the alveolar wall, it dissolves in plasma and then diffuses into red blood cells, where it is bound by hemoglobin. The oxygen-carrying capacity (C_{O_2}) of blood is far more dependent on the concentration of hemoglobin and percent saturation than the partial pressure of dissolved oxygen. One gram of hemoglobin can bind 1.36 mL of oxygen, and oxygen has a solubility coefficient of 0.0031 mL O_2/mmHg/dL blood. Thus,

$$C_{O_2} = 1.36 \, (Hgb) \, (Sa_{O_2}) + 0.0031 \, (P_{O_2})$$

Each molecule of hemoglobin has four binding sites for oxygen. With each binding of an oxygen molecule, there is an increased affinity for the next. This produces a sigmoidal relationship between the oxygen saturation of hemoglobin and the partial pressure of oxygen (Fig. 7). Such an arrangement facilitates hemoglobin loading with oxygen in the lungs with higher oxygen tension and unloading of oxygen in the periphery at lower oxygen tension. The affinity of oxygen for hemoglobin is also affected by other factors, such as temperature, P_{CO_2}, pH, and 2,3-diphosphoglyceric acid (2,3-DPG). Increased exertion and metabolic stress (as reflected by increased temperature, P_{CO_2}, and decreased pH) shift the curve to the right, decreasing the affinity of

hemoglobin for oxygen and facilitating oxygen unloading at the periphery. 2,3-DPG binds to the β chain of deoxyhemoglobin, decreasing the affinity for oxygen and also shifts the curve to the right. Chronic hypoxia stimulates increased synthesis of 2,3-DPG. Blood storage results in a marked decrease in 2,3-DPG.

Diffusion

The diffusion of gases across capillary surfaces is affected by the tissue solubility of the gas, dimensions of the alveolar–capillary interface, the driving pressure gradient of the gas, and the rate of equilibration of gas exchange.

Changes in the thickness and surface area dimensions of the alveolar–capillary interfaces affect diffusion. Reduction in the exchange surface area as with emphysema, or

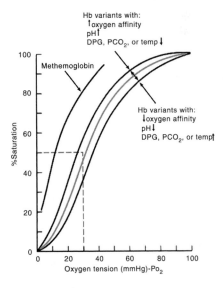

Figure 7 Oxygen–hemoglobin dissociation curve. *Note*: The percent saturation of hemoglobin with oxygen at different oxygen tensions is depicted by the middle sigmoidal curve. The P_{50} (i.e., oxygen tension at which the hemoglobin molecule is one-half saturated) is about 27 mmHg in normal erythrocytes (*dotted lines*). Heterotopic modifiers of hemoglobin function can shift the curve leftward by increasing or rightward by decreasing its oxygen affinity. *Source*: From Ref. 13.

increase in the thickness as with interstitial lung disease and pulmonary edema, decreases the diffusion of gases and limits gas exchange.

The variable affinity of hemoglobin for oxygen as described above, as well as the rate at which hemoglobin is circulated through the capillary bed (i.e., the cardiac output), has an effect on measuring oxygen-diffusing capacity. On average, a red blood cell takes approximately 0.75 second to cross the pulmonary capillary. Oxygen has a higher driving pressure gradient, while CO_2 has a higher solubility. Normally, it takes about 0.25 second for the pressure gradient across the alveolar–capillary interface to equilibrate. Thus, gas exchange is normally perfusion limited and the only way to increase gas exchange is to increase perfusion. However, as described above, many diseases can limit gas exchange such that there is no equilibration by the time blood crosses the capillary and gas exchange is diffusion limited.

Clinically, the diffusing capacity of carbon monoxide (DLCO, normal about 30–35 mL/min/mmHg) is usually measured as a surrogate with a single breath of a low concentration of carbon monoxide. Carbon monoxide has a molecular weight similar to oxygen but binds with a higher affinity to hemoglobin, creating a low partial pressure and essentially a constant pressure gradient for its diffusion, which simplifies measurement of diffusing capacity.

Ventilation/Perfusion

The relationship between ventilation and perfusion is important in the exchange of oxygen and carbon dioxide. Matching alveolar ventilation (V) to pulmonary blood flow (Q) is important for achieving ideal gas exchange and is measured by the V/Q ratio. Normally each liter of blood flow is matched with 0.8 L of ventilation. High V/Q ratios are produced by excessive ventilation or inadequate blood flow. At one extreme is dead space or ventilation that receives no perfusion for gas exchange, with a V/Q ratio of infinity. At the other extreme is shunt, or perfusion without ventilation, with a V/Q ratio of zero. Low V/Q ratios are generally caused by inadequate ventilation or excessive blood flow (Fig. 8). In the research setting, the V/Q ratio can be measured with the multiple inert gas elimination technique, although this is not practical clinically. Assessment of V/Q mismatch becomes clinically important when assessing the etiology of hypoxia.

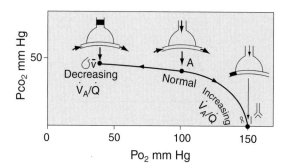

Figure 8 V/Q mismatch. *Note:* Oxygen–carbon dioxide diagram shows how the P_{O_2} and P_{CO_2} of a lung unit alter as the ventilation–perfusion ratio is changed. *Abbreviations:* I, inspired gas; v̄, mixed venous blood. *Source:* From Ref. 15.

Hypoxia

In general, hypoxia is caused by V/Q mismatch, shunt, alveolar hypoventilation, and increased diffusion gradient. V/Q mismatch is one of the most common causes of hypoxemia, but can be difficult to assess and is generally a diagnosis of exclusion. *Shunt* is the fraction of blood that enters arterial blood without gas exchange. Bronchial blood flow causes physiologic shunt. Normal shunt is about 5%. Pathologic intrapulmonary shunt occurs when portions of lung are perfused but not ventilated, as in lung consolidation from pneumonia or atelectasis. Extrapulmonary shunts also occur as in right-to-left cardiac shunts. Shunt can be measured by:

$$Q_S/Q_T = (Ci_{O_2} - Ca_{O_2})/(Ci_{O_2} - Cv_{O_2})$$

As defined by the following abbreviations:

Q_S/Q_T: (shunt flow/total flow)
Ci_{O_2}: ideal O_2 content or pulmonary capillary O_2 content
Ca_{O_2}: arterial O_2 content
Cv_{O_2}: mixed venous O_2 content

Alveolar hypoventilation can be caused by thoracic wall and neuromuscular disorders as well as by central respiratory depression. As described above, an increased diffusion gradient can be caused by changes in the dimensions of the alveolar–capillary interface, as in interstitial lung diseases and with pulmonary edema. Both alveolar hypoventilation and increased diffusion gradient can be treated with oxygen administration. True shunt will not be affected by additional oxygen administration. V/Q mismatch will respond partially to oxygen administration, depending on the amount of tendency toward shunt.

PERIOPERATIVE PULMONARY ASSESSMENT
Preoperative Assessment

Preoperative assessment of pulmonary risk begins with the history and physical examination. Obviously patients with a history of significant pulmonary disease, especially chronic obstructive pulmonary disease (COPD), are at increased risk, as are patients with significant heart disease and poor nutritional status. Preoperative counseling in patients with a smoking history has been demonstrated to have an impact as well. Physiologically, smoking cessation more than 48 hours has been demonstrated to decrease systemic carbon monoxide levels and improve mucosal ciliary function. Cessation of one to two weeks is associated with decreased sputum production. Cessation more than six weeks is associated with improved spirometry. Patients undergoing coronary artery bypass demonstrate a fourfold decrease in pulmonary complications with smoking cessation of two months. Smokers who stopped smoking for six months had a pulmonary complication rate equivalent to that of nonsmokers (16). Physical examination findings demonstrating use of accessory muscles, prolonged expiration, a barrel chest, cyanosis, heart failure, and pulmonary edema require further investigation.

In general, patients without evidence of pulmonary disease on history and physical examination do not require further preoperative testing if they are being prepared for operations not involving the thoracic cavity. Patients with pulmonary disease and/or patients undergoing thoracic surgery should have further testing as indicated. Preoperative arterial $P_{O_2} < 60$ mmHg, and arterial $P_{CO_2} > 45$ mmHg is associated with increased perioperative morbidity. In patients with known disease, a preoperative chest X ray can provide a useful baseline for comparison. PFTs can risk stratify high-risk patients and should be performed in all patients undergoing planned pulmonary resections. Pulmonary function testing indicators of high risk in non-thoracic surgery patients include an FVC < 2 L (or < 50% predicted), an FEV_1/FVC < 50% predicted, and a diffusing capacity < 50% predicted (17). In patients undergoing pulmonary resection, PFTs are used to define the risk for postoperative respiratory insufficiency. In general, pulmonary resections with a predicted postoperative FEV_1 of greater than 800 mL can be tolerated. Patients with an $FEV_1 > 2$ L can tolerate most resections, including pneumonectomy. Patients with an $FEV_1 < 2$ L may still be able to tolerate pulmonary resection, and ventilation perfusion studies can help predict how much the planned area of resection contributes to overall function. As experience with lung volume reduction surgery in patients with emphysema expands, it has been demonstrated that pulmonary resection of severely diseased tissue may even enhance postoperative pulmonary function (18).

In patients with borderline PFTs, physiological exercise testing with measurement of V_{O_2max} is predictive of outcomes. Patients who achieved V_{O_2max} of more than 20 mL/kg/min, even with poor PFTs, will generally tolerate pulmonary resection. Patients with an estimated postoperative V_{O_2max} of less than 10 mL/kg/min have prohibitively high rates of complication and are not surgical candidates (19).

Postoperative Pulmonary Complications

Postoperative pulmonary complications involving the lung are a leading cause of morbidity and mortality. In a review of 10,000 major operations, 10% of operative deaths occurred in patients who developed pneumonia (20). Stated another way, there was a 46% mortality in 1.3% of patients who got pneumonia.

Postoperative complications involving the lung can be broadly defined and studies differ in their approach to recording and reporting complications. Complications include a spectrum of disorders from dyspnea, atelectasis, and increased sputum production, to pneumonia, respiratory failure, and death. The risk for complications also depends on the anesthetic technique used as well as the surgical procedure. Thoracic incisions, upper abdominal incisions, and procedures lasting more than three hours are at increased risk of resulting in pulmonary complications. Minimally invasive surgery, such as laparoscopic cholecystectomy and video-assisted thoracoscopic surgery have been demonstrated to have fewer pulmonary complications (21).

Postoperative pain control techniques, such as patient-controlled analgesia and intercostal nerve blocks, have been demonstrated to decrease complications (22). Chest physiotherapy, incentive spirometry, and/or bronchodilators can prevent or reverse hypoxemia from atelectasis.

COMMON PULMONARY DISORDERS
Acute Respiratory Failure

In 1967, Ashbaugh et al. described a syndrome of dyspnea, hypoxemia, decreased pulmonary compliance, and diffuse alveolar infiltrates in 12 patients without a prior history of lung disease or congestive heart failure, which was termed adult respiratory distress syndrome or ARDS (23). In 1994,

the American–European Consensus Committee on ARDS redefined this acronym as *Acute Respiratory Distress Syndrome* to reflect its occurrence in children as well, and introduced the term *Acute Lung Injury* (ALI) to identify a similar but lower severity of respiratory failure. Both ALI and ARDS refer to a syndrome defined by inflammation and increased permeability associated with a constellation of clinical, radiologic, and physiologic abnormalities that cannot be explained by left atrial or pulmonary capillary hypertension (i.e., PCWP < 18 mmHg). ALI and ARDS are differentiated by the severity of hypoxemia as defined by the Pa_{O_2}/Fi_{O_2} (P/F) ratio. ALI is defined by a P/F ratio of 200 to 300, while ARDS is defined by a P/F ratio < 200 (24).

The reported incidence of ARDS has varied in part due to previous variations in definitions. A recent 2002 study of every admission to 21 adult Australian intensive care units over a two-month period, using the consensus definition, found an incidence of ALI and ARDS of 34 and 28 per 100,000, respectively. The 30-day mortality was 32% and 34%, respectively, for these conditions (25). Previous studies report a mortality of approximately 50%.

Multivariate analysis from multiple studies has demonstrated that the main risk factor for ARDS in patients is some type of systemic infection or sepsis. Blood transfusions, advanced age, and smoking have also been identified as independent risk factors. Recent epidemiologic studies have further found a genetic susceptibility associated with an angiotensin-converting enzyme (ACE) polymorphism. This polymorphism is associated with high circulating levels of ACE, which adversely affect pulmonary vascular tone, vascular permeability, epithelial survival, and fibroblast activation (26). Male sex and black race are also associated with a higher mortality in patients developing ARDS.

Clinically, ALI and ARDS present with an acute onset. Fifty percent of patients develop ARDS within 24 hours of the inciting event; 85% develop this condition within 72 hours (27). The earliest signs of ALI include tachypnea and anxiety. This is then followed with a progressively worsening dyspnea, tachycardia, mental status changes, rales, rhonchi, and ultimately consolidation that often requires mechanical ventilation to prevent pulmonary failure. While the degree of hypoxemia distinguishes ALI from ARDS, the initial P/F ratios and ventilatory parameters have not been predictive of outcome. Chest X-rays may reflect the initial inciting event or be normal. As lung injury progresses, X-rays demonstrate edema with bilateral diffuse infiltrates, followed by diffuse alveolar/reticular opacification (i.e., ground-glass opacification). Computed tomography (CT) imaging demonstrates diffuse pulmonary consolidation with air bronchograms and later cystic changes within the pulmonary parenchyma. However, imaging may not parallel the clinical spectrum of disease and often lags well behind the clinical course.

Histologically, three phases have been described. Initially there is an *exudative* phase. Damage to the alveolar epithelium and vascular endothelium allows leakage of fluid, protein, blood, and inflammatory cells into the interstitium and alveolar lumen. This is followed by a *proliferative* phase. Destruction of type I cells leads to accumulation of protein, fibrin, and other cellular debris forming hyaline membranes. Destruction of type II cells leads to alveolar collapse; type II cells then proliferate (fibroblastic reaction, remodeling, and differentiation to and regeneration of type I epithelium). Finally, there is a *fibrotic* phase. Fibroblastic remodeling can become irreversible with collagen deposition and development of microcysts (28).

Treatment of ALI/ARDS has been intensely studied (29). Treatment is focused on aggressive management of the initiating factors, appropriate control of underlying infection, aggressive nutritional support, and gentle mechanical ventilation management.

With mechanical ventilation, it is important to avoid both barometric and volumetric trauma. The ARDS network study demonstrated a 22% decrease in mortality with low volume ventilation (TV < 6 mL/kg) and low plateau airway pressure strategy (30). Insisting on a normal pH and P_{CO_2} by increasing minute ventilation may actually worsen lung injury, and strategies of gradual permissive hypercapnia allow lower volume ventilations. Arterial P_{CO_2} of 50 to 77 mmHg with a pH of 7.2 to 7.3 appear to be well tolerated. High concentrations of oxygen ($Fi_{O_2} > 60\%$) are also damaging and associated with increased edema, alveolar thickening, and fibrinous exudates. Adding positive end-expiratory pressure can help reduce Fi_{O_2}, although this may have the negative effect of impairing venous return and cardiac performance. Reverse inspiratory to expiratory (I:E) ratio ventilation has been proposed to decrease peak inspiratory and plateau pressures, but is associated with higher mean airway pressures that have not been shown to improve outcomes compared to conventional ventilation techniques (31).

Prognosis in ARDS is multifactorial. Death in ARDS is usually due to multisystem organ failure (MOF) and not simply respiratory failure itself. Increased age, immunocompromise, and chronic liver disease have also been demonstrated to increased mortality in ARDS (27). In patients who recover, pulmonary dysfunction can persist and present with a mix of obstructive, restrictive, and diffusion pulmonary impairments. Pulmonary function studies demonstrate that most patients will show general improvement at three to six months, with a plateau in improvement at one year (32). Neuropsychiatric testing has also demonstrated significant deficits that may persist beyond two years, associated with prolonged hypoxemia (33). Because MOF is commonly encountered in critically ill surgical patients and is intimately linked with ARDS, further discussion of this linkage can be found in the chapter on MOF (Chapter 11).

Atelectasis

Atelectasis is the term used to refer to a loss of lung volume. Depending on the cause, this volume loss may only involve a small portion of the lung that is not readily diagnosed on chest X-ray. In this circumstance, it is commonly called "micro" atelectasis. More substantial involvement can range from subsegmental, segmental, to involvement of an entire lobe. A wide variety of conditions may give rise to this disorder. For example, a space-occupying lesion within the lung parenchyma itself, such as a tumor, may compress adjacent lung tissue so that involved alveoli collapse. Similarly, a space-occupying abnormality in the pleural space, such as pneumothorax or hydrothorax, can also collapse adjacent lung. If a major bronchus or several secondary bronchi are occluded, an absorption-type atelectasis can occur due to resorption of air in the lung tissue distal to the obstruction. Examples of the obstructing agents include a foreign body, tumor, or mucus plug. Abnormalities in surfactant, which is a lipoprotein that is important in keeping alveoli open, may result in atelectasis in various inflammatory conditions such as pneumonia. In this setting, the surfactant may be inadequately synthesized, rapidly degraded, or become functionally suboptimal. The net result of any of these circumstances is alveolar collapse.

Atelectasis is a common postoperative problem that can be related to the effects of anesthesia, the underlying pulmonary status of the patient, and the type of incision used to carry out the operative procedure. Further, obesity, chronic bronchitis, pain, and advanced age are all predisposing factors. The pathophysiology of this condition in the postoperative period is related to various factors, all of which contribute to bronchial obstruction. These include a defective cough response so that retained secretions in the bronchus are not properly expectorated, and a reduction in the caliber of the bronchus, which may occur from direct airway trauma due to intubation, or result in edema and/or inflammation arising from this maneuver. Finally, the thickness of the bronchial secretions and the ability to clear them from the tracheal bronchial tree may prove difficult even when effective coughing seems adequate. Although the true incidence of atelectasis is unknown, most patients undergoing chest or abdominal procedures probably have some degree of microatelectasis. Involvement of segments or subsegments of the lung may occur in as many as 2% to 3% of all operations performed.

Atelectasis may be clinically manifested by fever, tachypnea, and tachycardia. The cause of the fever has been debated, but is probably related to secondary bacterial proliferation in the atelectatic areas of the lung (34). By the time these various clinical parameters become apparent, the atelectasis has usually been present for a day or more. Because prevention is always easier than cure, all patients undergoing a general anesthetic, regardless of the operative procedure, should be considered to be at risk for the development of postoperative atelectasis. Accordingly, such patients should be mobilized and encouraged to ambulate as quickly as possible after operation. Further, deep breathing, coughing, and nasotracheal suction should be instituted as appropriate. A bedside spirometer in a patient who has been extubated can be especially helpful in getting patients to maximally aerate their lungs. Pain management through the use of epidural catheters and intercostal nerve blocks can greatly minimize the splinting caused by pain, with resultant lobar collapse that is commonly seen in patients who have undergone upper abdominal and thoracic incisions. Marked global respiratory muscle dysfunction and deterioration are not uncommon following operations in which these incisions have been used.

Bronchial breathing or moist rales involving the lung bases are common clinical presentations of atelectasis. Aggressive pulmonary toilet, postural drainage, and nebulizer treatments are effective adjunctive therapies that may shorten the patient's hospitalization once atelectasis becomes a factor in management. Atelectasis caused by airway obstruction (tumor or foreign body) presents with wheezing and occasionally progresses to pneumonia. In such a patient, clearing secretions distal to the obstruction is often difficult and commonly results in pooling of secretions and bacterial overgrowth. Prompt mobilization with aggressive nasotracheal suctioning is necessary to overcome the tenacious sputum impactions that commonly occur. Flexible bronchoscopy should be utilized liberally to insure a rapid return to normal pulmonary function.

Parenchymal Lung Disease
Chronic Obstructive Pulmonary Disease (COPD)

COPD is a major source of morbidity and mortality worldwide, and is currently the fourth leading cause of these problems in the United States. Previous definitions of COPD have focused on chronic bronchitits and emphysema, reflecting a heterogeneous mix of airway disease and parenchymal destruction. In an effort to standardize terminology, an international consensus panel (Global Initiative for Chronic Obstructive Lung Disease) has produced a working definition of COPD as a disease state characterized by airflow limitation that is not fully reversible, usually progressive, and associated with an abnormal inflammatory response to noxious stimuli (35). With this broadened definition, emphysema, chronic bronchitis, and asthma are all variants of COPD, and all can evoke varying degrees of bronchospasm and increased airflow resistance. The common result of these abnormalities is an increased work of breathing and impaired gas exchange with enhanced difficulty in clearing the bronchial tree. This circumstance may express itself clinically as atelectasis, pneumonia, or even frank respiratory failure.

Because smoking is so commonly linked with COPD, cessation of this habit (as mentioned above) can greatly lessen perioperative complications in patients with obstructive lung disease. Bronchodilation therapy has also proved effective in improving pulmonary mechanics and secretion removal (36). Albuterol (a β_2-agonist) has been especially beneficial in this regard when administered as a wet nebulizer. As with other pulmonary conditions, deep breathing and coughing are effective adjunctive measures in the early postoperative period in patients with COPD, along with early ambulation to prevent complications such as atelectasis and pneumonia. Attention to such detail will result in a successful pulmonary outcome for most patients with COPD needing surgical intervention.

Idiopathic Pulmonary Fibrosis

Idiopathic pulmonary fibrosis (IPF) is the most commonly diagnosed diffuse lung disease seen in clinical practice (37). It is characterized by acute diffuse interstitial fibrosis of the lungs. Extrapulmonary involvement does not occur. It is heralded by progressive cough, dyspnea, and pulmonary infiltrates on chest X-ray. PFTs reveal a restrictive ventilatory pattern as the lung parenchymal destruction progresses. Peak onset occurs in the sixth decade and is more common in males who smoke. Possible etiologies of this disabling and frustrating disease are numerous and include exposure to various dusts and minerals, as well as being associated with other conditions, including collagen vascular disease, radiation therapy, and exposure to varied pharmacologic and cytotoxic agents. High-resolution CT scan reveals the ground-glass opacities with honeycombing that typifies IPF. From a physiologic standpoint, IPF patients demonstrate a restrictive defect on testing with impaired oxygenation and impaired gas exchange. Exercise is especially known to impair oxygenation and most patients experience hypoxemia at rest. Definitive diagnosis is made through surgical biopsy of the lung.

Unfortunately, this disease does not respond to treatment and is rapidly progressive (37). Although high-dose corticosteroids given in combination with immunosuppressive medications are used to modify its progression, there is little improvement in survival or quality of life. Survival is measured in years, with only 15% of patients surviving 10 years from the time of diagnosis. Selected patients with IPF may benefit from lung transplantation (see below). Because of the marked compromise in ventilatory function that exists in IPF, great caution should be exercised in operating on patients with this disease for elective problems that can be adequately managed otherwise.

Sarcoidosis

Sarcoidosis is a worldwide noncaseating granulomatous disease with multisystem involvement and a variable clinical course (37). This disease is more common in blacks and can affect any organ. While the lungs and mediastinal lymph nodes are most commonly involved, 25% of patients exhibit ocular and skin involvement as well. The diagnosis is established by clinical history and tissue confirmation. The differential diagnosis includes fungal diseases, tuberculosis, and malignancy. The cause of this disease is unknown. While infectious and environmental etiologies are suspected and the disease similarities to tuberculosis are remarkable, to date, no conclusive evidence supports any risk factors. The majority of patients are asymptomatic with hilar adenopathy. Symptomatic patients present with cough and dyspnea. Abnormal findings on chest X-rays are seen in 90% of patients, and the progression of sarcoidosis is easily seen as the hilar involvement advances to incorporate lung involvement. CT reveals the areas of mediastinal lymph node involvement; bronchoscopic biopsy is reliable (90%) in establishing the diagnosis. While 30% to 40% of patients undergo remission, many need corticosteroids to manage progressive involvement. Occasionally, cytotoxic and other alternative therapies are necessary, but responses to such therapy are inconsistent. Although the majority of patients with sarcoidosis who undergo an operation experience no untoward pulmonary problems, those with severe pulmonary fibrosis (approximately 10%) should be carefully screened as postoperative pulmonary sequelae are not infrequent.

Infectious Lung Disease
Pneumonia

Pneumonia is a condition in which the respiratory tract is colonized with substantial numbers of microorganisms so that neutrophils migrate to the locus of colonization, and along with alveolar macrophages, induce the development of a cellular alveolar inflammatory exudate (38). As the inflammatory process evolves, it is ultimately seen on the chest X-ray as an infiltrate. The lower respiratory tract is more typically involved with pneumonia than other parts of the lung. The usual signs of pneumonia include a purulent productive cough, fever ($>38°C$), and rales overlying the site of infection on auscultation. In the intubated patient, purulent debris is commonly noted on suctioning. In both situations, leukocytosis is usually present.

Pneumonia is a common problem in the postoperative surgical patient. The vast majority of pneumonias that occur in the surgical patient are nosocomial (i.e., hospital acquired). Most are related to endotracheal intubation or tracheostomy and mechanical ventilation. Ventilator-associated pneumonia is a serious issue in critically ill patients with an attributable mortality of 33% to 50% (39). Although the overall risk for nosocomial pneumonia varies between 5 to 10 cases per 1000 hospital admissions, it increases greatly in patients with chronic illness, prolonged malnutrition, advanced age, and conditions of immunodeficiency (e.g., HIV/AIDS). Other risk factors include patients receiving various drugs such as corticosteroids, cytotoxic agents, or inappropriate antibiotic agents, or possessing comorbid conditions such as coma, trauma, burns, and cirrhosis. Prolonged surgery can also be a risk factor. In patients requiring ventilatory support, pneumonia may occur in as many as 30% of those ventilated more than 48 hours (39).

Aspiration is a major risk factor for pneumonia in the surgical patient. It can result from inhalation of oropharyngeal secretions, which typically contain high concentrations of microorganisms, or inhalation of sterile gastric secretions that reflux up the esophagus from the stomach. Risk factors for aspiration include aberrations in the level of consciousness (e.g., head injury, stroke, or drug overdose), defective cough reflex (e.g., neuromuscular disorders), and problems with swallowing or esophageal function (e.g., tracheostomy, nasogastric intubation, or incompetent lower esophageal sphincter). Aspiration of oropharyngeal contents is particularly common in patients with altered or impaired consciousness, and is often seen in conditions of drug overdose or alcohol abuse. Aspiration of gastric contents is a frequent problem in patients with intestinal obstruction whether functional (e.g., postoperative ileus, dysmotility) or mechanical in nature. It is especially important to keep the head of the bed up and to monitor gastric residuals with some frequency to minimize the potential aspiration volume and protect those who are at highest risk for this complication (i.e., altered mental status). Although intubated patients and those with tracheostomy tubes are often thought to be protected from aspiration, in reality such patients are also at risk. Causative organisms for pneumonias resulting from orophyaryngeal aspiration include anaerobic and gram-negative bacteria. Although gastric fluids are usually sterile, bacterial colonization and secondary infection is not uncommon following aspiration of gastric contents.

Diagnosis can be difficult. Critically ill patients have many reasons for fever and elevated white blood cell counts. Pulmonary infiltrates on chest X-ray can represent pneumonia, but can also represent ALI/ARDS, pulmonary edema, and/or pulmonary contusions. Chest X-ray findings often lag behind the clinical presentation. The sensitivity of chest X-ray for pneumonia is only 62% and the specificity is even less at 28% (39). Quantitative bronchoalveolar lavage with a threshold of 10,000 cfu/mL is emerging as the test of choice in diagnosing pneumonia in the intubated patient with a sensitivity and specificity of 91% and 78%, respectively (40).

Several studies have looked at ways to reduce nosocomial pneumonia. Elevation of the head of the bed and avoidance of nasogastric tubes helps minimize the risk of aspiration. One randomized trial was stopped early when interim analysis demonstrated that semirecumbent positioning reduced the frequency of pneumonia from 23% to 5% compared to the supine position (41). Maintenance of gastric acidity may also reduce the incidence of pneumonia by preventing colonization of gastric contents, which can occur when acid-suppressing drugs are administered. Prophylactic systemic antibiotics have not been demonstrated to reduce nosocomial pneumonia. Multiple meta-analyses on selective decontamination of the digestive tract by oral antibiotics have shown that this can reduce infection rates and mortality. However, utility of such an approach is limited by development of antimicrobial resistance (42,43).

Treatment of pneumonia includes pulmonary toilet (local drainage) and specific tailored antibiotic therapy. Because most pneumonias in the surgical patient are related to intubation, aggressive weaning from the ventilator and extubation are important. Patients not easily weaned should be converted to a tracheostomy.

Patients who are suspected of aspiration present with cough, tachypnea, and tachycardia. Many immunocompetent patients mount a febrile response. Chest X-ray reveals atelectasis and infiltrates. Treatment of these patients requires early and repeated suctioning to clear the tracheobronchial tree. Prophylactic antibiotics are not usually indicated initially, but may be required if secondary infection develops. Steroids were previously used to treat aspiration, but many investigators now believe that they have no place in the management of aspiration because of their deleterious effects on pulmonary host defenses.

Lung Abscess

Lung abscesses are usually related to aspiration and typically occur in the superior segments of the right and left lower lobes as well as the posterior segment of the right upper lobe (44). The most common organisms are anaerobic bacteria from the oropharynx and gastrointestinal tract. The organisms stimulate fibroblastic proliferation, which can erode into adjacent bronchoalveolar spaces. Clinical findings include cough (especially hemoptysis, and/or productive of malodorous sputum), fever, and an air–fluid level on chest X-ray. Chest CT is the definitive study for diagnosing a lung abscess.

Treatment for lung abscess is generally conservative and basically follows the principles of pneumonia treatment, with focus on pulmonary toilet and tailored antibiotic therapy. Surgical therapy, including drainage and resection, is indicated in patients who fail to respond to conservative measures. Relative indications for surgery include patients with severe hemoptysis, bronchopleural fistula, empyema, and/or an abscess cavity more than 6 cm in diameter.

Tuberculosis

Pulmonary tuberculosis is the number one infectious disease resulting in death throughout the world. Despite advances in antibiotic treatment, tuberculosis has seen a recent resurgence due to HIV infections, and other increases in immunocompromised patients (cancer, transplant recipients, etc.). Treatment of pulmonary tuberculosis is primarily pharmacologic. The usual regimen is isoniazid, rifampin, pyrazinamide × 2 months + isoniazid and rifampin × 4 months, or isoniazid and rifampin × 9 months. Surgery is indicated for patients with positive sputum cultures and cavitary lesions greater than five months despite treatment; severe or recurrent hemoptysis; bronchopleural fistula not resolved by chest tube; mass-associated lesions; and disease due to drug resistant atypicals such as *Mycobacterium avium-intracellulare*.

Pulmonary Embolism

Blood clots from the systemic venous circulation can obstruct the pulmonary artery, causing significant morbidity and mortality. The differential diagnosis of acute pulmonary embolism (PE) is complex because PE can present in a variety of ways depending on the size of the clot, its location, and the underlying comorbidities of the patient. Myocardial infarction, pneumonia, and congestive heart failure may mimic PE. While there are known hypercoagulable states and genetic factor deficiencies, which contribute to PE formation, hospitalized patients have their own acquired risk factors that must be taken into consideration. Surgery and trauma are the key areas for surgical patients that may be impacted for prevention. Low-molecular-weight heparins administered preoperatively in addition to pneumatic compression sleeves for the legs significantly lessen, but do not eliminate, the clot risk.

The underlying pathophysiologic abnormality that occurs in PE is occlusion of the pulmonary arteries, so that alveoli subserved by this arterial system are ventilated but no longer perfused. This results in a ventilation–perfusion mismatch, the consequence of which is increased dead-space ventilation (45). Accompanying this event is a reflex airway constriction along with a vasoactive response that initiates a generalized pulmonary vasoconstriction. A variety of mediators have been proposed as possible etiologic agents, but the exact cause of the actions is poorly understood. The net result of these perturbations is an elevation in the pulmonary vascular resistance and a redistribution of pulmonary blood flow that often aggravates the *V/Q* mismatch triggered by the PE, and local atelectatsis and edema may eventuate in congestive atelectasis or pulmonary edema. It is quite understandable why patients with PE often present with hyperventilation and hypoxia in addition to chest pain in the region of the PE.

Clinical suspicion is the key to making the diagnosis of PE. Patients presenting with acute-onset dyspnea, tachypnea, and apprehension should be suspected of harboring a PE. Lab tests, EKG, and physical examination are unreliable and rarely are specific enough to document PE. Ventilation–perfusion scans, which historically were used to make the diagnosis, have generally been supplanted by CT angiography as the imaging modality of choice. Pulmonary angiography is the gold standard in the diagnosis of PE. In the patient suspected of having a PE, immediate anticoagulation with heparin should be administered. Supportive care with supplemental oxygen should also be rendered. These measures are quite efficacious in altering symptomatology and helping to reverse the aberrations induced by the PE.

Pleural Disease

Pneumothorax

Air in the potential space between the visceral and parietal pleurae is called pneumothorax. The loss of negative intrapleural pressure that occurs from this air collection allows the lung to collapse from elastic recoil. Pneumothorax usually occurs as a result of ruptured alveoli (from a congenital bleb, pneumatocele, or emphysematous bulla) or from small lacerations in the pulmonary parenchyma (rib fractures in blunt trauma, lacerations through the chest wall in penetrating trauma, or iatrogenic injuries such as needle injury during the placement of a central venous line). In most cases of pneumothorax, the damaged lung quickly seals so that the condition is not progressive. Thus, there is no shift in the mediastinal structures and the opposite lung is not adversely affected. A tension pneumothorax, on the other hand, occurs if the pressure of accumulated air in the pleural space exceeds the ambient pressure, resulting in net positive intrathoracic pressure. In this condition, the progressive accumulation of air within the thoracic cavity shifts the cardiomediastinal structures away from the affected lung. If the resultant tension pneumothorax is substantial, compression of the contralateral lung may occur. Tension pneumothorax can be conceived as a one-way valve in which air enters the pleural space during inspiration but cannot escape during expiration. It occurs from a ruptured bleb or lung laceration that has failed to seal. The resultant increase in pleural pressure can have profound effects on the venous return to the heart, usually by direct pressure on the low-pressure vena cava. If not recognized and rapidly treated, hypotension and complete circulatory collapse may promptly occur.

Pneumothorax can generally be diagnosed by auscultating the lungs. On the affected side, air movement is compromised to the extent that the pleural space has been replaced by air and the affected lung volume has been compromised. Often percussion of the chest wall will demonstrate hyper-resonance. If a tension pneumothorax has occurred, shifting of the trachea away from the affected side may be seen. There is usually pain in the hemithorax

involved. Profound dyspnea and panic may accompany tension pneumothorax.

Treatment of pneumothorax will depend on its clinical presentation. If diminished breath sounds and mild-to-moderate pain are major presenting clinical findings in the absence of severe dyspnea, pneumothorax probably is not progressive and the offending lung abnormality has sealed off. If marked dyspnea exists and little-to-no breath sounds can be heard on the affected side, irrespective of whether clear evidence of tracheal shift has occurred, a tension pneumothorax is probably responsible for the clinical situation. In this circumstance, immediate decompression of the affected hemithorax is required to obviate the respiratory and/or hemodynamic embarrassment. This is most readily achieved by needle thoracostomy to relieve the positive intrathoracic pressure. Tube thoracostomy after needle decompression constitutes definitive therapy. In the more common circumstance in which tension does not appear to be a component of the pneumothorax, the type of treatment will be dictated by the volume of lung parenchyma compromised. If less than a 30% pneumothorax appears to exist on chest X-ray, watchful waiting may be all that is needed. For a more substantial pneumothorax, tube thoracostomy is usually required. Once the affected lung injury seals (usually 2–3 days), the tube can be removed.

In interpreting X-ray findings of pneumothorax, Richardson (2) has emphasized that it must be remembered that the lung is a sphere and that the volume loss is calculated by the equation $V = \pi R^3$. Thus, if the diameter has been determined to have decreased from 20 to 16 cm on a chest radiograph, which assesses things from a two-dimensional frame of reference, the actual radius changes from 10 to 8 cm. This translates into a 50% net volume loss, rather than the 20% calculated by simple measurement of diameter loss from the radiograph itself (2).

Hemothorax

Hemothorax refers to a condition in which blood is present in the pleural space, usually resulting from trauma to the chest wall. Traumatic hemothorax represents a spectrum of clinical challenges. Most patients can be treated by tube thoracostomy and evacuation of the pleural space. However, a small subset of patients require operative intervention for hemorrhage control and adequate evacuation of the pleural space.

Posttraumatic hemothorax of sufficient size to be apparent on chest X-ray is most commonly due to laceration of the pulmonary parenchyma or chest wall vessels (intercostals or internal mammary artery). Standard treatment is large caliber–tube thoracostomy, which allows evacuation of the blood, reduces risk of clotted hemothorax, and provides accurate determination of the extent of ongoing bleeding. In the vast majority of cases, bleeding is self-limited, and operative intervention is unnecessary.

After tube thoracostomy, current guidelines recommend immediate surgery if 1500 mL of blood is evacuated initially or if drainage of 200 mL/hr for the ensuing two to four hours occurs (46). These guidelines coincide with the amount of blood loss expected to produce hemorrhagic shock in a previously healthy patient. Occasionally, despite early tube thoracostomy, the hemothorax is only partially evacuated. The residual blood then serves as a nidus for the development of empyema or fibrothorax, which ultimately may lead to thoracotomy and decortication to liberate the trapped lung. Advances in video-assisted thoracic surgery (VATS) have allowed the development of minimally invasive methods for draining retained hemothorax, and thereby have decreased the likelihood of developing empyema or fibrothorax. Clinical experience suggests that chest X-ray is insufficient to distinguish between retained hemothorax and contusion, and atelectasis or intraparenchymal hemorrhage that are not amenable to VATS treatment. Chest CT is much more useful in this scenario. Progressive clot organization and adherence leaves a window of three to five days postinjury when the semisolid clot and serum can be evacuated via VATS with a high degree of success. It may however, require persistence and multiple procedures to completely clear the pleural space. Repeated episodes of one-lung ventilation may actually increase the alveolar–arterial gradient and exacerbate relative hypoxemia.

Chylothorax

Chylothorax is the presence of lymph within the pleural space. It may be caused by congenital or primary lymphatic disease, but is usually due to intrathoracic malignancy with intrinsic or extrinsic obstruction, iatrogenic injury, or trauma. Postoperative chylothorax may complicate surgical procedures anywhere along the path of the thoracic duct between the diaphragm and the neck. Initial symptoms of dyspnea and exercise intolerance are the result of a large volume chylous effusion causing compressive atelectasis of the lung. Prolonged drainage leads to dehydration, malnutrition, and immunologic compromise due to loss of fluid, fat, protein, and lymphocytes, which make up the lymph fluid.

Nonoperative management may be appropriate as an initial strategy, particularly in the first few days after surgery or trauma, or in cases of malignancy that may respond to treatment of the primary disease (principally lymphoma). The components of initial management are drainage of the pleural space, reduction of chyle flow, and maintenance of hydration and adequate nutrition. Evacuation of the pleural space is most commonly achieved by tube thoracostomy, which facilitates pulmonary re-expansion and provides continuous drainage and accurate measurements of chyle flow. Chemical sclerotherapy is used to accelerate pleural symphysis and achieve obliteration of the pleural space.

Failed nonoperative management warrants surgical thoracic duct ligation. Lymphangiography provides useful information regarding the lymphatic anatomy and fistula site. Because it is quite challenging at times, it is usually only done in refractory chylothoraces that have failed initial surgical closure. Other methods to locate the leak include preoperative injection of Evans blue dye (1% subcutaneous in the thigh) or enteral administration of fat (cream or olive oil). Surgical options include direct ligation of the thoracic duct at the site of the leak, mass ligation of the thoracic duct and surrounding tissues, application of fibrin glue, or creation of a pleuroperitoneal shunt. If the chyle leak can be identified, direct ligation should be performed on either side of the leak. If the leak cannot be identified, mass ligation of all tissue between the aorta, spine, esophagus, and pericardium is best performed above the diaphragm in the right pleural space. This can be achieved either by thoracotomy or video-assisted thoracoscopy.

Traumatic Lung Injury
Smoke Inhalation and Pulmonary Dysfunction Following Burns

Burn injuries include smoke inhalation, direct thermal airway injuries, and pulmonary dysfunction caused by the products of combustion. The specific nature of the chemical products determines the lethality of the burn injury. Certain materials and chemicals are direct toxins to the airways and must be addressed aggressively if the burn victim is to survive. Edema formation and bronchoconstriction are early responses to released leukotrienes. Direct alveolar injury leads to increased lung water and difficulty in ventilation. Through the complement cascade, neutrophils migrate to the injured mucosa.

All patients with facial burns should be suspect for distal airway injuries. Upper airway edema and obstruction rapidly become life threatening and require bronchoscopy and intubation. This process progresses as high-volume fluid resuscitation and capillary leakage continues. While carbon monoxide levels are routinely obtained, many of the CNS manifestations are masked by intravenous narcotics needed for pain management.

Ventilatory support with the judicious use of fluids is critical if the patient is to survive. Pneumonias are expected with the prolonged need for pulmonary toilet and repeated bronchoscopy.

Chest Trauma

Chest trauma accounts for 10% to 12% of all trauma admissions to the hospital, but for nearly 25% of all deaths due to trauma (47). Chest wall injury is the most common thoracic injury, and rib fracture is associated with a 12% mortality. Chest trauma from penetrating sources is usually caused by knives or bullets, while blunt trauma injury usually comes from motor vehicle deceleration injuries. Fewer than 30% of all chest trauma patients require thoracotomy. In the immediate period, following a major motor vehicle collision, fatal injuries usually involve the thoracic aorta or heart and these patients typically die at the scene of the accident. Other life-threatening injuries can be managed effectively if they are recognized early.

The initial assessment of the trauma patient is the first priority. A patent airway must be confirmed and established rapidly. In certain instances, a surgical airway must be established when passage of an endotracheal tube is not possible or when upper airway obstruction exists. Hemodynamic control is the next priority and a large-bore intravenous access is mandatory for all patients. Most importantly, physical examination will reveal life-threatening injuries, which many times must be treated before obtaining diagnostic X-rays. These include tension pneumothorax, ruptured bronchus and diaphragm, and airway obstruction. While complete management algorithms of each of these entities are beyond the scope of this chapter, a basic understanding of these physiologic derangements is necessary to treat these patients. In many instances, chest tube insertion is the only interventional measure necessary for the management of these patients.

Tension pneumothorax must be recognized immediately during physical examination and treatment instituted with equal rapidity. The hallmarks of tension pneumothorax consist of complete lung collapse with concomitant tracheal deviation and mediastinal shift. Tachypnea, distended neck veins, and diaphoresis may be missed in a busy trauma bay. Because there is decreased venous return to the heart, hemodynamic instability in the form of hypotension and tachycardia occurs rapidly. Needle decompression followed by chest tube insertion is life saving and is warranted without X-ray examination.

Tracheobronchial injuries may be life threatening as well. Usually occurring within 2 cm of the carina, most injuries can be exposed and repaired through a right thoracotomy. Rarely is cardiopulmonary bypass necessary for the repair. These patients present with subcutaneous emphysema, pneumothorax, and massive air leak. Any patient with a pneumothorax that does not re-expand with chest tube insertion should be suspected of having a tracheobronchial injury. A definitive diagnosis requires careful bronchoscopy. Generally, repair consists of carefully placed interrupted absorbable sutures.

Fractures involving the upper six ribs are associated with life-threatening intrathoracic injuries, while fractures involving the lower six ribs are associated with life-threatening intra-abdominal injuries. Multiple rib fractures resulting in a flail segment have a significantly higher morbidity due to underlying pulmonary contusion. Elderly patients and/or patients with preexisting comorbidities and other underlying physiologic changes tend to have poorer outcomes.

Flail chest is the most serious chest wall injury encountered. Mechanically, it is the complete disruption of a portion of the chest wall by segmental fractures of two or more adjacent ribs (Fig. 9). It also may result from disruption of the ribs from the sternum at the costochondral cartilage and a fracture of the rib. Aside from the deleterious effects on chest wall mechanics and respiration, the force required to cause a flail chest places the patient at significant risk for other intrathoracic injuries.

Pain management is the most significant component to successful treatment of rib fractures and flail chest. The disruption of chest wall mechanics may decrease TV and impair the ability to generate an effective cough. This situation leads to the development of hypoventilation and subsequent atelectasis and pneumonia (48). Unless the affected segment is large, these alterations generally can be managed with incentive spirometry and aggressive pulmonary toilet, which require active patient participation. Oral narcotics rarely achieve effective pain control. Intravenous narcotics are able to provide adequate pain relief but at a degree of sedation that frequently will impair the patient's ability to effectively participate in pulmonary toilet. The preferred option for pain management is thoracic epidural anesthesia. A combination of narcotic and local anesthetic acts synergistically to provide excellent pain control without sedation. The patient can now breathe deeply and cough, and has increased mobility. This prevents hypoventilation, promotes clearance of secretions, and improves the chances of avoiding endotracheal intubation and mechanical ventilation.

Operative stabilization may be necessary for selected patients in whom adequate pain control cannot be achieved or who fail to be weaned from mechanical ventilation. Methods using either permanent or absorbable plates, screws, Kirschner wires, or Judet staples have been described. Stabilizing every other fractured rib is usually adequate to provide normalization of chest wall movement, decrease pain, and improve respiratory mechanics.

Pulmonary contusion is a diffuse hemorrhage into the lung parenchyma, resulting from either blunt or "blast injury" penetrating trauma (49). It commonly appears within several hours of the event as a patchy opacity on the chest X-ray, which then progresses over the next several days. Hemoptysis is a frequent manifestation of pulmonary contusion. Small peripheral contusions may produce only blood-tinged sputum, whereas injuries near the hilum may develop massive bleeding into the tracheobronchial tree that rarely may lead to life-threatening airway obstruction. In such circumstances, immediate resection of the damaged lung tissue and clearance of the airway is required.

Nonoperative management with attention to pulmonary toilet, incentive spirometry, and pneumonia surveillance is usually sufficient to treat the contusion (50). Strict attention to volume status is critical because over-resuscitation can contribute to pulmonary edema and hypoxia and volume depletion may result in hypotension and malperfusion syndromes. Monitoring central venous pressure and urine output is mandatory and some patients may require the use of pulmonary artery catheters. Effective drainage of effusions, hemothorax, or pneumothorax will greatly facilitate pulmonary expansion and maintain adequate oxygenation and ventilation.

NEOPLASTIC CONDITIONS
Mediastinum and Mediastinal Masses
The anatomy and the borders of the mediastinum predict the lesions that occur in this region. While surgical approaches were previously recommended for diagnosis of mediastinal masses, technological imaging advances have allowed greater noninvasive access to previously remote areas (Table 2). The anterior-superior mediastinum is the largest compartment and contains the greatest variety of pathology (50,51). Specific borders include the posterior sternum extending to the anterior pericardium. Typical components include the thymus gland, fat, and lymph nodes. The well-known mnemonic, the "4Ts" of the anterior mediastinum, includes thymoma, teratoma, terrible lymphoma, and thyroid. Access to this area can be readily obtained through anterior mediastinotomy and video thoracoscopy.

The middle mediastinum, also known as the visceral compartment, contains the heart, superior and inferior vena cava, ascending aorta and arch, main pulmonary arteries, phrenic and vagus nerves, trachea and main stem bronchi, and lymph nodes (50,51). Foregut duplication cysts originating from sequestrations of the ventral foregut are common. Bronchogenic cysts are the most common cysts followed by pericardial cysts. Mediastinoscopy is the most common

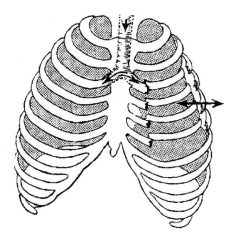

Figure 9 Fracture of chest wall in two locations is necessary for development of flail chest. Classic concept of altered mechanics causing "to-and-fro" movement of air between major bronchi (*double arrow*) has largely been dispelled. *Source*: From Ref. 2.

Table 2 Tumors of the Mediastinum

Anterior-superior compartment
   Parathyroid adenomas
   Thyroid tumors and cysts
   Thymic tumors and cysts
   Teratomas
   Pericardial cysts
   Germ cell tumors
   Bronchogenic cysts
   Lymphomas
Middle compartment
   Lymphatic tumors
   Lymphomas
   Foregut cysts
   Esophageal leiomyomas
   Pericardial cysts
   Bronchogenic cysts
Posterior compartment
   Neurogenic tumors
   Ganglioneuromas
   Gastroenteric cysts

access approach to this area. The posterior mediastinum extends from the posterior pericardium to the posterior chest wall and includes the esophagus, descending aorta, and the thoracic duct (50,51). Neurogenic tumors are the most common lesions in the posterior mediastinum. Typically, these lesions are malignant in children.

Clinically, the majority of mediastinal masses are asymptomatic and the physical examination is nondiagnostic. Lesions that are symptomatic have a higher likelihood of malignancy. While CT scan is the diagnostic test of choice, in certain circumstances, magnetic resonance imaging (MRI) is useful for delineating vascular and neuroanatomy relationships. Key tumor markers include LDH for lymphomas and seminoma differentiation. bHCG and alphafetoprotein levels should be obtained in all male patients and are complementary to a testicular examination and ultrasound.

Thymoma is the most common tumor of the anterior mediastinum. Thirty to fifty percent of patients have the autoimmune disease myasthenia gravis (MG). While many MG patients have muscle weakness, including diplopia and dysarthria, others present with paraneoplastic syndromes including agammaglobulinemia. CT is the diagnostic test of choice. Staging of thymoma is done at the time of surgery as determined by gross evidence of invasion. Surgical management of thymoma includes transcervical, median sternotomy, or VATS removal. The key surgical principle is complete surgical removal of the gland without leaving rests of residual tissue, precipitating recurrence. Adjuvant radiation therapy is used for frank invasion or residual tumor.

The anterior mediastinum is also the most common site of extragonadal germ cell tumors. Because they occur in young males (ages 20–35), all male patients should undergo testicular examination, including ultrasound and measurements of serum tumor markers. In general, cisplatin-based chemotherapy provides 50% five-year survival. Resection is reserved for teratomas and residual postchemotherapeutic tumor burden. Neurogenic tumors are the most common posterior mediastinal tumor, with most being exposed by thoracotomy or VATS. Dumbbell tumors extending into the spinal canal require MRI for delineation and neurosurgical assistance for removal.

Lymphomas commonly affect the mediastinum. Resection is rarely indicated or achievable; usually tissue

diagnosis, often utilizing flow cytometry, is all that is necessary. Once obtained, appropriate oncologic regimens are initiated. Substernal goiters cause compressive symptoms, including dyspnea and dysphagia and are more common in females. The majority (95%) can be removed through a cervical collar incision. Larger or deeper lesions may require partial sternal split for access and excision. Recurrent laryngeal nerve injury is rare despite the bulk of these lesions, due to the marked displacement of the normal anatomical structures.

Descending necrotizing mediastinitis must be considered when discussing the mediastinum. This rare polymicrobial infection commonly originates from an oropharyngeal source and carries a 50% mortality. The key to understanding this process is the realization that all three deep spaces of the neck (pretracheal, retrovisceral, and prevertebral) communicate with the chest and the mediastinum. Early aggressive drainage and debridement is needed with prolonged critical support if the patient is to survive. Many patients require additional drainage procedures because of developing loculations and empyema collections.

Tumors of the Lung

Lung cancer is the second most common malignancy in the United States. It is second in incidence to only prostate cancer in men and breast cancer in women. It is the leading cause of cancer-related deaths in men and women. The average age at diagnosis is 60 years. Despite some improvements in short-term survival, overall five-year survival remains at only 14%. The major cause of lung cancer has been clearly linked to smoking, with 80% to 90% of lung cancers occurring as a direct result of tobacco use.

Although both benign and malignant tumors occur in the lung, the vast majority (95–97%) of them are malignant. Malignant lung tumors are generally divided into non–small cell lung cancer (NSCLC) and small-cell lung cancer (SCLC) (52,53). NSCLC makes up about 80%, while SCLC makes up 10% to 15% of malignant lung tumors. Mixed tumor types are possible, and small cell carcinoma can be found with a non–small cell carcinoma in the same tumor, suggesting that both share a common precursor. With respect to benign neoplasia, hamartomas are the most common, followed by a variety of other tumors such as xanthomas, inflammatory pseudotumors, lipomas, myoblastomas, and fibrous mesotheliomas.

The vast majority of patients with lung tumors will present with symptomatic disease. Five percent of tumors are found incidentally on chest X-rays. The most common presenting symptoms are cough, weight loss, dyspnea, and chest pain; 30% of patients will present with hemoptysis. Occasionally, an unexplained solitary pulmonary nodule ("coin lesions") will be seen on chest X-ray in an asymptomatic patient. Most of these lesions are located in the lung periphery, are well circumscribed, are less than 5 cm in diameter, and occasionally exhibit calcifications. Half or more of these lesions will demonstrate malignancy on biopsy.

Advanced tumors invading the mediastinum may present with a wide range of findings depending on the structure involved (52,53). Vocal cord paralysis may result from invasion of the recurrent laryngeal nerve. Superior vena cava (SVC) syndrome results from SVC obstruction and may present with facial, neck, and upper extremity swelling, edema, cyanosis, headache, conjunctival injections, and occasionally orthopnea with a feeling of impending doom. Radiation therapy may alleviate some of these symptoms, but survival is usually measured in weeks to months. Extension of tumors into the thoracic inlet may result in shoulder and arm pain, Horner's syndrome (ptosis, miosis, exopthalmosis, and decreased sweating on the involved side due to involvement of the sympathetic ganglia), and Pancoast's syndrome (loss of upper-arm strength and ulnar paresthesisas due to involvement of the brachial plexus).

Ten to twenty percent of patients will present with a paraneoplastic syndrome in which various humoral agents are secreted by the tumor. Small-cell carcinoma and squamous cell carcinoma are the histologic subtypes commonly associated with these syndromes. Examples include the secretion of adrenocorticotrophic hormone–like substance that mimics Cushing's syndrome, a parathormone-like substance simulating hyperparathyroidism, and the manifestation of water retention and symptoms of hyponatremia due to secretion of an antidiuretic hormone–like substance. A particularly interesting extrapulmonary manifestation of lung cancer is hypertrophic pulmonary osteoarthropathy. This condition is characterized by clubbing of the fingers, diffuse bone (not joint) tenderness, and finger X-rays demonstrating linear calcium deposition along the periosteum. The precise mechanism responsible for this abnormality is unknown.

Diagnosis and staging of lung cancer is focused on early identification of patients with potentially curable tumors. In addition to the history and physical, imaging can help define tumor extent. In general, patients with X-ray findings of a suspicious pulmonary nodule should have a CT scan of the chest and upper abdomen. Patients with nonspecific neurologic or bony symptoms should have a head CT and/or radionuclide bone scan to assess for metastatic disease.

Histologic confirmation of lung cancer is not required prior to resection in an otherwise healthy patient with no evidence of advanced disease. If advanced disease is suspected and nonsurgical treatment is planned, histologic confirmation through bronchoscopy, transthoracic needle aspiration, and thoracoscopic and/or open biopsy should be obtained. Mediastinal lymph nodes larger than 1 cm seen on imaging should be biopsied by cervical mediastinoscopy or video-assisted thoracoscopic techniques.

Non–Small Cell Lung Cancer (NSCLC)

NSCLC can be divided into adenocarcinoma, squamous cell carcinoma, and large cell carcinoma. Adenocarcinoma is the most common type of lung cancer. Tumors are typically situated in the periphery and arise from subsegmental bronchioles. They can spread by both lymphatic and hematogenous routes. Squamous cell carcinoma is the next most common type of lung cancer. These tumors typically are centrally located. They can grow to a large size before metastasizing and can present with bronchus obstruction and central necrosis. They tend to metastasize to peribronchial or hilar lymph nodes. Large cell carcinoma is an undifferentiated aggressive tumor that can be difficult to distinguish from poorly differentiated adenocarcinoma or small cell carcinoma. Depending on the size of the tumor and its location, lobectomy or pneumonectomy is the usual surgical option.

Multiple genetic derangements have been described (54,55). The most common activated proto-oncogene in NSCLC is *k-ras*. In more than 50% of NSCLC, the tumor suppressor gene *p53* is overexpressed or mutated. Other genes implicated include *erbB*, *Rb*, and *bcl-2*. A genetic susceptibility to lung cancer has also been demonstrated, and the most common chromosomal abnormalities involve chromosomes 1, 3, 7, 9, and 17.

The TNM staging of NSCLC is shown in Figure 10. In general, tumors invading the mediastinum, those associated with a malignant pleural effusion, those with nodal metastasis to the contralateral side (stage IIIB), and those with metastasis to distant organ sites (such as brain, bone, kidneys, adrenals, etc.) represent advanced disease that will not be helped with aggressive surgical therapy.

Survival following surgical resection is shown below:

	1-yr survival (%)	5-yr survival (%)
Stage I	72–94	38–67
Stage II	55–89	22–55
Stage IIIa		23–25

Recent studies have shown a survival benefit for patients receiving adjuvant platinum-based chemotherapy after complete surgical resection. In the International Adjuvant Lung Cancer Trial, there was a 4.1% survival advantage in the surgery plus chemotherapy group (over surgery alone) for patients in stage I to stage III (57). In the Cancer and Leukemia Group B Protocol 9633, for patients with stage IB disease, chemotherapy after surgical resection conferred a 12% survival advantage (58). In the NCIC-BR10 study, a similar 15% overall survival advantage was seen for stage IB and stage II patients who received adjuvant chemotherapy (59). Recent trials regarding preoperative induction chemotherapy or chemoradiation therapy suggests there may be a benefit in a patient with stage II to IIIa disease.

Small Cell Lung Cancer (SCLC)

Approximately 15% of all lung cancers are SCLC. The vast majority present with advanced disease and surgery is generally not indicated (60). The overall five-year survival is 5% to 10%. One percent of patients with SCLC present with stage I or II disease. Five-year survival rates of approximately 50% have been reported in patients with SCLC with stage I or II disease, who underwent resection followed by chemoradiation.

LUNG TRANSPLANTATION

As of 2001, 12,000 lung transplants have been performed worldwide, with one-year survivals being in the 75% range for most patients requiring this form of treatment to manage their underlying pulmonary disease (61). Functional results are durable when the procedure is performed at experienced centers. Clinical indications for single- and double-lung transplantation are very specific and guidelines for both the donor and recipient must be adhered to because of the scarcity of available organs. Improvement in patient selection is the single most important factor responsible for the success of pulmonary transplantation. The majority of adult lung transplants are performed for emphysema due to COPD or alpha-1 antitrypsin deficiency. Other indications include cystic and pulmonary fibrosis. Operative mortality and long-term survival are directly associated with the patient's underlying diagnosis; patients with pulmonary hypertension and pulmonary fibrosis are typically more difficult to manage. Expected improvements in FEV$_1$ are well documented following successful surgery. Specific lung transplant complications include early allograft dysfunction, which may be caused by poor donor preservation or underlying lung pathology. Airway anastomotic complications have decreased as surgical anastomotic techniques

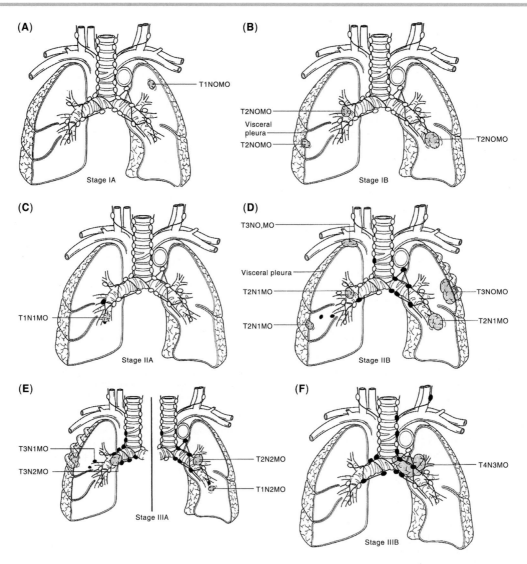

Figure 10   Staging of lung cancer. (**A**) Stage IA disease (T1 N0 M0) identifies a small ($<$ 3 cm) tumor surrounded by lung parenchyma. (**B**) Stage IB disease (T2 N0 M0) includes larger tumors that invade the visceral pleura or the main bronchi, or that have evidence of atelectasis/pneumonitis extending to the hilar regions. No metastatic disease is present with stage I tumors. (**C**) Stage IIA (T1 N1 M0) identifies small tumors with T1 characteristics ($<$ 3 cm) involving the peribronchial or hilar nodes by extension or metastasis. (**D**) Stage IIB disease includes larger tumors ($>$ 3 cm) involving the peribronchial or hilar lymph nodes (T2 N1 M0) or tumors with limited extrapulmonary extension such as involvement of the chest wall or the pericardium (T3 N0 M0) but no evidence of metastasis. (**E**) Stage IIIA describes tumors with localized extrapulmonary extension and involvement of peribronchial or hilar lymph nodes (T3 N1 M0) as well as any T1, T2, or T3 tumors with metastasis to the ipsilateral mediastinal and subcarinal lymph nodes (T1, T2, or T3 N2 M0). (**F**) Stage IIIB describes either extensive extrapulmonary tumor invasion (T4 any N M0) or metastasis to the contralateral mediastinal and hilar lymph nodes as well as ipsilateral and contralateral supraclavicular/scalene lymph nodes. *Source*: From Ref. 56.

and perioperative management have improved. Bronchiolitis obliterans with a decline in FEV$_1$ has continued to plague long-term lung transplantation results and survival. This form of chronic allograft dysfunction is undergoing aggressive research and may be related to the high frequency of gastroesophageal reflux in lung transplant patients.

SUMMARY

Oxygen delivery to meet tissue needs is critical to the survival of the human organism. The lungs make this possible by optimally matching ventilation to pulmonary arterial perfusion, so that inhaled oxygen is effectively diffused across the alveolar-capillary membrane in exchange for carbon dioxide, which is then removed from the body during exhalation. Disturbances in ventilation, perfusion, or alveolar-capillary membrane diffusion can drastically perturb the adequacy of tissue oxygenation and thereby directly influence not only the risk of undergoing an operative procedure, but also the likelihood that postoperative complications will occur. Accordingly, it is essential that the surgeon fully understand the basic mechanisms responsible for normal pulmonary function, and the way to optimize this function in patients with lung disease to insure a smooth perioperative course when surgical intervention is necessary. This chapter has summarized the basic mechanisms of lung function and how they are perturbed by a variety of insults, including intrinsic disease, infection, trauma, and neoplasia.

REFERENCES

1. Jackson CL, Huber JF. Correlated applied anatomy of the bronchial tree and lungs with a system of nomenclature. Dis Chest 1943; 9:319. [Adapted by Putnam JB Jr. Lung (including pulmonary embolism and thoracic outlet syndrome). In: Townsend CM Jr., et al., eds. Sabiston Textbook of Surgery. Philadelphia: Saunders WB and Co. 7th ed. 2001:1207].

2. Richardson JD. Common pulmonary derangements, respiratory failure, and adult respiratory distress syndrome. In: Miller TA, ed. Modern Surgical Care: Physiologic Foundations & Clinical Applications. 2nd ed. St. Louis: Quality Medical Pub, 1998:738–764.

3. West J. Pulmonary pathophysiology. Baltimore: Williams & Wilkins, 1982.

4. Whitcomb ME. The Lung, Normal and Diseased. St. Louis: Mosby, 1982:viii, 360.

5. Wright JR. Pulmonary surfactant: a front line of lung host defense. J Clin Invest 2003; 111(10):1453.

6. Wu H, Kuzmenko A, Wan S, et al. Surfactant proteins A and D inhibit the growth of Gram-negative bacteria by increasing membrane permeability. J Clin Invest 2003; 111(10):1589.

7. Richardson JD, Woods D, Johanson WG Jr, et al. Lung bacterial clearance following pulmonary contusion. Surgery 1979; 86(5):730.

8. Peters RM, et al. The Scientific Management of Surgical Patients. Little, Brown & Co, Boston: 1983.

9. Joost O, Wilk JB, Cupples LA, et al. Genetic loci influencing lung function: a genome-wide scan in the Framingham Study. Am J Respir Crit Care Med 2002; 165(6):795.

10. McKeever TM, Scrivener S, Broadfield E, et al. Prospective study of diet and decline in lung function in a general population. Am J Respir Crit Care Med 2002; 165(9):1299.

11. Crim C. Physiology of respiration. In: Miller TA, ed. Modern Surgical Care: Physiologic Foundations & Clinical Applications. 2nd ed. St. Louis: Quality Medical Pub, 1998, pp 729–737.

12. Scott–Conner C. Operative Anatomy, Lippincott.

13. West JB, Dollery CT, Naimark A. Distribution of blood flow in isolated lung: relation to vascular and alveolar pressures. J Appl Physiol 1964; 19:713.

14. Benz EJ Jr. Synthesis, structure and function of hemoglobin. In: Kelly WN, Devita VT, eds. Textbook of Internal Medicine. Vol. 1. Philadelphia, JB Lippincott, 1989:236.

15. West JB. Respiratory Physiology–The Essentials. 7th ed: Baltimore: Lippincott Williams & Wilkins, 2005.

16. Warner MA, Offord KP, Warner ME, et al. Role of preoperative cessation of smoking and other factors in postoperative pulmonary complications: a blinded prospective study of coronary artery bypass patients. Mayo Clin Proc 1989; 64(6):609.

17. Dunn WF, Scanlon PD. Preoperative pulmonary function testing for patients with lung cancer. Mayo Clin Proc 1993; 68(4):371.

18. Fessler HE, Scharf SM, Permutt S. Improvement in spirometry following lung volume reduction surgery: application of a physiologic model. Am J Respir Crit Care Med 2002; 165(1):34.

19. Weisman IM. Cardiopulmonary exercise testing in the preoperative assessment for lung resection surgery. Semin Thorac Cardiovasc 2001; 13(2):116.

20. Daly JM, Barie PS, Fahey TJ III. Preparation of the patient. In: Baker RJ, Fischer JF, eds. Mastery of Surgery. 4th ed. Philadelphia: Lippincott William & Wilkins, 2003:23–53.

21. Schauer PR, Luna J, Ghiatas AA, et al. Pulmonary function after laparoscopic cholecystectomy. Surgery 1993; 114:389.

22. Bonnet F, Marret E. Influence of anaesthetic and analgesic techniques on outcome after surgery. Br J Anaesth 2005; 95(1):52.

23. Ashbaugh DG, Bigelow DB, Petty TL, et al. Acute respiratory distress in adults. Lancet 1967; 2(7511):319.

24. Bernard GR, Artigas A, Brigham KL, et al. The American-European Consensus Conference on ARDS. Definitions, mechanisms, relevant outcomes, and clinical trial coordination. Am J Respir Crit Care Med 1994; 149(3 Pt 1):818.

25. Bersten AD, Edibam C, Hunt T, et al. Incidence and mortality of acute lung injury and the acute respiratory distress syndrome in three Australian States. Am J Respir Crit Care Med 2002; 165(4):443.

26. Marshall RP, Webb S, Bellingan GJ, et al. Angiotensin converting enzyme insertion/deletion polymorphism is associated with susceptibility and outcome in acute respiratory distress syndrome. Am J Respir Crit Care Med 2002; 166(5):646.

27. Luhr OR, Antonsen K, Karlsson M, et al. Incidence and mortality after acute respiratory failure and acute respiratory distress syndrome in Sweden, Denmark, and Iceland. The ARF Study Group. Am J Respir Crit Care Med 1999; 159(6):1849.

28. Tomashefski JF Jr. Pulmonary pathology of the adult respiratory distress syndrome. Clin Chest Med 1990; 11(4):593.

29. Dellinger PR. Adult respiratory distress syndrome: current consideration and future directions. New Horizons 1993; 1.

30. The Acute Respiratory Distress Syndrome Network. Ventilation with lower tidal volumes as compared with traditional tidal volumes for acute lung injury and the acute respiratory distress syndrome. N Engl J Med 2000; 342(18):1301.

31. Hirvela ER. Advances in the management of acute respiratory distress syndrome: protective ventilation. Arch Surg 2000; 135(2):126.

32. Aggarwal AN, Gupta D, Behera D, et al. Analysis of static pulmonary mechanics helps to identify functional defects in survivors of acute respiratory distress syndrome. Crit Care Med 2000; 28(10):3480.

33. Hopkins RO, Weaver LK, Collingridge D, et al. Two-year cognitive, emotional, and quality-of-life outcomes in acute respiratory distress syndrome. Am J Respir Crit Care Med 2005; 171(4):340.

34. Shields RT. Pathogenesis of postoperative pulmonary atelectasis. Arch Surg 1949; 58:489.

35. Calverley PM. The GOLD classification has advanced understanding of COPD. Am J Respir Crit Care Med 2004; 170(3):211; discussion 4.

36. Nelson HS. Beta-adrenergic bronchodilators. N Engl J Med 1995; 333:499.

37. Katzenstein AL, Myers JL. Idiopathic pulmonary fibrosis: current relevance of pathologic classification. Am J Respir Crit Care Med 1998; 157:1301.

38. Bowton DL. Nosocomial pneumonia in the ICU—year 2000 and beyond. Chest 1999; 115:28S.

39. Heyland DK, Cook DJ, Griffith L, et al. The attributable morbidity and mortality of ventilator-associated pneumonia in the critically ill patient. The Canadian Critical Trials Group. Am J Respir Crit Care Med 1999; 159(4 Pt 1):1249.

40. Chastre J, Fagon JY, Bornet-Lecso M, et al. Evaluation of bronchoscopic techniques for the diagnosis of nosocomial pneumonia. Am J Respir Crit Care Med 1995; 152(1):231.

41. Drakulovic MB, Torres A, Bauer TT, et al. Supine body position as a risk factor for nosocomial pneumonia in mechanically ventilated patients: a randomised trial. Lancet 1999; 354:1851.

42. Kollef MH. Selective digestive decontamination should not be routinely employed. Chest 2003; 123(suppl 5):464S.

43. Kollef MH. Prevention of hospital-associated pneumonia and ventilator-associated pneumonia. Crit Care Med 2004; 32(6):1396.

44. Pohlson EC, McNamara JJ, et al. Lung abscess: a changing pattern of the disease. Am J Surg 1985; 150:97.

45. Cina G, Marra R, Di Stasi C, Macis G. Epidemiology, pathophysiology and natural history of venous thromboembolism. Rays 1996; 21:315.

46. Peitzman AB, Puyana JC. Hemothorax. In: Cameron JL, ed. Current Surgical Therapy. 8th ed. Philadelphia: Elsevier Mosby, 679.

47. Mattox KL, Feliciano DV, Moore EE. Trauma. 4th ed. New York: McGraw-Hill, 1999.

48. Ahmed Z, Mohyuddin Z. Management of flail chest injury: internal fixation versus endotracheal intubation and ventilation. J Thoracic Cardiovasc Surg 1995; 110:1676–1680.

49. Trinkle JK, et al. Pulmonary contusion: pathogenesis and effect of various resuscitative measures. Ann Thorac Surg 1973; 16:569.

50. Davis RD, Oldham HN, Sabiston DC. Primary cysts and neoplasms of the mediastinum: recent changes in clinical presentation, methods of diagnosis, management and results. Ann Thorac Surg 1987; 44:229.

51. Cirino LM, Milanez de Campos JR, Fernandez A, et al. Diagnosis and treatment of mediastinal tumors by thoracoscopy. Chest 2000; 117:1787.

52. Depierre A, Milleron B, Moro-Sibilot D, et al. Preoperative chemotherapy followed by surgery compared with primary surgery in resectable stage I (except T1N0), II, and III A non-small cell lung cancer. J Clin Oncol 2002; 20:247.

53. Mountain CF, Dresler CM. Regional lymph node classification for lung cancer staging. Chest 1997; 111:1718.

54. Slebos RJC, Kibbelaar RE, Dalesio O, et al. K-ras oncogene activation as a prognostic marker in adenocarcinoma of the lung. N Eng J Med 1990; 323:561.

55. Rusch VW, Dmitrovsky E. Molecular biologic features of non-small cell lung cancer: clinical implications. Chest Surg Clin N Am 1995; 5:39.

56. Mountain CF. International system for staging lung cancer. Semin Surg Oncol 2001; 18:106.

57. Arriagada R, Bergman B, Dunant A, et al. Cisplatin-based adjuvant chemotherapy in patients with completely resected non-small-cell lung cancer. N Engl J Med 2004; 350(4):351.

58. Kato H, Tsuboi M, Kato Y, et al. Postoperative adjuvant therapy for completely resected early-stage non-small cell lung cancer. Int J Clin Oncol 2005; 10(3):157.

59. Winton T, Livingston R, Johnson D, et al. Vinorelbine plus cisplatin vs. observation in resected non-small-cell lung cancer. N Engl J Med 2005; 352(25):2589.

60. Lassen U, Hansen HH. Surgery in limited stage small cell lung cancer. Cancer Treat Rev 1999; 25:67.

61. Lau CL, Davis RD. Lung transplantation. In: Norton JA, et al., eds. Surgery: Basic Science and Clinical Evidence. New York: Springer-Verlag, 2001:1509.

32

Normal Cardiac Function

Andrew C. Fiore and Andrew S. Wechsler

INTRODUCTION

As a component of the cardiovascular system, the heart is responsible for maintaining adequate blood flow to meet the metabolic needs of the body. This is accomplished by the integration of neural, metabolic, anatomic, and physiologic subsystems that combine to form the intact, functioning human heart. An understanding of cardiac function must consider each of these factors, because a knowledge of only one, or even several, without an appreciation of the others gives an incomplete picture of the physiologic mechanisms responsible for this function. In discussing cardiac physiology, it is appropriate to begin with the molecular events underlying contraction and relaxation, to provide the basis for understanding the performance of the intact organ.

MOLECULAR MECHANISMS IN CONTRACTION AND RELAXATION

The basis of cardiac function is the relationship between the contractile proteins, actin and myosin. The nature of this relationship determines to a large extent the characteristics of activation and relaxation in individual muscle cells and in the intact heart. As in skeletal muscle, the functional unit of cardiac muscle is the sarcomere. The sarcomere is composed principally of four proteins (1). These are the previously mentioned contractile proteins, actin and myosin and the regulatory complex consisting of tropomyosin and troponin. In electron micrographs, the sarcomere appears as an arrangement of thick and thin filaments. This arrangement is shown schematically in Figure 1. The thick filament exists as an aggregate of myosin molecules. Myosin consists of a pair of heavy, coiled polypeptide chains, each of which is attached to a globular head region.

These head regions project from the axial core of the myosin aggregate and form cross-bridges to the thin filament (Fig. 2). The thin filament is made up of actin in association with troponin and tropomyosin. Actin is a globular molecule that polymerizes to form a double-stranded α-helical filament. Actin filaments attach to the Z line of the sarcomere and project inward as the thin filament. Here, they interact to various degrees with the thick filament. This interaction is regulated by troponin and tropomyosin.

Tropomyosin spans the length of the thin filament, and the troponin complex is normally located at every seventh actin site (4). Troponin consists of three subgroups that are responsible for binding calcium ions and for regulating the formation of attachments between actin and myosin by way of the cross-bridges (5). Troponin I hugs the myosin-binding site on actin and thereby prevents interaction with myosin, which is necessary to form the actin–myosin cross-bridge.

Troponin T anchors the three troponin subunits to tropomyosin, while troponin C is involved in the initiation of contraction through its calcium-binding site (6–8). In the resting state, tropomyosin blocks the binding sites on actin so that cross-bridge interaction is prevented. The presence of calcium bound to the troponin complex leads to a conformational change in tropomyosin, such that the actin–myosin association is no longer blocked. It is the specific binding of calcium to troponin C that removes the inhibitory effect of troponin I on the myosin-binding site of actin. Such removal allows formation of the actin–myosin cross-bridge (6–8).

The head region of myosin is the enzymatically active portion of the molecule (1). Adenosine triphosphate (ATP) binds here and is hydrolyzed to adenosine diphosphate and phosphorus (P). In this form, the affinity of myosin for actin is enhanced, such that if calcium is present, an actin–myosin complex is formed. As the hydrolysis products are released from the complex, the myosin head undergoes a conformational change that displaces the actin filament relative to the myosin. In this manner, force generation and shortening are accomplished. The addition of ATP to the actin–myosin complex results in dissociation of the filaments. The ATP is once again hydrolyzed, and the process repeats (6–10).

Force generation during activation depends to a large extent on the number of cross-bridge attachments that are formed (11). This number is a function of the degree of filament overlap and the level of calcium present. The rate of shortening is a measure of the ATPase activity of myosin (12). It has been established that myosin exists in several forms that are distinguished by the composition of their heavy chains (13). These various forms differ in their ATPase kinetics and thus in their rate of fiber shortening (14). The

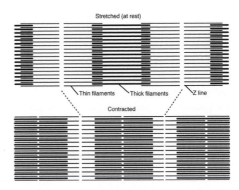

Figure 1 Schematic diagram showing the pattern of thick and thin filaments of one sarcomere. Degree of filament overlap varies with the phase of contraction. *Source:* From Ref. 2.

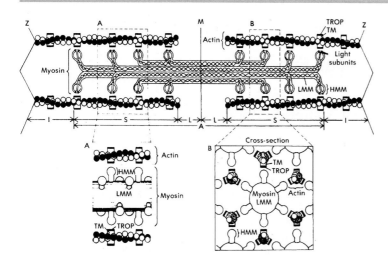

Figure 2 Detailed representation of filament structure. Helical tails of the myosin molecules form a rigid rod-like structure. Globular heads project from this toward the actin filament. (**A–B**) Three-dimensional relationships. Each myosin is seen to interact with six actin filaments (*B*). Note steric hindrance provided by troponin (*TROP*) and tropomyosin (*TM*). *Abbreviations*: HMM, heavy meromyosin; LMM, light meromyosin. *Source*: From Ref. 3.

composition of the myosin subunits is genetically determined; however, it has been shown to change in response to such hormones as thyroxin and to chronic elevations in the mechanical loading of the muscle (15,16).

The Cellular Basis of Cardiac Contraction

Cardiomyocytes may be considered to consist of three systems: (i) a sarcolemmal excitation system that participates in the spread of the action potential (AP) and functions as a switch that initiates the intracellular events giving rise to contraction, (ii) an intracellular excitation–contraction coupling (ECC) system that amplifies and converts the electrical excitation signal to a chemical signal that, in turn, activates the contractile system (iii) contractile system, a molecular motor based on formation of chemical cross-bridges between the two proteins, actin and myosin.

Excitation System

The cellular AP consists of a transient, local trans-sarcolemmal depolarizing current that raises the transmembrane potential from its normal resting value of negative 80 to 90 mV to slightly positive values, followed by a depolarizing current that returns the potential to its resting value. The AP is initiated within the specialized conduction tissue and is propagated to individual myocytes. It results from a series of coordinated changes in the conductance of specific ionic species through variably gated sarcolemmal channels. The earliest and largest component of membrane depolarization is caused by a rapid, inward Na current. The resting potential is established and maintained by the trans-sarcolemmal Na-K-ATPase, which uses energy from ATP hydrolysis to pump Na ions out of the cytoplasm.

With respect to initiation of contraction, the most important component of AP is a relatively slow, inward Ca current through voltage-sensitive, L-type (for long-lasting) Ca channels. These channels open, and the current begins to flow when transmembrane potential reaches −35 to −20 mV and, because of its slow kinetics, continues well after the Na current has ceased. The Ca current is mainly responsible for the AP plateau phase. It ceases when L-type channels become inactivated and regenerative currents (mainly K efflux) begin the repolarization process. L-type channels, also termed dihydropyridine receptors, are concentrated

in invaginations of the sarcolemma called the transverse-tubule system, in close proximity to the sarcoplasmic reticulum (SR) membrane–associated ryanodine receptor Ca release channels.

The AP results in a net movement of Ca ions into and Na ions out of the cytoplasm. Ionic balance is restored mainly by another sarcolemmal ion-transport mechanism, the Na–Ca exchanger. The exchanger is a shuttle that moves one Ca ion out of the cell against its concentration gradient while using energy from the Na gradient to move one Na ion into the cell. The exchanger also can function in the so-called reverse mode, moving a Ca ion into and a Na ion out of the cytoplasm. Normally, the reverse mode does not contribute significantly to inward movement of Ca ions.

Excitation-Contraction Coupling

Myocardial contraction is initiated following a rise in cytosolic calcium. During the plateau phase of the cardiac AP, a small number of calcium ions enter the muscle cell through slow channels. These ions do not significantly alter myoplasmic calcium (Ca^{2+}), but they do cause release of calcium stores from SR (17). This release significantly elevates myoplasmic Ca^{2+}. Calcium is now available to bind to troponin C, and muscle activation occurs. This process, in which calcium entry triggers intracellular calcium release and muscle activation, is called ECC (Fig. 3).

It is interesting to note the amplification of the effects of calcium in this process. The small number of ions entering the cell through the slow channel cause the release of intracellular stores that raise the myoplasmic Ca^{2+} from a resting value of 10^{-7} to 10^{-5} M (6). In turn, each calcium ion that binds to troponin C activates seven actin-binding sites. This two-step amplification illustrates the exquisite sensitivity of the muscle cell to calcium (18).

Muscle relaxation depends on the presence of adequate levels of ATP, which act to dissociate the actin–myosin complexes and provide energy for the restoration of myoplasmic Ca^{2+} to resting levels. The latter is accomplished primarily by a calcium-activated ATPase in the membrane of SR. In addition, smaller amounts of calcium are extruded from the cell through an Na^+/Ca^{2+} exchange mechanism that operates secondary to the Na^+, K^+-ATPase of the sarcolemma and is not voltage dependent, as are the slow

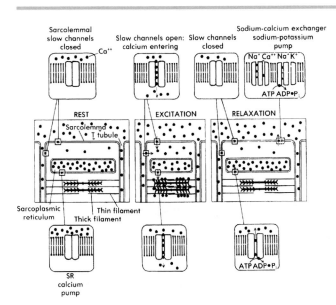

Figure 3 Representation of the transmembrane calcium movements during a contraction cycle. At rest, calcium concentration in the sarcoplasm is low when compared with that in the extracellular space and the interior of sarcoplasmic reticulum (SR). Slow channel is closed, and Ca^{2+} pumps are inactive. During excitation, the slow channel opens, allowing a small number of extracellular Ca^{2+} ions to enter the cell. This entry triggers a release of Ca^{2+} from SR, and the contraction proceeds. Relaxation is accomplished by the active restoration of resting gradients. *Abbreviations*: ADP, adenosine diphosphate; ATP, adenosine triphosphate; P_i, inorganic phosphate. *Source*: From Ref. 11.

channels (11,19,20). As calcium levels return to normal, troponin I reestablishes its cloaking of the myosin-binding site so that actin–myosin cross-bridging is again prevented.

Energy Metabolism

Myocytes are heavily dependent on oxidative metabolism and endowed with large numbers of mitochondria. Under basal conditions, myocytes preferentially take up and oxidize fatty acids to generate ATP. During stress, however, glucose uptake, glycogenolysis, and glycolysis become increasingly important. Certain ion pumps (e.g., SERCA2, see below) may be especially dependent on glycolytic ATP. Nitric oxide generated by vascular endothelium decreases myocardial oxygen consumption (VO_2) due to a direct effect on mitochondrial respiration, and may have a significant role in normal control of energy production and utilization.

The processes that account for the great majority of myocardial energy consumption are cross-bridge cycling (myosin ATPase), Ca reuptake by SR (SERCA2), and basal metabolism. Each cross-bridge cycle consumes one high-energy phosphate bond, although at very rapid cycling rates, it may be possible for one ATP to fuel more than one cycle. SERCA2 uses one high-energy phosphate bond for every two Ca ions pumped. As indicated earlier, the rate of energy consumption is heavily dependent on loading conditions, and resulting work and power generation. The thermodynamic efficiency of the heart muscle, its total mechanical energy output divided by its total chemical energy input, is uncertain, in large measure because of difficulties in quantifying total energy output. A more conventional approach is estimation of efficiency of external work production. External work efficiency is heavily dependent on loading conditions, ranging from a maximum under unloaded conditions to zero for an isometric contraction.

MECHANICS OF ISOLATED MUSCLE

Much of what is known about the nature of cardiac function has been learned from studies of isolated muscle. Under these conditions, it is possible to finely control the loading of the muscle while making accurate measurements of force

development and shortening characteristics. From these studies, three factors have arisen that determine the behavior of isolated muscle. They are muscle preload, afterload, and contractile state (21,22).

Preload is defined as the distending force, or load, that is placed on a muscle before contraction. The preload and the distensibility of the muscle are the determinants of the initial length of the muscle before contraction. The load encountered by the muscle after activation is defined as the afterload. The magnitude of the afterload determines the nature of the subsequent contraction. If the muscle is able to generate a force equivalent to the afterload, shortening occurs. Such a contraction is termed isotonic, because the force developed by the muscle is equal to the load and therefore remains constant during shortening. If the muscle is unable to generate force equal to the load, no external shortening occurs and the contraction is said to be isometric. Contractility refers to the intrinsic ability of the muscle to contract independently of loading conditions. This meaning will become clearer as the characteristics of muscle activation are explained.

Isotonic contractions are useful for studying the shortening characteristics of isolated muscle. From these studies, several fundamental principles of cardiac-muscle mechanics have been developed. The first of these defines the relationship between afterload and shortening. As the afterload is increased, the extent of muscle shortening and the velocity of shortening decrease (21). This effect is shown in isolated cat papillary muscle in Figure 4.

Cardiac muscle exhibits length-dependent properties: the length of the muscle before contraction affects the nature of the contraction. As initial muscle length is increased, there is an increase in both the extent and the velocity of shortening (Fig. 5). A third property of cardiac muscle involves the response of the muscle to inotropic agents. Positive inotropes enhance the contractility of the muscle, as defined by an increase in the rate and extent of shortening generated from a given preload. Figure 6 shows the effects of a positive inotrope on the velocity and extent of shortening. A unique feature of the force–velocity relationship is that it allows an estimation of the contractile state of the muscle. Theoretically, the velocity of muscle shortening at zero load should

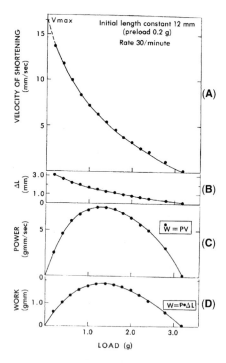

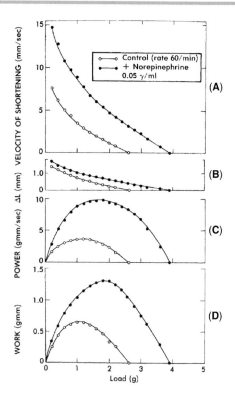

Figure 4 Force–velocity relations of isolated cat papillary muscle. **(A)** Velocity of the isotonic contraction is seen to be a decreasing function of load. Extrapolation of the velocity at 0 load (*dashed line*) provides an estimate of maximum velocity (V_{max}). **(B)** Extent of shortening (ΔL) also decreases with increasing load. **(C–D)** Concomitant effects of increasing load (*P*) on power and work (*W*). *PV*, load × velocity of muscle shortening. *Source*: From Ref. 21.

Figure 6 **(A)** Application of norepinephrine causes an increase in the shortening and maximum velocity. **(B)** Extent of muscle shortening is also increased at any shortening load. **(C)** and **(D)** show concomitant effects of load on power and work. *Source*: From Ref. 21.

be determined only by the kinetics of the actin–myosin association. Because any muscle contraction is necessarily loaded to some extent by the preload, the velocity of shortening at zero load (V_{max}) can be obtained only by extrapolation of

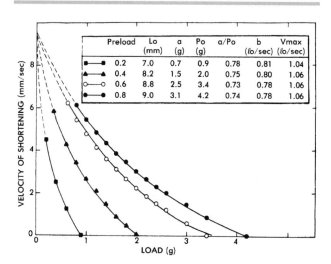

	Preload	Lo (mm)	a (g)	Po (g)	a/Po	b (ℓo/sec)	Vmax (ℓo/sec)
■	0.2	7.0	0.7	0.9	0.78	0.81	1.04
▲	0.4	8.2	1.5	2.0	0.75	0.80	1.06
○	0.6	8.8	2.5	3.4	0.73	0.78	1.06
●	0.8	9.0	3.1	4.2	0.74	0.78	1.06

Figure 5 Effects of varied preload on the force–velocity relations of cat papillary muscle. As the preload is increased, the velocity of shortening increases. However, the maximum velocity (V_{max}) does not change. *Source*: From Ref. 21.

the force–velocity curve to zero load. For the relationship shown in Figure 6, the addition of norepinephrine resulted in an increase in the extrapolated value of V_{max}. In contrast, Figure 5 demonstrates the required load independence of contractility as suggested by the stable estimates of V_{max} (21).

Isometric contractions provide a convenient means to study force development in isolated muscle. When a muscle is stimulated to contract isometrically, the amount of force (tension) developed depends only on the length before contraction and the inotropic state of the muscle. Variations in afterload are not a factor, because by definition, the magnitude of the afterload always exceeds the force-generating capability of the muscle. Increasing the initial length of the muscle at a given contractile state results in an increase in the level of resting tension borne by the muscle (Fig. 7). As the length of the muscle increases, the peak force generated from any given length also increases (Fig. 7), as does the rate of force development (dF/dt). The addition of Ca^{2+} has the effect of a positive inotrope on the isometric preparation. Specifically, resting tension is unaffected, but the peak force, time to peak force, and dF/dt are enhanced.

When a muscle fiber is distended, a point is reached at which force development is maximum. The length at this point is termed L_{max}. Further increases in muscle length beyond L_{max} result in a reduction in the amount of developed tension (6). This and other length-dependent properties of the muscle can be explained in part by relating the various muscle lengths to the degree of overlap in the thick and thin filaments of the sarcomere (Fig. 8). At rest, sarcomere length, defined as

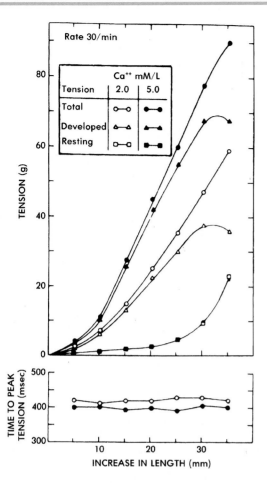

Figure 7 When a muscle contracts isometrically, the amount of tension that is developed depends on the length and inotropic state of the muscle. In this figure, the upward exponential curve (*squares*) represents the resting tension existing in the muscle as it is stretched to increasing lengths. Developed tension (*open triangles*) generated during isometric contraction from each length increases as the muscle is stretched. Addition of calcium does not affect the resting length–tension curve but does cause an upward displacement of developed tension. *Source*: From Ref. 23.

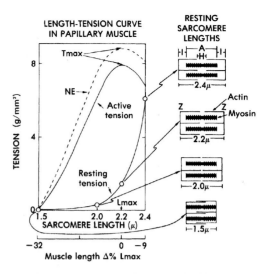

Figure 8 Representation of the relationship between active tension, resting tension, and filament overlap in the feline right ventricle. These relationships form the basis of the Frank–Starling principle as seen in the intact heart. Note that the degree of active tension that is developed depends on the extent of filament overlap. Maximum active tension (T_{max}) is developed at a sarcomere length of 2.2 μm (L_{max}), which also corresponds to the optimum length for filament interaction. *Abbreviation*: NE, norepinephrine. *Source*: From Ref. 3.

the distance between adjacent Z lines, averages 1.8 μm. As the muscle is lengthened, sarcomere length increases. More importantly, there is an increase in the degree of overlap between the chemically active portions of the thick and thin filaments. Because the potential for the formation of force-generating cross-bridges is increasing, there is a concomitant increase in the amount of force developed. The length of the sarcomere at L_{max} averages 2.2 μm. At this distance, the thick and thin filaments are arranged such that all myosin heads lie adjacent to actin filaments. In this state, the probability of interaction between the filaments is greatest; hence, force generation is greatest. With the application of large forces, cardiac muscle can be distended beyond L_{max}. Little change occurs in the amount of filament overlap, even though active tension declines sharply. This decline has been attributed to the damage of the myocytes as a result of the large deformations produced by the loading force (24). This relationship explains why overdistention of the heart (excessive filling) results in deterioration of cardiac function.

Examination of the resting force–length relationship reveals a nonlinear relationship between applied force and

deformation (25). This behavior is illustrated in the resting length–tension curves of Figures 7 and 8. At the lower ranges of preload, a given increment in applied force results in a relatively large degree of fiber deformation. In the upper range, the same increment in applied force results in a smaller deformation. This behavior is a manifestation of the mechanical properties of the tissue. The significance of this property will become evident when filling of the intact heart is discussed.

FUNCTION OF THE INTACT HEART

The heart is composed of a complex array of muscle fibers that are arranged to form the various cardiac chambers. Each of these fibers operates under the same basic principles as those that have been established for isolated muscle, namely a dependence on preload, afterload, and contractility. Heart rate is a fourth determinant of the heart's performance per unit of time. Each of these factors finds its analog at the organ level, and together they determine the ability of the intact heart to establish and maintain the circulation of blood in the body.

Wall Forces

The force relationships that govern the function of muscle fibers in the intact heart are determined by chamber pressures and geometries. At any point in the cardiac cycle, the pressure within a given chamber exerts a load on the wall of the chamber. This load (in dynes) is equivalent to the product of the pressure (dynes/cm^2) and the area over which the pressure acts (cm^2). In accordance with Newton's law of motion, this load must be precisely balanced by opposing forces in the wall. These forces, normalized to the areas over which they act, are known as wall stresses (26). Figure 9 shows the chamber pressure acting on a

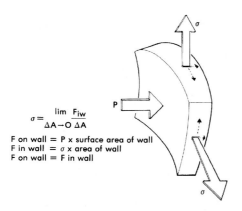

Figure 9 Section removed from the wall of the left ventricle is by a force (*F*) equal to the product of the chamber pressure (*P*) and the area over which it acts. For this element to be in equilibrium, opposing forces exist in the wall, which precisely balance this load. These forces are called wall stresses. This figure shows the loading pressure and the two principal resultant forces. *Source*: From Ref. 26.

section of the wall of the left ventricle and the two principal resultant forces. Assuming an ellipsoidal representation for the left ventricle, application of the Laplace relationship results in the following expression for the meridional (σ_1) and equatorial (σ_2) components of stress:

$$\frac{\sigma_1}{R_1} + \frac{\sigma_2}{R_2} = \frac{P}{h}$$

where, R_1 and R_2 represent the principal radii of curvature for the ellipsoid; P is the ventricular pressure, and h is the wall thickness. A number of expressions are available for independent solutions of σ_1 and σ_2 based on ventricular dimensions and pressure. These expressions and their limitations have been reviewed (27).

An alternative method of conceptualizing force considers only the net force existing in the wall rather than the normalized force (28). The net wall force at any level may be calculated by imagining that the ventricle has been transected by a plane (Fig. 10). The force necessary to hold the ventricle intact, then, is the net force acting on the wall at that level. This force is equal to the product of the ventricular pressure and the area of the chamber included in the plane. For a sphere, this force is constant at any level. For an ellipsoid, the net force depends on the plane of the section. If the section is made normal to the long axis of the ventricle, the pressure × area product is equivalent to the net force in the meridional direction. The magnitude of this force decreases as the plane of section is moved toward the poles of the ellipse, because chamber area is decreasing (29). Wall thickness also decreases toward the poles (30); therefore, stresses and deformation tend to remain uniform. If the plane of section is considered in the long axis, the pressure × area product approximates the equatorial component of wall force. Figure 11 shows pressure, equatorial wall stress, and net wall force for the left ventricle during one cardiac cycle.

Ventricular Geometry and the Cardiac Cycle

Efforts to quantify ventricular function often begin with the adoption of simplified geometric models. The normal left

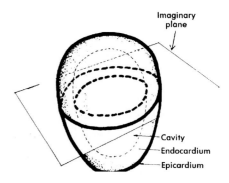

Figure 10 Net wall force concept considers that the ventricle is divided by an imaginary plane located at the level of interest. Net wall force is simply the force necessary to hold the ventricle together at the given level. It is equal to the ventricular pressure multiplied by the area of the chamber involved in the plane. *Source*: From Ref. 28.

ventricle has been represented as an ellipsoidal shell, a sphere, or a cylinder, with varying degrees of success. Even during the dynamic events of filling and ejection, accurate determinations of ventricular dimensions can be obtained with the appropriate use of these models. The elliptical model of left ventricular geometry is often used because it accurately represents the configuration of the left ventricle throughout the cardiac cycle (26,30). In this model, the left ventricle is considered as a general ellipse axisymmetric about its major axis, having a finite but varying wall thickness. The base-to-apex (major) axis is consistently greater than the transverse (minor) axis. The thickness of the ventricular wall is maximum in the equatorial minor axis plane and tapers to a minimum value at the poles of the ellipse (30). During the cardiac cycle, muscle shortening produces variations in ventricular dimensions, with the resultant generation of pressures and volume displacements. Figure 12 illustrates left ventricular chamber

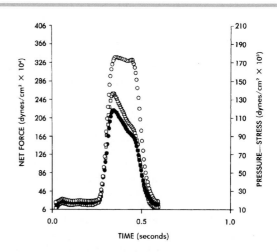

Figure 11 Left ventricular pressure and wall forces for one cardiac cycle in the canine heart. Shown here are pressure (*open circles*), equatorial wall stress (*open squares*), and net wall force (*closed circles*). Note the fall in stress and wall force as the ventricle unloads itself during ejection.

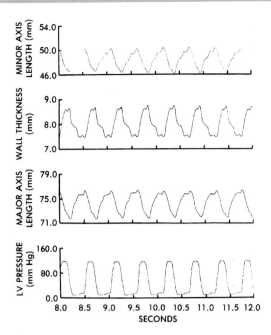

Figure 12 Left ventricular chamber dimensions and pressure in the conscious dog.

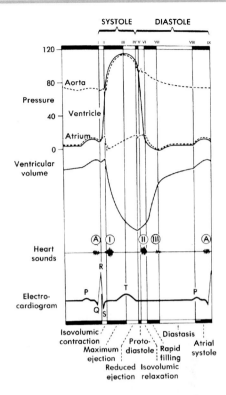

Figure 13 Phases of the cardiac cycle. Shown are left ventricular pressure and volume and the correlation of these measurements to left atrial and aortic pressures, heart sounds, and the electrocardiogram. A, Atrial sound; I, first heart sound; II, second heart sound; III, third heart sound. *Source*: From Ref. 31.

dimensions and pressure for several beats. The complex anatomy, configuration, and contraction pattern of the right ventricle have precluded efforts to model this chamber accurately with simple geometric reference figures. Accordingly, the remainder of this section describes the pattern of hemodynamic events in both chambers, with the inclusion of dimensional information for the left ventricle.

The cardiac cycle can be thought of as beginning with atrial contraction, as indicated by the P wave of the electrocardiogram (Fig. 13). Atrial contraction provides a final, active increment in ventricular filling before systole (32). With the onset of the QRS complex, the period of isovolumic ventricular contraction begins. This marks the beginning of ventricular systole. As ventricular pressures rise above atrial pressures, the AV valves close. The vibrations generated by the abrupt closure of these valves are responsible for the first heart sound. In the left ventricle, the minor axis dimension shortens, the major axis lengthens, and the thickness of the ventricular wall increases (30), resulting in an ellipsization of the chamber. During this period, there is a rapid rise in the rate of pressure generation (dP/dt). This parameter reaches a maximum value at the onset of the ejection phase. Ejection begins when pressure within each of the ventricles rises above the pressures in their respective outflow tracts. The higher ventricular pressures result in an opening of the semilunar valves, and the phase of rapid ejection ensues. Rapid ejection is followed by reduced ejection as pressures in the ventricles and great arteries fall.

In left ventricular ejection, the minor and major axes shorten, and the wall becomes thicker, resulting in a decrease in the internal chamber volume. In the canine heart, the major axis, minor axis, and wall thickness changes account, respectively, for 9%, 47%, and 44% of volume output during systolic ejection (30). In the right ventricle, contraction occurs in a peristaltic wave moving from the sinus region toward the conus (33). As ventricular and

arterial pressures fall, flows in the great vessels reverse. This point marks the end of systole and the beginning of the first phase of diastole, known as protodiastole. Protodiastole ends with the closure of the semilunar valves, which produces the second heart sound. Such closure is also marked by the incisura of the arterial pressure tracing. Protodiastole is followed by the period of isovolumic relaxation. During this period, the geometric patterns observed during isovolumic contraction generally are reversed, and the peak fall in dP/dt occurs. Ventricular pressures fall until they are less than pressures in the atria. The AV valves open, and diastolic filling begins.

Diastolic filling is composed of several phases. The first of these is the rapid filling phase, during which rapid volume expansion occurs. This phase is sometimes associated with an audible third heart sound. As the ventricles become full, the rate of filling slows, and the period of diastasis is approached. During diastole, the left ventricle becomes more spherical as the minor axis dimension increases with respect to the major axis, and the wall becomes thinner (30). The end of diastole is marked by atrial systole and the generation of the fourth heart sound.

At slow heart rates, the atrial contribution to ventricular filling is minimal. At more rapid heart rates or with stenosis of the AV valves, the contribution of atrial systole to ventricular filling becomes more important. In the failing heart, the contribution by atrial systole can result in a 20% to 30% increase in cardiac output.

Diastolic Behavior

Relaxation

Diastole represents the period of relaxation and filling in the cardiac cycle. During relaxation, the ion fluxes that occurred during the process of ECC are reversed, and the contractile proteins assume their resting configurations.

In the filling phases of diastole, the relaxed sarcomeres lengthen as the ventricles distend with blood and the initial muscle length for the next beat is determined. Relaxation is often thought of as a passive event, because pressures and flows are rapidly falling; however, it is a period of considerable metabolic activity, requiring the presence of ATP initially to dissociate the actin–myosin complexes and later to provide the energy for the active transport, which restores the resting ion gradients. For relaxation to occur, sarcoplasmic Ca^{2+} must be reduced to a level such that Ca^{2+} dissociates from the troponin complex. This activity is accomplished by pumps in the membrane of SR and to a lesser extent by transport mechanisms in the sarcolemma (11).

The common feature of these transport processes is the requirement for ATP. In light of this, abnormalities of relaxation have been explained in part on the basis of reduced ATP availability in the injured or diseased heart (34). An additional role has been suggested for ATP in the relaxation process. Adding ATP to a cell that has normal levels of ATP results in an enhancement of the uptake of Ca^{2+} by SR. Thus, ATP may act in a regulatory manner in controlling Ca^{2+} transport. Slight reductions in cellular levels as a result of moderate degrees of energy deprivation could result in impaired relaxation, even though sufficient levels are available to saturate the primary transport mechanisms (11).

Filling

The importance of the filling events of diastole as determinants of cardiac function was first noted by Frank in the late 19th century. Frank observed a direct relationship between end-diastolic volume (EDV) and the force of contraction in the isolated frog heart (35). Later, Starling made similar observations in the mammalian heart. This work culminated in the concept of the Frank–Starling relationship, which was simply stated as "the energy of contraction, however measured, is a function of the length of the muscle fiber" (36).

In the intact heart, diastolic filling determines the length of the muscle fibers before contraction and therefore influences the force of contraction. The nature and extent of this filling, in turn, are influenced by a number of factors; among these are the level of filling pressure, the material properties of the myocardium, the geometry of the chamber, and such external forces as pericardial and pleural pressures (34).

Within any of the cardiac chambers, the filling pressure produces distending forces within the wall of the chamber. These forces are a function of the magnitude of the pressure and the size and shape of the chamber. The resulting distention produced by a given increment of force is governed by the material properties of the myocardium. Because these forces act to determine the length of the muscle fibers before contraction, they may be considered analogs to the preload previously described for isolated muscle.

The "material properties" of the myocardium refer specifically to the elastic and viscous characteristics of the muscle. An elastic material deforms when acted on by an external force and recovers from the deformation when the force is removed. For a substance with linear elastic properties, deformation (e) is related to the force (f) as:

$$f = E(e)$$

where E, the slope of the relationship, is known as the coefficient of elasticity or Young's modulus (37). An increase in E reflects an increase in the stiffness of the material. In a viscoelastic material, force is a function of both deformation and the rate of deformation. Heart muscle is known to possess both elastic and viscous properties (38). The analysis of these properties and their influence on diastolic filling is complicated by the fact that the elastic properties, and possibly the viscous properties, are nonlinear entities (38).

When a force is applied along the long axis of an isolated papillary muscle, the deformation of the muscle obeys the following relationship, assuming that the rate of deformation is small so that viscous effects are not important (25).

$$F - \alpha[e^{\beta(x - x^*)} - 1]$$

where, x is the muscle length, x^* is the resting muscle length, and α and β are elastic constants analogous to the coefficient of elasticity of Eq. (2). F is the fiber stress. Stress is an expression of normalized force, here equal to the applied force divided by the cross-sectional area of the muscle specimen. This nonlinear elasticity of heart muscle is the principal factor affecting the relationship between diastolic pressure and volume in the intact left ventricle (39). Figure 14 shows the pressure–volume curve obtained by slowly filling a canine heart with saline.

Several important points are apparent from this illustration. First, even though the ventricle is composed of muscles that display exponential elastic behavior, the relationship between pressure and volume is not truly exponential. It is approximately linear in the lower pressure ranges and approaches exponentiality in the upper pressure ranges. Second, the elastic nature of the myocardium resists deformation above a filling pressure of about 20 mmHg. The significance of the second factor is that the increasing stiffness of the cardiac muscle prevents overextension of the individual sarcomeres, permitting the heart to function on the ascending limb of the Frank–Starling relationship, where increased volume results in increased output.

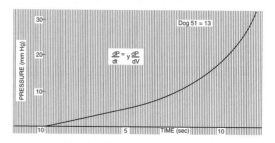

Figure 14 Relationship between pressure (d*P*) and volume (d*V*) [expressed as time (d*t*) of infusion of volume at a constant rate] in the isolated, arrested canine heart. The relationship is approximately linear in the lower pressure ranges and becomes exponential in the upper ranges. The increasing instantaneous slope of the pressure–volume curve reflects the increase in chamber stiffness that occurs as the ventricle is filled. *Source:* From Ref. 40.

Systolic Function

Normal pumping of the ventricles requires that they deliver appropriate amounts of blood to the tissues at acceptably low filling pressures (FPs). Thus, the most physiologically relevant means of characterizing the pump is to construct a function curve relating FP to a measure of mechanical output [stroke volume (SV), minute volume, work, and power]. Ventricular function curves display a prominent Frank–Starling effect, manifest as a curvilinear relationship between FP and output (once again, there is no descending limb in the normal ventricle). As discussed earlier, at the myocytes level, the Frank–Starling effect is mainly caused by increased myofilament Ca sensitivity at longer sarcomere lengths. Thus, a function curve relating EDV (ventricular preload) to mechanical output is a more accurate representation of the ventricular Frank–Starling effect. However, in the clinical setting, FP (pulmonary capillary wedge or right atrial pressure) is usually more readily available than volume. Whether FP or volume is employed, changes in intrinsic contractile performance result in upward or downward shifts of the ventricular function curve. However, characterization of ventricular performance in terms of function curves relating FP to output is a "black box" approach; alterations in diastolic compliance (see below) produce effects that are indistinguishable from alterations in contractile performance.

The normal heart can pump adequate amounts of blood to meet the needs of the body under the most stressful conditions. Indeed, maximal cardiac output (CO) normally is not limited by pumping capacity but by the ability of the systemic circulation, via venoconstriction and the systemic venous system of valves and muscular pumps, to return blood to the heart. Under pathologic conditions, pumping capacity may limit CO.

The peak force that can be generated at a given contractile state and EDV is attained in the isovolumically contracting heart (41). As EDV is raised, the peak developed force increases in a linear fashion (Fig. 15). This behavior demonstrates the operation of the Frank–Starling relationship in the intact ventricle, where force generation is an increasing function of fiber length, expressed here as EDV. The line that results from relating peak force to initial volume defines the limit of force generation for the ventricle. When the ventricle is permitted to eject, this line also defines the limit of systolic shortening (41).

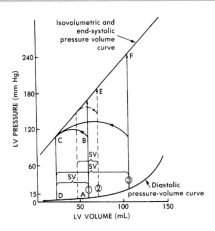

Figure 16 Schematic diagram of the pressure–volume loops for several beats under various loading conditions. Contraction 1 is considered control, contraction 3 shows the effects of increased preload, and contraction 2 shows the effects of increased afterload on SV and pressure generation. Points E and F represent the peak pressures that could be generated if the ventricle were to contract isovolumically from preloads at points 2 and 3, respectively. Note that points E and F define the limit for shortening in the ejecting heart. See text for further details. *Abbreviations:* SV, stroke volume; LV, left ventricular. *Source:* From Ref. 23.

Figure 16 depicts the pressure–volume relationships for an ejecting ventricle under changing conditions of preload and afterload. Contraction 1, originating from EDV A, contracts isovolumically to point B. At point B, the ventricular pressure just exceeds aortic pressure, and ejection begins. During ejection (points B to C), the force sustained by the muscle fibers in the wall of the ventricle represents the afterload. Ejection continues until a point is reached at which muscle force is maximum for a given volume (point C). This point contracts the isovolumic pressure–volume line and represents the end of systolic shortening. When preload is altered as in contraction 3, there is a change in SV, but the extent of fiber shortening does not change. Contraction 3 still proceeds to point C. Increasing the afterload by augmenting aortic pressure (contraction 2) results in both decreased SV and a change in the extent of fiber shortening. Thus the degree of fiber shortening in the ejecting heart is determined by the instantaneous load borne by the muscle, not by alterations in loading before contraction (41). The ability of the ventricle to generate force is influenced by the contractile state of the muscle. A change in contractility is represented by a change in the peak force.

Electrical Activity

Electrically excitable tissues communicate within themselves and with other structures through the generation of APs. Within the heart, there are certain cells that generate spontaneous APs, which propagate and serve as a stimulus to initiate contraction. This property is referred to as automaticity. A second property, intrinsic to the electrical activity of the heart, is conductivity. Conductivity describes the low-resistance intercellular connections that permit any depolarization to be spread throughout the mass of the heart.

Under normal circumstances, contraction of the heart is initiated by APs generated in the sinoatrial (SA) node (43). This structure, located at the junction of the right atrium and the superior vena cava, has the highest rate of intrinsic

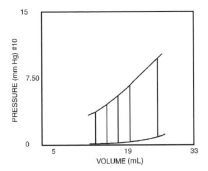

Figure 15 Development of pressure in the isovolumically contracting canine left ventricle. As resting volume is increased, the peak generated pressure increases. Line connecting the peak pressures defines the limit of force generation for the contracting ventricle. *Source*: From Ref. 42.

pacemaker activity found in the heart. APs generated here spread slowly over the right and left atria, with resultant atrial contractions. Excitation moves to the cardiac ventricles through the AV node. In contrast to the atria, impulse conduction through this structure is extremely slow. This delay permits the completion of atrial contraction before ventricular activation. Having passed through the AV node, the wave of excitation enters the bundle of His, a structure located in the subendocardium of the right surface of the interventricular septum. The bundle of His then divides into right- and left-sided branches, which ramify in the fibers of the Purkinje system. The Purkinje system extends over the subendocardial surfaces of both ventricles. Its electrical activity is characterized by a high conduction velocity, which permits near-simultaneous activation of the ventricles.

Many factors affect the nature of pacemaker activity and excitation in the heart. These include neural, hormonal, physicochemical, and pathologic influences. These influences often exert their effects by alterations of events occurring at the cellular level, specifically by inducing changes in the transmembrane electric potential and ion movement (44).

Transmembrane electric potential (V_m) in cardiac cells comes about as a result of an unequal distribution of ions across the cell membrane. In cardiac cells, as in most other cells of the body, the internal potassium concentration is high and the internal sodium concentration is low. The contribution of each of these ions to the net charge on the membrane can be estimated from the Nernst equation (45). For an unspecified ion X,

$$E = \frac{58}{Z} \log \frac{[X_{out}]}{[X_{in}]}$$

where, E is the equilibrium potential resulting solely from ion X, and Z is the charge number of the ion. If the membrane is permeable only to X, V_m equals E. When more than one ion is involved, V_m becomes a weighted average of the equilibrium potential of each ion. The weighting factors depend on the relative conductance of each ion. Conductance (g) is the reciprocal of resistance and is an expression of the ease with which an ion can cross the cell membrane. Thus, in general terms, for a cell permeable to ions A, B, and C, V_m could be approximated from the equation:

$$V_m = \frac{gA}{gA + gB + gC} E_A + \frac{gB}{gA + gB + gC} E_B$$
$$+ \frac{gC}{gA + gB + gC} E_C$$

where, in the case of cardiac tissue, the major ions involved in transmembrane flux are Na^+, K^+, and Ca^{2+} such that:

$$V_m = \frac{gNa}{gNa + gK + gCa} E_{Na} + \frac{gK}{gNa + gK + gCa} E_K$$
$$+ \frac{gCa}{gNa + gK + gCa} E_{Ca}$$

In the quiescent cardiac cell, K^+ permeability greatly exceeds Na^+ and Ca^{2+} permeability, or in terms of conductances, gK greatly exceeds gCa and gNa. Given this fact, Eq. (6) then reduces to the Nernst equation for K^+, and the resting V_m equals or approaches E_K.

APs in cardiac tissue result from changes in the relative conductances of the principal ions Na^+, K^+, and Ca^{2+}.

Ion concentrations across the membrane actually change very little. The arrival of an AP causes a rise in the resting V_m toward threshold value for the particular cell. Once threshold is achieved, a complex pattern of conductance changes ensues. Cardiac muscle cells and cells of the Purkinje system have a high relative gK at rest. Membrane potential is −80 to −90 mV, and threshold is approximately −60 mV. When cardiac muscle cells are stimulated, gNa becomes markedly elevated in what is known as phase 0 of the AP (Figs. 17 and 18). Sodium ions are now better able to cross the membrane. Note that this movement is favored by both chemical and electrical gradients; so it occurs quite rapidly. The net inward movement of positive charge causes depolarization of the cell; V_m moves toward and then past 0 mV. As the cell depolarizes, gNa falls, completing phase 0. Phase 1 is characterized by a rapid fall in V_m, thought to be the result of transient increase in membrane permeability to chloride (Cl^-). Phase 2 is the plateau phase of AP. This is brought about by a slow inward Ca^{2+} and Na^+ current balanced by an outward K^+ current. Repolarization occurs in phase 3 and is a result of a further increase in gK combined with an inactivation of the slow inward current of phase 2.

There are striking differences between APs seen in the nodal structures and those just described (Fig. 17). Recordings from cells of the SA node reveal a less negative resting potential, a decreased rate of phase 0 depolarization, no plateau, and a reduced rate of phase 3 depolarization. Perhaps most significant is the behavior that nodal tissue displays in phase 4. During this phase, V_m is not constant but moves steadily toward threshold. The basis for this

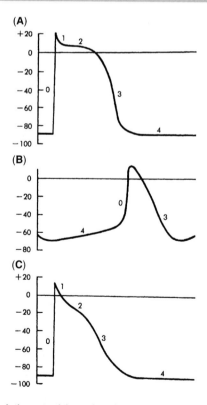

Figure 17 Action potential seen in various cardiac tissues. **(A)** Ventricular muscle cell, **(B)** sinoatrial node, **(C)** atrial muscle. Time base for **(B)** is half that of **(A)** and **(C)**. *Source:* From Ref. 46.

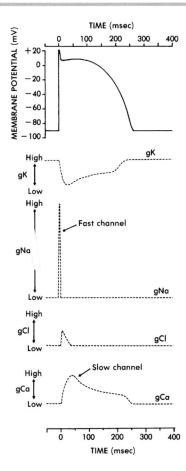

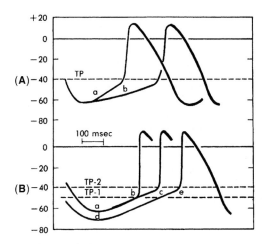

Figure 19 Altering the rate of pacemaker activity. **(A)** Altering the rate of firing by a decrease in the rate of phase 4 depolarization. Threshold potential (TP) is not changed. **(B)** Changing threshold at a given rate of phase 4 depolarization can alter heart rate by changing the time required to reach TP (tracings a–b and a–c). Hyperpolarization can also influence rate (tracings a–e). *Source*: From Ref. 46.

Figure 18 Conductance changes seen within a Purkinje fiber. Typical action potential is shown at the top, with the accompanying changes in conductance for potassium (gK), sodium (gNa), chloride (gCl), and calcium (gCa). *Source*: From Ref. 31.

behavior is believed to be a time-dependent decrease in the outward K^+ movement in the presence of a small, steady, inward movement of Ca^{2+}. The loss of the K^+ current disrupts the balance of charge and results in membrane depolarization. When the membrane potential reaches threshold, an AP is generated. In this manner, a nodal tissue serves as a pace generator for the heart. The rate of pacemaker activity depends on the minimum phase 4 V_m, the rate of depolarization, and the threshold potential (47). These factors are under neural and hormonal controls that act to vary the heart rate (Fig. 19) (15). For example, increased vagal activity results in the release of acetylcholine at the SA node. This has the effect of increasing gK, which hyperpolarizes the membrane and slows the heart rate. Conversely, catecholamines can increase the inward phase 4 Ca^{2+} current, which would increase both the rate of depolarization and the heart rate (see section on "Neural Control") (20,44,47,48).

Neural Control

The sympathetic and parasympathetic divisions of the autonomic nervous system act in concert to regulate cardiac function. Sympathetic effects are excitatory and are mediated through nerve fibers distributed to the atria, ventricles, and nodal tissue. Parasympathetic influences are generally inhibitory and act predominantly on atrial and nodal tissues.

The terminal regions of the sympathetic fibers synthesize and store norepinephrine, which is released as a result of nerve stimulation. Norepinephrine acts on β_1 adrenergic receptors imbedded in the membrane of the cardiac cell. β-receptors in the myocardium are of two types, β_1 and β_2. β_1-receptors are distributed exclusively to the ventricles, and their activation results in an increase in the ventricular contractility (49,50).

The mechanism of action is thought to involve increases in the level of cyclic adenosine monophosphate, which in turn promote the phosphorylation and activation of calcium channels in the membrane (51,52). The net effect of β_1-stimulation is an increase in calcium influx, which causes an increase in the contractile state of the muscle (14). β_2-receptors are found in the atria. The activation of these receptors results in an increased heart rate through their positive chronotropic effects (10). The stimulus for activation of β_2-receptors differs from that of β_1 types in that β_2 receptors are sensitive to epinephrine and norepinephrine.

Parasympathetic effects are mediated by fibers of the vagus nerve that are distributed to the atria, and, to a lesser extent, to the ventricles. Activation of these fibers results in a release of acetylcholine, which causes a depression of cardiac function characterized by a reduction in heart rate and atrial contractility. Ventricular contractility is affected to a lesser extent (53). The diminution in ventricular function seen during vagal stimulation can be explained in part by reduced ventricular filling, which occurs secondary to the fall in atrial contractility. Acetylcholine produces its negative chronotropic effects by hyperpolarizing the nodal tissue. Hyperpolarization is a consequence of the increase in potassium permeability caused by the application of acetylcholine. Acetylcholine also binds to muscarinic receptors on the sympathetic nerve fibers. Activation of muscarinic receptors results in reduced catecholamine release during sympathetic stimulation. Thus, the inhibitory influences of parasympathetic activity are more pronounced when sympathetic activity is high.

In recent years, an increasing emphasis on neural control of heart function has been evolving. Trauma, anesthesia, and anxiety evoke major alternations in cardiovascular function and may be the precipitants of arrhythmias or cardiac dysfunction.

Coronary Flow and Myocardial Oxygen Consumption

The energy imparted by the heart to the blood during the process of ejection is linearly related to three factors: heat rate, SV, and developed aortic pressure. A rise in any of these three variables leads to an increase in the myocardial oxygen consumption. Minute work of the heart is defined as the product of these three parameters. Changes in SV are associated with the greatest efficiency and the lowest energy cost to the heart, whereas increases in the heart rate and blood pressure are costly and require the greatest increase in myocardial oxygen delivery.

Because heart rate and blood pressure figure so much more prominently in the determination of myocardial oxygen consumption than SV, two clinical indexes based on heart rate and aortic pressure have been developed for estimation of myocardial oxygen consumption. These are the "double product" (the heart rate multiplied by the blood pressure) and the "tension time" index (the average ejection pressure of the left ventricle multiplied by the duration of ejection). Both of these indexes correlate well with cardiac oxygen consumption, but neither takes into account the effect of ventricular dilation or altered contractility. It is obvious from this discussion that myocardial oxygen consumption can be decreased and the efficiency of the heart improved by a reduction in heart rate and a decrease in mean arterial blood pressure (vasodilation).

The flow of oxygenated blood into the myocardium is controlled by the coronary circulation. Blood flow is regulated to ensure an environment of aerobic metabolism to support cardiac work. To accomplish this goal, the coronary circulation possesses two unique features:

- Under basal conditions, there is a high degree of oxygen extraction (coronary sinus oxygen saturation is 20–30%) so that the heart can adjust to changing oxygen needs by only a small increment in oxygen extraction.
- Accordingly, increasing oxygen requirements must be met by proportionate increases in coronary flow.

HEART FAILURE

Contraction 3 in Figure 20 represents a decreased contractile state, as might be seen in conditions of heart failure (32,54,55). Failure occurs when the heart can no longer pump blood commensurate with the needs of the body. This condition can occur as a result of depression in the intrinsic contractility of the muscle or as a result of the imposition of increased loading conditions on ventricular ejection (23). The heart can compensate in several ways. Contractile state can increase with endogenous catecholamine release. Also, muscle preload can be augmented by the increased filling pressure that often accompanies the reduced pumping ability of the failing ventricle. Hypertrophy and/or chamber dilation also can occur.

Associated with these compensatory mechanisms are certain detrimental factors that may contribute to the eventual failure of the heart. Increased preload results in an increased level of wall stress throughout diastole. Wall stress has been shown to be related to myocardial oxygen consumption (56); therefore, incorporation of this mechanism necessarily increases the flow requirements of the myocardium. As chamber

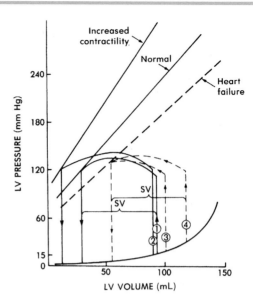

Figure 20 Conceptual pressure–volume loops for hearts at contractile states. Note the effect of the contractile state on the stroke volume (SV) generated from similar preloads at points 1, 2, and 3. During heart failure, SV may be decreased despite a slightly larger end-diastolic volume (EDV) at a comparable level of aortic pressure (see contraction 3). If EDV is further increased, SV may be restored (see contraction 4). *Abbreviation*: LV, left ventricular. *Source*: From Ref. 23.

enlargement occurs, several aspects of active force relations are affected. From the net wall force concept developed earlier, it is simple to see how an increase in the chamber size results in a decrease in the efficiency of the ventricular contraction. Recall that wall force (F) is equal to the product of chamber pressure (P) and area (A). Rearranged, this gives $P = F/A$. The generation of a given pressure within the large ventricle (larger A) then requires the existence of a greater wall force. A second aspect of chamber enlargement concerns the unloading of the ventricle during systole. In a normal heart, the muscle load (stress) peaks soon after the onset of ejection and then declines through the remainder of systole (Fig. 11). This occurs because the decrease in chamber size is more than the increase in pressure , resulting in a partial unloading of the ventricle. To generate a given SV, the enlarged heart undergoes a smaller degree of systolic shortening. It therefore unloads itself less than would a smaller heart ejecting the same volume. Worsened ejection resulting from prolonged high wall tension creates an afterload mismatch in the coupling of the heart to the periphery. Vasodilator therapy normalizes this loading of the heart and thereby facilitates ejection. At the same time, smaller volumes and wall tension decrease myocardial oxygen consumption.

A practical clinical index of global cardiac function is the ejection fraction (EF). EF is the percent of EDV that is ejected as the SV and is derived from the following equation:

$$EF = \frac{(EDV - ESV)}{EDV}$$

where ESV is the end-systolic volume. A normal functioning heart has an EF of 55% to 75%. In patients with severe compromise in myocardial reserve due to chronic heart failure and/or scarring from previous myocardial infarction,

EF may be as low as 15% to 20%. Although EF is not a perfect measure of cardiac function in that it is sensitive to preload, afterload, heart rate, and ventricular compliance, it is sufficiently reliable overall as to give an accurate index of the contractile capabilities of the heart. It can be measured in a variety of ways including echocardiography, cineangiography, and ventriculography.

SUMMARY

For many years, the complexity of the cardiovascular system prevented the systematic study of its properties. Although that complexity remains, several basic principles by which the heart functions have been determined. These principles include the dependence of myocardial performance on preload, afterload, and contractility. Preload is defined as the distending force, or load, that is placed on cardiac muscle before contraction. The preload and the distensibility of the muscle are the determinants of the initial length of the muscle before contraction. The load encountered by the cardiac muscle after activation is defined as the afterload. The magnitude of the afterload determines the nature of the subsequent contraction. Contractility refers to the intrinsic ability of the cardiac muscle to contract, independent of loading conditions. Heart failure occurs when the heart can no longer pump blood commensurate with the needs of the body. This condition can occur as a result of depression in the intrinsic contractility of the cardiac muscle or as a result of the imposition of increased loading conditions on ventricular ejection. Understanding the interplay among these various parameters and how their imbalance can be corrected or lessened, both medically and surgically, underlies the rationale for treatment in patients with cardiac dysfunction.

REFERENCES

1. Morkin E. Contractile proteins of the heart. Hosp Pract 1983; 18(6):97.
2. Murray J, Weber A. The cooperative action of muscle proteins. Sci Am 1974; 230(2):58.
3. Mason DT, et al. Mechanisms of cardiac contraction. In: Sodeman WA Jr, Sodeman TM, eds. Sodeman's Pathologic Physiology. 6th ed. Philadelphia: WB Saunders, 1979.
4. Bremel RD, Weber AM. Cooperation with actin filament in vertebrate skeletal muscle. Nature (New Biol) 1972; 238:97.
5. Weber A, Murray JM. Molecular control mechanisms in muscle contraction. Physiol Rev 1973; 53:612.
6. Opie LH. Mechanism of cardiac contraction and relaxation. In: Zipes DP, Libby P, Bonow RO, Braunwald E, eds. Braunwald's Heart Disease. 7th ed. Philadelphia: Elsevier Saunders, 2005:457–489.
7. Spudich JA. How molecular motors work. Nature 1994; 372:515.
8. Ebashi S. Excitation–contraction coupling and the mechanism of muscle contraction. Annu Rev Physiol 1991; 53:1.
9. Elliott GF, Worthington CR. How muscle may contract. Biochim Biophys Acta 1994; 1200:109.
10. Honerjager P. Pharmacology of bipyridine phosphodiesterase III inhibitors. Am Heart J 1991; 121:1939.
11. Katz AM, Smith VE. Relaxation abnormalities. I. Mechanisms. Hosp Pract 1984; 19(1):69.
12. Schwartz K, et al. Myosin isoenzymic distribution correlates with speed of myocardial contraction. J Mol Cell Cardiol 1981; 13:1071.
13. Samuel JL, et al. Distribution of myosin isozymes with single cardiac cells: An immunohistochemical study. Circ Res 1983; 52:200.
14. Van Breeman C, Aaronson P, Loutzenhiser R. Na–Ca interactions in mammalian smooth muscle. Pharmacol Rev 1979; 30:167.
15. Hoh JFY, McGrath PA, Hale PT. Electrophoretic analysis of multiple forms of rat cardiac myosin: effects of hypophysectomy and thyroid replacement. J Mol Cell Cardiol 1978; 10:1053.
16. Rupp H. The adaptive changes in the isoenzyme pattern of myosin from hypertrophied rat myocardium as a result of pressure overload and physical training. Basic Res Cardiol 1981; 76:79.
17. Fabiato A, Fabiato F. Calcium and cardiac excitation–contraction coupling. Annu Rev Physiol 1979; 41:473.
18. Barry WH, Bridge JHB. Intracellular calcium homeostasis. Circulation 1993; 87:1806.
19. Katz AM. Physiology of the Heart. New York: Raven Press, 1992.
20. Colucci WS, Braunwald E. Pathophysiology of Heart Failure. In: Zipes DP, Libby P, Bonow RO, Braunwald E, eds. Braunwald's Heart Disease. 7th ed. Philiadelphia: Elsevier Saunders, 2005:509–538.
21. Sonnenblick EH. Implications of muscle mechanics in the heart. Fed Proc 1962; 21(Suppl 12):975.
22. Katz AM. Regulation of cardiac contraction and relaxation. In: Willerson JT, Conn JN, eds. Cardiovascular Medicine. New York: Churchill-Livingstone, 1995:790.
23. Braunwald E. Pathophysiology of heart failure. In: Braunwald E, ed. Heart Disease. Philadelphia: WB Saunders, 1984.
24. Sonnenblick EH, et al. Redefinition of the ultrastructural basis of the cardiac length–tension relations. Circulation 1973; 48(suppl 4):65.
25. Glanz SA, Kernoff RS. Muscle stiffness determined from canine left ventricular pressure–volume curves. Circ Res 1975; 37:787.
26. Sandler H, Ghista DN. Mechanical and dynamic implications of dimensional measurements of the left ventricle. Fed Proc 1969; 28(4):1344.
27. Yin FCP. Ventricular wall stress. Circ Res 1981; 49(4):829.
28. Hefner LL, et al. Relation between mural force and pressure in the left ventricle of the dog. Circ Res 1962; 11:654.
29. Weber KT, et al. Contractile mechanics and the interaction of the right and left ventricles. Am J Cardiol 1981; 47:686.
30. Rankin JS, et al. The three-dimensional dynamic geometry of the left ventricle in the conscious dog. Circ Res 1976; 39(3):304.
31. Katz AM. Physiology of the Heart. New York: Raven Press, 1977.
32. Foex P, Leone BJ. Pressure–volume loops: a dynamic approach to the assessment of ventricular function. J Cardiothorac Vasc Anesth 1994; 8:84.
33. Meier GD, et al. Contractile function in canine right ventricle. Am J Physiol 1980; 239(8):H794.
34. Grossman W, Barry WH. Diastolic pressure–volume relations in the diseased heart. Fed Proc 1980; 38:148.
35. Frank O. On the dynamics of cardiac muscle. Am Heart J 1959; 58(2):282.
36. Starling EH. The Linacre lecture on the law of the heart. London: Longmans Green, 1918.
37. Mirsky I, Pasipoularides A. Elastic properties of normal and hypertrophied cardiac muscle. Fed Proc 1980; 39:156.
38. Pouleur H, et al. Diastolic viscous properties of the intact canine left ventricle. Circ Res 1979; 45:410.
39. Glantz SA. Computing indices of diastolic stiffness has been counterproductive. Fed Proc 1980; 39:162.
40. Diamond G, et al. Diastolic pressure–volume relationship in the canine left ventricle. Circ Res 1971; 29:267.
41. Weber KT, Janicki JS. The heart as a muscle-pump system and the concept of heart failure. Am Heart J 1979; 98(3):371.
42. Strauer BE, ed. The Heart in Hypertension. Heidelberg: Springer-Verlag, 1981.
43. DiFrancesco D. Pacemaker mechanisms in cardiac tissue. Annu Rev Physiol 1993; 55:455.
44. Naccarelli GV, Willerson JT, Blomqvist CG. Recognition and physiologic treatment of cardiac arrhythmias and conduction disturbances. In: Willerson JT, Cohn JN, eds. Cardiovascular Medicine. New York: Churchill-Livingstone, 1995:1282.

45. DeVoe RD, Maloney PC. Principles of cell homeostasis. In: Mount-castle VB, ed. Medical Physiology. 14th ed. St Louis: Mosby, 1980.

46. Berne RM, Levy MN, eds. Physiology. St. Louis: Mosby, 1983.

47. Campbell DL, Rasmusson RL, Strauss HC. Ionic current mechanisms generating vertebrate primary cardiac pacemaker activity at the single cell level: an integrative view. Annu Rev Physiol 1992; 54:279.

48. Zipes DP, Jalife J, eds. Cardiac Electrophysiology: From Cell to Bedside. 3rd ed. Philadelphia: WB Saunders, 2000.

49. Hedberg A, Minneman KP, Molinoff PB. Differential distribution of beta-1 and beta-2 adrenergic receptors in cat and guinea-pig heart. J Pharmacol Exp Ther 1980; 213:503.

50. Homcy CJ, Vatner ST, Vatner DE. Beta-adrenergic receptor regulation in the heart in pathophysiologic states: abnormal adrenergic responsiveness in cardiac disease. Annu Rev Physiol 1991; 53:137.

51. Feldman AM. Classification of positive inotropic agents. J Am Coll Cardiol 1993; 22:1223.

52. Leier CV. Current status of non-digitalis positive inotropic drugs. Am J Cardiol 1992; 69:120G.

53. Levy MN, Martin PJ. Neural control of the heart. In: Berne RM, ed. Handbook of Physiology. Section 2. The Cardiovascular System. Vol. 1. The Heart. Bethesda, Mary Land: American Physiological Society, 1979.

54. Folkow B, Svanborg B. Physiology of cardiovascular aging. Physiol Rev 1993; 73:725.

55. Klug D, Robert V, Swynghedauw B. Role of mechanical and hormonal factors in cardiac remodeling and the biologic limits of myocardial adaptation. Am J Cardiol 1993; 71:46A.

56. Braunwald E. 50th Anniversary Historical Article. Myocardial oxygen consumption: the quest for its determinants and some clinical fall out. J Am Coll Cardiol 2000; 35:45B.

Heart Failure and Resuscitation

Heinrich Taegtmeyer

When the patient thinks there is something amiss with his heart, he fears it may fail. It is therefore necessary that the doctor should understand what heart failure is and the signs by which it is made manifest.

Sir John Mackenzie, 1916 (1)

INTRODUCTION

Heart failure is a systemic disease caused by an impairment of efficient energy transfer in heart muscle. Clinically, heart failure exists when the heart fails in one or both of its primary functions: during diastole to receive blood into the ventricles under low pressure, during systole to propel blood into the systemic circulation under high pressure (Grossman W. Personal communication, 1995). Because the heart is both a consumer and provider of energy, a restriction in energy consumption (e.g., as it occurs in ischemic heart disease) results in impaired energy delivery to the rest of the body (2). Impaired energy delivery, in turn, causes adaptive and ultimately maladaptive responses of the organism as a whole.

This chapter focuses on aspects of heart failure most commonly encountered in the practice of surgery. The first part of the chapter reviews the etiology, pathophysiology, clinical manifestations, therapy, and prognosis of acute and chronic heart failure. A discussion of chronic heart failure is important, because it is often a comorbid condition in surgical patients and may significantly alter the care and prognosis of the patient. The second part of the chapter discusses the principles of cardiopulmonary resuscitation (CPR), because cardiopulmonary arrest (also termed "sudden death") is the extreme form of acute heart failure. The discussion includes the pathophysiology and etiology of cardiopulmonary arrest and techniques of resuscitation.

HEART FAILURE

Features of Heart Failure

Irrespective of the causes of heart failure, it is useful to distinguish its clinical features, which can occur either alone or in combination with one another. These features include acute and chronic, high-output and low-output, right ventricular and left ventricular, backward and forward, and systolic and diastolic heart failure (3).

The rapidity with which symptoms of heart failure develop depends on the underlying pathophysiology and on the time allowed for compensatory mechanisms to develop. Acute heart failure occurs within minutes or hours and may be caused by loss of cardiac muscle from acute myocardial infarction, volume overload, or arrhythmias. Chronic heart failure develops over months or years, and may be due to a slow loss of functional myocardium (e.g., as in hypertensive cardiomyopathy). In addition, a patient with chronic heart failure may achieve a well-compensated state, only to experience a superimposed acute exacerbation of heart failure, for example, caused by arrhythmias, volume overload, systemic infection, or noncompliance with medications.

In the hospitalized patient with symptoms and signs of pulmonary edema, it is often difficult to distinguish an acute exacerbation of chronic heart failure (i.e., acute on top of chronic heart failure) from a new presentation of acute heart failure. This is especially difficult in patients in the perioperative period, in patients with renal failure, and in those receiving blood products or intravenous fluids. Thus it is important to understand the etiology and pathophysiology of the various forms of acute and chronic heart failure so that effective diagnostic and therapeutic decisions may be made.

Etiology and Natural History of Heart Failure

Heart failure can occur as the result of three general derangements. First, mechanical or anatomic abnormalities may be present within the heart, in the coronary circulation, or in the pulmonary or systemic vascular bed and may result in inefficient pump function. Second, functional myocardial abnormalities may occur as a result of long-standing pressure or volume overload, primary myocardial disease, or myocarditis. Third, rhythm disturbances may bring the rhythmic function of the heart out of order and lead to inefficient pump action. In each situation, the development of heart failure may be acute or chronic. In addition, certain causes of cardiac dysfunction may lead to reversible disease, whereas others, especially those that are chronic and cause intrinsic myocardial changes, may lead to progressive, irreversible derangements. A list of the different causes of heart failure is shown in Table 1.

Mechanical or Anatomic Abnormalities Causing Heart Failure

A hallmark of chronic heart failure is an initial phase of adaptation to environmental changes, which is followed by deadaptation of the heart muscle (4). Adaptation is characterized by hypertrophy, which is brought about either by pressure overload or by volume overload of the heart. When presented with a patient whose main problem is heart failure, an important early step for the physician is to establish the cause of the compensatory hypertrophy. An increased pressure load on one or both of the ventricles may be due to systemic or pulmonary hypertension, aortic or pulmonary valve stenosis, pulmonary embolus, or coarctation of

Table 1 Cardiac and Systemic Abnormalities Resulting in Heart Failure

Structural myocardial abnormalities
   Cardiomyopathies (hypertrophic, dilated, restrictive)
   Inadequate myocardial mass (myocardial infarction, hypoplasia)
   Presbycardia (senile cardiomyopathy)
   Dysdynamic (ventricular aneurysm)
Metabolic
   Endocrine (thyroid dysfunction, acromegaly, pheochromocytoma,
     hypoparathyroidism, diabetes mellitus)
   Thiamine deficiency (beriberi)
   Ischemia
   Acidosis
Infections
   Viral, bacterial, rickettsial, parasitic, fungal
Inflammatory
   Connective tissue disease
   Rheumatic fever
Toxic
   Drugs [doxorubicin (Adriamycin), disopyramide, antituberculosis
     therapy, sulfonamides, heroin, cocaine, amphetamines, alcohol]
   Cobalt, iron, lead
   Radiation
Infiltrative
   Amyloidosis
   Glycogen storage disease
   Mucopolysaccharidosis
   Leukemia
   Wegener's granulomatosis
   Uremia
Cor pulmonale
   Acute (pulmonary embolus)
   Chronic (emphysema)
Arrhythmias

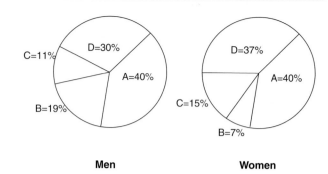

Men   **Women**

Figure 1 The prevalence of coronary artery disease and hypertension among 9405 male and female Framingham study subjects with congestive heart failure. *A* = Coronary artery disease plus hypertension; *B* = coronary artery disease alone; *C* = neither hypertension nor coronary artery disease; *D* = hypertension alone. *Source*: From Ref. 5.

the aorta. An increased volume load may be caused by a valvular regurgitant lesion, an increased filling pressure, or a shunt between the systemic and pulmonary circulation such as an arteriovenous fistula, an atrial septal defect, or a patent ductus arteriosus. Obstruction to ventricular filling leads to a volume overload upstream from the stenotic lesion. Examples are mitral or tricuspid valve stenosis or rare congenital abnormalities such as cor triatriatum. Pericardial constriction and tamponade cause an extrinsic mechanical force that may lead to a restrictive pattern of heart failure. Other mechanical causes of heart failure include endocardial or myocardial restrictive disease, ventricular aneurysm, and ventricular asynergy.

Intrinsic Myocardial Abnormalities Causing Heart Failure

Intrinsic myocardial abnormalities may cause heart failure either because of primary myocardial diseases, such as hypertrophic cardiomyopathy, or because of secondary influences such as viral infection. Although there are many primary and secondary causes of heart failure, the clinical presentation and treatment are very similar. Identification of the cause is crucial because treatment of the underlying disease may afford partial or complete reversal of the heart failure.

Rhythm and Conduction Disturbances Causing Heart Failure

Rhythm and conduction system abnormalities may lead to symptoms and signs of heart failure. Extreme tachycardia such as seen in sinus tachycardia greater than 150 beats/min,

ventricular tachycardia, atrial fibrillation or flutter, paroxysmal supraventricular tachycardia (atrioventricular nodal reentrant tachycardia), or multifocal atrial tachycardia may cause symptoms and signs of cardiac failure, often with a normal blood pressure. Electric asynchrony and conduction disturbances, as in atrial dysrhythmias and bundle branch blocks, cause a decrease in cardiac output and can lead to heart failure, especially in patients with underlying impaired ventricular function.

The most common underlying abnormalities that result in heart failure include systemic hypertension and coronary artery disease. When the different causes of heart failure were evaluated in a long-term follow-up of 9405 subjects in the Framingham study, it was found that nearly 90% of patients with heart failure have a history of hypertension, coronary artery disease, or both (5). Other causes, including the different forms of cardiomyopathies, make up the remaining 10%. These findings are shown in Figure 1.

Pathophysiology of Heart Failure

As stated earlier, heart failure is a systemic disease that begins and ends with the heart. Just as the causes of heart failure may be varied, there are different pathophysiologic mechanisms leading to the clinical entity of heart failure. Cellular biochemical mechanisms may be at work either as the precipitators of acute heart failure or as mediators of chronic heart failure. Pressure overload, volume overload, or both may be initiating factors. Heart failure may be due to loss of contractility from loss of heart muscle, abnormal muscle proteins, or impaired energy metabolism. Lastly, heart failure may also arise from extrinsic influences such as increased pericardial or pleural pressures.

Biochemical Derangements

The heart consumes energy locked in the chemical bonds of fuel molecules through their controlled combustion and converts chemical energy into physical energy (predominantly mechanical pump work) (2). When this ability is impaired, it results in functional and metabolic abnormalities in the rest of the body, commonly referred to as "heart failure." This may occur, for example, because of lack of supply of oxygen, as in coronary artery disease, or in inappropriate use of fuels, as in a cardiomyopathy. Ultimately, the increased energy demands and impaired energy production lead to a state of energy starvation, with subsequent further cardiac deterioration (decreased capillary density, decreased number of mitochondria, and increased connective tissue). Other organs deteriorate because the heart no longer effectively provides energy in the form of substrates and oxygen to the rest of the body.

Mechanical Derangements

Left ventricular function is dependent on the filling pressure of the ventricle (preload) and contractility (Fig. 2), as well as the resistance of blood flow out of the ventricle (afterload) (Fig. 3). The impedance is the sum of resistance in small arteries and arterioles (resistance vessels) and compliance in larger arteries (conductance vessels). The normal left ventricle is able to adjust to changes in resistance through an increase in contractility. This increase is caused by an increase in ventricular filling pressure (Frank–Starling mechanism). After the ventricle has faced increased loading conditions for some time, the Frank–Starling curve becomes depressed, such that a higher loading condition no longer elicits a comparable increase in contractility. Thus the now dysfunctional ventricle does not respond as well to changes in loading conditions or increases in resistance (6).

Abnormal Cardiac Contractility

The mechanism by which cardiac contractility becomes impaired is incompletely understood and may vary significantly depending on the cause. Loss of cardiac muscle may occur because of loss of myofibrillar protein, as seen in acute myocardial infarction. In chronic heart failure, muscular contraction may be compromised because of decreased activity of myofibrillar actinomyosin, or myosin adenosine-triphosphatase (ATPase) proteins (7,8). Additional abnormalities may occur because of decreased release or reuptake of calcium by the sarcoplasmic reticulum (9), decreased sodium/potassium exchange, or decreased cyclic adenosine monophosphate caused by decreased β-receptor activity

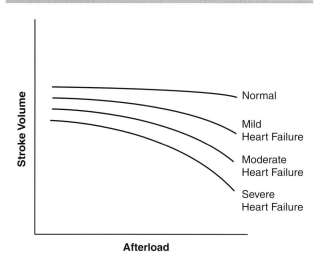

Figure 3 The relationship between ventricular function and afterload in the normal heart and in heart failure. Small increases in afterload may lead to a significant decline in ventricular function. Conversely, decreasing afterload improves the systolic performance of the failing heart.

(10) or decreased coupling with adenylate cyclase across the sarcolemma (6).

We have observed that heart failure can also be caused by impaired substrate flux through metabolic pathways. An example is the acute decrease in contractile function of the working rat heart perfused with ketone bodies as the only substrate, which is completely reversible on addition of glucose. This substrate-induced contractile dysfunction occurs because of inhibition of the Krebs citric acid cycle at the level of the enzyme α-ketoglutarate dehydrogenase and is reversed through replenishment of citric acid cycle intermediates by pyruvate carboxylation (2).

Extrinsic Mechanisms

In addition to abnormal loading conditions, other extra-cardiac factors influence cardiac performance. For example, pericardial disease may produce an extrinsic mechanical stress that may impair myocardial relaxation, leading to a restrictive pattern of heart failure. In a similar way, increased pleural pressures may affect contractility, as seen in tension pneumothorax or mechanically ventilated patients with positive end-expiratory pressure. All these factors may decrease cardiac output, leading to high filling pressures and poor forward flow, thus causing the clinical syndrome of heart failure.

Compensatory Mechanisms

In both the heart and the body, the responses to altered pathophysiology are initially adaptive and later maladaptive. As we discuss the adaptive compensatory mechanisms in both systems, we recognize that the maladaptive responses in the body lead to the clinical presentation of heart failure.

Myocardial Compensatory Mechanisms

It is well recognized that in heart failure there are alterations of myocardial structure, changes in the contractile function of myocytes, and changes in blood flow to the heart. The myocardial response to volume as well as to pressure overload, results in an increase of contractile units (hypertrophy) and

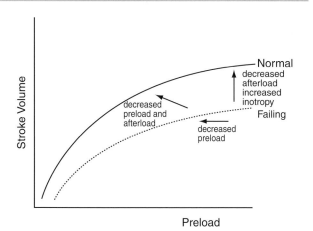

Figure 2 Frank–Starling curves in the normal heart and in heart failure. An improvement in inotropy or reduction in afterload improves the ventricular performance. Reducing the preload alone does not improve performance, because there is no physiologically relevant "descending limb" of the curve. Combining preload reduction with either a reduction in afterload or a direct inotropic stimulus provides better systolic function and a reduction in ventricular filling pressure.

thus a change in myocardial composition. This change leads to accelerated cell death with increased loading of the remaining normal cells (11).

The mediators of ventricular remodeling and hypertrophy are local (autocrine) and systemic (neuroendocrine). The autocrine mediators are angiotensin, endothelin, endothelin-derived relaxing factor, prostaglandin I_2, and prostaglandin E_2. The systemic mediators include the renin–angiotensin system (8), sympathetic stimulation (12), vasopressin, and atrial natriuretic peptide (ANP). Some of these mediators are vasoconstrictors, others are dilators, and it is the imbalance between these mediators that leads to decompensation and clinical manifestations in heart failure.

Overload on the ventricles causes changes in gene expression, altered synthesis of myocardial proteins, and abnormal membrane assembly, resulting in preferential synthesis of fetal isoforms of several proteins, which have a shortened life span. In addition, there is evidence of overexpression of cellular proto-oncogenes c-fos, c-myc, and c-jun in response to myocardial overload, leading to altered protein synthesis and thus an abnormal myocardial structure (11).

Pressure or volume overload on the ventricles results in an increase in the length of the sarcomeres and an increase in the total muscle mass. This mechanism allows maintenance of an elevated ventricular systolic pressure (in the case of volume overload) without depressed contractility. As heart failure advances, the alterations in contractility make this compensatory mechanism less and less efficient, ultimately resulting in depressed ventricular function (7).

Following the sustained increase in stroke volume, there is cardiac dilation and an increased rate of relaxation. The combination of the above leads to an adequate cardiac performance until a phase of "exhaustion" is reached, which is characterized by lysis of myofibrils, interstitial fibrosis, a decreased capillary density in relation to myocytes, impaired coronary flow reserve, and ultimately deterioration of cardiac performance.

Ventricular relaxation during diastole is also altered in the failing, hypertrophied heart (13). In this "diastolic dysfunction," the delay in relaxation with pressure overload interferes with diastolic filling and leads to elevated left ventricular filling pressures (Fig. 4). Sometimes this mechanism alone can be severe enough to cause clinically advanced heart failure.

Systemic Compensatory Mechanisms

Depressed systolic function of the heart leads to an inadequate effective arterial volume, which in turn triggers a series of humoral responses. Adrenergic stimulation, renin release, aldosterone secretion, and excessive release of vasopressin act to ensure adequate perfusion to vital organs.

The adrenergic system in heart failure is characterized by increased levels of circulating norepinephrine (12). These levels correlate inversely with the severity of ventricular dysfunction and with prognosis. For example, in acute heart failure following myocardial infarction, the compensatory increase in norepinephrine in the early stages later becomes deleterious because of increased afterload and arrhythmogenicity. In chronic heart failure, the prolonged increase of circulating norepinephrine leads to a downregulation of cardiac β-adrenergic receptors, with a decrease in their density and subsequent reduction in contractility. Reversal of this downregulation may be achieved with β_1-antagonists, which have been shown in some studies to be beneficial in low doses in the treatment of heart failure, possibly by restoring the responsiveness to adrenergic inotropic stimulation (14).

Aldosterone secretion is stimulated by decreased renal blood flow and increased sympathetic activity (12). The release of renin leads to increased production of angiotensin II, which causes increased afterload and stimulates myocardial hypertrophy. The increased production of aldosterone increases retention of sodium and water with a further increase in preload. This chain of events leads to the so-called "vicious cycle of heart failure" (Fig. 5). Reversal of these effects by angiotensin-converting enzyme (ACE) inhibitors has been shown to decrease mortality in heart failure of different etiologies (15–17).

Other systemic changes that occur in heart failure include changes in the levels of vasopressin, ANP, and peripheral oxygen delivery. The circulating levels of vasopressin are elevated in heart failure because of an abnormal response to serum osmolality. This causes systemic vasoconstriction and perhaps contributes to hyponatremia in the later stages of the disease. ANP is a counter-regulatory

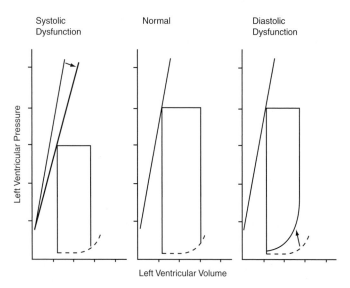

Figure 4 Pressure–volume loops comparing normal left ventricular function with impaired systolic and diastolic function. In systolic dysfunction, contractility is depressed and there is diminished capacity to eject blood into a high-pressure aorta. In diastolic dysfunction, there is diminished capacity to fill at low diastolic pressure. The left ventricular ejection fraction is low in systolic dysfunction and normal in diastolic dysfunction.

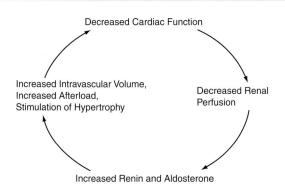

Figure 5 This "vicious cycle of heart failure" begins with an impaired cardiac function, leading to a low cardiac output and thus decreased renal perfusion. The subsequent release of renin and aldosterone causes an increased intravascular volume, increased afterload, and stimulation of left ventricular hypertrophy, all of which exacerbate cardiac dysfunction.

hormone opposing vasoconstriction and sodium and water retention, thus protecting the heart from volume overload. In acute heart failure, ANP inhibits the synthesis of renin, opposes the effects of angiotensin II, and stimulates renal excretion of sodium and water, thus, decreasing preload. Finally, there is a change in peripheral oxygen delivery in heart failure caused by the redistribution of cardiac output toward vital organs, an altered oxyhemoglobin dissociation curve, and an increased oxygen extraction by tissues.

The compensatory mechanisms in heart failure are a "double-edged sword," because they support myocardial performance in the early stages of heart failure but later cause undesirable effects leading to accelerated deterioration of the failing heart. Thus the goal in the treatment of heart failure is to modify these compensatory mechanisms using pharmacologic agents to break the cycle of maladaptive changes.

Clinical Manifestations of Heart Failure: A Series of Opposing Adjectives

Heart failure is characterized by a number of factors: sodium and water retention, dyspnea or fatigue (limitation of exercise tolerance), neurohormonal activation, decreased peripheral blood flow with subsequent lowering of end-organ metabolism, impaired systolic function, ventricular arrhythmias, and ultimately decreased survival (6).

In describing the clinical features of heart failure it is useful to consider a series of opposing adjectives (Table 2). These descriptions are useful particularly early in the course

Table 2 Clinical Adjectives Used in Describing Heart Failure

Acute vs. chronic
Right vs. left sided
High vs. low output
Forward vs. backward
Systolic vs. diastolic
Primary vs. secondary
Latent vs. overt
Reversible vs. irreversible
Compensated vs. refractory (intractable)
Stable vs. unstable

of the disease, but they do not necessarily signify fundamentally different disease states. Late in the course of the disease, the differences between these forms often become less distinct (4).

Right vs. Left Ventricular Failure

The distinction between right and left ventricular failure was first proposed by Harrison et al. (18) in 1932. Pure right ventricular failure is most commonly caused by cor pulmonale from chronic lung disease and increased pulmonary vascular resistance. The symptoms include edema, congestive hepatomegaly, systemic venous distention, weakness, fatigue, and central nervous system symptoms. The signs include an elevated central venous pressure, hepatojugular reflux, ascites, pleural/pericardial effusion, bowel edema (causing anorexia, nausea, vomiting, and malabsorption), and cachexia. Left heart failure is characterized by poor cardiac output, an increased left ventricular filling pressure, and pulmonary congestion. The symptoms include dyspnea, orthopnea, paroxysmal nocturnal dyspnea, cough, nocturia, and hemoptysis. The signs are tachycardia, auscultatory gallop, inspiratory rales, expiratory wheezes, and pulsus alternans. Many patients with advanced left ventricular failure develop right ventricular failure, and a combination of both left and right ventricular failure is a common clinical presentation. This is especially true for patients with mitral stenosis and patients with a dilated cardiomyopathy.

High-Output vs. Low-Output Heart Failure

The description, high output/low output, relates the cause to the typical clinical features. High-output heart failure is characterized by decreased peripheral resistance often in the absence of sodium and water retention. Etiologies known to cause high-output heart failure include hyperthyroidism, anemia, arteriovenous fistula, beriberi, Paget's disease of the bone, Albright's syndrome, multiple myeloma, hypernephroma with bone metastases, cirrhosis, and acute glomerulonephritis. Low-output heart failure is characterized by retention of sodium and water and often an elevated peripheral vascular resistance and is caused by anything that decreases the cardiac output, including left ventricular dysfunction, and restrictive influences on the heart.

Forward vs. Backward Heart Failure

The concepts of forward and backward heart failure date back to 1913 and 1832, respectively (19,20); although they are old concepts, they retain clinical utility today. Forward heart failure involves inadequate discharge of blood into the arterial system, which leads to decreased renal perfusion, activating the renin–aldosterone axis and causing sodium and water retention, mental obtundation, and hypotension. In backward heart failure, the ventricle fails to discharge its contents normally, and the end-diastolic volume and the pressure in the atria and ventricles are elevated, leading to pulmonary and venous congestion and sodium and water retention. The manifestations are hepatomegaly, ascites, and peripheral edema.

Systolic vs. Diastolic Dysfunction

Systolic dysfunction leads to increased filling pressures and pulmonary congestion, decreased cardiac output, redistribution of flow toward vital organs, decreased stroke volume, and increased left ventricular end-diastolic volume with dilation of the ventricle (21). There is a growing recognition of diastolic dysfunction (heart failure with normal heart size and ejection fraction) as a cause for impaired pump function of the heart (22). As seen in Figure 3, this diastolic dysfunction or "input failure" is characterized by the inability of the ventricle to relax and fill normally, leading to an increased filling pressure, increased ventricular end-diastolic pressure, and a decreased stroke volume because of decreased myofibrillar stretch and impaired diastolic filling. It is important to recognize that traditional therapy aimed at stimulation of systolic ejection may be ineffective or even deleterious in pure diastolic dysfunction (13,22).

Other Adjectives Used to Describe Heart Failure

There are other adjectives of value in describing heart failure, which may relate to cause, treatment, and prognosis. In "reversible heart failure," the manifestations disappear if the underlying cause is removed early in the course of the disease. Examples include ischemia, valvular lesions, constrictive pericarditis, infectious endocarditis, hypertension, and most of the causes of high-output heart failure. "Irreversible heart failure" occurs when the manifestations do not disappear after precipitating factors are eliminated; in fact, they are often progressive. The classic example is myocardial infarction with extensive myocardial necrosis. Other factors leading to irreversibility include isolated myocardial cell loss and interstitial fibrosis with plastic transformation of the adjacent myocardium.

The commonly used term "congestive heart failure" refers to abnormal circulatory congestion caused not only by impaired heart function but also by peripheral circulatory and sympathetic renal compensatory mechanisms. A "congested state" is an expanded intravascular volume with preserved ventricular function, for example, caused by vigorous volume infusions, anemia, beriberi, etc. It is often difficult to distinguish congestive heart failure from a congested state, especially in the postoperative patient and in patients with renal failure. It often becomes necessary to use invasive monitoring with determination of cardiac output and pulmonary capillary wedge pressure to make the distinction. If the precipitating factors persist, the congested state may become congestive heart failure (ventricular function becomes impaired).

"Primary heart failure" refers to diseases arising from the myocardium, such as congenital heart diseases, neuromuscular diseases, myocarditis, and presbycardia (senile heart). "Secondary heart failure" occurs because of other factors such as ischemic disease, systemic disorders, and metabolic and inflammatory diseases. "Unstable heart failure" means a severe circulatory derangement, which is life threatening if not aggressively treated, and includes acute pulmonary edema and cardiogenic shock. "Transient heart failure" (flash pulmonary edema) is often seen in patients with diastolic dysfunction resulting from hypertension and following cardiopulmonary bypass.

Special Considerations

Often a patient with chronic, well-compensated heart failure is hospitalized for a surgical procedure or other reasons and experiences an exacerbation of heart failure, leading to worsening of symptoms or signs of heart failure. There are many factors that may underlie the exacerbation, and most often it can be corrected by simply removing the offending cause (23); however, sometimes the cause leads to a direct worsening of ventricular function, which is irreversible and leads to unstable heart failure or a new level of compensation at a worsened functional class (Table 3).

Table 3 Events Precipitating or Exacerbating Heart Failure in Patients with Compensated Disease

Changes in environment or diet
Noncompliance with medical therapy
Arrhythmias
Myocardial ischemia
Anemia
Drugs: nonsteroidal anti-inflammatory drugs, corticosteroids, calcium channel blockers, β-blockers, etc.
Thyroid dysfunction
Metabolic deficiencies
Infections
Worsening renal function
Pulmonary embolism
Pregnancy
Emotional factors
Myocarditis
Endocarditis
Systemic hypertension
Myocardial infarction

The New York Heart Association classification of heart failure (Table 4) has gained broad acceptance as the standard clinicians use to communicate with one another regarding the severity of heart failure. It is based on subjective and objective findings, with the objective assessment being based not only on physical examination but also on noninvasive and invasive tests to evaluate cardiac status. It is accepted that the severity of symptoms may not necessarily be matched by equivalent degrees of impaired structure and function of the heart (24).

Therapy

Broad Objective: Correct the Deranged Physiology

The goal in the treatment of heart failure is to correct the deranged physiology while establishing and treating the underlying cause. Despite this, prevention of heart failure exerts far more salutary effect on public health than treatment. Prevention of the most common causes involves

Table 4 The New York Heart Association Classification of Heart Failure

Functional capacity
Class I: Patients with cardiac disease, but without resulting limitation of physical activity. Ordinary physical activity does not cause undue fatigue, palpitation, dyspnea, or anginal pain
Class II: Patients with cardiac disease resulting in slight limitation of physical activity. They are comfortable at rest. Ordinary physical activity results in fatigue, palpitation, dyspnea, or anginal pain
Class III: Patients with marked limitation of physical activity. They are comfortable at rest. Less-than-ordinary activity causes fatigue, palpitation, dyspnea, or anginal pain
Class IV: Patients with cardiac disease resulting in inability to carry on any physical activity without discomfort. Symptoms of heart failure or of the anginal syndrome may be present even at rest. If any physical activity is undertaken, discomfort is increased
Objective assessment[a]
A. No objective evidence of cardiovascular disease
B. Objective evidence of minimal cardiovascular disease
C. Objective evidence of moderately severe cardiovascular disease
D. Objective evidence of severe cardiovascular disease

[a]For example, physical examination, electrocardiogram, chest X-ray examination, cardiac catheterization, echocardiography, radiologic imaging, and stress testing.

early and vigorous treatment of hypertension, hyperlipidemia, diabetes, and the promotion of lifestyle changes to lower the risk of coronary artery disease. In addition, the early use of thrombolytic therapy in acute myocardial infarction decreases the risk of development of heart failure. Finally, the identification and management of the specific causes and precipitating factors in heart failure are important (Tables 1 and 3).

Once the diagnosis of heart failure is made, the therapeutic challenge is to alleviate symptoms and prolong life by correcting the abnormal physiology. The abnormal cardiac physiology involves both metabolic and mechanical derangements (25). The correction of mechanical derangements involves the increase in supply of energy substrates and blood flow to meet the increased energy demands. For example, coronary revascularization may improve ventricular performance in patients with coronary artery disease and depressed ventricular function. The treatment of the abnormal mechanical properties of the heart may include the reversal of maladaptive hypertrophy with ACE inhibitors or an increase in contractility with digoxin. The correction of systemic derangements involves lowering preload with salt restriction, diuretics, and venous vasodilators and lowering afterload with arterial vasodilators. The control of heart rate and rhythm is also important, and this can be achieved with β-blockers, antiarrhythmics, and pacemakers if needed. Lastly, in suitable patients with refractory heart failure, the treatment of choice may be cardiac transplantation; however, this option is limited by a supply of donor organs, which is only a fraction of the demand.

Treatment of Acute Heart Failure

General Principles

The therapy of acute heart failure and cardiogenic shock involves treatment modalities that are both similar and dissimilar to those used in chronic heart failure. The most prominent features include a clinical assessment of the intravascular volume status, invasive hemodynamic monitoring, inotropic pharmacologic therapy, and mechanical assist devices. The goal in treating hemodynamically unstable patients is to optimize oxygen delivery to vital organs by increasing cardiac output and decreasing pulmonary venous congestion. In the critical care setting, this therapy is assisted by a peripheral arterial catheter (for assessment of arterial pressure) and a balloon-tipped, flow-directed pulmonary artery catheter (for assessment of left ventricular filling pressure and cardiac output) (26,27).

Before considering invasive or complicated techniques to treat acute heart failure, it is important to remember that there are frequently simple derangements contributing to pump failure that may be easily corrected. For example, acid–base imbalances, electrolyte abnormalities, and hypoxia may directly contribute to myocardial depression and should be aggressively corrected. In addition, arrhythmias, such as sinus bradycardia or atrioventricular block or dissociation, may contribute to a low cardiac output. Finally, mechanical complications of acute myocardial infarction, such as mitral regurgitation caused by papillary muscle infarction, ventricular septal rupture, and ventricular free wall rupture may be the culprit in acute heart failure and require immediate surgical intervention.

Specific Measures

In the patient with acute heart failure, the inadequate cardiac output may be increased by the following means. First,

by increasing the end-diastolic volume or preload through volume expansion, one augments cardiac output by utilizing the Frank–Starling mechanism. Inotropic agents such as dopamine, dobutamine, norepinephrine, and digitalis increase cardiac output by directly increasing contractility. Lowering afterload with agents such as nitroprusside and ACE inhibitors improves cardiac output by decreasing resistance to ventricular ejection. Decreasing the degree of ischemia in patients with coronary artery disease may influence cardiac output by improving ventricular wall motion. When the stroke volume is fixed, cardiac output can be augmented by increasing the heart rate with a pacemaker or a positive chronotropic agent. When these measures are undertaken, it is important to weigh the possible negative effects on the myocardium, caused by an increase in oxygen demand with the need to improve the cardiac output (28).

An increase in pulmonary venous pressure is corrected by decreasing total circulating blood or fluid volume with diuretics or phlebotomy or by facilitating peripheral venous pooling with vasodilators or rotating tourniquets. In addition to decreasing the intravascular volume, diuretics also facilitate venous pooling (29).

Mechanical Assist Devices

In the setting of acute myocardial infarction, mechanical circulatory assistance devices such as the "intra-aortic balloon pump" (IABP) increase arterial pressure during diastole (diastolic augmentation) to maintain or enhance coronary arterial perfusion pressure and lower preejection and ejection pressures (systolic unloading) to reduce myocardial work and oxygen demand (28,30). In addition, the IABP improves the hemodynamic status and has been shown to reverse the shock syndrome. Despite these acute hemodynamic effects, the ultimate prognosis in patients using the IABP is not significantly improved. Indications for circulatory assistance using the IABP are cardiogenic shock secondary to myocardial infarction or myocardial depression following cardiac surgery, acute heart failure refractory to medical therapy, and recurrent life-threatening ventricular arrhythmias unresponsive to medication and/or pacing. In addition to these indications, the IABP is commonly used in the stabilization of patients who are hemodynamically compromised immediately after myocardial infarction while waiting for catheterization or cardiac surgery. Placement of an IABP is contraindicated in patients with irreversible brain damage, chronic end-stage heart disease, severe associated disease, or an incompetent aortic valve (26).

The "left ventricular assist device" (LVAD) is an extracorporeal or intracorporeal pump that provides the power to shunt oxygenated blood from the left ventricle to the ascending aorta, while reducing the workload of the ventricle. It is used most commonly in patients with end-stage heart failure as a bridge to cardiac transplantation and in patients with stunned myocardium, when cardiac function is slow to recover. Further discussion of the LVAD and IABP can be found in the chapter on Mechanical Support of the Failing Heart.

Metabolic Support

The concept of providing metabolic support for the ischemic myocardium with glucose, insulin, and potassium has stimulated new interest in the treatment of acute heart failure refractory to conventional therapy (31). The administration of a solution of high doses of glucose, insulin, and potassium (the latter to prevent hypokalemia) has demonstrated utility in improving ventricular function in patients with acute heart failure, especially after elective hypothermic ischemic arrest (31,32). Although it has been thought that the accumulation of glycolytic products worsens the functional effects of ischemia, the provision of glucose and insulin improves contractile function in myocardial infarction in the acutely ischemic, reperfused myocardium (33). It is thought that the glucose, insulin, and potassium solution preserves cell integrity (e.g., through preserving glycogen stores, activating ATP-sensitive potassium channels, and maintaining sodium and potassium ATPase activity).

Treatment of Chronic Heart Failure

The basic principles in the treatment of chronic heart failure are first to eliminate precipitating factors, second to determine if systolic dysfunction or diastolic dysfunction prevails and treat accordingly, and finally to identify and correct any other underlying cause. Patients may have purely systolic or diastolic dysfunction, but frequently they have some combination of the two (4,34). As stated earlier, the ultimate goal in treatment of chronic heart failure is the reduction of morbidity and mortality.

Approach to Asymptomatic Heart Failure

Irrespective of its cause, systolic dysfunction has an asymptomatic, a symptomatic, and a refractory stage. In the asymptomatic patient, the treatment consists of modification of risk factors for coronary artery disease, such as smoking, hypertension, hyperlipidemia, and obesity. Whereas strenuous physical activity may overtax the circulation of the patient with compensated heart failure, regular aerobic exercise can enhance the efficiency of the cardiovascular system, with a resultant increase in exercise tolerance (35). ACE inhibitors inhibit the maladaptive myocardial hypertrophy and may prevent progression to the symptomatic stage; thus, they are very important in the treatment of the asymptomatic patient (36). There is mounting evidence that ACE inhibitors influence intracellular signaling cascades, which have effects on growth and thus may inhibit growth of overloaded myocardial cells (36,37).

Approach to Symptomatic Heart Failure: Importance of Triple Therapy

In the symptomatic patient, the goals of therapy are to relieve symptoms and to prolong life. Specifically, the hallmarks of treatment involve lowering the workload of the heart, increasing contractility, controlling sodium and water retention, and controlling associated arrhythmias. The workload may be lowered by physical and emotional rest, treatment of obesity, and the use of preload- and afterload-reducing agents. ACE inhibitors have been shown to be of the greatest benefit; however, the combination of nitrates and hydralazine has also shown benefit (15,38,39). In addition, ACE inhibitors have been shown to affect favorably long-term outcome in patients who have heart failure as a result of myocardial infarction by decreasing adverse left ventricular remodeling (16). Digoxin continues to be the only positive inotropic agent available for oral administration. Long-term administration of digoxin has been shown to reduce morbidity and mortality when combined with afterload reduction and diuretics (15). Sodium and water retention can be modulated by the use of a low-sodium diet and diuretics. Precautions must be taken when using diuretics to avoid electrolyte imbalances. The combination of afterload reduction, digitalis, and diuretics forms the cornerstone of the management of chronic symptomatic heart failure. Finally, it is important to preserve or restore normal sinus rhythm (40).

Special Considerations

There are a number of special considerations in the treatment of heart failure, some of which have already been mentioned but are summarized once more here in context. First, the identification of diastolic dysfunction and pure right ventricular failure is important, because the treatment of these unique physiologic derangements is different from that of systolic left ventricular dysfunction (41). Second, in severe heart failure, the prevention of and treatment of thrombotic complications and arrhythmias is important. Lastly, the pharmacokinetics of many drugs may be altered in heart failure, even in the absence of renal impairment.

Diastolic Dysfunction

In contrast to the fundamental defect in systolic dysfunction, patients with isolated diastolic dysfunction have normal or often enhanced contractile function of the left ventricle (as measured by the ejection fraction). However, these patients also have dyspnea and fatigue and develop pulmonary edema in the same way as patients with systolic dysfunction. The key problem in this syndrome is that increased ventricular stiffness (or reduced compliance) leads to limitations on the use of preload reserve because of rapid increases in cardiac filling pressures at normal or slightly increased cardiac volume (13). Because the left ventricle contracts normally, there is no need to attempt to conserve or improve left ventricular function with inotropic agents. Similarly, there is no benefit from preload reduction, which may even worsen the situation. Treatment is instead directed at improving relaxation characteristics, mitigating the effects of an abnormal compliance, and prolonging diastole to allow for improved ventricular filling. Calcium channel–blocking agents and β-blocking agents have offered the best utility in this effort. ACE inhibitors cause regression of left ventricular hypertrophy and may have direct myocardial effects that improve diastolic function. Lowering of blood pressure into the normal range is of paramount importance and should be done with one of these three agents.

Arrhythmias

As ventricular performance deteriorates in chronic heart failure and the cardiac muscle is remodeling in response to overload, electrophysiologic abnormalities develop. The majority of patients with severe chronic heart failure have ventricular arrhythmias often manifested by ventricular tachycardia and ventricular fibrillation. It would be expected that patients with the most frequent or serious arrhythmias would be at the greatest risk for sudden death, but this does not seem to be the case. Complex ventricular arrhythmias are more a reflection of the severity of the patient's hemodynamic and functional status rather than a specific pathophysiologic event. Nonsustained ventricular tachycardia occurs in 40% to 60% of patients with the New York Heart Association class III and IV heart failure, and sudden death may occur in 40% of patients in class III and IV (Table 4). Antiarrhythmic therapy may suppress ventricular arrhythmias but does not prolong life in these patients (6). Furthermore, antiarrhythmic drugs appear to be most proarrhythmic in these myopathic ventricles. Some of these drugs were actually shown to increase mortality in certain circumstances (such as class IC agents following myocardial infarction) (42,43). Thus the jury is still out on the utility of antiarrhythmic therapy in patients with advanced heart failure.

Anticoagulation

Dilated atria and/or ventricular chambers can be the site of thrombi; however, because of its inherent morbidity, routine anticoagulation for prevention of thromboembolic events is not uniformly recommended. Patients with echocardiographic evidence for mural thrombi, presenting with a history of systemic or pulmonary embolism, or patients with a history of atrial fibrillation should be anticoagulated. Otherwise, the risks of complications from chronic anticoagulation, including intracranial or gastrointestinal hemorrhage, do not warrant the expected benefits (44).

Altered Pharmacokinetics

In heart failure, decreased gastric emptying delays absorption and decreases the peak plasma concentration of digoxin, furosemide, and bumetanide. Decreased first-pass metabolism in the liver increases the concentration of nitrates, morphine, and hydralazine. Decreased biotransformation to active forms causes diminished activity of ACE inhibitors. Thus the use of various medications necessitates frequent monitoring of blood levels, electrolytes, and clinical effects of the medication.

Right Ventricular Infarction

Right ventricular infarction, which occurs in less than 7% of patients with acute myocardial infarction, may lead to right ventricular failure. The hemodynamic picture in these patients is characterized by markedly elevated right atrial and right ventricular end-diastolic pressures with a normal or reduced right ventricular systolic pressure, normal or reduced pulmonary artery systolic pressure, and a normal or slightly elevated pulmonary capillary wedge pressure. Because of a markedly reduced right ventricular output, the left ventricle filling pressure becomes inadequate, and left ventricular output therefore decreases. Volume expansion to maintain right ventricular filling pressure and output has been the mainstay of treatment in the acute phase. Vasodilators may improve right ventricular output and, therefore, left ventricular filling pressure and output in the long term (26,27,43).

Therapy of Refractory Heart Failure:
Cardiac Transplantation

Refractory heart failure does not respond to conventional therapy, and thus more aggressive therapies must be used, usually in an inpatient setting. Inotropic support with parenteral inotropes such as dobutamine, dopamine, and the phosphodiesterase inhibitors amrinone and milrinone has been used widely to alleviate the symptoms and signs of heart failure temporarily. Removal of excess fluid by paracentesis, thoracentesis, or dialysis may be necessary. Mechanically assisted circulation with the IABP or the left or right ventricular assist device may become the last resort, but usually only as a bridge to transplantation. Cardiac transplantation has a greater than 60% five-year survival; however, the greatest hurdle is the timely procurement of donor organs, which limits this option to relatively few patients (45).

Future of Treatment Strategies for
Chronic Heart Failure

The future of treatment of chronic heart failure will involve the development of new high-technology devices to augment or supplant the pumping function of the heart and also the elucidation of the genetic basis of heart failure and attempts to alter this genetic destiny. In addition, as more knowledge about the complex neurohormonal interactions involved in heart failure becomes available, new therapies such as the use of low-dose β-adrenergic blocking

agents may come into use (20,46,47). Both modalities merit a brief mention.

Total Artificial Heart

A new emphasis on the concept of the total artificial heart (TAH) has emerged, and prototypes are being developed at institutions in the United States and Japan. The new generation of TAH will be totally implantable with no transcutaneous implements. Power will be supplied by transmission of energy through intact skin to a subcutaneous receiver from battery packs worn by the patient. The development teams believe that new technology in microminiaturization and computer-aided design will enable the new TAH to overcome the pitfalls of the existing Jarvic TAH, such as thrombosis and infection. It is hoped that this technology will supplant cardiac transplantation and become a therapeutic option for both chronic and acute heart failure (48). Effective devices have already been tested in humans, with limited short-term success (see chapter on Mechanical Support of the Failing Heart).

Gene Therapy

Gene therapy is aimed at correction of abnormal cardiac gene expression, and it is believed that the gene response to overload may lead to cell death. The target gene(s) has (have) not been identified; however, the genes responsible for some specific cardiac disease states have been found, and research is under way to develop treatments based on them (49,50). For example, it has been shown that a mutation on a specific site on chromosome 14 encoding the myosin heavy chain is associated with familial hypertrophic cardiomyopathy, and thus, theoretically, the reversal of this mutation could prevent the development of this disease (51).

RESUSCITATION

Cardiopulmonary arrest is the extreme form of acute heart failure. During cardiopulmonary arrest there is the cessation of systemic blood circulation and effective ventilation. Basic life support, or CPR, provides artificial ventilation and circulation until advanced cardiac life support (ACLS) can be initiated. Modern CPR has revolutionized the treatment of sudden death and began with the observation of Kouwenhoven et al. (52), in 1960, that rhythmic depression of the sternum in animals produced pulsations in arterial pressure and permitted successful closed-chest electric defibrillation after prolonged ventricular fibrillation. Since the introduction of this technique, many modifications have been proposed, but none have consistently been proven superior to the basic idea that to be successful the pump function of the heart must be maintained and/or restored. Because of the poor long-term survival rates of patients receiving CPR, it has been difficult to quantitate the survival benefit of traditional CPR or any newer techniques (53). The clinical scenarios in patients most likely to be successfully resuscitated using traditional CPR are outlined in Table 5.

Pathophysiology of Cardiopulmonary Resuscitation

Blood flow during CPR is maintained by a generalized increase in intrathoracic pressure, causing blood to move from the vascular structures of the thorax to the peripheral circulation. When the chest compression is released, blood flows back from the peripheral structures to the thorax. The flow is maintained in the antegrade direction by the valves in the heart and the veins and can reach 1.7 L/min (54). Some investigators have proposed that the increase in

Table 5 Clinical Scenarios of Patients Most Likely to Be Successfully Resuscitated with Traditional Cardiopulmonary Resuscitation

Witnessed sudden arrest caused by ventricular fibrillation outside the hospital, when electric countershock can be performed within 7–8 min

Hospitalized patients with primary ventricular fibrillation and ischemic heart disease

Cardiac arrest in the absence of life-threatening coexisting conditions

Primary respiratory arrest

Arrest caused by hypothermia, drug overdose, or airway obstruction

pleural pressures rather than compression of the heart results in blood flow to the periphery (55). It has been shown that mechanical ventilation alone increases intrathoracic pressures. Translocation of blood from the pulmonary bed into the systemic bed with forward flow can be achieved with the left heart chamber as a conduit (56). Forceful, rhythmic cough can also generate systolic pressures equivalent to normal cardiac activity and sustain cardiac output during asystole, maintaining cerebral blood flow and peripheral flow (57). Paradoxically, the compression of the heart and the increase in intrathoracic pressure with CPR can lead to pulmonary edema in one-third to one-half of patients, representing a major cause of hypoxemia during resuscitation. Some investigators have found that pulmonary artery mean pressure and pulmonary capillary wedge pressures increase within 5 to 10 minutes of CPR and return to baseline within five minutes of effective spontaneous circulation (58).

The experimental strategies to increase the effectiveness of CPR are aimed at making pleural pressures more positive during cardiac emptying and more negative during filling. The former can be achieved by inflation of the lungs during chest compressions and the use of a pneumatic vest. The latter is accomplished with chest cuirass, stimulation of the inspiratory muscles, negative airway pressure during the filling phase, and increasing the abdominal pressure during filling (59).

Cerebral Blood Flow During Cardiopulmonary Resuscitation

Irreversible brain damage occurs within four to six minutes of anoxia. Although isolated neurons show complete recovery after 20 to 60 minutes of anoxia, the postischemic damage is due to hypoperfusion secondary to vasospasm and the release of oxygen-derived free radicals from injured tissues and neuronal calcium overload. Experimental techniques used to preserve cerebral function during CPR include calcium channel blockers, free radical–scavenging agents, transient postresuscitation hypertension, retrograde arterial perfusion with low-viscosity solutions, anticoagulation, hypothermia, barbiturate coma, and hyperosmotic solutions (60). None of these have been shown to be consistently effective in clinical trials. Excessive volume loading is actually detrimental to cerebral perfusion because of cerebral edema or shunting of blood through extracerebral vessels (61).

Coronary Blood Flow During Cardiopulmonary Resuscitation

The basal myocardial oxygen consumption is 30% to 40% of normal during ventricular fibrillation; thus if coronary perfusion cannot meet this demand, the likelihood of successful defibrillation is low. Coronary blood flow decreases from

30% to 5% of normal within the first 20 minutes of CPR. This decrease in flow may be due to epinephrine, direct heart compression, abdominal compression, or negative pleural pressure during the filling phase.

Other methods employed to increase the effectiveness of CPR include vigorous volume infusion and the use of glucose-containing fluids. These methods are controversial because they may increase cerebral damage during ischemia or after reperfusion or may cause pulmonary edema (56). High doses of epinephrine may increase aortic pressure and coronary flow, and the α-receptor stimulation may restore a spontaneous heartbeat; however, the β-receptor activity increases oxygen consumption and may be detrimental (62,63). Calcium channel blockers theoretically would decrease intracellular damage and postischemic cerebral and coronary vasospasm, but their negative inotropic and chronotropic action precludes their use. Sodium bicarbonate corrects systemic acidosis, which may compromise cardiac function, suppresses spontaneous cardiac activity, decreases the threshold for ventricular fibrillation, and impairs cardiac and peripheral response to catecholamines. Despite these beneficial effects, bicarbonate may also exacerbate central nervous system acidosis, produce a paradoxic intracellular acidosis, change the oxygen dissociation curve so as to decrease oxygen delivery, increase osmolality, and cause hypernatremia. Studies have failed to show an improved outcome with its use in CPR.

Ventilation during CPR should be achieved with endotracheal intubation if at all possible. This method is the best at achieving oxygenation during arrest. Other less-effective methods are mouth-to-mouth ventilation, mouth-to-mask ventilation, esophageal obturator, or multiluminal airway device (64–66).

Advanced Cardiac Life Support

The initial objective of ACLS has been the treatment of life-threatening arrhythmias. The prototypical arrhythmias causing cardiopulmonary arrest are ventricular tachycardia and ventricular fibrillation, which are treated with a series of electric countershocks to achieve defibrillation to normal rhythm. This has been shown to be very successful, especially in patients in the intensive care unit setting when defibrillation can be accomplished early. If another rhythm is the cause of the arrest or if ventricular tachycardia or fibrillation persists after countershock, endotracheal intubation, chest compressions, intravenous access, and delivery of medications should take precedence over other measures (64,66).

When ventricular fibrillation is successfully electrically cardioverted, 70% to 80% of patients convert to a rhythm that is capable of supporting adequate perfusion if cardioversion is done within three minutes of onset (64). If ventricular fibrillation persists after the initial countershocks, epinephrine should be given prior to further attempts. Although the use of antiarrhythmic agents is encouraged, whether there are true benefits is controversial.

Asystole is frequently the initial rhythm identified in patients with cardiac arrest found outside the hospital and in critically ill inpatients. This rhythm carries the worst prognosis, with less than 2% of patients surviving hospitalization. In addition to epinephrine and atropine, the use of transcutaneous and transvenous pacing should be encouraged if they can be instituted in a short period of time.

Pulseless electric activity, formerly also termed "electromechanical dissociation," can be due to metabolic and mechanical derangements. This is a disturbance frequently encountered in the traumatized or burned patient where hypovolemia, cardiac tamponade, tension pneumothorax, acidosis, and hypoxia are prevalent. Other causes may include pulmonary embolus and a large myocardial infarction. After ACLS has been initiated, each of the possible causes should be investigated and treated immediately.

Cardiopulmonary Arrest Following Trauma

The approach to the patient with cardiopulmonary arrest as a result of trauma is different than that to the patient with arrest as a result of a primary cardiac or pulmonary event. The causes of arrest associated with trauma may include exsanguination with hypovolemia and diminished oxygen delivery, diminished cardiac output resulting from tension pneumothorax or pericardial tamponade from penetrating trauma, or direct trauma to the heart or great vessels. In addition, there may be causes that may not be as readily apparent as the purely mechanical causes, such as cardiovascular collapse or primary respiratory arrest resulting from a neurogenic response to severe central neurologic injury and trauma associated with a primary arrest, such as in the patient who suffers ventricular arrhythmias while driving a car.

The management of patients who suffer arrest associated with trauma begins with immediate evaluation of the airway and electrocardiographic rhythm. Ventilation should be accomplished as first priority because the tolerance of pulselessness may be extended in patients who have achieved adequate oxygenation. While establishing an adequate airway, in-line stabilization of the neck should be performed, and lateral neck supports, strapping, and backboards should be used to prevent worsening of a possible neck injury. If after airway control and defibrillation of dysrhythmias there is no pulse or blood pressure, chest compressions may have to be initiated. In penetrating injury to the chest, the thorax should be vented if there is asymmetry of breath sounds or an increase in airway resistance. A thorough survey of the body should be made for penetrating injury that may cause pneumothorax or tension pneumothorax. Once identified, a penetrating injury should be sealed, and immediate monitoring for (and relief of) tension pneumothorax should be performed. Emergency thoracotomy permits direct massage of the heart and allows relief of tamponade, control of thoracic and extrathoracic hemorrhage, and aortic cross-clamping (64). Open cardiac massage increases cardiac output and aortic pressures more than standard CPR; however, it has been shown that there is no benefit of this procedure if initiated after 30 minutes of standard CPR (56,64,66).

When a patient becomes pulseless as a result of intravascular volume loss, functional long-term survival is unlikely unless single-organ hemorrhage can be rapidly terminated, along with aggressive volume resuscitation, blood transfusions, and circulatory support. Patients with prehospital arrest caused by multiple-organ hemorrhage, as is commonly seen with blunt trauma, rarely survive neurologically intact, despite rapid prehospital and trauma-center response. Those who survive prehospital arrest associated with trauma are generally young, have penetrating injuries, have received early endotracheal intubation, and undergo rapid transport by highly skilled paramedics to a definitive care facility (64).

Monitoring the Effectiveness of Cardiopulmonary Resuscitation

CPR is most effective when the mean and diastolic aortic pressures are maintained continually at an adequate level.

These are the critical pressures that define perfusion of oxygenated blood to the coronary arteries and systemic circulation. In addition, adequate aortic pressures are needed to promote effective circulation of emergency medications such as catecholamines and antiarrhythmics. However, if the left atrial pressure is as high as the aortic pressures, there may not be forward flow even with adequate aortic pressures, and the result may be reverse flow and pulmonary edema. This situation may be encountered, for example, in patients with mitral or aortic valvular dysfunction.

Arterial pH and PO_2 do not correlate well with outcome in CPR except in the extreme. With a very high pH, for example, there may be failure of defibrillation. A very low pH portends a poor outcome. Arterial lactate levels are an indicator of perfusion with oxygenated blood and have an inverse correlation with outcome. Mixed venous or coronary venous pH and PCO_2 do not correlate with outcome; however, failure to eliminate carbon dioxide as measured by an increased mixed venous carbon dioxide and a low end-tidal carbon dioxide tension is associated with the onset of ventricular fibrillation (64,66,67).

Morbidity, Mortality, and Prognosis

With in-hospital cardiopulmonary arrest, there is a 55% rate of successful resuscitation; however, only 15% of the patients survive the hospitalization (64,66,68). The extent of prearrest morbidity plays an important role in the outcome of CPR. Approximately one out of five survivors suffers serious permanent brain damage, and this complication is most correlated to the amount of time in cardiopulmonary arrest prior to beginning CPR and ACLS.

The most important prognostic factors are a prolonged delay in the onset of CPR, a prolonged duration of CPR, age less than 40 or greater than 70, the presence of hypotension and lactic acidosis after arrest, severe hypoxia before arrest, azotemia, hyperglycemia, and comorbid conditions such as sepsis, renal failure, and malignancy (64).

SUMMARY

As the general population ages, acute and chronic heart failure is an increasingly important cause of morbidity and mortality in the adult surgical patient. While there are a large number of causes and exacerbating factors for heart failure, management issues may be similar. With this in mind, it is important to understand the pathophysiology of heart failure, because the treatment is aimed directly at influencing and hopefully reversing the maladaptive physiologic mechanisms both within the heart and systemically. Although there is great promise in the future for metabolic, molecular biologic, and sophisticated mechanical treatments for acute and chronic heart failure, early diagnosis and aggressive treatment while excluding reversible causes is and will remain the hallmark of treatment of heart failure.

After more than 40 years of use, CPR remains a desperate effort to treat cardiopulmonary arrest, and, unfortunately, the benefits are limited to only a small number of patients. It is interesting that despite many efforts at change, the original technique of CPR has changed little throughout the years. Perhaps the greatest impact in the future will be the development of improved measures at prediction and prevention of arrest and improvement in postresuscitation measures.

REFERENCES

1. Mackenzie J. Principles of Diagnosis and Treatment in Heart Affections. London: Oxford University Press, 1916:38.
2. Taegtmeyer H. Energy metabolism of the heart, from basic concepts to clinical applications. Curr Probl Cardiol 1994; 11:64.
3. Isselbacher K, ed. Harrison's Principles of Internal Medicine. New York: McGraw Hill, 1994:989.
4. Braunwald E, ed. Heart Disease: A Textbook of Cardiovascular Medicine. 4th ed. Philadelphia: WB Saunders, 1992:393.
5. Ho KK, et al. The epidemiology of heart failure, the Framingham study. J Am Coll Cardiol 1993; 22(suppl A):6A.
6. Willerson JT, ed. Treatment of Heart Diseases. London: Gower Medical Publishing, 1992:2.3.
7. Gerdes AM, et al. Structural remodeling of cardiac myocytes in patients with ischemic cardiomyopathy. Circulation 1992; 86:426.
8. Weber KT, Brilla CC. Pathological hypertrophy and cardiac interstitium: fibrosis and renin-aldosterone system. Circulation 1991; 86:426.
9. Langer GA. Calcium and the heart: exchange at the tissue, cell and organelle levels. FASEB J 1992; 6:893.
10. Ungerer M, et al. Altered expression of beta-1 adrenergic receptors in the failing human heart. Circulation 1993; 87:454.
11. Schwartz K, et al. Switches in cardiac muscle gene expression as a result of pressure and volume overload. Am J Physiol 1992; 262:364.
12. Goldsmith SR, Hasking GJ, Miller E. Angiotensin II and sympathetic activity in patients with CHF. J Am Coll Cardiol 1993; 21:1107.
13. Goldsmith SR, Dick C. Differentiating systolic from diastolic heart failure: pathophysiologic and therapeutic considerations. Am J Med 1993; 95:645.
14. Bristow MR. Pathophysiologic and pharmacologic rationales for clinical management of chronic heart failure with beta blocking agents. Am J Cardiol 1993; 71:12C.
15. The CONSENSUS Trial Study Group. Effects of enalapril on mortality in severe congestive heart failure. N Engl J Med 1987; 316:1429.
16. Pfeffer MA, et al. The effect of captopril on mortality and morbidity in patients with left ventricular dysfunction following myocardial infarction: Results of the survival and ventricular enlargement (SAVE) trial. N Engl J Med 1992; 327:669.
17. The SOLVD Investigators. Effect of enalapril on mortality and the development of heart failure in asymptomatic patients with reduced LV ejection fraction. N Engl J Med 1992; 327:685.
18. Harrison TR, et al. Congestive heart failure. The mechanism of dyspnea on exertion. Arch Int Med 1932; 50:690.
19. Hope JA. Treatise on the Diseases of the Heart and Great Vessels. London: Williams-Kid, 1832.
20. Mackenzie J. Diseases of the Heart. 3rd ed. London: Oxford University Press, 1913.
21. Carabello B. Clinical assessment of systolic dysfunction. ACC Curr J Rev 1994; 23:25.
22. Bonow RO, Udelson JE. Left ventricular diastolic dysfunction as a cause of congestive heart failure: mechanisms and management. Ann Intern Med 1992; 117:502.
23. Fleisher LA, Eagle KA. Lowering cardiac risk in noncardiac surgery. N Engl J Med 2001; 345:1677.
24. Dolgin M, ed. Nomenclature and Criteria for Diagnosis of Disease of the Heart and Great Vessels. 9th ed. New York: Little Brown, 1994:253.
25. Scheuer J. Metabolic factors in myocardial failure. Circulation 1993; 87(suppl 7):VII54.
26. Chatterjee K. Acute Heart Failure, Critical Care Management. Boston: Little Brown, 1975:203.
27. Passmore J Jr., et al. Hemodynamic Support of the Critically 111 Patient in Cardiopulmonary Critical Care. Orlando, Florida: Grune & Stratton, 1986:359.
28. Braunwald E, et al. Effects of drugs and of counterpulsation on myocardial oxygen consumption. Circulation 1969; 40 (suppl 4):220.
29. Dikshit K, et al. Renal and extrarenal hemodynamic effects of furosemide in congestive heart failure after acute myocardial infarction. N Engl J Med 1973; 288:1087.
30. Kantrowitz A, et al. Initial clinical experience with intra aorta balloon pumping in cardiogenic shock. JAMA 1968; 203:135.
31. Taegtmeyer H. The use of hypertonic glucose, insulin and potassium (GIK) in myocardial preservation. J Appl Cardiol 1991; 6:255.
32. Grandinak S, et al. Improved cardiac function with glucose-insulin-potassium after coronary bypass surgery. Ann Thorac Surg 1981; 48:484.
33. McElroy DD, Walker WE, Taegtmeyer H. Effects of glycogen on function and energy metabolism of the isolated rabbit heart after hypothermic ischemic arrest. J Appl Cardiol 1989; 4:455.
34. Hurst JW, ed. Current Therapy in Cardiovascular Diseases. Chicago: Mosby-Year Book, 1993.
35. Uren NG, Lipkin DP. Exercise training as therapy for chronic heart failure. Br Heart J 1992; 67:430.
36. Smith WHT, Ball SG. ACE inhibitors in heart failure: an update. Basic Res Cardiol 2000; 95(suppl 1):I8.
37. Katz AM. Treating heart failure: yesterday, today and tomorrow. Adv Cardiovasc 1994; Med 1:1.
38. Cohn JN, et al. Effects of vasodilator therapy on mortality in chronic congestive heart failure: results of a Veterans Administration Cooperative Study (V-HeFT). N Engl J Med 1986; 314:1547.
39. Goldman S, et al. Mechanisms of death in heart failure: the vasodilator-HF trials. Circulation 1993; 3(87 suppl 6):VI-24.
40. Hochleitner M, et al. Usefulness of physiologic dual-chamber pacing in drug resistant idiopathic dilated cardiomyopathy. Am J Cardiol 1990; 66:198.
41. Gaash WH. Diagnosis and treatment of heart failure based on LV systolic or diastolic dysfunction. JAMA 1994; 271:1276.
42. Armstrong PW, Moe GW. Medical advances in the treatment of congestive heart failure. Circulation 1993; 88:2941.
43. Parrillo JE. Current Therapy in Critical Care Medicine. 2d ed. Philadelphia: BC Decker, 1991.
44. Clinical Practice Guideline #11. Rockville, Maryland: Agency for HealthCare Policy and Research, 1994:11.
45. DEFIBRILAT Study Group. Actuarial risk of sudden death while awaiting cardiac transplantation in patients with atherosclerotic heartdisease. Am J Cardiol 1991; 68:545.
46. Sonnenblick EH, LeJemtel TH. Heart failure: its progression and its therapy. Hosp Pract Sept 1993; 75.
47. Reiken S, Gaburjakova M, Gaburjakova J. Beta-adrenergic receptor blockers restore cardiac calcium release channel (iyanodine receptor) structure and function in heart failure. Circulation 2001; 104:2843.
48. Lenfant C. Report of the task force on research in heart failure. Circulation 1994; 90:1118.
49. Watkins H, et al. Characteristics and prognostic implications of myosin missense mutation in familial hypertrophic cardiomyopathy. N Engl J Med 1992; 326:1108.
50. del Monte F, Hajjar RJ, Harding SE. Overwhelming evidence of the beneficial effects of SERCA gene transfer in heart failure. Circ Res 2001; 88:E66.
51. Hejtmancik JF, et al. Localization of the gene for familial hypertrophic cardiomyopathy to chromosome 14ql in a diverse US population. Circulation 1991; 83:1592.
52. Kouwenhoven WB, Jude JR, Knickerbocker GG. Closed-chest cardiac massage. JAMA 1960; 173:1064.
53. Tucker KJ, et al. Cardiopulmonary resuscitation: historical perspectives, physiology, and future directions. Arch Intern Med 1994; 154:2141.
54. Rudikoff MT, et al. Mechanisms of blood flow during cardiopulmonary arrest. Circulation 1980; 61:345.
55. Chandra N, et al. Contrasts between intrathoracic pressures during external clot compression and cardiac massage. Crit Care Med 1981; 9:789.
56. Schleien CL, et al. Controversial issues in cardiopulmonary resuscitation. Anesthesiol 1989; 71:133.
57. Criley YM, et al. Modification of cardiopulmonary resuscitation based on cough. Circulation 1986; 74(suppl 4):42.

58. Ornato JP, et al. Rapid changes in pulmonary vascular hemodynamics with pulmonary edema during CPR. Am J Emerg Med 1985; 3:237.

59. Einagle V, et al. Interposed abdominal compress and carotid blood flow during CPR. Chest 1988; 93:1206.

60. Safar P, Bricher NG. Cardiopulmonary Cerebral Recirculation. 3rd ed. Philadelphia: WB Saunders, 1988:229.

61. Lumpkin JR, Safar P. Brain resuscitation after cardiac arrest. In: Harwood AL, ed. CPR. Baltimore: Williams & Wilkins, 1982:55.

62. Stiell IG, et al. High-dose epinephrine in adult cardiac arrest. N Engl J Med 1992; 327:1045.

63. Behringer W, Kittler H, Sterz F, et al. Cumulative epinephrine dose during cardiopulmonary resuscitation and neurologic outcome. Ann Intern Med 1998; 129:450.

64. Kern KB, Halperin HR, Field J. New guidelines for cardiopulmonary resuscitation and emergency cardiac care: changes in the management of cardiac arrest. JAMA 2001; 285:1267.

65. Hallstrom A, Cobb L, Johnson E, et al. Cardiopulmonary resuscitation by chest compression alone or with month-to-month ventilation. N Engl J Med 2000; 342:1546.

66. International guidelines 2000 conference on cardiopulmonary resuscitation and emergency cardiovascular care. Circulation 2000; 102(suppl I):II36.

67. Gudipati CV, et al. Expired carbon dioxide: a noninvasive monitor of CPR. Circulation 1988; 77:234.

68. Burns R, et al. Prediction of in-hospital cardiopulmonary arrest outcome. Arch Intern Med 1989; 149:1318.

34

Mechanical Support for the Failing Heart:
Current Physiologic Concepts of Management

Sina L. Moainie and Bartley P. Griffith

INTRODUCTION

The development of the extracorporeal heart–lung machine, or cardiopulmonary bypass (CPB) circuit as it is sometimes called, made possible heart surgery as we know it today. Even with this technology, however, not all patients with cardiac disorders are suitable candidates for coronary bypass operations or valve replacement surgery due to the magnitude of the underlying disease. Fortunately, other technological advances have occurred so that devices are now available to support even the most profound circulatory failure. These include the intra-aortic balloon pump (IABP) for acute management of cardiac failure and the left ventricular assist device (LVAD) for chronic end-stage LV failure. While such devices are generally employed to salvage whatever cardiac function exists in anticipation for future cardiac transplantation, more recent technological approaches have aimed at the management of the failing heart from the standpoint of maintaining additional years of meaningful life even when transplantation is not a suitable alternative. This chapter reviews the technological strategies currently available to support the failing circulation and which patients are likely to benefit most from these approaches.

CARDIAC SUPPORT IN END-STAGE HEART FAILURE
Pathophysiology of Heart Failure

Heart failure is defined as the pathologic state in which the heart is unable to pump blood at a rate adequate to meet the physiologic requirements of the tissues despite normal cardiac filling pressures (1). This disease affects an estimated five million Americans, with approximately 550,000 new cases diagnosed each year (2). Coronary artery disease is the most common etiology of heart failure with only approximately 30% of cases of heart failure resulting from other causes including congenital malformations, valvular disease, or viral or idiopathic cardiomyopathy (3).

Following an initial event resulting in diminished cardiac function, a number of compensatory mechanisms are initiated to maintain normal organ perfusion. In response to the decrease in cardiac function, the sympathetic nervous system and the renin–angiotensin system are activated. Release of the neurotransmitter norepinephrine from cardiac adrenergic nerves results in increased vascular tone, leading to improved preload and increased myocardial contractility. Activation of the renin–angiotensin system not only increases preload via an increased renal fluid retention, but also results in vasoconstriction mediated by angiotensin II. The combined effect of the sympathetic and renin–angiotensin response is an increase in preload and myocardial contractility with an ensuing increase in stroke volume via the Starling mechanism.

While the activation of the sympathetic nervous system and rennin–angiotensin system are initially compensatory in response to diminished cardiac function, these responses ultimately become maladaptive.

The progressive decompensation in ventricular function following an index cardiac event is a consequence of adverse ventricular remodeling. The chronic increase in preload and vascular tone increases myocardial wall stress, which sets in motion a biochemical cascade resulting in regional and global myocardial dysfunction (4). Additionally, angiotensin II and aldosterone stimulate collagen synthesis and inhibit collagen degradation leading to interstitial fibrosis (5–7). Pathologic increases in myocardial interstitial collagen content reduce ventricular filling by increasing diastolic stiffness (8). The physiologic consequences of altered ventricular stiffness are manifest by increased central venous and pulmonary artery pressures as well as decreased cardiac output.

Another maladaptive consequence of ventricular remodeling is an increase in ventricular volume and sphericity (9,10). Increased ventricular sphericity, volume, and stiffness have all been demonstrated to result in increased ventricular wall stress with an ensuing increase in myocardial metabolic requirements (8). The mismatch between increasing myocardial metabolic requirements and decreasing cardiac output results in progressive myocardial ischemia. Because intramyocardial pressure has its most profound effects on the subendocardium, it is this region that is most affected by the decrease in blood flow. Several investigators have hypothesized that it is this mismatch between increasing myocardial oxygen demand and decreasing coronary perfusion that leads to the progressive decline in function in advanced heart failure (11,12).

Myocyte loss occurs in the failing heart not only due to necrosis from subendocardial ischemia, but also from myocardial apoptosis. Apoptosis, or programmed cell death via an energy-requiring enzymatic destruction of myocyte DNA, has been demonstrated in failing hearts (13,14). The exact mechanism by which myocardial apoptosis is initiated is as yet unclear, but factors that initiate cellular apoptosis such as upregulation of the gene p53, and increase of the cytokine tumor necrosis factor–alpha have been observed in failing hearts. Additionally, oxygen free-radical generation in response to increased ventricular wall stress has also been implicated in the induction of myocyte apoptosis (15).

The end result of the combined effects of increased myocardial metabolic need, diminishing cardiac function, and progressive myocyte loss lead to a heart that is unable to meet the metabolic needs of the body. Ongoing tachycardia and increasing sympathetic tone secondary to decreased cardiac output further exacerbate the vicious downward spiral resulting in advancing cardiac dysfunction ultimately leading to a heart that is unable to meet the resting metabolic requirements of the tissues. The disparity between the continually increasing population of patients with advanced heart failure and the fixed supply of donor organs for cardiac transplantation has fueled the interest in mechanical support for the failing heart.

Mechanical Circulatory Support

Currently, approximately 6000 patients per year in the United States receive some form of cardiac support following cardiac surgery. The hospital survival for these patients ranges between 20% and 40%. An additional 400 patients per year receive a cardiac support device as a bridge to transplantation, with a survival rate through transplantation ranging between 50% and 70% (16). With the approval of ventricular assist devices for permanent use or "destination" therapy of heart failure, the number of assist devices implanted is expected to increase significantly in the future. Cardiac support devices may be divided into two broad categories; those designed for acute use of days to two weeks and those for longer bridge-to-transplant (BTT) or permanent support.

Acute Support Devices

Intra-Aortic Balloon Pump

The easiest device to apply and the most commonly used remains intra-aortic balloon counterpulsation, which was introduced clinically in 1967 to support patients with acute cardiac decompensation (17). The IABP (Fig. 1) consists of a catheter-mounted inflation/deflation balloon that is positioned in the descending thoracic aorta just distal to the takeoff of the left subclavian artery. It is usually placed using percutaneous introduction into a femoral artery. Generally, the device is inserted in an intensive care unit, in a cardiac catheterization laboratory, or in a cardiac surgical suite. A patient supported by IABP must remain prone with the hip fully extended. This limits its use to less than a week. The indications for IABP support include (i) cardiogenic shock secondary to an ischemic event, (ii) acute treatment of intractable angina prior to planned coronary intervention, (iii) temporary cardiac support of a patient with perioperative cardiogenic shock, or (iv) periprocedural support during complex angioplasty (18,19). Chief in the decision to proceed with IABP placement is the assumption that the source of the cardiogenic shock and/or ischemia necessitating support is thought to be temporary (planned revascularization of ischemic myocardium or anticipated rapid ventricle recovery from post-CPB myopathy). Contraindications to placement of an IABP include aortic valvular insufficiency, aortic dissection, distal aortic occlusion, large aortic aneurysm, or severe peripheral vascular disease.

The IABP augments cardiac function by increasing diastolic blood pressure and reducing afterload. Using ECG, aortic pressure, or set pacing as a trigger, the balloon is set to inflate just after the aortic valve closes and to deflate just after the aortic valve opens. The effectiveness of the device is limited at heart rates above 120 bpm and when ventricular arrhythmia is common. Inflation begins just after the aortic valve closes (the start of diastole), and the increased pressure within the proximal aorta raises the diastolic pressure and thus the coronary perfusion. The augmentation of coronary perfusion pressure reduces myocardial ischemia, which then leads to an improvement in myocardial contractility. Given that the balloon functions in part by augmenting diastolic flow, aortic insufficiency is a

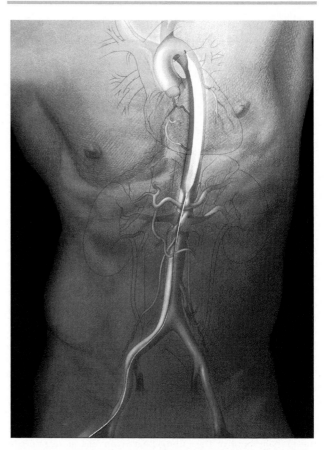

Figure 1 Illustration demonstrating correct positioning of intra-aortic balloon pump with proximal aspect just distal to branching of the left subclavian artery. *Source*: Courtesy of Arrow International, Reading, Pennsylvania, U.S.A.

contraindication to IABP placement because the increase in diastolic pressure would exacerbate aortic regurgitation and lead to increased LV distention. Deflation of the balloon immediately after the aortic valve opens (the start of systole) causes a decrease in the aortic volume (volume occupied by the inflated balloon). Because pressure is directly proportional to volume, deflation of the balloon leads to a resultant decrease in the systolic aortic pressure (afterload). Decreased afterload and increase in coronary perfusion combine to result in an increase in cardiac output of approximately 10% to 25%.

The IABP is most commonly introduced via the femoral artery using a percutaneous Seldinger technique. When extensive occlusive peripheral vascular disease prevents femoral arterial access, the IABP may be introduced directly into the thoracic aorta; this approach is rarely used because this mode of insertion would necessitate a thoracotomy. This approach has been used after cardiac surgery, but most surgeons opt for placement of a temporary ventricular assist device in lieu of an IABP in this circumstance (20). Fluoroscopy is generally not necessary for IABP placement but a chest radiograph should be obtained following placement to confirm correct positioning. The radiopaque tip of the balloon should be positioned just distal to the takeoff of the left subclavian artery, which can be identified radiographically using the second rib as a landmark. The complications of IABP use include visceral or limb ischemia, arterial perforation, retroperitoneal hemorrhage, aortic dissection, and thrombocytopenia resulting from platelet aggregation secondary to a foreign body reaction (21,22). Visceral ischemia may be the result of balloon malposition and may be treated with repositioning of the device. Daily chemistry profiles may alert the clinician to visceral malperfusion as evidenced by rising tests of liver function, serum creatinine or decreasing serum bicarbonate. Limb ischemia is the most common complication of IABP use occurring in 5% to 19% of patients (23). Often limb ischemia resolves with the removal of the IABP, but surgical intervention in the form of angiography, thrombectomy, or angioplasty is required in some cases. Any patient with a femorally placed IABP should have hourly assessment of distal perfusion by physical examination and bedside Doppler. Most physicians opt to anticoagulate patients with heparin to reduce the risk of arterial thrombosis and emboli. Daily complete blood count measurements can alert the clinician to the possibility of hemorrhage or the development of thrombocytopenia.

When the patient demonstrates recovery of ventricular function as evidenced by a cardiac index greater than $2.0 \, L/min/m^2$, a systolic blood pressure greater that 90, and an absence of metabolic acidosis while on minimal inotropic support, IABP support may be withdrawn. Weaning of the IABP is accomplished by decreasing the frequency of augmentation from 1:1 (in which the IABP augments every heart beat) to 1:2 and then 1:3 (IABP augments every third heart beat) in stepwise increments decreasing support every two to three hours. If the patient has continued stable hemodynamics with no increasing inotrope requirement with the IABP on 1:3 augmentation, the device may be removed (24).

Ventricular Assist Devices

While the IABP is relatively easy to use and can be applied within minutes, often the degree of cardiac dysfunction is more than can be supported with counterpulsation. Several devices have been approved to address this profound loss of cardiac function. These fully supporting blood pumps are identified commonly as ventricular assist devices. Several have been targeted for very short-term use of approximately one week, while others are designed with more durable components and have supported patients for up to several years (Table 1).

Short-Term Ventricular Assist Devices. Both the devices currently in use for short-term ventricular support are extracorporeal pulsatile systems. The Thoratec ventricular assist system (VAS) (Fig. 2) is a pneumatically powered device that may be used for univentricular or biventricular support. This pump is composed of a polyurethane compressible

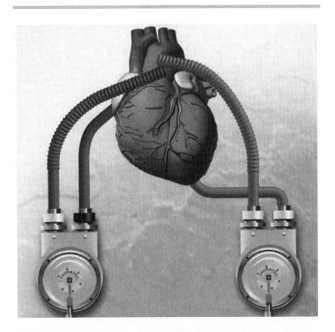

Figure 2 Illustration demonstrating biventricular support with Thoratec device. Right ventricular support utilizes right atrial inflow and pulmonary artery outflow. Left ventricular (LV) support is achieved using LV apical inflow and aortic outflow.

sac-like chamber that draws blood from and through inlet and outlet valves. It has been used as short-term postcardiotomy support for 7 to 10 days but also is durable for longer BTT type support, lasting months or even years. The device is approved for out-of-hospital use, and the pneumatic power source has a rechargeable battery and is packaged in a roll-on type suitcase. When used for LV support, the inflow (fill) cannula is placed either into the LV apex or via the right side interatrial groove into the left atrium. The outflow graft is sewn to the ascending aorta. The right atrium provides inflow and the main pulmonary artery is used for outflow in cases of right ventricular support. Bjork-Shiley mechanical tilting-disk valves are incorporated within the device housing to ensure unidirectional flow. The inlet and outlet cannulae are externalized subcostally and connected to the pump that is powered using pressurized air controlled by the external drive console. The Thoratec VAS has a maximum stroke volume of 65 cc and can provide 6.5 L/min of flow (25). When used for biventricular support, the right ventricular assist device (RVAD) is

Table 1 Mechanical Circulatory Assist Available in the United States

Device	Power	Type	Target indication	Duration of use	FDA approval
ABIOMED BVS5000	Pneumatic	Pulsatile extracorporeal	Postcardiotomy shock	24 hr to 10 days	+
AB5000® Ventricle	Pneumatic	Pulsatile extracorporeal	Postcardiotomy shock and BTT	1–6 mo	+
IAPB	Pneumatic	Pulsatile extracorporeal	Acute cardiac decompensation/ischemia	1–7 wk	+
Thoratec VAD	Pneumatic	Pulsatile extracorporeal	Postcardiotomy shock and BTT	1 wk to 1 yr	+ (BTT)
HeartMate VAD	Electric	Pulsatile intracorporeal	BTT permanent use	1 mo to 1.5 yr	BTT, destination
WorldHeart VAD	Electric	Pulsatile intracorporeal	BTT Permanent use	1 mo to 1 yr	+ (BTT)
CardioWest TAH	Pneumatic	Pulsatile intracorporeal	BTT	1 mo to 1 yr	BTT
MicroMed Axial VAD	Electric	Continuous flow intracorporeal	BTT	1 mo to 1 yr	−
Jarvik Axial VAD	Electric	Continuous flow intracorporeal	BTT	1 mo to 3 yr	−

Abbreviations: BTT, bridge-to-transplant; FDA, Food and Drug Administration; VAD, ventricular assist device; TAH, total artificial heart.

set at an output that is less than that of the LVAD to prevent pulmonary congestion. The Thoratec VAS may be programmed to operate in a fixed rate, volume, or synchronous mode. In the volume mode, the pump is triggered to contract when the sac is fully filled. The volume mode is most commonly utilized and provides maximum output. The synchronous mode uses the r-wave of the patient's electrocardiogram for triggering and is most effective for weaning from support. As with the IABP, assist device can be set from a range of 1:1 to 1:3, and weaning is accomplished in a similar manner as with the IABP by gradually reducing the number of assisted heartbeats (26–28).

The Thoratec is useful for acute cardiac decompensation usually associated with failed cardiac surgery. It is unique in that it is also durable enough to provide long-term BTT support as well. Because it is positioned paracorporeally, it can be used in patients of small body size (body mass index $\geq 1.25\,m^2$) and is the choice of most surgeons when severe biventricular failure indicates the need for combined left and right ventricular support. Because the patient's blood is in contact with the prosthetic material of the cannula, valves and pump sac that activate clotting, and anticoagulation are required. Generally, the circumstance requiring univentricular support is one in which the left ventricle has suffered an acute (ischemic) or chronic power failure. In this circumstance, the ability of the native right ventricle to deliver blood flow across the left heart is critical in determining the adequacy of univentricular versus biventricular support.

As with the Thoratec VAS, the Abiomed BVS5000 (Fig. 3) is a paracorporeal pulsatile ventricular assist device that may be used for left, right, or biventricular support. It is economical and thus is available in most cardiac surgical suites. It is easy to insert and operate, but it lacks durability and has a relatively high incidence of emboli within 10 days of use. Unlike the Thoratec device, the Abiomed BVS5000 requires the patient to remain recumbent. Cannulation for right and left ventricular support is identical to that for the Thoratec device. Like the heart itself, the Abiomed device contains a reservoir that receives blood from the inflow chamber. This chamber in turn loads the pumping chamber. The chambers are connected by a unique trileaflet polyurethane valve that assures unidirectional flow (29). Blood flows into the pump by gravity, and a drive console is used to pneumatically compress the pumping chamber. The device is designed for complete support of the left and/or right heart, and the system microprocessor manages the duration of pump systole and diastole to optimize pump function and maintain a targeted stroke volume of 83 mL after cardiac surgery. The Abiomed BVS5000 also requires the use of systemic anticoagulation as soon as mediastinal hemorrhage abates to prevent formation of device-related thrombus. Recently, the Abiomed company has introduced a pneumatic, sac-like ventricular assist devices (VAD) with polyurethane inlet and outlet valves that connect to the same cannulae for easy exchange. This device, like the Thoratec, is more durable and expensive than the ABVS5000, and permits patients to ambulate in the hospital.

Long-Term Ventricular Assist Devices. A number of devices have been developed to target the need for long-term LV support. Most of the systems use a similar cannulation schema with an LV apical conduit used for device inflow and the ascending aorta used for device outflow. Because the aim of all of the long-term assist devices is to provide outpatient support, these devices tend to use small electric

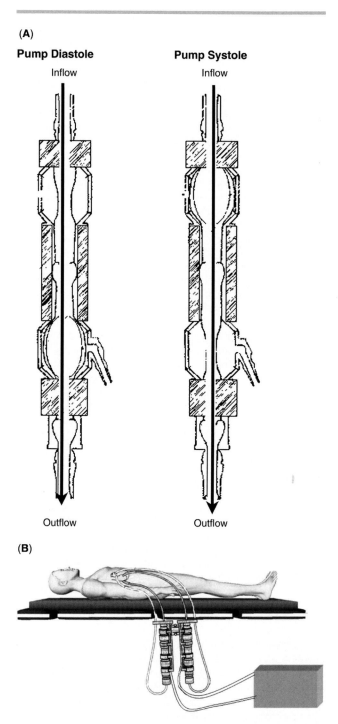

(A)

Pump Diastole   **Pump Systole**

Inflow   Inflow

Outflow   Outflow

(B)

Figure 3 **(A)** Illustration of Abiomed BVS5000 paracorporeal pulsatile ventricular assist device demonstrating position of chambers in pump diastole and systole. **(B)** In vivo positioning of Abiomed BVS5000.

AC battery power and controller modules. The newer flexible and small bore percutaneous power cords have been well tolerated and generally have not been a source of inevitable driveline infection that ascends along the subcutaneous track or seeds the intimal components of the device via homologous spread.

WorldHeart Novacor LVAS. The WorldHeart Novacor LVAS (Fig. 4) is placed via an extended median sternotomy with

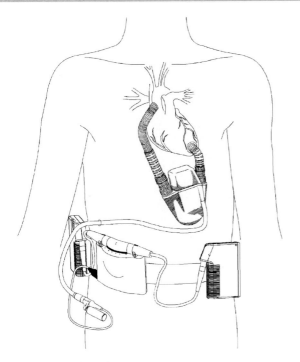

Figure 4 Illustration demonstrating left ventricular (LV) support with the Novacor LVAD. Inflow is via LV apex and outflow is via proximal aorta.

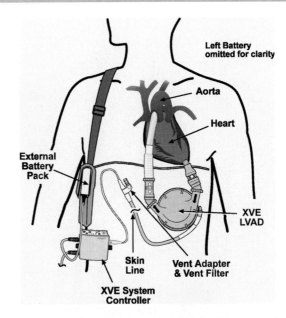

Figure 5 Illustration demonstrating left ventricular (LV) support with the Thoratec XVE. Inflow is via LV apex and outflow is via proximal aorta. *Abbreviations*: LVAD, left ventricular assist device.

the LV apex inflow and aortic outflow conduits connected to the pump that is positioned in the anterior abdominal wall. The pump utilizes two electrically powered opposing pusher plates to eject blood and bioprosthetic valves within the conduits to ensure unidirectional flow. A percutaneous cable connects the pump to the external controller and battery pack, both of which may be worn on a belt to provide for excellent patient mobility. The cable also contains the vent line for the pump. In addition to the fixed-rate mode, the device may also be operated in a synchronized mode that uses an electrocardiographic signal to time pump diastole to cardiac systole and vice versa. The synchronized mode thus provides the most effective means of cardiac unloading because the heart is ejecting into the low resistance pump hence limiting strain on the heart. Although the Novacor LVAS employs smooth, seamless blood-contacting surfaces and bioprosthetic valves to limit thrombogenicity, systemic anticoagulation is still required during the period of support.

Thoratec HeartMate VE LVAS. The Thoratec HeartMate VE LVAS (Fig. 5) is electrically powered. The motor drives a cam mechanism up and down to power the pusher-plate mechanism. An external vent is utilized to equalize air pressure and provide a means for emergency pneumatic device actuation. Should the electrical motor fail, the device may be pneumatically powered by a hand-held portable pump. The electrical motor is normally powered by two rechargeable batteries, delivering four to six hours of power per charge. The batteries may be worn on a vest or belt, thus allowing for high degree of mobility (30,31). A unique feature of the HeartMate device is that the blood-contacting surfaces of the device are designed to promote deposition of circulating cells creating a "pseudoneointimal" layer that discourages platelet adhesion and thrombosis. Additionally,

the device uses a pusher-plate blood pump that creates a central vortex of blood preventing stagnant flow. The combination of these features reduces the likelihood of thrombus formation and so lesser degrees of anticoagulation are required for use of the device, and in fact, the device may be used safely with no anticoagulation when used for long-term support (32).

Lionheart LVD2000 LVAS. The Lionheart System (Fig. 6) is similar in design to other long-term displacement pumps in that it includes an LV apex inflow conduit and aortic outflow conduit that are connected to a subdiaphragmatically placed VAD. The device uses an electrically powered roller screw mechanism to power a pusher plate that compresses the blood sac. Tilting-disk valves provide unidirectional flow. Uniquely, the Lionheart system utilizes a transcutaneous energy transmission system that transfers power from the external battery pack across intact skin using electromagnetic induction. By utilizing a transcutaneous power transfer mechanism, the Lionheart device eliminates the need for a transcutaneous driveline or cables, theoretically reducing the risk of infection (33). Because there is no percutaneous driveline to vent the displacement of the sac, the Lionheart includes an intrathoracically placed compliance chamber that allows air to be vented to the chamber during diastole and toward the pump during systole. The compliance chamber is placed in the left thorax. To counteract passive diffusion of gas out of the chamber and into the surrounding tissue, the chamber is recharged with atmospheric air every few weeks through a subcutaneous port.

Long-Term Nonpulsatile Ventricular Assist Devices. All of the implantable pulsatile LVADs share several disadvantages that include relatively large size, the need for valves to prevent reversal of flow, and the need for either a large bore percutaneous vent/driveline or a compliance chamber. Several continuous axial flow pumps currently under clinical

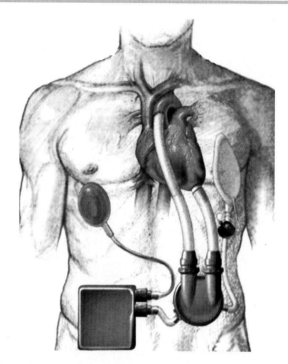

Figure 6 Illustration demonstrating left ventricular (LV) support with the Lionheart Left Ventricular Assist Device (LVAD). Inflow is via LV apex and outflow is via proximal aorta. The compliance is placed within the right chest. *Source*: Courtesy of Arrow International, Reading, Pennsylvania, U.S.A.

trial potentially overcome these limitations. Given the extremely small "D-cell battery" size of the axial flow pumps, the devices may be thought of essentially as "powered apicoaortic conduits" that can provide up to 5 to 6 L/min of nonpulsatile flow using the LV apex for inflow and the aorta for outflow. The devices currently undergoing investigation in the United States are the HeartMate II, Jarvik 2000 (Fig. 7),

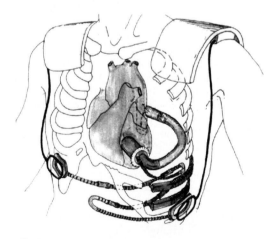

Figure 7 Illustration of the original concept for the Jarvik 2000 fully implanted system with the use of lithium polymer batteries and electronics implanted within the prosthetic ribs. Inflow is via left ventricular apex and outflow is via the descending thoracic aorta. *Source*: Courtesy of Rob Jarvik, M.D., Jarvik World Heart, New York, New York, U.S.A.

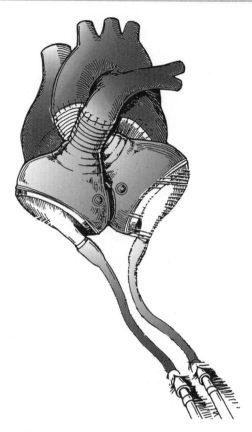

Figure 8 Illustration demonstrating replacement of native heart with the CardioWest Total Artificial Heart.

and DeBakey/NASA LVAD (34–36). These devices provide continuous flow and induce a reduced pulse pressure. Generally, most of these pumps have been used to assist the left ventricle as opposed to completely replacing its function. Most investigators tend to run their pumps at a speed that enables LV ejection and thus pulsatile flow.

Total Artificial Heart
The CardioWest C-70 Total Artificial Heart (Fig. 8) (formerly called the Symbion or Jarvik Total Artificial Heart) allows for total, biventricular cardiac support using a pulsatile pneumatically powered pump. The device is placed orthotopically and requires native cardiectomy for placement. Mechanical valves housed in the inflow and outflow orifices ensure unidirectional flow. The device is powered and controlled by an external console that is connected to the pump via a percutaneous driveline (37). The device does require anticoagulation to prevent thrombus formation.

Clinical Use of Mechanical Circulatory Support Devices
Currently, mechanical cardiac support is used both as a BTT and more recently as destination therapy. A recent study demonstrated significantly improved survival in transplant recipients who were supported with an LVAD versus those in a control group (71% vs. 36%, respectively, 90 days posttransplant) (38). The improved survival is most likely secondary to the superiority of mechanical support over

medical therapy in providing tissue perfusion thus enabling improved peritransplant organ function leading to improved survival. The benefits of mechanical circulatory support are balanced to some degree by the complications associated with device use. Bleeding and infection are the most prevalent complications associated with mechanical support devices. Bleeding rates are described as high as 60% and are more likely in patients requiring biventricular support as compared to those requiring univentricular support. The high rate of bleeding is related to coagulopathy due to heart failure–induced hepatic dysfunction, and the combined effects of CPB and device-related rheology resulting in platelet dysfunction (39). Infection rates range from 30% to 40% and this results in significant morbidity. The newer totally implantable devices eliminate percutaneous cables, which should theoretically reduce infection rates by eliminating the significant factor of a percutaneous portal of entry of infectious agents.

SUMMARY

This chapter has summarized the enormous advances that have been made in recent years to support the failing circulation due to underlying heart disease. Not only can survival from acute cardiac failure be anticipated in many patients using IABP, but chronic end-stage LV failure can also be now supported for months to years, if necessary, in anticipation of cardiac transplantation. Even when the latter approach is not a suitable option, the LVAD has been shown to afford meaningful life in patients who a decade ago would have been subjected to sudden death. While the total artificial heart is still in its infancy, models currently available have been shown to support the entire circulation satisfactorily for many months. It is only a matter of time until an artificial heart is developed, which can add years to the life of a cardiac cripple who without such technology would die.

REFERENCES

1. Braunwald E. Heart Disease: A Textbook of Cardiovascular Medicine. 6th ed. Philadelphia: WB Saunders, 2001.
2. American Heart Association. Heart Disease and Stroke Statistics—2004 Update. Dallas, TX: American Heart Association, 2003.
3. Gheorghiade M, Bonow RO. Chronic heart failure in the United States: a manifestation of coronary artery disease. Circulation 1998; 97:282–289.
4. Jackson BM, Gorman JH, Moainie SL, et al. Extension of borderzone myocardium in postinfarction dilated cardiomyopathy. JACC 2002; 40:1160–1167.
5. Tan LB, Jalil HE, Pick R, Janicki JS, Weber KT. Cardiac myocyte necrosis induced by angiotensin II. Circ Res 1991; 69:1185–1191.
6. Brilla CG, Maische B. Regulation of the structural remodeling of the myocardium: from hypertrophy to heart failure. Eur Heart J 1994; 15(suppl D):45–52.
7. Brilla CG, Matsubara L, Wber KT. Anti-aldosterone treatment and the prevention of myocardial fibrosis in primary and secondary aldosteronism. J Mol Cell Cardiol 1993; 25:563–575.
8. Beltrami CA, Finato N, Rocco M, et al. Structural basis of end-stage failure in ischemic cardiomyopathy in humans. Circulation 1994; 89:151–163.
9. Borow KM, Neumann A, Wynne J. Sensitivity of end-systolic pressure-dimension and pressure-volume relations to the inotropic state in humans. Circulation 1982; 65:988–997.
10. Lamas GA, Vaughan DE, Parisi AF, Pfeffer MA. Effects of left ventricular shape and captopril therapy on exercise capacity after anterior wall acute myocardial infarction. Am J Cardiol 1989; 63:1167–1173.
11. Unverferth D, Magorien R, Lewis R, Leier C. The role of subendocardial ischemia in perpetuating myocardial failure in patients with non-ischaemic congestive cardiomyopathy. Am Heart J 1983; 105:176–179.
12. Parodi O, De MR, Oltrona L, et al. Myocardial blood flow distribution in patients with ischemic heart disease or dilated cardiomyopathy undergoing heart transplantation. Circulation 1993; 88:509–522.
13. Narula J, Haider N, Virmani R, et al. Apoptosis in myocytes in end-stage heart failure. N Engl J Med 1996; 335:1182–1189.
14. Olivetti G, Abbi R, Quaini F, et al. Apoptosis in the failing human heart. N Engl J Med 1997; 336:1131–1141.
15. Mak S, Newton GE. Oxidative stress hypothesis of congestive heart failure: radical thoughts. Chest 2001; 120(6):2035–2046.
16. Stevenson LW, Kormos RL. Mechanical cardiac support 2000: current applications and future trial design. JACC 2001; 35(1):340–370.
17. Kantrowitz A, Tjonneland S, Freed PS, Phillips SJ, Butner AN, Sherman JL Jr. Initial clinical experience with the intraaortic balloon pumping in cardiogenic shock. JAMA 1968; 203:113–118.
18. McEnany MT, Kay HR, Buckley MJ, et al. Clinical experience with intraaortic balloon pump support in 728 patients. Circulation 1978; 58:I124–I132.
19. Kern MJ, Ahuirre F, Bach R, Donahue T, Siegel R, Segal J. Augmentation of coronary flow by intra-aortic balloon pumping in patients after coronary angioplasty. Circulation 1993; 87:500.
20. Gueldner GL, Lawrence Gh. Intra-aortic balloon assist through cannulation of the ascending aorta. Ann Thorac Surg 1975; 19:88–91.
21. Creswell LL, Rosenbloom M, Cox JL, Ferguson TB Sr, Kouchoukos NT, Spray TL. Intraaortic balloon counterpulsation: patterns of usage and outcome in cardiac surgery patients. Ann Thorac Surg 1992; 54:11–20.
22. Macoviak J, Stephenson LW, Edmunds LH Jr, Harken AH, Macvaugh H. The intraaortic balloon pump: an analysis of five years experience. Ann Thorac Surg 1980; 29:451–480.
23. Lefemine AA, Kosowsky B, Madoff I, Black H, Lewis M. Results and complications of intra-aortic balloon pumping in medical and surgical patients. Am J Cardiol 1977; 40:416–420.
24. Baumgartner WA, Owens SG, Cameron DE, Reitz BA. The Johns Hopkins Manual of Cardiac Surgical Care. St. Louis: Mosby-Year Book, 1994.
25. Hunt SA, Frazier OH. Mechanical circulatory support and cardiac transplantation. Circulation 1998; 97:2079–2090.
26. Körfer R, El-Banayosy A, Posival H, et al. Mechanical circulatory support with the Thoratec assist device in patients with post-cardiotomy shock. Ann Thorac Surg 1996; 61:314–316.
27. McBride LR, Naumheim KS, Fiore AC, et al. Clinical experience with 111 Thoratec ventricular assist devices. Ann Thorac Surg 1999; 67(5):1233–1238; discussion 1238–1239.
28. Körfer R, El-Banayosy A, Arusoglu L, et al. Temporary pulsatile ventricular assist devices and biventricular assist devices. Ann Thorac Surg 1999; 68(2):678–683.
29. Gray LA, Champsaur CG. The BVS 5000 biventricular assist device: the worldwide registry experience. ASAIOJ 1994; 40:M460–M464.
30. Oz MC, Argenziano M, Catanese KA, et al. Bridge experience with long-term implantable left ventricular assist device. Circulation 1997; 95:1844–1852.
31. McCarthy PM, Smedira NO, Vargo RL, et al. One hundred patients with the Heartmate left ventricular assist device: evolving concepts and technology. J Thorac Cardiovasc Surg 1998; 115:904–912.
32. Rose EA, Levin HR, Oz MC, et al. Artificial circulatory support with textured interior surfaces: a counterintuitive approach to minimizing thromboembolism. Circulation 1994; 90:II-87–II-91.

33. Pagani FD, Aaronson KD. Mechanical circulatory support. In: Greenfield LJ, Mulholland MW, Oldham KT, Zelenock GB, Lillemoe KD, eds. Surgery: Scientific Principles and Practice. 3rd ed. Philadelphia: Lippincott, 2001:1505–1528.

34. Westaby S, Katsumata T, Houel R, et al. The Jarvik 2000 Oxford System: increasing the scope of mechanical circulatory support. J Thorac Cardiovasc Surg 1997; 114:467–474.

35. Westaby S, Katsumata T, Houel R, et al. Jarvik 200 Heart: potential for bridge to myocyte recovery. Circulation 1998; 98:1568–1574.

36. DeBakey ME. A miniature implantable axial flow ventricular assist device. Ann Thorac Surg 1999; 68:637–640.

37. Copeland JG, Pavie A, Duveau D, et al. Bridge to transplantation with the CardioWest total artificial heart: an international experience 1993 to 1995. J Heart Lung Transplant 1996; 15(pt 1): 94–99.

38. Frazier OH, Rose EA, McCarthy P, et al. Improved mortality and rehabilitation of transplant candidates treated with long-term implantable left ventricular assist system. Ann Surg 1995; 222:327–336.

39. Goldstein DJ, Beauford RB. Left ventricular assist devices and bleeding: adding insult to injury. Ann Thorac Surg 2003; 75:S42–S47.

35

Congenital Heart Lesions

Ralph S. Mosca and Edward L. Bove

INTRODUCTION

The surgical treatment of congenital heart defects has progressed at a rapid rate since its beginning more than half a century ago. Numerous technical achievements have been made possible by advances in many fields. Precise knowledge of anatomy and physiology, detailed noninvasive diagnostic capabilities, better perfusion and myocardial preservation techniques, and improved neonatal intensive care have all played major roles in allowing the management of congenital heart disease to progress to this extent. Nearly all congenital heart defects are now amenable to surgical repair. This chapter discusses the pathophysiology underlying some of the cardiac defects more commonly encountered by the pediatric cardiac surgeon and covers the physiologic rationales behind their treatment.

ADJUSTMENTS IN THE CIRCULATION AFTER BIRTH

Although it is beyond the scope of this chapter to discuss in detail the physiology of the intrauterine circulation and its adaptation to extrauterine life, a brief description is included to aid in the understanding of the topics to follow.

Oxygen-enriched placental blood returns to the fetus through the umbilical vein and then passes through the liver. There it joins the inferior vena caval return and enters the right atrium. Much of this blood passes across the patent foramen ovale (PFO) by preferential streaming into the left atrium, left ventricle, and ascending aorta, from where it is distributed to the brain and coronary circulations (Fig. 1). Superior vena caval return is directed across the right atrium, tricuspid valve, and right ventricle to be ejected into the pulmonary artery. Nearly all this blood passes across the patent ductus arteriosus (PDA) into the descending aorta. Because the ductus is nonrestrictive, both ventricles essentially function as a unit and eject blood against the same overall resistance. However, systemic vascular resistance is low because of the placental circulation, and pulmonary vascular resistance (PVR) is high in the nonaerated fetal lung, resulting in less than 10% of the fetal cardiac output going to the lungs.

At birth, the placenta is eliminated from the circulation, resulting in an abrupt rise in the systemic vascular resistance. Expansion of the lungs leads to a fall in PVR. As arterial and alveolar partial pressure of oxygen (PO_2) increase, PVR falls further and pulmonary blood flow rises, resulting in an increase in the left arterial pressure and functional closure of the flap valve of the foramen ovale. The increase in arterial PO_2 also causes constriction of the smooth muscle in the wall of the ductus arteriosus, closing the duct and completing the separation of the two circulations. PVR falls to adult normal levels within two to four weeks in the term infant.

CONGESTIVE HEART FAILURE

Simply defined, congestive heart failure is the failure of myocardial oxygen supply to meet oxygen demand. The classic findings of congestive heart failure in infants include tachypnea, tachycardia, diaphoresis, and hepatomegaly. Peripheral edema and rales are not typically noted in infants. The neonatal myocardium is already functioning at maximal stroke volume and can only increase cardiac output by increasing heart rate. Further, the neonatal myocardium has a reduced density of contractile elements. For these reasons, the already stressed neonate with limited cardiac reserve is easily susceptible to congestive heart failure. Congenital heart disease typically results in congestive heart failure in either of two ways, volume overload or pressure overload.

Volume overload occurs with either a large communication between the systemic and pulmonary circulations or valvular regurgitant lesions (Fig. 2). When a left-to-right shunt occurs, the volume of shunted blood depends on

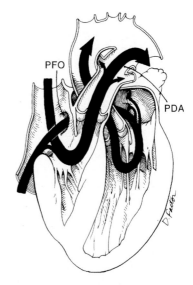

Figure 1 Course of the intracardiac circulation before birth. Most inferior vena caval blood passes across the PFO to the left atrium. The superior vena caval return is directed predominantly across the PDA. *Abbreviations*: PFO, patent foramen ovale; PDA, patent ductus arteriosus.

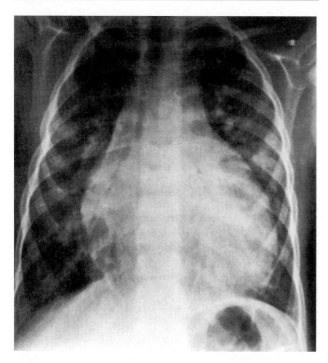

Figure 2   Chest radiograph of a patient with atrial septal defect. There is cardiomegaly and an increase in pulmonary vascular markings as a result of the large left-to-right shunt.

the relative resistances of the two vascular beds. As the PVR falls during the first few weeks of life, pulmonary blood flow may increase dramatically, producing a large volume overload of the left ventricle. Because this shunt depends on a falling PVR, congestive failure from volume overload is not usually seen until two or three weeks of age.

Pressure overload results from an obstruction to ventricular emptying. This obstruction is usually located at the level of the semilunar (pulmonary or aortic) valve, but it may be seen with subvalvular or supravalvular blockage. When the ventricle can no longer eject an adequate blood volume through the obstruction, pulmonary and systemic venous congestions with congestive heart failure result.

Cyanosis

Cyanosis is a blue discoloration of the skin and mucous membranes caused by the presence of at least 5 g/dL unsaturated circulating hemoglobin. When it is noted in infancy, the administration of 100% oxygen is a reliable test to establish the presence of intracardiac shunting related to congenital heart disease. If the PO_2 in the right radial artery rises above 250 mmHg, cyanotic heart disease is virtually eliminated. Although values less than 250 mmHg are not certain indicators of cardiac disease, a PO_2 less than 100 mmHg generally indicates a cardiac problem.

Cyanosis resulting from congenital heart disease may be caused by decreased pulmonary blood flow with intracardiac right-to-left shunting or by abnormalities of intracardiac mixing. When cyanosis is caused by decreased pulmonary blood flow, two conditions are necessary—obstruction to flow into the lungs and an intracardiac communication between the two circulations proximal to the obstruction. The obstruction may be located anywhere between the systemic venous atrium (tricuspid atresia)

and the branch pulmonary arteries (tetralogy of Fallot). Resistance to flow through the obstruction is at least that through the communication, allowing desaturated blood to enter the systemic circulation directly.

Cyanosis may also occur as a result of inadequate mixing of the blood between the systemic and pulmonary circulations. This situation is classically seen in transposition-type physiology. Although total systemic and pulmonary blood flow may be normal or increased, the effective flow is reduced. That is, the amount of desaturated blood actually reaching the lungs and the amount of fully saturated blood reaching the body are decreased. This condition is discussed in detail later in this chapter.

Finally, common mixing occurs when desaturated and saturated bloods freely mix, allowing some desaturated blood to reach the body. This can occur at atrial (common atrium), ventricular (common or single ventricle), or great vessel level (truncus arteriosus).

OBSTRUCTIVE LESIONS
Coarctation of the Aorta

Coarctation is a narrowing in the thoracic aorta most commonly located just distal to the left subclavian artery, opposite the insertion of the ductus arteriosus or ligamentum arteriosum (Fig. 3A). Obstruction to left ventricular emptying results in a pressure overload of the ventricle, which may lead to congestive heart failure. In infancy, associated defects often dictate the hemodynamic condition. When the ductus arteriosus is patent, blood may flow from the pulmonary artery across the duct into the descending aorta (Fig. 3B). In this situation, differential cyanosis is present, with desaturated blood perfusing the lower extremities and saturated blood perfusing the upper body. Approximately 20% of patients have an associated ventricular septal defect (VSD). The impedance to left ventricular emptying imposed by the coarctation increases the left-to-right shunt and results in severe congestive heart failure from combined pressure and volume overload. Other obstructive lesions in the left side of the heart may also be seen with coarctation; most common is aortic stenosis related to a bicuspid aortic valve.

When coarctation results in congestive heart failure in infancy, nonoperative treatment carries a high mortality rate. Most patients with coarctation, however, do not have symptoms, and the defect is not found until after infancy. The discovery of upper-extremity hypertension with diminished or absent femoral pulses typically leads to the diagnosis. Flow murmurs over the back and palpable pulsations in the subscapular area from prominent collaterals may be present. All extremity pulses must be carefully palpated. A decrease in the left-arm pulse may indicate the involvement of the origin of the left subclavian artery in the coarctation. Plain chest radiographs may show dilation of the aorta proximally and distally to the narrowed segment (3 sign) and notching of the ribs related to enlarged intercostal arteries. In the past, aortography was generally recommended to accurately define the anatomy of the coarctation before surgical repair. Today, noninvasive techniques, including Doppler echocardiography and magnetic resonance imaging, are generally adequate to delineate the anatomy. In rare cases, the coarctation may be in an unusual location.

The exact cause of hypertension in coarctation remains obscure. The etiology in older patients is apparently more than obstruction alone, because relief of coarctation in adulthood does not result in the restoration of normal blood

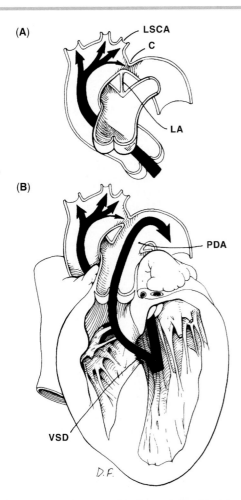

Figure 3 Hemodynamic abnormalities in coarctation (**C**) of the aorta. (**A**) Pathophysiology in the older child or adult. (**B**) In infancy, PDA allows blood flow to the descending aorta from the right ventricle. *Abbreviations*: LA, ligamentum arteriosum; LSCA, left subclavian artery; VSD, ventricular septal defect; PDA, patent ductus arteriosus.

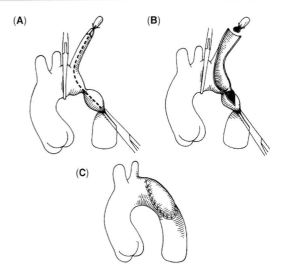

Figure 4 Repair of coarctation with the subclavian angioplasty technique. (**A**) Left subclavian artery is mobilized and divided distally. (**B**) Longitudinal incision through the artery and adjacent aorta is made. This incision must extend distally beyond the coarctation until normal aorta is reached. (**C**) Completed repair.

pressure in every case. It seems certain that in these cases, a renal mechanism is in part responsible. In a classic experiment performed by Scott et al. (1), coarctation was surgically created in dogs. The resultant hypertension was relieved by removal of one kidney and transplantation of the other above the level of the coarctation. When abnormal plasma renin activity is unmasked by volume depletion, abnormally high renin–angiotensin activity has been found in patients with coarctation (2).

Virtually all patients with hemodynamically significant coarctation of the aorta should undergo operative repair. The ideal age for repair in the child without symptoms is not well defined, but it has been moved earlier and earlier in recent years. Repair is probably best accomplished between the ages of one and three years. Earlier operation may increase the risk of recoarctation with growth of the aorta, whereas delaying repair beyond childhood increases the chance of persistent hypertension (3). The presence of congestive heart failure in infancy dictates operative intervention, regardless of age or size.

The classic surgical technique remains resection of the narrowed segment with end-to-end anastomosis. The

benefits of this technique include removal of all the ductal tissue, thus decreasing the risk of recoarctation. The potential disadvantages include the need for greater dissection, increased technical difficulty, and the possibility of tension at the repair site. Concerns about growth of the aorta in the face of a circumferential suture line have been minimized by the use of absorbable suture material and further alleviated by good results with other similar neonatal repairs, such as the arterial switch procedure.

We prefer the resection and end-to-end anastomosis in virtually all cases. However, the subclavian angioplasty procedure, first reported by Waldhausen in 1966 (Fig. 4) (4), is preferred by some groups. Although this technique does not remove all the ductal tissue and is not suitable for augmentation of more proximal aortic narrowing, it is technically easier and avoids suture line tension. Division of the subclavian artery can, on occasion, lead to disparate upper-extremity growth.

Synthetic patch aortoplasty retains abnormal ductal tissue and may lead to aneurysm formation on the aortic wall opposite the patch (also reported with subclavian flap technique). This technique should be used only in cases of discrete recoarctations in which mobilization for end-to-end repair is not feasible. Balloon angioplasty is being performed in several centers for both native and recurrent coarctation (5). Controversy continues regarding the safety and efficacy of angioplasty of native coarctation (6); however, new balloon-expandable and covered stents may be useful in older adolescents and adults (7). Results appear quite good for catheter-based treatment of recurrent stenosis (8).

Coarctation associated with a large VSD is best treated by a single-stage complete repair through a median sternotomy. During a period of circulatory arrest, the coarctation is resected and repaired with the mobilized distal aortic segment used to augment the transverse aortic arch if necessary. The VSD is then closed from a transatrial approach.

Aortic Stenosis

The most common cause of obstruction to left ventricular ejection is aortic stenosis. The obstruction is typically located at the level of the valve, but it may be subvalvular or supravalvular (Fig. 5). Valvular aortic stenosis is usually caused by a bicuspid aortic valve with varying degrees of fusion of the commissures, although fused tricuspid valves may also be found. A dome-shaped unicusp valve may result in significant obstruction in infancy. Subvalvular aortic stenosis may be discrete or diffuse. In the discrete form, a fibrous membrane is found just below the aortic valve leaflets. The diffuse form is seen in obstructive cardiomyopathies, such as idiopathic hypertrophic subaortic stenosis or muscular tunnel-type subvalvular hypoplasia. In supravalvular stenosis, the obstruction is most commonly caused by an hourglass deformity of the ascending aorta just above the valve.

Valvular aortic stenosis may be seen at any age. In infancy, severe stenosis may cause congestive heart failure (9). In most children, however, an asymptomatic heart murmur is detected on physical examination beyond the neonatal period. When symptoms are present in childhood, exertional dyspnea, syncope, and angina pectoris are the usual manifestations. Syncope is caused by the inability of the left ventricle to maintain adequate cerebral blood flow through a narrow, fixed orifice valve during exercise. Angina pectoris, although rare in childhood, may be seen when pressure overload results in significant left ventricular hypertrophy and myocardial blood flow does not adequately perfuse the thickened, hypertensive ventricular muscle.

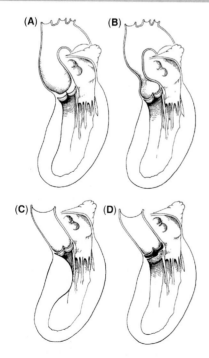

Figure 5 Anatomic types of left ventricular outflow tract obstruction. **(A)** Valvular stenosis related to a bicuspid aortic valve. Note the poststenotic dilation of the ascending aorta. **(B)** Hourglass narrowing of the ascending aorta, resulting in supravalvular stenosis. **(C)** Subvalvular stenosis resulting from diffuse hypertrophy of the ventricular septum. **(D)** Subvalvular stenosis resulting from a discrete subaortic membrane.

Indications for operation in patients with valvular aortic stenosis include syncope, congestive heart failure, or angina with a significant left ventricular outflow tract gradient. A significant gradient is usually considered to be at least 50 mmHg, unless cardiac output is greatly diminished. The timing of operative intervention in the child without symptoms who has moderate or severe obstruction is less well defined. Electrocardiographic changes indicating left ventricular strain or ischemia, either at rest or induced during exercise, are considered definite indications. Severe gradients, greater than 70 mmHg, are best treated promptly, even in the absence of symptoms or electrocardiographic changes.

Options for relief of critical aortic stenosis in the neonate include open valvotomy, transventricular dilatation, and transcatheter therapy. The standard approach has been open valvotomy with cardiopulmonary bypass. Relief of valvular aortic stenosis is accomplished by direct incision of fused commissures. The incision is stopped 1 to 2 mm from the annulus to avoid detaching all leaflet support and creating significant aortic regurgitation. In a true bicuspid valve, rudimentary commissures must not be incised, or a flail leaflet will result. Although satisfactory reduction of the gradient can usually be accomplished, it may be difficult to provide complete relief of obstruction in all cases (10). Certain bicuspid valves may not lend themselves to valvotomy and may remain obstructive despite lack of commissural fusion. Although a few studies have reported good results with open aortic valvotomy (11,12), the mortality rates have remained high in most series. This may be in part because congenital aortic stenosis is a heterogeneous, complex disorder in which the aortic valvular and annular substrates may not be conducive to direct operative intervention.

Transventricular dilatation, first described by Trinkle et al. (13) in 1975, provides a simple and effective technique of closed aortic valvotomy in infants. Through an apical left ventricular approach, progressive dilatation of the valve is accomplished with or without cardiopulmonary bypass. Transventricular dilatation provides effective relief of the obstruction without creating significant aortic insufficiency, and it avoids the myocardial ischemia inherent in open techniques (14).

Transcatheter therapy through the femoral, umbilical, or carotid arteries is also quite effective in the neonatal population. The risks of balloon aortic valvotomy continue to include inadvertent aortic cusp perforation, with resultant severe aortic insufficiency as well as arterial injury. Most centers believe that surgical and balloon valvotomy for critical aortic stenosis in the neonate have similar outcomes and therapy is program specific (15–17).

The goal of treatment of neonates' and infants' critical aortic stenosis is to establish an effective aortic orifice, thereby relieving the left ventricular pressure overload without inducing hemodynamically significant aortic insufficiency. Few of these patients are cured by their initial procedure. Because of the complexity of the disease (valvular stenosis, annular hypoplasia, varying degrees of subaortic stenosis, and the turbulent flow as a result of these), most patients require further operative intervention. Replacement of the aortic valve with a pulmonary autograft (Ross procedure) can be performed at any age, even in the neonate, and is the optimal procedure when more conservative treatment fails.

Operation for subvalvular stenosis is recommended for the same indications as in valvular obstruction. The required gradient may be somewhat less for discrete subvalvular stenosis, however, because resection of the membrane is more often curative (18). Many patients with untreated discrete subvalvular stenosis later have progressive aortic regurgitation related to turbulence beneath the valve. Early resection of the membrane, often combined with a septal myectomy, may prevent this complication. Diffuse, muscular left ventricular outflow tract obstruction is more difficult to relieve. Transaortic resection of hypertrophied septal muscle, an aortoventriculoplasty, or bypass of the obstruction by insertion of a valved conduit from the left ventricular apex to the aorta is often needed (19,20).

Supravalvular aortic stenosis is the least common site of left ventricular outflow tract obstruction. Isolated supravalvular aortic stenosis is rare in infants and may occur as part of the Williams syndrome in older children. This lesion is also highly variable, ranging from a membranous ring-like constriction, the classic hourglass deformity, to a diffuse form involving much of the aorta and brachio-cephalic vessels. The coronary arteries are exposed to high pressure, and degenerative changes may be seen early in life. Indications for operation include a gradient greater than 50 mmHg and evidence of coronary obstruction. Repair involves a longitudinal incision in the ascending aorta, extended proximally into both the noncoronary and right coronary cusps in an inverted Y configuration. The patch is then extended as far distally as necessary to relieve the obstruction.

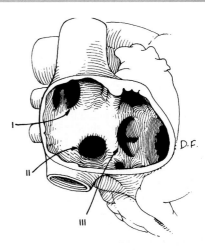

Figure 6 Locations of the three common types of atrial septal defect. The sinus venous defect is shown with anomalous drainage of the right upper lobe pulmonary vein (I). The ostium secundum defect is in the mid-portion of the septum (II). The ostium primum defect is located in the base of the septum, with its inferior edge formed by the continuity of the tricuspid and mitral valves (III). Note the cleft-like anomaly in the anterior leaflet of the mitral valve visible through the defect.

LEFT-TO-RIGHT SHUNTS

Atrial Septal Defect

Atrial septal defect (ASD) accounts for approximately 10% of all congenital cardiac lesions. The defect in the septum allows blood to flow from the left to the right atrium, producing a volume overload of the right ventricle and pulmonary circulation. The shunt is directed from left to right because of the greater diastolic compliance and lower diastolic pressure in the right-sided chambers. Moderate-sized defects result in pulmonary blood flow from one and one half to three times the systemic flow, whereas in large defects, the pulmonary to systemic flow ratio exceeds three to one. In most cases, pulmonary artery pressure and systemic blood flow remain normal.

ASDs often occur as isolated lesions and tend to remain asymptomatic until early adult life (21). When present, symptoms are often nonspecific and consist of fatigue or mild dyspnea on exertion. In the presence of a large left-to-right shunt, overt congestive heart failure can occur at any age. Most commonly, however, nearly normal activity is maintained until the third or fourth decade of life, when symptoms of congestive heart failure become manifest.

Any chronic left-to-right shunt may eventually produce changes of pulmonary vascular occlusive disease. Although these changes occur more frequently and earlier in life with defects that cause an increase in both pulmonary blood flow and pressure, uncomplicated ASDs may result in irreversible pulmonary occlusive changes. This problem is discussed in detail in the following section concerning VSDs.

Most ASDs occur in the center of the atrial septum and are referred to as *ostium secundum ASDs* (Fig. 6). In approximately 5% to 10% of patients, the defect is located high in the atrial wall, where the superior vena cava joins the right atrium. These defects, known as *sinus venosus ASDs*, are almost always associated with drainage of the right upper lobe pulmonary veins into the right atrium or

superior vena cava. About 5% of patients have another variety of defect, called *ostium primum ASDs*. These defects, which are located low in the septum, are part of a more complex anomaly referred to as *endocardial cushion defect*. In its simplest form, the ostium primum ASD is associated with a cleft in the anterior leaflet of the mitral valve. Mitral regurgitation may be present and can be severe.

Any ASD in which the ratio of pulmonary to systemic blood flow (Q_p/Q_s) is at least 1.5:1 should be closed. Operative correction prevents the long-term complications of congestive heart failure and pulmonary vascular occlusive disease. Studies on patients who did not undergo surgery indicated that life expectancy is significantly reduced, to the fourth or fifth decade of life. To prevent these complications, elective repair before school age is advised.

The technique of repair involves suture closure during cardiopulmonary bypass in most patients. Through an incision in the right atrium, the anatomy is easily exposed. In large defects, a patch of pericardium or polytetrafluoroethylene (Gore-Tex) may be necessary to avoid tension on the edges of the repair. In sinus venosus defects with partial anomalous pulmonary venous return, closure is achieved by modifying the patch to redirect the pulmonary veins to the left atrium. Ostium primum ASDs must also be repaired with a patch, because no lower rim of atrial septum is present. The lower edge of this defect is the junction of mitral and tricuspid valves on the crest of the ventricular septum. If significant mitral regurgitation is present before the operation, the valve should be studied carefully at operation and a valvuloplasty should be performed (22). Secundum ASDs of the appropriate size and location are now being closed routinely with transcatheter techniques. Results are good and continue to evolve (23).

Ventricular Septal Defect

Excluding bicuspid aortic valve, VSD is the most common congenital structural cardiac anomaly. It accounts for 20%

to 25% of all cardiac lesions and is estimated to occur in 2 of 1000 live-born infants. The hemodynamics, symptoms, and treatment depend on the size of the VSD and on the magnitude of the shunt. With a small VSD, right ventricular pressure remains normal, Q_p/Q_s is less than 1.5:1, and symptoms are usually absent. Moderate-sized defects have right ventricular pressure as great as half of systemic levels and a Q_p/Q_s as great as 2.5:1 or 3:1. Some degree of congestive heart failure is often present, but growth is usually normal. A large VSD is present when the Q_p/Q_s exceeds 3:1. Right ventricular pressure usually exceeds half that of the left ventricle, but it may be normal when PVR is low. Severe congestive heart failure and poor growth are often found.

Approximately 50% of VSDs discovered in infancy undergo spontaneous reduction in size or complete closure. Thus, all defects are initially managed medically, with early surgical intervention reserved for those with refractory congestive heart failure. Small VSDs usually do not require treatment, and nearly all eventually close. Spontaneous closure is less likely with larger defects but may still occur.

In response to the increasing pulmonary blood flow seen with moderate and large VSDs, pulmonary arteriolar resistance rises, and pulmonary artery pressure may also become elevated. Sustained increases in pulmonary artery flow and pressure can lead to early development of pulmonary vascular occlusive disease. Irreversible changes in resistance may become apparent by two years with an isolated large VSD or by six months in patients with associated trisomy 21. These changes have been classified by Heath and Edwards (24) on a histologic level. The early changes in the small pulmonary arteries and arterioles of medial hypertrophy (grade I) and intimal proliferation (grade II) are considered reversible. More advanced changes, consisting of intimal fibrosis (grade III) and progressive dilation lesions with eventual arterial necrosis (grades IV–VI), are irreversible.

Cardiac catheterization documents the magnitude of the shunt, right ventricular and pulmonary artery pressures, and PVR. Left ventricular cineangiography and two-dimensional echocardiography delineate the locations and number of VSDs. Associated defects, including coarctation, aortic stenosis, PDA, and pulmonary stenosis, are common and must be identified.

VSDs may be single or multiple. Most VSDs are single and located high in the membranous portion of the ventricular septum, just beneath the aortic valve. These defects are classified by their relationship to structures in the right ventricle (25,26). The typical high VSD, referred to as *infundibular* VSD, can be found beneath the anteroseptal commissure of the tricuspid valve (Fig. 7). Inlet VSDs are located more inferiorly, beneath the septal leaflet of the tricuspid valve, and subarterial VSDs occur high in the septum immediately below the pulmonary valve. When a VSD extends to the annulus of the tricuspid valve, it is referred to as *perimembranous*; otherwise, it is a muscular defect. Muscular defects occurring in the heavily trabeculated portion of the septum are more likely to be multiple.

The indications for surgery depend on the hemodynamic situation and presence of symptoms. With moderate and large VSDs, persistent, severe congestive heart failure (often with failure to thrive) despite medical management is an operative indication. When heart failure is well controlled medically, the primary factors influencing the decision to operate are the pulmonary arterial pressure and PVR. These should be assessed by 12 months of age. If the pulmonary arterial pressure is greater than half of systemic levels by this age, surgical intervention should be carried

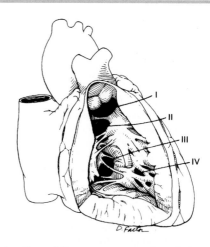

Figure 7 Locations of the common types of ventricular septal defect. Subarterial defects (**I**) are located in the infundibular portion of the septum, beneath the pulmonary valve. In the most common type, perimembranous infundibular (**II**), part of the defect edge is formed by the tricuspid valve. Inlet defects (**III**) are found more inferiorly, beneath the septal leaflet of the tricuspid valve. Muscular defects (**IV**) are remote from the valve annulus.

out to prevent progressive changes in PVR. Moderate defects with minimal symptoms and normal pulmonary artery pressure and PVR may continue to be observed, because late spontaneous closure could still occur. If VSDs do not close by three to five years of age, operative therapy is indicated.

If the PVR is severely elevated, above two-thirds of systemic resistance, VSD closure may be contraindicated. When PVR reaches this level, it will often progress further and eventually exceed that of the systemic circulation. Reversal of flow through the defect then occurs (Eisenmenger's syndrome), and cyanosis results. Closure of the VSD in this situation would result in right-sided heart failure and shortened life expectancy.

The optimal surgical treatment of VSDs consists of patch closure. In infants, deep hypothermia with reduced flow on cardiopulmonary bypass is used to facilitate exposure and reduce operative risk. The operative approach for most defects is through the right atrium and tricuspid valve. A patch of polytetrafluoroethylene (Gore-Tex) is sutured to the right ventricular side of the defect edge; care is taken not to injure the conduction tissue, which must be precisely located for each VSD (27). In complex lesions, the atrioventricular node and bundle of His may be identified with endocardial mapping. Subpulmonary defects are best closed through the right atrium or pulmonary artery. Anterior muscular VSDs can often be quite difficult to close because they are obscured by the heavy trabeculations of the right ventricle. Apical muscular defects may require a small apical left ventriculotomy for proper exposure. In each case, initial exposure and evaluation through the tricuspid valve allow the surgeon to plan the best approach.

Complete repair in infancy may not be advisable in all cases. When multiple defects are found, for example, palliation with pulmonary artery banding may be indicated. With constriction of the main pulmonary artery, the resistance to flow into the lungs is markedly increased, reducing the magnitude of the left-to-right shunt and controlling congestive heart failure. Further, the pulmonary vascular bed is protected against the development of pulmonary vascular occlusive disease, allowing complete repair to be done at less risk when the patient is older. Because of the good results of complete repair of most congenital heart defects in infants, multiple, complicated VSDs may be one of the few remaining indications for pulmonary artery banding in infants.

Patent Ductus Arteriosus

PDA is the most common cause of left-to-right shunting at the great artery level. Because aortic pressure is greater than pulmonary artery pressure throughout all phases of the cardiac cycle, shunting occurs in both systole and diastole. This gives rise to the typical continuous or machinery-like murmur. Additionally, the diastolic runoff into the low-resistance pulmonary circulation results in a wide pulse pressure and bounding arterial pulses. A large PDA may allow substantial left-to-right shunting and significant heart failure. Pulmonary artery pressure and PVR may be elevated as described in the previous section, resulting in eventual pulmonary vascular occlusive disease.

The anatomy of the duct is quite constant. Its aortic end originates just distal to the left subclavian artery, and it enters the pulmonary artery bifurcation or proximal left pulmonary artery.

Any duct that remains patent beyond infancy should be closed. Elective closure is usually recommended in early childhood. A large PDA in a patient with heart failure and pulmonary hypertension should be closed immediately. Small PDAs may be complicated by bacterial endarteritis, aneurysm formation, or calcification. Closure prevents these complications.

The operative approach is through a left thoracotomy. Exposure of the duct is easily accomplished after opening the mediastinal pleura. Care must be taken to avoid injury to the recurrent laryngeal nerve. Closure of the duct may be done by simple ligation, usually over a length of the duct, by division and suture, or by hemoclip occlusion in premature infants. Recently, new forms of therapy have been introduced, including transluminal placement of coils, umbrellas, or clamshell devices (28–30) and clipping of the PDA by means of video-assisted thoracoscopy (31).

RIGHT-TO-LEFT SHUNTS

Tricuspid Atresia

Tricuspid atresia is an uncommon defect in which the tricuspid valve is completely absent. The ASD that is invariably present shunts all vena caval blood directly to the left atrium. The degree of cyanosis depends on the amount of pulmonary blood flow. When no communication between left and right ventricles is present, the ductus arteriosus is the sole source of flow to the lungs (Fig. 8A). These patients are deeply cyanotic in early infancy, and emergency prostaglandin infusion may be necessary (32). Prostaglandins of the E type relax the smooth muscle in the wall of the duct and are used to maintain ductal patency before palliative surgery.

In some cases, a VSD allows blood to flow from the left ventricle directly to the hypoplastic right ventricle and then to the pulmonary circuit (Fig. 8B). Depending on the size of this communication, cyanosis may be mild. However, these VSDs often undergo spontaneous reduction in size, thus decreasing pulmonary blood flow as the child grows. Less commonly, the aorta and pulmonary artery are transposed,

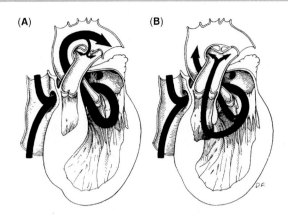

Figure 8 (**A**) Tricuspid atresia with normally related great vessels and without a ventricular septal defect. Pulmonary blood flow is duct dependent. (**B**) When a septal defect is present, forward flow across the pulmonary valve can occur.

and the pulmonary artery receives the direct output of the left ventricle, resulting in an increase in pulmonary blood flow and pressure.

The initial surgical treatment of tricuspid atresia with decreased pulmonary blood flow is aimed at increasing this flow by a systemic artery–to–pulmonary artery shunt (33,34). The modified Blalock–Taussig procedure, in which an interposition graft of polytetrafluoroethylene (Gore-Tex) is placed between the sides of the subclavian and pulmonary arteries, is the most commonly used operation (Fig. 9) (35). This procedure provides a source of pulmonary blood flow with minimum risk of increasing PVR or causing congestive heart failure. A relatively large graft (4 or 5 mm) is used, even in infants, because flow is limited by the smaller-sized native vessels. With growth of the subclavian and pulmonary arteries, flow can potentially increase and maintain effective palliation. Other shunt procedures are used much less commonly today. These include the Waterston (ascending aorta–to–right pulmonary artery), Potts (descending aorta–to–left pulmonary artery), and Glenn (superior vena cava–to–right pulmonary artery) anastomoses.

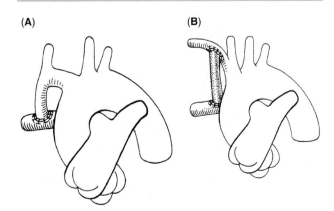

Figure 9 (**A**) Standard Blalock–Taussig anastomosis between the right subclavian and pulmonary arteries. (**B**) Modification of the procedure with an interposition polytetrafluoroethylene graft.

The shunt procedure is then followed in many circumstances by a bidirectional Glenn or hemi-Fontan procedure. This second stage removes the volume load imposed by the aortopulmonary shunt, improves the effective pulmonary blood flow, and may allow ventricular remodeling prior to the Fontan procedure.

The third stage, and the most satisfactory form of treatment for tricuspid atresia, was first reported in 1971 by Fontan and Baudet (36). Originally done by direct connection of the right atrium to the pulmonary artery or hypoplastic right ventricle, this procedure is now most commonly performed with the lateral tunnel technique (37). A tube of appropriately sized polytetrafluoroethylene (Gore-Tex) is opened longitudinally and sewn within the atrium to incorporate the orifices of the superior and inferior venae cavae without obstructing the pulmonary venous return (Fig. 10). Many centers now routinely incorporate a fenestration of the lateral baffle to allow a small degree of mixing of saturated and desaturated blood. This serves as a "pop-off" mechanism, limiting systemic venous pressures to an extent and preserving cardiac output, albeit with desaturated blood. Later, the fenestration is closed by means of a snare device or by transcutaneous umbrella occlusion, restoring normal systemic oxygenation and eliminating left ventricular volume overload. Although the early results with this procedure have been most gratifying, long-term follow-up is lacking and a late rise in the hazard function for survival has been noted (38–40). Specifically, the late

effects of chronic venous hypertension and lack of pulsatile pulmonary blood flow are unknown.

Tetralogy of Fallot

The most common congenital heart defect resulting in cyanosis is tetralogy of Fallot. In this abnormality, obstruction to pulmonary blood flow occurs at the level of the right ventricular outflow tract, usually as the result of a combination of infundibular and pulmonary valvular stenoses (Fig. 11). The basic anatomic defect is anterior and superior displacement of the infundibular (outlet) portion of the ventricular septum. This obstructs right ventricular outflow and results in a large malalignment VSD (Fig. 12). Overriding of the aorta above the VSD and right ventricular hypertrophy (related to obstruction) complete the tetrad.

The clinical status of patients with tetralogy of Fallot depends on the severity of the right ventricular outflow tract obstruction. In its severest form, pulmonary atresia may be present with duct-dependent pulmonary blood flow. More commonly, infundibular obstruction coexists with varying degrees of pulmonary valve hypoplasia, resulting in moderate cyanosis. Patients with tetralogy of Fallot may have hypercyanotic "tet" spells. These occur when the dynamic portion of the obstruction is transiently worsened as a result of increased contractility of the muscle in the right ventricular outflow tract, often in combination with a decrease in systemic vascular resistance. Pulmonary blood flow is dramatically reduced, with an increase in the right-to-left shunt across the VSD.

Complete repair is now possible with good results in the infant and neonate (41). It is believed that by early repair, the consequences of severe right ventricular hypertrophy (ventricular systolic and diastolic dysfunction) can be reduced or eliminated. In addition, early reestablishment of normal pulsatile pulmonary arterial blood flow may

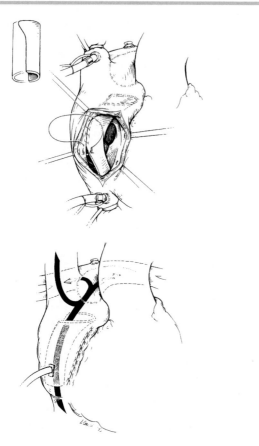

Figure 10   Fontan procedure (lateral tunnel technique). Following a hemi-Fontan reconstruction, the inferior vena caval blood is tunneled within the atrium to the confluent pulmonary arteries.

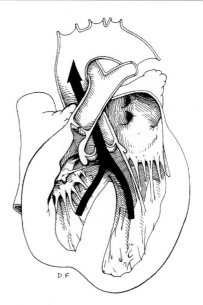

Figure 11   Typical anatomy in tetralogy of Fallot. The large ventricular septal defect (VSD) with overriding of the aorta is shown. The right ventricular outflow tract obstruction results in desaturated blood crossing the VSD directly into the aorta.

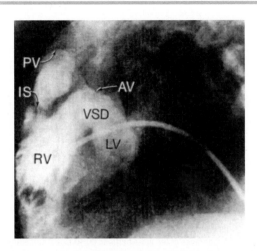

Figure 12 Cineangiogram from a patient with tetralogy of Fallot. *Abbreviations*: AV, aortic valve; IS, infundibular stenosis; LV, left ventricle; PV, pulmonary valve; RV, right ventricle; VSD, ventricular septal defect.

improve the development of alveoli and intraparenchymal pulmonary arteries (42). Contraindications to repair in infancy may include significant hypoplasia of the pulmonary arteries and the origin of the anterior descending coronary artery from the right coronary artery. Because relief of the obstruction in the latter situation may require the insertion of a valve-bearing conduit or allograft, repair may best be postponed until the patient reaches an age at which a larger conduit may be inserted.

Complete repair includes relief of right ventricular outflow tract obstruction and closure of the VSD. Relief of the obstruction is governed by the individual anatomy. Whenever possible, pulmonary valve function should be preserved and resection of right ventricular muscle should be minimized (43). In the past, the standard repair involved a right ventriculotomy to close the VSD and divide or resect the obstructing muscle bundles. Obstruction at the level of the pulmonary valve or annulus was dealt with by a commissurotomy or transannular patch as necessary. In the vast majority of patients, this can be performed through a transatrial approach across the tricuspid valve. In neonates and infants, obstructing muscle bundles need only be divided, not resected. If pulmonary valvular stenosis is present, a commissurotomy is performed. Pulmonary valvular hypoplasia is treated with a limited (<10 mm) transannular patch. Only in cases of true infundibular hypoplasia are a formal ventriculotomy and large outflow tract patch needed.

The operative mortality rate for repair of tetralogy of Fallot is 5% or less. Transatrial repair in the neonatal and infant period may improve the development of the pulmonary vascular bed and help to avoid the late sequelae of a right ventriculotomy (right ventricular dysfunction and ventricular dysrhythmias).

INADEQUATE MIXING

Transposition of the Great Arteries

In transposition of the great arteries (TGA), two separate and parallel circulations—systemic and pulmonary—are present. In the simplest form of TGA, the aorta arises from the right ventricle and receives the desaturated systemic venous return and the pulmonary artery arises from the left ventricle and receives oxygenated pulmonary venous blood (Fig. 13). Some exchange of blood between the two circulations (mixing) must be present to sustain life. This most commonly occurs by means of an interatrial communication allowing saturated blood to pass from the left to the right atrium and then to the right ventricle and aorta. An equal amount of desaturated blood must pass from right to left atrium to reach the pulmonary circulation. The adequacy of this mixing determines the amount of saturated venous blood reaching the aorta (effective systemic blood flow) and desaturated venous blood reaching the pulmonary artery (effective pulmonary blood flow), and thus the clinical status of the infant.

Even with adequate intracardiac mixing, the neonate with TGA has noticeable cyanosis. Quite often, the interatrial defect is restrictive, and profound cyanosis is detected within hours of birth. Arterial PO_2 may be less than 25 to 30 mmHg, and progressive acidosis during the first days of life can occur. The clinical presentation is also influenced by the presence of associated lesions. In approximately 10% of cases, a large VSD or hemodynamically significant pulmonary stenosis is present. When only a VSD is present, cyanosis is lessened because mixing occurs at both the atrial and ventricular levels. Because total pulmonary blood flow is elevated further, however, severe congestive heart failure usually results. If pulmonary stenosis is also present, volume overload is reduced, tending to lessen the effect of the VSD. When pulmonary stenosis is particularly severe, with or without a VSD, total pulmonary blood flow may be reduced to a level below normal, and cyanosis may be worsened. Finally, communication between the two circulations may also occur from a PDA. Similar to the situation with a large VSD, both effective and total pulmonary blood flows are increased, improving oxygenation but resulting in congestive heart failure.

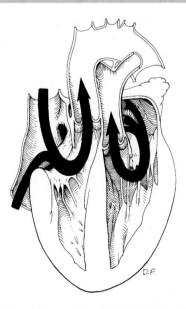

Figure 13 Anatomy of transposition of the great arteries. The aorta arises from the right ventricle, and the pulmonary artery arises from the left ventricle.

The initial treatment of an infant with TGA is aimed at improving the intracardiac mixing by enlarging the ASD. This is performed in the cardiac catheterization laboratory after the diagnosis has been established. The procedure, known as *balloon atrial septostomy* and originated by William Rashkind in 1966, involves passage of a balloon-tipped catheter from the right to the left atrium across the foramen ovale. The procedure can be performed in the catheterization laboratory or in the intensive care unit, with echocardiographic guidance used for accurate catheter placement. Once the catheter tip has been positioned in the left atrium, the balloon is inflated and the catheter is forcibly withdrawn to tear a portion of the atrial septum. This procedure is repeated two or three times to ensure a wide patency in the septum. Improvement in arterial oxygenation is usually noted immediately after the septostomy.

A few neonates may continue to have unsatisfactory oxygenation even with a large ASD (44). The poor mixing in these cases may be caused by the failure of the PVR to fall to its normally low level after birth. The diastolic compliances of the two ventricles remain about equal, and no mixing of blood between the two sides occurs. When this is coupled with closure of the ductus arteriosus, effective pulmonary blood flow may be poor. This situation may be treated temporarily by the administration of a prostaglandin infusion, maintaining ductal patency and allowing mixing at the great vessel level (45,46). This restores satisfactory oxygenation for a few days until PVR falls.

When TGA is associated with a large VSD, significant congestive heart failure and pulmonary hypertension may be apparent very early in life. Prior to the arterial switch repair, banding of the main pulmonary artery to reduce pulmonary blood flow and pressure was indicated. This procedure, however, invariably results in a drop in arterial PO_2 because pulmonary blood flow is reduced by the band. An adequate interatrial communication is mandatory. If severe pulmonary stenosis is present and pulmonary blood flow and pressure are below normal, a systemic artery–to–pulmonary artery (Blalock–Taussig) shunt may be performed.

Correction of TGA may be performed at the atrial, ventricular, or great vessel level, depending on the exact anatomy and associated defects. Prior to the 1980s, physiologic correction was achieved at the atrial level by redirecting venous inflow. This technique was first successfully performed by Senning in 1959 and revised by Mustard in 1964. Mustard's procedure involves the complete removal of the atrial septum, followed by the placement of a "baffle" (usually pericardium) to repartition the atria (Fig. 14). Vena caval blood drains behind the baffle into the mitral valve, left ventricle, and pulmonary artery, and the pulmonary veins drain into the tricuspid valve and then into the systemic circulation through the right ventricle. In the Senning procedure, little prosthetic material is used because redirection of venous inflow is done with the patient's own atrial tissue. Although more difficult to perform, Senning's operation may allow better growth and function of the atrial chambers. The operative mortality rates for both procedures are low (< 5%), even in infancy, and long-term results are good. Significant technical complications, such as obstruction to caval (usually superior vena caval) or pulmonary venous flow and troublesome atrial arrhythmias, continue to be a problem.

The major long-term difficulty with both the Mustard and the Senning procedures is the possible failure of the right ventricle to perform at systemic workloads for long periods (47). Late congestive heart failure, often with tricuspid insufficiency, has been recognized in a small percentage

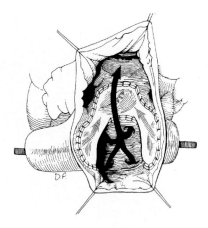

Figure 14   Appearance of the atrial baffle in the Mustard procedure. Superior and inferior vena caval blood passes behind the patch to the mitral valve. The pulmonary venous blood passes over the patch to the tricuspid valve.

of children. Careful studies of right ventricular function late after repairs have shown impaired performance even in patients without symptoms. The exact cause remains unclear. Most children, however, have excellent long-term results after Mustard or Senning operations.

During the last decade, the arterial switch has emerged as the procedure of choice in patients with TGA (Fig. 15). The arterial repair of TGA has the benefit of restoring the left ventricle as the systemic pump (48). Although early operative mortality rates were quite high, current techniques have reduced the risk to acceptable levels. These technical improvements include the refinement of coronary transfer, repair of the pulmonary artery with a pantaloon pericardial patch, and superior myocardial protection. Successful performance of this procedure seems to require that the left ventricle be prepared to pump against systemic resistance. Patients with TGA and a large VSD retain high pressure in the left ventricle and are ideal candidates for arterial repair. Banding of the pulmonary artery to raise

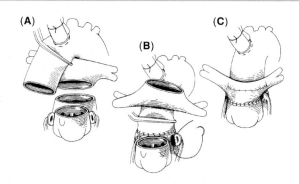

Figure 15   Steps in the performance of the arterial switch procedure. **(A)** The pulmonary artery is transected just proximal to its bifurcation. The aorta is transected at the same level. The coronary arteries are removed with wide buttons of adjacent aorta. **(B)** The distal aorta is brought behind the pulmonary artery confluence and anastomosed to the proximal pulmonary artery. The coronary arteries are then relocated to the new aorta. **(C)** The right ventricular outflow tract is reconstructed by anastomosing the distal pulmonary artery confluence to the proximal aorta.

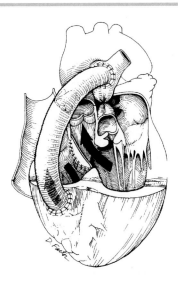

Figure 16 Repair of transposition of the great arteries with ventricular septal defect and pulmonary stenosis. The defect is patched to place both great vessels in continuity with the left ventricle. The pulmonary artery is ligated proximally. The right ventricle is then connected to the distal pulmonary artery with a valved conduit.

left ventricular pressure in some patients with TGA and intact ventricular septum has been advocated to prepare the left ventricle for an arterial switch procedure (49). When arterial repair is done within the first month of life, however, preliminary banding is unnecessary.

In patients with TGA, large VSD, and left ventricular outflow tract obstruction (pulmonary stenosis), repair can be carried out at both the ventricular and great vessel levels. The VSD is closed in a way that diverts left ventricular blood through the defect into the aorta (Fig. 16). The main pulmonary artery is ligated, and the right ventricle is connected to the pulmonary artery bifurcation with a valved extracardiac conduit. The left ventricle is restored as the systemic pump, and the coronary arteries do not require relocation (50). Recently, surgeons have been performing a modified Rastelli procedure utilizing a sleeve of autograft aorta to avoid the use of a prosthetic right ventricle to PA conduit. This approach allows for primary correction in the young patient and perhaps reduces the need for further operative intervention (51).

HYPOPLASTIC LEFT HEART SYNDROME

Hypoplastic left heart syndrome (HLHS) is a collective term referring to a spectrum of congenital heart defects with varying degrees of hypoplasia of left-sided cardiac structures. The vast majority of patients with HLHS (84%) have aortic and mitral atresia, hypoplasia, or stenosis (classic HLHS), whereas 16% have a malaligned atrioventricular canal defect (52). A coarctation is present in more than 80% of patients.

Patients with HLHS have complex cardiopulmonary physiology. The pulmonary arteries, ductus arteriosus, and descending aorta are arranged in parallel circulations. Q_p/Q_s depends on the balance between PVR and systemic vascular resistance.

Because of its hypoplasia and obstructed outflow, the left ventricle is essentially a nonfunctional structure.

Pulmonary venous return is directed across an ASD and mixes with the systemic venous return. The right ventricle provides both the pulmonary and systemic output. Coronary and systemic perfusion is maintained through the ductus arteriosus. In most cases, the PVR declines after birth, leading to excessive pulmonary blood flow. Although this produces good arterial oxygen saturations, the systemic perfusion may be poor, resulting in metabolic acidosis. Without intervention, HLHS is almost uniformly fatal in the first weeks of life. Initial therapy is directed at maintaining an adequate PDA with prostaglandin E. This allows the child's overall condition to stabilize.

Surgical options for the treatment of HLHS consist of neonatal cardiac transplantation or staged reconstruction. In the best of situations, neonatal cardiac transplantation is associated with a one-year survival of 80% to 90% (53). However, because of the limited availability of organ donors, approximately 15% to 25% of patients die while awaiting organ transplantation. In addition, the patient faces the need for lifelong immunosuppression, with its attendant risks.

For these reasons, many centers have opted to pursue palliative repair in this group of patients. The repair of HLHS involves three separate procedures: the Norwood, bidirectional Glenn, and Fontan procedures. The Norwood operation connects the right ventricle and pulmonary valve to the augmented ascending, transverse, and descending aorta and provides a limited amount of pulmonary blood flow through a modified Blalock–Taussig shunt. In the last two years, a modification of the Norwood procedure utilizing an RV-to-PA conduit for pulmonary blood flow has been revisited (54). The absence of a systemic artery–to–pulmonary artery shunt helps avoid the diastolic runoff inherent in this circulation and may prove beneficial in some patients early after the Norwood procedure (55). Performed at six months, the bidirectional Glenn procedure consists of division of the aortopulmonary shunt and connection of the superior vena cava to the cephalad portion of the right pulmonary artery. This decreases the volume load on the right ventricle and improves the effective pulmonary blood flow. A fenestrated Fontan procedure is then planned at 18 months to channel the desaturated inferior vena caval blood to the undersurface of the right pulmonary artery. First-stage reconstruction is now associated with an 85% to 90% in-hospital survival, and the actuarial survival for the three stages together is approximately 75% at two years (56).

Overall, the outlook for patients born with HLHS has improved dramatically during the past few years. Cardiac transplantation offers good intermediate results but is plagued by donor shortages and the need for immunosuppression. Results of palliative procedures have improved greatly, but three operative procedures are required, and the right ventricle is retained as the systemic ventricle. Further study is needed to better categorize which patients benefit most from these treatment modalities.

SUMMARY

Successful surgical treatment of most forms of congenital heart disease is now possible. However, the surgeon must be knowledgeable about more than just cardiac anatomy to achieve this success. In particular, a thorough understanding of cardiac physiology in infants and children is essential so that a well-conceived treatment plan can be devised for even the most complex of anomalies. In some cases, one or more palliative procedures may be necessary, either because no definitive repair is ultimately possible or because it is best postponed until the patient is older. These procedures must provide satisfactory immediate palliation and, in addition, must ensure that ultimate repair can be performed with the lowest possible risk to the patient.

Early corrective surgery, now routinely performed for many defects, is expected to significantly reduce the associated complications of congenital heart disease. The elimination of pulmonary vascular disease, chronic cyanosis, and long-standing congestive heart failure are only a few examples of the advantages of early correction. However, examining the benefits of surgical repair in light of the late results is increasingly important. The development of ventricular dysfunction and electrophysiologic abnormalities are examples of potentially serious consequences that may detract from an apparent early success. In some cases, a number of late studies have led to alterations in surgical technique designed to maintain excellent long-term functional results. These evaluations serve as a stimulus for cardiac surgeons to continue to strive for improvement in the treatment of congenital heart disease.

REFERENCES

1. Scott HW Jr, et al. Study of the renal pressure system in experimental coarctation of the abdominal aorta. Am Surg 1977; 43:771.
2. Parker FB, et al. Preoperative and postoperative renin levels in coarctation of the aorta. Circulation 1982; 66:513.
3. Simsolo R, et al. Long-term systemic hypertension in children after successful repair of coarctation of the aorta. Am Heart J 1988; 115:1268.
4. Waldhausen J. Repair of coarctation of the aorta with a subclavian flap. J Thorac Cardiovasc Surg 1966; 51:532.
5. Tynan M, Finley JP, Fontes V, et al. Balloon angioplasty for the treatment of native coarctation: results of Valvuloplasty and Angioplasty of Congenital Anomalies Registry. Am J Cardiol 1990; 65:790.
6. Hijazi ZM, Geggel RL, Marx GR, Rhodes J, Fulton DR. Balloon angioplasty for native coarctation of the aorta: acute and mid-term results. J Invasive Cardiol 1997; 9(5):344–348.
7. Macdonald S, Thomas SM, Cleveland TJ, Gaines PA. Angioplasty or stenting in adult coarctation of the aorta? A retrospective single center analysis over a decade. Cardiovasc Interventional Radiol 2003; 26(4):357–364.
8. Hijazi ZM, Fahey JT, Kleinman CS, et al. Balloon angioplasty for recurrent coarctation of the aorta. Immediate and long-term results. Circulation 1991; 84:1150.
9. Sandor CGS, et al. Long-term follow-up of patients after valvotomy for congenital valvular aortic stenosis in children. J Thorac Cardiovasc Surg 1980; 80:171.
10. Ankeney JL, Tzeng TS, Liebman J. Surgical therapy for congenital aortic valvular stenosis. J Thorac Cardiovasc Surg 1983; 85:41.
11. Buich M, et al. Open valvotomy for critical aortic stenosis in infancy. Br Heart, J 1990; 63:37.
12. Messina LM, et al. Successful aortic valvotomy for severe congenital valvular aortic stenosis in the newborn infant. J Thorac Cardiovasc Surg 1984; 88:92.
13. Trinkle JK, et al. Closed aortic valvotomy and simultaneous correction of associated anomalies in infants. J Thorac Cardiovasc Surg 1975; 69:758.
14. Mosca RS, Jannettoni MD, Schwartz SM, et al. Critical aortic stenosis in the neonate: a comparison of balloon valvuloplasty and transventricular dilation. J Thorac Cardiovasc Surg 1995; 109(1):147–154.
15. McCrindle BW, Blackstone BH, William WG, et al. Are outcomes of surgical versus transcatheter balloon valvotomy equivalent in neonatal critical aortic stenosis? Circulation 2001; 104(12, suppl 1):1-152–1-158.
16. Marasini M, Zannini L, Ussia GP, et al. Discrete subaortic stenosis: incidence, morphology and surgical impact of associated anomalies. Ann Thorac Surg 2003; 75(6):763–768.
17. McElhinney DB, Retrossian B, Tworetzkyw, et al. Issues and outcomes in the management of supravalvular aortic stenosis. Ann Thorac Surg 2000; 69(2):562–567.
18. Shem-Tov A, et al. Clinical presentation and natural history of mild discrete subaortic stenosis. Circulation 1982; 66:509.
19. Bjornstad PG, et al. Aortoventriculoplarty for tunnel subaortic stenosis and other obstructions of the left ventricular outflow tract. Circulation 1979; 60:59.
20. Sweeney MS, et al. Apioaortic conduits for complex left ventricular outflow obstruction: 10-year experience. Ann Thorac Surg 1986; 42:609.
21. Craig RJ, Selzer A. Natural history and prognosis of atrial septa defect. Circulation 1968; 37:805.
22. Losay J, et al. Repair of atrial septal defect primum. J Thorac Cardiovasc Surg 1978; 75:248.
23. Koenig P, Cao QL, Heitschmidt M, et al. Role of intra cardiac echocardiographic guidance in transcatheter closure of atrial septal defects and patent foramen ovule using the Amplatzer device. J Interventional Cardiol 2003; 16(1):51–62.
24. Heath D, Edwards JE. The pathology of hypertensive pulmonary vascular disease: a description of six grades of structural changes in the pulmonary arteries with special reference to congenital cardiac septal defects. Circulation 1958; 18:533.
25. Becker AE, Anderson RH. Classification of ventricular septal defects—a matter of precision. Heart Vessels 1985; 1:120.
26. Lincoln C, et al. Transatrial repair of ventricular septa defects with reference to their anatomic classification. J Thorac Cardiovasc Surg 1977; 74:183.
27. Milo S, et al. Surgical anatomy and atrioventricular conduction tissues of hearts with isolated ventricular septal defects. J Thorac Cardiovasc Surg 1980; 79:244.
28. Rashkind WJ, Cuaso CC. Transcatheter closure at patent ductus arteriosus. Pediatr Cardiol 1979; 1:3.
29. Sato K, et al. Transfemoral plug closure of patent ductus arteriosus: experience in 61 consecutive cases treated without thoracotomy. Circulation 1975; 51:337.
30. Rothenberg SS. Transcatheter versus surgical closure of patent ductus arteriosus. N Engl J Med 1994; 330:1014.
31. Laborde F, et al. A new video-assisted thoracoscopic surgical technique for interruption of patent ductus arteriosus in infants and children. J Thorac Cardiovasc Surg 1993; 105:278.
32. Freed MD, et al. Prostaglandin E$_1$ in infants with ductus arteriosus-dependent congenital heart disease. Circulation 1981; 64:899.
33. de Brux JL, et al. Tricuspid atresia. J Thorac Cardiovasc Surg 1978; 48:378.
34. Dick M, Fyler DC, Nadas AS. Tricuspid atresia: clinical course in 101 patients. Am J Cardiol 1975; 36:327.
35. Blalock A, Taussig HB. The surgical treatment of malformations of the heart. JAMA 1945; 128:189.
36. Fontan F, Baudet S. Surgical repair of tricuspid atresia. Thorax 1971; 26:240.
37. Jonas RA, Castaneda AR. Modified Fontan procedure: atrial baffle and systemic venous to pulmonary artery anatomic techniques. J Cardiac Surg 1988; 3:91.
38. Fontan F, et al. Repair of tricuspid atresia in 100 patients. J Thorac Cardiovasc Surg 1983; 85:647.
39. Fontan F, et al. Outcome after a "perfect" Fontan operation. Circulation 1990; 81:1520.
40. Sanders SP, et al. Clinical and hemodynamic results of the Fontan operation for tricuspid atresia. Am J Cardiol 1982; 49:1733.
41. Touati G, et al. Primary repair of tetralogy of Fallot in infancy. J Thorac Cardiovasc Surg 1990; 99:396.
42. Rabinovitch M, et al. Growth and development of pulmonary vascular bed in patients with tetralogy of Fallot with or without pulmonary atresia. Circulation 1981; 64:1234.
43. Bove EL, et al. The influence of pulmonary insufficiency on ventricular function following repair of tetralogy of Fallot. J Thorac Cardiovasc Surg 1983; 85:691.

44. Mair DD, Ritter DF. Factors influencing systemic arterial oxygen saturation in complete transposition of the great arteries. Am J Cardiol 1973; 31:742.

45. Benson LN, et al. Role of prostaglandin E₁ infusion in the management of transposition of the great arteries. Am J Cardiol 1979; 44:691.

46. Lang P, et al. Use of prostaglandin E₁ in infants with D-transposition of the great arteries and intact ventricular septum. Am J Cardiol 1979; 44:76.

47. Benson LN, et al. Assessment of right ventricular function during supine bicycle exercise after Mustard's operation. Circulation 1981; 65:1052.

48. Jatene AD, et al. Anatomic correction of transposition of the great vessels. J Thorac Cardiovasc Surg 1976; 72:364.

49. Yacoub M, et al. Clinical and hemodynamic results of the two-stage anatomic correction of simple transposition of the great arteries. Circulation 1980; 62(suppl 1):1190.

50. Marcelletti C, et al. The Rastelli operation for transposition of the great arteries. J Thorac Cardiovasc Surg 1976; 72:427.

51. Metras D, Kreitmann B. Modified Rastelli using an autograft: a new concept for correction of transposition of the great arteries with ventricular septal defect and left ventricular outflow tract obstruction. Pediatr Cardiac Surg Annu Semin Thorac Cardiovasc Surg 2000; (3):117–124.

52. Bharati S, Lev M. The surgical anatomy of hypoplasia of aortic tract complex. J Thorac Cardiovasc Surg 1984; 88:97.

53. Bailey L, et al. Pediatric heart transplantation: issues relating to outcome and results. The Loma Linda Pediatric Heart Transplant Group. J Heart Lung Transplant 1992; 11:5267.

54. Sano S, Ishino K, Kawada M, et al. Right ventricle-pulmonary artery shunt in first-stage palliation of hypoplastic left syndrome. J Thorac Cardiovasc Surg 2003; 126(2):504–509.

55. Mair R, Tulzen G, Sames E, et al. Right ventricular to pulmonary artery conduit instead of modified Blalock-Taussig shunt improves postoperative hemodynamics in newborns after the Norwood operation. J Thorac Cardiovasc Surg 2003; 126(5): 1378–1384.

56. Iannettoni MD, Bove EL, Mosca RS. Improving results with first-stage palliation for hypoplastic left heart syndrome. J Thorac Cardiovasc Surg 1994; 107:934.

FURTHER READING

Baue AE, et al., eds. Glenn's Thoracic and Cardiovascular Surgery. 6th ed. Norwalk: Conn. Appleton & Lange, 1996.

Castaneda AR, et al. Cardiac Surgery of the Neonate and Infant. Philadelphia: WB Saunders, 1994.

Garson A Jr, Bricker JT, McNonara DG, eds. The Science and Practice of Pediatric Cardiology. Philadelphia: Lea & Febiger, 1990.

36

Acquired Cardiac Disorders

Dipin Gupta, Andrew C. Fiore, and Glenn J. R. Whitman

INTRODUCTION

In contrast to congenital heart disease, in which surgical intervention is usually required to restore the underlying pathophysiology to normalcy, acquired cardiac disorders are often amenable to medical management. Notwithstanding this circumstance, several diseases are still best treated surgically and will probably remain so for many years to come. Acquired heart disease in which surgical management plays a prominent role forms the basis for this chapter. The first sections focus on ischemic heart disease and abnormalities of the cardiac valvular system, and on the role that surgery plays in correcting disordered physiology in these conditions. Heart failure—and the novel surgical therapies that are currently being developed—forms the basis of the next section. The final sections concentrate on diseases that require surgical attention less commonly, but in which the cardiac surgeon still renders important help in the delivery of optimal care. These disorders include cardiac dysrhythmias, pericardial disease, and cardiac tumors.

ISCHEMIC HEART DISEASE
The Coronary Circulation
Coronary Arteries

The right coronary artery (RCA) and left coronary artery originate from the aorta just above the aortic valve cusps (Fig. 1). In fact, the positions of these two arteries within the sinuses of Valsalva designate the right and left coronary cusps. The third cusp is referred to as the noncoronary cusp, because it does not have an associated coronary ostium. The left main coronary artery, which travels posterolaterally to the left behind the pulmonary artery, divides into two main branches, the left anterior descending coronary artery (LAD) and the left circumflex coronary artery. The LAD emerges from behind the pulmonary artery to course anteriorly within the interventricular groove. The initial tributary of the LAD is usually the first diagonal, which runs over the anterolateral surface of the left ventricle, followed by the first septal perforator, which emerges at a right angle from the LAD and penetrates into the interventricular septum. The LAD may then give off more diagonal and septal branches. The left circumflex coronary artery descends posteriorly from the left main coronary artery. In 80% to 85% of cases, it terminates with branches to the posterolateral wall of the left ventricle. In the remainder, it extends to the crux of the heart and then gives off the posterior descending coronary artery (PDA), which runs in the posterior interventricular groove. The branches of the circumflex artery are referred to as obtuse marginals and cover the lateral and posterolateral portion of the left ventricle.

The RCA runs in the right atrioventricular groove, where in 80% to 85% of cases it gives off the PDA, continuing with terminal branches to the posterior left ventricular wall. The RCA feeds the anterior surface of the right ventricle with acute marginal branches.

Coronary Veins

Three venous systems drain the coronary circulation. (i) The coronary sinus located in the posterior atrioventricular groove receives blood from the great, middle, and small cardiac veins. The great cardiac vein ascends along the LAD and then follows the circumflex artery to empty into the coronary sinus. The middle cardiac vein follows the PDA, again emptying into the coronary sinus. The small cardiac vein follows the RCA in the atrioventricular groove before it, too, joins the coronary sinus. (ii) The thebesian veins are tiny venous orifices that drain directly into any of the four chambers of the heart. (iii) The anterior cardiac veins drain the right ventricular coronary system, traversing the right ventricular free wall and crossing the atrioventricular groove to empty directly into the right atrium.

Coronary Blood Flow

The heart extracts a greater percentage of delivered oxygen than any other organ in the body. In fact, the heart uses 60% to 70% of the oxygen supplied, as opposed to only 25% for the body as a whole. Coronary sinus oxygen content is only 4 to 6 mL oxygen/dL blood, which corresponds to an oxygen tension of approximately 24 mmHg and a hemoglobin oxygen saturation of only 20% to 30%. Therefore, even at rest, the heart is extracting oxygen maximally, and, unlike in other organs, increased oxygen demand can only be met by increased delivery, rather than increased oxygen extraction.

The most important factor that regulates coronary blood flow is perfusion pressure. Myocardial blood flow occurs almost entirely during diastole, because during systole, cavitary left ventricular pressure equal to that of aortic pressure prevents coronary flow. Coronary flow also depends on coronary luminal diameter. In general, obstruction is considered clinically significant when luminal diameter decreases to two-thirds of baseline. Myocardial blood flow thus depends on diastolic pressure as well as coronary arterial patency. Tachycardia can therefore lead to ischemia not only by increasing oxygen demand, but also by limiting diastolic perfusion time.

A variety of metabolic factors regulate coronary circulation as well. In fact, these autoregulatory capabilities increase blood supply to the heart in response to increased myocardial oxygen requirements. The most important metabolic regulator of this phenomenon is the potent vasodilator adenosine (2). Increased oxygen demand increases

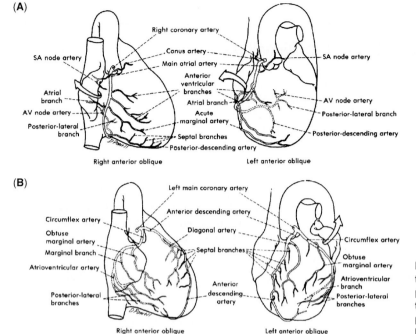

Figure 1 **(A)** Diagram of the right coronary artery circulation in the right anterior oblique and left anterior oblique projections. **(B)** Diagram of the left coronary arterial circulation in the right anterior oblique and left anterior oblique projections. *Abbreviations*: SA, sinoatrial; AV, atrioventricular. *Source*: From Ref. 1.

adenosine triphosphatase (ATP) use, with a resultant increase in adenosine concentration, because it is a direct breakdown product of ATP. This results in coronary vasodilation and increased oxygen delivery. Conversely, thromboxane A_2 is thought to play a crucial role in coronary vasoconstriction. Interestingly, it is released by platelets, particularly in the setting of platelet clumping, a situation that occurs almost universally in the setting of angina with myocardial infarction (MI) (3).

Coronary Atherosclerosis

The Lesion

Atherosclerotic lesions all have in common a mixture of proliferating smooth muscle with a tissue matrix consisting of collagen, elastin, and proteoglycans formed by these cells, as well as the accumulation of intracellular and extracellular lipid (Fig. 2). The lesions characteristically occur within the intima and progress from benign, fatty streaks to complicated, occlusive plaques. It is known that fatty streaks may occur as early as the first decade of life. With time, particularly in populations at risk, the fatty streaks develop into a fibrous plaque, a protruding lesion that may become obstructive. The subintimal smooth muscle cell proliferation that goes along with this fibrous plaque is the factor most responsible for this protrusion. With time, the fibrous plaque may enlarge, become calcified, and degenerate on its intimal surface, resulting in ulcerations that are thrombogenic. Organization of clot with platelet clumping on this surface not only causes increased obstruction to flow, but also, as stated previously, may release thromboxane A_2, further exacerbating the compromised delivery of blood and, therefore, oxygen to the myocardium.

Risk Factors

A number of established risk factors predispose patients toward atherosclerosis (5). These include a genetic predisposition, hypertension, diabetes mellitus, hyperlipidemia, and cigarette smoking. Genetic factors appear to have a direct effect on endothelial cell biology and predisposition toward the development of atherosclerosis. The risk of coronary artery disease increases with increasing blood pressure; among patients with blood pressure greater than 160/95 mmHg, the incidence of coronary disease is five times greater than among those who are normotensive. Of most importance is the fact that control of hypertension decreases this risk. Diabetes mellitus is clearly associated with coronary artery disease. The risk of coronary disease is increased at least twofold in patients with diabetes, with the risk even higher among those with juvenile-onset diabetes. Unfortunately, it is not certain that rigorous control of hyperglycemia decreases coronary mortality rate in this population. The Lipid Research Clinics Trial (6) demonstrated an unequivocal association between cholesterol level and morbidity and mortality from coronary artery disease. As with hypertension, decreasing the level of hyperlipidemia decreases the risk of coronary disease. Interestingly, high-density lipoproteins (HDLs), which contain approximately 20% of total plasma cholesterol, protect one from coronary disease. HDL level is known to be raised by exercise and estrogens and decreased by cigarette smoking. Cigarette smoking is one of the most important risk factors for the development of coronary artery disease, not simply because it is so clearly related to its development but because its cessation so clearly decreases the risk. In patients who smoke only one pack of cigarettes per day, the death rate from coronary artery disease is 70% higher than in nonsmokers. Furthermore, cigarette smoking appears to potentiate other risk factors.

Other factors postulated to contribute to the progression of coronary artery atherogenesis include increasing age, male gender, supranormal serum levels of homocysteine and lipoprotein A (7), and low-estrogen states such as menopause (8). Age has a complex association with the development of atherosclerosis, because many other risk factors are associated with aging. It is well documented that

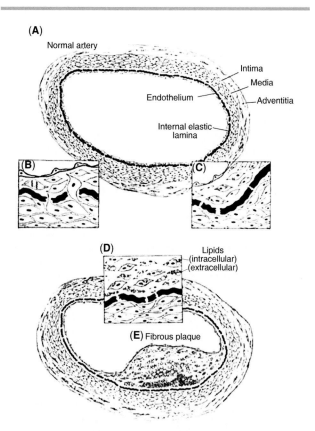

Figure 2 Developmental stages of the lesions of atherosclerosis. **(A)** The normal muscular artery consists of an internal intima with endothelium and internal elastic lamina. The smooth muscle of the vessel wall is in the media, and the thin adventitial layer contains connective tissue and vasovasorum. With age, the thin, sparsely muscled intima increases in thickness and smooth muscle cell content. **(B)** In the first phase of an atherosclerotic lesion, there is a focal thickening of the intima with smooth muscle cells and extracellular matrix. There is also initial accumulation of intercellular lipid deposits. **(C)** Extracellular lipid may also develop. **(D)** When both intracellular and extracellular lipids are present in the earliest phase, this is referred to as a fatty streak. **(E)** Fibrous plaque results from continued accumulation of fibroblasts covering proliferating smooth muscle cells laden with lipids and cell debris. The lesion becomes more complex as continuing cell degeneration leads to ingress of blood constituents and calcification. *Source*: From Ref. 4.

men are three times more likely than women to acquire coronary disease, and, in fact, the development of ischemic syndromes occurs, on the average, 10 years earlier in affected men than in affected women.

Because of the recognition that atherosclerosis may begin as early as the first or second decade of life, primary prevention of this disease must begin early. The importance of understanding the risk factors for coronary disease and eliminating or modifying those over which we have control cannot be overemphasized.

Clinical Presentation of Ischemic Heart Disease

The clinical presentation of ischemic heart disease can take many forms. As many as 25% of patients with positive stress test results due to coronary occlusive disease may have no symptoms. Similarly, some acute MIs may occur silently. In fact, in some patients sudden cardiac death is the first and only manifestation of this disease process. Another subset of patients without typical symptoms may have

progressive heart failure. This in general is caused by a slow, diffuse loss of ventricular function associated with increasing coronary obstructions. This entity is often referred to as ischemic cardiomyopathy. Most commonly, however, when significant coronary obstructive disease is present, angina pectoris results.

The typical description of angina is as a pressure or heaviness felt in the middle of the chest, radiating to the left shoulder and down the left arm. Abdominal pain, nausea, belching, jaw pain, and hand heaviness or numbness are less typical manifestations of cardiac ischemia. In almost all cases, however, stable angina pectoris is brought on by reproducible increases in myocardial demand for a pathologically limited oxygen supply. Emotional excitement or stress, exposure to cold, eating, and exercise are typical historical events that trigger demand-induced angina. In unstable angina, however, the symptom of chest pain may occur at rest, or even when the patient is sleeping. These patients are exhibiting a phenomenon of myocardial ischemia without demonstrable changes in myocardial oxygen demand. This reflects a situation in which the supply of blood to the myocardium is so marginal that spontaneous coronary vasoreactivity alone may lead to symptoms. Prinzmetal's or variant angina is a less typical form of angina that also may occur spontaneously without increasing myocardial oxygen demand. It is thought to result from spontaneous coronary arterial spasm, but it is almost always associated with underlying fixed atherosclerotic lesions. Patients may have ST-segment elevation, as opposed to the more typical ST-segment depressions associated with classical angina. Angina may be graded according to the Canadian Heart Classification scheme. Class I patients have no symptoms, class II patients have angina on significant exertion, class III patients have angina on mild exertion, and class IV patients have symptoms at rest.

On physical examination, there is usually no detectable sign of coronary artery disease. There may be evidence of associated peripheral vascular disease, however, with loss of pulses or presence of bruits in the carotid arteries, abdominal aorta, or femoral arteries. Xanthomas or hypertensive retinal changes provide evidence of the presence of risk factors for coronary disease.

Multiple studies are used to identify factors that may stress the heart. Anemia, of course, can exacerbate underlying coronary insufficiency. Results of electrocardiographic (ECG) examination are frequently normal, but some patients have evidence of old MIs, clearly indicating the presence of coronary disease. Stress testing is an ideal physiologic examination for assessing the functional significance of coronary disease. In this study, the patient undergoes graded exercise on a treadmill with continuous ECG monitoring. If the patient shows signs or symptoms of angina pectoris associated with typical ischemic ECG changes, this is considered a positive test result. Specificity of the test is improved dramatically if it is combined with the administration of thallium. Thallium is a radioactive isotope that is distributed in the intracellular space, like potassium. When thallium is injected during exercise, if a patient has coronary ischemia, the involved area of myocardium fails to pick up thallium and a defect is present on the scan. As the patient recovers from exercise and ischemia resolves, the myocardial defects fills in, suggesting the reversible nature of the problem. A defect on a thallium scan that never fills in is a sign of irreversibly scarred, nonviable myocardium.

Despite the specific and sensitive nature of thallium stress testing, coronary arteriography, although invasive, is the main modality used to make a definitive anatomic diagnosis of coronary artery disease. It is indicated in patients with atypical presentations in whom it is important to rule out a definitive diagnosis of coronary disease. Otherwise, patients with classic anginal symptoms and ECG changes in whom the diagnosis is not in question should undergo coronary arteriography; if the condition is refractory to medical therapy, they are candidates for revascularization, or both. If patients have suspected severe coronary disease, such as left main or severe proximal three-vessel disease, regardless of symptoms, coronary arteriography should be performed to document this condition in preparation for revascularization. Well-known survival benefits accrue to patients who undergo surgery after such documentation. Diagnostic coronary arteriography should also be performed in patients with other cardiac diseases such as valvular heart disease in whom valve surgery is planned but in whom there is a risk of concomitant coronary disease.

Less invasive means of detecting coronary artery disease are being developed, and will likely obviate the need for coronary angiography in some patients in the future. To date, multislice spiral computed tomography has been found to have a sensitivity and specificity of 95% and 86%, respectively, when compared to angiography (9). Similarly, magnetic resonance coronary angiography has been found to have a sensitivity of 76% and specificity of 91% compared to angiography (10). With evolution of this technology, these tests are likely to gain further accuracy.

The medical management of coronary disease includes the identification and reduction of controllable risk factors. Once the disease presents itself in the form of clinically significant ischemia, however, the focus for the clinician is on decreasing myocardial oxygen uptake and increasing myocardial oxygen supply. It therefore follows that patients with hyperthyroidism or anemia, one of which affects oxygen demand and the other supply, should have these underlying conditions corrected.

In general, though, there are five classes of drugs, in the armamentarium of the physician, which are useful for treating ischemic heart disease. Aspirin plays a critical role in prevention of platelet aggregation. Nitrates are the most commonly used agents. They primarily dilate venous capacitance blood vessels, with resultant decreases in preload, wall tension, and oxygen uptake. Although nitrates do not appear to increase coronary blood flow in the normal heart, improvement in coronary collateral blood flow does occur in patients with ischemic heart disease. β-adrenergic blocking agents reduce myocardial oxygen demand by decreasing both cardiac contractility and heart rate. These agents may also reduce blood pressure and systemic vascular resistance, further reducing the work of the heart. 3-hydroxy-3-methyl-glutaryl coenzyme A reductase inhibitors—also known as "statins"—have been shown to be effective in primary and secondary prevention of coronary artery disease by lowering serum concentration of low-density lipoprotein (11). Finally, calcium-channel–blocking agents such as nifedipine and diltiazem decrease myocardial oxygen uptake by decreasing ventricular contractility. By causing arterial dilation, they diminish systemic vascular resistance as well, and they are particularly effective in patients with a component of coronary vasospastic disease.

Acute Myocardial Infarction

MI is one of the most common diagnoses of hospitalized patients in the United States. Approximately 1.5 million MIs occur each year, with an early mortality rate of approximately 25%. More than half of these deaths occur before the patient ever reaches the hospital.

Acute MI is the direct result of interruption of blood supply to the myocardium. It almost always occurs as the result of coronary arterial thrombosis at the site of a significant stenosis over a complicated plaque. Although the acute event associated with acute MI is thrombosis, cardiac catheterization studies show that within days 20% to 30% of culprit coronary arteries are patent. This is more common in nontransmural MI than in transmural MI.

A major determinant of prognosis after an acute MI is the amount of ventricular myocardium that undergoes necrosis. In patients who have ejection fractions greater than 50% after MI, three-year survival is close to 90%, but when ejection fraction after MI falls to less than 37%, three-year survival is only 50%. Loss of 25% of ventricular myocardium leads to symptomatic cardiac dysfunction, whereas the loss of more than 40% is frequently associated with cardiogenic shock and death. Therefore, efforts to treat patients who are having an acute MI should be focused on decreasing myocardial loss by improving flow to the area at risk, as soon as possible. Interestingly, although well-developed collaterals may not prevent demand-induced angina, they may significantly diminish the loss of myocardium after an acute MI.

Presentation

Pain is the most common presenting complaint in patients with MI. It is by no means universally present, however, with 20% to 25% of patients having no symptoms. Interestingly, acute MIs associated with the LAD distribution frequently result in sympathetic hyperactivity, with tachycardia and hypertension, whereas inferior MIs involving the RCA frequently have parasympathetic activity with bradycardia and hypotension. The classic ECG picture of an acute MI is the development of Q waves and elevated coved ST segments in leads reflecting the affected areas (Fig. 3). In fact, the type of MI can frequently be characterized by the associated ECG changes. Transmural infarctions usually cause Q waves, whereas subendocardial or nontransmural MIs are usually characterized by transient ST-segment changes with inverted T waves, without the development of Q waves.

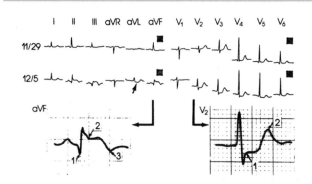

Figure 3 Acute inferior wall myocardial infarction (MI). The electrocardiogram of 11/29 shows minor nonspecific ST-segment and T-wave changes. On 12/5, an acute MI occurred. There are pathologic Q waves (**1**), ST-segment elevation (**2**), and terminal T-wave inversion (**3**) in leads II, III, and aVF, indicating the location of the infarct on the inferior walls. Reciprocal changes are seen in aVL (*small arrow*). Increasing R-wave voltage with ST depression and increased voltage of the T wave in V₃ is characteristic of true posterior wall extension of the inferior infarction. *Source*: From Ref. 12.

The most common modality used for diagnosing MI lies in the evaluation of specific cardiac isoenzymes released by necrotic myocytes in large enough quantities to be detected in the blood. In particular, serum levels of creatine kinase (CK), a cardiac enzyme involved with high-energy phosphate metabolism, are increased after MI, rising within 8 to 24 hours and returning to normal within one to two days. CK is found in brain (CK-BB) and skeletal muscle (CK-MM), and it can rise significantly after a variety of clinical scenarios such as stroke, surgery, cardiac catheterization, or simple intramuscular injection. It is therefore crucial to measure the cardiac-specific isoenzyme, CK-MB, when ruling out an MI. More recently, subunits of the troponin complex that regulates the calcium-mediated contractile process of striated muscle have been used in diagnosis of MI. Troponin T and troponin I have been observed to rise above the reference range within three hours of the onset of chest pain. These markers may persist in the serum for 10 to 14 days.

Medical Treatment

During the early phase of MI, principles of management are to maximize oxygen delivery to myocardium and to minimize oxygen consumption. In this regard, oxygen should be administered, heart rhythm and rate should be monitored, and pain should be controlled usually with intravenous morphine. Decreasing pain has a significant therapeutic benefit because it decreases myocardial oxygen demand, helping to limit infarct size. Intravenous nitroglycerin should be initiated, because it may diminish infarct size, decrease the risk of sudden cardiac death, and lower the incidence of congestive heart failure (CHF) (13). β-Blockers have also been shown to limit infarct size and decrease early mortality rates (14). Angiotensin-converting enzyme (ACE) inhibitors have been shown to reduce morbidity and reduce the incidence of chronic CHF following acute MI, and are now regarded as essential therapy (15).

In the mid-1970s, it was hypothesized that the administration of thrombolytic agents could lead to the dissolution of coronary thromboses, reversing the process precipitating the MI. A consequent European trial of streptokinase (SK) revealed a significant benefit when the drug was given within 12 hours of acute MI (16). Since then, thrombolytic trials have established without doubt the benefits of this approach, showing that thrombolysis reopens acutely occluded coronary arteries in most cases, restoring flow and reducing mortality rate (17). Four intravenous thrombolytic agents are currently approved by the Food and Drug Administration (FDA) for use in acute MI: SK, Anistreplase (APSAC), Alteplase (rTPA), and Reteplase. The most widely used is SK, which has been effective in several very large trials and is inexpensive. APSAC was developed to enable treating physicians to give one intravenous bolus dose in a few minutes, with maintenance of the effect for several hours because of its long half-life. However, APSAC has not been significantly better than SK, and its prolonged half-life has become a drawback rather than a benefit. rTPA produced by recombinant DNA techniques is more effective than SK. It also yields higher patency rates and generates less of a systemic fibrinolytic effect. However, rTPA is several times more expensive than SK, and it thus may not be cost-effective.

What is clear is that the earlier the thrombolytic treatment, the greater the impact on post-MI morbidity and mortality, with the greatest benefit accruing to those patients treated within one to two hours of the onset of symptoms. Heparin and antiplatelet drugs should be added to thrombolytic therapy, particularly to rTPA, which has a short half-life and exerts little antithrombin effect, because it does not generate excessive fibrin-degradation products. Hemorrhage is the major problem with all thrombolytic agents, occurring commonly at the site of vascular access. Strokes occur in fewer than 1% of patients but may be catastrophic because of their hemorrhagic nature (18).

Platelet membrane glycoprotein IIb/IIIa inhibitors are a new class of potent antiplatelet agents that block the final common pathway in platelet aggregation. FDA approval has been obtained for the following intravenous agents: Abciximab (ReoPro, a monoclonal antibody), Eptifibatide (Integrilin, a synthetic peptide), and Tirofiban (Aggrastat, a nonpeptide mimetic). These agents have been tested with and without percutaneous coronary interventions. In addition, clinical trials are underway involving a new group of oral glycoprotein IIb/IIIa inhibitors.

Ticlopidine (Ticlid) and Clopidogrel (Plavix) are a new class of antiplatelet agents, which act by irreversibly inhibiting the adenosine diphosphate receptor involved in platelet aggregation. Both have been shown to improve outcome in patients suffering acute coronary syndromes, though patients who received Clopidogrel plus aspirin suffered more bleeding complications than patients receiving aspirin alone (19).

Mechanical Intervention in Acute Myocardial Infarction

After thrombolytic therapy with early recanalization, the issue remains whether anything more needs to be done in the acute setting. Despite early reperfusion, significant residual stenoses remain in the culprit coronary arteries. The Thrombolysis in Myocardial Ischemia (TIMI)-II trial (20) compared immediate cardiac catheterization with percutaneous transluminal coronary angioplasty (PTCA) with elective cardiac catheterization and PTCA, only if ischemia developed during the hospital course. The more invasive approach failed to provide any increased benefit with respect to early or late mortality rates. As a result of this and other studies, cardiac catheterization and mechanical intervention should be withheld in most patients after acute MI unless patients exhibit ischemia during their hospital stay or have poor results of a predischarge low-level exercise stress test.

Indications for Surgery After Acute Myocardial Infarction

Postinfarction Angina

Recurrent chest pain occurs in 10% to 15% of patients after acute MI, an incidence that increases to 30% to 35% among patients who receive thrombolytic therapy. It is well recognized that after MI, the mortality rate may increase several fold if infarct extension occurs (21). Infarct extension is a powerful predictor of post-MI mortality risk, as seen by an increase in the average one-year mortality rate from approximately 18% to 65%, if infarct extension occurs. Thus, postinfarction angina is an indicator of continued myocardial ischemia and a harbinger of infarct extension. It should be regarded as an indication for cardiac catheterization with mechanical intervention, either PTCA or coronary bypass surgery.

Cardiogenic Shock

Cardiogenic shock after MI is uncommon, only occurring in approximately 7% of patients with acute MI. Shock after acute

MI is associated with a 65% mortality rate, compared with a mortality rate of only 4% if shock is not present. The risk factors for development of cardiogenic shock after acute MI are age greater than 65 years, ejection fraction less than 35% on admission, a large MI as evaluated by peak CK-MB serum concentration, a history of diabetes mellitus, and a history of previous MI. Because shock develops after hospitalization in more than 50% of patients, identifying patients with these risk factors is important because it might possibly allow early intervention to prevent development of shock.

Animal studies have shown that in cases of prolonged regional MI, intervention with emergency revascularization may decrease the amount of damage sustained by the myocardium. By focusing on ways to decrease myocardial energy expenditure during early reperfusion, as well as decreasing cell swelling and oxidant injury and improving intermediary cellular metabolism, a significant decrease in myocardial injury can be achieved. This has led to a prospective study evaluating the effect of coronary bypass surgery on patients in cardiogenic shock after MI (22). If surgery occurred within 18 hours of the onset of shock, mortality rate was reduced from 65% to 7%, whereas if surgery occurred after 18 hours, mortality rate was 31%, still a definite improvement from medical therapy. At centers capable of performing surgery of this kind, this may be an ideal approach to patients in shock after MI. However, these results have not been duplicated by other institutions. Until they are, they must be viewed as preliminary.

Ventricular Septal Defect

A ventricular septal defect (VSD) occurs in approximately 2% of patients after MI. This complication, which occurs when the myocardium is at its weakest, approximately three to five days after an MI, has an associated medical mortality rate of more than 90%. It is seen most frequently in elderly hypertensive female patients with anterior transmural infarcts. An increase in the right ventricular oxygen saturation is often observed. The initial medical therapy involves decreasing afterload as much as possible, invariably with the use of the intra-aortic balloon pump as well as vasodilator therapy. Preload is optimized and surgery is performed immediately. Early operation, before the complications of shock occur, appears to carry a much better survival rate (23).

Acute Mitral Regurgitation

As with VSD, acute papillary muscle rupture with mitral regurgitation occurs in only 2% of patients after acute MI. Posteroinferior MIs lead to this complication more frequently than do anterior MIs, almost certainly because the circumflex artery and PDA distributions are the most crucial blood supplies to the papillary muscles. This complication presents similarly to a VSD. As opposed to the pattern in patients with an acute VSD, however, the pulmonary capillary wedge pressure shows prominent V waves, and there is no right ventricular hemoglobin oxygen saturation step-up. Medical therapy involves maximizing afterload reduction through the use of an intra-aortic balloon pump. Early surgery, although it carries a high risk, decreases mortality rate from 90% to less than 50%. If the mitral valve apparatus can be preserved, mortality risk can be decreased even further.

Free Wall Rupture

Like the previous two complications, ventricular free wall rupture occurs at a time when the myocardium is at its weakest, three to five days after acute MI. The medical mortality rate is exceedingly high (>90%), because the patients die acutely in tamponade. Surgical case reports cite dramatic rescues of these patients, but in general, for successful treatment, free wall rupture must be small and contained, allowing time for diagnosis and operative intervention. Most commonly, free wall rupture leads to pericardial tamponade, cardiogenic shock, and death.

Revascularization

Angioplasty

In the mid-1970s, Gruentzig and Hoff designed a balloon dilatation catheter for use in the coronary arteries and initiated the important treatment option for patients with ischemic heart disease currently known as PTCA. Under fluoroscopic guidance, a catheter is directed into the coronary artery. A guide wire is then placed across the obstructing lesion, and a balloon catheter is then passed over the guide wire and positioned in the mid-portion of the lesion. Under fluoroscopic control, the balloon is inflated to 4 to 10 atm pressure for 20 to 60 seconds in an effort to reduce the degree of coronary obstruction. The indications for PTCA are the same as those for coronary artery bypass surgery, which is the main alternative revascularization technique. Patients with intractable symptoms and those with proximal coronary stenoses that place a large amount of myocardium at risk are potential candidates for angioplasty. The ideal lesion is a symmetric, focal stenosis in a proximal epicardial vessel. PTCA is contraindicated if there is significant disease in the left main coronary artery, if the target coronary artery is less than 2 mm in diameter, if there are multiple significant obstructive lesions in the same artery, or if there are complex obstructive lesions involving arterial bifurcations. The primary risk of angioplasty is the dissection of the coronary artery with acute closure, which occurs in approximately 3% of cases and usually requires emergency coronary bypass surgery. Otherwise, the risks are similar to those of coronary arteriography and include cerebral vascular accidents and local arterial trauma. Under development are atherectomy catheters that incorporate tiny rotating blades for lysis of atheromatous plaque, as well as laser-tipped catheters that vaporize intraluminal obstructions. Coronary stents are small, implantable cylindric devices designed to maintain patency of diseased arteries when more conventional balloon angioplasty is ineffective. Successful dilation of favorable coronary arterial obstructive lesions occurs in more than 90% of PTCA attempts, with an immediate complication rate of only 3%. The most significant long-term problem with PTCA is the high incidence of restenosis, which occurs in between 20% and 40% of patients within the first four to six months after the initial PTCA (24). Although redilatation of recurrent stenotic lesions may be carried out successfully, many of these patients ultimately require coronary bypass surgery.

The persistent problem of in-stent restenosis has yielded the development of coronary brachytherapy and drug-eluting stents. Radiation treatment using β-radiation or γ-radiation has been observed to effectively reduce the degree of in-stent restenosis and to prevent recurrent restenosis (25). Local delivery of specific agents via the stent is also possible. In this manner, sirolimus (rapamycin, an inhibitor of smooth muscle cell and lymphocyte proliferation) and paclitaxel (an inhibitor of cell division) have been seen to dramatically lower the incidence of adverse cardiac events after stenting. For example, at follow-up of one year, major cardiac events were seen in approximately 6% of patients receiving a sirolimus-coated stent versus approximately 30% of patients receiving a standard stent (26). Given these encouraging results, FDA approval was obtained for use of sirolimus-coated coronary stents in 2002. Furthermore, Clopidogrel (Plavix) has been shown to be effective in reducing in-stent stenosis, as an adjunct therapy to aspirin (27), and thus most patients are placed on both drugs after percutaneous interventions.

Coronary Artery Bypass Surgery

Coronary bypass surgery is among the most commonly performed operations in the United States today, with more than 250,000 procedures performed yearly. The goal, as with PTCA, is to treat ischemic heart disease by relieving the imbalance between myocardial oxygen supply and demand.

Indications

In general, data from clinical trials and retrospective studies show that as the number of diseased major coronary arterial segments increases, the greater the survival benefit from coronary bypass surgery. Three major prospective, randomized coronary bypass surgery studies—the Coronary Artery Surgery Study (CASS) (28), the Veterans Affairs Cooperative Study (29), and the European Cooperative Study (30)— are in large part responsible for how we treat patients with ischemic heart disease. Patients with intractable symptoms were not involved in these studies; those patients, in general, should undergo bypass surgery because it is the most successful way to relieve angina. These three studies have provided us with the anatomic indications for bypass surgery, which include left main stenosis and double- and triple-vessel disease involving the proximal LAD (Table 1). As stated previously, the most common indication for bypass surgery continues to be angina refractory to medical therapy. Bypass surgery can be expected to eliminate angina in more than 90% of patients at one year, with benefit continuing for 60% of patients at five years.

Patients being medically treated for unstable angina require aggressive therapy, including nitrates, platelet inhibitors, β-blockers, and ACE inhibitors. Often, heparin anticoagulation is necessary. If the patient continues to have angina while receiving maximal medical therapy, urgent revascularization is indicated. Finally, as noted before, emergency coronary bypass surgery is necessary in approximately 3% of patients who have coronary occlusive complications after PTCA. Most of these occlusions result from coronary dissections proximal or distal to the site of dilatation. Most patients in the midst of an evolving MI have some attenuation of the ischemic injury by the placement of

Table 1 Indications for Coronary Bypass Surgery

Anatomy
1. Left main disease
2. Triple-vessel disease involving the proximal LAD, with normal or diminished ejection fraction
3. Double-vessel disease involving the proximal LAD, with normal or diminished ejection fraction

Symptoms
1. Unstable (crescendo) angina
2. Post-MI angina
3. Acute coronary occlusion after PTCA
4. Symptoms unsuccessfully controlled with medical therapy
5. Controlled symptoms, but with unacceptable lifestyle

Abbreviations: LAD, left anterior descending coronary artery; MI, myocardial infarction; PTCA, percutaneous transluminal coronary angioplasty.

an intra-aortic balloon counter-pulsation device before transport to the operating room. If hemodynamic instability continues despite balloon pump support, portable cardiopulmonary bypass perfusion with femoral arterial and femoral venous cannulation may allow sufficient time to stabilize the patient's condition for an operation.

Surgical Technique

In coronary artery bypass surgery, the diseased portion of the coronary artery is bypassed by the creation of an alternative conduit for delivery of blood beyond the stenosis. Grafts are constructed by making an end-to-side anastomosis to the coronary artery distal to the obstruction. The proximal end of the vein graft is usually sutured end-to-side to the ascending aorta. Use of arterial grafts has increased in recent years. The most commonly used arterial graft is the left internal thoracic artery (LITA), which is used as a pedicle retaining its origin at the subclavian artery with a distal end-to-side anastomosis to the diseased coronary artery. Most commonly, this is the LAD. The right internal thoracic artery (RITA) may be used as either a pedicle graft or a free graft as well when more than one arterial graft is desired. In a much more limited fashion, the gastroepiploic artery, the radial artery, and the inferior epigastric artery have been used as conduits. The main benefit of these grafts is improved long-term patency; the 10-year patency of the internal thoracic artery is between 90% and 95%, whereas saphenous vein grafts have only a 50% 10-year patency. Use of the LITA has been shown to improve survival and reduce the incidence of late MI, recurrent angina, and the need for further cardiac interventions (31). Simultaneous use of both LITA and RITA is becoming more common, and has been reported to have beneficial effects in large single-center studies (32).

Traditionally, to maintain a quiet, bloodless field, cardiopulmonary bypass is employed for coronary bypass surgery (Fig. 4). With the patient on bypass and the heart empty, the distal ascending aorta is cross-clamped and potassium cardioplegic solution injected into the aortic root, causing nearly instantaneous cardiac arrest. The cardioplegic solution is usually between 4°C and 10°C, to induce rapid myocardial cooling. In addition, topical iced saline solution may be employed to provide surface cooling of the heart. The most important protective effects of cardioplegia are hypothermia and potassium, which causes arrest of the heart in diastole. Decreasing myocardial temperature to 10°C to 15°C, decreases the metabolic rate by as much as 80%, with mechanical arrest lowering the metabolic rate to as little as 5% of the normothermic, working heart.

A great deal of investigative effort has gone into determining the best type of cardioplegic solution. Again, though, the most important aspects of arresting the ischemic heart are maintaining hypothermia as well as mechanical arrest. Newer techniques employ initial warm induction of arrest followed by cold cardioplegia. Furthermore, on completion of the operation, administration of a warm dose of cardioplegic solution before removal of the cross-clamp has also been advocated. Both the techniques are used in an attempt to allow the metabolic machinery to perform reparative processes before asking the heart to perform any mechanical work. In fact, some surgeons prefer to do the entire operation with the patient and the heart warm, while cardioplegic solution is being administered continuously (34). During the past several years, retrograde cardioplegic administration has come into vogue. Delivery of cardioplegic solution through the coronary sinus and the coronary veins may

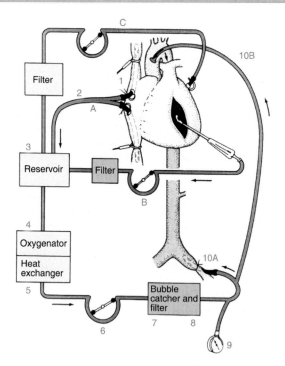

Figure 4 Schematic diagram of a typical cardiopulmonary bypass circuit. Blood is drained by gravity from the venae cavae (**1**) through venous cannula (**2**) into a venous reservoir (**3**). Blood from surgical field suction and from a ventricular vent (if used during operation) is pumped (B, C) into a cardiotomy reservoir (not shown) and then drained into a venous reservoir (**3**). Venous blood is oxygenated (**4**), temperature adjusted (**5**), raised to arterial pressure (**6**), filtered (**7,8**), and returned to the patient by way of a cannula in either the aorta (**10B**) or femoral artery (**10A**). Arterial line pressure is monitored (**9**). *Source*: From Ref. 33.

yield enhanced myocardial protection, because significant coronary stenoses can prevent the homogeneous antegrade delivery of cardioplegic solution. Retrograde cardioplegia is also useful in the presence of significant aortic insufficiency, because effective delivery of cardioplegic solution in an antegrade fashion is severely hindered by an incompetent aortic valve.

The distal anastomoses are generally performed with the aid of optical magnification. In addition to individual vein or thoracic artery graft anastomoses, two or more distal anastomoses can be constructed from a single vein or thoracic artery. These sequential grafts are favored when multiple distal sites are planned for anastomoses, or when there is a shortage of suitable conduit material. Sequential grafting is achieved by performing side-to-side anastomoses between the conduit and recipient artery and ending the graft with an end-to-side anastomosis to the most distal coronary artery. After completion of the distal anastomoses and initiation of reperfusion, a partially occluding side-biting clamp is placed on the ascending aorta, and the proximal anastomoses are constructed.

Rarely, if the recipient coronary artery is diffusely diseased with no available site for the distal anastomoses, the surgeon may be required to perform an endarterectomy to allow a reliable graft-to-artery anastomosis. Coronary endarterectomy sites are more vulnerable to early thrombosis and reocclusion, and this should be performed only if there is no alternative. Because patients with such diffuse disease are already likely to have poor outcomes, it has been difficult to demonstrate a beneficial effect from coronary endarterectomy.

New Developments
In the last few years, increasing attention has been paid to coronary artery bypass grafting without use of the cardiopulmonary bypass circuit and its inherent need for systemic heparinization, its propensity for inducing a systemic inflammatory reaction, and its known generation of microemboli to the brain. After widespread retrospective reports of improved perioperative morbidity and mortality (35) after "off-pump" coronary artery bypass grafting (OPCABG), a prospective, randomized trial was recently completed. Patients undergoing OPCABG received a similar number of bypass grafts, had equivalent 30-day mortality and stroke rate, required fewer blood transfusions, and had a shorter postoperative hospital length of stay when compared to patients undergoing conventional CABG using cardiopulmonary bypass (36). This technique has been greatly enhanced by the use of cardiac stabilization devices. Current generation devices employ two instruments that contact the epicardium: an apical suction device to retract the heart in various angles, and stabilization plate to isolate a single area of epicardium for suturing (Fig. 5).

Minimally invasive direct coronary artery bypass is a new technique that aims to avoid complications associated with a full sternotomy. Using a thoracic approach, all epicardial vessels can potentially be accessed. In addition, femoral artery and vein can be used for cardiopulmonary bypass cannulation sites, and the heart can be arrested and opened through this approach.

Upon unclamping of the aortic cross-clamp during the weaning of cardiopulmonary bypass, atheromatous debris is released from the intimal surface, and is often of a significant enough quantity to cause cerebral ischemic or stroke. New intra-aortic filters are being tested, which slide through an additional lumen in the aortic cannula, and open after being placed inside the aortic lumen. These filters have been shown in preliminary trials to reduce the incidence of post-CABG neurologic complications.

Aortocoronary anastomotic devices are being developed and tested, which will allow complete anastomoses to be constructed without the need for aortic cross-clamping. This device expands once the tip has been introduced into the aortic lumen, and deploys a radially shaped metallic structure, which contains hooks and attaches to the intimal surface of the aorta. Trials are underway to assess orifice patency, operative times, ease of deployment, and potential effect on operative mortality.

Postoperative Management
After the operation, cardiac surgical patients are monitored in an intensive care unit, with careful hemodynamic evaluation. Arterial blood pressure, central venous pressure, pulmonary artery pressures, cardiac output (CO), mixed venous oxygen saturation, and urinary output all provide valuable information regarding the adequacy of tissue perfusion and organ function. Mediastinal and chest tube drainage should be monitored hourly and, in fact, can be transfused to minimize the use of banked blood products. All patients have a capillary leakage syndrome and fluid accumulation after cardiopulmonary bypass, with a marked increase in total body sodium, such that patients typically gain between 5 and 10 kg. Most patients are able to be extubated within 4 to 12 hours of surgery,

(A)

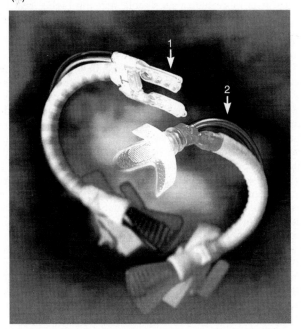

(B)

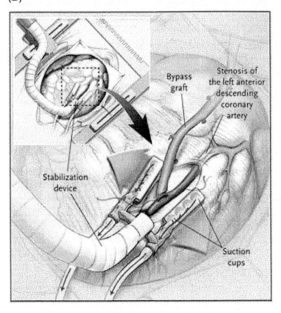

Figure 5 **(A)** Cardiac stabilization device used during off-pump coronary bypass surgery. Newer devices use suction cups on the stabilization platform **(1)** as well as the apical cup **(2)** to pull the epicardium into the instrument. Use of suction avoids the need for pressure to accomplish coronary stabilization, thereby minimizing hemodynamic instability during the anastamosis. **(B)** Diagram of stabilization platform use during bypass of left anterior descending artery. *Source:* From Ref. 37.

and thereafter can be transferred to a step-down unit, where continuous monitoring for arrhythmias, gentle diuresis to attain preoperative weight, and early ambulation are achieved.

Compared with other populations, the patient after cardiac surgery provides an opportunity for sophisticated

management and optimization of CO. In the early postoperative period, hypovolemia, increased systemic vascular resistance, hypothermia, and arrhythmias (both bradycardic and tachycardic) may all contribute to low CO. Management of these patients is both challenging and rewarding, because the cause of low CO is almost always reversible.

Low CO. When the calculated cardiac index (CI and CO divided by body surface area) is less than $2 \, L/min/m^2$, despite optimization of heart rhythm, preload, and afterload, use of an inotropic agent is invariably indicated (Table 2). If a patient remains in cardiogenic shock, despite significant inotropic support, consideration should be given to placement of an intra-aortic balloon pump. The balloon, which may be inserted percutaneously through the femoral artery, is positioned just beyond the subclavian artery takeoff of the aorta. Balloon inflation and deflation are timed so that intra-aortic balloon counter pulsation increases coronary artery perfusion pressure during ventricular diastole and, as a result of active deflation, maximally decreases afterload during ventricular systole. Rarely, if shock persists, a left ventricular-assist device (VAD) should be considered. However, the cause of persistent low CO in the early postoperative period should be pursued aggressively, with any reversible cause identified. Left VAD support is extremely labor intensive and costly, and it should only be considered if myocardial failure is considered to be reversible, or if the patient needs a bridge to transplantation.

Postoperative Complications. The major complications after open-heart surgery include bleeding, tamponade, infection, and stroke. Platelet function and blood clotting factors are severely altered after bypass and may not return to normal for as long as 36 hours. Average postoperative blood loss is between 400 and 800 mL and, as stated previously, may be reinfused to decrease the need for homologous blood transfusions. When bleeding exceeds a rate of 200 mL/hr for four hours or longer, return to the operating room for correction of any surgical cause of the bleeding should be considered. Before then, all medical causes of coagulopathy should be corrected aggressively. It is simple and safe to give additional protamine to reverse the residual heparin used during bypass, but transfusions of platelets, fresh-frozen plasma, or cryoprecipitate should be considered only if indicated by coagulation studies.

Cardiac tamponade is a potentially lethal cause of low CO early after operation. Clinically, one sees decreased CO increasing filling pressures and a narrowed pulse pressure. Pulsus paradoxus and a widened mediastinal silhouette on chest radiographs are frequently seen. Transesophageal echocardiography has made this diagnosis more easily established and should be used without hesitation when faced with this possible diagnosis.

Table 2 Causes of Low Cardiac Output After Coronary Bypass

1. Inadequate preload
2. Excessive afterload
3. Poor ventricular contractility
    a. Perioperative ischemia
    b. Poor myocardial preservation
4. Arrhythmia
5. Severe acidosis
6. Tension pneumothorax
7. Tamponade

The major wound complication facing surgeons after coronary bypass is sternal infection with mediastinitis, dehiscence, or both. This complication occurs in as many as 2% to 4% of patients, with the incidence increased when bilateral thoracic arteries are used, particularly in elderly patients and those with diabetes. Staphylococci are the most common organisms, and because of the devastating nature of this complication, most patients receive antistaphylococcal prophylaxis in the perioperative period. Mortality after development of this complication is between 20% and 30% (38).

Cerebral vascular accidents may be the most tragic of postoperative complications. Stroke is usually caused by atherosclerotic emboli that probably originate from the aorta, loosened by cannulation, cross-clamping, or the construction of the proximal anastomoses. Underlying cerebral vascular disease combined with hypotension during bypass contributes to this problem. Strokes occur in 1% to 2% of patients at low risk, but may occur in as many as 10% of octogenarians. No data suggest that the investigation of asymptomatic carotid bruits, prior to open-heart surgery with subsequent combined coronary bypass and carotid endarterectomy, would reduce the incidence of stroke after surgery. In patients who have both symptomatic carotid and coronary disease with significant stenosis of the carotid, however, a combined procedure is usually carried out.

Risk Factors for Operative Death

The assessment of the patient's mortality risk after bypass surgery is an important component of the preoperative evaluation in coronary artery disease. Furthermore, as issues regarding quality assurance and the delivery of efficient, cost-effective health care loom ever larger in our society, scrutiny of the benefits and risks associated with this most expensive of medical procedures has come increasingly in vogue (Table 3). Clearly, patients with concurrent medical problems such as cerebral vascular disease, pulmonary or renal insufficiency, diabetes, and morbid obesity are at higher risk for development of postoperative complications. Poor ventricular function is among the most important factors increasing the mortality rate after bypass surgery (39). Operative risk is also increased when patients require additional operative intervention such as valve repair or replacement. It is well documented that increasing age itself increases mortality rate. In the CASS study (28), the mortality rate among patients older than 70 years was nearly 8%, compared with an overall mortality rate of 3%. It has also been stated that women have a higher mortality rate after bypass surgery than do men. The explanation for this is not exactly clear, but may be related to the fact that women undergoing coronary bypass surgery are on average 10 years older than men and have a higher incidence of unstable angina, preoperative CHF, hypertension, and diabetes. It is more than conceivable that the higher risk for women is related to the higher incidence of these risk factors (40).

Long-Term Results

Most series show elimination of angina in 90% of patients at one year, with approximately 70% of patients remaining free of any cardiac event at three years. Although relief from symptoms is unquestioned, controversy exists regarding the long-term functional benefit of bypass surgery. However, functional improvement in left ventricular ejection fraction has been documented after bypass surgery and can be attributed to improved contractility in the myocardial regions in which there had been demonstrable ischemia prior to surgery.

Clinical improvement obviously depends at least in part on short- and long-term graft patency. The overall occlusion rate for saphenous vein bypass grafts is 5% to 20% during the first operative year and 2% to 4% annually thereafter, for an occlusion rate of approximately 30% at 5 years and 50% at 10 years. Use of the internal thoracic graft has become increasingly favored because of its 95% one-year and 90% 10-year patency rates. Excellent late internal thoracic artery graft patency clearly correlates with increased patient survival, reduced symptoms, and fewer reoperations. In a study at the Cleveland Clinic, where internal thoracic artery grafts have been used extensively, the 10-year survival rate among patients with saphenous vein grafts for triple-vessel disease was 71%, compared with 83% in a comparable group of patients who had an internal thoracic artery graft to the LAD. Approximately 80% of all patients undergoing primary coronary bypass surgery survive for 10 years, and use of the internal thoracic artery graft improves 10-year survival to close to 90%. Furthermore, about one in seven patients who have had only vein grafts require reoperation at 15 years, twice the reoperation rate for those patients who received at least one thoracic artery bypass.

Patients who undergo reoperation have approximately twice the primary operative mortality rate, because the operation is technically more difficult and because the patients are older, with more severe atherosclerotic disease (41). In addition, total revascularization is more difficult for technical reasons, and symptomatic relief is therefore usually of shorter duration as well.

Transplantation vs. High-Risk Coronary Surgery

In deciding whether to recommend transplantation or bypass surgery to a patient at high risk as a result of severely depressed left ventricular function, it is important to assess whether the myocardium is viable. In patients with ischemic but viable myocardium, ventricular function may improve after bypass surgery once adequate blood flow is restored. The term "hibernating myocardium" has been used to describe ventricular dysfunction caused by inadequate coronary flow (42). This condition should be distinguished from an ischemic cardiomyopathy, which implies irreversible myocardial dysfunction. Anginal symptoms suggestive of reversible ischemia are often a useful measure of myocardial viability.

Patients whose only symptom is heart failure should be approached with caution. Currently, myocardial viability may best be assessed by thallium scanning, either with exercise or at rest. Myocardium that takes up thallium either early or late is presumed to be viable. In this way, one may be able to estimate the possibly dramatic potential

Table 3   Prediction of the Risk for Operative Death

	Low	Medium	High
Age (yr)	60	75	75
Sex	Male	Female	Female
Diabetes	No	Yes	Yes
Unstable angina	Yes	No	Yes
Ejection fraction (%)	65	35	25
Three-vessel disease	Yes	Yes	Yes
Operative incidence	First	First	Redo
Predicted mortality rate (%)	0.8	3.4	12

Source: Based on The Society of Thoracic Surgery National Cardiac Database Risk Stratification Algorithm. Summit Medical Systems, Minneapolis, Minnesota, U.S.A.

for improved ventricular function with revascularization in the patient who has severely depressed ventricular function but viable myocardium. In a patient with these findings, especially if angina is present, surgery rather than transplantation is indicated if there is operable coronary disease. In patients with CHF and no evidence of viable myocardium, however, bypass surgery clearly carries high risk and little benefit, and transplantation should be considered.

Transmyocardial Revascularization

For those patients burdened with angina but whose coronaries are not anatomically approachable, transmyocardial revascularization is a new technique with promising initial results. This procedure employs a CO_2 laser, a needle, or high frequency ultrasound to create transmural channels in the myocardium and allow oxygenated blood to reach previously ischemic regions of the heart. Nearly four years after this procedure, patients have been found to have fewer anginal symptoms, require fewer hospitalizations, and have equivalent ventricular ejection fraction and mortality compared to patients receiving medical therapy alone (43).

VALVULAR HEART DISEASE
Aortic Valve Disease
Aortic Valvular Stenosis

The normal aortic valve consists of three equal-size leaflets attached to the aortic wall, forming the three aortic sinuses. As mentioned in the section on coronary artery disease, the coronary arteries arise from two of these sinuses, thereby defining the left, right, and noncoronary cusps.

Pathologic Anatomy

The most common cause of left ventricular outflow tract obstruction is aortic valvular stenosis. Supravalvular and subvalvular obstructions occur much less commonly. Aortic stenosis is the most common isolated valvular abnormality found in humans. Although congenital valvular stenosis may cause symptoms immediately, a congenital bicuspid valve is usually asymptomatic at birth and becomes symptomatic in the sixth to eighth decade of life. The turbulent flow across the bileaflet valve leads to fibrosis and calcification, so that stenosis develops with time. Rheumatic aortic stenosis, initially an inflammatory lesion, leads to fusion of the leaflet commissures, with thickening and calcification of the cusps themselves. Retraction of the leaflet borders, which occurs commonly, leads to regurgitation as well. In rheumatic aortic valvular disease, mitral involvement is invariably also present. In degenerative or senile aortic stenosis, normal leaflet stress leads to calcification and cusp immobility. This calcification can extend either interiorly onto the anterior mitral leaflet or upward along the aorta, occasionally causing coronary osteal stenosis (Fig. 1).

Pathophysiology

Narrowing of the left ventricular outflow tract becomes important when it obstructs flow, causing a transvalvular pressure gradient. In the presence of a normal CO, a transvalvular gradient of 60 mmHg or a calculated valve area of less than $0.7 \, cm^2$ is considered severe aortic stenosis. The normal response to aortic stenosis, a process that in itself can take years, is the development of left ventricular hypertrophy. This hypertrophy initially leads to a decrease in compliance, with an elevation in the left ventricular end-diastolic pressure. With progressive hypertrophy and loss of ventricular compliance, atrial contraction plays an

increasingly important role in left ventricular filling, so loss of a normal sinus mechanism [such as atrial fibrillation (AF)] can cause acute decompensation in these patients. Furthermore, with severe aortic stenosis, prolongation of the systolic ejection time and a concomitant elevation in left ventricular end-diastolic pressure act to decrease diastolic coronary blood flow, with a resultant oxygen debt. The subendocardium may become chronically ischemic, with cell death and fibrosis. In this situation, the left ventricle begins to fail as stroke volume decreases and CO falls. Paradoxically, follow-up of a patient with aortic stenosis may reveal a low or a decreasing aortic gradient during a period of years, which should not be confused with resolving or stable aortic valvular disease but rather indicates a failing left ventricle with a decreased stroke volume and therefore a decreased transvalvular gradient.

The clinical course of aortic stenosis may be divided into two phases. The initial phase involves hypertrophy of the left ventricle because it compensates for increasing afterload. Angina, the hallmark of this stage of aortic stenosis, results from the imbalance of myocardial oxygen demand and myocardial oxygen delivery. The second stage involves the onset of left ventricular dysfunction, which is the result of a progressively stiffening ventricle that requires increasing preload for adequate filling, with resultant pulmonary hypertension, shortness of breath, and dyspnea on exertion.

Diagnosis

Although auscultation of the patient with aortic stenosis reveals a systolic murmur best heard at the base of the heart at the left sternal border radiating up into the neck, this murmur can also be associated simply with normal systolic ejection. However, a slow, prolonged rise in the arterial pulse, as opposed to a sharp upbeat, is a palpable indicator that significant ventricular outflow tract obstruction is present. Doppler echocardiography has become an invaluable tool in the noninvasive detection of aortic stenosis. The peak aortic valvular gradient can be calculated by the following formula (44):

$$\Delta = 4V^2$$

where Δ is the peak gradient and V is the maximal measured blood velocity (in meters per second) across the valve. The most accurate measure of left ventricular outflow tract obstruction is determined invasively by cardiac catheterization, where a simultaneous aortic and ventricular pressure measurement can determine the exact aortic gradient (in the case of AF, this is the only acceptable means of determining this number). The aortic valve area (AVA, in square centimeters) may then be determined by the Gorlin formula (45):

$$AVA = AVF/44.5 \, (gradient)^{1/2}$$

where AVF is aortic valve flow, which equals CO in milliliters per minute divided by the systolic ejection period (in seconds per minute), and 44.5 is the empiric orifice constant (obtained by comparing calculated with measured AVA at operation or postmortem). For quick calculations, this simplifies to

$$AVA = CO/(gradient)^{1/2}$$

Patients frequently have symptoms when the AVA is less than $1 \, cm^2$, whereas they invariably have symptoms when the area is less than $0.7 \, cm^2$ (46). Angina is usually

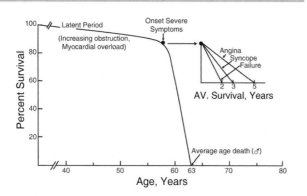

Figure 6 Average course of medically treated valvular aortic stenosis in adults (postmortem data). Although one can understand the difficulty in operating on the patient without symptoms, the severe slope of the curve mandates that patients be seriously considered for surgery at the onset of symptoms. *Source*: From Ref. 47.

the earliest symptom in patients with aortic stenosis. The mean survival after its onset is 4.7 years. However, when a patient has syncope, survival is typically decreased to less than three years, whereas when a patient has dyspnea and CHF, survival is on the order of one to two years (Fig. 6) (48).

Treatment
The only effective therapy for symptomatic aortic stenosis is operative. Symptoms alone are an indication for aortic valve replacement. Occasionally, a patient with aortic stenosis may have no symptoms. The appropriate timing of surgery in such patients is not clear. Timely surgery provides the opportunity for resolution of left ventricular hypertrophy, whereas allowing the condition to persist may lead to irreversible myocardial fibrosis with dysfunction. In general, patients without symptoms with progressive left ventricular hypertrophy should be offered surgical therapy because survival is superior to that with medical therapy (49). An unwritten dictum is that all patients with aortic stenosis should be given the opportunity for surgical therapy because it is so effective in leading to reversal of symptoms. With progressive fibrosis and irreversible myocardial dysfunction, however, an occasional patient may have a decrease in ejection fraction out of proportion to the increase in wall stress caused by the aortic stenosis. With this "end-stage aortic stenosis" (in which contractility has decreased out of proportion to the increase in wall stress), patients derive little benefit from surgical therapy (50,51).

In patients with good ventricular function, aortic valve replacement has an associated mortality rate of 2% to 8%. Perioperative risk factors include age, left ventricular function, preoperative New York Heart Association functional classification, and pulmonary function. The projected five-year survival for patients after aortic valve replacement is 80% to 85%. Although symptoms are generally relieved in all patients, improvement in ejection fraction with resolution of left ventricular hypertrophy may require months to occur (52,53). In patients with aortic stenosis as well as coronary artery disease, valve replacement and myocardial revascularization should be performed concurrently (54).

Percutaneous aortic balloon valvuloplasty is a "noninvasive" alternative to surgical therapy for aortic stenosis. In this procedure, either one or two balloon catheters are placed

in a retrograde fashion through the aortic orifice and inflated in an effort to crack the calcium that is retarding valvular motion. The immediate results show an increase in the AVA of 50%, with a 3% to 10% mortality rate and a similar stroke rate (55). Long-term results are abysmal, with a one-year mortality rate of 25% and a 30% to 35% symptomatic recurrence rate during that period. With recurrence of symptoms, death, hemodynamic evidence of restenosis, or a combination of these occuring in more than 50% of patients at six months after percutaneous aortic balloon valvuloplasty, surgical valve replacement will remain the mainstay of therapy. If valvuloplasty has a role at all, it should be limited to the aged and frail patient whose long-term prognosis is also abysmal.

Aortic Insufficiency

Pathologic Anatomy
Incompetence of the aortic valve may be the result of either primary valvular or aortic root disease (56). Rheumatic fever is a major cause of aortic insufficiency. As discussed with aortic stenosis, it causes retraction of the cusps, which prevents adequate apposition and leads to a central leak. Congenital bicuspid valves with time become calcified and generally lead to aortic stenosis. Ocasionally, however, bicuspid valves have a redundant leaflet that leads to regurgitation. Myxoid degeneration of the aortic valve, as seen in Marfan syndrome, Ehlers–Danlos syndrome, and cystic medial necrosis, may lead to redundancy, prolapse, and regurgitation. Infective endocarditis with bacterial destruction of the leaflets may also lead to valvular insufficiency. Ascending aortic dissection as a result of either trauma or hypertensive atherosclerotic disease often leads to loss of commissural suspension, with resultant leaflet prolapse. Furthermore, severe aortic dilation causes annular stretching (as seen in annuloaortic ectasia, syphilis, and ankylosing spondylitis), which leads to annular dilatation and central valvular incompetence.

Pathophysiology
With aortic regurgitation, there is a significant increase in preload, where end-diastolic volume is the result of both normal left ventricular filling through the mitral valve as well as left ventricular filling through the incompetent aortic valve. At the expense of an increase in left ventricular wall stress, ejection fraction remains normal as stroke volume and end-diastolic volume increase. Left ventricular dilatation increases wall tension, which increases myocardial oxygen demand. To counteract this, left ventricular wall thickness increases to maintain a wall thickness to cavity radius ratio that preserves myocardial efficiency. With time, however, left ventricular volume may become enormous. Increasing wall thickness does not keep pace with this increasing left ventricular dilation. Sharply increased wall tension develops, with resulting systolic dysfunction. At this point, an elevation in left ventricular end-diastolic pressure occurs and patients have symptoms (Fig. 7). Acute aortic regurgitation, on the other hand, such as occurs with dissections or endocarditis, leads to extremely high left ventricular end-diastolic pressures as a result of the acute increase in end-diastolic volume in the unconditioned ventricle. In these patients, symptoms develop immediately.

Diagnosis
Patients with aortic insufficiency have a characteristic pattern on physical examination that results from the wide pulse

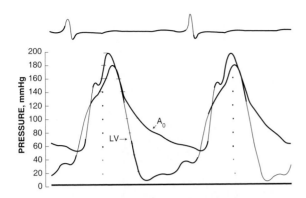

Figure 7 Simultaneous left ventricular and aortic pressure–time curves in a patient with severe aortic insufficiency. Note that in this patient with extremely severe aortic insufficiency, the left ventricle has become less and less compliant, and at end-diastole, the aortic pressure and left ventricular end-diastolic pressure have nearly equalized. *Abbreviation*: LV, left ventricle. *Source*: From Ref. 57.

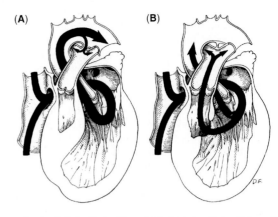

Figure 8 Survival of patients with medically treated aortic insufficiency. Unlike with aortic stenosis, cardiac failure from aortic insufficiency occurs much more gradually. Consequently, it is much more difficult to discern where one should intervene, particularly in the patient without symptoms. *Source*: From Ref. 59.

pressure associated with this disease. The peripheral pulses rise and fall abruptly (Corrigan's or water-hammer pulse), the head may bob with each systolic stroke (Musset's sign), and the capillaries visibly pulsate (Quincke's sign). Auscultation reveals a soft S_2 with a high-frequency, diastolic, regurgitant murmur best heard at the left sternal border. A mid-to-late diastolic rumble can be heard (Austin Flint murmur); this represents rapid diastolic flow across the mitral valve that is becoming narrowed as a result of rapid ventricular filling caused by the aortic insufficiency.

Clinical Course

In chronic aortic regurgitation, symptoms occur late after left ventricular dilatation and myocardial dysfunction (58). Symptoms occur as a result of elevation in left ventricular end-diastolic pressure, again a situation that occurs later in the course of the disease, because early on, left ventricular volumes increase to maintain compliance. Interestingly, nocturnal angina can occur as the result of a slow heart rate, so that diastolic pressure in the coronary arteries is low, and left ventricular end-diastolic pressure is high, compromising blood flow and oxygen delivery to the endocardium. Acute aortic regurgitation, however, is poorly tolerated, and patients have symptoms almost immediately. This is the result of extremely poor compliance of the ventricle and an excessively high diastolic volume.

Management

Patients with symptomatic aortic insufficiency require surgical therapy, because survival with medical therapy is only a few years from the onset of symptoms. The patient with no symptoms or mild symptoms but with moderate to severe aortic insufficiency presents a dilemma. Frequently, diuretics and afterload reduction may be able to maintain these patients for a considerable period before they experience symptoms. Without surgery, 75% of patients survive five years from the time of diagnosis, and 50% of patients survive 10 years (Fig. 8) (59). Despite the lack of symptoms, however, irreversible myocardial dysfunction occurs. The goal of the clinician should be to intervene before this happens. When end-systolic volume is less than $30 \, mL/m^2$, prognosis after surgical therapy is still excellent. With progressive systolic

dysfunction, however, end-systolic volumes may rise above $90 \, mL/m^2$, a situation that frequency portends permanent postoperative disability. End-systolic volumes between 30 and $90 \, mL/m^2$ have intermediate short- and long-term-results (60). Indications for surgical therapy in the patient without symptoms thus should rest on serial echocardiography or radionuclide ventriculography to discern systolic dysfunction or decreasing ejection fraction. Despite good exercise tolerance, when systolic dysfunction occurs, surgery should be recommended.

The mortality rate associated with aortic valve replacement for aortic insufficiency is approximately 4% to 6%, somewhat higher than that seen in aortic stenosis (61–63). As discussed, long-term survival depends on preoperative left ventricular function.

Choice of Prosthetic Aortic Valve Type

The Department of Veterans Affairs trial randomized patients between 1982 and 1997 to receive mechanical or bioprosthetic valves. At average follow-up of 15 years, mechanical values were associated with lower mortality and lower reoperation rate. These differences became apparent after 10 years. In addition, the mechanical valves displayed no structural value deterioration, and use of the bioprosthetic valve was associated with fewer bleeding complications. Thus, bioprosthetic valves are at risk for late reoperation, but the avoidance of necessary long-term anticoagulation makes them an attractive option for some subgroups. Generally speaking, patients aged at least 65 to 70 years undergoing only valve replacement should receive a bioprosthetic valve. Patients aged at least 60 years undergoing concomitant procedures such as coronary bypass should also receive a bioprosthetic valve (64).

Mitral Valve Disease

Surgical Anatomy

The mitral valve appartus is composed of the left ventricular papillary muscles, the mitral valve chordae tendineae, the mitral valve leaflets, and the mitral valve annulus. By means of the chordae tendineae, the mitral leaflets are connected to the apical region of the left ventricle. Normal function of the valve depends on the coordinated interaction of these components. The mitral valve has two leaflets joined at two commissures. The anterior leaflet (also called the aortic leaflets) is broad and relatively square in shape. It is attached to the anterior one-third circumference of the mitral valve annulus and is in fibrous continuity with the aortic valve annulus. The posterior leaflet (also called the mural leaflet) is narrower and relatively rectangular. It is attached to the posterior two-thirds circumference of the mitral annulus. Each leaflet is attached by chordae to each of two papillary muscles arising from the luminal surface of the left ventricle, the anterior-lateral and the posterior-medial papillary muscles. The blood supply of the anterior-lateral papillary muscle is from the diagonal branches of LAD or by obtuse marginal branches of the circumflex coronary artery. The posterior-medial papillary muscle is supplied by the PDA coronary artery, which is usually the terminal branch of the RCA.

The mitral valve functions to permit antegrade blood flow from the left atrium into left ventricle during diastole and to prevent reflux of blood from left ventricle into the left atrium during systole. Blood flows antegrade through the mitral valve when the left atrial pressure exceeds left ventricular pressure. As the ventricle contracts during systole, closure of the valve is affected by several mechanisms. Once the left ventricular pressure exceeds left atrial pressure, leaflet closure is initiated, and the rate of blood flow from the atrium into the ventricle is decelerated. At the same time, contraction of the left ventricular muscle at the base of the heart serves to narrow the mitral annulus; echocardiographic data suggest that the annular area decreases by approximately one-third from end-diastole to mid-systole (65). This reduction in annular area helps achieve leaflet approximation. During systolic contraction, papillary muscle contraction pulls the chordae taut, preventing prolapse of the leaflets. Any disease process that interferes with the normal function of any portion of the mitral valve apparatus may result in mitral stenosis or regurgitation.

Mitral Stenosis

Rheumatic fever is the primary cause of mitral stenosis (66). Other etiologies of mitral stenosis are rare and include congenital mitral stenosis and stenosis resulting from collagen vascular diseases such as systemic lupus erythematosus and rheumatoid arthritis. Two-thirds of patients with rheumatoid mitral stenosis are female. After resolution of acute rheumatic fever, most patients remain free of symptoms for at least two decades before development of symptoms of mitral valve disease. Thereafter, patients have progressively worse symptoms (67).

The normal mitral valve orifice measures 4 to 6 cm^2 in cross-sectional area. A mitral valve area (MVA) of 2 cm^2 is considered moderate mitral stenosis. At this degree of narrowing, flow across the mitral valve may be accomplished only by generation of an abnormally high-pressure gradient across the valve. An MVA of 1 cm^2 is considered critical mitral stenosis, because flow across the valve (CO) is relatively fixed; even extremely high-pressure gradients across the valve are unable to increase flow (Fig. 9). As with the aortic valve, the MVA may be calculated according to the Gorlin formula (for the mitral valve, the constant is 38 rather than the 44.5 used for the aortic valve):

$$MVA = \text{(Flow rate across valve)}/$$
$$38\text{(mean gradient across valve)}^{1/2}$$

For any given MVA, the magnitude of the transvalvular gradient is proportional to the square of the transvalvular

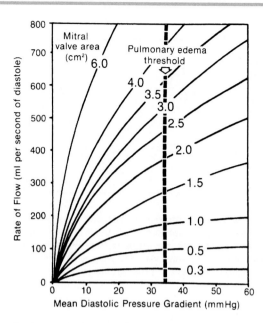

Figure 9 The relationship between mean diastolic gradient across the mitral valve and the rate of flow across the mitral valve per second of diastole. When the valve area is ≤1.0 cm^2, little additional flow can be achieved, despite an increased pressure gradient. *Source*: From Ref. 68.

flow rate; doubling the CO quadruples the transvalvular pressure gradient. Increased left atrial pressure results in increased pulmonary venous pressure, and in turn increased pulmonary capillary pressure. Should the transvalvular gradient culminate in a left atrial pressure greater than 25 mmHg, pulmonary edema may result. For this reason, exertional dyspnea is commonly the first symptom of mitral stenosis.

Patients frequently first have symptoms with the onset of AF. Chronically elevated left atrial pressure produces left atrial distention, ultimately producing AF. With the onset of AF, diastolic time is shortened; the same volume of blood must flow from left atrium to ventricle in less time, which further increases left atrial pressure. The atrial kick contributes approximately 30% to the presystolic transvalvular gradient in patients with mitral stenosis. Its loss with the onset of AF eliminates this mechanical advantage, and left atrial pressure rises and CO declines (69).

The contractile function of the left ventricle is typically well preserved in mitral stenosis. The hemodynamic features of mitral stenosis are notable for a reduced CO at rest (because of the mechanical obstruction of the stenotic valve), which rises subnormally with exercise along with pulmonary hypertension. The pulmonary hypertension is derived from retrograde transmission of elevated left atrial pressure, pulmonary arterial vasoconstriction, and obliterative structural changes in the pulmonary circulation produced by chronic left atrial hypertension. Pulmonary hypertension may become severe, resulting in impaired right ventricular function and tricuspid regurgitation.

Diagnosis
Patients with mitral stenosis typically are seen with easy fatigue, dyspnea on exertion, and orthopnea. As noted previously, symptoms may develop with the onset of AF.

A history of rheumatic fever is noted in approximately one half of cases. If the left atrial enlargement is sufficient to compress surrounding structures, patients may report dysphagia or hoarseness.

On cardiac auscultation, an opening snap of the mitral valve is common as a result of sudden tensing of the valve leaflets by the chordae, as the valve leaflets achieve their opening excursion. The opening snap may be heard within the first 100 msec after the second heart sound. Mitral stenosis produces a low-pitched, rumbling diastolic murmur best heard at the apex. The murmur is often difficult to appreciate, but may be provoked by maneuvers that increase CO. Pulmonary hypertension is suggested by a loud pulmonary component of the second heart sound. With pulmonary hypertension, an enlarged right ventricle may shift the left ventricle posteriorly, making the murmur extremely difficult to hear (silent mitral stenosis).

The chest roentgenogram is significant for left atrial enlargement. There may be elevation of the left main stem bronchus and posterior displacement of the esophagus on the lateral radiographic view. Pulmonary venous hypertension typically results in cephalization of pulmonary blood flow.

Two-dimensional echocardiographic evaluation of mitral stenosis reveals thickened mitral valve leaflets and restricted leaflet motion as the valve opens. The left atrium is typically enlarged, and the left ventricular cavity is usually reduced in size. Mitral annular calcification and left atrial thrombus are identifiable on echocardiography. Doppler echocardiography provides a functional estimate of the severity of mitral stenosis. The peak velocity of blood flow across the valve is increased, allowing an estimate of the transvalvular gradient (see the section on the Aortic Valve).

Medical Treatment

Medical treatment of mitral stenosis is of limited efficacy. The focus of medical treatment is to minimize pulmonary edema with diuretics and to control the ventricular rate with digoxin. Because left atrial thrombus may form, patients in AF should have anticoagulation with warfarin.

Surgical Treatment

Because of the efficacy of surgical treatment, the natural history of mitral stenosis is now unclear. However, after acute rheumatic fever, most patients remain free of symptoms for 20 to 25 years. Once these patients experience symptoms, at least five years is required for the progression of symptoms from mild to severe. According to the study of Olesen (70) of patients in the presurgical era, 40% of symptom-free patients with mitral stenosis had a significantly worsened condition or were dead within 10 years. Among patients with mild symptoms, the number was 80%. Munoz et al. (71) reported a 45% five-year survival rate for medically treated patients with mitral stenosis and mitral regurgitation. In a comparable population undergoing mitral commissurotomy, five-year survival rate was 80%.

The first report of successful surgical correction of mitral stenosis appeared in 1923; Cutler and Levine (72) reported successful relief of mitral stenosis by incision of the valve with a knife introduced through an apical left ventriculotomy. In 1925, Souttar (73) performed the first successful closed mitral commissurotomy through the left atrial appendage. After the reports of Harken et al. (74) in 1948 and Bailey (75) in 1949, closed mitral commissurotomy became widely used for mitral stenosis. Despite excellent long-term results after closed mitral commissurotomy (76), by the mid-1970s, this technique was supplanted by open

mitral commissurotomy. Closed mitral commissurotomy is now of historical interest only.

Although closed mitral commissurotomy offered good palliation of mitral stenosis, open mitral commissurotomy offers several advantages (77). First, the valvuloplasty may be performed under direct vision. The primary reason for failure of closed mitral commissurotomy was residual stenosis, not restenosis (78,79). In as may as 75% of patients, the subvalvular apparatus of the mitral valve contributes significantly to the stenosis (80). The open technique allows precise and maximal division of fused commissures as well as of fused chordae (81). In addition, calcium may be sharply debrided from the valve, and any residual mitral insufficiency may be corrected at the time of operation. Finally, the closed technique offers the disadvantages of potentially dislodging a left atrial thrombus, resulting in intraoperative embolization and stroke. The results of open mitral commissurotomy are excellent. Operative mortality rate is usually reported as 0.2% to 2%, and in most series, the need for reoperation is reported to be 2% per year (81).

Balloon Mitral Valvuloplasty

Inoue et al. (82) reported the first successful percutaneous balloon mitral valvuloplasty in 1984. The valvular pathology of mitral stenosis makes the valve unsuitable for balloon dilation. Nonetheless, this procedure is now an alternative to surgical relief of mitral stenosis in a small, select group of patients. After creation of a hole in the interatrial septum, a balloon catheter is introduced through the mitral valve and inflated within its orifice. The procedure is based on the idea that the inflated balloon will split fused commissures. As noted previously, however, the subvalvular apparatus contributes significantly to the stenosis, and this region is not addressed by balloon dilation. Immediate hemodynamic improvement is noted in most patients, with a significant reduction in transvalvular gradient, improved CO, and reduction in pulmonary arterial pressure (39). However, these hemodynamic benefits are not long standing, and the complication rate is significant. Reported mortality rates range from 0% to 4% (83), comparable to that of open mitral commissurotomy. Approximately 30% of patients are left with a significant atrial septal defect (84). Stroke is reported as a complication of the procedure in 3% to 4% (85). Recurrence of mitral stenosis is noted in as many as 30% to 40% of patients within one year (86). The small subset of patients with the best results from balloon mitral valvuloplasty are those with soft, pliable leaflets without calcification and without stenosis of the subvalvular apparatus. Such patents are, of course, rare. Thus, although balloon mitral valvuloplasty attempts to spare the patient a more invasive procedure, the patient is actually exposed to greater risk of complication and death. At the same time, the results are inferior to open mitral commissurotomy, which must be considered the procedure of choice.

Mitral Regurgitation

Structural abnormalities of any component of the mitral valve apparatus (mitral leaflets, chordae tendineae, and papillary muscles) may result in mitral regurgitation. Rheumatic fever remains the most common cause of mitral regurgitation; it results in deformity and retraction of the leaflets and shortening of the chordae. Other causes include perforation by trauma and infective endocarditis. Calcification of the mitral annulus may result in annular rigidity, preventing valve closure, and mitral annular dilation resulting from left ventricular dilation may likewise preclude leaflet apposition during systole. Chordal rupture may result from trauma, endocarditis, rheumatic fever, or diseases of collagen formation. Chordae to the posterior leaflet rupture more frequently than do those to the anterior. Coronary arterial disease may produce infarction of the papillary muscle, resulting in initial regurgitation. Infarction in distribution of the anterior descending coronary artery may be associated with necrosis of the anterior-lateral papillary muscle, whereas the posterior-medial muscle may infarct if blood flow through the PDA artery is interrupted. Mitral regurgitation caused by MI typically is seen as a new murmur several days after infarction.

Pathophysiology

The regurgitant mitral valve offers an alternative route by which blood may exit from the left ventricle. During both isovolumetric contraction and systole, blood is preferentially ejected into the low-pressure left atrium. The volume of the regurgitant flow (regurgitant fraction) depends on the size of the regurgitant orifice and the afterload against which the left ventricle must work to pump blood through the aortic valve. The regurgitant fraction is increased with increased left ventricular preload and increased afterload, both of which dilate the left ventricle, thereby enlarging the mitral annulus and regurgitant orifice. Because the valve leaks during systole, the volume of regurgitant flow also increases as heart rate (number of systoles per minute) increases. To maintain an adequate systemic blood flow (CO), the left ventricle becomes volume overloaded; it must pump the combined volume of systemic and regurgitant flows. Because the left ventricle is able to beat against the reduced resistance of the left atrium, parameters of systolic function (ejection fraction) are increased in mitral regurgitation. However, as with aortic insufficiency, the left ventricle ultimately fails, with chronic volume overload. In fact, normal values of systolic function indicate significant contractile dysfunction of the left ventricle. An ejection fraction of 40% to 50% in the setting of mitral regurgitation indicates severe left ventricular contractile dysfunction (66).

As in mitral stenosis, left atrial hypertension results from mitral regurgitation. This pressure is transmitted in a retrograde fashion into the pulmonary circulation; if high enough, it produces pulmonary hypertension. The magnitude of the left atrial pressure is a function of the compliance of the left atrium (Fig. 10). A normal or low compliance of the left atrium, such as may occur in acute mitral regurgitation, results in a relatively rapid rise in left atrial pressure. On the other hand, chronic, slowly developing left atrial volume overload may create significant enlargement of a compliant left atrium, with relatively low left atrial pressure.

Diagnosis

Symptoms result from the degree of mitral regurgitation, the rate of its progression, the degree of pulmonary hypertension, and the magnitude of left ventricular contractile dysfunction. Symptoms in patients with chronic mitral regurgitation typically do not occur until the left ventricle begins to fail. Patients with mild mitral regurgitation may remain free of symptoms for most of their lives (88). The onset of AF does impair the patient's functional status, but not to the same degree as with mitral stenosis. With moderate to severe chronic mitral regurgitation, patients may be free of symptoms for long periods. However, this lack of symptoms may be deceptive, because the contractile function of

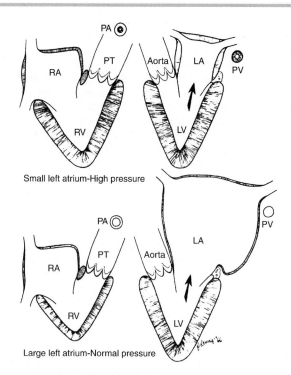

Figure 10 Syndrome of mitral regurgitation. When mitral regurgitation occurs abruptly in patients with previously normal heart, left atrial compliance is normal. This results in a rapid increase in left atrial pressure. On the other hand, the insidious development of mitral regurgitation allows the left atrial compliance to increase along with its size, attenuating the rise in left atrial pressure. *Abbreviations*: LA, left atrium; LV, left ventricle; PA, pulmonary artery; PT, pulmonary trunk; PV, pulmonary vein; RA, right atrium; RV, right ventricle. *Source*: From Ref. 87.

the left ventricle may be slowly deteriorating. Once symptoms occur, left ventricular contractile dysfunction may be irreversible.

The natural history of mitral regurgitation is obscure, because surgical intervention has effectively altered this history. In the presurgical era, however, approximately 80% of patients with severe mitral regurgitation survived five years and 60% survived 10 years (59).

On cardiac auscultation, a holosystolic murmur is best heard at the apex and radiates to the axilla and left scapular region. The ECG is notable for left atrial enlargement and, frequently, AF. The chest roentgenogram is significant for cardiomegaly and left atrial enlargement. Pulmonary venous hypertension may be manifested by cephalization of pulmonary blood flow and pulmonary edema.

Echocardiography is extremely valuable in confirming the diagnosis and severity of mitral regurgitation. Transesophageal echocardiography is particularly effective in providing an anatomic explanation for the regurgitation, such as perforated leaflets, poor leaflet coaptation, or ruptured chordae. Doppler echocardiography reveals a high-velocity jet of regurgitant blood flow into the left atrium during systole. The severity of the valve regurgitation is a function of the distance from the mitral annulus that the jet can be visualized (into the pulmonary veins) and the size of the left atrium. Contrast ventriculography performed at cardiac catheterization likewise demonstrates regurgitation during systole.

Management

The cornerstone of medical management is diuresis and afterload reduction with ACE inhibitors (66). The importance of afterload reduction cannot be overemphasized. Because blood leaving the left ventricle travels the path of least resistance, lowering systemic vascular resistance increases systemic CO.

The indications for surgical intervention are (i) symptoms despite medical management or (ii) evidence of deteriorating left ventricular contractile function, as determined by echocardiography or contract ventriculography. Surgical correction of mitral regurgitation should be undertaken before left ventricular contractile dysfunction becomes irreversible; the operative mortality rate increases substantially as the ventricle fails.

The two surgical options are repair and replacement of the valve. The final decision regarding which of these options to employ is made during the operation after inspection of the valve. There are several advantages to mitral valve repair rather than replacement. First, with mitral valve replacement, there is loss of the mitral valve apparatus connecting the mitral annulus to the apex of the left ventricle by means of the chordae and papillary muscles. In the long term, this may lead to left ventricular dysfunction. Mitral valve repair preserves this apparatus. Second, the risks associated with a prosthetic valve, such as prosthetic valve endocarditis and thromboembolic complications, are avoided. Third, the operative mortality rate associated with mitral valve repair is 0% to 4%, which is lower than the 2% to 8% reported for mitral valve replacement (80).

Finally, mitral valve repair can now be accomplished using minimally invasive techniques with robotic assistance, so that a median sternotomy incision is no longer required. In contrast, median sternotomy is still needed for mitral valve replacement.

HEART FAILURE
Epidemiology

CHF is the leading cause of hospitalization and death in the developed world, affecting 0.4% to 2% of the general adult population (89). Approximately 550,000 new cases of heart failure are diagnosed each year, and cause approximately 300,000 deaths per year. In the United States alone, over 34 billion dollars are spent on the medical care of patients with CHF. Among patients in the Framingham Study Group, the mean age at diagnosis was 63 years in the period from 1950 to 1969, and 80 years in the period from 1990 to 1999 (90). The most common cause of heart failure in men is MI, and in women, the most common cause is hypertension (91). Despite recent improvements in medical therapy for this disease, the Framingham Study showed that after the time of diagnosis there was a one-year survival of only approximately 75% and 50% at five years.

Medical Therapy

Medical therapy of CHF involves many of the same agents that are used in acute MI. ACE inhibitors are used for chronic unloading of the left ventricle. Chronic use of β-blockers causes myocardial upregulation of β-adrenergic receptors, making the heart more responsive to adrenergic stimulation. The addition of both to the medical regimen of CHF patients is now standard of care with an improvement in survival of

roughly 18% for ACE inhibitors and 35% for β-blockers compared to control, untreated patients. In patients with extremely poor myocardial function, outpatient inotropes may be used chronically via rate-controlled infusion into a large central vein. In this manner, Milrinone, a cyclic adenosine monophosphate–specific phosphodiesterase inhibitor or Dobutamine (a synthetic catecholamine), may be used to chronically support patients who otherwise would be hospitalized and unable to complete most activities of daily living due to such severe ventricular dysfunction.

Surgical Therapy

In patients with a maximal oxygen consumption less than 14 mL/kg/min (normal 30–50), heart transplantation provides the greatest survival advantage (68% 10-year survival) to patients with CHF, but its epidemiologic impact is limited by a severe shortage of donor organs. According to the registry of the International Society for Heart and Lung Transplantation, the number of heart transplants in the United States peaked in 1994 at approximately 4300, and has since fallen to the range of 2000 to 2500 transplants per year. Current efforts to increase the potential number of donor organs for heart transplantation are aimed at increasing public awareness, refinement of end-of-life donation consent policies, improvements in organ preservation techniques, and acceptance of organs previously considered marginal.

At least in some part due to the growing shortage of donor organs, a multitude of nontransplantation surgical techniques are being used more frequently to ameliorate CHF. These include cardiac revascularization, mitral valve reconstruction (92), and even left ventricular reconstruction using techniques such as the Batista and Dor procedures. Pathologic geometric remodeling of the left ventricle has been prevented by the CorCap cardiac support device (ACORN Cardiovascular, Inc., St. Paul, Minnesota, U.S.A.) or Myosplint (Myocor, Lie, Maple Grove, Minnesota, U.S.A.). The ACORN device (Fig. 11) is an elastic mesh sleeve that slides

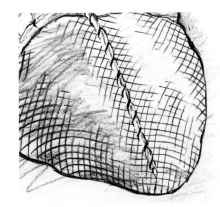

Figure 11 Diagram of ACORN device. During implantation, seam is placed anteriorly and oversewn to allow for the adjustment of circumferential tension, depending on heart size. Holes can be created in the jacket to allow for coronary bypass surgery. One can imagine the potential for postoperative scarring and adhesions making reoperative surgery extremely hazardous. *Source*: Courtesy of Acorn Cardiovascular, Inc., St. Paul, Minnesota, U.S.A.

(A)   **(B)**

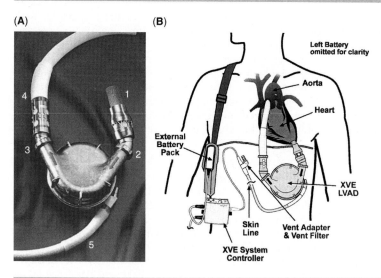

Figure 12 **(A)** Picture of Thoratec HeartMate© left ventricular assist system. This device is available as either a vented electric (XVE, shown) or an implantable pneumatic LVAD. Both devices are approved for use as bridge to transplantation, and the XVE is also approved for use as destination therapy. During implantation, the in-flow cannula is sewn to the ventricular apex and the out-flow cannula is sewn to the aorta. In-flow and out-flow valves as well as internal surfaces are covered with a material which alleviates the need for systemic anticoagulation. The driveline is the only portion of the device that is external to the body. **(B)** Schematic demonstrating necessary components of portable ventricular assist devices system. This device is capable of pumping up to 10 L/min, and its pump rate can be adjusted to either a fixed-rate mode or a variable-rate mode, depending on the body's needs. Each battery lasts up to six hours, and patients carry multiple batteries at a time. The device weighs approximately 1200 g (2.6 pounds). *Abbreviation*: LVAD, left ventricular assist device. *Source*: Courtesy of Thoratec Corporation, Pleasanton, California, U.S.A.

to cover all surfaces of the heart, and provides passive support to help reduce stress on the ventricular wall with prevention of subsequent ventricular dilatation. Biventricular pacing has been shown to improve quality-of-life measures, New York Heart Association functional class, and maximal exercise performance at follow-up of six months in patients with severe heart failure (93). Novel techniques in gene transfection are being developed to improve myocardial cellular dysfunction. Likewise, muscle cells have been injected into damaged myocardium to improve cardiac function (94).

Mechanical VADs have gained widespread popularity, used both as a bridge to transplantation for patients *in extremis* as well in nontransplant candidates as end therapy (referred to as *destination therapy*). This type of mechanical support is expected to assume an even larger role in the management of heart failure in the future. Initially developed in the 1960s, VADs have undergone significant evolution to gain their current FDA approval. A multicenter trial in the early 1990s demonstrated a 65% survival to transplantation in CHF patients after implantation of VAD compared to 50% survival to transplantation in medically treated patients (95). On the basis of this and other studies, the FDA approved the use of left VADs as a "bridge" to transplantation in 1994. Encouraging initial results of the Randomized Evaluation of Mechanical Assistance Therapy as an Alternative in Congestive Heart Failure trial—in which VADs were placed into CHF patients as "destination" therapy—led to the 2002 FDA approval for VADs to be used for this indication, no longer just as a bridge to transplantation (Fig. 12). Current areas of improvement in VAD design focus on minimizing risk of thromboembolism, reducing postoperative VAD-related infections, and prevention of mechanical device failure. In the arena of heart replacement therapy, the Abiocor (ABIOMED, Danvers, Massachussets, U.S.A.) totally implantable total artificial heart has achieved good initial results, but more widespread, long-term use is dependent on further reduction in the thromboembolism risk.

CARDIAC DYSRHYTHMIAS

Cardiac function can be adversely influenced by changes in both cardiac rhythm and cardiac rate, but in actuality,

perturbations in CO are more commonly rate related. Healthy individuals in sinus rhythm have a frequency of cardiac contraction that can vary considerably. In optimally physically conditioned individuals, resting heart rates may be as low as 40 to 50 beats/min (bpm), although most healthy persons range from 60 to 90 bpm. Cardiac rate can vary across a wide range (40 to 150 bpm) without eliciting symptoms. With the induction of exercise, however, symptoms generally occur at each end of this spectrum, and especially in individuals with underlying cardiovascular pathology. Although dysrhythmias can generally be managed medically, certain situations may necessitate surgical intervention.

Bradycardias

In patients with symptomatic bradycardia, implantation of a pacemaker may be indicated to increase the heart rate. The common types of symptomatic bradycardia include (i) congenital heart block, (ii) acquired heart block, (iii) iatrogenic heart block, (iv) sick sinus syndrome, (v) AF, and (vi) bradycardia–tachycardia syndrome.

Patients with congenital heart blocks are frequently free of symptoms because the heart is in other respects structurally and functionally normal. As the child enters adolescence and early adulthood, maintenance of adequate exercise tolerance may require pacemaker implantation. In elderly patients, in whom acquired heart block usually occurs, ischemic heart disease is commonly the underlying etiology. Symptoms may be evoked with minimal exercise and occasionally arise even under resting conditions. Acquired heart block is a common cause of syncope (Stokes–Adams attacks). Sudden cardiac death may occur in this situation as the rhythm degenerates into asystole as a result of the development of ventricular escape beats from the block and the resultant ventricular tachycardia and fibrillation.

Because the arterial supply to the atrioventricular node is derived from a branch of the RCA, acute MI resulting from occlusion of this artery may give rise to heart block. This occurs because the resultant ischemia from the coronary occlusion alters the normal function of the atrioventricular node. Although the heart block associated with acute MI usually resolves, these patients are candidates for prophylactic, temporary pacemakers. Occasionally, permanent pacing is required.

In patients undergoing repair of damaged valves or septal defects, or complex intra-atrial repairs associated with congenital heart disease, postoperative heart block may occur. Not uncommonly, such blockade does not manifest immediately after operation. Because cardiac surgeons have encountered this situation with sufficient frequency, temporary pacing wires are routinely placed in these patients at the time of surgery, so that external pacing can be administered rapidly should circumstances necessitate this approach.

Chronic sinus bradycardia is typically referred to as the sick sinus syndrome. In this condition, heart rates in the range of 30 to 40 bpm are characteristic. Although sudden cardiac death is much less likely than with complete heart block, the symptoms are essentially the same. The bradycardia is usually regular but can on occasion be irregular, and it typically occurs in older patients, many of whom have ischemic heart disease, although this is not a requirement for the syndrome to occur. Permanent pacing is usually required in patients with this condition.

Although chronic AF is effectively managed medically in most patients, significant bradycardia can at times occur, necessitating pacemaker placement. It must be confirmed, however, that the bradycardia is not related to digitalis toxicity before a pacemaker is placed. This can be determined by stopping the digoxin therapy to see whether the bradycardia is resolved.

In patients with the bradycardia–tachycardia syndrome, profound episodes of supraventricular tachycardia requiring digoxin prophylaxis produce profound symptomatic bradycardia related to the digoxin therapy necessary to manage tachycardia. The explanation for this effect is not clear, but the treatment of this syndrome requires the placement of a pacemaker to enable the administration of sufficient doses of digoxin to manage the tachycardia.

Pacemaker Placement

When pacemakers were first introduced approximately 40 years ago to manage cardiac dysrhythmias, they were placed in the left side of the chest through a formal thoracotomy. The pacemakers were large and heavy, and the pacing leads were sutured to the ventricular myocardium. Furthermore, the batteries needed to operate these pacemakers were generally short lived and required replacement at least every two years, often more frequently. In addition, the lead systems were undependable. Much progress has been made in the development of pacemakers during the last several decades, so that current pacemakers approach the size and weight of a silver dollar, use lithium batteries that have life spans of 10 or more years, and possess lead systems that are remarkably dependable.

Current pacemaker management makes use of both epicardial and endocardial methodologies. Epicardial insertion employs a subxiphoid approach to the pericardium in which the lead is screwed into the undersurface of the right ventricle, and the battery box itself is implanted subcutaneously, usually in the left upper abdominal quadrant. This technique requires general anesthesia for the lead placement, but the battery box can easily be replaced with local anesthesia. The endocardial approach employs a catheter system that uses the cephalic, subclavian, or jugular vein, through which the catheter tip is advanced and impacted into the apex of the right ventricle. In this circumstance, the battery box is implanted in a subcutaneous pocket inferior to the clavicle. Compared with the epicardial approach, this strategy of pacemaker management is less dependable,

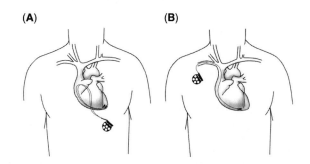

Figure 13 Schematic representation of the two approaches currently used for pacemaker placement. **(A)** Epicardial approach employs subxiphoid access in which pacemaker lead is secured to undersurface of right ventricle, and battery box is implanted subcutaneously in left upper abdominal quadrant. **(B)** Endocardial approach uses subclavian (or cephalic or jugular) vein for access, in which pacemaker tip is impacted into apex of right ventricle, and battery box is implanted subcutaneously inferior to clavicle.

requires more time to position the pacemaker, and is associated with a small but real hazard of perforating the right ventricle. Its major advantage with respect to the epicardial approach is that it can be carried out entirely with local anesthesia. These two approaches are schematically represented in Figure 13.

A wide variety of pacemakers are presently available. Despite their current level of sophistication compared with older models, they all fire on "demand" when they do not sense a QRS complex. They all have the capability to be programmed for such modalities as rate, size of electrical impulse, and sensing level after implantation. In recent years, there has been a trend toward dual-chamber pacemakers that pace the atria and ventricles sequentially, as well as pacemakers that sense changes in the native sinus rate (in response to a stimulus such as exercise), and thereby change the rate of ventricular firing. These newer systems, although expensive, have been demonstrated to be extremely beneficial in the vast majority of pacemaker candidates, particularly for patients with exercise intolerance or chronic CHF.

Not all patients with dysrhythmias require cardiac pacemaker implantation. Absolute indications for pacemaker implantation include third-degree or advanced second-degree AV block associated with symptomatic bradycardia, asystolic episodes greater than three seconds or an escape rate less than 40 bpm, or following catheter ablation of AV node (96,97). Relative indications include asymptomatic third-degree bloc and asymptomatic type II second-degree AV block with a narrow QRS complex (96,97). Guidelines for the use of pacemakers are summarized in Table 4.

Tachycardias

In addition to problems with bradycardia, tachycardias can also pose difficulties that may require surgical intervention, if medical management is not efficacious.

Supraventricular Tachycardias

Supraventricular arrhythmias, the most common rhythm disturbances encountered in surgical practice, usually occur in the postoperative period. Typical arrhythmias of this variety include atrial flutter, paroxysmal atrial tachycardia, and

Table 4   Guidelines for Cardiac Pacemaker Implantation

Accepted
In patients with symptoms and chronic conditions
    Atrioventricular block
        Complete (third-degree)
        Incomplete (second-degree)
            Mobitz type I (rare indication)
            Mobitz type II
        Incomplete with 2:1 or 3:1 block
    Sinus node dysfunction (symptomatic)
        Sinus bradycardia
        Sinoatrial block, sinus arrest
        Bradycardia–tachycardia syndrome
Controversial
In patients with symptoms
    Bifascicular/trifascicular intraventricular block
    Hypersensitive carotid sinus syndrome
In patients without symptoms
    Third-degree block
    Second-degree atrioventricular block Mobitz type II
    Transient complete or Mobitz type II atrioventricular block with
        bundle-branch block in selected situations (e.g., acute myocardial
        infarction)
    Congenital atrioventricular block
    Sinus bradycardia with heart rates < 45 beats/min, with long-term drug
        therapy necessary
    Overdrive pacing for ventricular tachycardia
Not warranted
    Syncope of undetermined cause
    Sinus bradycardia, sinoatrial block, or sinus arrest without symptoms
    Bundle-branch blocks
    Mobitz type I block (asymptomatic)

Source: From Ref. 98.

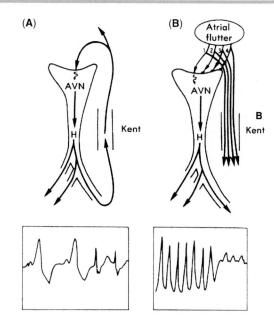

Figure 14   Two tachycardias found in patients with Wolff-Parkinson-White syndrome are shown. (**A**) Reentry type. The wide QRS of preexcitation changes to a narrow QRS during the reentry tachycardia (*box*). (**B**) Fast ventricular response during atrial flutter. The rhythm strip shows the rapid ventricular response progressing to ventricular fibrillation (*box*). *Source*: From Ref. 99.

AF. The diagnosis of these dysrhythmias is made with ECG testing. Most of these disturbances can be managed medically with drugs such as digoxin, β-blockers, calcium channel blockers, and amiodarone, or with combinations of these agents. On rare occasions, such medical management does not prove efficacious, and because of the rapid ventricular rate emanating from these dysrhythmias, emergency cardioversion is required.

A more worrisome supraventricular tachycardia that does not respond as well to medical management is the Wolff-Parkinson-White (WPW) syndrome. This disorder is caused by reentry of cardiac excitation impulses through an anomalous muscle bundle, known as the bundle of Kent, which connects the atrial and ventricular myocardia, that are normally electrically separate (Fig. 14). This bundle has been demonstrated in a variety of positions in the atrioventricular groove or junction of the atrial and ventricular septa, having been previously mapped experimentally. The seriousness of this condition is that the Kent bundle can conduct as many as 400 bpm with degeneration into ventricular responses characterized by tachycardia or fibrillation, with the potential for cardiac arrest. On ECG, patients with the WPW syndrome demonstrate a short PR interval (< 0.12 seconds) and small delta waves at the beginning of the QRS complex. Although a wide variety of antiarrhythmic drugs have been used to manage this syndrome (including procaine, quinidine, propranolol, verapamil, and amiodarone), such therapy has not proved especially successful. Fortunately, a means of ablating the Kent bundle surgically is now available. First introduced at Duke University in 1968, this modality has proved efficacious, and many patients treated with interruption of the Kent bundle have

had successful outcomes and have gone on to live normal lives (100). Recent experience with catheter-delivered radiofrequency ablation of the Kent bundle has also proved effective and has supplanted the surgical approach (101).

The success encountered with treating the WPW syndrome surgically has been extended to other mechanisms of tachycardia, such as concealed accessory connections, nodal and atrial tachycardia, and even refractory AF. Treatment of this last arrhythmia, the Cox-Maze procedure, consists of a series of atrial incisions to prevent atrial reentry and allow sinus node impulses to activate the entire atrial myocardium. In so doing, this procedure restores atrioventricular synchrony. This procedure has been reported to have an operative mortality of 2% and to have cured AF in 99% of cases (102). There is a significant occurrence of temporary postoperative AF (38%) and need for pacemaker implantation (15%). More recently, microwave energy and radiofrequency energy have been used intraoperatively in the treatment of AF to create lines of conduction blockade, which mimic the standard Maze incisions, but without the degree of morbidity seen with that procedure. These newer procedures have been observed to cure AF in 70% to 80% of cases (103). Perioperative AF occurs in over 60% of cases, and 30% to 40% of patients leave the hospital in AF, but this does not appear to be long-lasting and patients subsequently convert to sinus rhythm over the ensuing three to four postoperative months. Instrumentation is currently being tested, which will allow these procedures to be performed with less morbidity in an epicardial, thoracoscopic fashion.

Ventricular Tachycardia

Ventricular dysrhythmias are much more serious than supraventricular tachycardias because of the rate-induced depression of CO that can degenerate into life-threatening ventricular fibrillation. Most patients with sustained ventricular tachycardias have significant ischemic heart disease and have had one or more MIs, resulting in varying degrees of both reversible and nonreversible ischemic damage. Among patients surviving MI, significant ventricular tachycardias may occur in as many as 5%. Despite the recent development of new antiarrhythmic drugs, approximately one-third of patients with ventricular tachycardia do not have adequate control with them.

In this subset of patients, "mapping" the various areas of the epicardium and endocardium, which induce ventricular tachycardias electrically, and then resecting this area has proved efficacious in controlling the ventricular dysrhythmias (104–106). The mapped areas usually comprise subendocardial scar tissue that, from a surgical standpoint, are relatively easy to resect unless vital structures such as the mitral apparatus, membranous septum, and aortic annulus are involved in the scarred area. In such cases, local cryoablation has been substituted and proved useful.

Although the risk associated with this type of surgery is substantial, it is directly related to the degree of left ventricular function. The less dysfunction, the better is the outcome. As many as 70% to 80% of patients surviving this type of surgery have relief of their tachycardia without the need for further drug therapy or have substantial reduction in the drug requirements to manage their ventricular dysrhythmias.

Implantable Cardioverterdefibrillator

Patients who have had a documented cardiac arrest (sudden cardiac death syndrome) in the absence of a documented MI within the preceding 48 hours and who are not candidates for antiarrhythmic drug therapy, as documented by electrophysiologic study, should have an implantable cardioverter-defibrillator (ICD) implanted (106–108). This device, which is similar in size to a pacemaker, is implanted to sustain any cardioversions for several years.

Candidates for ICD placement usually have severe coronary artery disease and prior MI. The infarction zone provides the scarring and slow conduction needed for the re-entrant arrhythmias (ventricular tachycardia or ventricular fibrillation). As expected, this patient population is in extremely debilitated condition, with low ejection fractions and chronic CHF. Consequently, these patients are good candidates for ICD insertion, rather than long-term antiarrhythmic drug therapy, which is associated with negative inotropic effects and other morbid drug reactions. This type of therapy is extremely expensive ($12,000 to $20,000 per generator; $2000 to $8000 per lead system). It is, however, worthwhile for selected individuals at high risk, as it has been shown in selected patients to decrease one-year mortality from 90% to 10%.

Evaluation of Pacemakers Before Attempting Surgery

In patients about to undergo general anesthesia and surgery, it is mandatory that the surgical and anesthesia teams determine that the pacemaker is sensing and functioning normally. After the pacemaker has been properly identified, the currently active program can be retrieved by interrogation with the manufacturer's programmer. The first issue is to identify whether the patient is pacemaker dependent. If the pacemaker fails, does it have a dependable and adequate intrinsic rhythm? If the answer to this question is no or cannot be determined because the pacemaker is not programmable, a backup method of maintaining a heart rate must be defined. This is particularly important because electrocautery can induce pacemaker failure. Most pacemaker manufacturers recommend against the use of electrocautery in any patient without an adequate intrinsic rhythm. Unipolar cautery is far more hazardous than bipolar cautery. Electrocautery can, by its noise level, be misinterpreted by the pacemaker and cause inhibition of the pacemaker that is reversible when the cautery is turned off. Thus, frequently, electrocautery can cause the pacemaker to revert to a backup mode. This usually is a ventricular demand mode. The most severe problem the electrocautery may cause is complete and permanent loss of pacing. The best way to manage a pacemaker during the use of electrocautery is to program the generator to ventricular demand mode at a rate sufficient to minimize competition with the intrinsic heart rate (109). The simplest way to achieve this is to place a permanent magnet over the pacemaker. This prevents inhibition by electrocautery.

If a permanent loss of pacemaker function occurs in the operating room, with no intrinsic heart rate, the quickest and most efficient method of inducing an intrinsic rate is to begin intravenous infusion of a β-stimulant such as isoproterenol. After this maneuver, a temporary transvenous pacemaker should be inserted.

PERICARDIAL DISEASE

The pericardium is a fibrous sac that surrounds and envelops the heart. Its purpose is to fix the heart anatomically within the mediastinum, act as a barrier to the spread of infection from surrounding structures such as the lungs, and reduce friction between the enclosed heart and surrounding organs (110). In the nondiseased state, the pericardium has little or no effect on cardiac hemodynamics. Two specific pericardial disorders, however, may necessitate surgical intervention. These include pericardial effusion with tamponade and chronic constrictive pericarditis.

Pericardial Effusion with Tamponade

Pericardial effusion by itself is not uncommon. It can occur in response to acute viral pericarditis, MI, CHF, and various immune disorders such as rheumatoid arthritis and lupus erythematosus. In these conditions, the effusion is usually moderate and self-limited, and it abates with treatment of the underlying condition. In patients with chronic uremic pericarditis or malignant involvement of the pericardium, such as may occur from neoplastic spread of bronchogenic carcinoma, excessive amounts of effusion may collect in the pericardial sac so that adverse stresses are placed on the contracting heart, and cardiac dynamics are severely impaired. This state of pericardial tamponade can significantly compress the heart, not only by compressing the great veins and atria with substantial reduction of venous return to the ventricles but also by impeding the optimal filling of the ventricles during diastole, so that CO is severely depressed despite normal systolic function.

The fluid accumulating in the pericardial sac that gives rise to tamponade may be serous or sanguineous, depending on the underlying cause. Inflammatory disorders, such as viral infections or immune diseases, usually result in a serous fluid. Liquid or clotted blood within the pericardium is commonly associated with uremic pericarditis as well as with malignant pericardial involvement. Occasionally, the pericardial sac fills with blood after cardiac surgery, but this is rare with modern cardiovascular procedures if proper postoperative drainage techniques are employed. Cardiac trauma from penetrating injury, and rarely from blunt trauma, may also produce pericardial tamponade. In these settings, the pericardium is normal and a relatively small volume of blood (as little as 150–200 mL) may produce the tamponade, in contrast to those sustaining tamponade from more chronic pericardial disease, in which the volume may approach 1 L or more of fluid before symptoms develop. Although uncommon, trauma from within the heart as a result of a perforating transvenous pacemaker lead, the placement of a central venous pressure, or Swan–Ganz catheter can produce unsuspected tamponade. Thus, any patient who becomes hypotensive for unknown reasons in the presence of one of these devices may have a cardiac perforation.

The clinical presentation of pericardial tamponade is usually characterized by a triad of physical signs, including arterial hypotension, increased jugular venous pressure, and distant (or muffled) heard sounds. Facial cyanosis may also be present, as well as a paradoxic pulse. This latter sign is a drop in arterial blood pressure of 10 mmHg or more with inspiration. It is usually an exaggeration of the normal response to ventilation and is distinctly more prominent in individuals subjected to positive-pressure ventilation.

In patients with suspected pericardial tamponade, management depends on "how tight" the effusion is. This tightness is reflected in the degree of hypotension and elevation of venous pressure from the tamponade. In individuals with only moderate tamponade, a Valsalva maneuver is helpful in determining its seriousness. If palpable radial pulses are not lost with a Valsalva maneuver, the situation is not critical. Another useful approach to determine the seriousness of the tamponade is to test a patient's blood pressure response to a rapid infusion of intravenous fluid. If the tamponade is only moderate, a significant rise in arterial blood pressure should occur from this fluid bolus; in contrast, more serious degrees of tamponade blunt this response. The presence of an unexplained supraventricular dysrhythmia is a sign of significant tamponade and of the potential for incipient circulatory failure, especially if intermittent sinus arrest exists. It is essential in the analysis of suspected pericardial effusion that an echocardiogram be obtained. This modality is extremely useful in patients with pericardial effusions and potential pericardial tamponade. An echocardiogram can determine the location and characteristics of the fluid (loculated or free floating) and also ascertain to a reasonable extent whether the pericardial tamponade is of physiologic significance. In addition, it can be used to guide the insertion of a needle into the pericardial space to aspirate fluid, especially if this is deemed to be the appropriate treatment.

Once significant tamponade has been deemed to exist, fluid drainage may be accomplished percutaneously by pericardiocentesis with either a needle or catheter placement (Fig. 15). Alternatively, surgical intervention through a subxiphoid pericardial window can be performed. Situations in which traumatic hemopericardium exists require a sternotomy or thoracotomy for optimal management. It needs to be emphasized that if the tamponade is considered to be of only modest proportions and is not life threatening, great care should be taken to determine the benefit of the pericardiocentesis. This technique, although useful in urgent tamponade, can result in cardiac puncture and actually worsen the situation.

An important principle in managing a patient with tamponade is that endotracheal intubation should be

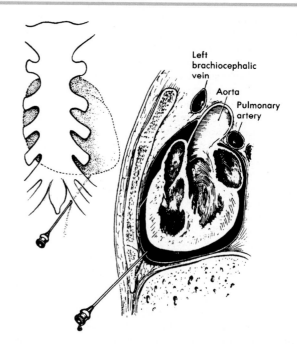

Figure 15 For pericardiocentesis, a 16-gauge plastic-sheathed needle is introduced beneath the costal margin and passed through the properitoncal fat and into the pericardial cavity through the tendinous part of the diaphragm. *Source*: From Ref. 111.

avoided. The reason for this is that positive-pressure ventilation frequently causes cardiac arrest in individuals with significant tamponade. Consequently, preparation and draping in the operating room should be carried out prior to induction of anesthesia and intubation, so that rapid decompression may be achieved in the event that it becomes necessary.

A generous subxiphoid window, instead of formal pericardiectomy, is usually adequate to decompress the pericardial sac in patients with uremic or malignant pericardial tamponade. After removal of the xiphoid cartilage, the pericardium is opened between two silk stitches and the window is created. The fluid is aspirated and sent for appropriate cultures, while the pericardium is formally sampled for biopsy. An angled chest tube is placed within the pericardial cavity along the diaphragmatic surface and exits through a separate stab-wound incision in the skin. This tube is removed when the drainage ceases. Although pericardial effusions can recur after subxiphoid window, this is distinctly uncommon.

Chronic Constrictive Pericarditis

Chronic constrictive pericarditis is the other condition of surgical significance involving the pericardium. This form of pericarditis is produced in response to chronic infectious tuberculosis and histoplasmosis, various collagen-vascular diseases, and, less commonly, after what appears to be uncomplicated cardiac surgery or MI, with the development of Dressler's syndrome (characterized by fever, pericardial friction rub and pain, and often pericardial effusion). The pericardial–epicardial scarring can be severe, with obliteration of the pericardial space, thickening of the pericardium (sometimes as much a 1 in. or more), and severe fibrosis and calcifications in which calcific deposits may actually grow in the myocardium. Pathophysiologically, this massive pericardial thickening induces several aberrations, including obstruction of venous return with severe diastolic cardiac dysfunction. Physical signs attendant on this condition are similar to those of severe CHF with elevated venous pressure, edema, hepatomegaly, and ascites. If calcification is not apparent on chest radiography, the diagnosis may not be evident. Cardiac catheterization is usually diagnostic. This latter modality usually shows small ventricular cavities, diastolic pressures within 5 mmHg of each other, jugular venous distention with measured mean arterial pressures above 10 mmHg, and the typical "dip and plateau" pattern of diastolic right ventricular pressure (the square-root sign).

Because surgical management of chronic constrictive pericarditis can be difficult and dangerous, and it may tax the skill of the most accomplished cardiac surgeon, a median sternotomy incision should be used with cardiopulmonary bypass (112). The absence of an epicardial–pericardial plane can make this procedure bloody. Therefore, a cell saver and aprotinin should be employed. Careful attention must be paid to freeing the atria and vena cavae as well as the ventricles, with recognition of the fact that the visceral pericardial layer may be as important as the parietal layer. This visceral pericardiectomy is complicated by the occasional "invasion" of the ventricular myocardium itself by calcific deposits. The pericardium should be removed from the phrenic nerve anteriorly, but it also should be removed posterior to the phrenic nerve. Complete removal of the constricting pericardium restores the left ventricular pressure–volume loop to normal or nearly normal. Operative mortality rate for this procedure ranges between 10% and 20%, and is adversely influenced by the severity of heart failure, elevation of right atrial pressure, and comorbid disease. Long-term results are poorest in patients with radiation pericarditis, and in all cases results vary primarily in proportion to the preoperative severity of heart failure.

CARDIAC TUMORS

The most common tumor of the heart is a metastatic neoplasm. Approximately 10% to 20% of patients who die of disseminated cancer have cardiac metastases (113,114). The most common tumors to metastasize to the heart are from leukemia (50% of the patients have cardiac metastases), breast cancer, lung cancer, lymphoma, and melanoma. Metastatic disease to the heart usually does not warrant surgical intervention, except if it is associated with pericardial effusion and tamponade. Pericardial drainage is best accomplished in these terminally ill patients through subxiphoid pericardiotomy. This operation is performed with local anesthesia and provides reliable relief of symptoms, a recurrence rate of 3%, and minimal morbidity.

Primary tumors of the heart are rare. The incidence ranges between 0.002% and 0.19%. Approximately 75% of primary cardiac tumors are benign, and 15% of these are myxomas (113,114). Although myxomas can arise in any cardiac chamber, 90% occur in the atria; 75% are observed in the left atrium, and 15% to 20% are found in the right atrium. Myxomas are distinctly rare in children. The peak incidence is the third to fourth decade of life, they are more common in women than in men, and 94% are solitary. About 5% of myxomas are familial, with an autosomal dominant inheritance. Familial patients tend to be younger, are equally likely to be male or female, and frequently have multicentric tumors. Most important, familial myxomas have the highest recurrence rate (20–60%).

Atrial myxomas arise from the interatrial septum near the oval fossa. Right atrial myxomas are most common in women and are broad based. Left atrial tumors are round, lobulated, gelatinous, and frequently pedunculated with a stalk. Consequently, they are quite mobile. Their color is usually white or yellow–brown, and they frequently are covered with thrombus. The average size is 5 cm. Myxomas arise from endocardium, not from a thrombotic origin as was formerly speculated. Myxomas have developed after cardiac trauma, especially atrial septal defect closure.

Constitutional symptoms include weight loss, fever, and lethargy. This clinical presentation is associated with leukocytosis, elevated sedimentation rate, thrombocytopenia, and elevated C-reactive protein. Immunoglobulin G levels and interleukin-6 are also elevated.

Clinical presentation is related most commonly to obstruction to blood flow within the heart. Left atrial myxomas mimic mitral stenosis or, less commonly, mitral regurgitation. Right atrial myxomas produce features of right heart failure, including venous distention, ascites, hepatomegaly, and peripheral edema.

Systemic embolization, the second most common mode of presentation, occurs in 30% to 40% of patients. Most commonly the tumor embolus goes into an intracranial vessel, producing a transient ischemic attack or complete stroke. Less commonly, embolization to the lower extremity occurs. Histologic examination of surgically removed peripheral emboli can establish a diagnosis of an otherwise unsuspected tumor.

The most useful diagnostic test is echocardiography, which establishes a diagnosis in nearly every case (115). Transesophageal echocardiography is particularly sensitive to detect small tumors, and it can be useful in the operating room to make certain that the entire mass has been removed.

Surgical resection employs cardiopulmonary bypass and bicaval cannulation, with care taken to avoid manipulation of the heart because myxomas are friable and can embolize (116,117). After aortic cross-clamping and cardioplegic arrest, the left atrium is opened widely, and the location of the myxoma is determined. In most cases, it is attached with a stalk to the interatrial septum. A second incision in the right atrium allows excision of the stalk with the atrial septum, followed by gentle removal of the mass through the left atrium. The surgically created atrial septal defect is closed with autologous pericardium. The operative mortality rate is 1% to 3%, and the recurrence rate in nonfamilial cases is 1% to 5%.

SUMMARY

Aberrations in normal cardiac function can occur when disease adversely affects cardiac rate and rhythm, the efficiency of cardiac pumping, and the optimization of cardiac loading. Acting either alone or in various combinations, derangements in each of these physiologic mechanisms can seriously affect circulatory dynamics, affecting the entire process whereby adequate delivery of oxygen and nutrients maintains cellular health and function. Although some acquired cardiac defects lend themselves to nonsurgical management strategies, in many situations the cardiac surgeon plays a key role in restoring normal cardiac physiology. As reviewed in this chapter, in most instances, ischemic heart disease, valvular heart disease, and heart failure are managed initially through medical therapy but with a reliance on surgical approaches when the initial approach fails or when the pathophysiology dictates an initial surgical approach as with left main coronary artery disease in ischemic syndromes or acute valve failure as seen with papillary muscle rupture. In addition, new technologies are emerging, which will prove increasingly useful in the surgical management of virtually all acquired cardiac disorders, from the realm of arrhythmias to ischemic heart disease, to valvular heart disease, and perhaps most dramatically, now in the treatment of end-stage CHF, where immunology and technical advances can add years to the lives of people who previously faced a terminal prognosis. Whether through a medical or surgical approach, the goal of the cardiac specialist is to restore cardiac function to enable adequate delivery of oxygen to the body. Increasingly, the treatment of cardiac disorders is involving a partnership among all disciplines with the traditional lines between surgery and medicine becoming increasingly blurred.

REFERENCES

1. Peter RH. Coronary arteriography. In: Sabiston DC Jr, Spencer FC, eds. Gibbon's Surgery of the Chest. 4th ed. Philadelphia: WB Saunders, 1983.
2. Berne RM. The role of adenosine in the regulation of coronary blood flow. Circ Res 1980; 47:807.
3. Robertson RM, et al. Thromboxane A2 in vasotonic angina pectoris. N Engl J Med 1981; 304:998.
4. Glomset JA, Ross R. Atherosclerosis and the arterial smooth muscle cell. Science 1973; 180:1332.
5. McGill H. Risk factors for atherosclerosis. Adv Exp Med Biol 1977; 104:273.
6. The Lipid Research Clinics Program. The Lipid Research Clinics coronary primary prevention trial results: II. The relationship of reduction in incidence of coronary heart disease to cholesterol lowering. JAMA 1984; 251:365.
7. Scheuner MT. Genetic predisposition to coronary artery disease. Curr Opin Cardiol 2001; 16(4):251–260.
8. Dimitrova KR, DeGroot K, Myers AK, Kim YD. Estrogen and homocysteine. Cardiovasc Res 2002; 15(3):577–588.
9. Nieman K, Cademartiri F, Lemos PA, et al. Reliable non-invasive coronary angiography with fast submillimeter multislice spiral computed tomography. Circulation 2002; 106(16): 2051–2054.
10. Yang PC, Meyer CH, Terashima M, et al. Spiral magnetic coronary angiography with rapid real-time localization. J Am Coll Cardiol 2003; 41(7):1134–1141.
11. Vaughan CJ, Gotto AM, Basson CT. The evolving role of statins in the management of atherosclerosis. J Am Coll Cardiol 2000; 35(1):1–10.
12. Wilson JD, et al. Harrison's Principles of Internal Medicine. New York: McGraw-Hill, 1990:957.
13. Flaherty JT, et al. A randomized prospective trial of intravenous nitroglycerin in patients with acute myocardial infarction. Circulation 1976; 54:766.
14. ACE Inhibitor Myocardial Infarction Collaborative Group. Indications for ACE inhibitors in the early treatment of acute myocardial infarction: systemic overview of individual data from 100,000 patients in randomized trials. Circulation 1998; 97:2202–2212.
15. Ryan TJ, Antman EM, Brooks NH, et al. 1999 Update: ACC/AHA guidelines for the management of patients with acute myocardial infarction, executive summary and recommendations. A report of the American College of Cardiology/American Heart Association Task Force on Practice Guidelines (Committee on Management of Acute Myocardial Infarction). Circulation 1999; 100:1016–1030.
16. European Cooperative Study Group for Streptokinase Treatment in Acute Myocardial Infarction. Streptokinase in acute myocardial infarction. N Engl J Med 1979; 301:797.
17. Fry ETA, Sobel BE. Coronary thrombosis. Prog Cardiol 1990; 2:199.
18. Tiefenbrunn AJ, Sobel BE. The impact of coronary thrombolysis on myocardial infarction. Fibrinolysis 1989; 3:1.
19. CURE trial investigators. Effects of clopidogrel in addition to aspirin in patients with acute coronary syndromes without ST-segment elevation. N Engl J Med 2001; 345:494–502.
20. TIMI Study Group. Results of thrombolysis in myocardial infarction (TIMI) phase II trial. N Engl J Med 1989; 320:618.
21. Maisel AS, et al. Prognosis after extension of myocardial infarct: the role of W wave on non-Q wave infarction. Circulation 1985; 71:211.
22. Allen BS, et al. Studies on prolonged acute regional ischemia IV. Myocardial infarction with left ventricular failure. J Thorac Cardiovasc Surg 1989; 98:691.
23. Daggett WM, et al. Improved results of surgical management of postinfarction ventricular septal rupture. Ann Surg 1982; 196:269.
24. King SB III, Talley JD. Coronary arteriography and percutaneous transluminal coronary angioplasty: changing patterns of use and results. Circulation 1989; 79(suppl 1):19.
25. Teirstein PS, Massuillo V, Jani S, et al. Catheter-based radiotherapy to inhibit restenosis after coronary stenting. N Engl J Med 1997; 336:1697–1703.
26. Morice MC, Serruys PW, Sousa JE, et al. A randomized comparison of a sirolimus-eluting stent with a standard stent for coronary revascularization. N Engl J Med 2002; 346: 1773–1780.
27. Steinhubl SR, Berger PB, Mann JT III, et al. Early and sustained dual oral antiplatelet therapy following percutaneous coronary intervention: a randomized controlled trial. JAMA 2002; 288:2411–2420.
28. Myers WO, et al. Medical versus early surgical therapy in patients with triple-vessel disease and mild angina pectoris: a CASS registry study of survival. Ann Thorac Surg 1987; 44:471.
29. Detre KM, et al. Long-term mortality and morbidity results of the Veterans Administration randomized trial of coronary artery bypass surgery. Circulation 1985; 72(suppl 5):84.
30. Varnauskas E. The European Coronary Surgery Study Group. Twelve-year follow-up of survival in the randomized European coronary surgery study. N Engl J Med 1988; 319:332.
31. Cameron A, Davis KB, Green G, et al. Coronary bypass surgery with internal thoracic artery grafts—effect on survival over a 15 year period. N Engl J Med 1996; 334:216–219.
32. Lytle BW, Blackstone EH, Loop FD, et al. Two internal thoracic artery grafts are better than one. J Thorac Cardiovasc Surg 1999; 117:855–872.
33. Nose Y. The Oxygenator. Vol. 2. St. Louis: Mosby, 1973.
34. Gundry SR, et al. Retrograde continuous warm blood cardioplegia: maintenance of myocardial homeostasis in humans. Ann Thorac Surg 1993; 55:358.
35. Whitman GJ, Hart JC, Crestanello JA, et al. Uniform safety of beating heart surgery using the octopus tissue stabilization system. J Card Surg 1999; 14(5):323–329.
36. Puskas JD, Williams MH, Duke PG, et al. Off-pump coronary artery bypass grafting provides complete revascularization with reduced myocardial injury, transfusion requirements, and length of stay: a prospective randomized comparison of two hundred unselected patients undergoing off-pump versus conventional coronary artery bypass grafting. J Thorac Cardiovasc Surg 2003; 125(4):797–808.
37. Rose EA. Are there advantages to off-pump coronary artery bypass surgery? N Engl J Med 2003; 348(5):379–380.
38. Gardlund B, Bitkover CY, Vaage J. Post-operative mediastinitis in cardiac surgery—microbiology and pathogenesis. Eur J Cardiothorac Surg 2002; 21(5):825–830.
39. Grove FL, et al. Factors predictive of operative mortality among coronary artery bypass subsets. Ann Thorac Surg 1993; 56:1296.

40. Barbir M, et al. Coronary artery surgery in women compared with men: analysis of coronary risk factors and in-hospital mortality in a single centre. Br Heart J 1994; 71:408.

41. Lyde BW, et al. The effect of coronary reoperation on the survival of patients with stenoses in saphenous vein bypass grafts to coronary arteries. J Thorac Cardiovasc Surg 1993; 105:605.

42. Braunwald E, Rutherford JD. Reversible ischemic left ventricular dysfunction: evidence for the hibernating myocardium. J Am Coll Cardiol 1986; 8:1467.

43. Aaberge L, Rootwelt K, Blomhoff S, et al. Continued symptomatic improvement three to five years after transmyocardial revascularization with CO_2 laser. J Am Coll Cardiol 2002; 39:1588–1593.

44. Yeager M. Comparison of Doppler derived pressure gradient to that determined at cardiac catheterization in adults with aortic valve stenosis: implications for management. In: Weyman AE, ed. Principles and Practice of Electrocardiography. Philadelphia: Lea & Febiger, 1994:525.

45. Gorlin R, Gorlin SG. Hydraulic formula for calculation of area of stenotic mitral valve, other cardiac valves, and central circulatory shunts. Am Heart J 1951; 41:1.

46. Lombard JT, Selzer A. Valvular aortic stenosis. Clinical and hemodynamic profile of patients. Ann Intern Med 1987; 106:292.

47. Ross J, Braunwald E. Aortic stenosis. Circulation 1968; 38(suppl 5):v61.

48. Olesen KH, Warburg E. Isolated aortic stenosis—the late prognosis. Acta Med Scand 1957; 160:437.

49. Copeland JB, et al. Long-term follow-up after isolated aortic valve replacement. J Thorac Cardiovasc Surg 1977; 74:875.

50. Carabello BA, et al. Hemodynamic determinants of prognosis or aortic valve replacement in critical aortic stenosis and advanced congestive heart failure. Circulation 1980; 62:42.

51. Fifer MA, et al. Myocardial contractile function in the aortic stenosis as determined from the rate of stress development during isovolumic systole. Am J Cardiol 1979; 44:1318.

52. Kennedy JW, Doces J, Stewart DK. Left ventricular function before and following aortic valve replacement. Circulation 1977; 56:944.

53. Pantely G, Morton M, Rahimtoola SH. Effects of successful, uncomplicated valve replacement on ventricular hypertrophy, volume and performance in aortic stenosis and in aortic incompetence. J Thorac Cardiovasc Surg 1978; 75:383.

54. Miller DS, et al. Surgical implications and results of combined aortic valve replacement and myocardial revascularization. Am J Cardiol 1979; 43:494.

55. Safian RD, et al. Balloon aortic valvuloplasty in 170 consecutive patients. N Engl J Med 1988; 319:169.

56. Olson LJ, Subramanian R, Edwards WD. Surgical pathology of pure aortic insufficiency: a study of 225 cases. Mayo Clin Proc 1984; 59:835.

57. Grossman W. Cardiac Catheterization, Angiography, and Intervention. Philadelphia: Lea & Febiger, 1991.

58. Alpert JS. Chronic aortic regurgitation. In: Dalen JE, Alpert JS, eds. Valvular Heart Disease. 2nd ed. Boston: Little, Brown, 1987:283.

59. Rapaport E. Natural history of aortic and mitral valve disease. Am J Cardiol 1975; 35:221.

60. Borrow K, et al. End-systolic volume overload from valvular regurgitation. Am J Med 1980; 68:655.

61. Bonow RO, et al. Survival and function results after valve replacement for aortic regurgitation from 1976 to 1983: impact of preoperative left ventricular function. Circulation 1985; 72:1244.

62. Greves J, et al. Perioperative criteria predictive of late survival following valve replacement for severe aortic regurgitation. Am Heart J 1981; 101:300.

63. Lytle BW, et al. Replacement of aortic valve combined with myocardial revascularization: determinants of early and late risk for 500 patients, 1967–1981. Circulation 1983; 68:1149.

64. Rahimtoola SH. Choice of prosthetic heart valve for adult patients. J Am Coll Cardiol 2003; 41:893–904.

65. Rankin JS. Mitral and tricuspid valve disease. In: Sabiston DC Jr, ed. Textbook of Surgery: The Biological Basis of Modern Surgical Practice. 13th ed. Philadelphia: WB Saunders, 1992: 2026.

66. Braunwald E. Valvular heart disease. In: Braunwald E, ed. Heart Disease. A Textbook of Cardiovascular Medicine. Philadelphia: WB Saunders, 1992:1007.

67. Bowe JC, et al. Course of mitral stenosis without surgery: 10 and 20 year perspectives. Ann Intern Med 1960; 52:741.

68. Wallace AG. Pathophysiology of cardiovascular disease. In: Smith LH Jr. Thier SO, ed. Pathophysiology: The Biological Principles of Disease. The International Textbook of Medicine. Vol. 1. Philadelphia: WB Saunders, 1981:1192.

69. Thompson ME, Shaver JA, Leon DT. Effect of tachycardia on atrial transport in mitral stenosis. Am Heart J 1977; 94:297.

70. Olesen KH. The natural history of 271 patients with mitral stenosis under medical treatment. Br Heart J 1962; 24:349.

71. Munoz S, et al. Influence of surgery on the natural history of rheumatic mitral and aortic valve disease. Am J Cardiol 1975; 35:234.

72. Cutler EC, Levine SA. Cardiotomy and valvulotomy for mitral stenosis: experimental observations and clinical notes concerning an operated case with recovery. Boston Med Surg J 1923; 188:603.

73. Souttar HS. The surgical treatment of mitral stenosis. Br Med J 1925; 2:603.

74. Harken DE, et al. The surgical treatment of mitral stenosis. N Engl J Med 1948; 239:801.

75. Bailey CP. The surgical treatment of mitral stenosis (mitral commissurotomy). Dis Chest 1949; 15:377.

76. Ellis LB, Harken DE. Closed valvuloplasty for mitral stenosis. A twelve-year follow-up of 1571 patients. N Engl J Med 1964; 270:643.

77. Montoya A, et al. The advantages of open mitral commissurotomy for mitral stenosis. Chest 1979; 75:131.

78. Higgs LA, et al. Mitral restenosis: an uncommon cause of recurrent symptoms following mitral commissurotomy. Am J Cardiol 1970; 26:34.

79. Harken DE, et al. Reoperation for mitral stenosis. A discussion of postoperative deterioration and methods of improving mitral and secondary operation. Circulation 1961; 23:7.

80. Kirklin JW, Barrett-Boyes BG. Mitral valve disease without tricuspid valve disease. In: Cardiac Surgery. 2nd ed. New York: Churchill Livingstone, 1993:425.

81. Smith WM, et al. Open mitral valvotomy: effect of preoperative factors on result. J Thorac Cardiovasc Surg 1981; 82:738.

82. Inoue K, et al. Clinical application of transvenous mitral commissurotomy by a new balloon catheter. J Thorac Cardiovasc Surg 1984; 87:349.

83. Nishimura RA, Holmes DR Jr, Reeder GS. Percutaneous balloon valvuloplasty. Mayo Clinic Proc 1990; 65:198.

84. Tuzcu EM, Block PC, Palacios IF. Comparison of early versus late experience with percutaneous mitral balloon valvuloplasty. J Am Coll Cardiol 1991; 17:1121.

85. Block PC. Early results of mitral balloon valvuloplasty (MBV) for mitral stenosis: reports from the NHLBI Registry. Circulation 1978; 78(suppl 2):11489.

86. Nobuyoshi M, et al. Indications, complications and short-term clinical outcomes of percutaneous transvenous mitral commissurotomy. Circulation 1989; 80:782.

87. Roberts WC, et al. Nonrheumatic valvular cardiac disease. A clinicopathologic survey of 27 different conditions causing valvular dysfunction. Cardiovasc Clin 1973; 5:403.

88. Stapleton JF. Natural history of chronic valvular disease. In: Frankl WS, Brest AN, eds. Cardiovascular Clinics. Valvular Heart Disease: Comprehensive Evaluation and Management. Philadelphia: FA Davis, 1986:105.

89. Levy D, Kenchaiah S, Larson MG, et al. Long-term trends in the incidence of and survival with heart failure. N Engl J Med 2002; 347:1397–1402.

90. Sutton JCS. Epidemiologic aspects of heart failure. Am Heart J 1990; 120:1538–1540.

91. Levy D, Larson MG, Vasan RS, et al. The progression from hypertension to congestive heart failure. JAMA 1996; 275:1557–1562.

92. Bach DS, Boiling SF. Improvement following correction of secondary mitral regurgitation in end-stage cardiomyopathy with mitral annuloplasty. Am J Cardiol 1996; 78:966–969.

93. Ahbraham WT, Fisher WG, Smith Al, et al. Cardiac resynchronization in chronic heart failure. New Engl J Med 2002; 346:1845–1853.

94. Menasche P, Hagege AA, Vilquin JT, et al. Autologous skeletal myoblast transplantation for severe post-infarction left ventricular dysfunction. J Am Coll Cardiol 2003; 41(7):1078–1083.

95. Frazier OH, Rose EA, Macmanus Q, et al. Multicenter clinical evaluation of the Heartmate 1000 IP left ventricular assist device. Ann Thorac Surg 1992; 53:1080–1090.

96. American College of Cardiology/American Heart Association/NASPE Heart Rhythm Society. 2002 Guideline update for implantation of pacemakers and antiarrhythmia devices. J Am Coll Cardiol 2002; 40(9):1703–1719.

97. Belott PH, Reynolds DW. Permanent pacemaker implantation. In: Ellenbogen KA, Kay GN, Wilkoff BL, eds. Clinical Cardiac Pacing. Philadelphia: WB Saunders, 1995:447.

98. AMA Council on Scientific Affairs. The use of cardiac pacemakers in medical practice. JAMA 1985; 254:1952.

99. Sealy WC, Selle JG. Surgical treatment of supraventricular arrhythmias. In: Roberts AJ, Conti CR, eds. Current Surgery of the Heart. Philadelphia: JB Lippincott, 1987.

100. Sealy WC, Anderson RW, Gallagher JJ. Surgical treatment of supraventricular tachyarrhythmias. J Thorac Cardiovasc Surg 1977; 73:511.

101. Ellenbogen KA, Kay GN, Wilkoff BL, eds. Clinical Cardiac Pacing. Philadelphia: WB Saunders, 1995; Furman S, Schwedel JB. An intracardiac pacemaker for Stokes-Adams seizures. N Engl J Med 1959; 261:948.

102. Cox JL, Ad N, Palazzo T, et al. Current status of the Maze procedure for the treatment of atrial fibrillation. Semin Thorac Cardiovasc Surg 2000; 12:15–19.

103. Williams MR, Stewart JR, Boiling SF, et al. Surgical treatment of atrial fibrillation using radiofrequency energy. Ann Thorac Surg 2001; 71:1939–1944.

104. Guiraudon GM, et al. Encircling endocardial ventriculotomy: a new treatment for life-threatening ventricular tachycardia. Ann Thorac Surg 1977; 26:438.

105. Harken AH, Josephson ME, Horowitz LN. Surgical endocardial resection for the treatment of malignant ventricular tachycardia. Ann Surg 1979; 190:456.

106. Bocker D, et al. Do patients with an implantable defibrillator live longer? J Am Coll Cardiol 1993; 21:1638; Lowe JL, Sabiston DC. The surgical management of cardiac arrhythmias. J Cardiovasc Surg 1986; 1:1.

107. Kim SG, et al. Long-term outcomes and modes of death of patients related with nonthoracotomy implantable defibrillators. Am J Cardiol 1995; 75:1229.

108. May CD, et al. The impact of implantable cardioverter defibrillator on quality of life. PACE Pacing Clin Electrophysiol 1995; 18:1411.

109. Levine PA, et al. Electrocautery and pacemakers. Management of the paced patient subject to electrocautery. Ann Thorac Surg 1996; 41:313.

110. Shabetai R. The Pericardium. New York: Grune & Stratton, 1981.

111. Edwards EA, Malone PD, Collins JJ Jr. Operative Management of the Thorax. Philadelphia: Lea & Febiger, 1972.

112. Seifer FC, et al. Surgical treatment of constrictive pericarditis: analysis of outcome and diagnostic error. Circulation 1985; 72(suppl 2):II264.

113. Harvey WP. Clinical aspects of cardiac tumors. Am J Cardiol 1968; 21:328.

114. Heath D. Pathology of cardiac tumors. Am J Cardiol 1968; 21:315.

115. Ensherding R, et al. Diagnosis of heart tumors by transesophageal ochocardiography. Eur Heart J 1993; 14:1223.

116. Miralles A, et al. Cardiac tumors: clinical experience and surgical results in 74 patients. Ann Thorac Surg 1991; 52:886.

117. Murphy MC, et al. Surgical treatment of cardiac tumors: a 25 year experience. Ann Thorac Surg 1990; 49:612.

37

Urine Formation: From Normal Physiology to Florid Kidney Failure

Akinsan Dosekun, John R. Foringer, and Bruce C. Kone

INTRODUCTION

The kidney fulfills several major functions. First, the organ regulates the excretion of several important inorganic and organic ions and participates in the regulation of acid–base balance. Second, the kidneys work in an integrated manner with the cardiovascular and central nervous systems to regulate body fluid osmolality and volume. The control of body fluid osmolality is central to the maintenance of normal cell volume in virtually all tissues. Third, the kidney excretes metabolic by-products and exogenous substances, including certain drugs. Finally, the kidney is an important endocrine organ, producing key hormones involved in the regulation of blood pressure and erythropoiesis, as well as calcium, phosphate, and bone metabolism. The kidney has remarkable functional reserve and, through adaptive changes, can maintain fluid, electrolyte, metabolic, and acid–base balance as the number of functioning nephrons is reduced by injury or disease. However, in response to significant injury, the kidney may undergo maladaptive changes that lead to acute irreversible and/or progressive renal disease. The incidence of acute and chronic kidney failure continues to rise, and despite extensive investigation into the pathophysiology of these disorders, major preventive or therapeutic advances have been infrequent. This chapter examines the anatomy and physiology of the normal kidney and then reviews the pathophysiology, diagnosis, and management of acute and chronic kidney failure, with special emphasis on clinical scenarios commonly encountered in modern surgical practice.

OVERVIEW OF RENAL PHYSIOLOGY

Renal Anatomy and Microanatomy

The cut surface of a bisected kidney reveals two major regions: the outer region, termed the cortex, in which the glomeruli reside, and the inner region, termed the medulla. The medulla is divided into 8 to 18 renal pyramids, whose bases begin at the corticomedullary junction and form an apex in a minor calyx of the papilla. The minor calyces drain into major calyces and then into the renal pelvis, an expanded region of the ureter. Smooth muscle contractions by the walls of the calyces, pelvis, and ureters drive the urine to the urinary bladder.

Macro- and Microcirculation

Although comprising only 0.5% of the total body mass, the kidneys receive roughly 25% of the cardiac output. This disproportionately high rate of blood flow facilitates glomerular filtration. The blood flow is distributed principally to the renal cortex, and diminishes progressively toward the cortex. The renal arteries branch successively into interlobular arteries, which divide at the level of the cortico-medullary junction to form the arcuate arteries (Fig. 1). The arcuate arteries lead to interlobar arteries, which branch into the afferent arterioles. The afferent arterioles give rise to the glomerular capillaries that coalesce to form the efferent arteriole. The efferent arterioles become a second capillary network, the peritubular capillaries, which surround the proximal tubules and successive tubular segments of the nephron (Fig. 2). The vasa recta arise from the juxtamedullary efferent arterioles and give rise to the descending vasa recta, which form a dense network of anastomosing, looping vessels that descend in parallel with Henle's loops to supply the outer and inner medulla. The venous system runs in parallel to the arterial vessels, with blood from the peritubular capillaries flowing sequentially through the stellate vein, the interlobular vein, arcuate vein, interlobar vein, and renal vein, which tracks beside the ureter. Blood from the ascending vasa recta enters the interlobular and arcuate veins. Despite receiving less than 1% of the renal blood flow (RBF), the vasa recta subserve several critical functions, including the return of reabsorbed solutes and water to the systemic circulation, the delivery of oxygen, nutrients, and substances for secretion to nephron segments, and the concentration and dilution of the urine. The total vascular resistance along the renal vascular tree is estimated to be about 25% before the afferent arteriole, 50% along the length of the afferent arteriole, and 30% along the efferent arteriole (1).

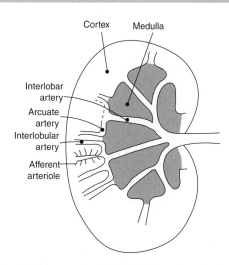

Figure 1 Organization of the arterial vascular system of the human kidney.

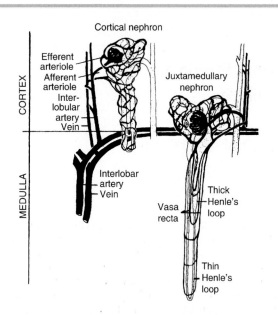

Cortical nephron

CORTEX

Efferent arteriole
Afferent arteriole
Inter-lobular artery
Vein

Juxtamedullary nephron

MEDULLA

Interlobar artery
Vein

Vasa recta

Thick Henle's loop

Thin Henle's loop

Figure 2 Postglomerular circulation of superficial and juxtameduillary nephrons. Note that the efferent arteriole gives rise to the peritubular capillaries in both classes of nephrons, but also the vasa recta in juxtameduillary nephrons. The vasa recta form capillary networks that surround the collecting ducts and ascending limbs of Henle's loop.

Nephron Structure

The functional unit of the kidney is the nephron, which consists of the renal corpuscle (containing the glomerulus and Bowman's capsule), the proximal tubule, Henle's loop, distal tubule, and the collecting ducts (Fig. 3). The proximal tubule comprises an initial convoluted segment followed by a straight segment that descends to the medulla. The proximal straight tubule then gives rise to the descending thin limb of Henle, which ends at a hairpin turn to become the ascending thin limb of Henle (in long-looped nephrons), which ascends through the medulla to form the medullary and cortical thick ascending limbs (cTAL) of Henle. A specialized portion of the cTAL, termed the macula densa segment, courses between the afferent and efferent arterioles of the same nephron. The distal tubule begins beyond the macula densa segment and continues to the junction of two or more nephrons at the cortical collecting duct. The cortical collecting duct descends to become the outer medullary collecting duct and inner medullary collecting duct. Nephrons are further subdivided into superficial and juxtamedullary types. For superficial nephrons, the renal corpuscle resides in the outer regions of the cortex, its Henle's loop is short, and its efferent arteriole branches into peritubular capillaries that form a network around neighboring nephrons. In contrast, juxtamedullary nephrons have renal corpuscles located in the cortex near the medulla, Henle's loop extends deep into the medulla, and the efferent arteriole forms not only the peritubular capillary network, but also the vasa recta.

The glomerular capillaries are lined by the fenestrated endothelium. The endothelium and epithelium are anchored by the continuous glomerular basement membrane (Fig. 4). The foot processes of the podocytes, also termed visceral epithelial cells, cover the outer segment of the capillary wall. The glomerular filtration barrier is formed by the glomerular

basement membrane itself, the foot processes of the podocytes, and the fenestrae of the glomerular endothelium (Fig. 4). The normal glomerular filtration barrier will allow the passage of molecules with molecular weight <58,000 Da. In addition to molecular size, electrical charge also strongly influences glomerular permselectivity. The glomerular basement membrane carries with it a net negative charge that tends to repel anionically charged proteins such as albumin. Multiple disease states result in the disruption of the glomerular filtration barrier and result in proteinuria. The glomerular capillary network is anchored and organized around the mesangium, a central zone that comprises mesangial cells and extracellular matrix. The capillary lumen is separated from the mesangium by the endothelium, without an interposed glomerular basement membrane. The juxtaglomerular apparatus comprises the macula densa, the extraglomerular mesangial cells, and the rennin-producing granular cells of the afferent arteriole. The juxtaglomerular apparatus participates in the tubuloglomerular feedback (TGF) system, which is involved in autoregulation of RBF and the glomerular filtration rate (GFR).

Innervation

Sympathetic nerves arising principally from the celiac plexus innervate the kidney and participate in the regulation of RBF, GFR, and the reabsorption of salt and water (3). Adrenergic fibers course adjacent to the smooth muscle cells of the interlobar, arcuate, and interlobular arteries, and the afferent and efferent arterioles. The renin-producing granular cells of the afferent arteriole are also innervated and activated by sympathetic nerves. In addition, the proximal tubule, Henle's loop, distal tubule, and collecting duct are innervated, so that activation of these nerves promotes sodium reabsorption by these segments. There is no parasympathetic innervation.

Lymphatics

Lymphatic capillaries form a superficial network just inside the renal capsule and a deeper network between and around the renal vasculature (4). The lymphatic networks inside the capsule and around the renal blood vessels drain into lymphatic channels coursing with the interlobular and arcuate blood vessels. The main lymph channels run in parallel with the main renal arteries and veins to drain into periaortic lymph nodes and lymph nodes near the origin of the renal arteries. While there are a few lymphatic capillaries present in the renal parenchyma, associated with connective tissue, the glomeruli contain no lymphatics.

Urine Formation

Urine formation involves the integration of three processes: glomerular ultrafiltration, tubular reabsorption of solutes and water, and tubular secretion of endogenous and exogenous substances.

Renal Blood Flow

RBF to each kidney is about 600 mL/min or about 25% of the cardiac output in resting individuals. Roughly 90% of the total renal plasma flow is directed to the cortex, about 9% to the outer medulla, and only about 1% to the inner medulla and papilla. The differences in blood flow among the renal parenchymal zones are under metabolic, hormonal, and sympathetic control. The RBF subserves several important roles: it indirectly sets the GFR, modifies the rate of solute

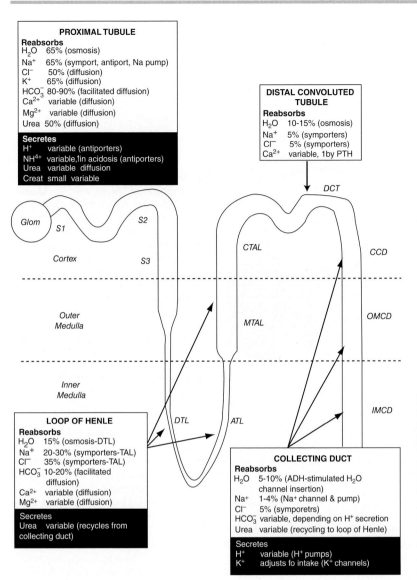

PROXIMAL TUBULE
Reabsorbs
H_2O 65% (osmosis)
Na^+ 65% (symport, antiport, Na pump)
Cl^- 50% (diffusion)
K^+ 65% (diffusion)
HCO_3^- 80-90% (facilitated diffusion)
Ca^{2+} variable (diffusion)
Mg^{2+} variable (diffusion)
Urea 50% (diffusion)

Secretes
H^+ variable (antiporters)
NH^{4+} variable,↑in acidosis (antiporters)
Urea variable diffusion
Creat small variable

DISTAL CONVOLUTED TUBULE
Reabsorbs
H_2O 10-15% (osmosis)
Na^+ 5% (symporters)
Cl^- 5% (symporters)
Ca^{2+} variable, ↑by PTH

LOOP OF HENLE
Reabsorbs
H_2O 15% (osmosis-DTL)
Na^+ 20-30% (symporters-TAL)
Cl^- 35% (symporters-TAL)
HCO_3^- 10-20% (facilitated diffusion)
Ca^{2+} variable (diffusion)
Mg^{2+} variable (diffusion)

Secretes
Urea   variable (recycles from collecting duct)

COLLECTING DUCT
Reabsorbs
H_2O 5-10% (ADH-stimulated H_2O channel insertion)
Na^+ 1-4% (Na+ channel & pump)
Cl^- 5% (symporetrs)
HCO_3^- variable, depending on H+ secretion
Urea   variable (recycling to loop of Henle)

Secretes
H^+ variable (H+ pumps)
K^+ adjusts fo intake (K+ channels)

Figure 3 Microanatomy and major segmental functions of of an isolated nephron. The nephron is the functional unit of the kidney and consists of the renal corpuscle, proximal tubule, Henle's loop, distal tubule, and collecting system. The human kidney typically has more than one million nephrons, which function to filter and modify the blood to produce the final urine. Not drawn to scale. *Abbreviations*: GLOM, glomerulus; DCT, distal convoluted tubule; S1, S2, S3, segments of the proximal tubule; CCD, cortical collecting duct; MTAL, medullary thick ascending limb of Henle; CTAL, cortical thick ascending limb of Henle; DTL, descending thin limb of Henle; OMCD, outer medullary collecting duct; ATL, ascending thin limb, IMCD, inner medullary collecting duct.

and water reabsorption in the proximal tubule, delivers oxygen, nutrients, and hormones to cells of the nephron, and removes carbon dioxide and reabsorbed fluid and solutes to the circulation, delivers substrates for urinary excretion, and participates in urinary concentration and dilution. The RBF represents the pressure difference between the renal artery and the renal vein, divided by the renal vascular resistance. RBF and GFR remain relatively constant as mean arterial blood pressure changes over the range of bout 70 to 180 mmHg, a phenomenon known as autoregulation (Fig. 5). At least two mechanisms are responsible for autoregulation: a myogenic mechanism and TGF. There appears to be a dynamic interplay between these two mechanisms. The myogenic mechanism is a pressure-sensitive mechanism intrinsic to the vascular smooth muscle in which stretching promotes contraction (1). Thus, elevations in arterial pressure stretch the renal afferent arteriole and the smooth muscle contracts. This increase in resistance offsets the increase in pressure so that RBF and GFR remain constant. TGF is a process in which the NaCl concentration (or another factor) in the tubular lumen is sensed by the macula densa, which transmits a signal that adjusts in an opposite manner afferent arteriolar resistance and, thereby, GFR. Thus, elevations in NaCl delivery to the macula densa prompt the afferent arteriole to constrict and return RBF and GFR to normal. Conversely, reduced NaCl delivery to the macula densa elicits signals that result in vasodilation of the afferent arteriole so that RBF and GFR increase to normal levels. Adenosine-1 receptors are absolutely required for eliciting. TGF responses in animals, and the background level of angiotensin II (Ang II) appears to be an important determinant for the efficiency of adenosine-1 receptor–induced vasoconstriction. The adenosine source remains unclear, but adenosine may be generated extracellularly from released adenosine triphosphate (ATP) by the action of ectonucleotidases. ATP may also activate P2 receptors in preglomerular vessels, which may contribute to autoregulation of renal vascular resistance. Finally, nitric oxide (NO) generated in macula densa cells opposes the constrictor effect of adenosine, but its exact role in states of TGF-induced hyperfiltration is still unclear (5). In addition to these influences, sympathetic nerves, vasoconstrictor

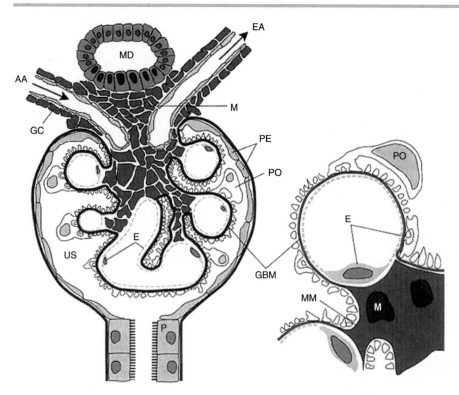

Figure 4 Microanatomy of the renal corpuscle and the juxtaglomerrular apparatus. The AA enters and the EA leaves the glomerular capillary tuft. The glomerular filtration barrier comprises the GBM, the fenestrae of the glomerular capillary endothelium (E), and the foot processes of the PO. The primary ultrafiltrate enters the US, which is continuous with the lumen of the proximal tubule (P). The juxtaglomerular apparatus consists of the MD segment, the rennin-producing granular cells of the AA, and the extraglomerular mesangial cells (M). *Abbreviations*: AA, afferent arteriole; EA, efferent arteriole; GBM, glomerular basement membrane; PO, podocytes; MM, mesangial matrix; PE, parietal epithelium; US, urinary space; MD, macula densa. *Source*: From Ref. 2.

molecules such as Ang II and endothelin, and vasodilator molecules such as NO, bradykinin, and prostaglandins (particularly prostaglandins E2 and I2) act on the vascular tone of the afferent and efferent arterioles and thus contribute to the regulation of RBF. Ang II plays a key role in the regulation of whole-kidney blood flow, cortical and medullary blood flow, and renal autoregulation. Ang II potently constricts both the afferent and the efferent arterioles, with responses modulated by paracrine and autocrine factors arising from endothelial cells and the macula densa. Ang II promotes vasoconstriction of the efferent arteriole via

calcium release from intracellular stores and calcium entry through voltage-independent calcium channels. The hormone promotes comparatively less constriction of the afferent arteriole, which occurs primarily by stimulation of calcium entry via voltage-sensitive L-type channels.

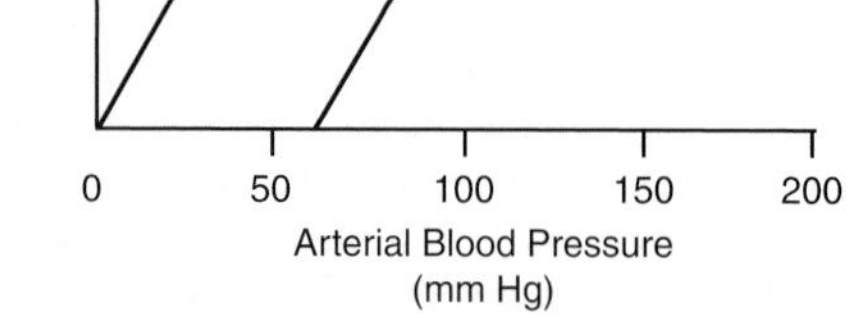

The relative changes in resistance of the afferent and/or efferent arterioles dictate the effects on RBF and GFR. For example, hemorrhage leading to hypotension results in accentuated activity of renal sympathetic nerves, which act by direct actions, and indirectly, through the activation of renin secretion and Ang II production, to constrict the renal arterioles. This results in reduced RBF and GFR and enhanced tubular reabsorption of sodium and water. Importantly, autoregulation is often impaired in patients with severe hypertension and in ischemic acute kidney failure (AKF). In these settings, the kidney is even more vulnerable to subsequent hypotensive or hypertensive insults.

Glomerular Filtration

The initial step in urine formation is the production of an ultrafiltrate by the glomerulus. The ultrafiltrate is virtually devoid of cells and proteins and has concentrations of ions and organic molecules similar to that of plasma. Normally, only 15% to 20% of the plasma entering the glomerulus is actually filtered: the filtration fraction. The remainder courses on through the glomerulus to the efferent arteriole and eventually returns to the circulation via the renal vein. Thus, if the RBF is 600 mL/min per kidney and GFR is roughly 120 mL/min, the filtration fraction would be 0.2. Starling forces (i.e., hydrostatic and oncotic pressures) across the glomerular capillary membrane dictate ultrafiltration; hence, changes in these forces result in altered GFR (6). Because the glomerular filtration barrier excludes substances greater than 70,000 Da, the ultrafiltrate is essentially protein free as it arrives in Bowman's space, and thus

Figure 5 Relationships among renal blood flow, glomerular filtration rate, and arterial blood pressure. Autoregulation maintains GFR and RBF relatively constant over a wide range of blood pressures.

contributes little oncotic pressure (π_{BS}). Accordingly, the glomerular capillary hydrostatic pressure (P_{GC}) is the only force favoring filtration. It is opposed by the minor hydrostatic forces in Bowman's space (P_{BS}) and the oncotic pressure of the blood in the glomerular capillary (π_{GC}):

$$\text{SNGFR} = K_f[(P_{GC} - P_{BS}) - (\pi_{GS} - \pi_{BS})]$$

where SNGFR is the single-nephron GFR, K_f is the product of the intrinsic permeability of the glomerular capillary and the glomerular capillary surface area available for filtration. The net ultrafiltration pressure gradient, representing the difference between the hydrostatic and oncotic pressure gradients, is greatest nearest the afferent arteriole, where the oncotic pressure is the lowest, and becomes progressively lower as the oncotic pressure increases along the glomerular capillaries to the efferent arteriole. Disease states that result in changes in these latter properties result in a reduction in GFR. Similarly, reduction in P_{GC}, as might occur in AKF, or increases in P_{BS}, as might occur in acute urinary tract obstruction, result in reduced GFR. In normal humans, GFR is regulated primarily by alterations in P_{GC} that result from changes in glomerular arteriolar resistance. Therapy to prevent progression of chronic kidney disease (CKD) [i.e., angiotensin-converting enzyme (ACE) inhibitors or Ang II receptor antagonists] is directed at lowering P_{GC} in glomeruli of the remaining functional nephrons to minimize thickening and fibrosis of the glomerular capillary wall.

As noted above, GFR is regulated in parallel with RBF, exhibiting autoregulation that is principally controlled by TGF. Factors that influence the vascular tone of the afferent and/or efferent arterioles or the TGF mechanism itself will cause alterations in GFR. Given the prime importance of Ang II, bradykinin, and prostaglandins in controlling vascular tone, pharmacologic interruption of these pathways with ACE inhibitors, Ang II receptor antagonists, or cyclooxygenase inhibitors can disrupt autoregulation and the regulation of GFR.

Tubular Functions

Epithelial Transport Mechanisms

Because membranes are generally impermeable to ions distributed across them, ion pumps are used to interconvert chemical energy derived from ATP hydrolysis into electrochemical gradients to drive ion transport against a concentration gradient in a process termed "primary active transport" (Fig. 6). In the kidney, the Na^+-K^+-ATPase is the primary mechanism for primary active transport,

functioning to maintain the low concentration of Na^+ and high concentration of K^+ in the intracellular environment. In secondary active transport, solutes are transported along an electrochemical gradient, without direct energy consumption (Fig. 6). Thus the energy stored in the steep Na^+ gradient generated by the Na^+-K^+-ATPase can direct Na^+-coupled transport of sugars, amino acids, and other solutes along the nephron. Finally, in tertiary active transport, the energy stored in the Na^+ gradient generated by the Na^+-K^+-ATPase can be indirectly used to drive the transport of other ions and organic molecules. For example, the Na^+/H^+ exchanger, a secondary active transporter driven by the transmembrane Na^+ gradient generated and maintained by the Na^+-K^+-ATPase, couples Na^+ influx with the H^+ efflux, and is thus principally responsible for the existence of this H^+ gradient (Fig. 6). This H^+ gradient can then drive the tertiary active transport of Cl^- across the brush border membrane via a Cl^-/HCO_3^- exchanger (Fig. 6).

NaCl and Water Reabsorption Along the Nephron

Under normal conditions, less than 1% of the filtered salt and water are excreted in the urine. In the absence of pharmacological interference, urinary excretion of Na^+ can vary between less than 0.1% and no more than 3% of the filtered load. Because spontaneous changes in GFR can dramatically alter the filtered load of Na^+, rapid adjustments in Na^+ reabsorption must occur along the nephron to prevent wide fluctuations in urinary Na^+ excretion and body Na^+ balance. The reabsorption of several important solutes is coupled directly or indirectly to Na^+ transport. The proximal tubule reabsorbs about 65% of the filtered Na^+, K^+, Cl^-, and water, as well as nearly all of the glucose and amino acids filtered by the glomerulus (Fig. 3). About two-thirds of the Na^+ is reabsorbed across the cells (transcellular), with the remainder reabsorbed by paracellular routes. Electrochemical gradients established by the Na^+-K^+-ATPase in the basolateral membrane of the proximal tubule drive the transport of Na^+ coupled with H^+ or organic solutes (Fig. 6) (7). The principal mechanisms of Na^+ entry across the apical membrane are the Na^+-H^+ exchanger. The exact amounts of Na^+ reabsorbed are determined by many regulatory factors such as glomerulotubular balance, Ang II, endothelin, sympathetic input, acid–base status parathyroid hormone (PTH), dopamine, and others. Starling forces across the peritubular capillaries also influence solute and water transport across the proximal tubule.

About 25% of the filtered NaCl is reabsorbed in the thick ascending limb, principally via secondary active

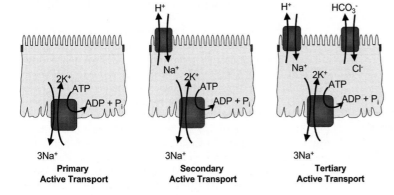

Figure 6 Modes of active solute transport in renal epithelial cells. Models illustrating the different modes of active transport are shown. Primary active transport (in this example, the Na^+-K^+-ATPase) uses adenosine triphosphate (ATP) hydrolysis to power the transport of solutes across the plasma membrane against their electrochemical gradients. Secondary active transport utilizes the energy inherent in the electrochemical gradient (in this case, the Na^+ gradient) generated by the primary active transporter to drive the influx or efflux of a coupled solute. Tertiary active transport couples the transport of a solute (in this example, Cl^-) to the gradient (in this example, H^+) created by the secondary active transport process. *Abbreviations:* ATP, adenosine triphosphate; ADP, adenosine diphosphate.

transport mediated by the apical Na$^+$-K$^+$-2Cl$^-$ cotransporter and driven by the Na$^+$-K$^+$-ATPase (Fig. 3). Because the thick ascending limb is impermeable to water, NaCl reabsorption in this segment reduces the osmolality of ("dilutes") the tubular fluid. The transport rate is determined by the Na$^+$ load and by several hormones and neurotransmitters, including prostaglandins, PTH, glucagon, calcitonin, antidiuretic hormone (ADH), and adrenaline. The distal tubule reabsorbs about 4% to 5% of the remaining NaCl by the actions of the apical thiazide-sensitive NaCl cotransporter and the basolateral Na$^+$-K$^+$-ATPase. The rate of transport is again determined by the delivered load and by several hormones and neurotransmitters. The collecting duct is the final arbiter of Na$^+$ reabsorption, with Na$^+$ channels mediating Na$^+$ entry.

Water reabsorption is a highly integrated and regulated process that can vary between 0.3% and 15% of the amount filtered under physiological conditions. About two-thirds of the filtered water is passively reabsorbed in the proximal tubule (Fig. 3). The driving force for water reabsorption in this segment is the osmotic gradient across the tubule established by solute reabsorption Roughly 15% is then passively reabsorbed in the descending thin limb of Henle (Fig. 3). The remainder of the loop of Henle and the distal tubule do not reabsorb significant amounts of water. The late distal tubule and collecting duct reabsorb variable amounts of the remaining water via constitutive and ADH-regulated water channels, termed aquaporins (Fig. 3). Changes in plasma osmolality and blood volume or pressure stimulate ADH release and thirst (Fig. 7). ADH acts on and binds to vasopressin (V2) receptors on the basolateral membrane of collecting duct cells. Receptor binding evokes an increase in cyclic adenosine monophosphate (cAMP) levels, which ultimately results in the insertion of vesicles containing aquaporin-2 in the apical membrane of the cell (8). Water is absorbed through these apical aquaporin-2 channels and through the basolateral membrane via aquaporin-3 channels, driven by the osmotic gradient built up by the countercurrent concentrating system. With ADH removal, the water channels are again internalized into the cell, rendering the apical membrane impermeable to water (8). The shuttling of the water

channels in response to ADH provides a rapid means to regulate membrane water permeability.

Potassium Handling

Roughly 98% of total body K$^+$ content in humans is distributed in the intracellular compartment, the result of active K$^+$ uptake by the Na$^+$-K$^+$-ATPase. The remaining 2% of K$^+$ normally resides in the extracellular pool (9). Excretion balances K intake even when intake increases more than 10-fold in normal humans. Normal individuals on a typical Western diet absorb about 90% of intake and excrete an equivalent amount of K$^+$ in the urine. The remaining 10% of K$^+$ excretion occurs principally in the stool. K$^+$ is freely filtered at the glomerulus. The proximal tubule reabsorbs about 67% of the filtered K$^+$, and the medullary thick ascending limb of Henle's loop (mTAL) reabsorbs another 20% as a constant fraction of the amount filtered (Fig. 3). In contrast, cells of the distal tubule and collecting duct have the dual ability to reabsorb and secrete K$^+$, processes that are highly regulated by multiple hormones and other factors (Fig. 3). Indeed, the principal mechanism for urinary K$^+$ excretion is the action of principal cells of the distal tubule and collecting duct to secrete excess K$^+$ from the blood into the tubular fluid (9). During states of K$^+$ deficiency, the outer and inner medullary collecting ducts reabsorb K$^+$ to reclaim all but 1% filtered K$^+$ before it is lost in the urine. However, the reabsorptive processes are less efficient than they are for Na$^+$, so that hypokalemia can ensue in states of K$^+$ restriction.

Calcium, Magnesium, and Phosphorus Handling

The kidney works in concert with the gastrointestinal (GI) tract and bones to regulate the balance of Ca^{2+} and inorganic phosphorus. Under normal conditions, 99% of the filtered Ca^{2+} is reabsorbed by the nephron. Ca^{2+} excretion by the kidney is determined by the net Ca^{2+} reabsorption by the intestine, the balance between bone formation and resorption, and the net transport rates by the distal tubule and thick ascending limb (Fig. 3). Calcitonin, calcitriol, and PTH also regulate urinary Ca^{2+} excretion, with PTH contributing the greatest control. PTH stimulates Ca^{2+} reabsorption by the thick ascending limb and the distal tubule (10,11). Calcitonin stimulates Ca^{2+} reabsorption by these segments, but to a quantitatively less degree. Calcitriol enhances Ca^{2+} reabsorption by the distal tubule. The proximal tubule reabsorbs 70%, and the thick ascending limb of Henle an additional 20% of the filtered Ca^{2+} (Fig. 3). The distal tubule and collecting duct reabsorb about 9% and 1%, respectively. Ca^{2+} reabsorption by the proximal tubule occurs via transcellular and paracellular pathways. Changes in Na$^+$ reabsorption result in coordinate changes in Ca^{2+} reabsorption by the proximal tubule and the thick ascending limb of Henle. Changes in Na$^+$ and Ca^{2+} reabsorption are not always in parallel in the distal tubule.

Mg^{2+} is the second most common cation in the intracellular fluid. About 80% of the total serum Mg^{2+} is filtered through the glomerular membrane. The proximal tubule reabsorbs about 10% to 15% of the filtered Mg^{2+} (Fig. 3). The bulk (approximately 60%) of the filtered Mg^{2+} is reabsorbed in the cTAL by passive means driven by the trans-epithelial voltage through the paracellular pathway (Fig. 3) (12,13). The distal tubule reabsorbs significant amounts of Mg^{2+} via an active transcellular process. Several hormones and nonhormonal factors influence renal Mg^{2+} reabsorption to variable extent in the cTAL and distal tubule. In states of dietary magnesium restriction, urinary Mg^{2+} excretion decreases through the adaptation of magnesium transport

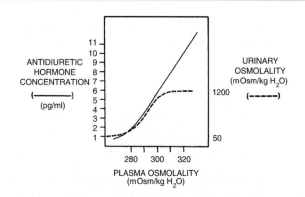

Figure 7 Relationships among antidiuretic hormone (ADH) concentration, the plasma osmolality, and the urine osmolality. As plasma osmolality increases above normal, ADH levels increase, which permits maximal urinary conservation of water up to a urine osmolality of about 1200 mOsm/kg water. Further increments in ADH concentration do not increase urine osmolality above this maximum.

in both the cTAL and the distal tubule. Elevation of plasma Mg^{2+} or Ca^{2+} concentration is sensed by an extracellular Ca^{2+}/Mg^{2+}-sensing receptor located on the peritubular side of cTAL and distal tubule cells and acts to inhibit Mg^{2+} and Ca^{2+} reabsorption. Metabolic acidosis, potassium depletion, or phosphate restriction results in diminished Mg^{2+} reabsorption within the cTAL and distal tubule (13).

Phosphate excretion is determined principally by glomerular filtration and by regulated reabsorption in the proximal tubule. All but about 10% of the filtered load of inorganic phosphorus (P_i) is reabsorbed, primarily by the proximal tubule (approximately 80%) and the distal tubule (approximately 10%) (14). A secondary active P_i transport mechanism—the brush-border membrane type IIa Na–Pi cotransporter—is the key player in proximal tubular P_i reabsorption, and PTH is the major regulator of P_i excretion. PTH inhibits P_i reabsorption by the proximal tubule, thereby enhancing urinary P_i excretion. Acidosis, volume expansion, and glucocorticoids also stimulate P_i excretion. In contrast, volume contraction, alkalosis, and growth hormone are known to limit P_i excretion in the urine (15).

Bicarbonate Reabsorption/Proton Secretion

Normal humans on a Western diet of normal caloric intake will generate approximately 20,000 mEq of acid/day in the form of CO_2 through fat and carbohydrate metabolism. The lungs eliminate this CO_2. Protein catabolism generates about 50 to 60 mEq/day of inorganic, nonvolatile acids (e.g., sulfuric, phosphoric, or hydrochloric acids) that must be excreted by the kidney. In addition, the kidney must reclaim filtered HCO_3^- to maintain acid–base balance.

HCO_3^- reabsorption of the filtered load is virtually complete along the nephron under normal conditions (Fig. 3). About 80% of the filtered load is reabsorbed in the proximal tubule in a process critically dependent on Na^+–H^+ exchanger isoform NHE3 and carbonic anhydrase at the apical membrane. H^+ secreted into the lumen in exchange for Na^+ combines with filtered HCO_3^-, and converted via the action of carbonic anhydrase into CO_2 and H_2O. The CO_2 freely diffuses across the luminal membrane into the cell, where it is hydrated in the presence of carbonic anhydrase to H_2CO_3. The intracellular H_2CO_3 then dissociates into HCO_3^-, which is reabsorbed across the basolateral membrane, and H^+, which is secreted into the luminal fluid. Thus, the bicarbonate actually reabsorbed is not that which was originally in the filtrate, but the net effect is the same as if this were the case. Because of their interdependence, HCO_3^- reabsorption generally parallels the rate of proximal tubule Na^+ reabsorption. An H^+-ATPase in the apical membrane of the proximal tubule participates in Na^+-independent HCO_3^- reabsorption. The thick ascending limb of Henle reabsorbs another 15% of filtered HCO_3^-, by transport mechanisms similar to those operating in the proximal tubule (16). The distal tubule and collecting duct reabsorb the small amount of HCO_3^- that escapes the more proximal segments (17,18). A number of factors, including extracellular fluid volume, Ang II, aldosterone, and plasma K^+ concentration, regulate HCO_3^- reabsorption along the nephron.

Other bases besides HCO_3^- may buffer H^+ secreted into the distal tubules, and H^+ may combine with ammonia also secreted by the tubules. The principal non-HCO_3^- base in the tubular fluid is dibasic sodium phosphate (Na_2HPO_4), which can accept H^+ to form monobasic sodium phosphate (NaH_2PO_4). Titratable acidity of the urine refers to the amount of urinary H^+ buffered by bases such as HCO_3^- and phosphate. It is measured by titrating the urine with strong base until the pH of the plasma from which the filtrate is derived is reached.

Under physiologic conditions, about two-thirds of the H^+ to be secreted in the urine is in the form of ammonium salts. Ammonia (NH_3) is absent from the plasma and glomerular ultrafiltrate, but is formed, along with glutamic acid, from the hydrolysis of glutamine by the enzyme glutaminase. A further molecule of ammonia arises from the deamination of glutamic acid to form glutaric acid, which is then metabolized. The NH_3 so formed passes into the lumen where it combines with secreted H^+ to form NH_4^+, which, as a charged molecule, is then trapped in the lumen. The NH_4^+ is excreted in the urine as ammonium salts of excess anions (e.g., chloride, sulfate, and phosphate). Increasing acid accumulation stimulates production of NH_4^+ by the tubular cells. Thus, H^+ secretion can be considered as the integration of three processes: reabsorption of filtered HCO_3^- in the proximal tubule, reabsorption of filtered HCO_3^- in the distal nephron, and formation of monobasic phosphate and ammonium salts. Accordingly, the total tubular H^+ secretion represents the sum of the amount of HCO_3^- reabsorbed, the amount of titratable acid, and the amount of NH_4^+ excreted.

Secretion of Organic Anions and Cations

The proximal tubule secretes a number of endogenous and exogenous (typically drugs) compounds. Anionic compounds include metabolic products such as bile salts, urate, and oxalate, and commonly used drugs, including furosemide, penicillin, and hydrochlorothiazide. Cationic organic molecules secreted by the proximal tubule include creatinine, dopamine, and epinephrine, as well as atropine, morphine, and other drugs. All organic compounds compete for the same transporter in the proximal tubule, so that high plasma levels of one organic ion can limit the secretion of the others (19–21).

A transport system for net transepithelial secretion of various hydrophobic organic anions has been described in the proximal tubule. This tertiary active transport process involves an organic anion/α-ketoglutarate exchange process in the basolateral membrane, Na^+–dicarboxylate cotransporters at both membranes, and an inwardly directed Na^+ gradient driving α-ketoglutarate uptake generated and maintained by the basolateral Na^+-K^+-ATPase. The transport of the organic anion into the cells against its electrochemical gradient occurs in exchange for α-ketoglutarate moving out of the cells down its electrochemical gradient. The outwardly directed gradient for α-ketoglutarate is maintained by metabolism and by transport into the cells by Na^+–dicarboxylate cotransporters. The inward Na^+ gradient driving α-ketoglutarate uptake is in turn generated and maintained by the basolateral Na^+-K^+-ATPase. The basolateral organic acid/α-ketoglutarate exchange process appears to be regulated by peptide hormones, growth factors, and the autonomic nervous system (22,23).

Sites and Mechanisms of Diuretic Action

A number of diuretic agents and other drugs target specific transport proteins or enzymes to effect their action (Table 1). Osmotic diuretics such as mannitol inhibit fluid reabsorption by altering the osmotic driving forces along the nephron (24). These agents are filtered at the glomerulus and are generally not reabsorbed by the tubules, so that they remain in the tubular lumen to exert an osmotic pressure to oppose

Table 1   Classes and Mechanisms of Diuretic Actions

Class	Site of action	Transport process inhibited	% Filtered Na^+ excreted
Thiazide diuretics (e.g., hydrochlorothiazide)	Early distal tubule	NaCl cotransporter	5–10
Loop diuretics (e.g., furosemide)	MTAL	Na^+-K^+-$2Cl^-$ cotransporter	20–25
Potassium-sparing diuretics [e.g., (a) amiloride, (b) spironalactone]	Collecting ducts	(a) apical Na^+ channels; (b) aldosterone-stimulated transepithelial Na^+ transport	1–2
Osmotic diuretics (e.g., mannitol)	Proximal tubule, TDL	Opposes osmotic gradient for NaCl reabsorption	10
Carbonic anhydrase inhibitors (e.g., acetazolamide)	Proximal tubule	Na^+-H^+ exchange indirectly	5–10

Abbreviations: MTAL, medullary thick ascending limb of Henle; TDL, thin descending limb of Henle.

water reabsorption. This effect is most prominent in the segments that are constitutively water permeable (i.e., the proximal tubule and the thin descending limb of Henle). Other classes of diuretics act on specific membrane transport proteins or enzymes coupled to salt and water transport. Carbonic anhydrase inhibitors (i.e., acetazolamide) inhibit proximal Na^+ reabsorption. HCO_3^- reabsorption depends to a large extent on Na^+ (the Na–H exchanger in the proximal tubule apical membrane) (25,26). This enzyme facilitates the formation of H^+ and HCO_3^- from CO_2 and H_2O. About one-third of all proximal tubule Na^+ reabsorption is related to this process of HCO_3^- reabsorption. Carbonic anhydrase inhibitors inhibit only 5% to 10% of the filtered Na^+ load, in part because more distal segments, in particular the thick ascending limb, increase Na^+ reabsorption when Na^+ delivery is increased. Loop diuretics (e.g., furosemide, bumetanide, torsemide, and ethacrynic acid) potently inhibit Na^+ absorption by blocking the Na-K-2Cl cotransporter of the apical membrane of the thick ascending limb of Henle (27). This action not only inhibits Na^+ reabsorption but also limits the kidney's ability both to concentrate and to dilute the urine. Loop diuretics promote an increase in Na^+ excretion that may reach 25% of the filtered load. Thiazide diuretics (e.g., chorothiazide, metolazone, and hydrochlorothiazide) inhibit Na^+ reabsorption by blocking the NaCl cotransport in the apical membrane of the early distal tubule (28). Thiazides also reduce the ability to dilute the urine, but because they do not interrupt the countercurrent multiplication system, they do not impair urinary concentration. Natriuresis with thiazides may approach 5% to 10% of the filtered load. By blocking sequential steps in Na^+ reabsorption along the nephron, the combined use of a loop diuretic and a thiazide diuretic results in even greater diuretic and natriuretic effect than either agent alone. K^+-sparing diuretics act on the late distal tubule and cortical collecting duct and work by either antagonizing aldosterone's action on the principal cells of the collecting duct (e.g., spironolactone) or by inhibiting apical membrane Na^+ channels in these cells (e.g., amiloride and triamterene). Accordingly, these agents produce a natriuresis of only about 3% of the filtered load, but concomitantly inhibit K^+ secretion in the collecting duct and thereby limit urinary K^+ wasting (29–31).

The ability of a diuretic to promote urinary Na^+ excretion is dependent on the diuretic dose, the amount of Na^+ typically reabsorbed by the nephron segment it targets, and the capacity of more distal segments to compensate, by increasing reabsorption, for the excess amounts of Na^+. Most diuretics act at the apical membrane of the tubules to impair Na^+ entry mechanisms, so that there is a dose-dependent relationship between the rate of presentation of the diuretic to its site of action and the Na^+ absorption it inhibits. Loop diuretics are more potent than thiazide or K^+-sparing diuretics because they target a segment that reabsorbs much more Na^+. Finally, when counter-regulatory responses of more distal segments are fully activated, as they are in congestive heart failure, for example, a given dose of loop diuretic will provoke less natriuresis than in normal subjects because of increased Na^+ reabsorption by the distal tubule and collecting duct. Provided the diuretic dose is constant, these counter-regulatory responses typically lead to the establishment of a new steady-state in which Na^+ intake balances Na^+ excretion within the first two weeks of diuretic therapy. In general, fluid and electrolyte complications associated with diuretics occur within this adaptive two-week period.

Physiologic Compensation for Nephron Loss

Progressive loss of renal function, proteinuria, and glomerulosclerosis has been seen in humans with a variety of renal disorders, even after correction of the primary abnormality. In addition, studies of kidney transplant donors, followed for more than a decade, have shown that, while the overall GFR is maintained, there is an increased incidence of proteinuria and hypertension. The kidney maintains near complete regulation of plasma concentrations of Na^+, K^+, and plasma osmolality until 75% to 90% of the nephrons are lost. HCO_3^-, Ca^{2+}, and P_i regulation are maintained adequately until 50% to 70% of the nephrons are lost. For these solutes, excretion is not solely a function of the GFR, but also reflects tubular transport. In contrast, plasma concentrations of creatinine and urea increase progressively as nephrons are lost. According to the intact nephron hypothesis (32), remaining nephrons function as intact units within an otherwise diseased kidney. That is, glomeruli do not filter fluid to nonfunctioning tubules, and normal tubules are nonfunctional in the absence of a corresponding functioning glomeruli. As the number of functioning nephrons becomes fewer, the range of solutes and water over which the kidney can regulate excretion is more limited. In addition, the ability of the kidney to respond rapidly to changes in dietary intake may be limited. These factors predispose patients with renal disease to fluid, electrolyte, and acid–base disturbances. Homeostasis for many solutes and water can be maintained, provided intake is restricted to match the limited excretion. Renal disease tends to be progressive when a critical number of nephrons have been destroyed. Brenner and colleagues (33–35) proposed that, following nephron loss from renal disease, surviving nephrons "hyperfilter" to compensate and normalize single nephron GFR. This hemodynamic change results in glomerular capillary hypertension, which is the most studied and most

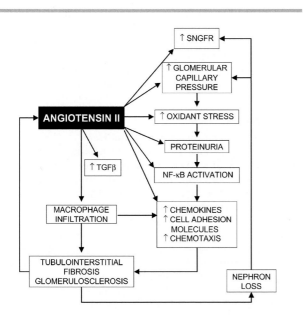

Figure 8 Mechanistic roles of angiotensin II in the progression of chronic kidney disease. *Abbreviations*: TGF-β, transforming growth factor-β; SNGFR, single nephron GFR.

consistent factor in the progression of CKD. High intracapillary pressures damage the capillary wall and generate powerful proinflammatory signals and growth factors that result in mesangial cell proliferation, excessive extracellular matrix production, the recruitment of T-lymphocytes and macrophages, and ultimately glomerular sclerosis and interstitial fibrosis. Unfortunately, however, these adaptations prove to be maladaptive in that they initiate and perpetuate glomerular injury. This vicious cycle, uninterrupted, may end in kidney failure (36). The pace of this injury is determined by the degree of nephron loss. Glomerular capillary hypertension is mediated in large part by Ang II–dependent mechanisms. Besides its hemodynamic effects, several nonhemodynamic effects of Ang II are also important in this process (Fig. 8).

Clinical Assessment of Renal Function
Urine Output
The volume of urine can vary widely from day to day, even in healthy individuals, as a result of food and fluid intake and extrarenal fluid losses. The daily volume averages 1.5 L, but after exercise in warm weather, it may fall as low as 500 mL, and after excess fluid intake, it may reach three or more liters. Within a 24-hour period, urine output is less in the early hours, is maximal during the first few hours after rising, and peaks after meals. Measurement of urine volume and of the rate of urine output is useful adjuncts in clinical management of fluid volume and the diagnosis of kidney injury. Because many patients may be unable to void spontaneously, bladder catheterization may be needed to assess accurately the urine volume. Anuria refers to the absence of urine output and is relatively uncommon in clinical practice. When anuria is present, however, complete bilateral urinary obstruction or bilateral cortical necrosis from severe ischemic insults is the most common etiology. Oliguria is commonly defined as a urine volume less that 400 mL/24 hr, and it suggests a reduced

GFR. Such a reduction in urine volume may present a normal adaptive response to hypovolemia, tubular injury, or urinary tract obstruction. Conversely, the absence of oliguria does not necessarily imply normal kidney function.

Polyuria, or excessive urination, may be caused by diverse etiologies and may be related to severe underlying disorders. Polyuria related to primary water diuresis may be indicative of primary disorders of water balance (central diabetes insipidus, nephrogenic diabetes insipidus, and psychogenic polydipsia) (37). In these settings, there is either a pathological lack of (central diabetes insipidis) or unresponsiveness to (nephrogenic diabetes insipidus) ADH or pathologic water gluttony (psychogenic polydipsia). The two forms of diabetes insipidus are commonly encountered in surgical settings, where brain injury or surgery, or renal tubule injury from nephrotoxic agents may be present. In contrast, solute diuresis may be caused by electrolytes (e.g., sodium chloride and sodium bicarbonate), organic molecules (e.g., glucose and urea), or both (38), or by exogenous agents (e.g., mannitol and certain radiocontrast agents). These solutes produce an osmotic diuresis.

Urinalysis
Urine Specific Gravity and Osmolality
The specific gravity is the weight of the solution compared to the weight of an equal volume of distilled water and is used as an estimate of urine osmolality. Plasma is 0.8% to 1.0% heavier than water, so that its specific gravity is 1.008 to 1.010. Normal urine specific gravity values range from 1.002 to 1.028. Specific gravity differs from the more accurate measurement of urine osmolality, because it is proportional to both the number and the weight of solute particles present in the solution. Hence, excessive amounts of heavier solutes such as glucose or radiocontrast medium will yield urine specific gravity values disproportionately higher than the true osmolality. In these instances, urine specific gravity can exceed 1.030 even when the urine osmolality is 300 mOsm/kg. Thus a random urine specific gravity is of little value as an index of urinary concentration unless it is correlated with plasma osmolality and/or volume status.

Urine osmolality determinations may be helpful in determining whether the kidney's ability to handle water is appropriate in states where plasma osmolality is abnormal. During hypo-osmolar states, urinary water excretion should be maximal and, hence, urine osmolality should be maximally dilute (Fig. 7). If urine osmolality is not low as predicted in this setting, urinary dilution is impaired. Conversely, if isosmolar urine is detected in the presence of plasma hyperosmolality, urinary concentration is impaired.

Urinary pH
Urinary pH can vary over a wide range (4.4–8.0) depending on the demands of the body to excreted acid or base. An alkaline urine (pH > 7) is commonly encountered in metabolic alkalosis or when urea-splitting organisms are infecting the urinary tract. Mildly alkaline urine with concomitant hyperchloremic metabolic acidosis may reflect renal tubular acidosis.

Proteinuria
Under normal conditions, the urine contains only very small amounts of protein (< 50 mg/24 hr). However, the amount of protein in the urine may be increased after exercise, in pregnancy, and in some persons when standing (orthostatic

proteinuria). A large amount of protein, particularly if in the nephrotic range ($>3.5\,g/24\,hr$), is typically indicative of glomerular disease, for which there are many etiologies. However, chronic tubulointerstitial disease, polycystic kidney disease, renal vein thrombosis, and other disorders may also present with significant proteinuria. In addition, protein overproduction such as in multiple myeloma may overwhelm the capacity of the proximal tubule to reabsorb protein and escape into the urine.

Pigmenturia

The urinary dipstick test for heme detects both hemoglobin and myoglobin. With hematuria, erythrocytes are observed on microscopic examination of the urine, and the dipstick test for heme gives a positive reaction. With hemoglobinuria from massive hemolysis (e.g., major blood transfusion reaction), however, no erythrocytes are apparent in the urine but the dipstick is still positive for heme. Similarly, with myoglobunuria resulting from muscle breakdown (e.g., rhabdomyolysis), the dipstick heme test is reactive, and no erythrocytes are evident in the urine. These possibilities can be distinguished by the appearance of the plasma or urine supernatant (clear in myoglobinuria and pink or red in hemoglobinuria) or by the measured urinary myoglobin or hemoglobin.

Glycosuria

The proximal tubule has a fixed capacity to reabsorb filtered glucose. When this capacity is exceeded as a consequence of hyperglycemia, increased GFR, or proximal tubule injury, glycosuria results. In individuals on normal carbohydrate loads, glycosuria typically indicates that the patient has diabetes mellitus. In some healthy persons, however, there may also be an abnormal amount of glucose in the urine because of a low threshold for tubular reabsorption, without any disturbance of glucose metabolism. Ketone bodies (acetone and acetoacetic acid) may be present in traces in normal urine, but may be present in larger quantities in severe untreated diabetes and in carbohydrate starvation.

Urine Microscopic Examination

Examination of the urinary sediment may provide not only information on the presence of an underlying renal disorder but clues as to its specific etiology. White blood cells, particularly as casts, commonly indicate infectious (e.g., pyelonephritis) or inflammatory acute tubulointerstitial nephritis (ATIN) disease. Urinary eosinophils detected by Hansel's stain may be found in acute interstitial nephritis, but have also been found in several other disorders. Red blood cells may arise from either upper or lower tract bleeding. However, the presence of dysmorphic red blood cells or red blood cell casts in a freshly voided urine sample is much more suggestive of glomerulonephritis. Cellular casts derived from the renal tubules may indicate injury, and are commonly present in acute tubular necrosis (ATN). Finally a number of crystals may be apparent in the urine. Calcium oxalate dihydrate crystals typically are colorless squares resembling an envelope. In some cases, they result from increased calcium related to disorders of calcium metabolism. These crystals can also be seen in cases of ethylene glycol intoxication. If seen in large numbers in the urine of a patient with AKF, this diagnosis should be entertained. Uric acid crystals may be seen in gout and uric acid stone formation. They appear and often occur in a diamond shape, but may also be prism or hexagon shaped, or simply as amorphous material. Amorphous phosphates and urates cannot be distinguished by routine microscopy. Struvite crystals (magnesium ammonium phosphate and triple phosphate) usually appear as colorless, three-dimensional, prism-like crystals ("coffin lids"). Urinary tract infection with urease-positive bacteria promotes struvite crystalluria by raising urine pH and increasing free ammonia.

Renal Function Tests

Serum Creatinine Concentration and GFR

Creatinine is a product of creatine metabolism in muscle. A less significant source of creatinine is dietary meat intake. Creatinine generation therefore directly correlates with muscle mass. Individuals with larger muscle mass, such as a young, muscular males have greater creatinine production; at a given level of glomerular filtration, such individuals will have higher levels of serum creatinine. Individuals with smaller muscle mass (e.g., females, the elderly, malnourished patients with muscle wasting, and patients with chronic liver disease) have lower levels of serum creatinine. In particular, patients with CKD with anorexia, weight loss, and muscle wasting, as well as dietary protein restriction will have serum creatinine levels that underestimate the degree of loss of renal function. Factors that interfere with renal tubular secretion of creatinine or with extrarenal excretion of creatinine also change the relationship of serum creatinine and GFR. Extrarenal elimination of creatinine occurs in the gut by colonic secretion into the lumen followed by its degradation by colonic bacteria. Creatinine clearances by this route vary from 1 to $7\,mL/min$. Although negligible at near-normal levels of renal function, this becomes a significant fraction of creatinine clearance in severe kidney failure.

The relationship between serum creatinine concentration and GFR is valid only in the steady state. In the extreme case in which GFR halts, plasma creatinine will still remain normal for several hours until nonexcreted creatinine has accumulated. The relationship between true GFR and serum creatinine is important to consider. During initial reductions in GFR to about $60\,mL/min$, enhanced tubular secretion of creatinine maintains serum creatinine levels at near normal levels (Fig. 9). With further reductions in GFR corresponding to plasma creatinine concentrations of 1.5

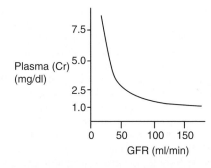

Figure 9   Correlation between plasma creatinine concentration and glomerular filtration rate (GFR). The amount of creatinine that is filtered (GFR $\times P_{Cr}$) is equivalent to the amount that is excreted ($U_{Cr} \times V$). Because creatinine production by skeletal muscle is also relatively constant, creatinine excretion must be constant to maintain equilibrium. Thus, as GFR falls, P_{Cr} must increase proportionately to keep the filtration and excretion of creatinine equal to the creatinine production rate.

to 2.0 mg/dL, however, the tubular secretion of creatinine is saturated, and creatinine concentrations rise proportionate to the fall in GFR. Thus, significant disease progression can occur, while serum creatinine levels remain in the normal or near-normal range. Careful consideration of these factors is needed when attempting to deduce renal functional status from the creatinine level. Two empiric formulae are frequently used to estimate renal function from the serum creatinine level, which are as follows:

The Cockroft–Gault equation (39, 40): creatinine clearance (mL/min) = [140−age (years)] × weight (kg)/72 × serum serum Cr (mg/mL) for men, and corrected by a factor of 0.85 for women The MDRD study formula (41): GFR (mL/min per 1.73m^2) = 186 × (Scr)$^{-1.154}$ × (age)$^{-0.203}$ × (0.724 if female) × (1.210 if African-American), which predicts GFR and not creatinine clearance and takes into consideration race, albumin, and blood urea nitrogen (BUN) levels.

Serum creatinine measurements and estimates of creatinine clearance or GFR provide quick and convenient information about renal function. Serial measurements give an idea of the course of disease and the impact of treatment, provided caution is exercised in their interpretation (42).

BUN and GFR

Like serum creatinine, BUN is excreted by glomerular filtration and tends to vary inversely with GFR. The BUN level is a much less reliable as a marker of GFR than serum creatinine. BUN is greatly influenced by factors other than glomerular filtration. Urea generation is far more variable than creatinine generation: it is elevated with increased protein intake and in states of excessive catabolism—infections, febrile states, and trauma—or decreased during anabolism, as with corticosteroid and tetracycline therapy. Gastrointestinal hemorrhage is of particular clinical importance as a cause of markedly increased urea generation. Conversely, low protein intake, malnutrition, severe liver parenchymal disease, and myxedema are associated with decreased urea generation.

Renal handling of urea is more complex than that of creatinine. Urea is freely filtered at the glomerulus, and 35% to 40% of filtered urea is obligatorily reabsorbed in the proximal tubule. Urea is secreted into the tubular lumen in the loop of Henle, and reabsorbed in the medullary collecting duct via urea transporters that are regulated by vasopressin. The state of hydration, RBF rate, and urine flow rates all influence the rate of urea excretion. In states of dehydration or volume depletion, only 35% to 40% of filtered urea appears in the urine, because of increased proximal reabsorption, while in states of volume repletion or diuresis, this proportion may be higher than 80%. Despite these limitations, analysis of BUN can be clinically helpful. A high BUN: serum creatinine ratio (>20) is suggestive of volume depletion (prerenal azotemia), if renal ischemia, obstruction, or excessive urea generation has been excluded.

Clinical Measurement of GFR

The GFR is measured by assaying the clearance of creatinine or exogenously administered substances. The most frequently used exogenous substances used in clinical practice are iodinated iothalamate and technetium-labeled diethylene-triaminepentaacetic acid, but several nonradionuclide compounds (e.g., nonradioactive iothalamate) and nonionic iodinated contrast media (e.g., iohexol and iopental) are also used in some instances. The most commonly used method for the routine measurement of GFR is the determination of creatinine clearance. A timed collection of urine is required, which must necessarily be accurate, because an incomplete collection can lead to an underestimation of the GFR. The adequacy of the urine collection can be judged by measuring the total creatinine excretion of the patient, which should approximate 10 to 15 mg/kg/day in women and 15 to 20 mg/kg/day in men.

The creatinine clearance is calculated according to the following equations:

$$\text{Assumption: Amount filtered} = \text{Amount excreted}$$
$$P_{Cr} \times \text{GFR} = U_{Cr} \times V$$
$$\text{GFR} = \frac{U_{Cr}}{P_{Cr}} \times V$$

(P_{Cr} and U_{Cr} are the serum and urinary concentrations of creatinine, respectively, and V is the urine flow rate.)

Creatinine clearances always overestimate GFR, because they do not take into account the contribution of tubular secretion of creatinine to urinary creatinine excretion. The contribution of tubular secretion is negligible at normal levels of renal function and serum creatinine; creatinine clearance overestimation of GFR in this setting is in the range of 5% to 10% approximately. Drugs that block the tubular secretion of creatinine (e.g., cimetidine) can produce an elevated plasma creatinine concentration without affecting GFR. With severe degrees of kidney failure, however, creatinine clearance overestimation of GFR may be in excess of 100%. Because creatinine clearances markedly overestimate GFR in advanced stages of renal failure, while urea clearances underestimate GFR, the mean of creatinine and urea clearances may sometimes be used to estimate more accurately GFR in advanced stages of renal failure.

Clinical Estimation of RBF

The measurement of RBF is often required in the management of the post–renal transplant patient and occasionally in the evaluation of renovascular disorders. The renal clearance of substances excreted by both glomerular filtration and tubular secretion is used to estimate effective renal plasma flow. Most commonly used are the radionuclides mercaptoacetyltriglycine, chelated to technetium, and iodohippurate. Doppler ultrasonographic methods are also used to estimate RBF.

ACUTE KIDNEY FAILURE

AKF is a common clinical problem associated with considerable morbidity and mortality. AKF is primarily a hospital-acquired disease, occurring in approximately 5% of hospitalized patients, 5% to 15% of patients following coronary artery bypass grafting, and up to 25% of patients in an intensive care unit (ICU). Mortality in AKF is greatly influenced by comorbid events. The high mortality associated with AKF is well described and reaches 65% in ICU patients (43–45). Of the patients who experience AKF requiring dialysis, 5% to 30% will require long-term dialysis therapy, without renal recovery (46). Importantly, AKF is an independent risk factor for morbidity and mortality. AKF is associated with a 5.5 odds ratio of dying (47). Thus AKF should not be viewed solely as a treatable complication of a serious illness.

AKF can be defined by a decrease in the GFR that occurs over days to weeks. Commonly used definitions include an increase of serum creatinine >0.5 mg/dL over baseline, an increase of serum creatinine over 50% of baseline, or a reduction in creatinine clearance of 50%. However, no standardization of the definition of AKF has been adopted, and the true magnitude of the problem is likely unrecognized. The GFR can decline rapidly with only small changes in the serum creatinine. Understanding the significance of the relationship between early declines in GFR and changes in serum creatinine may help in the early recognition and treatment of AKF.

Classification of AKF

It is useful to subcategorize renal disorders based on clinical and pathologic features. AKF has traditionally been divided into prerenal, renal, or postrenal according to the etiology of the insult (Table 2). Distinguishing these three causes of kidney failure is important to the diagnostic and therapeutic strategy. The majority of hospital-acquired AKF is secondary to prerenal azotemia and ischemic or toxic ATN, an intrinsic renal cause of AKF.

Prerenal Azotemia

Prerenal azotemia accounts for approximately 70% of AKF cases in hospitalized patients (48,49). Prerenal azotemia is a normal physiologic response to decreased renal perfusion and rapidly resolves with restoration of glomerular ultrafiltration pressure. The decrease in glomerular ultrafiltration pressure may be secondary to a true reduction in circulating blood volume from bleeding or cutaneous, GI, or urinary losses, or from renovascular disease or dysfunction (Fig. 10). Cirrhosis, congestive heart failure, and sepsis produce effective circulating volume depletion with similar hypoperfusion of the glomerulus. Mean arterial pressures (MAP) below 80 to 90 mmHg will induce a fall in RBF. If the fall in the MAP is promptly corrected, renal parenchymal damage does not typically ensue. If the prerenal state is allowed to continue, however, renal pathology may occur, and ATN can develop. Sustained reduction in RBF results in cellular hypoxia leading to pathologic tubular changes and ATN. Prerenal azotemia and ischemic ATN are opposite extremes of a continuum related to renal hypoperfusion: the

Table 2   Common Causes of Acute Kidney Failure: Urinary Findings and Confirmatory Tests

Cause of acute kidney failure	Typical urinalysis	Confirmation
Prerenal azotemia		
Volume depletion	No cellular elements or proteinuria	Rapid resolution of ARF with correction of renal hypoperfusion
Decreased EABV		Invasive monitoring—CVP or PCWP
NSAIDs		
ACE-I or ARB		
Postrenal azotemia		
Abdominal or flank pain	Hematuria without dysmorphic red blood cells, casts, or proteinuria	Abdominal X-ray
Palpable bladder		Renal ultrasound
Enlarged prostate		IVP
Nephrolithiasis		Retrograde pyelography
Urinary frequency, oliguria, or anuria		
Intrinsic renal azotemia		
Acute tubulointerstitial nephritis	WBCs	Systemic eosinophilia
	Urine eosinophils	Renal biopsy
	White cell cast	Biopsy of skin rash
	Red blood cells	
	Rarely red blood cell casts	
Hemolysis	Urine supernatant is pink and heme +	Elevated serum K+, PO4, uric acid, LDH
	Hemoglobinuria	Hypocalcemia
	No red blood cells	Peripheral smear with fragmented red blood cells
Hemolytic uremic syndrome and thrombotic thrombocytopenic purpura	Urine red blood cells Heme +	Renal biopsy Peripheral smear with schistocytes and fragmented red cells
		Thrombocytopenia
Glomerulonephritis	Proteinuria	Renal biopsy
	Red blood cell casts	Serum antibody test
	White blood cell casts	
Radiocontrast	May have granular, coarse, or tubule epithelial cell casts	Temporal relationship to the contrast infusion
Rhabdomyolysis	Urine supernatant Heme + without red blood cells	Elevated serum myoglobin, creatine phosphokinase, PO4, uric acid, K+
	Myoglobinuria	Hypocalcemia
Tumor lysis syndrome	Urate crystals	Elevated serum K+, PO4, uric acid
		Decreased serum Ca2+
Ischemia	Muddy brown granular, coarse, or tubule epithelial cell casts	Clinical assessment and urine findings usually sufficient

Abbreviations: EABV, effective arterial blood volume; NSAIDs, nonsteroidal anti-inflammatory drugs; ACE-I, angiotensin-converting enzyme inhibitor; ARB, angiotensin receptor blocker; LDH, lactate dehydrogenase; PCWP, pulmonary capillary wedge pressure; CVP, central venous pressure.

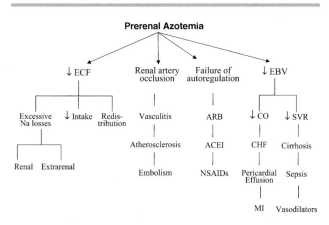

Figure 10 Pathogenesis and etiologies of prerenal azotemia. *Abbreviations*: ARB, angiotensin II receptor blocker; ACEI, angiotensin converting enzyme inhibitor; NSAIDs, nonsteroidal anti-inflammatory drugs; CO, cardiac output; SVR, systemic vascular resistance; EBV, effective blood volume; ECF, extracellular fluid; CHF, congestive heart failure; MI, myocardial infarction.

severity of the insult will dictate the progression from the normal physiologic response to ischemic tubular damage. Less commonly, prerenal AKF can result from diseases of renal microvasculature, including inflammatory (glomerulonephritis and vasculitis) and noninflammatory insults (malignant hypertension) of the vessel wall, thrombotic microangiopathies, and, rarely, hyperviscosity syndromes (Fig. 10). In many instances, the renal hypoperfusion caused by these disorders progresses from prerenal azotemia to ischemic ATN.

Common causes of prerenal azotemia are listed in Table 2 and Fig. 10. The common mechanism leading to a decrease in the GFR is a reduction in the circulating arterial blood volume in the renal vasculature. A reduction in the systemic arterial volume or perfusion pressure causes afferent arteriolar dilation, with concomitant increases in the vasomotor tone of the efferent arteriole. This is accomplished through activation of the renin-angiotensin-aldosterone system. Release of norepinephrine and ADH from the sympathetic nervous system completes the basic neural–hormonal attempt to restore the MAP and circulating blood volume (50,51). The early recognition and correction of prerenal azotemia is paramount in preventing progression to tubular damage from prolonged renal hypoperfusion.

In patients with severe hepatic disease, splanchnic vasodilation and reductions in systemic vascular resistance lead to prerenal azotemia. In these patients, however, the decline in GFR is commonly masked by low production rates of urea (from liver disease) and creatinine (from reduced muscle mass). As a result, plasma creatinine concentrations and BUN levels may remain in the "normal" range despite progressive kidney failure. Hepatorenal syndrome is an otherwise unexplained development of AKF in patients with advanced hepatic disease. Mortality is high, unless hepatic function can be improved, as with liver transplantation.

Postrenal Azotemia

Postrenal azotemia is defined as AKF secondary to urinary tract obstruction. Postrenal azotemia accounts for less than 5% of all cases of AKF, though the frequency is more common in specific patient populations such as elderly men

and certain surgical patients. Obstruction can occur at any level of the urinary collecting system from intratubular to bladder outlet obstruction. Common causes of intrinsic tubular obstruction include nephrolithiasis, blood clots, myoglobinuria, hyperuricosuria, drug crystallization, tumors, and papillary necrosis (Table 2). External retroperitoneal disease processes can cause ureteral obstruction including retroperitoneal fibrosis or abscess, cancers, and retroperitoneal hemorrhage. Accidental surgical ligation of a ureter is also a possibility. The most common cause of postrenal azotemia arising from the lower urinary tract is bladder outlet obstruction, usually from prostatic disease or neurogenic bladder. With timely resolution of the obstruction, there is often complete resolution of the azotemia.

Intrinsic Renal Azotemia

The most common cause of renal azotemia is a direct ischemic insult to the kidney usually resulting in ATN. Other common injuries encountered in the surgical patient include pigmented nephropathy from myoglobinuria or hemoglobinuria, direct nephrotoxic insults from medications and intravenous iodinated contrast, and acute interstitial nephritis (Table 2) typically from medications. ATN accounts for approximately 75% of AKF episodes among hospitalized patients. As discussed earlier, ATN differs from prerenal azotemia in that renal hypoperfusion has been severe enough to injure renal parenchymal cells, particularly tubule epithelium, and AKF does not resolve immediately after restoration of RBF as it does in prerenal azotemia. If the ischemic episode is prolonged, cortical necrosis can ensue and lead to irreversible renal failure.

Hemoglobinuria and myoglobinuria can lead to direct tubular injury through a pigmented cast nephropathy. Extensive trauma resulting in rhabdomyolysis or mismatched blood transfusions leading to massive hemolysis are two common causes of the pigmented nephropathies. In either circumstance, the myoglobinuria or hemoglobinuria results in accumulation of pigmented cast in the proximal tubular lumen and direct injury to tubular cells. With the proximal tubular obstruction, there is also renal vasoconstriction, and both processes contribute to the decline in GFR (52). Renal atheroembolic disease, often following invasive arterial procedures, can also produce AKF (53). Livido reticularis, peripheral and urinary eosinophilia, hypocomplementemia, and thrombocytopenia are classic clinical manifestations of this disorder. Intravenous iodinated contrast promotes an intense renal vasoconstriction and direct tubular cell injury leading to a prerenal azotemia then progression to an intrinsic renal azotemia and ATN. Patients with preexisting renal disease and/or diabetes mellitus are at greatest risk for developing contrast nephropathy (54,55). The temporal relationship between the decrease in GFR and the exposure to the contrast is the most helpful clinical clue to this diagnosis: decrements in GFR are typically seen within 24 to 48 hours of radiocontrast exposure. Recovery from radiocontrast nephropathy often occurs within two weeks of the insult.

Nephrotoxic injury from medications can be caused by a wide array of insults that promote direct tubular damage or injury related to renal vasoconstriction. Common offending agents are the aminoglycoside antibiotics, which can cause a decrease in GFR through multiple mechanisms, including renal vasoconstriction, alterations in glomerular capillary permeability, and direct tubular cell disruption (56). Amphotericin and its lipid-based derivatives cause similar changes in the kidney (57–59). Some medications can cause a change in the serum creatinine with or without an acute change in the GFR; two classic examples of this are cimetidine and trimethoprim-sulfamethoxazole. Both drugs can block the secretion of creatinine, resulting in an elevated serum creatinine level despite preserved GFR. However, both can also cause an interstitial nephritis and a true renal azotemia (60–62).

ATN can be divided into initiation, maintenance, and recovery phases, the pathophysiology and management of which differs (63). In the initiation phase (hours to days), ischemic injury is evolving. GFR falls because of impaired RBF and glomerular ultrafiltration pressure, disrupted integrity of tubule epithelium with backleak of glomerular filtrate, and obstructed urine flow due to intra-tubular formation of casts comprising detached epithelial cells and cellular debris. The terminal portion of the prox-imal tubule and the mTAL are the nephron segments most vulnerable to ischemic injury. Both have high rates of active solute transport and oxygen consumption. Furthermore, both of these segments are located in the outer medulla, an ischemic zone even under basal condition by virtue of the unique countercurrent arrangement of the medullary vasculature. Importantly renal injury can be limited by restoration of RBF during this period. In the maintenance phase (typically 1–2 weeks), during which epithelial cell injury is established, GFR stabilizes at its nadir despite correction of systemic hemodynamics, and uremic compli-cations may arise. In the recovery phase, kidney function is restored to a degree by regeneration and/or repair of kid-ney parenchymal cells.

Diagnosis

In distinguishing prerenal, renal, and postrenal azotemia, the most useful early clinical indices include the timing of the changes in serum creatinine, BUN, and urinary volume following in relation to other clinical events, the urine specific gravity, examination of the urinary sediment, and assessment of the urine electrolytes. In certain circum-stances, evaluation of the urine osmolality and special stains for urine eosinophils are valuable. In determining hemody-namic changes from cardiac failure or sepsis, central hemo-dynamic monitoring is often incorporated into the evaluation of critically ill patients with renal failure.

Hourly urine output can be used as a measure of ade-quate renal perfusion. In a prerenal state with inadequate glomerular perfusion pressure, the urine output will often drop to less than 0.5 mL/kg of body weight. Oliguria, defined by a urine output of less than 400 mL/day, is pre-sent in about 50% of AKF cases. In the evaluation of prerenal azotemia, urine indices are predictable based on the effect of norepinephrine, ADH, and Ang II on urine flow rate and sodium and water reabsorption. The BUN-to-creatinine ratio is usually elevated to greater than 20:1 in a prerenal state; it is common to see an elevated BUN in the face of a normal creatinine early in the coarse of glomerular hypoperfusion. In differentiating prerenal azotemia from ATN, the urine sodium and specific gravity are often used, the typical clinical indices are illustrated in Table 3. However, urine sodium, osmolality, and specific gravity, as well as the serum BUN-to-creatinine ratio are relatively insensitive measures for the differential diagnosis of AKF. An alternative method of evaluating the kidneys ability to handle sodium is the fractional excretion of sodium (FE_{Na}). The FE_{Na} has been adopted to help differentiate, in the oliguric patient, prerenal azotemia from intrinsic renal failure. The FE_{Na} utilizes the urine sodium and creatinine

Table 3 Urinary Indices in the Differential Diagnosis of Acute Kidney Failure

Index	Normal value	Prerenal azotemia	Acute tubular necrosis	Obstruction
Urinary volume	≥ 0.5 mL/kg/hr	≤ 0.5 mL/kg/hr	Variable	Variable
Urine specific gravity	1.003–1.025	≥ 1.020	1.010	Variable
Urinary sodium	Variable	< 20 mEq/L	> 40 mEq/L	< 40 mEq/L early > 40 mEq/L late
FE_{Na}[a]	< 1%	< 1%	> 3%	< 1% early > 3% late
BUN: creatinine	10:1	> 20:1	Variable	Variable

[a]$Fena\ (\%) = \frac{U/PNa}{U/PCr} \times 100$

Abbreviation: BUN, blood urea nitrogen.

with simultaneous measurements of serum sodium and creatinine (Table 3).

In the normal kidney, the FE_{Na} is less than 1%, indicat-ing that less than 1% of the filtered sodium is excreted in the urine. The same is true in prerenal azotemia in which case the tubules are sodium avid in the face of volume depletion and suppressed atrial natriuretic peptide (ANP) release. In contrast, intrinsic kidney failure from ischemic or nephro-toxic injury typically has a FE_{Na} greater than 1% (64,65). However, many confounding factors and conditions can alter the FE_{Na} much like the other urine indices mentioned above, including saline infusion, diuretics, or bicarbonaturia rendering it of limited value in the differential diagnosis of AKF (66).

The urinalysis can often give clues to the underlying etiology of AKF. Hemoglobinuria and myoglobinuria, as well as infectious causes of AKF are easily identifiable by a posi-tive test for large blood on the urine dipstick, despite mini-mal or no red blood cells in the urine on microscopic exam. A large amount of protein (> 3 g/day) is suggestive of an intrinsic kidney, and typically glomerular, injury. Pyuria and white blood cell casts can be secondary to infection, glo-merulonephritis, or ATIN; with the latter, urine eosinophilia may be present but is not a specific finding restricted to ATIN. Red blood cell casts suggest glomerulonephritis. ATN is associated with tubular epithelial cells, epithelial cell casts, and coarse granular cast, whereas prerenal azotemia is associated with fine granular and hyaline casts (Table 2).

Prevention

Given the limited therapeutic options currently available, a clear understanding of which patients are at risk is the best defense against AKF. Patients at the greatest risk for AKF are those with preexisting kidney disease and diabetes mel-litus with or without overt signs of nephropathy. It is also paramount to understand the relationship of measured serum creatinine to GFR. A 75-year-old woman who weighs 55 kg with a "normal" serum creatinine of 1.0 mg/dL actu-ally has a calculated GFR of 44 mL/min and moderate kidney failure. Despite her preexisting kidney disease, it is relatively common for a patient like this with a normal serum creatinine value to receive intravenous iodinated con-trast or other nephrotoxic agents.

A common theme in the prevention of AKF is fluid resuscitation. Often presurgical patients are placed on restricted fluid intake prior to procedures. Adequate intravenous hydration is important especially if intravenous contrast will be used during radiographic studies, if bowel preparation is needed, or if insensible losses are high from bowel surgery or in burn patients. Medications that interfere with the autoregulation of renal perfusion, such as amphotericin, nonsteroidal anti-inflammatory medications, or ACE inhibitors put the patient at a greater risk for prerenal azotemia and ATN.

Specific Measures

N-Acetylcysteine

Newer means of protecting against specific injuries such as contrast-induced nephropathy have become commonplace in the clinical setting. Intravenous contrast can cause AKF by a direct reduction in glomerular perfusion pressure through hemodynamic changes and by exerting a direct toxic effect on the tubular epithelial cells. A proposed mechanism of this action is mediated through the production of oxygen free-radical species. Animal models have shown that free-radical scavengers can reduce the oxidant injury in the kidney and prevent AKF (67). N-acetylcysteine is an antioxidant that promotes renal vasodilation by increasing the bioavailability of NO. Based on these properties and the fact that it is generally well tolerated, N-acetylcysteine has been used for the prevention of AKF from radiocontrast agents in high-risk individuals. Several small clinical trials have shown that its administration prior to radiocontrast significantly reduces the rise in serum creatinine values from baseline as compared to the placebo group (68,69). However, whether N-acetylcysteine prevents severe AKF or the need for dialysis has not been determined. In patients at high risk for radiocontrast nephropathy, it is reasonable to provide N-acetylcysteine given the low potential for harm from the therapy. The most important factors in limiting kidney injury from radiocontrast agents, however, still appear to be providing adequate hydration and minimizing contrast dose (70–73). At the time of this writing, there is no evidence to advocate its routine use in preventing other forms of AKF. There is currently no consensus on its benefit in preventing contrast-induced nephropathy.

Low-Dose Dopamine

In normal human subjects, low-dose (1–3 μg/kg/min) dopamine increases RBF and GFR and acts on the proximal tubule to promote natriuresis. Numerous studies have used low-dose dopamine either to treat or to prevent AKF resulting from radiocontrast administration, repair of aortic aneurysms, orthotopic liver transplantation, unilateral nephrectomy, renal transplantation, and chemotherapy with interferon (INF) (74,75). However, prevention trials have been small, inadequately randomized, and of limited statistical power. Furthermore, low-dose dopamine has been associated with potentially harmful side effects, including tachyarrhythmias, myocardial ischemia, decreased mesenteric blood flow, and suppressed T-cell function (74–76). In diabetic patients treated with low-dose dopamine to prevent radiocontrast nephropathy, there is an associated increase risk of AKF (77). Therefore, it is generally recommended that the use of low-dose dopamine for the prevention of AKF be abandoned.

Low-Dose Fenoldopam

Fenoldopam is a pure dopamine type-1 receptor agonist that has similar renal vascular hemodynamic effects as dopamine, but without the α- and β-adrenergic stimulation. Animal data have shown that a pure dopamine-1 receptor agonist has the potential to reduce the renal injury induced by hypoperfusion of the kidney. In a hypovolemic dog model, infusion studies with fenoldopam mesylate, a selective dopamine-1 receptor agonist, increases cortical and medullary blood flow and preserves GFR (78). The limited clinical trials available suggest that fenoldopam reduces the occurrence of AKF associated with radiocontrast and aortic aneurysm repairs (79,80). However, there is limited clinical data and, as yet, no large randomized controlled trials to support its indiscriminate use.

Diuretics

Furosemide is a loop diuretic and vasodilator that may decrease oxygen consumption in the loop of Henle by inhibiting secondary active transport of sodium (69,81). By increasing urine volume, furosemide may reduce intratubular obstruction from cellular debris and reduce backleak of filtrate. This combination of actions in the kidney may lessen the ischemic potential. Clinical studies have shown furosemide to be ineffective in preventing AKF after cardiac surgery (82), but it may actually increase the risk of AKF in patients given radiocontrast (81). Mannitol acts as an osmotic diuretic that can scavenge free radicals. It may have some benefit when added to solutions to preserve organs for transplantation and to protect against AKF associated with rhabdomyolysis (83,84). Like furosemide, mannitol may actually worsen AKF associated with radiocontrast (77).

Atrial Natriuretic Peptide

ANP increases GFR by causing vasodilatation of the afferent arteriole and constriction of the efferent arteriole, and inhibits tubular sodium reabsorption. Two studies have examined the efficacy of ANP for the prevention of renal dysfunction in renal transplant recipients and found no benefit (85,86). Otherwise, most studies have focused on the treatment of established AKF and found little therapeutic benefit (87). As with low-dose dopamine, furosemide, and mannitol, ANP infusion has been associated with an increased risk of AKF with radiocontrast administration in diabetics (77).

Management

Management is directed at prevention of ATN in high-risk patients and control or uremic complications with established ATN until spontaneous recovery of renal function (63). In the early management of AKF, quick recognition of the renal insult and resolution of the potential cause are most important. If the patient is volume depleted, volume resuscitation is indicated. It is widely held that the degree of renal injury may be minimized in patients with optimized effective intravascular volume. However, the definition of adequate volume expansion has yet to be determined. Also open to question is the type of fluid that should be utilized. Randomized trials evaluating colloids versus crystalloids have revealed conflicting results (88). Albumin is frequently used for volume expansion, with no clinical evidence of its benefit in critically ill patients. A recent meta-analysis of studies involving albumin use in critically ill patients suggested that albumin infusion actually increases mortality (89). Medications that may inhibit the kidney's normal ability to autoregulate glomerular filtration pressure, such as ACE inhibitors and Ang II receptor blockers, should be discontinued if possible when AKF is recognized.

Current evidence suggests that nonoliguric renal failure has a better prognosis than oliguric renal failure. In the nonoliguric patient, volume overload and the potential for prolonged ventilation and poor wound healing are reduced. Volume resuscitation and nutritional support have less potential for complications. Clinical trials have attempted to elucidate if converting oliguric AKF to nonoliguric AKF with pharmacologic measures improves outcome. The use of high doses of loop diuretics early in AKF is common. The potential beneficial effects of loop diuretics include the reduction of intratubular obstruction with cellular debris and limiting oxygen consumption in tubular cells, and thus potentially reducing ischemic tubular damage. The available evidence suggests that using loop diuretics as a continuous infusion will produce a better diuresis than intermittent bolus administration and help manage volume overload (38). While diuretics may simplify patient management, there is no evidence that converting oliguric AKF to nonoliguric AKF with loop diuretics improves renal recovery or patient survival (90,91).

Fluid, Acid–Base, and Electrolyte Abnormalities

Oliguric AKF is often complicated by derangements in electrolytes and fluid balance. In AKF, water intoxication with resultant hyponatremia is a potential complication if hypotonic solutions are used. If the hyponatremia is significant enough, exacerbation of the effects of uremia on the central nervous system can occur. The critically ill patient is often catabolic; so acute hyperkalemia can arise. Serum potassium levels near 6 mEq/L require therapy, particularly if the patient is symptomatic with muscle cramps or weakness, or has electrocardiographic changes that may be a harbinger of life-threatening cardiac arrhythmias. Immediate temporizing maneuvers should include glucose and insulin infusion (start with 25 g, 50% glucose solution plus 10 U of intravenous regular insulin). If the patient is acidotic, intravenous sodium bicarbonate can be infused. Both the insulin and the bicarbonate are temporary measures to redistribute the potassium into the intracellular space, not to eliminate the potassium from the body. After institution of the acute temporizing measures, attempts should be made to eliminate the total body potassium overload. Ion exchange resins such as sodium polystyrene sulfonate (Kayexalate, 30–60 g given orally or rectally) are effective. Kayexalate acts in the intestinal tract through cationic exchange to increase potassium elimination in the stool. In the postoperative patient, it is advisable to administer sorbitol with Kayexalate to prevent constipation and promote catharsis, especially if the patient is receiving narcotic pain medications.

The management of AKF can also be complicated by hypocalcemia, hypermagnesemia, and hyperphosphatemia. Early in AKF, phosphorous levels will rise. The goal of the acute management of hyperphosphatemia is to keep the calcium × phosphate product less than 70. As the calcium × phosphate product rises above 70, the risk of cardiac conduction abnormalities, vascular endothelial damage, and central nervous system injury increases. Phosphorous binders (calcium carbonate, aluminum hydroxide, or cationic polymers such as sevalamer hydrochloride) given with meals can be used to control dietary phosphorous absorption. The phosphate content of enteral feedings or total peripheral nutrition should be reduced. Hypocalcemia is a rare complication of AKF except in the setting of tumor lysis syndrome or rhabdomyolysis, and ionized calcium levels should be monitored in critically ill patients.

AKF is associated with loss of renal acid–base regulation typically resulting in metabolic acidosis. Sodium bicarbonate infusion can help alleviate the metabolic acidosis, but often the associated volume and sodium load is rate limiting. Common solutions for bicarbonate infusion include D5W with 3 amps $NaHCO_3$, 0.25% NaCl with 2 amps $NaHCO_3$, or 0.45% NaCl with 1 amp $NaHCO_3$. It is important to keep the bicarbonate infusion as near to an isotonic solution as possible to limit infusion of excessive Na. In the face of an organic acid such as lactic acid or ketoacids, bicarbonate infusion will produce carbon dioxide, and in a postoperative patient with poor ventilation, this may produce a respiratory acidosis. Frequently the oliguric patient will be unable to tolerate the volume load associated with sodium bicarbonate infusions, so that dialysis is necessary to control the acidosis.

CHRONIC KIDNEY DISEASE

CKD results from the loss of normal renal function arising from any of a wide variety of causes. Table 4 lists the major causes of chronic kidney failure. Whatever the original cause of renal disease, whether primarily glomerular or primarily nonglomerular, CKD tends to worsen because of a progressive loss of functioning nephrons. These processes result in the gradual development of a clinical state of uremia. The rate of progression of renal failure may or may not be predictable depending on the nature of the primary renal disease; however several known "progression" factors—hypertension, tubulointerstitial nephritis, proteinuria, hyperlipidemia, tobacco smoking—are known to influence strongly the process. There is a close correlation between clinical symptoms and the GFR; the GFR has therefore become the clinical marker of the stage of CKD. A clear understanding of the relationship of serum creatinine and GFR is needed so as to make right deductions about the degree of CKD.

Uremic Toxins

Traditionally, the uremic state has been viewed as a "toxic" state, the result of retained "uremic toxins" that would otherwise be excreted by normally functioning kidneys. This view received strong support from the early successes of dialysis therapy in improving uremic symptoms, presumably by the removal of such toxins (92–94). More recently, the uremic state has also been viewed as a chronic inflammatory condition. There are ongoing efforts to identify the triggers for this inflammation, its mediators and consequences. Uremic "retention" of toxic compounds or solutes are arbitrarily classified according to molecular weight into low

Table 4 Causes of Chronic Kidney Failure

Glomerular diseases—primary (idiopathic) and secondary
Tubulointerstitial diseases
Diabetes mellitus
Hypertension
Obstructive nephropathies
Renal cystic diseases
Renovascular diseases
Renal involvement in multisystem diseases, including diabetes mellitus and hypertension
Renal involvement in congenital and heredofamilial diseases
Renal injury secondary to medications, chemicals, drug abuse, radiation, heavy metal

($M_W < 300$ Da; e.g., urea, uric acid, xanthine, and methylguanidine), middle [e.g., β_2-microglobuni, complement factor D, leptin, interleukin-6 (IL-6)], and high-molecular-weight molecules ($M_W > 500$ Da). These are further subdivided into non–protein-bound and protein-bound molecules. Dialysis procedures clear the non–protein-bound, low-molecular-weight solutes predominantly by diffusive and convective forces. There is some clearance of larger molecules by hemodialysis filters, by the process of adhesion. Middle-molecular-weight-molecules are hypothesized to contribute to some of the features of uremia, though specific toxins have not yet been identified (95). Laboratory abnormalities associated with retention of middle-molecular-weight-molecules include disturbances of lymphocyte proliferation, cell growth, interleukin production, osteoblast mitogenesis, and apolipoprotein (apo) A-1 secretion, while clinical abnormalities such as anorexia, polyneuropathy, and carpal tunnel syndrome may occur (96). In addition, a number of protein-bound molecules have been suggested to account for some of uremic toxicity.

Pathophysiology of CKD

Glomerular and tubulointerstitial scarring characterize the renal histopathology of patients with chronic renal failure. These lesions often are similar in appearance, regardless of the nature of the primary renal disease. Decreased glomerular filtration is the result of atubular glomeruli and of increased backleak of filtrate through denuded tubular basement membranes. In all forms of renal disease, both the degree of interstitial infiltration with inflammatory cells and the interstitial fibrosis predict subsequent renal failure more accurately than does glomerular scarring or sclerosis. Interstitial fibrosis therefore represents the final common pathway of response to injury in the kidney, irrespective of the nature of the initial injury (97). Tubulointerstitial fibrosis is characterized by tubular atrophy, tubular dilatation, increased interstitial matrix deposition, and loss of capillaries. Matrix accumulating in the interstitium contains proteins such as collagens l, lll, and V, fibronectin, and laminin. An important phenomenon is the appearance of myofibroblasts, highly fibrogenic and contractile cells that may originate from tubular cells by "transdifferentiation." Tubulointerstitial fibrosis is initiated by tubular epithelial cell injury and activation, and by the recruitment of inflammatory cells such as CD4$^+$ lymphocytes and macrophages into the interstitium (98,99). Some of the factors known to activate tubular cells include proteinuria, cytokines, ischemia, and reactive oxygen species. Activated tubular cells release cytokines such as macrophage chemoattractant protein-1 (MCP-1), regulated on activation, normal T expressed and secreted (RANTES), TGF-β1 and PDGF, and cell adhesion molecules such as integrins, vascular cell adhesion molecule (VCAM), intercellular adhesion molecule (ICAM), E-selectin, and osteopontin that attract more inflammatory cells into the interstitium. After this initial phase of acute interstitial inflammation, a second phase of inflammatory matrix synthesis ensues with the local release of profibrogenic cytokines and tissue inhibitors of matrix metalloproteinase (TIMPs). Finally, the process of persistent matrix synthesis occurs resulting from sustained action of profibrogenic cytokines and epithelial-mesenchymal transformation (transdifferentiation). The appearance of myofibroblasts in the interstitium is the single worst prognostic predictor of later development of interstitial fibrosis (100,101). The origin of these cells is uncertain. There is evidence to suggest that they are derived from resident interstitial fibroblasts, pericytes, or

from transdifferentiated tubular epithelial cells. The major issue awaiting clarification is the mechanism whereby the process of scarring, once initiated, continues even after the original or primary insult is in remission.

Of the cytokines produced by resident glomerular, tubular, and interstitial cells, as well as by infiltrating lymphocytes, macrophages, fibroblasts, and myofibroblasts, TGF-β1 is the predominant fibrogenic molecule involved in tubulointerstitial scarring (99). TGF-β1 production is stimulated by a variety of vasoactive compounds (e.g., Ang II and endothelin-1), circulating peptides, shear stress, and ischemia. It promotes transcription of genes encoding matrix components, inhibits matrix-degrading enzymes, promotes the evolution of myofibroblasts, and enhances chemotaxis of fibroblasts and monocytes. The fibrinolytic system (and plasmin) plays a major role in degrading fibrin and extracellular matrix, and its inhibition by plasminogen activator inhibitor (PAI) impairs the repair process while promoting interstitial fibrosis. TGF-β1 stimulates and upregulates the gene expression of PAI. Downstream signaling pathways for TGF-β1 have not been fully characterized. TGF-β1 is thought to bind to the type II receptor on the cell membrane, which in turn phosphorylates the type I receptor. This complex activates Smad proteins and the mitogen-activated kinase pathway (99). In addition to glomerular capillary hypertension, significant, positive correlation is observed between the magnitude of proteinuria and the degree of tubulointerstitial fibrosis. Proteinuria itself is toxic to the renal tubules. Candidate plasma proteins that may be toxic to renal epithelial cells are albumin, complement components, transferrin, and lipoproteins.

Clinical Course of CKD

Given the large renal functional reserve and slow progression of most renal diseases, most patients remain asymptomatic until 85% to 90% of renal function is lost. Thus, in its early stages, CKD is a subclinical condition, and represents a loss of renal reserve. Excretory and other functions are well maintained, despite a diminution of GFR up to 50%. The usual clinical laboratory parameters—BUN and serum creatinine—may remain in the normal range. Kidney insufficiency ensues at more severe reductions in GFR. Azotemia, impaired concentrating ability resulting in nocturia, anemia, and an easy vulnerability of the kidneys to hemodynamic insults such as volume (salt) depletion, dehydration, hypotension, congestive heart failure, the administration of ACE inhibitors, NSAIDs, and to catabolic drugs and potassium loads, diagnosed as acute-on-chronic renal failure. The stage of clinically overt kidney failure is characterized by severe anemia, fluid overload, hypertension, hyperphosphatemia, hypocalcemia, metabolic acidosis, hyponatremia, isosthenuria, and hyperchloremia. Hyperkalemia still is generally absent unless the patient is receiving large loads of potassium. At end stage, in uremia, there is a constellation of signs and symptoms that involve all the systems—the uremic syndrome (Table 5). Ideally, the full-blown uremic syndrome should not occur, because renal replacement therapy with dialysis or transplantation has already been initiated.

The National Kidney Foundation published "Clinical Practice Guidelines for Evaluation, Classification, and Stratification of Chronic Kidney Disease" in 2002 (102). In this scheme, CKD is defined as (i) kidney damage for more than three months, as defined by structural or functional abnormalities of the kidney, with or without decreased GFR, manifested by either (a) pathologic abnormalities or (b) markers of kidney damage, including abnormalities in the

Table 5 Uremic Manifestations

System	Clinical manifestations
Cardiovascular	Hypertension
	Pericarditis
Gastrointestinal	Anorexia
	Nausea, vomiting
Neurologic	Encephalopathy
	Peripheral neuropathy
Hematologic	Anemia
	Platelet dysfunction
Endocrine	Insulin resistance
	Hyperlipidemia
	Decreased fertility
Musculoskeletal	Renal osteodystrophy
	Myopathy
	Uremic arthropathy

composition of the blood or urine, or abnormalities in imaging tests; and (ii) GFR < 60 mL/min per 1.73 m^2 for more than three months, with or without kidney damage. These guidelines propose specific functional stages of CKD (Table 6) and clinical action plans to pursue depending on the stage.

Clinical Manifestations of CKD
Gastrointestinal System
Gastrointestinal symptoms occur frequently and are prominent in CKD (103) (Table 5). Most common among these are anorexia, nausea vomiting, metallic taste, hiccups, and diarrhea. Additional complications include stomatitis, gastritis, duodenitis, esophagitis, parotitis, and gastroparesis.

Acid–Base, Fluid, and Electrolyte Abnormalities
Metabolic acidosis occurs uniformly in CKD. At GFRs in the 20 to 50 mL/min range, there is usually already a mild drop in serum bicarbonate concentration. The main cause of the metabolic acidosis is decreased ammonia synthesis by the surviving nephrons, which occurs despite the fact that there is an adaptive increase in ammonia synthesis per nephron. This diminution of total ammoniagenesis limits the capacity to excrete acid loads. Sustained metabolic acidosis has a number of potential adverse effects for which the clinical evidence remains controversial.

In CKD, limitation of the capacity to excrete potassium results in hyperkalemia. Hyperkalemia is usually mild (5.0–5.5 mEq/L), even at GFRs as low as 20 mL/min, and requires only dietary potassium restriction and close monitoring as management. With worsening renal failure, however, hyperkalemia becomes more severe and requires definitive treatment. However, there are a number of diseases that are associated with a tendency to hyperkalemia,

Table 6 Stages of Chronic Kidney Disease

Stage	Description	GFR (mL/min/1.73 m^2)
1	Kidney damage with normal or increased GFR	> 90
2	Kidney damage with mild decrease in GFR	60–89
3	Moderate decrease in GFR	30–59
4	Severe decrease in GFR	15–29
5	Kidney failure	< 15/dialysis

Abbreviation: GFR, glomerular filtration rate.

such that hyperkalemia occurs earlier and with more severity in the course of progressive renal failure. These conditions, in particular diabetic nephropathy, are mostly associated with the syndrome of hyporenninemic hypoaldosteronism. Table 7 lists some of the conditions that are commonly associated with the syndrome of hyporenninemic hypoaldosteronism as well as additional clinical situations that predispose to hyperkalemia in CKD. Patients with CKD are at risk of hyperkalemia when these conditions are present. Hyperkalemia needs close monitoring and anticipation in these patients.

With mild-to-moderate degrees of CKD, there is a limitation of sodium excretory capacity despite adaptive compensatory sodium wasting in surviving nephrons. This is manifested mainly as hypertension. Only in severe kidney failure (GFR < 10–15 mL/min) does edema become evident, provided there are no other causes of edema such as nephrotic syndrome or congestive heart failure. Peripheral pitting edema is the most common finding. But with the often co-existing hypertension and left ventricular hypertrophy (LVH) and dysfunction, pulmonary congestion and edema can supervene. Treatment is by dietary sodium restriction (usually 2 g daily), along with the judicious use of diuretics. With moderate CKD, thiazide diuretics are no longer effective. Because of resistance to diuretic therapy, increasing doses of the loop diuretics may be needed before the required dose is determined. Because of their short duration of action (4–6 hours), loop diuretics often need to be dosed frequently. Torsemide, a long-acting (24 hours) loop diuretic, is more convenient and is effective in a once-a-day regimen. The diuretic effect of loop diuretic therapy may be augmented by concomitant administration of hydrochlorothiazide or metalozone.

Table 7 Clinical Conditions That Predispose to Hyperkalemia

Diseases
   Diabetic nephropathy
   Obstructive nephropathy
   Sickle cell nephropathy
   Tubulointerstitial nephropathies
   Systemic lupus erythematosis
   Renal transplantation
   Elderly patients
   Amyloidosis

Drugs
   Potassium chloride, including K$^+$-containing salt substitutes
   Angiotensin-converting enzyme inhibitor; angiotensin II receptor blocker
   Nonsteroidal anti-inflammatory drugs
   Spironolactone
   Amiloride and triamterene
   β-Adrenergic antagonists
   Digoxin, particularly in digoxin toxicity
   Heparin
   Cyclosporine and tacrolimus
   Trimethoprim and pentamidine
   Succinylcholine
   Arginine chloride
   Mannitol
   Glycerol

Other clinical conditions
   Acidosis
   Hyperglycemia
   Volume depletion
   Internal bleeding, especially gastrointestinal bleeding
   Tissue damage, especially rhabdomyolysis

This potent combination should be used with caution because it can rapidly be complicated by volume depletion and acute-on-chronic renal failure, as well as severe hypokalemia.

With progressive CKD, there is the loss of the capacity to dilute or concentrate urine, termed isosthenuria. The individual is prone to excessive and inappropriate water loss and therefore hypernatremia, if water intake is restricted or if the patient is unable to have access to water. Conversely excessive water intake or injudicious administration of hypotonic solutions readily leads to water excess and hyponatremia. Elderly patients are particularly prone to these complications.

Abnormalities of Calcium, Phosphate, and Bone Metabolism

Several alterations of calcium, phosphate, and bone metabolism occur in CKD. The major bone pathologic lesions are described as uremic osteodystrophy. Modifications of this primary bone lesion arise from the different therapeutic interventions and nutritional factors, as a result of which there is a spectrum of bone abnormalities in uremia. Bone disease is mainly attributed to severe secondary hyperparathyroidism, which is characterized by elevated serum PTH levels and parathyroid gland hyperplasia and hypertrophy. Several possible "primary" abnormalities have been postulated as responsible for secondary hyperparathyroidism: phosphate retention, hypocalcemia, deficiency of 1,25 dihydroxy vitamin D (calcitriol), parathyroid gland resistance to calcitriol and calcium, and bone resistance to PTH (104). The principal skeletal and extraskeletal consequences of secondary and tertiary hyperparathyroidism in the CKD patient are presented in Table 8.

Calcitriol deficiency arises not only as a result of loss of nephrons but also by inhibition of its synthetic enzyme, 1α-hydroxylase, by uremic toxins (105). Calcitriol exerts its biologic action by binding to the vitamin D receptor (VDR), the hormone–receptor complex then binding to vitamin D response elements in the DNA. In uremia, parathyroid resistance to calcitriol results in part from reduced expression of VDR as well as altered binding of the hormone–receptor complex to DNA. Similarly, there is parathyroid resistance to calcium associated with reduced expression of the calcium-sensing receptor. Initial diffuse parathyroid hyperplasia and hypertrophy may transform to nodularity of the gland with monoclonal cellular expansion. Allelic loss at loci on chromosome 11 at the location of the MEN-1 gene, which is associated with primary parathyroid hyperplasia, has been described (106). Other mechanisms

of this transformation include somatic mutation and decreased expression of cell cycle regulatory genes.

The principles of treatment and prevention of secondary hyperparathyroidism and renal osteodystrophy derive from the following goals: (i) control of hyperphosphatemia—dietary phosphate restriction: phosphate binders to be taken with meals; (ii) replacement therapy of calcitriol with synthetic 1,25 dihydroxy vitamin D or any of its new analogs; (iii) modulation of dialysate calcium for more effective control of PTH levels; (iv) close monitoring of calcium, phosphate, and PTH levels; and (v) parathyroid surgery or percutaneous ablation for uncontrollable "tertiary" hyperparathyroidism. Ablation can be accomplished by total or subtotal parathyroidectomy, total parathyroidectomy with immediate autotransplantation, total parathyroidectomy with cryopreservation of parathyroid tissue, ultrasound-guided percutaneous ethanol injection directly into the enlarged glands, or ultrasound-guided percutaneous calcitriol injection directly into the enlarged glands.

Calcific uremic arteriolopathy (calciphylaxis) is a rare condition involving the calcification of subcutaneous vessels and infarction of the adjacent skin and tissues. Its pathogenesis is not understood, and morbidity and mortality are very high (107,108). Risk factors may include: high calcium × phosphate products, severe hyperparathyroidism, adynamic bone disease, excessive doses of calcitriol, hypercoagulable state, and intravenous iron therapy. Debridement of necrotic tissue, control of infection, skin grafting, and hyperbaric oxygen therapy may aid management.

Uremic Arthropathy

Monoarticular and polyarticular arthritides and tendinitis are common in uremic patients (108). The causes of articular disease may be classified into crystal-related, related to secondary hyperparathyroidism, related to dialysis therapy (particularly β_2-microglobulin amyloid-associated arthropathy), related to underlying or concomitant systemic diseases, and septic arthritis. Diagnosis usually requires diagnostic joint aspiration. Commonly used arthritic medications such as NSAIDs and colchicine need to be avoided or carefully dosed.

Anemia of CKD

Anemia is a leading cause of morbidity and mortality in CKD (109). Erythropoietin deficiency is the most common cause of anemia in these patients. Adequate treatment of anemia is essential in CKD, in particular, because of its role in the development of LVH with all of its attendant complications. Recombinant human erythropoietin (r-HuEPO and epoietin) is the mainstay of anemia management, not only in end-stage kidney disease but also in the predialysis patient. Adequate treatment of anemia has been shown to improve morbidity, quality of life, and mortality. It is therefore essential to screen vigorously for anemia and treat in a cost-efficient manner in view of the high cost of this medication. Iron deficiency is the most common cause of a lack of response (resistance) to erythropoietin action, so that iron status needs to be closely monitored and corrected. Other mechanisms that contribute to anemia include blood loss, shortened RBC survival, inhibition of erythropoiesis by uremic toxins, chronic inflammation, and severe hyperparathyroidism.

Subcutaneous administration of r-HuEPO is usually more efficient than intravenous, and target hemoglobin levels are about 12 to 13 g/dL. The uremic patient requires iron administration to maintain adequate erythropoiesis

Table 8 Clinical Consequences of Secondary/Tertiary Hyperparathyroidism

Skeletal	Extraskeletal
High turn-over bone disease	Metastatic calcifications (skin, myocardial, vascular, valvular, pulmonary)
Osteitis fibrosa	Bone marrow fibrosis (resistance to erythropoietin)
Mixed osteodystrophy	Myocardial hypertrophy and fibrosis
Bone pain	Encephalopathy, electroencephalographic changes
Osteopenia	Peripheral neuropathy
Fractures	Hypertension, hyperlipidemia, glucose intolerance

and responsiveness to epoietin. Transferrin saturations need to be maintained above 20%. A level of transferrin saturation below 20% is considered to represent iron deficiency in this setting. This level of transferrin saturation is often difficult to achieve with oral iron agents, so that intravenous administration is the preferred route (110). Guidelines for intravenous iron therapy and monitoring of iron stores and availability are provided in the DOQI guidelines of National Kidney Foundation (111).

Cardiovascular Complications

There is excessive cardiovascular morbidity and mortality in uremia (112,113). In the most recent report of the United States Renal Data System (USRDS) data, all-cause mortality in patients with end-stage kidney disease is about 20% per year; of these, cardiovascular complications account for approximately 50%. Among cardiovascular complications, atherosclerotic events (acute myocardial infarction, ischemic cardiomyopathy, peripheral vascular disease, cerebral infarctions, and mesenteric infarctions) account for at least 50% of deaths. The proportion of atherosclerotic events is even greater if account is taken of the ischemic component of congestive heart failure and sudden death. Cardiac death rates are 10 to 15 times higher in uremic patients than in age-matched controls of both genders. Twenty to thirty percent of cardiac deaths are due to myocardial infarctions. Besides the high prevalence rates of coronary artery disease in uremic patients, there is a high fatality rate in these patients, possibly a reflection of poor coronary perfusion reserve. Mortality rates of first myocardial infarctions are higher and of recurrent myocardial infarctions even more so. There is a higher rate of restenosis after PTCA. These data suggest that uremia further exaggerates the risks of coronary artery disease (112,113).

Atherosclerosis in uremic patients is thus particularly severe and aggressive. Although there is controversy whether it progresses at an accelerated pace, the term "accelerated atherogenesis or atherosclerosis" is commonly used to describe this phenomenon. The use of these terms is best reserved, for the present, for the observation that atherogenesis is noted at a very early age in uremic patients. More than 80% of young chronic dialysis patients (age 20–30 years) already have severe and progressive coronary artery calcifications as detected by electron beam computed tomography. In the 20 to 40 years age group, coronary artery disease rates are up to 40 times the background population (112,113). There is evidence that the uremic state per se and not dialysis is the major causative factor in accelerated atherosclerosis. Incidence rates and age at first myocardial infarction are similar in predialysis and end-stage kidney disease (ESKD) patients. Nearly 40% of patients have coronary artery disease and congestive heart disease at the start of dialysis. Some of these observations may be attributed to the high incidence of diabetes, and the older age of patients in the ESKD population.

LVH and Uremic Cardiomyopathy

LVH and an increased left ventricular mass index are highly prevalent in CKD and ESKD patients (114). In the general population and in uremic patients, LVH is the strongest predictor of adverse cardiovascular events. In the general population, vigorous control of hypertension and the use of ACE inhibitors result in a decline in LVH and cardiovascular morbidity. Unfortunately LVH is frequently underdiagnosed, and hypertension is inadequately treated in CKD and ESKD. Both concentric and eccentric LVH occur in combination in

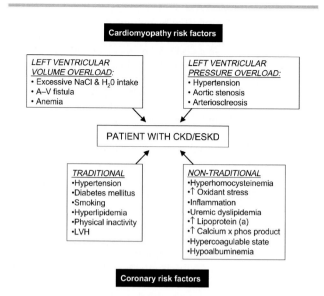

Figure 11 Risk factors for cardiovascular disease in chronic kidney disease and ESKD patients. *Abbreviations*: CKD, chronic kidney disease; ESKD, end-stage kidney disease.

CKD. Concentric LVH is mainly secondary to hypertension and aortic stenosis; remodeling of the arterial tree with arterial dilatation, wall thickening, and stiffening also results in pressure overload and concentric hypertrophy. On the other hand, volume overload results in eccentric hypertrophy with enlargement of the left ventricular chamber (Fig. 11). The three main factors contributing to volume overload are sodium and water excess, anemia, and the arterio-venous (A-V) access. Myocardial cells are overloaded and have an increased rate of energy expenditure in the presence of impaired coronary circulation and diminished coronary reserve resulting in myocardial cell death. Abnormal induction of proto-oncogenes, which promote and regulate cell proliferation and differentiation, and activation of growth factors that stimulate the proliferation and activity of cardiac fibroblasts result in cardiomyopathy and myocardial fibrosis: a rapid increase in collagen synthesis and extracellular matrix. Myocardial fibrosis is more marked in pressure overload than in volume overload and is favored by factors such as senescence, ischemia, catecholamines, Ang II, and aldosterone. Other factors such as endothelin, PTH, and sympathetic nerve discharge contribute to myocardial fibrosis. Delayed relaxation resulting from slower uptake of calcium by the sarcoplasmic reticulum contributes to diastolic dysfunction and arrhythmias, which are also favored by conduction abnormalities resulting from myocardial fibrosis and hypertrophy. In ESKD patients without preexisting cardiac disease, systolic function is usually well preserved; diastolic function is usually abnormal as a result of LV stiffness and delayed relaxation. Diastolic dysfunction is characterized by marked sensitivity to changes in left ventricular volume. A small increase in LV volume can cause pulmonary congestion, while a small decrement can lead to systolic hypotension and hemodynamic instability.

Coronary Artery Disease

The prevalence of ischemic heart disease in ESKD patients on chronic hemodialysis is 10 to 20 times that in the general population (115). According to the USRDS, 42% of chronic hemodialysis patients have had an acute myocardial infarction or a coronary revascularization procedure: 20% of cardiovascular deaths in ESKD patients is due to acute myocardial infarction, the excessive risk being highest in the elderly and diabetics. In addition to traditional risk factors, a number of uremia-specific risk factors contribute to coronary atherosclerosis and myocardial ischemia (116) (Fig. 11). In nonuremic patients with suspected myocardial damage, serum levels of myoglobin, creatinine kinase (CK)-MB, and troponins are reliable markers for early diagnosis and risk stratification.

In chronic hemodialysis patients, there is a high prevalence of silent myocardial ischemia, significant coronary artery disease occurring in 30% to 50% of asymptomatic or mildly symptomatic patients (115). Thus, symptoms of angina pectoris are unreliable. Conversely, because of small-vessel disease and microcirculatory dysfunction, 25% of hemodialysis patients with angina pectoris have no significant stenosis of epicardial coronary arteries. Electrocardiographic findings are often confounded by nonspecific changes due to LVH, electrolyte abnormalities, and uremic pericarditis. Noninvasive ECG stress testing is limited by nonspecific baseline ECG changes, poor exercise tolerance, and excessive hypertension during exercise. Both exercise thallium scintigraphy and pharmacologic stress testing have poor sensitivity and specificity. Dobutamine stress echocardiography is independent of exercise tolerance, and appears to be the most valuable noninvasive test currently available. Coronary angiography is therefore frequently indicated, but with careful consideration of attendant risks. The CKD patient, especially if advanced, is at high risk of contrast nephropathy and acute-on-chronic kidney failure that may require dialysis. Dialysis patients are also at risk of volume overload, pulmonary edema, and bleeding complications.

Revascularization Procedures

There is a high complication rate associated with coronary bypass surgery. Complications include arrhythmias, myocardial infarction, low-output congestive heart failure, bleeding, and infection. Preoperative risk factors include older age, emergency surgery, LVH and dysfunction, myocardial and coronary calcification, and New York Heart Association class IV. Long-term outcome in dialysis patients undergoing coronary artery bypass surgery is poor. According to the USRDS, in dialysis patients who underwent bypass surgery between 1978 and 1995, five-year survival was 26.5% compared with 90% in nonuremic patients.

Balloon angioplasty (PTCA) in dialysis patients is characterized by higher complication rates as well as high rates of recurrent ischemia, myocardial infarction, restenosis, and death (117,118). The lesions are more complex and diffuse; there is extensive vascular calcification and small vessel disease; vessel diameters are smaller; there is more multivessel involvement; there is a higher proportion of diabetes mellitus and hypercoaguability. New techniques may offer particular benefit in these complicated patients, such as coronary artery stenting, newer antiplatelet therapies—the thienopyridines and glycoprotein IIb/IIIa-receptor antagonists—rotational atherectomies, and brachytherapy (117,118).

Hypertension

It is established that hypertension is a major risk factor for cardiovascular disease in the general population. There is an extremely high incidence of hypertension in CKD (119). Even when hypertension is not currently present, there may have been a prior history with the fall in blood pressure coinciding with the development of severe left ventricular systolic dysfunction. After adjusting for age, diabetes mellitus, ischemic heart disease, hemoglobin, and albumin level, each 10 mmHg rise in MAP was independently associated with a progressive increase in concentric LVH, development of de novo congestive heart failure, and new-onset ischemic heart disease (119). Thus hypertension is a major risk factor for the development of cardiac disease in CKD. Impaired coronary perfusion coupled with ventricular hypertrophy leads to a vicious cycle of impaired left ventricular contraction, left ventricular dilatation, progressive alteration of left ventricular geometry, and systolic dysfunction. Vigorous treatment of hypertension is advocated, and the guidelines for target blood pressure as well as for recommended choice of medications are under intense study. No single class of antihypertensive medication is superior to the other in dialysis patients.

Pericarditis

Before the advent of chronic dialysis therapy, uremic pericarditis was an agonal development in the course of the disease. With chronic dialysis, uremic pericarditis is less common and is treatable. It however remains a significant cause of morbidity and mortality in CKD. In dialysis patients, uremic pericarditis is associated with inadequate dialysis often in relation to a dysfunctioning vascular access or poor compliance with dialysis prescriptions (120). Pericarditis also frequently occurs in hypercatabolic states such as severe infections, postsurgery. Volume overload has been proposed as a risk factor. Clinical presentation is highly variable and most importantly the patient may be asymptomatic. Dialysis patients with pericarditis often present with fluid retention, an increasing difficulty with fluid removal (ultrafiltration) during dialysis treatments and hypotension. Pleural effusions often accompany uremic pericarditis, considered to be part of a diffuse serositis. The pericardial fluid is exudative and frequently hemorrhagic with a lot of organized fibrin; the fluid is often loculated. Uremic pericarditis is usually successfully treated with intensified dialysis. Pericarditis occasionally occurs in patients who are considered to be adequately dialyzed. This appears to be a dialysis-associated pericarditis, for which heparin used in dialysis anticoagulation may be a risk factor. Much less commonly, a constrictive pericarditis occurs. The mainstays of therapy are a high index of suspicion, intensified dialysis for uremic pericarditis, and close monitoring. Patients with dialysis-associated pericarditis do not respond well to intensive dialysis. Heparin should not be administered with dialysis. NSAIDs or steroids are not effective. Pericardiotomy or pericardiectomy is indicated for the persistent or enlarging effusion or at the earliest sign of hemodynamic compromise (120). Other causes of pericarditis should be in the differential diagnosis—viral, bacterial, and mycobacterial infections, autoimmune diseases, malignancies, and drugs.

Lower Extremity PAOD

Peripheral arterial occlusive disease (PAOD) is a major cause of morbidity and mortality in end-stage renal disease patients on dialysis (121). In ESKD patients, PAOD confers additional risks for hospitalizations, death within six months of the initiation of chronic dialysis, and death following a myocardial infarction, and poor outcomes following renal transplantation—prolonged hospitalizations, poor allograft survival, and increased mortality rates. The incidence of nontraumatic lower extremity amputations after renal transplantation is 10 times higher in ESKD patients than in non-ESKD patients even after correction for diabetes mellitus. Lower extremity amputation is the most common vascular complication following renal transplantation. Septicemia secondary to PAOD is one of the leading causes of death among ESKD patients. Risk factors for PAOD include advancing age, diabetes mellitus, hypertension, hyperlipidemia, smoking (tobacco), coronary artery disease as well as numerous novel, nontraditional atherosclerosis risk factors. Vascular calcification is very common.

With "noncritical ischemia," patients are either asymptomatic or present with claudication. With more advanced disease, "critical stenosis," patients present with rest pain, ischemic ulceration, and gangrene. Diagnostic testing needs to be performed early because history and physical examination are not reliable. Because of heavily calcified peripheral arteries, ankle brachial index may be falsely negative. Other noninvasive screening tests such as toe brachial index, transcutaneous partial pressure of oxygen measurements, and toe pulse volume recording are not affected by lower leg arterial calcifications. Digital arterial calcifications occur in ESKD patients, and this may interfere with the toe brachial, and toe pulse volume tests. Duplex scanning, conventional angiographic studies, and, more recently, peripheral magnetic resonance angiography and CO_2 angiography are alternative tests in these settings. Because a high proportion of patients progress to critical stenosis and require surgical intervention, preventive and conservative measures should be vigorously pursued (121).

Uremia-Associated Immune Deficiency

The uremic state is associated with an immunodeficiency state, the mechanisms of which await full elucidation. This immune abnormality is characterized by a chronic state of activation of all the key components of the immune system—T-cell, B-cell, monocyte/macrophage, and polymorphonuclear neutrophil systems—which paradoxically result in immune deficiency (122). The abnormalities occur early in the predialysis stage and are not reversed by dialysis. Therefore, it is postulated that this abnormally activated immune state is triggered by metabolic derangements resulting from uremia or by nondialyzable "uremic toxins." Additional factors contributing to the immunodeficiency include malnutrition, vitamin deficiencies, anemia, use of drugs such as intravenous iron especially in the presence of iron overload, and vitamin D, known for its immunosuppressive activity, and hemodialysis therapy especially when bioincompatible dialyzer membranes are used. In summary, in uremia, T-lymphocytes exist in a state of activation but exhibit impaired response capacity; B-lymphocytes are in an activation state but are not capable of sustaining an adequate antibody response; monocytes are activated and produce abnormally high levels of interleukin 1 (IL-1), IL-6, and tumor necrosis factor-α (TNF-α), while polymorphonuclear neutrophils are activated, with increased generation of reactive oxygen species and the increased release of their cytoplasmic proteases. CKD patients are susceptible to a high frequency of bacterial, viral (including hepatitis B and C), and mycobacterial infections, and may exhibit cutaneous anergy.

Abnormalities of Coagulation

A bleeding tendency is the most common abnormality in uremia (123). Numerous laboratory abnormalities of coagulation have been described in uremia, but platelet dysfunction appears to be the most dominant defect. The bleeding diathesis improves with dialysis, suggesting that retained dialyzable compounds or toxins may play an important role. Minor or major epistaxis, hematuria, menorrhagia, melena, retroperitoneal hemorrhage, and hemorrhagic pleural or pericardial effusions may be encountered. There is a diminution in number and binding affinity of the platelet membrane glycoprotein receptors llb and llla. Possible mediators of the bleeding diathesis include NO, cAMP, urea, phenols, and guanidinosuccinic acid. Altered blood rheology secondary to a low hematocrit may also contribute to bleeding. CKD appears to be a risk factor for postoperative bleeding in patients undergoing coronary artery bypass graft surgery. Even mild levels of renal impairment were associated with increased risk for postoperative bleeding: patients with a GFR of 40 mL/min or less had six times the odds of postoperative bleeding than patients with a GFR greater than 100 mL/min (124).

Thrombosis is uncommon in uremia. However, thrombosis occurs frequently in dialysis A-V grafts as well as in the coronary and cerebrovascular circulations (125). Risk factors for thrombosis include smoking, trauma, immobilization, thrombocytosis, antiphospholipid antibodies, resistance to activated protein C (the factor V Leiden mutation), and hyperhomocysteinemia.

Abnormalities of Carbohydrate and Lipid Metabolism

Hypertriglyceridemia and hypercholesterolemia with decreased HDL levels and elevated Lp(a) levels are common in ESKD patients (126,127). Hyperinsulinemia is secondary to reduced renal catabolism of insulin and insulin resistance (128). As renal failure progresses, insulin requirements fall. Failure to recognize this can result in severe hypoglycemic episodes. Oral hypoglycemics are prone to cause hypoglycemia. Additional abnormalities include altered peripheral glucose utilization.

Neurologic Complications

Neurologic complications in uremia are a common cause of morbidity and mortality (129–131). The central nervous system as well as peripheral and autonomic nervous systems are affected. Uremic encephalopathy describes central nervous system dysfunction secondary to chronic renal failure. Differential diagnosis includes electrolyte derangements, particularly of sodium and calcium, drug toxicities, hypertensive disorders, ischemic cerebrovascular syndromes, sepsis, and coexisting hepatic neurologic or other multisystemic diseases.

Dialysis dementia is a severe, fatal neurologic complication of dialysis first noted in epidemic form and characterized by difficulties of speech with rapid progression and deterioration and death occurring within months of diagnosis (132). There is strong evidence that dialysis dementia is associated with aluminum exposure and toxicity. This devastating complication is now rare and has been largely controlled by the use of reverse osmosis (RO) in deionization of dialysis water. Dialysis disequilibrium syndrome is a complication of hemodialysis comprising headaches, nausea, vomiting, muscle cramps, tremors disorientation, and seizures during hemodialysis, possibly related to rapid fluxes of urea or other solutes and/or disturbances of brain intracellular pH (133).

Uremic peripheral neuropathy is usually distal, symmetric, and mixed (sensory and motor) (134). Autonomic neuropathy is characterized by loss of baroreceptor sensitivity resulting in postural hypotension, hypotension during dialysis unresponsive to volume repletion, paroxysmal hypertension during dialysis, arrhythmias, gastroparesis and other GI motility problems, and sexual dysfunction (135).

Management of Progressive CKD

There is currently no convenient, inexpensive method of measuring progression of renal failure. Serial creatinine measurements are unreliable because creatinine levels do not rise until renal failure is quite advanced. The reciprocal of serum creatinine or logarithm of serum creatinine over time has a more linear relationship with GFR, and these are sometimes used, but intermittent estimations of GFR with creatinine clearance measurements or other methods are often required. The mainstays of management include the assessment of severity and stage of renal failure; reno-protection—monitoring and control of progression factors; control of complications, including appropriate drug dosing; and timely recognition of the need to initiate renal replacement therapy (97) (Tables 9 and 10). All of these goals require effort to inform and educate patient and family of the nature of disease and benefits of adherence to the treatment plan.

Diagnostic Use of Renal Imaging in CKD

Diagnostic imaging may be of value in the diagnosis and management of CKD (136–138). Renal ultrasonography is an integral part of the evaluation of chronic renal failure and is now available in many renal clinics. The renal ultrasound is used to assess (i) renal size, position, and number; (ii) parenchymal disease (echogenicity); (iii) obstruction; (iv) tumors, cysts, inflammation, and abscesses; (v) trauma; (vi) renovascular diseases; (vii) abnormalities of the transplanted kidney; (viii) nephrocalcinosis; and (ix) in ultrasound-guided interventional procedures. Computed tomography (CT) scanning is used in evaluation of (i) renal masses, cysts, inflammation, and cysts; (ii) obstruction and site of obstruction; (iii) perinephric hematomas, abscesses, or other collections; and (iv) renal stones and nonopaque filling defects. Magnetic resonance imaging provides additional anatomic information in the evaluation of renal diseases. MR arteriography is now the diagnostic test of choice in the evaluation of renal artery stenosis in many centers. MR venograms are also useful in detecting renal vein thrombosis.

Perioperative Management of the CKD Patient

Because of their limited capacity to maintain fluid, electrolyte, and acid–base homeostasis, CKD and ESKD patients experience increased perioperative morbidity and mortality

Table 9 Management of Chronic Kidney Disease

Control of hypertension, with attention to evidence-based optimum
Blood pressure reduction and choice of antihypertensive agent
Dietary restrictions—phosphate, sodium, potassium, protein, lipid, and fluid
Glycemic control in diabetics
Control of:
  Anemia
  Hyperparathyroidism
  Dyslipidemia
  Hyperhomocysteinemia
  Increased oxidant stress
Attention to atherosclerosis, coronary artery and peripheral vascular disease, and left ventricular hypertrophy
Timely recognition of need to initiate renal replacement therapy
Education of patient regarding treatment modalities and early planning of dialysis access

Table 10 Indications for the Initiation of Chronic Dialysis

Absolute indications
  Progressive advanced chronic kidney failure with:
    Pericarditis/pericardial effusions
    Severe encephalopathy—confusion, asterexis, coma, myoclonus
    Severe, difficult-to-control hypertension
    Refractory volume overload, anasarca, pulmonary congestion and edema
    Intractable nausea
    Bleeding diathesis
    Malnutrition
    BUN levels > 100 mg/dL (if primarily reflective of reduced GFR)
    Serum creatinine levels > 10 mg/dL
Relative indications
  Somnolence (daytime)
  Inability to concentrate
  Poor memory
  Restless leg syndrome
  Anorexia, nausea, vomiting, weight loss
  Pruritus
  Increased vulnerability to infection
  Depression

Abbreviations: BUN, blood urea nitrogen; GFR, glomerular filtration rate.

rates compared to patients with normal renal function (139,140). In CKD and ESKD patients, cardiac arrhythmias and sepsis are the most frequent causes of perioperative mortality. ESKD patient who undergo cardiac surgery tends to require longer postoperative vasopressor support, mechanical ventilation, and ICU and hospitalization stays than patients who do not have kidney disease (141). Meticulous evaluation and management is required in the perioperative period to avoid acute and often catastrophic clinical problems. Previously undetected cardiac or pulmonary disease must be identified and compensated for or corrected in the preoperative period. Preoperative testing may be necessary in patients with cardiac risk factors. The patient must be adequately dialyzed, preferably receiving hemodialysis within 12 to 24 hours of the operative procedure. In the case of CAPD or CCPD, dialysis can generally continue until called to the operating room, at which time the peritoneal cavity is drained. Plasma electrolyte levels, in particular potassium concentrations, must be optimized before surgery, particularly because electrolyte fluxes can be problematic during anesthesia. Preoperative hyperkalemia in ESKD patients is common (142) and can be temporarily improved by the intravenous administration of an insulin–dextrose combination or bicarbonate, and polystyrene-binding resins or dialysis can remove excess stores of potassium. CKD and ESKD patients commonly experience preoperative and intraoperative hypertension. With few exceptions, CKD and ESKD patients with chronic hypertension should continue antihypertensive drug therapy throughout the surgical period. Transdermally administered clonidine two to three days before surgery or intravenously administered agents can potentially substitute for oral agents that cannot be given intravenously. If future vascular access grafting is contemplated, intravenous line placement and blood draws should be avoided in a patient's nondominant arm.

Anesthetics have multiple effects on the renal microcirculation and the release of certain hormones. The volatile anesthetic drugs (e.g., halothane) can reduce cardiac output and blood pressure resulting in glomerular hypoperfusion and prerenal azotemia. The inhaled anesthetics do not appear to directly alter renal autoregulation (143). Renal hypoperfusion from volatile anesthetics and increased ADH release associated with surgical procedures may result in intraoperative oliguria. However, in the absence of surgical manipulation, anesthetics are not associated with increased ADH release (144). In addition, halothane and enflurane have been shown to increase renin levels in sodium-depleted animals (145). Preoperative hydration with normal saline attenuates the prerenal azotemia, and the release of ADH and renin in these clinical settings.

Whether inhalation anesthetics cause direct nephrotoxicity is controversial. However, a concentrating defect in the kidney, which can lead to polyuria with dilute urine and associated hypernatremia, has been described with the metabolism of anesthetics such as methoxyflurane, enflurane, and sevoflurane to fluoride (146–149). Patients with CKD have been reported to be at increased risk for worsening renal dysfunction after enflurane inhalation (150). However, there is no evidence that fluoride levels are increased in patients with depressed GFR's in this circumstance, presumably because of bone uptake of the metabolite. Halothane and isoflurane are not known to be nephrotoxins (151).

CKD reduces the clearance of long-acting nondepolarizing muscle relaxants (e.g., pancuronium). The duration of action of vecuronium is unpredictable (152). The clearance of atracurium and mivacurium is not affected by a low GFR, and these agents are safe choices in patients with CKD requiring anesthesia (152). The acetylcholinesterase inhibitors neostigmine, pyridostigmine, and edrophonium are more than 50% excreted in the urine, and CKD may prolong their clearance (153). Careful attention to drug selection and dosing is therefore critical.

Because of the increased risk of bleeding related to uremic platelet dysfunction, the ESKD patient should be well dialyzed, and medications with antiplatelet effects should be avoided close to the time of surgery. Bleeding time is the most sensitive indicator of the extent of platelet dysfunction, although test results are variable across laboratories. Bleeding times of greater than 10 to 15 minutes may be associated with a high risk of hemorrhage (154), but a precise correlation between prolonged bleeding times and surgical risk in the ESKD patients has not been clearly established. The synthetic ADH analog, 1-deamino-8-D-arginine vasopressin (DDAVP; 0.3 mcg/kg IV one hour before surgery) (155), cryoprecipitate [10 units over 30 minutes IV; effects generally apparent in one hour (156)], or conjugated estrogens [0.6 mg/kg/day IV or orally for five days; some effect should be apparent in six hours, with peak effect in five to seven days (157,158)] can be administered to improve the bleeding time. Cryoprecipitate can be given repeatedly to effect improvements in bleeding risk, but DDAVP is subject to tachyphylaxis with repeated dosing. Intensive dialysis or transfusion of packed red blood cells to raise the hematocrit to at least 30% may also reduce bleeding risk. Nonetheless, packed blood cell transfusion should generally be reserved for patients with clinically significant anemia, to avoid the potential for antibody formation that may limit the prospects for successful renal transplantation in the future. Many patients with CKD or ESKD receive prophylactic antibiotics for surgical procedures, especially dialysis A-V graft procedures (159), and minor procedures [e.g., dental care (160)]. To avoid bacterial seeding of the grafts before epithelialization occurs, antibiotic prophylaxis using standard endocarditis regimens is recommended for the first several months after synthetic vascular access are placed.

In the postoperative period, strict attention must be paid to volume and hemodynamic status and drug dosing, as well as fluid, electrolyte, and acid–base balance. Surgical trauma, blood product transfusions, and acidosis may promote significant hyperkalemia, which may require emergent treatment. Postoperative hypokalemia is generally not treated unless signs, symptoms, or cardiac dysrhythmias referable to hypokalemia supervene, or the patient requires digitalis therapy. Operative blood losses, third-space volume losses, and fluid losses from drains and fistulae must be carefully evaluated to optimize postoperative care in the renal patient.

Dialysis

Different types of dialysis modalities are in clinical use. These can be broadly categorized as intermittent hemodialysis, continuous renal replacement therapy (CRRT), and peritoneal dialysis. The relative advantages and disadvantages of these modalities in various clinical settings are presented in Table 11.

Hemodialysis

Hemodialysis became standard treatment for kidney failure in the 1960s. In this process, the blood is circulated through a machine containing a dialyzer (also called an artificial kidney). The dialyzer has two spaces separated by the thin, semipermeable dialysis membrane. Blood passes on one side of the membrane, and dialysis fluid passes on the other. The wastes and excess water pass from the blood through the membrane into the dialysis fluid, which is discarded. The dialyzed blood is returned to the circulation. The process of removing excess fluid is known as ultrafiltration. The blood is circulated and diffused numerous times during a dialysis session. Chronic hemodialysis is commonly performed three or more times a week for four hours or more.

Physical Process of Solute and Water Transport Across the Dialyzer Membrane

The dialyzer membrane is a semipermeable membrane. Solute molecules and water, the solvent, move across this

Table 11   Comparative Advantages (+) and Disadvantage (−) of Dialysis Modalities

Clinical variable	Intermittent hemodialysis	Peritoneal dialysis	CRRT
Continuous renal replacement	−	+	+
Hemodynamic stability	−	+	+
Superior attainment of fluid balance	−	−	+
Unlimited nutritional support	−	−	+
Superior metabolic control	−	−	+
Continuous removal of toxins	−	+	+
Limited anticoagulation	+	+	−
Stable intracranial pressure	−	+	+
Rapid removal of poisons, drugs	+	−	−
Need for intensive care nursing support	−	+	+
Need for hemodialysis nursing support	+	+	−
Ease of operation	−	+	+/−
Patient mobility	+	−	−

Abbreviation: CRRT, continuous renal replacement therapy.

membrane under the influence of three physical processes—diffusion, convection, and ultrafiltration. Diffusion is the process of solute movement down a concentration gradient across the membrane. The flux of solute molecules depends on the size and shape of the solute molecule (characteristics that are described in a term called the diffusion coefficient of the solute); the porosity of the membrane, as well as its thickness, and surface area; and the concentration gradient and temperature of the solution. Whereas these factors enable a close prediction of solute fluxes or clearance in simple solutions, protein binding and electrical charge further influence solute flux in vivo.

A second mechanism of the movement of solute molecules is convection. Water (solvent) is moved across the membrane by filtration; the flux of water is determined by the balance of hydrostatic and oncotic pressures across the membrane (the transmembrane pressure), and the permeability of the membrane to water molecules (hydraulic permeability) defined in the term, "coefficient of hydraulic permeability" (K_f). Convective movement of solute is the movement of solute molecules with water, a phenomenon known as solvent drag. The convective flux depends on the ultrafiltration rate and the solute concentration, as well as the sieving coefficient of the membrane for the solute. Sieving coefficients of membranes to solutes are determined by a characteristic of the membrane, the reflection coefficient. Dialysis membranes are classified according to ultrafiltration coefficient and solute sieving profiles into high-flux and low-flux membranes. Low-flux membranes are called dialyzers and clear solute mainly by diffusion, while high-flux membranes are called hemofilters and clear solute mainly by convection.

The Dialyzer Membrane and Dialyzer Design

Several important characteristics are required of the dialyzer membrane. These include adequate clearance of small molecules such as urea; adequate removal of water; retention of large molecules; biocompatibility (i.e., nonthrombogenic, nontoxic, and noninflammatory); capable of sterilization by steam, gamma irradiation, or ethylene oxide; and possessing microscopic structure that confers strength to the high transmembrane pressures required for ultrafiltration. Dialyzer membranes are classified into categories depending on their method of production. Semisynthetic membranes are cellulose derived or modified/regenerated cellulose (cellulose acetate, cellulose diacetate, and cellulose triacetate). Synthetic membranes include those composed of polysulfone, polyamide, polyacrylonitrile, or polymethylmethacrylate. The dialyzer membranes are assembled or bundled in two main designs—hollow fiber and parallel plate. Modern dialyzers are constructed of hollow fiber filters.

Hemodialysis Vascular Access

A well-functioning, dependable vascular access is needed for hemodialysis. For chronic hemodialysis, the ideal, permanent access is a "native" A-V fistula: the alternative is a synthetic A-V graft. However, in several clinical situations, temporary vascular access is needed. Percutaneous central venous hemodialysis catheters (CVCs) are available for such situations.

Central Venous Catheters. The ability of CVCs to provide high blood flow rates (300–400 mL/min) is compromised by the development of very negative pressures at the catheter tip and pores as a result of high blood velocities in the area—the Bernoulli effect. This effect is worsened by additional obstruction from thrombosis and fibrin sheaths and results in the collapse of the venous wall around the catheter. To minimize this problem, catheters are positioned in the right atrium; they are made with a wide internal diameter, multiple pores placed in all directions around the catheter, and the arterial port placed away from the wall of the vein. The ideal CVC should provide adequate blood flows with minimum resistance, pressure drop, and Bernoulli effect; its placement should cause minimal trauma to the vein and its intimal lining; and minimal activation of the coagulation cascade, white cells and platelets, and infection by the migration of bacteria from skin, along the sides of the catheter or through the catheter lumen. The material of the CVC should be able to withstand the negative pressures without collapsing and should not kink, break, or deteriorate with use of antiseptic agents (161,162).

The materials of which dialysis CVC catheters are made need to fulfill certain requirements for clinical safety and performance as well as for manufacturing purposes (162). The material should be biocompatible and nonthrombogenic; the body of the catheter must be strong so as not to crack or break easily; it should be able to withstand repeated exposure to alcohol, iodine, and other cleaning and antiseptic chemicals; it should be sufficiently rigid as to enable threading over a guidewire or splitsheath during placement, but not too rigid as to cause injury to the vessel wall; it should resist kinking and collapsing under very negative pressures; it should be flexible so as to negotiate bends, especially in the tunnel; the catheter itself should have as large as possible an internal diameter without being too large so as to minimize trauma to the vessel. For manufacturing purposes, it should be moldable, and bondable for use with other materials used in making of the other parts of components of the catheter. Most catheters in current use are polyurethane. Polyurethane has high material strength—catheters can be made with a very thin wall; it is flexible and can be made very rigid or soft; it is moldable and bonds well with other materials. A main disadvantage is that it is damaged by alcohol and antibiotic ointments such as mupirocin and betadine ointment that contain polyethylene glycol.

Common femoral vein cannulation is relatively easy and is preferred in the critically ill patient, where rapid and safe cannulation is required (163). Thus, in the emergency room or ICU, to minimize the risk of pneumothorax in the mechanically ventilated patient, cardiac arrhythmias, hemothorax, and pericardial tamponade, there is a high incidence of catheter-associated bacteremia. Ultrasound guidance or fluoroscopy are usually not required but may be useful in the morbidly obese or where there have been multiple prior cannulations and severe scarring; this may also be useful to determine catheter tip position where there is poor catheter function and high recirculation rates. In this situation, long catheters (>20 cm) are needed with X-rays to ensure catheter tip placement in the right atrium. Attempts at subclavian vein cannulation are associated with a high rate of severe acute complications—subclavian artery puncture, hemothorax and pneumothorax, and a high rate of subclavian vein stenosis in long-dwelling catheters (164), which will compromise the arm for subsequent placement of A-V accesses. Subclavian vein dialysis catheters are no longer recommended. For internal jugular (IJ) vein cannulation, the right IJ vein is preferred, because it runs straight inferiorly to the superior vena cava. Thus, the risk of malposition and malfunction is minimized, and endothelial injury is minimized so that chronic stenoses and occlusion are less common. There is great anatomic variability in the diameter of the vein and in its relations to the internal carotid artery, hence IJ vein placement is preferably done with ultrasound or fluoroscopic guidance or by surgical implantation (where there has been prior extensive neck surgery or multiple cannulations of the IJ with scarring) easily done under local anesthesia to minimize trauma to the vein, and the risk of injury to the IJ artery. The left IJ vein has a tortuous course, and catheters in this vein are complicated more frequently by malfunction, intimal injury, and chronic central venous stenosis, injury to the thoracic duct, pneumothorax, and hemothorax (163).

Inadequate Dialysis from Catheter Malfunction and Unreliability. Adequate dialysis delivery requires adequate blood flow (Q_b) in the 350 to 400 mL/min range. Access malfunction is therefore not to be tolerated. Blood flow rates as read by the machine tend to overestimate true blood flow rates, more so at more negative pressures. CVCs generate very negative pressures around their ports as a result of direct sucking and of the Bernoulli effect. Thus, machine blood flow readings with CVCs often greatly overestimate the actual blood flow. This, coupled with the fact that CVCs provide blood flows much lower than A-V accesses and have high recirculation rates, explains why CVCs are frequently associated with inadequate dialysis.

CVCs are vulnerable to thrombosis, fibrin sheath formation, primary malposition, secondary displacement or dislocation of the catheter tip. Adherence of the catheter tip to the vein wall can be corrected by reversing catheter ports, but this leads to higher recirculation rates. These CVC complications can be successfully managed by interventional radiologic procedures such as changing of the catheter over a guidewire, thrombolysis with tissue plasminogen activator, or fibrin sheath stripping (163). Where chronic hemodialysis has to be done using a CVC, meticulous monitoring of dialysis adequacy with aggressive use of these procedures to optimize catheter function is mandatory (161,165).

Hemodialysis Catheter-Related Infections. Catheter-related bacteremia and septicemia are a major cause of morbidity and mortality in hemodialysis patients (166–170). The majority of infections are due to *Staphylococcus aureus* and coagulase-negative *staphylococcus*. Coagulase-negative *S. aureus* most commonly colonizes the catheter exit site, but less frequently accounts for sepsis, whereas *S. aureus* colonization of the exit site is associated with a high incidence of bacteremia. Hemodialysis catheter-related bacteremia is less frequently caused by gram-negative bacteria such as *Escherichia coli*, *Pseudomonas* spp., *Klebsiella* spp., *Proteus* spp., and *Serratia* spp. Hemodialysis catheter-related infections due to fungi are not common in chronic dialysis patients; however this complication occurs in long-dwelling dialysis catheters in acute renal failure in hospitalized patients. Adherence of bacteria to the catheter surface is determined by an interplay of host, bacterial, and catheter-related factors. A layer of thrombin, rich in fibrin and fibronectin, forms around the catheter. *S. aureus* adheres tightly to fibrin, while coagulase-negative staphylococci adhere tightly to fibronectin and not to fibrin. The bacteria produce a fibrous glycocalyx called extracellular slime; coagulase-negative staphylococci are particularly slime producing. The thrombin and slime are components of a biofilm layer that supports further bacterial adherence and growth and also acts as a barrier protecting the organisms from antibiotics, antibodies, phagocytic neutrophils, and macrophages. The nature of the catheter material also plays a role in biofilm

Table 12   Risk Factors for Catheter-Related Bacteremia

Nasal carriage of *S. aureus* usually associated with skin carriage
Catheter hub colonization
Duration of catheterization
Frequency of catheter manipulation
Procedure of dialysis itself, which involves several exposures
The conditions of catheter placement and postinsertion catheter care
Patient's personal hygiene
Adherence by medial staff to universal precautions, including hand washing, wearing of gloves and masks when catheter is manipulated
Catheter clotting
Diabetes mellitus
Frequent skin needle punctures (e.g., diabetics or drug users)

formation. Following bacterial adherence to the dialysis catheter surface, biofilm organizes into a complex structure regulated by the exchange of chemical signals between bacterial cells, a process known as quorum sensing. This "multicellular" cell–cell communication leads to the emergence of virulence phenotypes. Two quorum-sensing systems are identified in *S. aureus*, the autoinducer RNAIII-activating protein (RAP) and its target molecule TRAP; and the peptide pheromone AIP and its receptor AgrC. More understanding of these mechanisms of biofilm formation may lead to novel approaches to the management of CVC. The risk factors for the development of catheter-related bacteremia are presented in Table 12.

The Native AVF.   The arteriovenous fistula (AVF) is the first choice of hemodialysis vascular access, using the patient's own artery and vein (171,172). Time, sometimes up to three months, is needed for the vein to arterialize or "mature." Every effort should be made to create an AVF, in spite of the fact that an increasing proportion of patients needing dialysis are surgically challenging. More dialysis patients are diabetic and elderly, with more severe diffuse atherosclerosis and more venous damage or injury resulting from multiple prior venipuncture for blood draws and intravenous infusions, as well as central vein catheterizations.

The radiocephalic AVF, first described by Brescia and Cimino in 1966 (173), is the classical AVF, created at the wrist using the radial artery and the forearm cephalic vein (174) (Fig. 12). In individuals with severe atherosclerosis, the radial artery may not provide adequate blood inflow, and thus it is necessary to use the brachial artery in the antecubital fossa, connected to the lateral upper arm cephalic vein. Careful preoperative evaluation of artery and vein is essential for successful AVF creation. The radial artery usually has a blood flow rate of 20 to 30 mL/min, which increases to 200 to 300 mL/min after AVF creation; by the time of maturation of the AVF, typical blood flows are 600 to 1200 mL/min. This marked increase in blood flow requires a distensible inflow artery, thus the atherosclerotic, thick-walled and calcified artery is a poor candidate for successful AVF creation. The greatest threats to successful maturation of the vein are prior multiple venipunctures, with resulting venous sclerosis, multiple venous tributaries draining blood flow, hypertrophic venous valves, and central venous stenosis or thrombosis, often subclinical or asymptomatic. Preoperative evaluation should include a history taking and physical examination, with careful palpation of arteries and veins, auscultation and blood pressure measurements on both arms, ultrasonographic study of the arteries and veins to evaluate their caliber, wall structure and flow characteristics (this has replaced the Allen test),

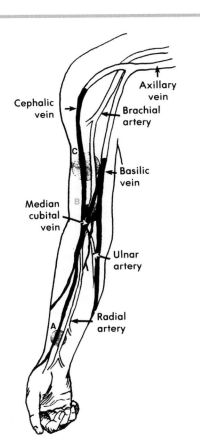

Figure 12   Potential vascular sites for creation of an endogenous arteriovenous fistula for hemodialysis vascular access. The preferred access site is created at the wrist by anastomosing the radial artery and cephalic vein (**A**). Other potential sites for access creation include the brachial artery with either the medial cubital vein at the elbow (**B**) or the cephalic vein at the upper arm (**C**).

and contrast or magnetic resonance venography in selected cases. Recently, the surgical procedure of transposition of the basilic vein in the upper arm has allowed the use of proximal upper arm vessels for AVF creation (175).

The NKF-DOQI Clinical Practice Guidelines for Vascular Access has recommended an AVF rate of approximately 50% in new ESRD patients (176). The high prevalence of diabetic, obese, and elderly patients in the ESRD population in the United States demands particular effort to reach this goal. Most AVFs require approximately three months to mature (cf 2–3 weeks for A-V grafts). Fistulas have a high primary failure rate due to a failure to mature or early thrombosis. A common problem in the dialysis center is that of the patient waiting for long durations for their AVF to mature or having successive AVFs thromboses. These patients are forced to continue with CVCs for long periods, which is not ideal. In order to increase the chances of achieving successful AVF placement, maturation, and function, preoperative vein mapping by sonography, contrast, or magnetic resonance venography is needed. Absolute contraindications to A-V access are severe congestive heart failure with low ejection fraction that may be worsened by the A-V shunt, symptomatic steal syndrome, morbid obesity, chronic and intradialytic hypotension, hypercoagulable states, skin disease, and severe venous hypertension leading to severe edema of the arm.

Arteriovenous Graft. The arteriovenous graft (AVG), introduced in mid-1970, is the second option for vascular access. Graft material may be autogenous, heterogenous, or synthetic. Expanded polytetrafluoroethylene is the most commonly used graft material (177). Grafts may be placed in the upper or lower extremities and may be straight or looped, and the anastomosis may be end-to-end, end-to-side, or side-to-side. The end-to-side anastomosis is the most commonly used. Graft thrombosis is the most common complication of AVGs (70%); of these, 90% are associated with venous anastomotic stenosis, the result of neointimal hyperplasia. As a consequence, there is a high incidence of access malfunction and poor outcomes in patients with AVGs. In the United States, AVGs account for approximately 70% of all vascular accesses. Recent studies reveal that chronic AVGs are associated with a chronic inflammatory state with higher levels of inflammatory markers such as C-reactive protein (178). In diabetics, AVGs were associated with an overall mortality risk of 1.41; cause-specific relative risks are significantly higher, and the relative risk of death from infection is more than twice that of diabetics with AVFs (179). AVGs develop an aggressive form of venous anastomotic intimal hyperplasia characterized by smooth muscle cell proliferation, extracellular matrix synthesis and deposition, and neointimal and adventitial angiogenesis. There is no effective pharmacological therapy as yet for this lesion. In view of the high rates of graft dysfunction and thrombosis, and the lack of specific therapy, attempts have been made to develop simple and reliable tests of graft function that will give early warning of dysfunction and impending thrombosis. These methods include dynamic pressure measurements, static intra-access pressure measurements, access blood flow measurements using Doppler ultrasound and ultrasound dilution methods, and recirculation measurements using urea-based methods, ultrasound dilution or thermodilution methods. These programs of graft surveillance have proven useful in prolonging graft survival and have ensured adequate delivery of dialysis. Using well-validated criteria of access function, dysfunctioning vascular accesses are then referred for fistulography or graftography and further interventional procedures (172).

Management of AVG Dysfunction. Interventional radiology, interventional nephrology, or vascular surgery departments primarily manage the management of graft thrombosis. Procedures can be performed more promptly, and thus with minimal interruptions of the patients' dialysis treatment schedules, and they are less invasive and they do not require general anesthesia. These procedures allow access sites to be preserved better for future use and also provide more precise anatomic diagnosis of lesions within the access and on both arterial and venous side, up to the central venous system. This more precise diagnosis makes it possible to develop the appropriate treatment plan, and this should be done in a multidisciplinary approach involving the interventionist, nephrologist, and surgeon. More AV accesses are salvaged in this way, longevity of the access is increased, accesses that are not salvageable are more clearly identified and referral to surgery and outcomes are improved. The usual interventional procedures are thrombolysis, usually mechanical, but occasionally with the aid of thrombolytic agents, and angioplasty of venous anastomotic stenotic lesions as well as venous stenotic lesions that may occur all the way up to the central veins (180). Occasionally lesions are detected on the arterial anastomotic region, which may be amenable to angioplasty, and stenting of stenotic venous segments is performed where indicated. Surgery is indicated when the interventional approach has failed or is not feasible and is usually carried out with more detailed anatomic data and with a view to preserve access sites for the future and to address the underlying lesion. Surgical procedures include thrombectomies, placement of patch angioplasties, interpositional or jump grafts, or the creation of new AV accesses. Additionally, surgical intervention is required for the management of bleeding, infections, and pseudoaneurysms.

Anticoagulation. Activation of the hemostatic system as a result of contact between blood and the foreign surfaces of extracorporeal circulatory systems is a challenge in hemodialysis dialysis therapies. Clotting occurs within the blood compartment of the dialyzer and/or at different vulnerable points along the dialysis blood lines or circuitry. Filter clotting results in treatment interruptions and inefficiency, nursing difficulties, increased cost of treatment, and, most important, inadequacies of clearances and ultrafiltration capacity. Anticoagulation is therefore usually required for the effective delivery of the dialysis prescription. The anticoagulation regimen must be individualized for the needs of each patient. Hospitalized patients, acutely ill with infection, sepsis, post-trauma, surgery, strokes, or myocardial infarctions and such conditions may be hypercoagulable or coagulopathic. Careful consideration of these factors must go into the determination of the requirements for anticoagulation for dialysis. Anticoagulation is usually systemically administered, but where there are serious bleeding risks, it may be done locally or regionally, across the dialyzer only. Regional anticoagulation is particularly preferred with continuous dialysis therapies in the severely ill intensive care patients and also because of the potential for anticoagulants to accumulate with continuous administration. Treatment characteristics that affect clotting include vascular access—catheter diameter, traumatic catheter placement, catheter malposition, and kinking; blood flow rates; ultrafiltration rates; dialyzer membrane material and geometry; and nursing attention to alarms and other warning signs of impending thrombosis. Anticoagulation may be systemic or regional. Sometimes no anticoagulation is used or required. Patients with liver failure, uremic bleeding diathesis, severe thrombocytopenia, consumptive coagulopathy, or patients receiving medications with anticoagulant effect such as the recently introduced activated protein C may require only intermittent saline flushes to maintain patency of the extracorporeal circuit.

Water for Dialysis and Dialysate Composition. Water for dialysis is usually municipal water; occasionally only well water is available. The water undergoes a number of filtration steps to remove particles, dissolved organic compounds, chloramines, and chlorine, after which it is pumped through a water softener, and an ion exchange resin to remove calcium and magnesium ions (181,182). Municipal water is allowed to contain up to 100 colony-forming units of microorganisms per mL. Ion exchange resins promote bacterial growth. Next, the water filtered and softened is pumped through an RO unit, for the elimination of up to 99% of all ions present. The hemodialysis machines are connected to the water purification system by polyvinyl chloride tubing. Water stagnation in the tubing promotes bacterial overgrowth as well as biofilm formation, especially from *Pseudomonas* species, which are a constant source of endotoxins

and other pyrogenic bacterial products. Failure of the water treatment system results in incorrect electrolyte composition of the final dialysate, patient exposure to unwanted chemical contents such as chloramines, fluorides, nitrates, copper, and aluminum, as well as to microorganisms and their products. Salt concentrates, particularly bicarbonate concentrate, are prone to heavy contamination with microorganisms, especially *Pseudomonas* species. Solid bicarbonate in powder form is now available. Bacterial products back filtrate from dialysate side to the blood side. There is a current effort to provide pyrogen-free (ultra-pure) dialysate by adding pyrogen-adsorbing membranes, or ultraviolet radiation to the water treatment system. The final dialysate is mixed in a proportioning system from dialysate concentrates and the dialysate water. Dialysate composition is individualized according to clinical requirement. The main variables are dialysate sodium, potassium, calcium, and, more uncommonly, bicarbonate and magnesium. It is easy to imagine that errors of dialysate composition from a faulty proportioning system or human error can have severe deleterious clinical effects. Monitoring of ionic conductivity is used as a safety measure against this possibility.

Measurement of Dialysis Adequacy. The effort to quantify dialysis adequacy has engaged the interest of nephrologists for many years. Among the first choices of uremic toxins selected for such analysis was urea, representative of small solutes. Several parameters need consideration—dialyzer membrane transport characteristics, blood and dialysate flow rates, duration of treatment, vascular access performance, in particular blood flow recirculation within the access, ultrafiltration rates, hematocrit, etc. These in turn are factored to a measure of patient size. The most successful parameter to date, dialysis dose, and which has been validated as predictive of patient outcome, is the K_t/V urea index (183). This is the clearance of urea factored to total body water. A K_t/V of one indicates urea clearance equal to the volume of total body water. The NKF/DOQI Clinical Practice Guidelines give evidence-based targets of dialysis dosing to be delivered to patients so as to ensure adequate dialysis (184–186).

Continuous Renal Replacement Therapies

CRRT have become the most effective treatment modality in critically ill patients (187,188). Several features of these modalities explain their advantages: 24-hour treatment provides continuous removal of toxic compounds that are presumed to be continuously generated; there is a marked overall increase in dialysis clearances; and small hemofilters and small volume extracorporeal circuits are used to minimize blood volume reduction in the hemodynamically unstable patient. The hemofilters have large pore-size with high hydraulic permeability permitting large volume ultrafiltration [continuous veno-venous hemofiltration (CVVHF) and continuous veno-venous hemodiafiltration (CVVHDF)], as well as the passage of middle and some high–molecular-weight toxins (up to 30–50 Da): this enables the clearance of inflammatory cytokines, anaphylatoxins (C3 and C5), platelet-activating factor, and substance such as myocardial depressant factors. The capacity for high volumes of ultrafiltration also enables the safe administration of large volumes of fluid required for administration of medications, nutrition, and blood products. Additionally, these techniques offer gradual and continuous correction of electrolyte, acid–base and osmolality abnormalities, as well as the capacity to cope with the severe azotemia of the severely ill and

Table 13 Potential Indications for Continuous Renal Replacement Therapy

Acute renal failure with:
    Severe hypercatabolism
    Cerebral edema
    Cardiovascular failure
    Acute or chronic liver failure
Adult respiratory distress syndrome
Tumor lysis syndrome
Lactic acidosis
Cardiopulmonary bypass
Sepsis syndrome
Refractory congestive heart failure
Acute necrotizing pancreatitis
Rhabdomyolysis
Acute intoxications
Hyperammonemia associated with inborn errors of metabolism

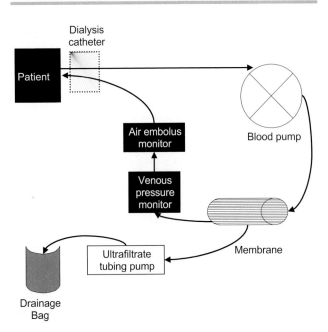

Figure 13 Continuous venovenous hemofiltration (CVVH) circuit. CVVH offers large-volume ultrafiltration in critically ill patients with specific indications. Blood moves from and to the patient via a dual-lumen central venous catheter, with the filtration pressure being provided by a blood pump.

hypercatabolic patient. It has recently been demonstrated that adsorption is an important mechanism of solute clearance in CRRT. In many cases the clinical significance of such clearances is yet to be understood. Table 13 lists some of the renal failure and nonrenal conditions that have been reported to benefit from CRRT (189). CRRT may be particularly advantageous when AKF is accompanied by refractory volume overload, hypercatabolism, intracerebral edema, hemodynamic instability, or uncontrollable hyperkalemia or metabolic acidosis.

    The first continuous therapies were continuous arteriovenous, requiring arterial cannulation, with the force for blood flow provided by the arterial blood pressure. With the introduction of a blood pump into the extracorporeal circuit, and the availability of single dual-lumen catheters, continuous veno-venous therapies became possible and are much preferred. The modalities of continuous therapies can now be classified into three categories: convective therapies, dialysis therapies, and continuous ultrafiltration.

Convective Therapies: CVVHF and CVVHDF
The convective therapies are hemofiltration (CVVHF) and hemodiafiltration (CVVHDF) (Fig. 13) (187,188). The dialyzing membrane is highly permeable to solutes and water. In CVVHF, there is no dialysis fluid, while in CVVHDF, there is a dialysis fluid flow. In both CVVHF and CVVHDF, very large volumes of ultrafiltration are the goal, far in excess of ultrafiltration required for the purposes of volume balance; therefore, in both procedures there is a need for replacement or substitution fluid. Typical ultrafiltration rates are about 30% of blood flow rates; at blood flow rates of 200 to 300 mL/min, typical ultrafiltration rates are 60 to 90 mL/min. CVVHF and CVVHDF achieve very high clearances of both small and large-molecular-weight solutes. With CVVHF, clearances of small-molecular-weight-solutes depend mainly on ultrafiltration volume; therefore to achieve high small-solute clearances, high blood-flow rates (approximately 500 mL/min) are required. With the availability of online production of substitution fluid, it is possible to achieve such a high blood flow into the hemofilter (e.g., 250 mL/min actual blood flow and 250 mL/min predilution substitution fluid). With CVVHDF, small solute clearance depends not only on ultrafiltration rates but also on diffusion down a concentration gradient; predilution with substitution while increasing ultrafiltration rates also dilutes concentrations of these solutes, thereby reducing diffusive clearances.

Predilution therefore reduces clearance of small solutes in CVVHDF. Substitution fluid is administered postfilter.

    Both CVVHF and CVVHDF can only be accomplished by the availability of large volumes of substitution fluid made possible by its online production. There is currently great interest in the development of the continuous convective therapies, for the treatment of acute renal failure in the setting of sepsis or the multiple organ dysfunction syndrome (MODS). Besides the improved small solute clearances, hemodynamic stability, metabolic control, and nutritional support that can be provided, it is suggested that there is improved clearances of middle and large molecules, especially inflammatory mediators and endotoxins (by convection and adsorption), the removal of which will aid the management of sepsis. This has led to novel therapies aimed at the treatment of sepsis or MODS as opposed to AKF. In principle, two main approaches are being pursued: high volume hemofiltration with filtration rates averaging 35 mL/kg/hr or more and ultrahigh-efficiency clearance using plasma filtration and adsorption.

The Dialysis Therapies: CVVHD and SLED
CVVHD and sustained low-efficiency dialyis (SLED) are diffusion (dialysis)-based techniques as in regular hemodialysis (187,188,190), but unlike routine hemodialysis, dialysate flow rates are lower, rendering the procedure less efficient. With CVVHD, the dialysate flow rates are in the range of 1 to 2 L/hr (17–35 mL/min); blood flow rates are also slowed, averaging 200 mL/min. The dialysate is completely saturated in its passage through the dialyzer, and dialysate flow rate is the limiting factor to clearance. Small solute clearance is the objective in CVVHD. At this rate of dialysate flow, the dialysate is supplied in bags from the manufacturer or custom-mixed in the hospital pharmacy. Because

of the undesirability of leaving bicarbonate solution sitting for long periods, the alkalinizing agent in these dialysate solutions has been more commonly citrate than bicarbonate, though both types of solution are in use. With SLED, higher dialysate flows can be achieved using bicarbonate for alkalinization as in regular hemodialysis.

Ultrafiltration: SCUF

Slow continuous ultrafiltration (SCUF) provides low water and sodium removal continuously and can be useful in the management of refractory congestive heart failure, sometimes as a bridging procedure to cardiac transplantation.

Complications of CRRT

The major complications of CRRT are related to anticoagulation and metabolic disturbances (191). Continuous therapies often require continuous anticoagulation (192,193). This, in the presence of kidney failure, carries the high risk of excessive anticoagulation and bleeding, more so in critically ill patients with other bleeding risks. The trend therefore is to do regional, rather than systemic, forms of anticoagulation. Citrate anticoagulation is the most commonly used of these methods. Recent increased interest in alternatives to heparin is the result of increasing reports of the devastating complication of heparin-induced thrombocytopenia.

Pharmacokinetics and Drug Dosing Adjustments During CRRT

Drugs are cleared during CRRT mainly by convection and adsorption (194). Drugs that are normally cleared by the kidneys are usually also removed by CRRT. The critically ill patient already has major abnormalities of drug handling from altered absorption, distribution, metabolism, and excretion. Drug dosing in CRRT is best guided by measuring levels where this is applicable. CRRT drug clearances can be measured or estimated; where this is not feasible, drug dosing can be adjusted (according to reference guidelines) using measured CRRT creatinine clearances. With nontoxic drugs, dosing may be done in excess of estimates (approximately 30%), to ensure adequate levels.

Peritoneal Dialysis

In peritoneal dialysis, the intra-abdominal peritoneal microcirculation, with its large surface area, blood flow, and the solute and fluid exchange properties of the capillary network, is exploited. Dialysate is injected into the peritoneal space through a two-way catheter. The peritoneal membrane allows waste and fluid to pass from the blood into the dialysate, which is drained out. The peritoneal dialysate contains electrolytes in physiologic concentrations to facilitate correction of acid–base and electrolyte abnormalities. The dialysate glucose concentration can be increased or decreased depending on the desire to promote or restrict, respectively, osmotic movement of fluid from the peritoneal capillaries into the peritoneal space. Urea clearances of 10 to 15 mL/min can be achieved using this method. The amount of solute removal is a function of the degree of its concentration gradient, the molecular size, membrane permeability and surface area, duration of dialysis, and charge. Peritoneal dialysis must be performed everyday and fluid must be in the abdomen at all times to clean the blood adequately. Advantages of peritoneal dialysis over acute intermittent hemodialysis include the fact that in peritoneal dialysis, fluid removal is more gradual and less hemodynamically stressful, dialysis is slower and more continuous so that

electrolyte shifts may be less dramatic, anticoagulation is not required, and less specialized equipment and personnel are required. In the AKF setting, acute peritoneal dialysis is not as efficient as acute intermittent or continuous hemodialysis in correcting metabolic, fluid, and electrolyte abnormalities. Continuous ambulatory peritoneal dialysis (CAPD) exchanges approximately 2 L of dialysate three to six times a day while the patient is active. The patient connects a bag of dialysate fluid to the peritoneal catheter and allows it to infuse into the abdomen. After the dialysate filters for four to six hours (the "dwell" time), the patient drains the fluid and exchanges it for fresh fluid. In automated peritoneal dialysis, also termed "continuous cyclic peritoneal dialysis" (CCPD), a machine exchanges the fluid while the person sleeps. Over the 8- to 12-hour night, the machine exchanges fluid four to eight times. Upon waking, the patient's fluid is exchanged and used throughout the day. Some patients require a mid-day exchange.

Early peritoneal dialysis fluids composed of solutions varying from normal saline to 5% dextrose. Sodium concentrations were varied as required to correct hypo- or hypernatremia. To correct acidosis, bicarbonate, acetate or lactose was used as base. Dextrose in high concentrations (up to 7%) was used as the osmotic agent to provide ultrafiltration. These high concentrations of glucose posed a problem owing to caramelization during sterilization. With the advent of commercially prepared peritoneal fluid, two problems arose. One was the inability of keeping calcium and bicarbonate in solution in storage for long durations (precipitation of calcium carbonate); the second was that bicarbonate solutions are difficult to keep sterile. Thus modern peritoneal dialysis fluids remain buffered with lactate.

The technique, in its early history, was hardly suitable for the chronic treatment necessary for ESKD. The first efforts required repeated catheterization of the peritoneum for each treatment. This "periodic" peritoneal dialysis was extremely painful and uncomfortable for the patient, and had a high rate of infections and peritoneal adhesions. Unsuccessful attempts were made to develop devices such as abdominal buttons or other conduits to facilitate the repeated catheterizations. The earliest peritoneal dialysis catheters were made from tubing easily available on the hospital ward—stainless steel sump drains, trochars, and rubber catheters—all of which were unsuitable for long-dwelling use. Polyvinylchloride and polyethylene tubing became available in the early 1950s, but these were limited by their tendency to kink, leak, and get blocked. Catheter placement initially required a trochar, but later designs had pointed stylets for convenience of placement. In 1968, Tenckhoff (195) introduced his catheter, a silicone rubber catheter with two Dacron cuffs, designed to be used as a long-term indwelling dialysis catheter. All other peritoneal dialysis catheters designed since have been modifications of the Tenckhoff catheter. The Tenckhoff catheter is, arguably, the single most important device that has made chronic peritoneal dialysis a reality. Peritoneal dialysis catheters can now be placed laparoscopically at the bedside or in the operating room, or by open surgery. Straight, coiled, single- or double-cuffed, Swan Neck, Ash T-fluted, and presternal catheters are all in use. The coil of the catheter gives it weight in its pelvic location, which minimizes the possibility of migration from the pelvis. The Swan Neck design allows a downward direction of the exit site, which markedly reduces the risk of exit site infection. The Dacron cuffs on the catheter are highly fibrogenic and help to secure the catheter in position and minimize the possibility of pericatheter leak and infection. The internal cuff, placed within the rectus abdominus muscle, helps to prevent catheter leak or migration. The coiled intraperitoneal segment helps to prevent catheter migration and minimizes pain from infusion of fluid. Presternal catheters are suitable for the morbidly obese and patients with abdominal ostomies. A variety of peritoneal catheter-related complications may occur (Table 14).

At the same time as the indwelling catheter was evolving, efforts in the area of fluid delivery led to the introduction of automatic cycling machines—machines capable of delivering fluid to the patient's peritoneal cavity in cycles, with varying volume and composition of fluid, duration of inflow, dwell, and outflow. At first, the dialysate was premixed and provided in large containers. Later, the dialysate was available in plastic bags of different dextrose concentrations or strengths, with the possibility of being mixed or matched to provide a final composition appropriate for the patient. Over the years, peritoneal dialysis cyclers have become smaller and more portable. The next major development in peritoneal dialysis was the concept of CAPD proposed by Popovich and Moncrief in 1973 (196). They hypothesized that peritoneal dialysis could be performed on a principle of "equilibration" dialysis: that is, if each exchange of fluid introduced into the peritoneum was allowed to "dwell" there until it equilibrated with the blood and then was drained; they calculated that only a relatively small amount of peritoneal fluid, in a relatively small number of exchanges would be required to provide the necessary amount of solute and fluid clearance. Specifically, they calculated, for example, that exchanges of 2 L, each with an ultrafiltration of 500 mL and thus a drain volume of 2500 mL, four times in the course of a 24-hour period, would result in a 12 L drain volume or effluent. If it is assumed that this volume of dialysis fluid effluent achieved equilibration with blood, then the amounts of urea and creatinine cleared, which can be calculated should be adequate to treat ESKD. The patient in this way achieves steady state chemistries, with minimal fluctuation of serum creatinine or BUN levels. The developments in peritoneal dialysis described thus far formed the basis of modern peritoneal dialysis technique. Further developments have only been the modifications of these principles.

Because CAPD requires exchanging peritoneal dialysis fluid four to five times daily, the potential for contamination of fluid and resulting peritonitis is high. Numerous devices and techniques to achieve and maintain sterile connections with minimal risk of contamination have since been developed. Automated cycling machines that can automatically

Table 14 Peritoneal Dialysis Catheter-Related Complications

Exit-site infections
Extrusion of the external cuff
Catheter obstruction by:
   Clot
   Bowel (constipation)
   Omentum
   Adhesions
   Full bladder
   Kinks
Pericatheter leaks
Infusion or drainage pain
Peritonitis
Migration
Cuts, material deterioration and breakdown, organ erosion, and allergic
   reactions (rare)

Table 15 Peritoneal Dialysis as Chronic Renal Replacement Therapy

Advantages
   More liberal diet with less fluid intake restrictions
   Minimal fluctuation of blood chemistries
   Better anemia control
   Better hypertension control
   Improved sense of well-being
   Suitable for children in school and employed patients
   Less cost
Disadvantages
   Catheter malfunction
   Weight gain
   Patient fatigue with the procedure
   Development of abdominal hernias
   Peritonitis

provide the needed dialysis exchanges, usually at night during sleep, have been developed and are in common use. Evidence-based standards for quantification of peritoneal dialysis, guidelines for adequacy of treatment, and protocols for the diagnosis and treatment of peritonitis, exit site infections, and tunnel infections have also been established. Catheter design and placement techniques and peritoneal dialysis fluid composition and biocompatibility have been improved. As a result of these developments, peritoneal dialysis is now widely available for the treatment of ESKD in most parts of the world, and its use is growing much faster than that of hemodialysis. The advantages and disadvantages of peritoneal dialysis, as well as the indications and contraindications for peritoneal dialysis and factors that influence the choice of hemodialysis versus peritoneal dialysis are presented in Table 15.

RENAL TRANSPLANTATION

Kidney transplantation is the treatment of choice for ESKD, and the number of kidney transplants (both cadaveric and living donor) performed in the United States has dramatically increased in the past decade. This reflects an increased availability of living kidney donation, the result of increased public education and awareness. Living unrelated kidney donation is the area of greatest increase in the United States. Although cadaveric kidney donation has not substantially increased, there has been a lowering of the threshold of acceptable cadaveric kidney transplantation, which has been largely responsible for the increase in cadaveric kidney transplantation. Donor organ availability continues to fall short of demand, resulting in long transplant waiting lists.

Transplantation Immunobiology

The major barrier to successful allotransplantation is immunologic. Renal allograft rejection remains the major cause of graft loss. The delineation of molecular mechanisms of allograft rejection has led to new classes of biologic agents for the abrogation and control of allograft rejection. Additionally, there is the increasing prospect of achieving transplantation tolerance and of successful xenotransplantation.

Central to the question of transplantation immunology are the facts of self-identity of the organism and the ability to differentiate self from nonself and mount an immune response to destroy the non–self-"invader." Most of the proteins of the body are oligomorphic or nonpolymorphic, and as such, lack the necessary variation to distinguish individual members of the species, one from the other.

The vast polymorphism, of almost limitless extent, that is needed to achieve this "self-identity," is to be found in the major histocompatibility complex (MHC) structure. Unlike any other region of the chromosome, the MHC gene is highly polymorphic, as are its products, the MHC class I and class II cell surface proteins. Individuals with identical MHC proteins [other than identical (monozygotic) twins] are extremely rare. Histocompatibility antigens can be divided into a single MHC or system and numerous minor histocompatibility (miH) systems. Incompatibility for either MHC or miH antigens between donor and recipient leads to an immune response against the graft, although more vigorous reaction occurs with MHC differences.

MHC class I glycoproteins are expressed on the surface of most nucleated cells, although at different levels. They are responsible for activating T-cells bearing the CD8 surface protein (CD8$^+$ cells). MHC class II proteins, which are also membrane-anchored glycoproteins, stimulate T-cells bearing CD4 surface protein (CD4$^+$ cells). Under basal conditions, class II proteins are expressed only in B-lymphocytes, dendritic cells, and some endothelial cells. During an immune or inflammatory response, however, many other cell types may be induced to express MHC class II proteins.

Both class I and II proteins form a similar three-dimensional structure at the cell surface. Within this structure is a groove flanked by two alpha helices; the amino acids in the groove show the highest polymorphism within a species. During the synthesis and transport of MHC class I and II proteins to the cell surface, they become associated with small peptides that fit into the groove. Class I proteins bind peptides derived from the intracellular compartment, while class II proteins bind peptides derived from the extracellular compartment. The combination of MHC protein and peptide is recognized by the antigen receptor on the T-cell, the T-cell receptor (TCR). Thus, antigenic peptides are recognized by T-cells only when they are presented in the groove of (i.e., in the context of) the MHC; antigen recognition is said to be "MHC restricted." When the renal allograft is placed, host-specialized antigen-presenting cells take up foreign protein from the graft, process them, and load some of the resulting "foreign" peptides onto their MHC grooves. These are then presented at the cell surface to host T-cell. The class III region of the MHC is large and contains many uncharacterized genes. Genes that have been characterized encode proteins with a variety of functions important in immunity, such as TNF-α and TNF-β. miH antigens (e.g., the male antigen or H-Y) may play a prominent role in graft rejection in a recipient who is given an MHC-compatible graft but in whom preexisting sensitization to miH antigens exists. It may, for example, explain graft rejection and loss in renal transplants performed between human leukocyte antigen (HLA)-identical siblings. Multiple miH differences have been shown to represent an immunogenic stimulus that can be equivalent to that of the MHC.

The process of graft rejection begins when recipient CD4$^+$ T-cells are activated by graft alloantigen (197). Graft alloantigen is presented to the recipient T-cells by either of the processes of direct antigen presentation or indirect antigen presentation. The transplanted kidney contains bone marrow–derived leukocyte-like cells called passenger leukocytes. These passenger leukocytes rapidly traffic (migrate) out of the graft, via the lymphatic drainage, to the recipient's lymphoid organs. Here, they rapidly mature into potent antigen-presenting cells (dendritic-like cells). Non–self MHC class II molecules expressed on these specialized, antigen-presenting cells of the graft, directly activate recipient CD4$^+$ cells. The peptide-binding grooves of these non–self-MHC molecules may contain peptides derived from graft or recipient proteins. Non–self-MHC are extremely potent transplantation antigens, which activate large numbers of T-cell clones in the recipient. Up to 5% of all clones in the body may respond to a non–self-MHC molecule (198).

This process of presentation of donor MHC by donor "dendritic" cells is described as direct antigen presentation. In similar fashion, non–self-MHC class I molecules expressed on many cells in the graft may directly activate recipient CD8$^+$ T-cells. Another example of direct antigen presentation is when recipient T-cells react with endothelial cells of the donor (allograft), which in an activated state express MHC molecules. Direct antigen presentation results in powerful stimulation of the immune system and is thought to be mainly responsible for acute allograft rejection. Direct antigen presentation bypasses antigen processing by recipient antigen-presenting cells.

The second mechanism of host T-cell activation involves indirect antigen presentation. In this mechanism, antigen-presenting cells of the recipient migrate into the transplanted kidney, take up graft alloantigens, process the molecules, and present the resulting peptides on self-MHC molecules to T-cells, stimulating and activating them.

Conversely donor cells could traffic out of the allograft and interact with recipient APCs in the lymphoid organs. Recipient APCs may also react with soluble "circulating" donor proteins that have been released into the bloodstream as a result of processes within the allograft, e.g., ischemia and inflammation that result in cell injury and/or cell death. Following the binding of antigenic protein by the APC, the protein is taken up into intracellular proteolysosomes and digested into peptide fragments. A relatively small number of these peptide fragments, and which are immunogenic, are selected, placed in the groove of the MHC molecule, and transported as the MHC–peptide complex to the cell surface to be presented to T-cells. With indirect antigen presentation, donor antigen-presenting cells such as dendritic cells and macrophages are involved as intermediaries between recipient T-cells and transplanted donor cells. The results of CD4$^+$ and CD8$^+$ activation, whether by direct or indirect mechanism of antigen presentation, are the generation of cytokine synthesis, and the proliferation and differentiation of T-cells into cytotoxic T-cells (CTLs).

Tests for Histocompatibility Antigens

Tissue typing consists of the analysis of histocompatibility antigens of donor and recipient so as to determine the degree of foreignness between the two individuals and thus to predict the outcome of the transplantation. There are several ways to determine the degree of parity or disparity between transplantation antigens: (i) serologic detection of cell surface antigens (lymphocytotoxicity test); (ii) measurement of the reaction between leukocytes from the donor and recipient in the mixed lymphocyte reaction; and (iii) genotyping of transplantation epitopes.

T-Cell Antigen Recognition, Processing, and Signaling

The TCR expressed on the surface of the T-cell interacts with the antigenic peptide located in the groove of the MHC molecule on the surface of the APC, but does not transduce a signal. The TCR is associated with a transmembrane coreceptor, the CD4 or CD8 molecule; CD4 and CD8 molecules act as adhesion molecules tightening the binding of T-cells with APCs, and also transduce signals into the cell. Additional costimulatory molecules expressed on APCs bind with their respective ligands on the T-cell, thereby enhancing and sustaining T-cell activation. Other adhesion molecules, the accessory molecules interact in pairs between APC and T-cells, resulting in the formation of the immunological synapse, which allows full activation of the T-cell. Activation of the CD4$^+$ cell results in proliferation, cytokine synthesis and secretion, migration of T-cells from lymphoid tissue into the allograft and differentiation into memory cells, while activation of CD8$^+$ cells results in their differentiation into cytotoxic T-lymphocytes (T-killer cells).

Interaction of the TCR and alloantigen brings results in a complex-signaling cascade that lead to the activation of at least two major signaling pathways: the Ca^{2+}–calcineurin cascade and the protein kinase C (PKC)–Erk cascade. Calcineurin is a serine/threonine phosphatase that dephosphorylates and functionally inactivates key transcription factors such as nuclear factor of activated T cells (NFAT) involved in IL-2 gene transcription. PKC activation, in a multistep signaling pathway, leads to phosphorylation of Erk, which then phosphorylates and activates transcription factors such as c-fos and Elk-1, leading to the initiation of gene transcription.

Cytokines and Chemokines

Graft rejection involves interactions among many cells involved in the immune and inflammatory responses and other cells such as endothelial and parenchymal cells. These cells communicate through direct contact using recognition molecules located on their cell surfaces (e.g., MHC, TCR CD4, CD8, CD40L, and FasL). In addition to the numerous cell–cell-based interactions required for T-cell activation, important signals are also delivered through the binding of soluble proteins, the cytokines, to specific cell surface cytokine receptors. A cascade of cytokines is produced that amplifies immune and inflammatory processes after transplantation (199). Cytokines such as IL-1 and IL-12, derived mainly from antigen-presenting cells, sensitize T-cells, by upregulating their expression of receptors for other cytokines, mainly T-cell derived, such as IL-2 and IL-4, which cause proliferation and differentiation. Many of the phenomena observed in the immune response to a transplant are mediated by several cytokines, acting redundantly and synergistically. On the other hand, calcineurin induces many cytokines, including CD40L, calcineurin, cytokine γ_c chain, and tyrosine-protein kinase receptor torso precursor (TOR), which all serve nonredundant functions. Activation of the calcineurin pathway results in the activation of transcription factors that regulate the transcription of genes encoding for several key cytokines (e.g., IL-2 and IFN-γ) and cytokine receptors.

Cytokines regulate MHC expression and the peptide generation and processing pathways. Under basal conditions, parenchymal cells express MHC antigens, adhesion molecules, and costimulatory molecules at levels too low to allow T-cell recognition. Certain cytokines may increase the antigenicity of an allograft by inducing the expression of MHC class I and II, adhesion and signaling molecules, and cytokine receptors. Costimulatory signals are also regulated by cytokines. IFN-γ increases the transcription of the large mutifunctional protease genes and the genes for transporters associated with antigen processing, which are encoded in the class II region of the MHC, and could influence the peptides available for binding to the class I grooves. The growth factor cytokines such as IL-2 mediate the triggering, commitment, and clonal expansion of T- and

B-lymphocytes and the emergence of their effector functions. T-cell receptor triggering is dependent on the presence of costimulatory factors (such as CD28 engaging B7-1/B7-2) and may be promoted by the binding of certain cytokines produced by the APC to their cognate receptors (e.g., IL-2, IL-6, and IL-12) on the T-cell (200). The subsequent lymphocyte differentiation and clonal expansion also require that certain cytokines produced by T-cells (e.g., IL-2, IL-4, IL-7, and IL-13) engage their receptors on T-cells, producing paracrine or autocrine effects. The aggregate strength of those signals may be a rate-limiting step in the immune response.

Cytokines also play a crucial role in the organization of inflammation in a rejecting allograft. Cytokines can activate endothelial cells and affect their interactions with leukocytes and platelets, as well as their regulation of vasomotor tone and fluid movement. The primary role of cytokines in an immune response is to initiate proliferation, differentiation, and homing of leukocytes in the generation of immunity. However, certain cytokines also may directly damage tissue acutely or chronically. TNF-α produced by CTLs and macrophages may damage a graft, and blocking the effects of TNF with neutralizing antibodies can prolong organ graft survival.

Several chemokines have been identified, which modulate help to determine the extent and kinetics of immune-related transplantation injury and rejection (201). The chemokines are classified into two major groups based on their structure: the cysteine-X-cysteine (CXC) or alpha chemokines (e.g., IL-8 and IFN-γ-inducible protein), which primarily attract neutrophils and T-cells, and the CC or beta chemokines (e.g., macrophage inflammatory protein-1α/β (MIP-1α/β, RANTES and MCP-1), which attract T-cells, monocyte/macrophages, dendritic cells, natural killer cells, and some polymorphs. Chemokines orchestrate the trafficking of leukocytes to sites of inflammation. Chemokines and their receptors are important in the development of graft infiltrates as well as in reperfusion injury. They act not only as attractants for various leukocyte populations but also by augmenting the effector functions of leukocytes within the graft.

Migration of Activated Leukocytes into the Graft

To enter the site of inflammation or immune response, leukocytes must migrate across the vascular endothelium. This migration process is controlled by the elaboration of chemokines and by cell–cell interactions between leukocytes and the endothelium. The adhesion of leukocytes to the endothelium is a complex multistep process that involves a series of interactions between the surface of the leukocyte and the endothelial cell or its extracellular matrix (202). Activated cells bear adhesion proteins, chemokine receptors, and addressins, which allow homing to and migration into the graft. The expression of many adhesion proteins involved in these interactions is upregulated by proinflammatory cytokines. Ischemic damage alone results in increased expression of several cytokines, and of these, IL-1 upregulates the expression of members of the selectin family. Other adhesion proteins such as ICAM-1, VCAM-1, and E-selectin (endothelial-specific selectin) are known to be upregulated by the type of cytokines also induced after the trauma of transplantation. Antigen-activated lymphocytes may show tissue-specific homing and show preference for sites in which they are most likely to reencounter their specific antigen. This process seems to be facilitated by recognition by the T-cell of MHC class II/peptide complexes on the vascular endothelium. It may be possible to hide the proteins involved in leukocyte extravasation, thereby slowing or preventing the rejection process. Blocking the adhesion proteins by using antibodies or inhibiting their expression has been attempted in experimental and clinical transplantation. In general, cocktails of antibodies are more potent than single antibodies.

Destruction of the Graft

The immune system generates many different effector mechanisms, most of which are involved in the destruction of the graft. Patients who have been exposed to MHC antigens through transplant, blood transfusions, or pregnancy often develop antibodies reactive to those MHC antigens. These antibodies can cause hyperacute rejection. The conventional cross-match test, however, detects not only harmful MHC-directed cytotoxic antibodies, but also harmless autoantibodies. In most cases, it is now possible to distinguish autoreactive from alloreactive antibodies, and it is now possible to transplant patients across an apparent positive crossmatch, but in whom the reactivity is due to autoantibodies. Many of the changes associated with acute rejection, including arteriolar thrombosis, interstitial hemorrhage, and fibrinoid necrosis of the arteriolar walls, may result from the deposition of antibody and fixation of complement.

MHC-mismatched lymphocytes proliferate and produce cytokines that allow the differentiation of precursor CTLs into effector cells that lyse target cells bearing the mismatched MHC antigens. Furthermore, through the elaboration of high levels of IFN-γ and other cytokines or chemokines, CTLs are able to recruit and activate cells involved in delayed type hypersensitivity (DTH) lesions, initiating acute or chronic rejection. Macrophages also participate by elaborating proinflammatory and profibrogenic cytokines that may result in the atherosclerotic and fibrotic changes associated with chronic rejection.

Renal Injury During Transplantation

Injury to the kidney frequently occurs during transplantation and often manifests clinically as delayed graft function (DGF) (Table 16) (203) or transplant acute tubular necrosis (TxATN). This injury can occur at many stages and also has short- and long-term consequences for the graft. Factors that participate in renal injury include donor hypertension and aging; brain death in the cadaveric donor; injury arising from harvesting, preservation, and implantation; prolonged warm ischemic time; and anastomosis time or rewarm time. The pathology of transplant ATN is not identical to that of native kidney ATN. The extent of tubular necrosis is usually more widespread in transplant ATN, which may be related to the presence of endothelial injury and disseminated intravascular coagulation (DIC) in the brain-dead donor as well as the exposure of the transplant kidney to cold flush and storage. Ischemia/reperfusion injury causes direct injury to the kidney, but also induces an inflammatory response during the phase of healing.

Delayed graft function is associated with an increased rate of acute rejection and irreversible graft rejection. Transplant ATN adversely affects survival, while total preservation time and sharing between centers do not predict transplant ATN. Transplant ATN is associated not only with graft loss, but also with patient death and irreversible rejection. These adverse effects of DGF are manifested in the first six months. Pulsatile perfusion is associated with a reduction in DGF. In this era of stronger and improved immunosuppressive therapy, DGF is assuming greater

Table 16 Differential Diagnosis of Delayed Graft Function

Prerenal azotemia (e.g., hemorrhage, overdiuresis)
Acute tubular necrosis
Urologic complications
  Ureteral anastomotic obstruction
  Obstruction of the bladder catheter
  Urine leak, urinoma
Vascular complications
  Hemorrhage
  Renal artery thrombosis
  Renal vein thrombosis
  Renal artery stenosis
Calcineurin inhibitor nephrotoxicity (cyclosporine, tacrolimus)
  Vasoconstriction
  Thrombotic microangiopathy
Other nephrotoxic agents
  Amphotericin B
  Aminoglycosides
  Acyclovir
  Contrast media
  Angiotensin-converting enzyme inhibitors
  Nonsteroidal anti-inflammatory drugs
Infection
  Septicemia
  Graft pyelonephritis
  Cytomegalovirus infection
Acute rejection
Recurrent disease
  Focal segmental glomerulosclerosis
  Hemolytic uremic syndrome
  Other glomerulopathies

importance in graft outcomes. Risk factors for DGF include anastomosis time, total preservation time, black race, donor cerebrovascular accidents, as well as immunological variables such as panel reactive antibodies (PRAs), donor-related mismatches, and high cytotoxic antibodies. The failure of DGF to recover usually represents severe rejection in an injured transplant. The worst one-year survival rate is recorded in grafts that had both DGF and acute rejection. Evidence suggests that DGF causes an increased frequency of acute rejection, and the real cause of the impaired graft survival is the rejection. Living donor kidneys with extensive HLA mismatching have excellent graft survival, perhaps lacking the injury associated with brain death and prolonged cold storage that accompanies cadaver donation. Several renal syndromes may affect the transplanted kidney (Table 17).

Allograft Rejection

Hyperacute rejection is characterized by the sudden, irreversible cessation of graft function minutes to hours after revascularization. Preformed antibodies against donor

Table 17 Renal Syndromes Affecting the Transplanted Kidney

Hyperacute rejection
Accelerated rejection
Acute rejection
Delayed graft function/transplant acute tubular necrosis
Cyclosporine nephrotoxicity
Chronic allograft nephropathy
Chronic rejection
De novo glomerulopathy
Recurrent glomerulopathy

antigens present on the endothelium mediate this form of rejection (204). One setting for hyperacute rejection is ABO incompatibility, wherein circulating antidonor ABO blood group hemagglutinins bind to glycolipid determinants on endothelial cells. A second setting is the attachment of preformed recipient antidonor HLA antibodies to the vascular lining of the graft. Histologically, there is extensive glomerular and vascular thrombosis. However, routine pretransplant cross-match testing minimizes the risk of hyperacute rejection.

Accelerated rejection is characterized by anamnestic responses that occur within five days posttransplant. These responses may include the production of generally low-affinity antidonor antibodies by presensitized B-cells or the generation of CTLs from memory elements. The immune elements bind to the donor endothelium without the involvement of complement (Type II endothelial activation), leading to disruption of the vascular layer and interstitial hemorrhage. Parenchymal rupture may result in acute pain, tenderness, and swelling of the graft and life-threatening hemorrhage. Accelerated rejection is uncommon with current immunosuppressive strategies, and can often be reversed by antilymphocyte globulin (ALG), plasmapheresis, and cyclophosphamide.

Acute rejection is the most common type of rejection in clinical practice, affecting up to 40% of patients. It usually occurs between 7 and 90 days posttransplant, but it may occur later. In the early posttransplant period, there is the activation of alloantigen-specific T-cells, which initiate acute rejection or subclinical graft injury (197). It is often responsive to steroid therapy, but sometimes there is an antibody component, in which cases there is resistance to steroids and a partial response to ALG. Histologically, acute rejection is characterized by intimal arteritis and tubulitis (205). Uncontrolled acute rejection can result in graft swelling, vascular occlusion, and necrosis. Acute rejection episodes that are not completely reversed (to serum creatinine < 1.6 mg/dL) increase the probability of graft loss.

Chronic rejection occurs in about half of all renal allografts within 10 years. In contrast to acute rejection, chronic rejection does not respond to immunosuppressive therapy (206). Histopathologically, there is arterial narrowing and hyalinization and interstitial fibrosis. Chronic kidney rejection is often associated with the presence of antidonor antibodies, which correlates with the presence of arterial hyalinization. In addition to these antigen-dependent factors, the development of chronic rejection seems to be influenced by nonimmunological factors associated with ischemia/reperfusion injury, including evidence of cardiovascular compromise in the donor, prolonged cold ischemia time prior to transplantation, and impaired RBF in the recipient. The incidence of chronic rejection may be minimized by aggressive treatment of acute rejection episodes with the goal of achieving complete resolution (207); the use of surveillance biopsies to diagnose subclinical rejection, which if treated could result in better long-term outcomes; matching of HLA antigens; effective maintenance immunosuppression; and vigorous control of hypertension, hyperlipidemia, and diabetes mellitus.

Late Graft Dysfunction

In addition to chronic rejection, several disorders can potentially cause graft dysfunction remote from the time of initial transplant: recurrent primary disease, infectious, calcineurin inhibitor–related, and mechanical disorders. Some primary renal diseases recur at a high and predictable rate and may be a relative contraindication to transplantation (e.g., oxalosis). Others recur at a rate that is acceptable for transplantation but sufficient to be seriously considered as a differential diagnosis of late graft dysfunction (e.g., hemolytic uremic syndrome and diabetes mellitus). Immunoglobulin A nephropathy recurs in up to 50% of cases, but is rarely a cause of graft dysfunction. Membranoproliferative glomerulonephritis (especially Type I) also recurs but also rarely causes graft dysfunction. Recurrent focal segmental glomerulosclerosis can occur within minutes of establishing the transplant arterial anastomosis. Acute urinary tract infections may be complicated by transplant pyelonephritis causing allograft dysfunction. Fever, graft tenderness and swelling, rising serum creatinine, and high-ultrasound resistive indices resemble acute graft rejection. Cytomegalovirus (CMV) infection in its most common form presents with fever, malaise, leukopenia, pancytopenia, myalgia, and occasionally renal dysfunction. More severe forms include pulmonary infiltrates, respiratory failure, hepatitis, and renal failure. CMV may directly involve the graft and cause a CMV glomerulopathy (208). The calcineurin inhibitors, cyclosporine and tacrolimus, are nephrotoxic. Chronic interstitial fibrosis in a striped pattern is the classic histologic finding in chronic calcineurin inhibitor nephropathy. Finally, obstructive uropathy can occur by mechanisms that afflict native kidneys, including renal stone disease, but also those peculiar to the transplanted kidney, including ureteral anastomotic stenosis, lymphoceles, and BK virus infection.

Evaluation and Selection of the Living Donor

The living donor evaluation begins with education regarding the process of evaluation and donation, followed by a thorough history, physical examination, and psychosocial evaluation. A comprehensive laboratory screening is performed, including complete blood count, chemistry panel, HIV, HBsAg, antihepatitis C virus, CMV, glucose tolerance test (for diabetic families), urinalysis, urine culture, pregnancy test, and two 24-hour urine determinations for creatinine clearance and protein excretion. Chest X ray, electrocardiogram, and exercise treadmill test are performed for patients aged 50 years and older. Psychosocial evaluation, and intravenous pyelogram, renal angiogram, and/or helical CT urogram are performed. Potential donors are tissue typed and cross-matched. Prospective donors are generally excluded if they are less than 18 or more than 65 years of age, or have hypertension, diabetes, proteinuria, reduced GFR, microscopic hematuria, urologic abnormalities, or significant medical or psychiatric conditions (including active substance abuse).

Evaluation of Prospective Kidney Transplant Recipients

An extensive pretransplant evaluation of the prospective recipient is performed to detect and treat reversible medical and surgical conditions that might increase the risk of transplantation if left untreated. Ischemic heart disease substantially increases the risk of transplantation. Cancer screening is directed at common cancers for the age group and gender. Screening for colorectal malignancy is accomplished with a stool occult blood test as well as sigmoidoscopy or colonoscopy in older patients. Chest X rays are used to screen for lung cancer. Digital prostate exam and possibly prostate-specific antigen determinations are performed to detect prostate cancer. Women should undergo pelvic exam and a

Table 18   Contraindications to Renal Transplantation

Disseminated malignancy
Refractory cardiac failure
Chronic respiratory failure
Advanced hepatic disease
Extensive vascular disease: coronary, cerebral, or peripheral
Severe congenital urinary tract abnormality
Chronic infection, refractory to therapy
Persistent coagulation disorder
Severe mental retardation
Psychosocial problems: severe psychosis, alcoholism, or drug addiction

Pap smear. Women over 40 years or younger women with a family history of breast cancer should have a mammogram. In patients with a history of cancer, it is generally recommended that a two-year interval for the most invasive cancers elapse before transplantation. Smoking cessation should be accomplished. Screening for esophagitis and peptic ulcer disease can be reserved for patients with symptoms. Evidence for tuberculosis, CMV, or HIV infection should be established. Pulmonary function studies may be indicated in patients with chronic lung disease. Urologic evaluation can generally be reserved for patients with chronic bladder dysfunction or recurrent infection. Renal ultrasound, computerized tomography, or magnetic resonance imaging study is probably needed to screen for renal malignancies or other structural problems. Psychosocial evaluation is obtained to ensure that the patient is capable of providing informed consent and can comply with the posttransplant immunosuppression regimen. Despite these potential contraindications (Table 18), selection criteria are generally less restrictive than in past, and more patients with significant comorbidity and older patients are receiving renal transplants.

The donor and recipient should be ABO blood group compatible and have no preformed antibodies. Antibodies directed against a random panel of lymphocytes from the general population are assayed, and the percentage of these lymphocytes that incite a reaction from the recipient—termed the percent PRA—is measured. Transplant recipients with a high PRA are more likely to have preformed antibody against a donor kidney and thus more susceptible to hyperacute rejection. When a potential donor kidney becomes available, the recipient's serum is tested for reaction against cells from the potential donor. If the potential recipient's serum reacts with the donor, transplantation is usually contraindicated. MHC antigens are also measured on cells from both the donor and the recipient. In the United Network for Organ Sharing protocol for organ allocation, highest priority is given to kidneys with no MHC antigen mismatches. Because the average waiting time currently exceeds two years, periodic reevaluation of the recipient may be needed in the interval.

Immunosuppressive Agents

The search for the optimal chronic immunosuppression regimen for renal transplant patients continues to evolve as new immunosuppressive agents are introduced and new combinations of therapies tried. All of these agents have therapeutic effects, toxicities related to immunodeficiency (i.e., increased infection and malignancies), and nonimmune toxicities (e.g., nephrotoxicity, hyperlipidemia, and diabetes). The initial period after transplantation requires intense immunosuppression. During the "induction" period, high doses of combinations of calcineurin inhibitors,

mycophenolate mofetil (MMF), rapamycin, or azathioprine, and glucocorticoids are often used. The reversal of acute rejection also requires intense immunosuppression with high doses of glucocorticoids, but also in more severe cases, with anti-CD3 of polyclonal ALG or ATG. Maintenance immunosuppression can generally be achieved after three to six months, and now usually involves cyclosporine or tacrolimus in combination with MMF, rapamycin or azathioprine, and/or steroids. However, drug regimens and treatment guidelines are constantly evolving.

Corticosteroids downregulate the expression of several genes that encode for inflammatory cytokines, inhibit leukocyte migration to sites of inflammation, promote apoptosis of lymphocytes and eosinophils, and reduce expression of MHC class II molecules, thereby inhibiting T-cell activation and function. Azathioprine blocks RNA and DNA synthesis by inhibiting inosinic acid, the precursor for the purines adenylic and guanidylic acids. Chlorambucil and cyclophosphamide alkylate DNA and interfere with DNA metabolism. These compounds are cytotoxic to lymphocytes and are thus immunosuppressive. The cytotoxic effects of these compounds are not limited to the immune system; however, they have a wide range of side effects (e.g., anemia, leukopenia, thrombocytopenia, intestinal damage, and hair loss) that may limit the dosage and duration of therapy. Cyclosporine and tacrolimus exert their pharmacologic effects by inhibiting the activity of calcineurin, an intracellular phosphatase essential for transcriptional activation of IL-2 gene, and ultimately T-cell activation. In contrast, sirolimus inhibits a different pathway required for full T-cell activation by blocking the phosphorylation of p70(s6) kinase and the eukaryotic initiation factor-4E-binding protein, PHAS-1 (209). Cyclosporine is effective before transplantation, but is ineffective in suppressing ongoing rejection. Both cyclosporine and tacrolimus are nephrotoxic and associated with a higher risk of cancer in patients who take the drugs long term. Sirolimus is minimally nephrotoxic when given alone; thrombocytopenia and severe dyslipidemia are its major side effects. Leflunomide blocks T-cell activation by inhibiting the activity of tyrosine kinases associated with cytokine receptors. This agent also prevents T-cell proliferation by inhibiting de novo pyrimidine synthesis (210). ALG, prepared in horses immunized with human lymphocytes, has been used to treat acute rejection. It can cause serum sickness. Monoclonal antibodies are less immunogenic than ALG and can be more specifically targeted. *OKT3* is a "humanized" mouse antibody directed against CD3 that is in common use. Antibodies to the IL-2 receptor (CD25) on activated T-cells, and to CD4 are also in use. *MMF* inhibits the de novo synthesis of purines, crucial to cell cycling of T- and B-cells. It thus blocks clonal expansion of T- and B-cells, preventing antibody production and the generation of CTLs, as well as other effector T-cells (211). In contrast to other immunosuppressive drugs, MMF also inhibits antibody production by B-cells. There seems to be a trend toward better graft survival at three years post-transplant (211).

Complications of Renal Transplantation

Transplant patients are at risk of numerous medical and surgical complications (Table 19). Infectious complications, arising mainly as a result of immunosuppressive therapy, are among the most common and significant. Infections may be classified according to duration after transplantation, or by organism or system involved. The main risk factors for

Table 19 Complications of Renal Transplantation

Surgical complications	Medical complications
Urologic	Cardiovascular
Obstruction	Coronary artery disease
Stricture	Hypertension
Edema	Metabolic
Blood clot	Hyperparathyroidism
Stone	Hyperkalemia
Excess ureter redundancy	Hypomagnesemia
Tumor	Hyperuricemia and gout
Infection (fungus ball, viral)	Posttransplant diabetes mellitus
Indwelling ureteric stent	Hepatic
Fluid collections	Viral hepatitis (hepatitis B and C)
Lymphocele	Drug-induced liver dysfunction (e.g.,
Hematoma	cyclosporine, azathioprine, and,
Urinoma	rarely, mycophenolate mofetil;
Abscess	antimicrobials)
Urine leaks	Hematologic
Calyceal	Anemia
Renal pelvic	Polycythemia (usually associated
Ureteral	with transplant renal artery stenosis)
Ureteroneocystostomy	Leukopenia (azathioprine, mycophenolate
Vesical	mofetil, ganciclovir, and
	cytomegalovirus infection)
Vascular	Infectious
Renal artery thrombosis	Intravenous catheter associated
Renal artery stenosis	Pulmonary
Renal vein thrombosis	Gastrointestinal infections
Complications of	Central nervous system infections
percutaneous	Neurologic
allograft biopsy	Diffuse encephalopathies
Arteriocalyceal fistulas	Focal neurological disorders
Arteriovenous fistulas	Seizure disorders
Iliac or mesenteric	Peripheral nerve disorders
vascular	Cancer
lacerations	Skin cancers
Perirenal hematomas	Posttransplant lymphoproliferative disease
Pseudoaneurysms	Sarcomas
Gross hematuria	Carcinomas of the vulva, anus, cervix, liver
Intra-abdominal	
organ injury	

infection are immunosuppressive therapy, the immuno-compromised state of uremia, and major surgery involving urologic and vascular procedures. Other risk factors include DGF and acute rejection, hyperglycemia, diabetes, splenectomy, and hepatitis B infection. Infections may be transmitted from the donor. Pretransplant screening for infections is critical as are prophylactic measure post-transplant. The timing of infections posttransplant is of diagnostic importance. Infections within the first month posttransplant are associated with the surgical procedure, usually bacterial infections of the urinary tract, respiratory tract, perinephric space, surgical wound, and vascular access sites (line sepsis). Herpes simplex virus (HSV) infections may occur at this time. From one to six months, the most common infection is due to CMV; other infectious agents during this interval include opportunistic organisms such as pneumocystis carinii, cryptococcus, aspergillus and other fungal infections, nocardia, toxoplasma, listeria, nontyphoid salmonella, tuberculosis, and viral infections, including primary or reactivated CMV, Epstein–Barr virus (EBV) varicella-zoster virus, and adenovirus. After six months, community-acquired infections predominate. Persistent viral infections (e.g., CMV, HSV, EBV, hepatitis B and C, and HIV) can assume great importance in the transplant patients.

SUMMARY AND CONCLUSIONS

The kidney is an extremely complex organ with tightly integrated functions that are critically involved in the maintenance and restoration of normal physiology of humans over a wide range of clinical conditions. Perhaps more than any other organ, the physiology and pathophysiology of the kidney is directly tied to numerous, significant clinical disorders. The kidney is vulnerable to both acute and chronic injury, which poses a multitude of potential problems for the management of fluid, mineral, electrolyte, acid–base, and metabolic balance, blood pressure, and anemia, particularly in critically ill surgical patients experiencing acute renal decompensation or in ESKD patients undergoing surgery. The trend toward increasingly aggressive resuscitation and life support measures, growing numbers of trauma victims, and the growth in the rate of surgical procedures performed on patients with significant comorbidities will continue to increase the incidence of AKF in the surgical setting. Given the explosive growth in the incidence rates for CKD and ESKD, surgeons will also encounter an increasing proportion of patients with chronically impaired renal function presenting for surgical interventions of other organ systems. Unfortunately, no therapies to date have been shown to reverse renal injury, so that emphasis must be placed on prevention, early detection, prompt correction of precipitating, contributing, or exacerbating factors, and appropriate timing and choice of renal replacement therapy when indicated. Fortunately, continuous dialysis therapies are evolving, which will continue to facilitate advanced therapeutic options for critically ill surgical patients with AKF, and advances in kidney transplantation have allowed it to become applicable to a much broader population of ESKD patients. The Holy Grail, of course, remains the discovery of methods for therapeutic recovery of renal function.

REFERENCES

1. Just A, Arendshorst WJ. Dynamics and contribution of mechanisms mediating renal blood flow autoregulation. Am J Physiol Regul Integr Comp Physiol 2003; 285:R619–R631.
2. Venkatachalum MA, Kriz W. Anatomy. In: Heptinstall RH, ed. Pathology of the Kidney. 4th ed. Boston: Little, Brown and Co., 1992:35.
3. DiBona GF, et al. Neural control of the kidney: functionally specific renal sympathetic nerve fibers. Am J Physiol Regul Integr Comp Physiol 2000; 279:R1517–R1524.
4. Cockett AT. Lymphatic network of kidney. I. Anatomic and physiologic considerations. Urology 1977; 9:125–129.
5. Schnermann J, Levine DZ. Paracrine factors in tubuloglomerular feedback: adenosine, ATP, and nitric oxide. Annu Rev Physiol 2003; 65:501–529.
6. Navar LG. Renal autoregulation: perspectives from whole kidney and single nephron studies. Am J Physiol 1978; 234: F357–F370.
7. Aronson PS. Ion exchangers mediating NaCl transport in the renal proximal tubule. Cell Biochem Biophys 2002; 36:147–153.
8. Nielsen S, Frokiaer J, Marples D, et al. Aquaporins in the kidney: from molecules to medicine. Physiol Rev 2002; 82:205–244.
9. Giebisch GH. A trail of research on potassium. Kidney Int 2002; 62:1498–1512.
10. Loffing J, Kaissling B. Sodium and calcium transport pathways along the mammalian distal nephron: from rabbit to human. Am J Physiol Renal Physiol 2003; 284:F628–F643.
11. Hoenderop JG, Nilius B, Bindels RJ. Molecular mechanism of active Ca2+ reabsorption in the distal nephron. Annu Rev Physiol 2002; 64:529–549.

12. Yu AS. Evolving concepts in epithelial magnesium transport. Curr Opin Nephrol Hypertens 2001; 10:649–653.

13. Quamme GA, de Rouffignac C. Epithelial magnesium transport and regulation by the kidney. Front Biosci 2000; 5: D694–D711.

14. Murer H, Hernando N, Forster I, et al. Proximal tubular phosphate reabsorption: molecular mechanisms. Physiol Rev 2000; 80:1373–1409.

15. Friedlander G. Autocrine/paracrine control of renal phosphate transport. Kidney Int Suppl 1998; 65:S18–S23.

16. Good DW. The thick ascending limb as a site of renal bicarbonate reabsorption. Semin Nephrol 1993; 13:225–235.

17. de Mello-Aires M, Malnic G. Distal tubule bicarbonate transport. J Nephrol 2002; 15(suppl 5):S97–S111.

18. Hamm LL, Hering-Smith KS. Acid-base transport in the collecting duct. Semin Nephrol 1993; 13:246–255.

19. Russel FG, Masereeuw R, van Aubel RA. Molecular aspects of renal anionic drug transport. Annu Rev Physiol 2002; 64:563–594.

20. Masereeuw R, Russel FG. Mechanisms and clinical implications of renal drug excretion. Drug Metab Rev 2001; 33:299–351.

21. Berkhin EB, Humphreys MH. Regulation of renal tubular secretion of organic compounds. Kidney Int 2001; 59:17–30.

22. Dantzler WH. Renal organic anion transport: a comparative and cellular perspective. Biochim Biophys Acta 2002; 1566: 169–181.

23. Dresser MJ, Leabman MK, Giacomini KM. Transporters involved in the elimination of drugs in the kidney: organic anion transporters and organic cation transporters. J Pharm Sci 2001; 90:397–421.

24. Lang F. Osmotic diuresis. Ren Physiol 1987; 10:160–173.

25. Brater DC. Pharmacology of diuretics. Am J Med Sci 2000; 319:38–50.

26. Preisig PA, Toto RD, Alpern RJ. Carbonic anhydrase inhibitors. Ren Physiol 1987; 10:136–159.

27. Prandota J. Furosemide: progress in understanding its diuretic, anti-inflammatory, and bronchodilating mechanism of action, and use in the treatment of respiratory tract diseases. Am J Ther 2002; 9:317–328.

28. Velazquez H. Thiazide diuretics. Ren Physiol 1987; 10:184–197.

29. Ryan MP. Magnesium and potassium-sparing diuretics. Magnesium 1986; 5:282–292.

30. Doggrell SA, Brown L. The spironolactone renaissance. Expert Opin Investig Drugs 2001; 10:943–954.

31. Suki WN. Use of diuretics in chronic renal failure. Kidney Int Suppl 1997; 59:S33–S35.

32. Bricker NS. On the meaning of the intact nephron hypothesis. Am J Med 1969; 46:1–11.

33. Anderson S, Brenner BM. The role of intraglomerular pressure in the initiation and progression of renal disease. J Hypertens Suppl 1986; 4:S236–S238.

34. Brenner BM. Nephron adaptation to renal injury or ablation. Am J Physiol 1985; 249:F324–F337.

35. Brenner BM, Lawler EV, Mackenzie HS. The hyperfiltration theory: a paradigm shift in nephrology. Kidney Int 1996; 49:1774–1777.

36. Brenner BM, Mackenzie HS. Nephron mass as a risk factor for progression of renal disease. Kidney Int Suppl 1997; 63: S124–S127.

37. Halperin ML, Bohn D. Clinical approach to disorders of salt and water balance. Emphasis on integrative physiology. Crit Care Clin 2002; 18:249–272.

38. Oster JR, Singer I, Thatte L, et al. The polyuria of solute diuresis. Arch Intern Med 1997; 157:721–729.

39. Robertshaw M, Lai KN, Swaminathan R. Prediction of creatinine clearance from plasma creatinine: comparison of five formulae. Br J Clin Pharmacol 1989; 28:275–280.

40. Vervoort G, Willems HL, Wetzels JF. Assessment of glomerular filtration rate in healthy subjects and normoalbuminuric diabetic patients: validity of a new (MDRD) prediction equation. Nephrol Dial Transplant 2002; 17:1901–1913.

41. Levey AS, Bosch JP, Lewis JB, Greene T, Rogers N, Roth D. A more accurate method to estimate glomerular filtration rate from serum creatinine: a new prediction equation. Modification of Diet in Renal Disease Study Group. Ann Intern Med 1999; 130:461–470.

42. Manjunath G, Sarnak MJ, Levey AS. Estimating the glomerular filtration rate. Dos and don'ts for assessing kidney function. Postgrad Med 2001; 110:55–62; quiz 11.

43. van Bommel EF, Leunissen KM, Weimar W. Continuous renal replacement therapy for critically ill patients: an update. J Intensive Care Med 1994; 9:265–280.

44. Brivet FG, Kleinknecht DJ, Loirat P, Landais PJ. Acute renal failure in intensive care units—causes, outcome, and prognostic factors of hospital mortality; a prospective, multicenter study. French Study Group on Acute Renal Failure. Crit Care Med 1996; 24:192–198.

45. Albright RC Jr. Acute renal failure: a practical update. Mayo Clin Proc 2001; 76:67–74.

46. Silvester W. Outcome studies of continuous renal replacement therapy in the intensive care unit. Kidney Int Suppl 1998; 66:S131–S141.

47. Levy EM, Viscoli CM, Horwitz RI. The effect of acute renal failure on mortality. A cohort analysis. JAMA 1996; 275: 1489–1494.

48. Hou SH, Bushinsky DA, Wish JB, Cohen JJ, Harrington JT. Hospital-acquired renal insufficiency: a prospective study. Am J Med 1983; 74:243–248.

49. Anderson RJ, Linas SL, Berns AS, et al. Nonoliguric acute renal failure. N Engl J Med 1977; 296:1134–1138.

50. Yared A, Kon V, Ichikawa I. Mechanism of preservation of glomerular perfusion and filtration during acute extracellular fluid volume depletion. Importance of intrarenal vasopressin-prostaglandin interaction for protecting kidneys from constrictor action of vasopressin. J Clin Invest 1985; 75:1477–1487.

51. Guazzi MD, Agostoni P, Perego B, et al. Apparent paradox of neurohumoral axis inhibition after body fluid volume depletion in patients with chronic congestive heart failure and water retention. Br Heart J 1994; 72:534–539.

52. Slater MS, Mullins RJ. Rhabdomyolysis and myoglobinuric renal failure in trauma and surgical patients: a review. J Am Coll Surg 1998; 186:693–716.

53. Scolari F, Tardanico R, Zani R, et al. Cholesterol crystal embolism: a recognizable cause of renal disease. Am J Kidney Dis 2000; 36:1089–1109.

54. Porter GA. Contrast-associated nephropathy. Am J Cardiol 1989; 64:22E–26E.

55. Parfrey PS, Griffiths SM, Barrett BJ, et al. Contrast material-induced renal failure in patients with diabetes mellitus, renal insufficiency, or both. A prospective controlled study. N Engl J Med 1989; 320:143–149.

56. Alexandridis G, Liberopoulos E, Elisaf M. Aminoglycoside-induced reversible tubular dysfunction. Pharmacology 2003; 67:118–120.

57. Kaloyanides GJ, Pastoriza-Munoz E. Aminoglycoside nephrotoxicity. Kidney Int 1980; 18:571–582.

58. Porter GA, Bennett WM. Nephrotoxic acute renal failure due to common drugs. Am J Physiol 1981; 241:F1–F8.

59. Deray G. Amphotericin B nephrotoxicity. J Antimicrob Chemother 2002; 49(suppl 1):37–41.

60. Richman AV, Narayan JL, Hirschfield JS. Acute interstitial nephritis and acute renal failure associated with cimetidine therapy. Am J Med 1981; 70:1272–1274.

61. Dutt MK, Moody P, Northfield TC. Effect of cimetidine on renal function in man. Br J Clin Pharmacol 1981; 12:47–50.

62. Berglund F, Killander J, Pompeius R. Effect of trimethoprim-sulfamethoxazole on the renal excretion of creatinine in man. J Urol 1975; 114:802–808.

63. Esson ML, Schrier RW. Diagnosis and treatment of acute tubular necrosis. Ann Intern Med 2002; 137:744–752.

64. Espinel CH, Gregory AW. Differential diagnosis of acute renal failure. Clin Nephrol 1980; 13:73–77.

65. Miller ED Jr, Ackerly JA, Peach MJ. Blood pressure support during general anesthesia in a renin-dependent state in the rat. Anesthesiology 1978; 48:404–408.

66. Zarich S, Fang LS, Diamond JR. Fractional excretion of sodium. Exceptions to its diagnostic value. Arch Intern Med 1985; 145:108–112.

67. Bakris GL, Lass N, Gaber AO, Jones JD, Burnett JC Jr. Radiocontrast medium-induced declines in renal function: a role for oxygen free radicals. Am J Physiol 1990; 258:F115–F120.

68. Durham JD, Caputo C, Dokko J, et al. A randomized controlled trial of N-acetylcysteine to prevent contrast nephropathy in cardiac angiography. Kidney Int 2002; 62:2202–2207.

69. Mueller C, Buerkle G, Buettner HJ, et al. Prevention of contrast media-associated nephropathy: randomized comparison of 2 hydration regimens in 1620 patients undergoing coronary angioplasty. Arch Intern Med 2002; 162:329–336.

70. Briguori C, Manganelli F, Scarpato P, et al. Acetylcysteine and contrast agent-associated nephrotoxicity. J Am Coll Cardiol 2002; 40:298–303.

71. Boccalandro F, Amhad M, Smalling RW, Sdringola S. Oral acetylcysteine does not protect renal function from moderate to high doses of intravenous radiographic contrast. Catheter Cardiovasc Interv 2003; 58:336–341.

72. Tepel M, van der Giet M, Schwarzfeld C, Laufer U, Liermann D, Zidek W. Prevention of radiographic-contrast-agent-induced reductions in renal function by acetylcysteine. N Engl J Med 2000; 343:180–184.

73. Kay J, Chow WH, Chan TM, et al. Acetylcysteine for prevention of acute deterioration of renal function following elective coronary angiography and intervention: a randomized controlled trial. JAMA 2003; 289:553–558.

74. Denton MD, Chertow GM, Brady HR. "Renal-dose" dopamine for the treatment of acute renal failure: scientific rationale, experimental studies and clinical trials. Kidney Int 1996; 50:4–14.

75. Segal JM, Phang PT, Walley KR. Low-dose dopamine hastens onset of gut ischemia in a porcine model of hemorrhagic shock. J Appl Physiol 1992; 73:1159–1164.

76. Burton CJ, Tomson CR. Can the use of low-dose dopamine for treatment of acute renal failure be justified? Postgrad Med J 1999; 75:269–274.

77. Weisberg LS, Kurnik PB, Kurnik BR. Risk of radiocontrast nephropathy in patients with and without diabetes mellitus. Kidney Int 1994; 45:259–265.

78. Halpenny M, Markos F, Snow HM, et al. Effects of prophylactic fenoldopam infusion on renal blood flow and renal tubular function during acute hypovolemia in anesthetized dogs. Crit Care Med 2001; 29:855–860.

79. Tumlin JA, Wang A, Murray PT, Mathur VS. Fenoldopam mesylate blocks reductions in renal plasma flow after radiocontrast dye infusion: a pilot trial in the prevention of contrast nephropathy. Am Heart J 2002; 143:894–903.

80. Sheinbaum R, Ignacio C, Safi HJ, Estrera A. Contemporary strategies to preserve renal function during cardiac and vascular surgery. Rev Cardiovasc Med 2003; 4(suppl 1):S21–S28.

81. Solomon R, Werner C, Mann D, D'Elia J, Silva P. Effects of saline, mannitol, and furosemide to prevent acute decreases in renal function induced by radiocontrast agents. N Engl J Med 1994; 331:1416–1420.

82. Lassnigg A, Donner E, Grubhofer G, Presterl E, Druml W, Hiesmayr M. Lack of renoprotective effects of dopamine and furosemide during cardiac surgery. J Am Soc Nephrol 2000; 11:97–104.

83. Better OS, Rubinstein I, Winaver JM, Knochel JP. Mannitol therapy revisited (1940–1997). Kidney Int 1997; 52:886–894.

84. Bonventre JV, Weinberg JM. Kidney preservation ex vivo for transplantation. Annu Rev Med 1992; 43:523–553.

85. Ratcliffe PJ, Richardson AJ, Kirby JE, Moyses C, Shelton JR, Morris PJ. Effect of intravenous infusion of atriopeptin 3 on immediate renal allograft function. Kidney Int 1991; 39: 164–168.

86. Sands JM, Neylan JF, Olson RA, O'Brien DP, Whelchel JD, Mitch WE. Atrial natriuretic factor does not improve the outcome of cadaveric renal transplantation. J Am Soc Nephrol 1991; 1:1081–1086.

87. Allgren RL, Marbury TC, Rahman SN, et al. Anaritide in acute tubular necrosis. Auriculin Anaritide Acute Renal Failure Study Group. N Engl J Med 1997; 336:828–834.

88. Choi PT, Yip G, Quinonez LG, Cook DJ. Crystalloids versus colloids in fluid resuscitation: a systematic review. Crit Care Med 1999; 27:200–210.

89. Human albumin administration in critically ill patients: systematic review of randomised controlled trials. Cochrane Injuries Group Albumin Reviewers. BMJ 1998; 317:235–240.

90. Kellum JA. The use of diuretics and dopamine in acute renal failure: a systematic review of the evidence. Crit Care (Lond) 1997; 1:53–59.

91. De Vriese AS. Prevention and treatment of acute renal failure in sepsis. J Am Soc Nephrol 2003; 14:792–805.

92. Deppisch RM, Beck W, Goehl H, Ritz E. Complement components as uremic toxins and their potential role as mediators of microinflammation. Kidney Int Suppl 2001; 78: S271–S277.

93. Miyata T, Sugiyama S, Saito A, Kurokawa K. Reactive carbonyl compounds related uremic toxicity ("carbonyl stress"). Kidney Int Suppl 2001; 78:S25–S31.

94. Dhondt A, Vanholder R, Van Biesen W, Lameire N. The removal of uremic toxins. Kidney Int Suppl 2000; 76:S47–S59.

95. Vanholder R, De Smet R, Vogeleere P, Ringoir S. Middle molecules: toxicity and removal by hemodialysis and related strategies. Artif Organs 1995; 19:1120–1125.

96. Ringoir S. An update on uremic toxins. Kidney Int Suppl 1997; 62:S2–S4.

97. Yu HT. Progression of chronic renal failure. Arch Intern Med 2003; 163:1417–1429.

98. Stahl PJ, Felsen D. Transforming growth factor-beta, basement membrane, and epithelial-mesenchymal transdifferentiation: implications for fibrosis in kidney disease. Am J Pathol 2001; 159:1187–1192.

99. Bottinger EP, Bitzer M. TGF-beta signaling in renal disease. J Am Soc Nephrol 2002; 13:2600–2610.

100. Badid C, Vincent M, Fouque D, Laville M, Desmouliere A. Myofibroblast: a prognostic marker and target cell in progressive renal disease. Ren Fail 2001; 23:543–549.

101. Norman JT, Fine LG. Progressive renal disease: fibroblasts, extracellular matrix, and integrins. Exp Nephrol 1999; 7: 167–177.

102. K/DOQI clinical practice guidelines for chronic kidney disease: evaluation, classification, and stratification. Kidney Disease Outcome Quality Initiative. Am J Kidney Dis 2002; 39: S1–S246.

103. Krawiec DR. Managing gastrointestinal complications of uremia. Vet Clin North Am Small Anim Pract 1996; 26:1287–1292.

104. Drueke TB. Abnormal skeletal response to parathyroid hormone and the expression of its receptor in chronic uremia. Pediatr Nephrol 1996; 10:348–350.

105. Ho LT, Sprague SM. Renal osteodystrophy in chronic renal failure. Semin Nephrol 2002; 22:488–493.

106. Sato K, Obara T, Yamazaki K, et al. Somatic mutations of the MEN1 gene and microsatellite instability in a case of tertiary hyperparathyroidism occurring during high phosphate therapy for acquired, hypophosphatemic osteomalacia. J Clin Endocrinol Metab 2001; 86:5564–5571.

107. Wilmer WA, Magro CM. Calciphylaxis: emerging concepts in prevention, diagnosis, and treatment. Semin Dial 2002; 15:172–186.

108. Bardin T. Musculoskeletal manifestations of chronic renal failure. Curr Opin Rheumatol 2003; 15:48–54.

109. Obrador GT, Pereira BJ. Anaemia of chronic kidney disease: an under-recognized and under-treated problem. Nephrol Dial Transplant 2002; 17(suppl 11):44–46.

110. Agarwal R, Warnock D. Issues related to iron replacement in chronic kidney disease. Semin Nephrol 2002; 22:479–487.

111. Bickford AK. Evaluation and treatment of iron deficiency in patients with kidney disease. Nutr Clin Care 2002; 5: 225–230.

112. Jaradat MI, Molitoris BA. Cardiovascular disease in patients with chronic kidney disease. Semin Nephrol 2002; 22:459–473.

113. Paparello J, Kshirsagar A, Batlle D. Comorbidity and cardiovascular risk factors in patients with chronic kidney disease. Semin Nephrol 2002; 22:494–506.

114. Levin A. Anemia and left ventricular hypertrophy in chronic kidney disease populations: a review of the current state of knowledge. Kidney Int 2002; 80(suppl):35–38.

115. Goldsmith DJ, Covic A. Coronary artery disease in uremia: etiology, diagnosis, and therapy. Kidney Int 2001; 60: 2059–2078.

116. Uhlig K, Levey AS, Sarnak MJ. Traditional cardiac risk factors in individuals with chronic kidney disease. Semin Dial 2003; 16:118–127.

117. Logar CM, Herzog CA, Beddhu S. Diagnosis and therapy of coronary artery disease in renal failure, end-stage renal disease, and renal transplant populations. Am J Med Sci 2003; 325:214–227.

118. Elsner D. How to diagnose and treat coronary artery disease in the uraemic patient: an update. Nephrol Dial Transplant 2001; 16:1103–1108.

119. Levin A. Identification of patients and risk factors in chronic kidney disease—evaluating risk factors and therapeutic strategies. Nephrol Dial Transplant 2001; 16(suppl 7):57–60.

120. Alpert MA, Ravenscraft MD. Pericardial involvement in end-stage renal disease. Am J Med Sci 2003; 325:228–236.

121. O'Hare A, Johansen K. Lower-extremity peripheral arterial disease among patients with end-stage renal disease. J Am Soc Nephrol 2001; 12:2838–2847.

122. Cohen G, Haag-Weber M, Horl WH. Immune dysfunction in uremia. Kidney Int Suppl 1997; 62:S79–S82.

123. Weigert AL, Schafer AI. Uremic bleeding: pathogenesis and therapy. Am J Med Sci 1998; 316:94–104.

124. Winkelmayer WC, Levin R, Avorn J. Chronic kidney disease as a risk factor for bleeding complications after coronary artery bypass surgery. Am J Kidney Dis 2003; 41:84–89.

125. Casserly LF, Dember LM. Thrombosis in end-stage renal disease. Semin Dial 2003; 16:245–256.

126. Crook ED, Thallapureddy A, Migdal S, et al. Lipid abnormalities and renal disease: is dyslipidemia a predictor of progression of renal disease? Am J Med Sci 2003; 325:340–348.

127. Prinsen BH, de Sain-van der Velden MG, de Koning EJ, Koomans HA, Berger R, Rabelink TJ. Hypertriglyceridemia in patients with chronic renal failure: possible mechanisms. Kidney Int 2003; 84(suppl):S121–S124.

128. Hall JE, Brands MW, Henegar JR, Shek EW. Abnormal kidney function as a cause and a consequence of obesity hypertension. Clin Exp Pharmacol Physiol 1998; 25:58–64.

129. Brown TM, Brown RL. Neuropsychiatric consequences of renal failure. Psychosomatics 1995; 36:244–253.

130. Fraser CL, Arieff AI. Metabolic encephalopathy as a complication of renal failure: mechanisms and mediators. New Horiz 1994; 2:518–526.

131. Fraser CL, Arieff AI. Nervous system complications in uremia. Ann Intern Med 1988; 109:143–153.

132. Mach JR Jr, Korchik WP, Mahowald MW. Dialysis dementia. Clin Geriatr Med 1988; 4:853–867.

133. Arieff AI. Dialysis disequilibrium syndrome: current concepts on pathogenesis and prevention. Kidney Int 1994; 45:629–635.

134. Pirzada NA, Morgenlander JC. Peripheral neuropathy in patients with chronic renal failure. A treatable source of discomfort and disability. Postgrad Med 1997; 102:249–250, 255–247, 261.

135. Kurata C, Uehara A, Sugi T, et al. Cardiac autonomic neuropathy in patients with chronic renal failure on hemodialysis. Nephron 2000; 84:312–319.

136. Herts BR. Imaging for renal tumors. Curr Opin Urol 2003; 13:181–186.

137. Prasad S, Bannister K, Taylor J. Is magnetic resonance angiography useful in renovascular disease? Intern Med J 2003; 33:84–90.

138. Ather MH, Noor MA. Role of imaging in the evaluation of renal trauma. J Pak Med Assoc 2002; 52:423–428.

139. Kellerman PS. Perioperative care of the renal patient. Arch Intern Med 1994; 154:1674–1688.

140. Horst M, Mehlhorn U, Hoerstrup SP, Suedkamp M, de Vivie ER. Cardiac surgery in patients with end-stage renal disease: 10-year experience. Ann Thorac Surg 2000; 69:96–101.

141. Lissoos I, Goldberg B, Van Blerk PJ, Meijers AM. Surgical procedures on patients in end-stage renal failure. Br J Urol 1973; 45:359–365.

142. Deutsch E, Bernstein RC, Addonizio P, Kussmaul WG III. Coronary artery bypass surgery in patients on chronic hemodialysis. A case-control study. Ann Intern Med 1989; 110: 369–372.

143. Bastron RD, Perkins RM, Pyne JL. Autoregulation of renal blood flow during halothane anesthesia. Anesthesiology 1977; 46:142–144.

144. Philbin DM, Coggins CH. Plasma antidiuretic hormone levels in cardiac surgical patients during morphine and halothane anesthesia. Anesthesiology 1978; 49:95–98.

145. Miller TR, Anderson RJ, Linas SL, et al. Urinary diagnostic indices in acute renal failure: a prospective study. Ann Intern Med 1978; 89:47–50.

146. Cousins MJ, Mazze RI. Methoxyflurane nephrotoxicity. A study of dose response in man. JAMA 1973; 225:1611–1616.

147. Cousins MJ, Greenstein LR, Hitt BA, Mazze RI. Metabolism and renal effects of enflurane in man. Anesthesiology 1976; 44:44–53.

148. Creasser C, Stoelting RK. Serum inorganic fluoride concentrations during and after halothane, fluroxene, and methoxyflurane anesthesia in man. Anesthesiology 1973; 39: 537–540.

149. Behne M, Wilke HJ, Harder S. Clinical pharmacokinetics of sevoflurane. Clin Pharmacokinet 1999; 36:13–26.

150. Loehning RW, Mazze RI. Possible nephrotoxicity from enflurane in a patient with severe renal disease. Anesthesiology 1974; 40:203–205.

151. Cousins MJ, Skowronski G, Plummer JL. Anaesthesia and the kidney. Anaesth Intensive Care 1983; 11:292–320.

152. Hunter JM, Jones RS, Utting JE. Comparison of vecuronium, atracurium and tubocurarine in normal patients and in patients with no renal function. Br J Anaesth 1984; 56: 941–951.

153. Morris RB, Cronnelly R, Miller RD, Stanski DR, Fahey MR. Pharmacokinetics of edrophonium in anephric and renal transplant patients. Br J Anaesth 1981; 53:1311–1314.

154. Steiner RW, Coggins C, Carvalho AC. Bleeding time in uremia: a useful test to assess clinical bleeding. Am J Hematol 1979; 7:107–117.

155. Chen KS, Huang CC, Leu ML, Deng P, Lo SK. Hemostatic and fibrinolytic response to desmopressin in uremic patients. Blood Purif 1997; 15:84–91.

156. Davenport R. Cryoprecipitate for uremic bleeding. Clin Pharm 1991; 10:429.

157. Vigano GL, Mannucci PM, Lattuada A, Harris A, Remuzzi G. Subcutaneous desmopressin (DDAVP) shortens the bleeding time in uremia. Am J Hematol 1989; 31:32–35.

158. Livio M, Mannucci PM, Vigano G, et al. Conjugated estrogens for the management of bleeding associated with renal failure. N Engl J Med 1986; 315:731–735.

159. Manian FA. Vascular and cardiac infections in end-stage renal disease. Am J Med Sci 2003; 325:243–250.

160. Werner CW, Saad TF. Prophylactic antibiotic therapy prior to dental treatment for patients with end-stage renal disease. Spec Care Dentist 1999; 19:106–111.

161. Work J. Hemodialysis catheters and ports. Semin Nephrol 2002; 22:211–220.

162. Ash SR. The evolution and function of central venous catheters for dialysis. Semin Dial 2001; 14:416–424.

163. Trerotola SO. Hemodialysis catheter placement and management. Radiology 2000; 215:651–658.

164. Okadome K, Komori K, Fukumitsu T, Sugimachi K. The potential risk for subclavian vein occlusion in patients on haemodialysis. Eur J Vasc Surg 1992; 6:602–606.
165. Akoh JA. Central venous catheters for haemodialysis: a review. Niger Postgrad Med J 2001; 8:99–103.
166. Saad TF. Central venous dialysis catheters: catheter-associated infection. Semin Dial 2001; 14:446–451.
167. Kovalik EC, Schwab SJ. Treatment approaches for infected hemodialysis vascular catheters. Curr Opin Nephrol Hypertens 2002; 11:593–596.
168. Berns JS. Infection with antimicrobial-resistant microorganisms in dialysis patients. Semin Dial 2003; 16:30–37.
169. Kuti J. Antibiotic treatment of catheter-related bacteremia in the hemodialysis patient. Conn Med 2003; 67:85–88.
170. Sandroni S, McGill R, Brouwer D. Hemodialysis catheter-associated endocarditis: clinical features, risks, and costs. Semin Dial 2003; 16:263–265.
171. Cooper SG, Sofocleous CT. Dialysis access. Semin Roentgenol 2002; 37:327–342.
172. Konner K. Vascular access in the 21st century. J Nephrol 2002; 15(suppl 6):S28–S32.
173. Brescia MJ, Cimino JE, Appel K, Hurwich BJ. Chronic hemodialysis using venipuncture and a surgically created arteriovenous fistula. N Engl J Med 1966; 275:1089–1092.
174. Burkhart HM, Cikrit DF. Arteriovenous fistulae for hemodialysis. Semin Vasc Surg 1997; 10:162–165.
175. Paulson WD, Ram SJ, Zibari GB. Vascular access: anatomy, examination, management. Semin Nephrol 2002; 22:183–194.
176. NKF-DOQI clinical practice guidelines for vascular access. National Kidney Foundation-Dialysis Outcomes Quality Initiative. Am J Kidney Dis 1997; 30:S150–S191.
177. Santoro TD, Cambria RA. PTFE shunts for hemodialysis access: progressive choice of configuration. Semin Vasc Surg 1997; 10:166–174.
178. Nassar GM, Fishbane S, Ayus JC. Occult infection of old nonfunctioning arteriovenous grafts: a novel cause of erythropoietin resistance and chronic inflammation in hemodialysis patients. Kidney Int 2002; 80(suppl):49–54.
179. Konner K. Increasing the proportion of diabetics with AV fistulas. Semin Dial 2001; 14:1–4.
180. Cynamon J, Pierpont CE. Thrombolysis for the treatment of thrombosed hemodialysis access grafts. Rev Cardiovasc Med 2002; 3(suppl 2):S84–S91.
181. Levin R, Hoenich NA. Running water: measuring water quality in a dialysis facility. Part 2. Nephrol News Issues 2003; 17:25–26, 78.
182. Levin R, Miller L. Running water: designing the dialysis clinic water room. Part 1. Nephrol News Issues 2003; 17:65, 68–70.
183. Oreopoulos DG. Beyond Kt/V: redefining adequacy of dialysis in the 21st century. Int Urol Nephrol 2002; 34:393–403.
184. I. NKF-K/DOQI Clinical Practice Guidelines for Hemodialysis Adequacy: update 2000. Am J Kidney Dis 2001; 37:S7–S64.
185. DOQI guidelines/fourth in a series. Adequacy HD dose, reuse, compliance. NKF-Dialysis Outcomes Quality Initiative. Nephrol News Issues 1997; 11:52–53.
186. NKF-DOQI clinical practice guidelines for hemodialysis adequacy. National Kidney Foundation. Am J Kidney Dis 1997; 30:S15–S66.
187. Gibney RT, Kimmel PL, Lazarus M. The Acute Dialysis Quality Initiative—part I: definitions and reporting of CRRT techniques. Adv Ren Replace Ther 2002; 9:252–254.
188. Ronco C, Bellomo R. Continuous renal replacement therapy: evolution in technology and current nomenclature. Kidney Int Suppl 1998; 66:S160–S164.
189. van Bommel EF. Should continuous renal replacement therapy be used for 'non-renal' indications in critically ill patients with shock? Resuscitation 1997; 33:257–270.
190. Kes P. Slow continuous renal replacement therapies: an update. Acta Med Croatica 2000; 54:69–84.
191. Locatelli F, Pontoriero G, Di Filippo S. Electrolyte disorders and substitution fluid in continuous renal replacement therapy. Kidney Int Suppl 1998; 66:S151–S155.
192. Davenport A, Mehta S. The Acute Dialysis Quality Initiative—part VI: access and anticoagulation in CRRT. Adv Ren Replace Ther 2002; 9:273–281.
193. Hidalgo N, Hynes-Gay P, Hill S, Burry L. Anticoagulation in continuous renal replacement therapy. Dynamics 2001; 12:13–17.
194. Bugge JF. Pharmacokinetics and drug dosing adjustments during continuous venovenous hemofiltration or hemodiafiltration in critically ill patients. Acta Anaesthesiol Scand 2001; 45:929–934.
195. Tenckhoff H, Schechter H. A bacteriologically safe peritoneal access device. Trans Am Soc Artif Intern Organs 1968; 14:181–187.
196. Moncrief JW, Popovich RP, Nolph KD. The history and current status of continuous ambulatory peritoneal dialysis. Am J Kidney Dis 1990; 16:579–584.
197. Divate SA. Acute renal allograft rejection: progress in understanding cellular and molecular mechanisms. J Postgrad Med 2000; 46:293–296.
198. Kamoun M. Cellular and molecular parameters in human renal allograft rejection. Clin Biochem 2001; 34:29–34.
199. Bunnapradist S, Jordan SC. The role of cytokines and cytokine gene polymorphism in T-cell activation and allograft rejection. Ann Acad Med Singapore 2000; 29:412–416.
200. Dai Z, Lakkis FG. The role of cytokines CTLA-4 and costimulation in transplant tolerance and rejection. Curr Opin Immunol 1999; 11:504–508.
201. Inston NG, Cockwell P. The evolving role of chemokines and their receptors in acute allograft rejection. Nephrol Dial Transplant 2002; 17:1374–1379.
202. Solez K, Racusen LC, Abdulkareem F, Kemeny E, von Willebrand E, Truong LD. Adhesion molecules and rejection of renal allografts. Kidney Int 1997; 51:1476–1480.
203. Shoskes DA, Halloran PF. Delayed graft function in renal transplantation: etiology, management and long-term significance. J Urol 1996; 155:1831–1840.
204. Bohmig GA, Exner M, Watschinger B, Regele H. Acute humoral renal allograft rejection. Curr Opin Urol 2002; 12:95–99.
205. Robertson H, Kirby JA. Post-transplant renal tubulitis: the recruitment, differentiation and persistence of intra-epithelial T cells. Am J Transplant 2003; 3:3–10.
206. Joosten SA, Van Kooten C, Paul LC. Pathogenesis of chronic allograft rejection. Transpl Int 2003; 16:137–145.
207. Knight RJ, Burrows L, Bodian C. The influence of acute rejection on long-term renal allograft survival: a comparison of living and cadaveric donor transplantation. Transplantation 2001; 72:69–76.
208. Soderberg-Naucler C, Emery VC. Viral infections and their impact on chronic renal allograft dysfunction. Transplantation 2001; 71:SS24–SS30.
209. Brunn GJ, Hudson CC, Sekulic A, et al. Phosphorylation of the translational repressor PHAS-I by the mammalian target of rapamycin. Science 1997; 277:99–101.
210. Pascual J, Orte J, Marcen R, Burgos J, Ortuno J. Use of leflunomide in human renal transplantation. Transplantation 2001; 72:1709.
211. Mele TS, Halloran PF. The use of mycophenolate mofetil in transplant recipients. Immunopharmacology 2000; 47:215–245.

38

Urinary Tract Obstruction

J. Robert Ramey and Deborah T. Glassman

INTRODUCTION

Urinary tract obstruction may result from numerous etiologies and at various levels within the urinary system. Sources may be congenital or acquired, benign or malignant. Moreover, patients' presenting symptoms will vary not only by the location of obstruction, but also with the time course over which the blockage has developed. This chapter systematically addresses the physiologic alterations to renal and bladder function that result from obstruction of normal urinary flow, the pathologic processes that may produce obstruction, and the varied options for restoring proper drainage of the urinary tract.

THE UPPER URINARY TRACT
Normal Physiology of the Renal Pelvis and Ureter

The upper urinary tract is a closed drainage system that functions to deliver urine from the kidney to the bladder. It begins at the level of the minor calyces. Each minor calyx receives urine from a single renal papilla and drains via an infundibulum into one of the major calyces (Fig. 1). These major calyces, usually numbering two to three, fuse to form the renal pelvis. The ureter and renal pelvis join at the ureteropelvic junction (UPJ), and the ureter then courses inferiorly through the retroperitoneum to empty into the bladder. These anatomic divisions do not exist on a functional basis; however, they do provide a useful framework for understanding upper tract obstruction (1) and planning correctional interventions.

The contractile force that propels each bolus of urine downstream to the bladder is provided by the smooth muscle cells enveloping the mucosa of the upper tract. The smooth muscle of the ureter is arranged into inner longitudinal and outer circumferential layers. Individual

cells are connected via intermediate junctions (2,3), producing a functional syncytium (4) that allows the conduction of electrical signals down the ureter. Specialized pacemaker cells are found at the pelvicalyceal junction (5). Action potentials generated by these cells are propagated downstream via diffusion. These waves of depolarization produce peristaltic contractions of the renal pelvis and ureter, which serve to propel urine into the bladder (4).

Unilateral vs. Bilateral Ureteral Obstruction

Complete unilateral ureteral obstruction (UUO) has been well studied in a variety of animal models and produces consistent alterations in renal hemodynamics and ureteral function (6–8). There is a triphasic response consisting of an acute increase in both renal blood flow (RBF) and ureteral pressure resulting from preglomerular vasodilation followed by a period of decreasing RBF, during which ureteral pressures remain elevated. Chronically, both ureteral pressure and RBF are maintained at below normal levels secondary to preglomerular vasoconstriction (6,9). These changes are mediated by intrarenally produced prostaglandins, with prostaglandin E (PGE_2) producing the initial vasodilation and thromboxane A_2 responsible for the subsequent vasoconstriction (10).

Bilateral ureteral occlusion (BUO) produces slightly different alterations in RBF as well as ureteral pressure. Initially, rapid increases in both RBF and ureteral pressure occur as with unilateral obstruction; however, unlike UUO, chronic BUO results in decreased RBF with persistently elevated ureteral pressures (10–12). These chronically elevated ureteral pressures are responsible for the reduction in glomerular filtration rate (GFR) during BUO rather than the preglomerular vasoconstriction seen in phase 3 of UUO (12).

These divergent responses to BUO and UUO are mediated by elevated levels of atrial natriuretic peptide (ANP) present during BUO, but not UUO (13–15). ANP is secreted in response to atrial stretch that occurs in volume-overloaded states (13). In an unobstructed system, ANP increases GFR by producing afferent arteriolar vasodilation along with efferent arteriolar constriction (16). During BUO, ANP counteracts the thromboxane A_2–mediated preglomerular vasoconstriction seen in phase 3 of UUO, while maintaining efferent arteriolar vasoconstriction, thereby producing the elevated ureteral pressures seen with BUO (10,11,13).

Chronic obstruction of one or both ureters results in hydroureteronephrosis proximal to the level of obstruction. The degree of dilation that develops varies depending on the duration and degree of obstruction, as well as the anatomy of the collecting system. The ureteral walls become unable to coapt due to the dilation, thus rendering peristaltic contractions ineffective. Subsequently, urine must drain from the obstructed system in a passive fashion via gravity or

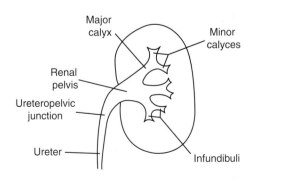

Figure 1 Anatomy of the renal collecting system.

pyelovenous backflow (17). Histologically, obstructive nephropathy results in obliterative interstitial fibrosis, with subsequent loss of functional cortex (18).

Presentation and Diagnosis of Upper Tract Obstruction

Signs and Symptoms of Ureteral Obstruction

The signs and symptoms of upper tract obstruction vary greatly with the time course over which the obstruction occurs. Acute obstruction produces flank pain on the affected side due to distension of the collecting system and renal capsule. The common innervation of the distal urinary tract and genitalia often results in radiation of the pain to the patient's ipsilateral testicle/labia. Similarly, obstruction in the proximal urinary tract can radiate to the shoulder or across the abdomen due to shared innervation with the gastrointestinal tract. Generally colicky in nature, the pain is often accompanied by nausea and vomiting. Patients are restless and on physical examination have extreme costovertebral angle tenderness on the affected side. If the urine becomes infected, fevers may develop along with bacteremia and even overt sepsis. Gross hematuria may accompany intrinsic obstructing lesions, such as calculi or transitional cell carcinomas. Complete BUO, or UUO of a solitary kidney, will produce anuria.

Chronic obstruction often develops asymptomatically. Some patients may have signs of uremia, or vague complaints of lethargy or abdominal discomfort. It may be discovered serendipitously as hydronephrosis seen on abdominal imaging performed for unrelated complaints, or during investigation of previously unrecognized renal failure. Patients may also present with complaints of recurrent urinary tract infections (UTI) or pyelonephritis.

Laboratory analysis should include serum chemistries, complete blood count, and urinalysis with culture. Blood urea nitrogen and creatinine allow monitoring of renal function, while leukocytosis may accompany systemic infection. Specific gravity on urinalysis reveals the kidneys' concentrating ability, while white blood cells and bacteria may indicate a UTI. Crystals may be present on microscopic examination of the urine from patients with renal calculi. Empiric antibiotics may be initiated; however, all infections should be confirmed with a culture.

Diagnostic Studies

Renal ultrasonography is often the initial study performed in the evaluation of renal failure. Due to the absence of ionizing radiation, ultrasound is also frequently used during pregnancy and with pediatric patients, as well as for patients with iodinated contrast allergies. It provides anatomic detail of the renal parenchyma and is fairly accurate in detecting the presence of hydronephrosis, especially in the setting of chronic obstruction. However, unless one of the above conditions exists, ultrasound is not the diagnostic study of choice in obstruction because its sensitivity as well as specificity is less than that of intravenous urography (IVU) (19). Duplex Doppler interrogation with calculation of resistive indices improves the ability of ultrasound to diagnose obstruction, yet this technique still falls short of IVU (20).

For years, IVU has been the "gold standard" for diagnosing ureteral obstruction, providing both anatomic and functional information. In the setting of acute obstruction, delayed uptake and excretion of contrast by the kidney, along with dilation of the collecting system, are seen. If present, extravasation of contrast indicates the presence of

forniceal rupture. IVU will often reveal cortical thinning, along with a dilated collecting system and tortuous ureter containing a standing column of contrast in chronically obstructed systems (17).

Unenhanced computed tomography (CT) scans provide the most sensitive study for the detection of calculi (21,22). Hydroureteronephrosis, perinephric stranding, and periureteral edema indicate the presence of ureteral obstruction (23). CT scans provide excellent anatomic detail of the entire abdomen, and IV contrast may be given following the acquisition of unenhanced images to perform a CT urogram, producing a functional study of the kidneys and making it an ideal study for potentially complex cases.

Nuclear medicine renal scans may also be employed in the evaluation of potentially obstructed urinary systems. Using radiolabeled tracers that are given intravenously and excreted by the kidney, the drainage of each system may be assessed by the half-life ($t_{1/2}$) for tracer transit from renal pelvis to bladder during diuresis. A prolonged $t_{1/2}$ (more than 20 minutes) is diagnostic of obstruction.

Prior to the development and refinement of noninvasive diuretic nuclear renography, the Whitaker test was routinely utilized to demonstrate obstruction. The study is performed by measuring the pressure within the renal pelvis during the infusion of a saline and contrast solution via a percutaneously placed cannula with a Foley catheter in place to drain the bladder. A pressure difference between renal pelvis and bladder greater than $22\,cmH_2O$ at a flow rate of $10\,cc/min$ is diagnostic of obstruction. The addition of contrast to the infusate allows fluoroscopic images to be obtained during the study revealing anatomic information regarding the level and degree of obstruction (17). The test remains useful in patients with poor renal function or marked hydronephrosis, because both of these hinder the interpretation of diuretic renograms (24).

Relieving Obstruction

Once a renal unit is determined to be obstructed, the physician must decide whether to temporarily drain the system or proceed directly with definitive repair. Indwelling ureteral stents or catheters may be placed endoscopically, while nephrostomy tubes can be inserted percutaneously for temporary relief of ureteral obstruction. Patients with signs of infection should undergo drainage and antibiotic therapy prior to proceeding with definitive repair. Ureteral stents function well in cases of intrinsic obstruction from such etiologies as calculi and strictures; however, in the face of extrinsic compression from retroperitoneal fibrosis (RPF) or malignant lesions, percutaneous nephrostomy tubes usually provide more reliable drainage (25).

Etiologies of Upper Urinary Tract Obstruction

Numerous processes may ultimately result in either UUO or BUO. Table 1 lists various sources of urinary tract obstruction, while Figure 2 depicts the locations of common lesions. Determining whether obstruction is due to extrinsic compression or internal blockage is vital in planning definitive correction. The following section addresses some of the more common sources of ureteral occlusion and the surgical options for management.

Extrinsic Compression

Retrocaval Ureter

During normal embryologic development, the infrarenal inferior vena cava (IVC) arises from the supracardinal vein.

Table 1 Common Causes of Urinary Obstruction

Intrinsic diseases of the urinary tract	Extrinsic obstruction of the ureter
Congenital disorders	Vascular lesions
Ureteropelvic junction lesions	Accessory vessels
Primary megaureter	Aortic, Iliac aneurysms
Ectopic ureter	Ovarian vein syndrome
Ectopic ureterocele	Circumcaval (retrocaval) ureter
Neuropathic bladder disease	Pelvic and retroperitoneal masses
Urethral valves	Pregnancy
Detrusor-sphincter dyssynergia	Enlarged uterus—benign, malignant
Ureteral dysplasia (prune-belly	disorders
syndrome)	Hydrometrocolpos
Metabolic and inflammatory	Ovarian lesions
disorders	Embryologic remnants (cysts of
Urinary calculi	Gartner's duct)
Blood clots	Pelvic and retroperitoneal tumors,
Fungus balls	primary and metastatic
Sloughed papillae (papillary	Pelvic lipomatosis
necrosis)	Lymphocele
Renal, ureteral, or vesical	Uterine prolapse
tuberculosis	Inflammatory diseases
Urethral strictures	Retroperitoneal fibrosis
Prostatic inflammatory diseases	Retroperitoneal abscess
Meatal stenosis	Retroperitoneal hemorrhage
Foreign body	Tubo-ovarian abscess; pelvic
Neoplastic disorders	inflammatory disease
Benign prostatic hyperplasia	Appendiceal or diverticular abscess
Renal pelvic and ureteral tumors	Endometriosis
Bladder tumors	Granulomatous (Crohn's) disease
Prostatic tumors	of the bowel
Urethral tumors	
Traumatic disorders	
Ureteral stricture (postsurgical)	
Urethral stricture	

When this segment forms from the subcardinal vein instead, a portion of the ureter comes to lie in a retrocaval position where the IVC exerts extrinsic compression producing partial obstruction. Contrast-enhanced CT scan is the study of choice for evaluation of this anomaly. Surgical correction involves transection of the ureter with reanastomosis anterior to the IVC, though cases with severe obstructive nephropathy and a nonfunctional kidney may require nephrectomy (26).

Arterial Aneurysm
Acquired aneurysmal lesions of the abdominal aorta and iliac arteries may also result in ureteral obstruction. Perianeurysmal fibrosis involving the ureter produces occlusion of the lumen (27). CT scan is a valuable tool to evaluate the ureter's anatomic relationship to vascular structures prior to surgery. If necessary, ureterolysis may be performed prior to aneurysm repair, or concomitantly (17).

Idiopathic Retroperitoneal Fibrosis
RPF is a benign inflammatory process that produces an intense fibrotic infiltrate that may encompass and compress one or both ureters, and the great vessels. Radiographic imaging will reveal a large retroperitoneal mass in addition to hydronephrosis. Excretory urography (IVU or CT urogram) often reveals medial deviation of the involved ureter(s) (28). Biopsy of the mass to rule out malignancy should be performed. This may be accomplished surgically via either an open or laparoscopic approach, or percutaneously under CT or ultrasound guidance (17). Once the diagnosis of RPF

has been established pathologically, definitive therapy may be initiated. Surgical ureterolysis provides the best long-term results for correction of ureteral obstruction (29). Successful medical management utilizing corticosteroids (30) and tamoxifen has been reported in patients who are poor surgical candidates (28,31–33). Long-term indwelling ureteral stents or nephrostomy tubes may be employed for relief of obstruction in patients unfit for surgery.

Malignancy
Various malignancies may produce ureteral obstruction via extrinsic compression from the primary tumor (carcinoma of the prostate, cervix, ovaries, or bladder) or retroperitoneal lymphadenopathy due to metastatic disease (leukemia, lymphoma, and testicular neoplasm). Regardless of tumor origin, malignant ureteral obstruction portends a poor prognosis because median survival is less than seven months (34). Percutaneous nephrostomy tube placement is often required for palliation of malignant obstruction, because more than half of patients with pelvic malignancies will fail internal drainage with ureteral stents (25).

Intrinsic Obstruction
UPJ Obstruction
Obstruction at the UPJ may present at any age, though it represents the most common cause of upper urinary tract obstruction in children (35). Patients frequently complain of flank pain that may be intermittent or chronic in nature. Additionally, there may be a history of UTI or stones. The etiology of UPJ obstruction (UPJO) remains an area of some dispute with both congenital and acquired conditions implicated (36).

IVU and diuretic renal scan are typically utilized in the diagnosis and treatment planning of UPJO (37). Surgical correction via open pyeloplasty has a 90% success rate, while antegrade endopyelotomy via percutaneous nephrostomy tract produces equivalent results initially (37). Advances in ureteroscopic and laparoscopic instrumentation and techniques have allowed these minimally invasive approaches to yield similar success without the morbidity of open incisions or nephrostomy tubes (36,38).

Ureteral Stricture
Ureteral strictures may develop in response to numerous insults including ischemia, instrumentation, radiation, and calculi. While a diuretic renogram confirms obstruction, it does not provide anatomic detail as to the length or level of the stricture. This information is easily obtained with either an IVU or retrograde pyelogram. Distal and mid-ureteral strictures may be managed endoscopically with balloon dilation or endoluminal incision. Mid-ureteral strictures occasionally require ureteroureterostomy, while distal lesions not amenable to minimally invasive techniques can be corrected via ureteroneocystotomy.

Calculi
When a given solute reaches supersaturation in the urine, it precipitates out of the solution, forming a calculus. Calcium stones are most common, but uric acid, struvite, and cystine stones are also seen in humans. A nonenhanced helical CT scan is the study of choice when considering the diagnosis of stone disease (21,22), because it provides details regarding the size, location, and number of stones, all vital information for planning intervention. Extracorporeal shock wave lithotripsy (ESWL) produces excellent results for renal stones less than 2.0 cm, and proximal ureteral stones less than

(A)

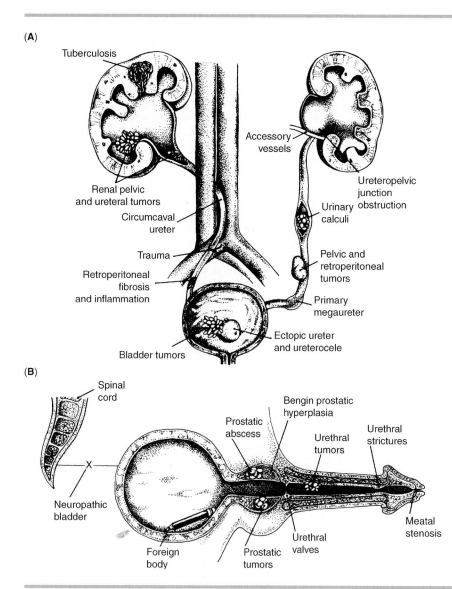

(B)

Figure 2 **(A)** Causes of upper urinary tract obstruction. **(B)** Causes of lower urinary tract obstruction. *Source*: Courtesy of J. N. Corriere Jr., from Chapter 43 in the Second Edition.

1.0 cm that do not pass spontaneously (39). Distal ureteral calculi, proximal calculi larger than 1.0 cm, and residual fragments from calculi previously treated with ESWL should be treated with ureteroscopic lithotripsy, because patients undergoing ESWL in these cases are more likely to require multiple procedures to be rendered stone free (39,40).

THE LOWER URINARY TRACT
Normal Anatomy of the Urinary Bladder and Urethra

The detrusor muscle of the bladder overlies a transitional cell mucosa. Its myofibrils are arranged into fasicles oriented in random directions, in contrast to the more organized smooth muscle of the ureter (41). At the lateral aspect of the bladder base, the ureters tunnel through the detrusor obliquely, producing functional antireflux valves. The ureteral orifices then open into the bladder at the posterolateral corners of the trigone.

Arising from the bladder neck, the urethra extends to the external meatus. In women, the urethra is relatively short and runs within the distal one-third of the anterior vaginal wall, while the male urethra covers a much longer

course and is comprised of four segments: prostatic, membranous, bulbous, and penile urethra. The smooth muscle of the urethra is arranged into a thick inner layer of longitudinal fibers and a sparse outer layer of circumferential muscle (42). The external sphincter also encircles the urethra; however, it comprises striated muscles and is thus under volitional control.

The Micturition Cycle

The intact bladder provides a highly compliant reservoir for urine storage during the filling phase of the micturition cycle. Emptying requires the coordination of detrusor contraction with relaxation of the internal and external sphincters. The pons, located within the brainstem, houses the micturition center responsible for organizing the normal voiding reflex. Spinal sympathetic and somatic reflex arcs are initially inhibited producing relaxation of the internal and external sphincters, respectively. Parasympathetic stimulation subsequently results in the coordinated contraction of the detrusor leading to complete emptying of the intact, unobstructed lower tract (43). Thus, pathologic processes that increase resistance to the outflow of urine or decrease bladder contractility may result in voiding dysfunction. The remainder of this chapter focuses on the diagnosis and treatment of common lesions that produce increased resistance to urine flow, and thus lower urinary tract obstruction.

Bladder Outlet Obstruction
Benign Prostatic Hyperplasia
As men age, the prostate gland undergoes hyperplasia, with the prevalence of benign prostatic hyperplasia (BPH) increasing from 0% in those below 30 years of age to 88% in men in their 80s (44). Common complaints include urinary frequency and urgency, hesitancy and intermittency of urinary stream, incomplete voiding, and nocturia. This symptom cluster is frequently referred to as the lower urinary tract syndrome, or LUTS. Traditionally, patients with enlarged prostates and significant LUTS have been treated with transurethral resection of the prostate (TURP). However, over the past decade, this "gold standard" has been challenged by the introduction of medical therapies and novel surgical procedures.

Medical therapies target alpha$_1$-adrenergic receptors in the smooth muscle of the prostate and bladder neck or the 5-alpha-reductase enzyme. Alpha-blockers relax the smooth muscle within the prostate, prostatic capsule as well as periurethral fibers, thereby decreasing outlet resistance. Meanwhile, 5-alpha-reductase inhibitors prevent the conversion of testosterone to dihydrotestosterone (DHT), the principal active androgen in the prostate. Reduced DHT levels result in decreased prostate volume with long-term therapy (45).

Various transurethral techniques have also been introduced to challenge TURP. All aim to produce equivalent reduction in LUTS, with decreases in TURP-associated morbidities (bleeding, infection, and hospitalization). Radio frequency [transurethral needle ablation (TUNA)], microwave energy [transurethral microwave thermal therapy (TUMT)], and various laser media have been utilized to destroy hyperplastic prostate tissue in a minimally invasive fashion (45,46). Smaller glands (prostate volume < 50–60 cc) may be treated effectively with transurethral incision (TUI), rather than formal resection (46). Prostate glands larger than 80 cc may best be treated with open simple prostatectomy.

Bladder Neck Contracture
Resection of the prostate via open or endoscopic techniques may result in scarring and contracture of the bladder neck, which subsequently produces bladder outlet obstruction (BOO). Bladder neck contracture (BNC) occurs in 0.48% to 32% of patients undergoing radical prostatectomy (47) versus 0.14% to 20% with TURP (48). Transurethral dilation and endoscopic incision of the contracture are equally effective treatment options (47).

Detrusor–External Sphincter Dyssynergia
During normal voiding, the pontine micturition center coordinates relaxation of the striated muscle of the external sphincter with contraction of the detrusor. Lesions between the pons and sacral spinal cord resulting from traumatic spinal cord injury, transverse myelitis, multiple sclerosis, etc. may interfere with this coordination (49). The uncoupling of detrusor contraction and external sphincter relaxation is termed dyssynergia and is commonly referred to as DESD.

DESD produces a functional obstruction that often results in elevated voiding pressures and decreased bladder compliance. Chronically, this may lead to vesicoureteral reflux and renal parenchymal deterioration, especially in patients with voiding pressures greater than 40 cmH$_2$O (50). Urodynamic evaluation consists of cystometrography and external sphincter electromyography (EMG). Uninhibited detrusor contractions with concomitant increased EMG activity in the external sphincter confirm the diagnosis. Treatment options include anticholinergics and self-catheterization, transurethral external sphincterotomy, and stenting of the external sphincter (49,51,52).

Urethral Obstruction
Posterior Urethral Valves
With an estimated incidence between 1:3000 and 1:8000, posterior urethral valves (PUV) are the most common congenital cause of lower urinary tract obstruction. Renal insufficiency and failure due to renal dysplasia are common, while pulmonary hypoplasia with respiratory failure may be seen in neonates with a history of oligohydramnios secondary to obstruction (53). Neonates classically presented with palpable abdominal masses from either a distended bladder or hydronephrotic kidneys, or in pulmonary distress secondary to hypoplasia of the lungs. Later in life, UTI or obstructive voiding symptoms are often the presenting complaint. Presently, most cases are discovered as bilateral hydronephrosis seen on prenatal ultrasonography (54). Voiding cystourethrogram (VCUG) is the diagnostic test of choice for PUV.

In addition to upper tract damage, PUV result in a hypertrophied, trabeculated, and noncompliant detrusor that may produce vesicoureteral obstruction as well (53). Thus, initial management should consist of temporary drainage with a Foley catheter, and patients who fail to reach a serum creatinine nadir of less than 2 mg/dL should be considered for upper tract diversion via nephrostomy tube or cutaneous ureterostomy (54). Primary transurethral endoscopic valve ablation is currently the treatment of choice, though patients with significant bilateral reflux may benefit from temporary cutaneous vesicostomy prior to valve ablation (55).

Urethral Stricture
Urethral strictures represent scar formation in response to injury of the urethral mucosa and corpus spongiosum (56). Prior to the advent of effective antibiotic therapy, the vast majority of stricture disease was secondary to gonococcal urethritis; however, presently, most strictures result from trauma due to straddle injury, or iatrogenic instrumentation (57–59). Patients present with obstructive voiding complaints such as straining to void, decreased stream, and terminal dribbling. Radiographic evaluation should include dynamic fluoroscopic retrograde urethrogram and VCUG. Some urologists advocate transperineal ultrasonography because they feel it provides further information regarding stricture length, location, and degree of fibrosis within the corpus spongiosum (59).

A myriad of treatment options exist for stricture disease including dilatation, endoscopic internal urethrotomy, and open urethroplasty. Ultimately, the procedure of choice is determined by the characteristics of the given stricture (i.e., length, location, and degree of fibrosis). Various models of rigid dilators exist; however, balloon-dilating catheters provide the least traumatic dilatation (57). Unfortunately, with strictures other than the most superficial, membrane-like lesions, dilation is rarely curative. In selected patients with short strictures (1.0–1.5 cm) of the bulbous urethra and relatively little spongiofibrosis, internal urethrotomy provides cure rates in excess of 90% (58). Bulbous urethral strictures of slightly longer length (< 2.0–3.0 cm) may be successfully managed via excision with a spatulated primary anastomosis (56). Longer strictures and those of the penile urethra require more complex open urethroplasty techniques, which employ various onlay grafts or tissue flaps to reconstruct the urethra (57,58).

Post-Obstructive Diuresis

Following the relief of bilateral upper tract obstruction or urinary retention due to lower tract obstruction, patients should be closely monitored for postobstructive diuresis (POD). The tubular dysfunction resulting from obstruction results in an inability to excrete acid and concentrate urine; thus prior to release of obstruction, patients typically present with a hyperchloremic, hyperkalemic metabolic acidosis (9). Signs of volume overload and severe renal impairment with encephalopathy should alert the clinician to the potential for significant POD (60). Retained sodium and urea may both provoke POD. Urea-provoked diuresis is usually self-limited, whereas salt-induced POD may perpetuate into a pathologic state with ensuing dehydration, hypotension, electrolyte disturbances, and death if not recognized and treated appropriately (61). ANP has also been implicated in POD because levels are elevated in patients with obstructive uropathy and return to normal following relief of obstruction with ensuing natriuresis and diuresis (13,62).

Recognition and management of POD requires that clinicians maintain a high index of suspicion. Based on clinical examination and serum studies, patients may be categorized as low, medium, or high risk for developing POD (61). The low- and medium-risk patients have minimal to no signs of volume overload, azotemia, or encephalopathy and may be managed with oral rehydration alone unless urine output exceeds 200 cc/hr or signs of hemodynamic instability or mental status changes develop. Patients with significant volume overload, mental confusion, or chronic BOO are at high risk for developing POD. Their urine output should be replaced 1/2 cc:cc with hypotonic saline solution containing 20 mEq KCl/L. If hyponatremia is present on initial serum chemistry, normal saline should be used for replacement of urine output (9,60). Serum electrolytes should be monitored closely and any derangements corrected appropriately. Excessive fluid replacement should be avoided because this may iatrogenically prolong diuresis following recovery of renal function.

SUMMARY

Urinary tract obstruction can occur at any age and in either sex, but is most commonly encountered in pediatric patients and those 60 years or older. Symptoms can be acute or chronic and have minimal or significant adverse effects on underlying renal function. The most serious complication of obstruction is renal failure with its attendant life-threatening effects. Fortunately, the refinement in current imaging techniques has enabled early diagnosis of this condition and exact determination of the site of obstruction so that optimal therapy can be rendered in a timely fashion. In the unfortunate subset of patients in whom significant renal dysfunction has occurred, relief of obstruction may still enable recovery of enough function so that dialysis is not needed. Even when intermittent dialysis becomes essential, current approaches to this treatment option will make possible longer life and better quality of living.

REFERENCES

1. Kabalin JN. Surgical anatomy of the retroperitoneum, kidneys, and ureters. In: Walsh PC, Retik AB, Vaughn ED, Wein AJ, eds. Campbell's Urology. 8th ed. Philadelphia: Saunders, 2002:3–40.
2. Uehara Y, Burnstock G. Demonstration of "gap junctions" between smooth muscle cells. J Cell Biol 1970; 44:215–217.
3. Libertino JA, Weiss RM. Ultrastructure of human ureter. J Urol 1972; 108:71–76.
4. Weiss RM. Physiology and pharmacology of the renal pelvis and ureter. In: Walsh PC, Retik AB, Vaughn ED, Wein AJ, eds. Campbell's Urology. Philadelphia: Saunders, 2002:377–409.
5. Dixon JS, Gosling JA. The fine structure of pacemaker cells in the pig renal calices. Anat Record 1973; 175:139–153.
6. Vaughn ED, Sorenson EJ, Gillenwater JY. The renal hemodynamic response to chronic unilateral complete ureteral occlusion. Investig Urol 1970; 8:78–90.
7. Moody TE, Vaughn ED, Gillenwater JY. Relationship between renal blood flow and ureteral pressure during 18 hours of total unilateral ureteral occlusion. Investig Urol 1975; 13:246–251.
8. Dal Canton A, Stanziale R, Corradi A, Andreucci VE, Migone L. Effects of acute ureteral obstruction on glomerular hemodynamics in rat kidney. Kidney Int 1977; 12:403–411.
9. Bruce RG, Waid TH, Lucas BA. Understanding postobstructive diuresis. Contemp Urol 1997; 9:53–66.
10. Wilson DR. Pathophysiology of obstructive nephropathy. Kidney Int 1980; 18:281–292.
11. Moody TE, Vaughn ED, Gillenwater JY. Comparison of the renal hemodynamic response to unilateral and bilateral ureteral occlusion. Investig Urol 1977; 14:455–459.
12. Dal Canton A, Corradi A, Stanziale R, Maruccio G, Migone L. Glomerular hemodynamics before and after release of 24-hour bilateral ureteral obstruction. Kidney Int 1980; 17:491–496.
13. Gulmi FA, Matthews GJ, Marion D, Von Lutterotti N, Vaughn ED. Volume expansion enhances the recovery of renal function and prolongs the diuresis and natriuresis after release of bilateral ureteral obstruction: a possible role for atrial natriuretic peptide. J Urol 1995; 153:1276–1283.
14. Purkeson ML, Blaine EH, Stokes TJ, Klahr S. Role of atrial peptide in the natriuresis that follows relief of obstruction in rat. Am J Physiol 1989; 256:F583–F589.
15. Fried TA, Lau AT, Ayon MA, Stein JH. Elevation of atrial natriuretic peptide (ANP) in ureteral obstruction in the rat. Clin Res 1986; 34:596A.
16. Cogan MG. Renal effects of atrial natriuretic factor. Annu Rev Physiol 1990; 52:699–708.
17. Gulmi FA, Felsen D, Vaughn ED. Pathophysiology of urinary tract obstruction. In: Walsh PC, Retik AB, Vaughn ED, Wein AJ, eds. Campbell's Urology. Philadelphia: Saunders, 2002:411–462.
18. Nagle RB, Bulger RE. Unilateral obstructive nephropathy in the rabbit. II. Late morphologic changes. Lab Investig 1978; 38:270–278.
19. Laing FC, Jeffrey RB, Wing VW. Ultrasound versus excretory urography in evaluating acute flank pain. Radiology 1985; 154:613–616.
20. Deyoe LA, Cronan JJ, Breslaw BH, Ridlen MS. New techniques of ultrasound and color Doppler in the prospective evaluation of acute renal obstruction. Do they replace the intravenous urogram? Abdominal Imaging 1995; 20:58–63.
21. Smith R, Rosenfield A, Choe K, et al. Acute flank pain: comparison of non-contrast-enhanced CT and intravenous urography. Radiology 1995; 194:789–794.
22. Yilmaz S, Sindel T, Arslan G, et al. Renal colic: comparison of spiral CT, US, and IVU in the detection of ureteral calculi. Eur Radiol 1998; 8:212–217.
23. Youssefzadeh M, Katz DS, Lummerman JH. Unenhanced helical CT in the evaluation of suspected renal colic. Am Urol Assoc Updates 1999; 28:203–207.
24. Whitaker RH, Buxton-Thomas MS. A comparison of pressure flow studies and renography in equivocal upper urinary tract obstruction. J Urol 1984; 131:446–449.

25. Feng MI, Bellman GC, Shapiro CE. Management of ureteral obstruction secondary to pelvic malignancies. J Endourol 1999; 13:521–524.

26. Rubinstein I, Cavalcanti AG, Canalini AF, Freitas MA, Accioly PM. Left retrocaval ureter associated with inferior vena caval duplication. J Urol 1999; 162:1373–1374.

27. Lindblad B, Almgren B, Bergqvist D, et al. Abdominal aortic aneurysm with perianeurysmal fibrosis: experience from 11 Swedish vascular centers. J Vasc Surg 1991; 13:231–239.

28. Bourouma R, Chevet D, Michel F, Cercueil JP, Arnould L, Rifle G. Treatment of idiopathic retroperitoneal fibrosis with tamoxifen. Nephrol Dial Transplant 1997; 12:2407–2410.

29. De Luca S, Terrone C, Manassero A, Rocca-Rossetti S. Aetiopathogenesis and treatment of idiopathic retroperitoneal fibrosis. Ann Urol 1998; 32:153–159.

30. Kadar AH, Kattan S, Lindstedt E, Hanash K. Steroid therapy for idiopathic retroperitoneal fibrosis: dose and duration. J Urol 2002; 168:550–555.

31. Frankhart L, Lorge F, Donckier J. Tamoxifen for retroperitoneal fibrosis. Postgrad Med J 1997; 73:653–654.

32. Owens LV, Cance WG, Huth JF. Retroperitoneal fibrosis treated with tamoxifen. Am Surgeon 1995; 61:842–844.

33. Clark CP, Vanderpool D, Preskitt JT. The response of retroperitoneal fibrosis to tamoxifen. Surgery 1991; 109:502–506.

34. Russo P. Urologic emergencies in the cancer patient. Semin Oncol 2000; 27:284–298.

35. Snyder HM, Lebowitz RL, Colodny AH, Bauer SB, Retik AB. Ureteropelvic junction obstruction in children. Urol Clin North Am 1980; 7:273–290.

36. Streem SB, Franke JJ, Smith JA. Management of upper urinary tract obstruction. In: Walsh PC, Retik AB, Vaughn ED, Wein AJ, eds. Campbell's Urology. 8th ed. Philadelphia: Saunders, 2002: 463–512.

37. Meretyk I, Meretyk S, Clayman RV. Endopyelotomy: comparison of ureteroscopic retrograde and antegrade percutaneous techniques. J Urol 1992; 148:775–783.

38. Soroush M, Bagley DH. Ureteroscopic retrograde endopyelotomy. Tech Urol 1998; 4:77–82.

39. Lam JS, Greene TD, Gupta M. Treatment of proximal ureteral calculi: holmium: YAG laser ureterolithotripsy versus extracorporeal shock wave lithotripsy. J Urol 2002; 167:1972–1976.

40. Pace KT, Weir MJ, Tariq N, Honey RJD. Low success rate of repeat shock wave lithotripsy for ureteral stones after failed initial treatment. J Urol 2000; 164:1905–1907.

41. Donker PJ, Droes JP, Van Alder BM. Anatomy of the musculature and innervation of the bladder and urethra. In: Chisolm GO, Williams DI, eds. Scientific Foundations of Urology. Chicago: Year Book Medical, 1982:404–441.

42. Chancellor MB, Yoshimura N. Physiology and pharmacology of the bladder and urethra. In: Walsh PC, Retik AB, Vaughn ED, Wein AJ, eds. Campbell's Urology. 8th ed. Philadelphia: Saunders, 2002:831–886.

43. Wein AJ. Pathophysiology and categorization of voiding dysfunction. In: Walsh PC, Retik AB, Vaughn ED, Wein AJ, eds. Campbell's Urology. 8th ed. Philadelphia: Saunders, 2002: 887–899.

44. Berry SJ, Coffey DS, Walsh PC, Ewing LL. The development of human benign prostatic hyperplasia with age. J Urol 1984; 132:474–479.

45. Holtgrewe HL. Current trends in management of men with lower urinary tract symptoms and benign prostatic hyperplasia. Urology 1998; 51(suppl 4A):1–7.

46. Jepsen JV, Bruskewitz RC. Recent developments in the surgical management of benign prostatic hyperplasia. Urology 1998; 51(suppl 4A):23–31.

47. Borboroglu PG, Sands JP, Roberts JL, Amling CL. Risk factors for vesicourethral anastomotic stricture after radical prostatectomy. Urology 2000; 56:96–100.

48. Kulb TB, Kamer M, Lingeman JE, Foster RS. Prevention of post-prostatectomy vesical neck contracture by prophylactic vesical neck incision. J Urol 1987; 137:230–231.

49. Kim YH, Kattan MW, Boone TB. Bladder leak point pressure: the measure for sphincterotomy success in spinal cord injured patients with external detrusor-sphincter dyssynergia. J Urol 1998; 159:493–497.

50. McGuire EJ, Woodside JR, Borden TA, Weiss RM. Prognostic value of urodynamic testing in myelodysplastic patients. J Urol 1981; 126:205–209.

51. Rivas DA, Chancellor MB, Bagley D. Prospective comparison of external sphincter prosthesis placement and external sphincterotomy in men with spinal cord injury. J Endourol 1994; 8:89–93.

52. Chancellor MB, Kaplan SA, Blaivas JG. Detrusor-external sphincter dyssynergia. Ciba Foundation Symp 1990; 151:195–206.

53. Yohannes P, Hanna M. Current trends in the management of posterior urethral valves in the pediatric population. Urology 2002; 60:947–953.

54. Gonzales ET Jr. Posterior urethral valves and other urethral anomalies. In: Walsh PC, Retik AB, Vaughn ED, Wein AJ, eds. Campbell's Urology. 8th ed. Philadelphia: Saunders, 2002:2207–2230.

55. Walker RD, Padron M. The management of posterior urethral valves by initial vesicostomy and delayed valve ablation. J Urol 1990; 144:1212–1214.

56. Jezior JR, Schlossberg SM. Excision and primary anastomosis for anterior urethral stricture. Urol Clin North Am 2002; 29:373–380.

57. Jordan GH, Schlossberg SM. Surgery of the penis and urethra. In: Walsh PC, Retik AB, Vaughn ED, Wein AJ, eds. Campbell's Urology. 8th ed. Philadelphia: Saunders, 2002:3886–3954.

58. Jezior J, Jordan GH. Management of the bulbous urethral stricture. AUA Update Ser 2002; 22(1):1–7.

59. Gallentine ML, Morey AF. Imaging of the male urethra for stricture disease. Urol Clin North Am 2002; 29:361–372.

60. Vaughan ED, Gillenwater JY. Diagnosis, characterization and management of post-obstructive diuresis. J Urol 1973; 109: 286–292.

61. Baum N, Anhalt M, Carlton CE, Scott R. Post-obstructive diuresis. J Urol 1975; 114:53–56.

62. Gulmi FA, Mooppan UMM, Chou SY, Kim H. Atrial natriuretic peptide in patients with obstructive uropathy. J Urol 1989; 142:268–272.

39

Neurogenic Lower Urinary Tract Dysfunction

Hari Siva Gurunadha Rao Tunuguntla and Unyime O. Nseyo

INTRODUCTION

The normal function of the urinary bladder is to store and expel urine in a coordinated, controlled fashion. This coordinated activity is regulated by the central and peripheral nervous systems. *Neurogenic bladder* is a term applied to a malfunctioning urinary bladder due to neurogenic dysfunction or insult emanating from internal or external trauma or disease. *Neurogenic lower urinary tract dysfunction* (NLUTD) is the new term currently applied to "neurogenic bladder dysfunction". NLUTD is a multi-facetted pathology and an important clinical as well as public health problem that is associated with complex management issues. Therefore, knowledge of the anatomy and pathophysiology of NLUTD remains the prerequisite for the safe and appropriate surgical–medical management of this disorder.

ANATOMY AND PHYSIOLOGY OF CONTINENCE AND MICTURITION

Anatomy and Physiology of the Bladder Outlet

Functionally, the lower urinary tract (LUT) (bladder and its outlet, the urethra) works in an integrated fashion for a normal voiding cycle to occur. The normal voiding cycle includes bladder filling and storage at a low pressure and without urinary incontinence. The subsequent voluntary and active voiding also occurs at a relatively low pressure. The bladder is one of the most compliant organs in the body, and allows normal filling to occur with only a gradual rise in intravesical pressure independent of large urine volumes. Increased tension in the external urethral sphincter, the so-called rhabdosphincter or striated sphincter (SS), occurs during the bladder filling and ensures continence even with increased intra-abdominal pressure. Urine storage ends when sensory tracts transmit to the central nervous system (CNS) the sensation of bladder fullness. Under appropriate sociocultural environment control, micturition occurs by coordinated neural activities leading to detrusor contraction, funneling of bladder neck, and relaxation of the bladder outlet. Cessation of neural activity leads to relaxation of the external SS during the micturition phase. As voiding ends, neural activities and tension return to the bladder outlet and relaxation of detrusor muscle occurs and a new urine storage cycle begins.

Embryologically, the bladder is derived from the urogenital sinus, the anterior portion of the cloacal membrane. The urogenital sinus is further divided into upper and lower segments at the level of the insertion of the fused distal portion of the mullerian ducts. In the male the ventral or pelvic segment forms the bladder and the prostatic urethra above the verumontanum, whereas in the female this portion forms the bladder and the entire urethra. Anatomically,

the bladder may be divided into the detrusor and trigone. However, neuropharmacologically the bladder may be conceived as comprising both a body and base, which differ substantially (1). The urinary bladder wall is organized into three layers: inner epithelial layer, or "mucosa" lined by specialized transitional epithelium called the urothelium, which is impervious to fluids and ions; smooth muscle layer (detrusor); and the outer serosal layer comprising of connective tissue. The urothelium characteristically unfolds and expands during bladder filling. The detrusor smooth muscle layer has a heterogeneous composition of smooth muscle cells, fibroblasts, elastin, collagens, and proteoglycans. The actual smooth muscle composition ranges from 50% to 60% and may diminish during bladder outlet obstruction (1). The bundles of the detrusor muscle merge into the trigone and bladder base. These bundles lack uniform orientation during the resting phase. However, reorientation occurs during stretch. Also, at rest and during passive bladder filling, these smooth muscle bundles occlude the bladder outlet. Realignment and coordinated relaxation of these smooth muscle bundles must occur to allow efficient opening of the bladder outlet and the low voiding pressure of less than 40 cm of H_2O.

The adult female urethra averages 5 cm in length and 6 mm in diameter. Its wall is composed of an outer muscular layer and an inner epithelial layer. The inner epithelial layer forms internal folds, which then form a mucosal *seal* and contribute to the continence mechanism. The outer longitudinal muscle extends the entire length of the inner epithelial layer. Most investigators have accepted the existence of an inner longitudinal smooth muscle layer. However, the notion by Tanagho of the outer longitudinal layer representing a direct continuation of the detrusor remains controversial (2–4). The middle third of the female urethra contains the intrinsic striated skeletal muscle, which loops around the urethral lumen, probably in an oblique fashion as in the male. Both the intrinsic and extrinsic components of the SS surround the inferior aspect of the female urethra. The distal end of the intrinsic rhabdosphincter aborts in the bulky skeletal muscle of the so-called "external urinary sphincter." Future research may offer succinct explanation for the presence of a very robust urethral muscle tone that contributes to urinary continence in the female.

Anatomically, the male urethra is divided into the anterior component, which contains a penile and bulbar urethra. The posterior urethra contains the membranous and the prostatic urethra, which measures 3 to 4 cm in length. Inner longitudinal and outer circular layers of smooth muscle comprise the wall of the male posterior and membranous urethra. These two layers of smooth muscle extend beyond the apex of the prostate to the bulbar urethra distally. Many investigators believe that the smooth muscles of the trigone extend into the urethra (Fig. 1). Consequently, these proponents

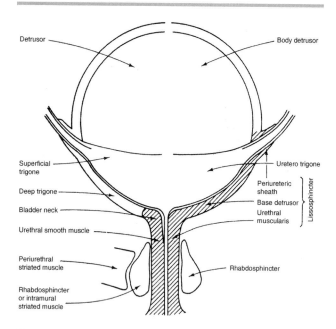

Figure 1 Anatomy of the bladder and its outlet as defined by Gosling and Dixon versus El badawi and co-workers. *Source*: From Ref. 5.

hypothesize that this anatomic arrangement facilitates funneling of the urethrovesical angle for efficient micturition. The contraview is that the trigone is physiologically and neuropharmacologically unique to allow functional funneling of the opening of the bladder neck during micturition.

The striated muscle component of the urethra has an intrinsic layer (the so-called "rhabdosphincter") within the urethra, and also tends to wrap around the lumen of the urethra in an obliquely spiral fashion. The rhabdosphincteric fibers interdigitate with fibers of the external component of the extrinsic skeletal muscle intimately to the levator ani muscle group and separate from the urethral wall (3).

Anatomically no "sphincter" is observable at the bladder neck, which remains rich with collagen and elastin that co-mingle with smooth muscle bundles. The patency and closing of the bladder neck at rest depends heavily on the passive forces of the components of the extracellular matrix (ECM) and active tone of the smooth muscle. The intrinsic tone in the bladder neck region and the proximal urethra leads to higher urethral pressure than intravesical pressure during bladder filling. The decrease in the internal urethral pressure occurs at the onset of micturition and leads to voiding at a low detrusor pressure. The competence of this "internal sphincteric mechanism" of the smooth muscle is very essential for continence. The external SS works in concert with the so-called internal sphincter of the bladder neck to ensure urinary continence. Unlike in the female urethra, both the intrinsic and extrinsic components of the SS surround the proximal male urethra. The involuntary contraction of the striated external sphincter during bladder contraction leads to striated detrusor–sphincter dyssynergia (DSD) (Fig. 2) common among patients with neurologic disease. This condition manifests also in the presence of a lesion between the brain and sacral cord. The only non-neurologic condition associated with DSD is the so-called Hinman Syndrome, common in children (6).

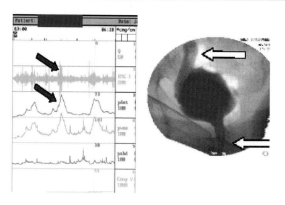

Figure 2 Detrusor–external sphincter dyssynergia. Note the increased activity of the external urethral sphincter on electromyogram during detrusor contraction; video showing detrusor contracting against contracting external urethral sphincter, the resulting high detrusor pressure leading to bilateral (right > left) vesicoureteral reflux.

Innervation of the Urinary Bladder

Voiding is an autonomic reflex and involuntary in the infant. However, normal neural maturation leads to somatic control of the LUT in due course. Central and peripheral nervous systems (Figs. 3 and 4) coordinate the complex interactions between the smooth muscle of the detrusor, bladder neck, and urethra during micturition. The contemporary literature supports the "urogenital short nervous system" (USNS), which contains postganglionic neurons that innervate the LUT (1). The USNS arises from the ganglia within or intimately proximal to the bladder wall. Classically, the sympathetic autonomic system leaves the preganglionic neurons of the thoraco-lumbar spinal segment to reach the first synapse in the following ganglia: (i) adjacent to the vertebral bodies (paraganglia), (ii) between the vertebral bodies and the organ (preganglia), and (iii) within the end organ (peripheral ganglia) (1). There is some evidence that urogenital neuronal fibers may connect the muscle with efferent neurons via the peripheral ganglion, which allows function that is

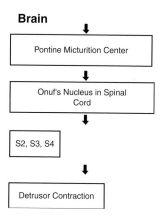

Figure 3 Micturition pathway.

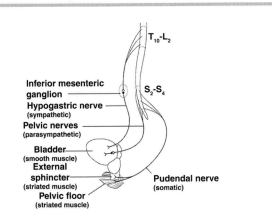

Figure 4 Innervation of the lower urinary tract.

independent of the spinal cord. Also the sympathetic system may affect the parasympathetic ganglia via alpha-receptors, which modulate motor activity to the bladder.

In addition to the traditional autonomic neurotransmitters of acetylcholine and norepinephrine, the noncholinergic and nonadrenergic neurotransmitters include adenosine triphosphate, serotonin, histamine, prostaglandins, peptides, and nitric oxide (1). These transmitters most certainly play a critical role in autonomic neurotransmission most likely through the principle of "cotransmission," with one molecule/peptide altering the postjunctional cell for the primary neurotransmitter (1). The postsynaptic cell membrane of the smooth muscle contains receptors that recognize the neurotransmitter. The resulting specific binding generates the process of excitation–contraction in the effector cell, accompanied by a rise in the free cytosolic calcium concentration. The cholinergic receptor membrane proteins that bind acetylcholine predominate in neurons of somatic fibers, all preganglionic autonomic fibers, and all postganglionic parasympathetic fibers. The cholinergic receptors are divided into nicotinic (nicotine, a mimicry of acetylcholine) and muscarinic (alkaloid muscarinic inhibitor of acetylcholine). The nicotinic receptors abound in skeletal muscle motor end plates and autonomic ganglia. They may also have control over bladder function. The muscarinic receptors are widely distributed in all autonomic effector cells in sweat glands, large and small bowel, gall bladder, and urinary bladder. Molecular biochemists have defined five subtypes of the muscarinic receptors based on the type of protein, "M," and mRNA's (1). Structural differences are difficult to delineate; however, their functions are distinct. The urinary bladder contains only 20% of the muscarinic receptor density. The muscarinic receptor subtype, M2, predominates in the urinary bladder. Nevertheless, activation of M3 subtypes initiate bladder contraction, and activation of M2 subtype inhibits adrenergic pathway, which leads to force generation (1,7). The conditions that affect the density of the muscarinic cholinergic receptors of the bladder include pregnancy (downregulation), estrogen (upregulation), spinal cord injury, acute urinary tract obstruction, and diabetes.

The adrenergic receptors bind to the catecholamines (e.g., norepinephrine) and predominate in most postganglionic sympathetic fibers. Classification of the adrenergic receptors is based on physiologic functions referred to as alpha or beta. The alpha-receptors mediate nasal congestion and smooth muscle contraction. Stimulation of beta-adrenergic receptors leads to increased myocardial contractility and smooth muscle relaxation. The alpha-receptors have well-characterized subtypes, alpha-1 (postsynaptic) and alpha-2 (pre- and postsynaptic). Adrenergic sites in the bladder are predominantly beta-subtypes (1,7,8). They also are localized in the trigone, with sparse distribution in the bladder body. Adrenergic innervation predominates in the smooth muscle of the bladder neck and the proximal urethra. The beta-adrenergic receptors exist in several major forms: beta-1, -2, and -3. Affinity of beta-1 receptors remains high for norepinephrine, whereas epinephrine has a greater affinity for beta-2 receptors. Beta-2 receptors predominate in the presynaptic and postsynaptic membranes and in the urinary bladder. Stimulation of beta-2 receptors results in relaxation of the smooth muscle in the urinary bladder.

The SS is innervated by the pudendal nerves, which originate from the S2 to S4 spinal cord segments. Somatic control of the SS is responsible for the physiologic increase in activity during bladder filling and abortion of this activity at the initiation of and throughout micturition. Supratrigonal mechanoreceptors control somatic activity of the SS, which explains the failure of the external sphincter in paraplegic patients. The cholinergic receptors for smooth muscle are muscarinic whereas those associated with SS contraction are nicotinic. Anticholinergic agents such as oxybutynin act at muscarinic sites, and therefore, have no effect on SS. The muscarinic receptors of SS can be blocked by endoscopic injection of botulinum toxin to treat refractory voiding dysfunction or as an alternative to sphincterotomy.

Less is known about the sensory innervation of the LUT. Afferent nerve fibers have been demonstrated in the pelvic, pudendal, and hypogastric nerves. Sensation of distention originates in the bladder wall and travels in the pelvic nerves. Mechanoreceptors are present in the hypogastric nerves. These nerves carry afferent nociceptive stimuli. The afferent neurons from the sphincter (SS) and urethra carry sensations of pain, temperature, and urinary distention.

Denervation leads to increased sensitivity of smooth muscle to neuro-humoral stimuli. This supersensitivity is often associated with injury involving the postganglionic fibers. Injury involving the preganglionic nerve fibers leads to decentralization. Neuronal injuries during radical hysterectomy or abdominal perineal resection constitute examples of decentralization injuries. In summary, the adrenergic efferent neurons modulate the bladder storage function as follows: (i) stimulation of alpha-receptors of the bladder base and urethra increase bladder outlet resistance and facilitate urinary storage, (ii) stimulation of beta receptors in the bladder body engenders increase in bladder compliance and facilitates storage, and (iii) adrenergic fibers and involved alpha-receptors suppress parasympathetic transmission in the pelvic ganglia and inhibit bladder contractions.

The classic concept of deGroat maintains that the role of the adrenergic system favors urinary storage at low pressures (9). McGuire (10) and El Badawi (4) endorse the concept, and emphasize that the storage phase of micturition is controlled principally by the sympathetic system and the voiding phase by parasympathetic vesicourethral innervation. The challenge to deGroat's classic concept centers on the observations that patients on alpha-blockers for hypertension do not loose bladder capacity; and retroperitoneal lymphadenectomy for testicular cancer in normal individuals does not result in urinary incontinence/voiding dysfunction (2).

CNS Control of Urinary Storage and Micturition

Normal voiding essentially is a spinal reflex that is modulated by the CNS (brain and spinal cord) (Fig. 3), which coordinates the functions of the bladder and urethra. The bladder and urethra are innervated by three sets of peripheral nerves arising from the autonomic nervous system (ANS), the somatic nervous system, and the CNS, which comprises the brain, brain stem, and the spinal cord (Figs. 5 and 6).

Brain

The brain is the master control of the entire urinary system. The micturition control center is located in the frontal lobe of the brain. The primary activity of this area is to send inhibitory signals tonically to the detrusor muscle to prevent the bladder from emptying (contracting) until a socially acceptable time and place to urinate are available. The signal transmitted by the brain is routed through two intermediate centers (the brainstem and the sacral spinal cord) prior to reaching the bladder. Certain cerebral lesions or diseases, such as stroke, cancer, and dementia, often derange the control of the normal micturition reflex.

Brainstem

The brainstem is located at the base of the skull. Within the brainstem is a specialized area known as the pons, a major relay center between the brain and the bladder. The pons is responsible for coordinating the activities of the urinary

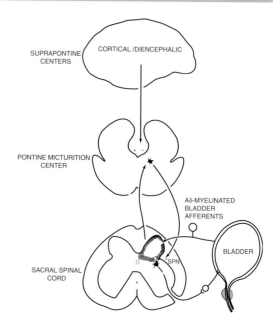

Figure 6 Schematic of supraspinal micturition reflex pathway. Bladder distention activates unmyelinated Aδ fiber afferents. Ascending input is relayed to a region of the pons termed the pontine micturition center. Depending on cortical input, excitatory descending input activates neurons in the sacral parasympathetic nucleus, which cause bladder contraction. Evidence for a spinobulbospinal pathway exists in the cast (de Groat and Ryall, 1969) and rat (Mallory et al, 1989).

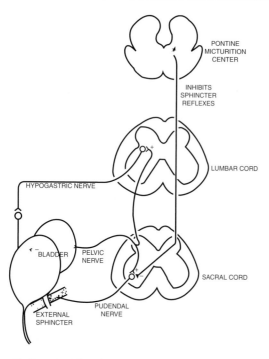

Figure 5 Representation of sphincter reflexes. Distention of bladder during filling produces low-level afferent firing, which triggers (1) hypogastric outflow to the bladder, and (2) pudendal outflow to the external urethral sphincter. Hypogastric pathways may promote urine storage by mediating relaxation (−) of the bladder body via beta-adrenegic receptors and contraction (+) of the bladder base and urethra via alpha adrenoceptors. Hypogastric input may also inhibit ganglionic transmission in some species. During voiding, inhibition of hypogastric and pudendal pathways promotes complete bladder emptying. *Source*: From Ref. 11.

sphincters and the bladder so that they work in synergy. The mechanical process of urination is coordinated by the pons in the area known as the pontine micturition center (PMC). The PMC coordinates the urethral sphincter relaxation and detrusor contraction to facilitate urination.

The conscious sensations associated with bladder activity are transmitted to the pons from the cerebral cortex. The PMC controls a variety of excitatory and inhibitory neuronal systems and functions as a relay switch in the voiding pathway. Stimulation of the PMC causes the urethral sphincters to open, while facilitating the detrusor to contract and expel the urine. When the bladder becomes full, the stretch receptors of the detrusor muscle send a signal to the pons, which in turn notifies the brain. Patients perceive this signal (bladder fullness) as a sudden desire to go to the bathroom. Under normal situations, the brain sends an inhibitory signal to the pons to inhibit the bladder from contracting until a bathroom is found. Deactivation of the PMC leads to disappearance of the urge to urinate, allowing the patient to delay urination until locating a suitable bathroom. Within the appropriate environment, the brain sends excitatory signals to the pons, allowing the urinary sphincters to open and the detrusor to contract for bladder emptying.

Spinal Cord

The spinal cord extends from the brainstem down to the lumbosacral spine. It is located in the spinal canal and is protected by the cerebrospinal fluid, meninges, and the vertebral column. It is approximately 14-inches long in an adult. Along its course, the spinal cord sprouts off many nerve branches to different parts of the body. The spinal cord functions as a long communication pathway between the brainstem and the sacral spinal cord (Figs. 5 and 6). When the sacral cord receives the sensory information from the bladder, this signal travels up the spinal cord to the pons and then ultimately to the brain. The brain interprets this signal and sends a reply via the pons that travels down the spinal cord via the sacral cord to the bladder.

In the normal cycle of bladder filling and emptying, the spinal cord acts as an important intermediary between the pons and the sacral cord. An intact spinal cord is critical for normal micturition. If the spinal cord is severely injured or severed, the affected individual will exhibit constant urinary leakage because of uncontrollable detrusor contracture with bladder spasms, a condition called detrusor hyper-reflexia (Table 1).

In a condition of complete spinal cord transection, the patient will demonstrate symptoms of urinary frequency, urgency, and urge incontinence, but will be unable to empty his or her bladder completely. This occurs because the urinary bladder and the external urethral SS are both overactive, a condition termed DSD with detrusor hyper-reflexia (DSD–DH) (Fig. 2; Table 1).

The sacral spinal cord is the terminal portion of the spinal cord situated at the lower back in the lumbar area. This is a specialized area of the spinal cord known as the sacral reflex center, which is responsible for bladder contractions. The sacral reflex center (Fig. 3) is the primitive voiding center and the only functional "micturition center" in the infant.

In infants, the higher center of voiding control (the brain) is not mature enough to command the bladder, which is why control of urination in infants and young children comes from signals sent from the sacral cord. The full infant bladder triggers an excitatory signal that goes to the sacral cord. The sacral cord responds by signaling the spinal reflex center to automatically trigger detrusor contraction, which results in involuntary coordinated voiding.

A continuous cycle of bladder filling and emptying occurs, which is why infants and young children are dependent on diapers until they are toilet trained. As the child's brain matures and develops, it gradually dominates the control of the bladder and the urinary sphincters to inhibit involuntary voiding until complete control is attained. Voluntary continence usually is attained by age three to four years. By this time, control of the voiding process has been relinquished by the sacral reflex center of the sacral cord to the higher center in the brain. If the sacral cord becomes severely injured (e.g., spinal tumor and herniated disc), the bladder may not function. Affected patients may develop urinary retention, termed "detrusor areflexia"

Table 1 Neurogenic Bladder Dysfunction According to the Neurologic Abnormality

Level of the lesion	Type of neurogenic bladder dysfunction
Brain	Detrusor hyper-reflexia[a]
Pontine micturition center; S2; lumbar, thoracic, cervical spinal cord lesions	Detrusor hyper-reflexia[a]/detrusor sphincter dyssynergia
Pontine micturition center	Detrusor hyper-reflexia[a]/detrusor sphincter dyssynergia
S3,4 spinal cord lesions	Detrusor hyporeflexia (hypocontractile detrusor)
S2,3,4 peripheral nerves	Detrusor hyporeflexia (hypocontractile detrusor)

[a]Neurogenic detrusor overactivity, according to the current International Continence Society (ICS) nomenclature.

(Table 1). The detrusor lacks the ability to contract, resulting in inability to urinate and urinary retention.

Peripheral Nerves

Peripheral nerves form an intricate network of pathways for sending and receiving information throughout the body. The nerves originate from the main trunk of the spinal cord and branch out in different directions to cover the entire body. Nerves convert the internal and external environmental stimuli to electrical signals so that the human body can understand stimuli as one of the ordinary senses (i.e., hearing, sight, smell, touch, taste, and equilibrium). The bladder and the urethral sphincters are under the influence of their corresponding nerves. The ANS lies outside of the CNS, and regulates the actions of the internal organs (e.g., intestines, heart, and bladder) under involuntary control. The ANS is divided into the sympathetic and the parasympathetic nervous system. Under appropriate conditions, the bladder and the internal urethral sphincter (bladder outlet) primarily are under sympathetic nervous system control (7,8). When the sympathetic nervous system is active, it causes the bladder to increase its capacity without increasing detrusor resting pressure (accommodation) and stimulates the internal urinary sphincter/bladder neck to remain tightly closed. The sympathetic activity also inhibits parasympathetic stimulation, that is, detrusor contraction.

The parasympathetic nervous system functions in a manner opposite to that of the sympathetic nervous system. In terms of urinary function, the parasympathetic nerves stimulate the muscarinic (M) receptors that mediate detrusor contraction, leading to bladder emptying (1,7). Immediately preceding parasympathetic stimulation, the sympathetic influence, that is, the activity of the adrenergic receptors on the internal urethral sphincter, becomes suppressed so that the internal sphincter relaxes and opens. In addition, the activity of the pudendal nerve is inhibited to cause the external urethral SS to open, resulting in the facilitation of voluntary urination.

Like the ANS, the somatic nervous system is a part of the nervous system that lies outside of the central spinal cord. The somatic nervous system regulates the actions of the muscles under voluntary control. Examples of these muscles are the external urethral SS and the pelvic diaphragm. The pudendal nerve originates from the nucleus of Onuf and regulates the voluntary actions of the external urinary sphincter and the pelvic diaphragm. Activation of the pudendal nerve causes contraction of the external sphincter and the pelvic floor muscles, which occurs with activities such as Kegel exercises. Difficult or prolonged vaginal delivery may cause temporary neuropraxia of the pudendal nerve and stress urinary incontinence. Conversely, suprasacral-infrapontine spinal cord trauma can cause overstimulation of the pudendal nerve that results in urinary retention.

Physiology of LUT

Normal bladder function consists of two phases—filling and emptying. The normal micturition cycle requires that the urinary bladder and the urethral sphincter work together as a coordinated unit to store and empty urine. During urinary storage, the bladder acts as a low-pressure receptacle, while the urinary sphincter maintains high resistance to urinary flow to keep the bladder outlet closed. During urine elimination, the bladder contracts to expel urine while the urinary sphincter opens (low resistance) to allow unobstructed urinary flow and bladder emptying.

Filling Phase

During the filling phase, the bladder accumulates increasing volumes of urine while the pressure inside the bladder remains low. As the bladder initially fills, a small rise in intravesical pressure, which is never greater than 10 cm of H_2O, occurs (Fig. 7) (12). The filling of the urinary bladder depends on the inherent viscoelastic properties of the bladder and the inhibition of the parasympathetic nerves. Thus, bladder filling primarily is a passive event. However, the sympathetic nerves also facilitate urine storage by (i) inhibiting the parasympathetic nerves from triggering bladder contractions, (ii) directly causing relaxation and expansion of the detrusor muscle, and (iii) causing the closure of the bladder neck by constricting the inner urethral SS. This sympathetic input to the LUT remains very active during bladder filling.

As the bladder fills, the pudendal nerve becomes excited. Stimulation of the pudendal nerve results in contraction of the external urethral SS. Contraction of the external sphincter, coupled with that of the internal smooth muscle sphincter, maintains the urethral pressure (resistance) higher than normal bladder pressure. The combination of both urinary sphincters constitutes the purported continence mechanism. The pressure gradients within the bladder and urethra play an important functional role in normal micturition and continence. As long as the urethral pressure is higher than the bladder pressure, urinary continence is ensured. However, abnormally low urethral pressures or abnormally high intravesical pressures result in urinary incontinence.

Physical activities, coughing, sneezing, or laughing often result in the sharp rise of pressure within the abdomen, which is transmitted to both the bladder and urethra. As long as the pressure is evenly transmitted to the bladder and urethra, urine will not leak. However, when the pressure transmitted to the bladder is greater than that transmitted to the urethra, stress urinary incontinence results.

Emptying Phase

The storage phase of the urinary bladder can be switched to the voiding phase either involuntarily (reflexly) or voluntarily. Involuntary reflex voiding occurs in an infant when the volume of urine exceeds the voiding threshold. When the bladder is filled to capacity, the stretch receptors within the bladder wall signal the sacral cord. The sacral cord, in turn, sends a message back to the bladder indicating that it is time to empty the bladder. Concurrently, the pudendal nerve causes relaxation of the levator ani so that the pelvic floor muscles relax. The pudendal nerve also signals the external sphincter to open. The sympathetic nerves send a message to the internal sphincter to relax and open, resulting in a lower urethral resistance. As the urethral sphincters relax and open, the parasympathetic nerves trigger contraction of the detrusor. The bladder contracts and the detrusor pressure overcomes the urethral pressure, resulting in urinary flow. These coordinated series of events allow automatic and unimpeded emptying of the bladder. A repetitious cycle of bladder filling and emptying occurs in newborn infants. The bladder empties as soon as it fills because the brain of an infant has not matured enough to regulate the urinary system. Because urination is unregulated by the infant's brain, predicting when the infant will urinate is difficult.

As the infant brain develops, the PMC also matures and gradually assumes voiding control. During childhood (usually at the age of three to four), this primitive voiding reflex becomes suppressed and the brain dominates the control of bladder function, which is why toilet training usually is successful at ages three to four. However, this primitive voiding reflex may reappear in people with spinal cord injuries.

PATHOPHYSIOLOGY OF LUT DYSFUNCTION

The bladder appears to be the only human visceral organ that requires an intact central neural system for function and survival of the individual. Any abnormality within the nervous system affects the entire voiding cycle, and any part of the nervous system may be affected, including the brain, pons, spinal cord, sacral cord, and peripheral nerves. Consequently, voiding dysfunction occurs with different symptoms, which range from acute urinary retention to an overactive bladder, or a combination of both.

Urinary incontinence results from a dysfunction of the bladder, the sphincter, or both. Bladder hyperactivity (spastic bladder) is associated with the symptoms of urge incontinence, whereas urethral sphincteric hypoactivity (decreased resistance) results in symptomatic stress incontinence. A combination of detrusor hyperactivity and sphincteric deficiency (hypoactivity) may result in mixed symptoms of urge and stress incontinence in the same individual.

Brain Lesions

Lesions of the brain above the pons may destroy or impair the primary cortical micturition center, resulting in the complete or variable loss of voiding control. However, the voiding reflexes of the LUT—the primitive voiding reflexes—remain intact. Affected individuals show signs of urge incontinence, or spastic bladder (detrusor hyper-reflexia) (Table 1). The bladder empties too quickly and too often, with relatively low volumes. Consequently, the storage function of the bladder is deranged, marked clinically by day- and night-time (nocturia) urinary frequency, urgency, and urge incontinence. Typical brain lesions include stroke, brain tumor, Parkinson's disease, hydrocephalus, cerebral palsy, and Shy–Drager syndrome. The latter disorder is a rare condition associated with open bladder neck, and is discussed later in this chapter.

Lesions of the Spinal Cord

Diseases or injuries of the spinal cord between the pons and the sacral spinal cord also result in spastic bladder or

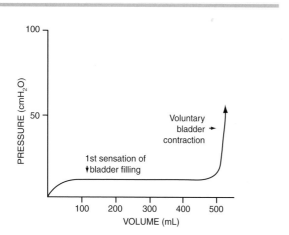

Figure 7 Normal cystometrogram.

overactive bladder (neurogenic detrusor overactivity) (Table 1). People who are paraplegic or quadriplegic have lower extremity spasticity. Acute spinal cord trauma results in the acute spinal shock syndrome; the patient enters a spinal shock phase which the nervous system shuts down the vesical–neural axis. After 6 to 12 weeks, the nervous system gradually reactivates. This reactivation results in heightened stimulation of the affected organs. For example, the legs become spastic. The bladder suffers a voiding disorder, primarily urinary frequency and urge incontinence, which is similar to that of the brain lesion except that the external SS may have paradoxical contractions as well. If both the bladder and external sphincter become spastic at the same time, the affected individual will sense an overwhelming desire to urinate but only a small amount of urine may dribble out. This is DSD because the bladder and the external SS function in discordance. Spinal cord injury may result from a motor vehicle accident, diving accidents, and gun-shot wounds. Multiple sclerosis (MS) is a common systemic cause of spinal cord disease in young women. Children born with myelomeningocele may have spastic bladders and/or an open urethra. Conversely, some children with myelomeningocele may have hypotonic instead of a spastic bladder.

Sacral Cord Injury

Selected injuries of the sacral cord and the corresponding nerve roots arising from the sacral cord may prevent the bladder from emptying. A sensory neurogenic bladder presents with a loss of sense of bladder fullness. In the case of a motor neurogenic bladder, the patient retains the sense of bladder fullness; however, the detrusor may not contract, a condition known as detrusor areflexia (acontractile detrusor). Consequently, there is the failure to empty with associated overflow urinary incontinence and bladder decompensation. Typical causes include sacral cord tumor, herniated disc, crush pelvic injuries, lumbar laminectomy, radical hysterectomy, and abdominoperineal resection. Tethered cord syndrome must be ruled out in a teenager with sudden onset of voiding dysfunction. The spinal cord injury in this syndrome is marked by the tip of the sacral cord being stuck near the sacrum and hence being unable to stretch as the child grows taller. Ischemic changes of the sacral cord associated with the tethering cause the manifestation symptoms of dysfunctional voiding.

Peripheral Nerve Injury

Diabetes mellitus and AIDS cause peripheral neuropathy that results in dysfunctional voiding (Table 1). These diseases destroy the nerves to the bladder, resulting in a silent, painless distention of the urinary bladder. Patients with chronic diabetes first lose the sensation of bladder filling and fullness, prior to bladder decompensation. Similar to the case of injury to the sacral cord, affected individuals will have difficulty urinating, with the attendant problems of overflow incontinence and bladder decompensation. Other diseases manifesting this condition are poliomyelitis, Guillain–Barre syndrome, genitoanal herpes, pernicious anemia, and neurosyphilis (tabes dorsalis).

DEFINITION OF COMMON TERMS IN NEUROGENIC VOIDING DYSFUNCTION

Neurogenic bladder is a malfunctioning bladder due to any type of neurologic disorder.

Detrusor overactivity refers to overactive bladder symptoms due to a neurologic (suprapontine upper motor neuron neurologic)/non-neurologic disorder. In neurologic detrusor overactivity, the external sphincter functions normally. There is functional synergy between the bladder and the external urethral SS. However, the patient often presents with frequency, urgency, and urge incontinence.

DSD–DH refers to overactive bladder symptoms due to neurologic upper motor neuron disorder of the suprasacral spinal cord. Paradoxically, the patient is in urinary retention. Both the detrusor and the SS are contracting at the same time, that is, synchronous activation of both parasympathetic and pudendal nerves, which act in dyssynergia (lack of coordination).

Detrusor overactivity with impaired contractility refers to overactive bladder symptoms, but the detrusor cannot generate enough pressure to allow complete emptying. The external sphincter is in synergy with detrusor contraction. The detrusor is too weak to mount an adequate contraction for proper voiding to occur. The condition is similar to urinary retention, but irritating voiding symptoms are prevalent.

Acontractile/hypocontractile detrusor is a complete inability of the detrusor to empty due to a lower motor neuron lesion (e.g., sacral cord and peripheral nerves).

Urinary retention is the inability of the urinary bladder to empty, and the problem of failure to empty may have neurologic or non-neurologic etiology.

SPECIFIC NEUROLOGIC LESIONS

Supraspinal lesions

Supraspinal lesions refer to those lesions of the CNS above the pons, which include cerebrovascular accidents, brain tumors, Parkinson's disease, and Shy–Drager syndrome (13).

Cerebrovascular Accidents

After a stroke, the brain may enter into a temporary acute cerebral shock phase. During this time, the urinary bladder will be in retention due to detrusor areflexia. About 25% of stroke victims develop acute urinary retention. Following the cerebral shock phase, the bladder demonstrates detrusor overactivity with coordinated urethral sphincter activity, because the PMC is released from the cerebral inhibitory center. The symptoms of detrusor overactivity/hyperactivity/ hyper-reflexia often include urinary frequency, urgency, and urge incontinence. The treatment for the cerebral shock phase is indwelling Foley catheter or clean intermittent catheterization (CIC). The resultant hyper-reflexic bladder is often managed with anticholinergic medications to facilitate bladder filling and storage. Detrusor hyper-reflexia (Fig. 8) with coordinated urethral SS is the most commonly observed urodynamic pattern associated with a brain tumor (Fig. 8). Any associated hyper-reflexia is managed similarly with anticholinergic medications.

Parkinson's Disease

This is a degenerative disorder of pigmented neurons of the substantia nigra of the cerebrum, associated with dopamine deficiency and increased cholinergic activity in the corpus striatum. Patients with Parkinson disease manifest symptoms of bradykinesia, skeletal muscle tremor, cogwheel rigidity, and masked facies. Symptoms specific to the urinary bladder include urinary frequency, urgency, nocturia, and urge incontinence. Typical urodynamic findings are

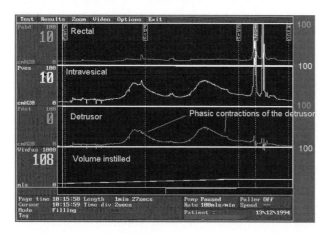

Figure 8   Detrusor overactivity/hyper-reflexia. Note the phasic detrusor over-activity reflected in the detrusor pressure curve (P_{det}); this may or may not be associated with urinary leak (incontinence). Detrusor overactivity is of two types: neurogenic (spinal cord injury) and non-neurogenic. Terminal detrusor overactivity with leak is characterized by end-filling detrusor overactivity.

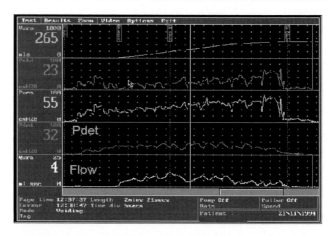

Figure 9   Pressure–flow study in hypocontractile/acontractile bladder (detrusor hyporeflexia). Note the low detrusor-voiding pressure with low urinary flow rate; one of the patterns in spinal cord injury.

consistent with detrusor hyper-reflexia (Fig. 8) and urethral SS bradykinesia, that is, the striated urethral sphincter often demonstrates poorly sustained contraction. Similar to other supraspinal lesions, the treatment of voiding dysfunction associated with Parkinson disease is to facilitate bladder filling and promote urinary storage with anticholinergic agents. If Parkinson disease coexists with symptoms of bladder outlet obstruction due to benign prostatic hyperplasia (BPH), the diagnosis of BPH must be confirmed by multichannel urodynamic studies (UDS). The most common cause of postprostatectomy incontinence in the patient with Parkinson disease is detrusor hyper-reflexia. If transurethral resection of the prostate (TURP) is performed without urodynamic confirmation of obstruction, the patient may become totally incontinent after the TURP procedure.

Shy–Drager Syndrome

Shy–Drager syndrome is a rare, progressive, and degenerative disease affecting the ANS with multisystem organ atrophy. In addition to Parkinson-like symptoms, cerebellar ataxia and autonomic dysfunction are common. Affected individuals demonstrate orthostatic hypotension, anhidrosis, and urinary incontinence. Degeneration of the nucleus of Onuf results in denervation of the external SS. Sympathetic nerve atrophy causes a nonfunctional bladder and an open bladder neck. Urodynamic evaluation often reveals neurogenic detrusor overactivity (Fig. 8), although a few individuals may have acontractile detrusor (Fig. 9) or poorly sustained bladder contractions. Often, the bladder neck (internal smooth sphincter) will be open at rest, while there is SS denervation. The treatment for Shy–Drager syndrome is to facilitate urinary storage with anticholinergic agents coupled with CIC or indwelling catheter. Patients with Shy–Drager syndrome should avoid undergoing TURP, because the risk of total incontinence is high.

Spinal Cord Lesions
Spinal Cord Injury

A spinal cord injury from a diving accident or motor vehicle injury results in the initial response of acute spinal shock.

During this acute spinal shock phase, the patient experiences flaccid paralysis below the level of injury, and the somatic reflex activity is either depressed or absent. The anal or bulbocavernosus reflex is typically absent. The autonomic activity is depressed, resulting in acute urinary retention and constipation. Urodynamic findings are consistent with acontractile detrusor (Fig. 9). The internal smooth and external urethral striated sphincteric activities, however, are normal. The spinal shock phase typically lasts for 6 to 12 weeks; it may be prolonged in some cases. The urinary bladder is managed either by indwelling urethral catheter or by CIC. The bladder function returns with reflex excitability and detrusor hyper-reflexia following the spinal shock phase (Fig. 8). Depending on the level of the lesion, the individual may develop DSD–DH and urinary leakage between CIC. Periodic UDS is indicated to monitor the effect of this alteration on detrusor behavior. During UDS, intravesical instillation of cold saline may indicate return of reflex activity or help better characterize the lesion. Suprasacral lesions may result initially in acontractile detrusor, which progresses to detrusor overactivity over time. Conversely, sacral cord lesions are associated with acontractile bladders, which may become hypertonic over time.

Spinal Cord Lesions (Above the Sixth Thoracic Vertebrae)

A complete cord transection above the sixth thoracic vertebrae (T6) most often will result in urodynamic findings of neurogenic detrusor overactivity and striated and smooth muscle sphincter dyssynergia (Fig. 2). A unique complication of T6 injury is *autonomic dysreflexia*. Autonomic dysreflexia is an exaggerated sympathetic response to any stimuli below the level of the lesion. This occurs most commonly with lesions of the cervical cord. Often, the inciting event is instrumentation of the urinary bladder or the rectum, causing visceral distention. Symptoms of autonomic dysreflexia include sweating, headache, hypertension, and reflex bradycardia. Acute management of autonomic dysreflexia is to decompress the bladder or rectum. Decompression usually will reverse the effects of unopposed sympathetic outflow. If additional measures are required, parenteral ganglionic or adrenergic blocking agents, such as chlorpromazine, may be used. Oral blocking agents, including terazosin, may be used for prophylactically treating patients with autonomic dysreflexia. Alternatively, a spinal anesthetic may be used as a prophylactic measure whenever bladder instrumentation is considered.

Spinal Cord Lesions (Below T6)

Spinal cord lesions below T6 level reveal urodynamic findings of detrusor hyper-reflexia (Fig. 8), SS dyssynergia (Fig. 2), and smooth sphincter dyssynergia but no autonomic dysreflexia. Neurologic evaluation reveals skeletal muscle spasticity with hyper-reflexic deep tendon reflexes, extensor plantar response, and positive Babinski sign, and above all, incomplete bladder emptying secondary to DSD, or loss of facilitatory input from higher centers. The cornerstone of treatment involves CIC and anticholinergic medications.

Multiple Sclerosis

MS is caused by focal demyelination of the CNS. It most commonly involves the posterior and lateral columns of the cervical spinal cord. Usually, poor correlation exists between the clinical symptoms and urodynamic findings. Thus, using UDS to evaluate patients with MS is critical. The most common urodynamic finding is detrusor hyper-reflexia (Fig. 8), occurring in as many as 50% to 90% of MS patients. About 50% of these patients will demonstrate DSD–DH. Detrusor areflexia occurs in 20% to 30% of cases. The optimum therapy for a patient with MS and neurogenic voiding dysfunction must be individualized, based on the urodynamic findings.

Peripheral Nerve Lesions

Peripheral nerve lesions due to diabetes mellitus, tabes dorsalis, herpes zoster, herniated lumbar disk disease, and radical pelvic surgery result in detrusor areflexia.

Diabetic Cystopathy

Usually, neurogenic bladder dysfunction occurs 10 or more years after the onset of diabetes mellitus. Neurogenic bladder occurs because of autonomic and peripheral neuropathy. A metabolic derangement of the Schwann cell results in segmental demyelination and impaired nerve conduction. The first symptoms of diabetic cystopathy are loss of sensation of bladder fullness followed by loss of motor function. Classic urodynamic findings associated with this condition are elevated residual urine, decreased bladder sensation, impaired detrusor contractility, and, eventually, acontractile detrusor (Fig. 9). Paradoxically, DHIC may occur. Treatment of diabetic cystopathy is CIC, long-term indwelling catheterization, or urinary diversion.

Tabes Dorsalis (Neurosyphilis)

In tabes dorsalis, central and peripheral nerve conduction is impaired, resulting in decreased bladder sensation and increased voiding intervals. The most common urodynamic finding associated with neurosyphilis is detrusor areflexia with normal striated sphincteric function.

Herpes Zoster

Herpes zoster is a neuropathy associated with painful vesicular eruptions in the dermal distribution of the affected nerve. The herpes virus lies dormant in the dorsal root ganglia or the sacral nerves. Sacral nerve involvement leads to impairment of detrusor function. The early stages of herpes infection are associated with LUT symptoms of urinary frequency, urgency, and urge incontinence, whereas the late stage is characterized by decreased bladder sensation, increased residual urine, and urinary retention. Urinary retention is self-limited and will resolve spontaneously with resolution of the herpes infection.

Herniated Disc

Slow and progressive herniation of the lumbar disc may cause irritation of the sacral nerves resulting in detrusor hyper-reflexia. Conversely, acute compression of the sacral roots associated with deceleration trauma or pathologic fracture impairs nerve conduction, which results in detrusor areflexia. A typical urodynamic finding of sacral nerve injury is acontractile detrusor with intact bladder sensation (Fig. 9). Association with internal sphincter denervation may occur. Damage of the peripheral sympathetic nerves results in an open and nonfunctional internal sphincter. Peripheral sympathetic nerve damage often occurs in association with detrusor denervation. The SS, however, is preserved.

Pelvic Surgery

Major pelvic surgery such as radical hysterectomy, abdominoperineal resection, proctocolectomy, or total exenteration will usually result in varying degrees of bladder dysfunction postoperatively. Most commonly, postsurgical symptoms of acontractile detrusor occur. However, spontaneous recovery of function occurs within six months after surgery in about 80% of the patients.

CLASSIFICATION OF NLUTD

Numerous schemes have been proposed to classify neurological voiding dysfunction (Table 2) (14–20). Neurourological classifications are predicated based upon descriptive detrusor pathophysiology as well as the site of the neurologic disease. Table 2 summarizes the historic six classification schemes, from the "neurologic" of Bradley to the "functional" of Wein. We have adopted for this chapter the functional classification proposed by Wein (20), which is based on the ability of the patient to either store urine in the bladder or empty the bladder completely. This classification must depend on the technological advances in modern urodynamics including videofluoroscopy and electromyography (EMG), which allow descriptive urodynamic interpretation of McClellan–Lapides nomenclature (1,20). The specific urodynamic interpretation enables appropriate therapeutic intervention for the patient with NLUTD.

DIAGNOSIS OF NLUTD

History

Both in congenital and acquired NLUTD, early diagnosis and treatment are essential because irreversible changes may occur in children with myelomeningocele, but also in patients with traumatic spinal cord injury. Symptoms of neurogenic bladder range from detrusor underactivity to overactivity, depending on the site of neurologic insult. The striated urinary sphincter also may be affected, resulting in sphincter underactivity or overactivity and loss of coordination with bladder detrusor function. The appropriate therapy and a successful outcome are predicated upon accurate diagnosis through thorough history and physical

Table 2   Major Classification Schemes

Bradley (14)	Gibbon (15)	Bors/Comarr (14)	McClellan/Lapides (17,18)	Krane/Siroky (19)	Wein (20)
Loop 1: Frontal lobe Brainstem	Suprasacral lesion	Upper motor neuron lesion—complete vs. incomplete; balanced vs. imbalanced	Uninhibited NB Reflex NB	Detrusor hyper-reflexia (or normoreflexia) Coordinated sphincters Striated sphincter dyssynergia Smoother sphincter dyssynergia	Failure to store bladder outlet
Loop 2: Brainstem–detrusor nucleus (sacral cord)					
Loop 3: Detrusor–pudendal nucleus (sacral cord)	Sacral lesion Motor sensory	Lower motor neuron lesion—complete vs. incomplete; balanced vs. imbalanced	Autonomous NB Motor paralytic bladder Sensory NB	Detrusor areflexia Coordinated sphincters Nonrelaxing striated sphincter	Failure to empty bladder outlet
Loop 4A: Frontal lobe–pudendal nucleus 4B: Pudendal-pudendal	Mixed lesion	Mixed lesion		Denervated striated sphincter	

Abbreviation: NB, neurogenic bladder.

examination with a variety of clinical evaluations, including urodynamics and selective radiographic imaging studies. The general history should include questions relevant to neurological and congenital abnormalities, information on the previous occurrence and frequency of urinary infections, and on relevant past surgery. Specific urinary history consists of symptoms related to both the storage and emptying functions of the LUT. The onset and the nature of the NLUTD (acute or insidious) should be determined. Specific symptoms and signs must be assessed in NLUTD and, if appropriate, be compared with the patient's condition before the NLUTD developed. Voiding symptoms of hesitancy, stranguria, decrease in the force and caliber of urinary stream, incomplete bladder emptying, or frank urinary retention suggest differential diagnosis that must include bladder outlet obstruction due to benign prostatic enlargement, prostate cancer, or urethral stricture and neurologic bladder disease. Specific signs such as pain, dysuria, infection, hematuria, or fever may justify further specialized work-up. The history must rule out congenital anomalies or metabolic disorders with possible neurological implications. Also, the history must include present medications, particularly those with known or possible effects on the LUT, and lifestyle factors such as smoking, alcohol, or addictive drug use. The general history should also include the assessment of menstrual, sexual, and bowel function, and obstetric history. Importance of bowel history must be stressed here because patients with NLUTD may suffer from a related neurogenic condition of the lower gastrointestinal tract. The bowel history also must address symptoms related to the storage and the evacuation functions and specific symptoms and signs including anorectal symptoms, previous defecation pattern, fecal incontinence, and rectal sensation. Mode and type of defecation must be compared with the patient's condition before the neurogenic dysfunction developed. Hereditary or familial risk factors should be recorded. Like the bowel function, the sexual function may also be impaired because of the neurogenic condition. The details of this history of course differ between men and women. However, such a focused evaluation should elicit information on genital or sexual dysfunction symptoms, previous sexual function, sensation in the genital area, and

for sexual functions and erectile, orgasmic, or ejaculatory dysfunction. Specific neurologic history should concentrate on eliciting information regarding acquired or congenital neurologic conditions, neurological symptoms (somatic and sensory), with onset, evolution, and therapy, as well as spasticity or autonomic dysreflexia (lesion level above T6).

Physical Examination

A complete and thorough general physical examination must be performed with special emphasis on the urologic and neurologic systems. Performance of a general urological and, when appropriate, gynecological examination is expected in every case.

Attention should be paid to the patient's physical and possible mental handicaps with respect to planned diagnostic investigations. Impaired mobility, particularly in the hips, or extreme spasticity may lead to problems in patient positioning in the urodynamics laboratory. Patients with very high neurological lesions may suffer from a significant drop in blood pressure when moved in a sitting or standing position. Subjective indications of bladder-filling sensations may be impossible in retarded patients. Prostate palpation or observation of pelvic organ descensus is made. The neurourologic examination should investigate the motor and sensory functions of the body and —the limbs, and the hand function. The examination should include the assessment of perineal sensation, the perineal reflexes supplied by the sacral segments S2 to S4, and anal sphincter tone and control.

Laboratory and Radiologic Evaluation

In the patient with LUT dysfunctional voiding, laboratory evaluation must include urinalysis and urine culture to rule out urinary tract infection (UTI) that can cause irritative voiding symptoms and urge incontinence. Urine cytology must exclude the diagnosis of carcinoma-in-situ of the urinary bladder, particularly in those patients with hematuria and/or irritative voiding symptoms that are out of proportion to the overall clinical presentation. Cystoscopy is also indicated in the evaluation of this subset of patients. Determination of serum creatinine and blood urea nitrogen allows important assessment of renal function, which could be impaired in the patient with neurologic bladder dysfunction. Fasting blood glucose may be necessary to rule out diabetes mellitus, and serum serologic test for syphilis may be indicated. Intravenous urogram (IVU) has remained the standard imaging modality to assess the upper urinary system for changes due to neurologic bladder disease. Renal sonogram, which is the screening modality of choice in children, and magnetic resonance imaging (MRI) can be utilized in the patients who may have a contraindication to IVU or impaired renal function. Imaging study is indicated to rule out hydronephrosis, urinary tract stones, and renal scarring from chronic pyelonephritis. Voiding cystourethrogram (VCUG) is indicated to rule out vesicoureteral reflux in children with congenital neurological defect such as myelodysplasia. Additional specialized neurological studies such as head or spine computed tomography scan, MRI, myelogram, or EMG may be indicated to rule out or confirm specific neurological disease. However, long-term follow-up of these patients should include regular periodic imaging of the kidneys and the bladder to rule out stones, hydronephrosis, or masses.

Voiding Studies

Uroflometry (UFR) (Fig. 10) with assessment of postvoid residual (PVR) urine remains a useful test to rule out bladder obstruction in the differential diagnosis of LUT dysfunction. This test gives a first impression of the voiding function and is mandatory before any invasive urodynamics is planned. For reliable information, it should be repeated at least two to three times. Possible pathologic findings include low flow rate, low voided volume, intermittent flow, hesitancy, and elevated PVR urine (Fig. 11). Care must be taken in judging the results in patients who are not able to void in a normal position. Both the flow pattern and the flow rate may be modified by inappropriate position and by any construction to divert the flow.

More often, UFR and PVR are performed as a part of the complex UDS, which generates other useful clinical parameters such as intravesical pressure, pelvic floor EMG, and VCUG monitored with fluoroscopy.

Urodynamic Studies

UDS (Fig. 12) objectively assesses the LUT function. It is important to know that during UDS patients with spinal

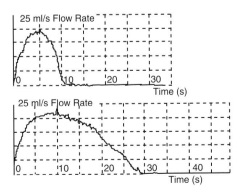

Figure 10 Normal free uroflow curve ("bell-shaped"). The uroflow curve is bell shaped; important parameters to note include maximum flow rate (Q_{max}), voided volume, and postvoid residual volume.

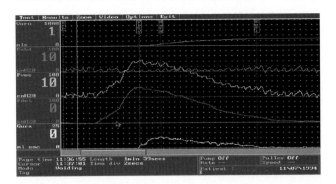

Figure 11 Pressure–flow study in bladder outlet obstruction. Note the high detrusor-voiding pressure and low urinary flow rate; the computer-generated graph is compared to the *International Continence Society Standards* and *Schafer's Nomograms* to objectively document the degree of obstruction.

cord injury above T6 may exhibit autonomic dysreflexia, which is characterized by hypertension, bradycardia, sweating, pounding headache, and piloerection among others following certain stimuli such as bladder distension and stimulation of lower portions of the body. Such patients should have blood pressure monitored during the study.

The rectal ampulla should be empty of stool before the UDS. Drugs that influence the LUT function should be discontinued, if feasible, at least 48 hours before the investigation or otherwise be taken into account for the interpretation of the data. All urodynamic findings must be reported in detail and performed according to the International Continence Society technical recommendations and standards.

Urodynamic Tests

Cystometry

Cystometry is the method by which the pressure–volume relationship of the bladder is measured and is used to assess

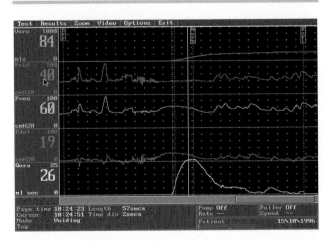

Figure 12 Normal pressure–flow study. P_{det} is normally very low until the end-filling stage of the pressure–flow study, and there is a sustained and effective detrusor contraction with the command to void resulting in urinary flow and relaxation of the external urethral sphincter.

detrusor activity, sensation, capacity, and compliance (Figs. 7 and 12).

Filling Cystometry. An average adult bladder holds approximately 350 to 500 mL of urine. During the test, provocative maneuvers help to unveil bladder instability (Fig. 13A and B). Filling cytometry is important if combined with bladder pressure measurement during micturition (pressure–flow study) and videourodynamics. The latter is necessary to document the status of the LUT function during the filling phase. The bladder should be empty at the start of filling. A relatively physiologic filling rate (< 35 mL/min) should be used with body-warm saline, because fast-filling and room-temperature saline are provocative. Possible pathologic findings during filling cystometry include detrusor overactivity, low detrusor compliance, abnormal bladder sensation, and incontinence and incompetent or relaxing urethra.

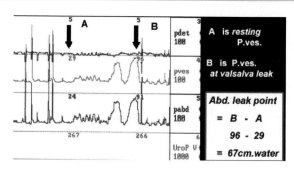

Figure 14 Valsalva (abdominal) leak point pressure measurement. The lowest abdominal pressure (P_{abd}) at which leak is noted with Valsalva maneuver during bladder filling is called valsalva (abdominal) leak point pressure; VLPP of less than 20–30 cmH$_2$O indicates severe intrinsic sphincter deficiency and results in stress urinary incontinence. *Abbreviation*: VLPP, Valsalva leak point pressure.

LPP Measurements

Abdominal or Valsalva Leak Point Pressure. The abdominal pressure (P_{abd}) at which leak is noted during bladder filling is known as abdominal (or Valsalva) leak point pressure (VLPP) (Fig. 14). This test is useful in patients with urinary incontinence and helps to assess intrinsic sphincter dysfunction. In addition, VLPP of more than 70 to 80 cmH$_2$O carries the risk of upper tract damage. However, there is currently no uniform consensus regarding the methodology of measurement LPP.

Detrusor Leak Point Pressure (DLPP). This specific investigation is important to estimate the risk for the upper urinary tract or for secondary bladder damage. The DLPP greater than 40 cmH$_2$O places the upper tract at risk of damage. The DLPP is only a screening test, because it lacks information on the duration of the high pressure that might have more impact on the upper urinary tract. A high DLPP warrants further testing, including videourodynamics to document any associated vesicoureteral reflux.

Pressure–Flow Study

Pressure–flow study reflects the coordination between the detrusor and the urethra or pelvic floor during the voiding phase. This is the only test that can assess bladder contractility and the severity of a bladder outlet obstruction. Pressure–flow study simultaneously records the voiding detrusor pressure and the rate of urinary flow (Fig. 9). Pressure–flow studies can be combined with voiding cystogram and videourodynamics for complicated cases of urinary incontinence. It is even more powerful in combination with filling cystometry and videourodynamics. Possible pathologic findings include detrusor underactivity/contractility, DSD, nonrelaxing urethra, and residual urine. Most types of bladder obstruction caused by NLUTD are due to DSD or static/nonrelaxing urethra or bladder neck. Pressure–flow analysis mostly assesses the severity of the mechanical obstruction caused by the urethra's inherent mechanical or anatomic obstruction, and has limited value in patients with NLUTD.

Sphincter EMG

The cystometrogram may be performed simultaneously with EMG to assess the activity of the external urethral SS, the periurethral striated musculature, the anal sphincter, or

(A)

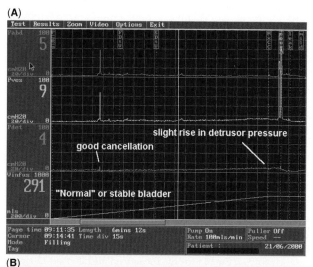

(B)

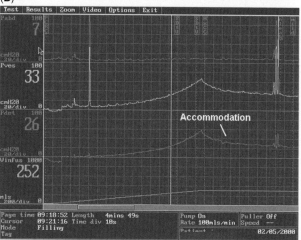

Figure 13 **(A)** Normal stable detrusor with normal compliance during filling cystometry. Note the stable detrusor during the filling stage with low detrusor pressure and normal compliance. **(B)** Poor detrusor compliance. Note the rise in the detrusor pressure (P_{det}) during the filling stage; this may be seen in spinal cord injury and interstitial cystitis and may coexist with detrusor overactivity.

the striated pelvic floor muscles during micturition (Fig. 2). Normally, the pelvic floor striated muscle electromyographic activity diminishes at the onset of bladder detrusor contraction. Bladder outlet obstruction due to detrusor–external sphincter dyssynergia is diagnosed by persistence of the activity on the EMG during voiding or attempt to void.

Video Urodynamics

This combination of filling cystometry and pressure–flow study with LUT imaging is the gold standard urodynamic investigation in NLUTD. This complex testing combines VCUG and multichannel urodynamics (Fig. 2). The procedure enables documentation of the anatomic and functional integrity of the LUT, as well as the functional pressure–flow relationship between the bladder, the bladder outlet, and urethra. The VCUG can identify a bladder diverticulum, urethral diverticulum, urethral obstruction, and vesicoureteral reflux.

Provocative Tests During Urodynamics

Coughing, triggered voiding, or anal stretch can provoke LUT dysfunction. Fast-filling cystometry with cooled saline (the "ice water test") is considered a discriminative test between an upper motor neuron lesion (UMNL) and a lower motor neuron lesion (LMNL). Patients with UMNL with intact detrusor muscle will exhibit detrusor contraction, whereas patients with LMNL will not. The test gives false-positive results in young children (21) and may not be fully discriminative in other patients (21). A positive bethanechol supersensitivity test (detrusor contraction more than 15 cmH$_2$O over baseline) was presumed to prove detrusor denervation hypersensitivity, the intactness of the motor innervation of the bladder, and the muscular integrity of an acontractile detrusor. The test often gives equivocal results, and other clinical conditions such as cystitis magnify its false positivity. A recent variation of this method was reported with intravesical electromotive administration of the bethanechol (8). This test turned out to be both selective and predictive for successful oral bethanechol treatment.

MANAGEMENT OF NLUTD

The primary aims for treatment of NLUTD include protection of the upper urinary tract, improvement of urinary continence, improvement of the patient's quality of life, and restoration of the normal LUT function. Preservation of the upper urinary tract function is of paramount importance. Until 25 years ago, renal failure remained the primary long-term cause of mortality in the spinal cord–injured patient surviving the initial trauma. This has led to the *golden rule* in the treatment of NLUTD: assure that the detrusor pressure remains within safe limits during both the filling phase and the voiding phase. This approach has indeed significantly reduced the mortality and morbidity from urological complications in this patient group. Bladder dysfunction can result in hydronephrosis, vesicoureteral reflux, infections, or stones. In patients with high detrusor pressure during the filling phase (detrusor overactivity, low detrusor compliance, etc.) or during the voiding phase (DSD and other causes of bladder outlet obstruction), therapy is aimed primarily at the conversion of an active, aggressive high-pressure bladder into a passive low-pressure reservoir despite the resulting residual urine, which can be managed by CIC. Therapy of urinary incontinence is important for the social rehabilitation of the patient and thus contributes substantially to the quality of life, but is

also pivotal in the prevention of UTI and perineal area skin infections.

Despite the varied neuropathies detected in the patient with NLUTD, a simple practical scheme for their management is based on the premise that NLUTD results primarily in failure to either empty or store urine.

Failure to Empty

Assisted Bladder Emptying

Incomplete bladder emptying is a serious risk factor for UTI, for developing high intravesical pressure during the filling phase, and for incontinence. The method of choice to improve the voiding process should be based on practicality, the subject's compliance, and, most importantly, on long-term clinical impact.

Third-Party Bladder Expression (Credé Maneuver)

Regretfully, this method is still applied, foremost in infants and young children with myelomeningocele and sometimes in tetraplegics. The suprapubic downward compression of the lower abdomen leads to an increase in the intravesical pressure, but also causes a compression of the urethra and thus a functional obstruction that may reinforce an already existing high bladder outlet resistance and lead to inefficient emptying. Because of the high pressures that may be created during this maneuver, it is potentially hazardous for the urinary tract, and thus is contraindicated. Although it is a noninvasive method, its use should be discouraged unless urodynamics shows intravesical pressures to stay within the safe range.

Abdominal Straining (Valsalva)

In recommending voiding by abdominal straining, the considerations mentioned under Credé above also hold for the Valsalva maneuver. Most of these patients are unable to scale the pressure they exert on the bladder during Valsalva; therefore, there is the inherent risk of exceeding the safe range.

Triggered Reflex Voiding

Stimulation of the sacral or lumbar dermatomes in patients with UMNL can elicit reflex contraction of the detrusor. Morbidity occurs more often during the first decades of treatment. This method may be used in patients in whom it is urodynamically safe.

Catheter Drainage

Indwelling Continuous Catheter Drainage

Indwelling continuous catheter drainage (urethral or suprapubic), in general, remains attractive for practicality and effectiveness in the short term. The most common use of a suprapubic catheter is in individuals with spinal cord injuries (paraplegic and quadriplegic) and a malfunctioning bladder. A long-term suprapubic catheter remains an attractive alternative to a long-term indwelling urethral catheter. However, use of smaller (e.g., 14F and 16F) tubes is recommended for either drainage method. In male patients, long-term continuous urethral catheterization is associated with high complication rates of urethral strictures, fistulas, bladder stones, and infection. Although rare, malignancy can also occur with chronic indwelling urethral catheters. This is especially true in paraplegic women (21). In 6 out of 59 patients who had a chronic indwelling urethral catheter

(22), squamous cell carcinoma developed. In another study, squamous metaplasia and leukoplakia developed in 11 out of 81 spinal cord–injured patients with a chronic indwelling catheter (23). Bacteriuria occurs within 72 hours of placement of a continuous indwelling urethral catheter, and consequently chronic inflammation can result in a contracted fibrotic bladder. Finally, urinary incontinence associated with bladder spasms often is treated by increasing the balloon size with some traction on the catheter, which predisposes to erosion of the bladder neck.

Potential complications with chronic suprapubic catheterization are similar to those associated with indwelling urethral catheters, including leakage around the catheter, bladder stone formation, UTI, and catheter obstruction. However, with a suprapubic catheter, the risk of urethral damage is eliminated; because the catheter comes out of the lower abdomen rather than the penis or vaginal area, a suprapubic tube is more patient-friendly. Bladder spasms occur less often because the suprapubic catheter does not irritate the trigone, as does the urethral catheter. In addition, suprapubic tubes are more sanitary for the individual, and bladder infections are minimized because the tube is away from the perineum. Nonetheless, suprapubic tube neither prevents bladder spasms from occurring in unstable bladders nor improves the urethral closure mechanism in an incompetent urethra. If the suprapubic tube falls out inadvertently, the exit hole of the tube will seal up and close quickly within 24 hours if the tube is not replaced with a new one. Regardless of the method employed, the catheter should be changed very regularly, at least once a month.

Management with chronic continuous catheter drainage is a risk factor also for renal deterioration. Investigators have reported significant differences in renal scarring and caliectasis in spinal cord–injured patients managed by chronic catheterization versus those using a reflex avoiding method (24,25). Because of the deleterious effects of chronic continuous catheter drainage in this particular patient subgroup, it should be avoided at all costs.

Intermittent Catheterization

Intermittent catheterization or self-catheterization is a mode of draining the bladder at timed intervals, as opposed to continuous bladder drainage. Intermittent catheterization has become a healthy alternative to indwelling catheters for individuals with chronic urinary retention due to an obstructed bladder, a hypocontractile bladder, or a nonfunctioning bladder. Of the three possible options, i.e., urethral catheter, suprapubic tube, and intermittent catheterization, the latter is the best solution for bladder decompression of a motivated individual who is not physically handicapped or mentally impaired. A prerequisite for self-catheterization is the patient's ability to use their hands and arms; however, in a situation in which a patient is physically or mentally impaired, a caregiver or health professional can perform intermittent catheterization for the patient. Many studies of young individuals with spinal cord injuries have shown that intermittent catheterization is preferable to indwelling catheters (i.e., urethral catheter and suprapubic tube) for both men and women, including young children with myelomeningocele. Intermittent catheterization may be performed using a soft red-rubber catheter or a short, rigid, plastic catheter. The use of plastic catheters is preferable to red rubber catheters, because they are easier to clean and last longer. The bladder must be drained on a regular basis, either based on a timed interval (e.g., on awakening, every three to six hours during the day, and before bed) or based

on bladder volume, which must be kept at less than 400 to 500 cc during each session. CIC results in lower rates of infection than the rates noted with indwelling catheters. However, all patients should be placed on an antibiotic prophylaxis using an agent such as nitrofurantoin for the initial few weeks, to allow the LUT acclimatization to the bacterial colonization.

Pharmacologic Therapy

Aiding Bladder Emptying

Acetylcholine mediates the stimulation of the muscarinic, M3-subtype receptors of the detrusor smooth muscles, which results in physiologic bladder contraction and voiding. Activation of the M2-subtype receptor inhibits bladder relaxation through inhibition of the signal transduction pathways, leading to accumulation of cyclic adenosine monophosphate (1,12). Neural injury or denervation leads to upregulation of the M2 receptors. Pharmacologic manipulation involving direct stimulation of the muscarinic receptors would enhance detrusor contraction and bladder emptying. Therefore, useful agents would seem to be those that mimic the action of acetylcholine. Bethanechol chloride is the most commonly recommended acetylcholine-like drug for those patients with failure to empty due to impaired detrusor contractility. Bethanechol exhibits relative selectivity in the bladder, with minimal effect at the level of neural ganglia and cardiovascular targets. Furthermore, bethanechol in doses of 5 to 10 mg has been employed in the treatment of patients with postoperative or postpartum urinary retention. Although, it has remained for many decades the primary therapy in those patients with atonic or hypotonic bladders (26), doubts have continually persisted about its clinical efficacy in aiding bladder emptying. Controversy has also surrounded the use of bethanechol for inducing reflex bladder contraction in patients with supraspinal spinal cord injury, and experience has shown that this agent should not be recommended in those patients with overactive bladder associated with poor compliance, because of the potential deterioration of the upper tract by the rising intravesical pressure. Overall, there is no solid clinical evidence to support the use of bethanechol as a parasympathomimetic agent to aid in the physiologic emptying of the neurogenic bladder.

Decreasing Bladder Outlet Resistance

In contrast to using a parasympathomimetic agent to stimulate bladder emptying, alpha-blockers have been used with partial success in an attempt to decrease bladder outlet resistance in patients with neurovesical dysfunction. The rationale for these drugs is that increased bladder outlet resistance occurs in response to the stimulation of sympathetic reflexes, and the alpha-adrenergic receptors primarily inhibit the pelvic parasympathetic ganglionic transmission with a resultant increased relaxation of the bladder body and efficient urine storage. Prazosin hydrochloride, terazosin, doxazosin, and alfuzosin are antihypertensive agents with affinity for the postsynaptic α_1-adrenergic receptors. These α_1-receptor antagonists relax the smooth muscle of the bladder outlet and urethra, and thus lower the outlet resistance. Terazosin and doxazosin are the commonly used alpha-blockers for lowering the outlet resistance and aiding in bladder emptying. Further, these drugs have longer half-lives (12 hours), which improve compliance, and are thus well tolerated. The commonest side effects include asthenia, orthostatic hypotension, and dizziness.

The doses are usually titrated from 1 to 10 mg with the average dose at 5 mg; the patients are usually instructed to take it at bedtime to minimize the side effects.

Decreasing Outlet Resistance at the SS

The centrally acting muscle relaxants such as chlordiazepoxide, methocarbamol, orphenadrine, and diazepam are oral agents that cause relaxation of the striated muscles of the pelvic floor. Dantrolene sodium, which is the most commonly used skeletal muscle relaxant in patients with classic detrusor–SS dyssynergia, has been successful in facilitating voiding in these patients. The recommended adult therapy begins with the dose of 25 mg twice daily, and slowly titrated to the maximum daily divided doses of 400 mg. Sedation is the most common side effect; however, potential adverse events include euphoria, dizziness, diarrhea, and hepatitis. The later is related to high dosage and long-term use.

Baclofen, a gamma-amino-amino butyric acid agonist has been used commonly as a centrally acting agent to relax the external urethral sphincter. The purported mode of action is the inhibition of the primary afferent fibers terminal in the spinal cord, thereby abolishing any monosypnatic or polysynaptic spinal reflex activity. Treatment is usually started with a dose of 5 mg, three times a day, and titrated to a total daily dose of 60 mg. The reported benefits of baclofen in the management of neurogenic voiding dysfunction include reduction in SS activity, decrease in residual urine, abolition of hyper-reflexia and nocturia, and increase in bladder compliance. Side effects include lower extremity flaccidity (at the therapeutic doses), respiratory depression, erectile dysfunction, and constipation. Drowsiness, insomnia, rash, pruritus, dizziness, weakness, hallucination, and seizures are other potential complications of baclofen therapy.

Electrical Stimulation

Currently, direct electrical stimulation to aid in complete bladder emptying in a patient with neurogenic urinary retention remains an attractive alternative to intermittent catheterization, but clinical application has been limited because of poor results and unwanted side effects. Fifty to sixty percent of patients have been reported to exhibit low residual urine volumes following application of direct electrical stimulation to treat their hypotonic or acontractile bladders. However, the collateral spread of electrical current to other pelvic organs with a low stimulus threshold often results in abdominal, pelvic, and perineal pain, desire to defecate, contraction of pelvic and leg muscles, and erections and ejaculations, making this approach less than ideal. To overcome such undesirable effects, investigators have designed devices to stimulate individual sacral nerve roots (27,28), or employ a tripolar electrode in the differential stimulation of large and small fibers with low current, e.g., *anode* blockade (29). Development of a patient-friendly device, low morbidity, and nearly complete bladder emptying remain the elusive goals of electrostimulation in the management of incomplete bladder emptying in patients with NLUTD. Sacral anterior root stimulation (SARS) is aimed at producing a detrusor contraction. The urethral sphincter efferents are also stimulated, but as the striated muscle relaxes faster than the smooth muscle of the detrusor, the so-called "poststimulus voiding" will occur. This approach has only been successful in highly selected patients. Unfortunately, by changing the stimulation parameters, this method can also induce defecation or erection.

Surgical Management

External Sphincterotomy

The therapeutic destruction of the external urethral SS is primarily indicated in males with incomplete bladder emptying due to suprasacral lesions, and when other management methods have failed or are impractical. The prerequisites are that there is an adequate involuntary detrusor contraction and an adequate penile shaft to anchor the external collection device, usually a condom catheter. Many patients, particularly paraplegics, with detrusor–SS dyssynergia can be successfully managed with CIC; however, recurrent episodes of UTI and upper urinary tract deterioration warrant recommendation for external sphincterotomy. External sphincterotomy has replaced pudendal neurectomy as the surgical treatment of choice for these patients. A successful acute sphincterotomy will result in a substantial improvement in bladder emptying in 70% to 90% of cases, a stable upper urinary tract, resolution of existing vesicoureteral reflux, and maintenance of sterile urine in patients with low volumes and without indwelling catheters.

External sphincterotomy is usually performed endoscopically with a knife or loop electrode, or laser, preferably with laser evaporization. Tissue destruction should occur preferably at the 12 o'clock position deep through the bulk of the SS anterior-laterally from the level of verumontanum to the bulbomembranous junction. To minimize the chance of penile (paired carvenosal nerves) nerve injury with resultant impotence, the incision must avoid the 2 to 3 o'clock position on the right and the 9 to 10 o'clock position on the left urethra. Complications of this procedure include impotence in 5% to 30% of patients and urinary extravasation (30). Hemorrhage is unlikely to occur with high-powered (40–60 W) laser evaporization (Nseyo, unpublished data, 2003).

Long-term complications include failure of the procedure in 50% of patients, including renal deterioration, condom catheter problems, and decreased bladder compliance. This long-term failure rate of external sphincterotomy has diminished its appeal and engendered interest in urinary diversion in the management of neurogenic urinary retention in many NLUTD patients.

Cutaneous Vesicostomy

CIC remains the most widely used and attractive method for the management of failure to empty in young children with neurogenic bladders. However, cutaneous vesicostomy has been an effective alternative to CIC in managing those children with a poorly emptying bladder and persistent UTIs and upper tract deterioration. The decision to perform vesicostomy should be individualized and based on clinical grounds and a satisfactory radiographic response to catheterization. In children, the dome of the bladder is easily mobilized through a small transverse skin incision; a button of the detrusor is excised and the bladder wall is sutured to the skin. This Blocksom technique, popularized by Duckett (31), has replaced the old technique, which involved a skin flap that was internalized and sutured to the bladder. The Blocksom technique has fewer complications including stromal stenosis and vesical herniation.

Vesicostomy is managed with drainage of urine into the diaper and prophylactic antibiotics. At an appropriate age, when the patient can perform CIC, the vesicostomy can be closed.

Failure to Store

Patients with NLUTD who fail to store urine and therefore are incontinent tend to exhibit either uninhibited bladder contractions or decreased resistance in the bladder neck and urethra. Generally, this group of patients is more difficult to treat than those whose primary problem is failure to empty.

Pharmacologic Therapy

Acetylcholine is the principal neurotransmitter that mediates bladder detrusor contractions; therefore, uninhibited bladder contractions associated with reflex NLUTD can be treated with anticholinergic agents. Clinically, the commonly used anticholinergic agents are nonselective for the muscarinic receptors, M2 and M3 subtypes, which are functionally important in the human bladder (1,12). All available anticholinergic agents with atropine-like actions bind with equal effectiveness to all subtypes of the muscarinic receptors. Treatment leads to an atropine-like response against detrusor hyperactivity with urodynamic evidence of increased volume at first sensation, decreased amplitude and uninhibited contractions, and increased total bladder capacity or compliance with attendant reduction in symptoms of urgency and urgency incontinence. Anticholinergic agents generally do not cure patients of their underlying neurogenic symptoms. In some spinal cord injury patients with decreased detrusor compliance, these agents are often used in combination with intermittent catheterization. Such a strategy may prevent loss of bladder compliance due to change in the ECM secondary to chronic urinary retention. The commonly used anticholinergic agents include oxybutynin, which has both short- and long-acting formulations, tolterodine (standard and extended releases), probantheline, and hyoscyamine. The newer formulations in recent years (darefenacin, solefenacin, trospium) have not eliminated the common side effects of anticholinergic therapy, namely dry mouth (inhibition of secretions of salivary glands), pupillary dilatation (blockade of the ocular iris sphincter muscle), blurred vision (dysfunction of the ciliary muscle of the ocular lens), tachycardia, drowsiness, and decreased gut motility. These agents also exhibit a central effect by inducing confusion in the elderly and restlessness in children. Dental problems, especially in the elderly, are attributable to dry mouth caused by the anticholinergic agents. In an effort to improve effectiveness and minimize side effects, an intravesical formulation of oxybutynin is being investigated. It should be noted that all antimuscarinic agents are contraindicated in patients with narrow-angle glaucoma and symptomatic benign prostatic enlargement.

Drugs that increase bladder outlet resistance, such as the alpha-adrenergic receptor agonists, phenyl propanolamine, ephedrine, and pseudoephedrine have been used with variable results to increase adrenergic activities to achieve urine storage. The tricyclic antidepressants, such as imipramine hydrochloride, have been used to facilitate urine storage. This agent has three pharmacologic actions: (i) exhibits central and peripheral anticholinergic effects at some selective sites, (ii) blocks, at the presynaptic nerve terminals, the reuptake of neurotransmitters serotonin and noradrenaline, and (iii) binds to glutamate receptors in the CNS. The net effect of these actions is the enhancement of adrenergic activity peripherally, which leads to increased sympathomimetic action. This results in increased bladder outlet resistance (α-adrenergic receptor stimulation) and relaxation of bladder body (β-adrenergic receptor stimulation).

Clean Intermittent Catheterization

As discussed above, often the patient with neurogenic urinary incontinence secondary to NLUTD can be treated with anticholinergic agents to induce urinary retention (failure to empty). CIC is then initiated to empty the bladder and prevent the bladder from ever reaching a volume that exerts the high reflex activity leading to urinary incontinence.

Continuous Catheter Drainage

As discussed previously, chronic long-term continuous catheter drainage should not be the treatment of choice for dysfunctional voiding irrespective of the underlying pathophysiology. When indicated, as in the elderly, the principles and catheter care program outlined previously should be practiced.

Artificial Urinary Sphincter

Selection of appropriate patients for implantation of an artificial urinary sphincter (AUS) requires a thorough neurourologic work-up to discern the uniqueness of the patient's incontinence. The patient should appropriately meet the specific criteria of intrinsic sphincteric deficiency with normal detrusor contractility and compliance. The most commonly used AUS consists of an inflatable cuff placed around the bulbous urethra of the adult male or the bladder neck with the pressure balloon reservoir placed beneath the fascia of the abdominal muscle or in the space of Retzius (Fig. 15). The pump control is placed in the scrotum or labia. Activation occurs by compressing the pump chamber, and deactivation can be achieved by pressing the button on the side of the control assembly. Significant rises in intra-abdominal pressure during vigorous exercises or lifting will trigger urinary leakage. Overall, the success rate is reported at 97% for social dryness, with a reoperation rate of approximately 30%. However, this rate is about 55% in patients with a history of prior radiation (32).

Bladder Augmentation or Substitution (Augmentation or Substitution Cystoplasty)

Bladder augmentation, by procedures such as the clam cystoplasty, is a valid option to decrease detrusor pressure and increase bladder capacity whenever more conservative approaches have failed (12,32). The results of the various procedures are very good and comparable. Scaffolds, probably of tissue-engineered material for bladder augmentation or substitution or alternative techniques are promising

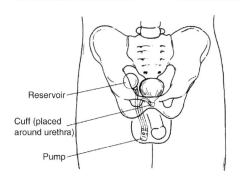

Figure 15 Artificial urinary sphincter. *Source*: Courtesy of George S. Benson, MD, from Chapter 45 of the Second Edition.

future options. Replacing or expanding the bladder by intestine or other passive expandable coverage will increase the detrusor compliance and reduce the pressure effect of the detrusor overactivity. Therefore, patients with NLUTD who develop a noncompliant bladder and are at high risk for vesicoureteral reflux, hydronephrosis, and deterioration of renal function are potential candidates when conservative measures fail. Bladder substitution to create a low-pressure reservoir may be indicated in patients with a severely thick and fibrotic bladder wall. The surgical technique includes resecting most of the anterior hemisphere of the bladder and sparing the trigone, ureteric orifices and the bladder neck. The "augmentation patch" could be an isolated piece of ileum (ileocystoplasty), colon (colocystoplasty), or stomach (gastrocystoplasty, particularly in children) (Table 3), which is then sutured onto the residual bladder (Fig. 16). Another method known as the detrusor myectomy (auto-augmentation) is aimed at improving the shrunken bladder that is enlarged by removal of lateral detrusor tissue to free the entrapped ureter in a nonfunctional fibrotic detrusor. This procedure reduces the detrusor overactivity and increases the compliance. The augmented bladder must be emptied by CIC. Contraindications for augmentation cystoplasty include renal insufficiency, bowel disease, and inability or lack of resources to perform CIC.

The inherent complications associated with these procedures include recurrent infection, stone building, perforation, diverticulum formation, possible malignant changes, and intestinal metabolic abnormalities such as mucus production and impaired bowel function.

Neural Manipulation

Electrical stimulation, neuromodulation, denervation, and deafferentation constitute various neural manipulations to achieve urinary storage in patients with NLUTD and urinary incontinence. A strong contraction of the urethral sphincter and/or pelvic floor, as well as anal dilatation, manipulation of the genital region, and physical activity reflexly inhibit micturition. Whereas the first mechanism is affected by activation of efferent fibers, the latter ones are produced by activation of afferents. Electrical stimulation of the pudendal nerve afferents produces a strong inhibition of the micturition reflex and the detrusor contraction. This stimulation then might support the restoration of

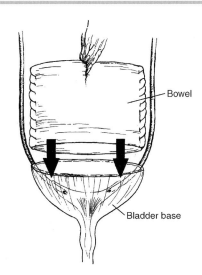

Figure 16 Augmentation cystoplasty. An isolated segment of bowel is opened along its antimesenteric border and used as a "patch" to reconstruct the bladder. *Source*: Courtesy of George S. Benson, MD, from Chapter 45 of the Second Edition.

the balance between excitatory and inhibitory inputs at the spinal or supraspinal level, and it might imply that patients with incomplete lesions will benefit, but patients with complete lesions will not. Stimulation of the tibial nerve afferents has not been applied in patients with NLUTD. Sacral rhizotomy, also known as sacral deafferentation, has achieved some success in reducing detrusor overactivity, but it is used nowadays mostly as an adjuvant to SARS (27,28).

Sacral Nerve Neuromodulation (Interstim™) (33)

During sacral nerve stimulation or sacral neuromodulation, the bladder afferents are stimulated, which probably restores the correct balance between excitatory and inhibitory impulses from and to the pelvic organs at a sacral and suprasacral level, thus reducing the detrusor overactivity. It is used either as a temporary procedure using foramen electrodes with an external stimulator, with the expectation of perseverance of the changes after treatment, or as a chronic procedure with an implanted stimulator. In the latter case, a test procedure, the percutaneous nerve evaluation, with an external stimulator is performed before the implant to judge the patient's response. This procedure also has considerable success in selected patients.

DEVICE THERAPY

Inflow Device to Empty the Bladder

A rare cause of incontinence is a situation where the bladder never empties completely and overflows. This problem is seen most commonly with nerve problems affecting the bladder, such as MS and spinal cord injury. Thus far, the most effective treatment to empty the bladder is CIC, three to four times per day. The inflow device, an alternative approach, sits in the urethra and allows the bladder to empty with a pump design activated by an external controller without having to catheterize to empty the bladder. The early results with this device are quite encouraging in selected patients.

Table 3 Bowel Segments Used in Various Urinary Diversion Techniques

Type of urinary diversion	Bowel segment used
Incontinent diversion	Ileum (Bricker's conduit), colon (transverse colon, sigmoid colon)
Continent diversions	
Indiana pouch	Cecum, ascending colon, and terminal ileum
Kock pouch	Ileum
Reddy pouch	Colon
Mainz pouch	Cecum, ascending colon, and terminal ileum
UCLA pouch	Right colon, hepatic flexure, and terminal ileum
Neobladder	Ileum (Studer pouch, Camey procedure, "S" pouch, and "M" pouch), colon
Ureterosigmoidostomy	Sigmoid colon
Sigma-rectum pouch	Sigmoid colon and rectum

URINARY DIVERSION

When no other therapy has been successful, urinary diversion must be considered for the protection of the upper tracts and for the patient's quality of life.

Continent Diversion

This should be the first choice for diversion. In patients for whom indwelling catheterization or suprapubic catheterization is the only feasible treatment option, the change to a continent diversion may be a better prospect. Some patients with limited dexterity prefer a cutaneous stoma above using the urethra for catheterization. The continent cutaneous stoma is created following various reservoir techniques (Table 3). They are constructed to create a low-pressure reservoir for urine storage and contain antireflux and continence mechanisms. The patients empty the reservoirs by periodic catheterization of the continent cutaneous stoma. The continent reservoirs are created generally from segments of ileum or colon, or combination of the segments that have been detubularized and folded into a cistern to obtain the low-pressure systems. The detubularization helps to eliminate the unidirectional peristalsis. An example of an ileal-based diversion is the Studer's diversion (Table 3), which uses 50 to 60 cm of terminal ileum, which results in the creation of a low-pressure reservoir of 300 cc and an antireflux limb. The Indiana pouch consists of the detubularized segment of the proximal colon (cecum, ascending and a portion of the transverse), which is folded into the low-pressure reservoir (Table 3). The ureters are tunneled into the colon with an antireflux technique, whereas the ileocecal valve provides the continent mechanism, and the ileal segment is doubly imbricated or stabled over a 14-French catheter to configure the catheterizable stoma. All of the forms of continent diversion do show frequent complications, including leakage or stenosis of the ureterointestinal anastomosis or the stoma. The short-term continence rates are over 80%, and good protection of the upper urinary tract is achieved. For cosmetic reasons, the umbilicus is often used for the stoma site, but this may have a higher risk of stomal stenosis. An example of continent urinary diversion is shown in Figure 17.

Incontinent Diversion

If catheterization is impossible, incontinent diversion with a urine-collection device is indicated. Fortunately, nowadays, this indication is seldom needed because many appropriate alternatives can be offered. Ultimately, it could be considered in patients who are wheelchair bound or bed-ridden with intractable and untreatable incontinence, in devastated LUTs, and when the upper urinary tract is severely compromised, and in patients who refuse other therapy.

Various techniques have been described for creating an incontinent urinary diversion; however, several basic principles must be observed in their construction (Table 3). The ureters are first mobilized from the deep pelvis and detached from the bladder, and one ureter is tunneled behind the colonic mesentery to lie next to the contralateral ureter. An adequate ileal or colonic segment is used for the conduit that contains the ureters implanted by the ureteral mucosa–to–bowel mucosa technique into the distal ileal portion, whereas in the colonic conduit, the ureters are tunneled to create antireflux. The proximal end of the conduit is then exteriorized and sutured to the skin to mature the cutaneous intestinal stoma. The continuity of the bowel that was chosen as the conduit is reestablished by bowel–bowel anastomosis. Urine drains continuously into a collection device over the stoma, so the surrounding skin must be protected from urine contact to prevent the aggravation of squamous metaplasia and bleeding. In ureterosigmoidostomy, the ureterointestinal anastomosis is performed similar to the colonic procedure with tunneling of the ureters and the creation of antireflux. Example of these various types of supravesical urinary diversion are shown in Figure 18.

QUALITY OF LIFE

The issue of quality of life should remain a paramount consideration in the global scheme of managing patients with NLUTD. Apart from the limitations that relate directly to the neurologic pathology, the NLUTD can be treated adequately in the majority of patients and must not interfere with social independence. The life expectancy of the patient does not need to be impaired by the NLUTD. With appropriate and adequate treatment, and consequent neurourological care over the patient's lifetime, the quality of life can be assured.

FOLLOW-UP

NLUTD is an unstable condition and can vary considerably even within a relatively short period. Meticulous follow-up

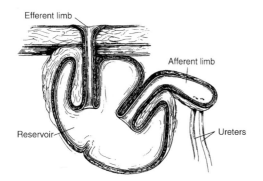

Figure 17.   Continent urinary diversion. A low-pressure reservoir is created and is emptied by intermittent catheterization of the efferent limb. *Source:* Courtesy of George S. Benson, MD, from Chapter 45 of the Second Edition.

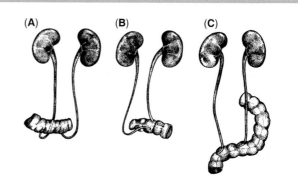

Figure 18.   Types of supravesical urinary diversion. (**A**) ileal conduit. (**B**) colon conduit. (**C**) ureterosigmoidostomy. *Source:* Courtesy of George S. Benson, MD, from Chapter 45 of the Second Edition.

and regular evaluation are necessary. Depending on the type of the underlying neurological pathology, the current clinical condition, and the stability of the NLUTD, the interval between the specific follow-up investigations should not exceed one to two years. In patients with MS and acute spinal cord injury, this interval is, of course, much shorter. Urine dipsticks should be available for the patient, and urinalysis should be performed at least every second month to check for signs of infection. The upper urinary tract, the bladder shape, and residual urine should be checked every six months. Physical examination and laboratory assessments of blood and urine should take place every year. Any sign indicating a risk factor warrants specialized investigation and/or referral to a specialist.

SUMMARY

Neurogenic bladder dysfunction comprises a spectrum of diseases that can be categorized into two broad subgroups: (i) failure to empty urine properly, and (ii) failure to store urine adequately. With careful history taking and physical examination, and the prudent use of UDS, the specific abnormality in a given patient can usually be identified. Previously, supravesical urinary diversion was the common means of managing most patients with complicated neurogenic bladder disease. Newer therapeutic modalities have obviated the need for this approach except under the most unusual of circumstances. For patients with bladder emptying problems, intermittent self-catheterization and/or pharmacotherapy have offered effective therapy for most conditions. When these approaches have failed, external sphincterotomy has proved useful in selected adults, and cutaneous vesicostomy in children. In patients with bladder storage dysfunction, intermittent self-catheterization has again proved useful in many, either alone or in combination with various forms of pharmacologic manipulation. When these approaches have failed or proved inadequate, artificial urinary sphincter (AUS) implantation or augmentation cystoplasty are often warranted.

REFERENCES

1. Zderic SA, Chacko S, DiSanto ME, Wein AJ. Voiding function: relevant anatomy, physiology and molecular aspects. In: Gillenwater JY, Grayback JT, Howards SS, Mitchell ME, eds. Adult and Pediatric Urology. Philadelphia: Lippincott, Williams and Wilkins, 2002:1061.
2. Tanagho TA. The anatomy, and physiology of micturition. Clin Obstet Gynecol 1978; 5:3.
3. Gosling JA, Chilton CP. The anatomy of the bladder, urethra and pelvic floor. In: Mundy AR, Stephenson TP, Wein AJ, eds. Urodynamics: Principles, Practice and Application. London: Churchill Livingston, 1984:3.
4. El Badawi A. Autonomic muscular innervation of the vesical outlet and its role in micturition. In: Himnam F Jr, ed. Benign Prostatic Hypertrophy. Berlin: Springer-Verlag, 1983:330.
5. Torrens M, Morrison JFB. The physiology of the urinary bladder. Berlin: Springer-Verlag, 1987:1.
6. Hinman F Jr. Syndromes of vesical incoordination. Urol Clin North Am 1980; 7:311.
7. Gosling JA, Dixon JS. The structure and innervation of smooth muscle in the wall of the bladder neck and proximal urethra. Br J Urol 1975; 47(5):549.
8. Bharia NN, Bradley WE. Neuroanatomy and physiology: innervation of the urinary tract:. In: Raz S, ed. Female Urology. Philadelphia: WB Saunders, 1989:12.
9. deGroat WC. A neurologic basis for the overactive bladder. Urology 1997; 50(6A):36.
10. McGuire EJ, Herlihy E. Bladder and urethral responses to sympathetic stimulation. Invest Urol 1979; 17:9.
11. de Groat WC, Booth AM: In: Dyck PK, et al., eds: Peripheral Neuropathy, 2d ed. Philadelphia: WB Saunders, 1984:289.
12. Benson GS. Neurogenic bladder and urinary diversion. In: Miller TA, 2nd ed. Physiology Basis of Surgical Practice.
13. Steers WD, Barrett O, Wein AJ. Voiding dysfunction: diagnosis, classifications and management. In: Gillenwater JY, Grayback JT, Howards SS, Mitchell ME, eds. Adult and Pediatric Urology. Philadelphia: Lippincott, Williams and Wilkins, 2002:1061.
14. Bors E, Comarr AE. Neurologic Urology. Baltimore: University Park Press, 1971.
15. Gibbon NOK. Nomenclature of neurogenic bladder. Urology 1976; 8:423.
16. Krane RJ, Siroky MB. Classification of neuro-urologic disorders. In: Clinical Neuro-Urology. Boston: Little, 1979: Brown.
17. Lapides J. Neuromuscular vesical and urethral dysfunction. In: Campbell MF, Harrison JH, eds. Urology. Vol. 2. 3rd ed. Philadelphia: WB Saunders, 1970.
18. McClellan FC. The Neurogenic Bladder. Springfield, IL: Charles C. Thomas, 1979.
19. Krane RJ, Siroky MB. Classification of neuro-urologic disorders. In: Krane RJ, Siroky MB, eds. Clinical Neuro-Urology. Boston: Little, Brown, 1979:143.
20. Wein AJ. Classification of neurogenic voiding dysfunction. J Urol 1981; 125:605.
21. Baldew J, Van Gelderen HH. Urinary retention without a cause in children. Br J Urol 1985; 55:200.
22. Dolin P, Darby S, Beral V. Paraplegia and squamous cell carcinoma of the bladder in the young women: findings from a case control study. Br J Cancer 1984; 70:167.
23. Jacobs SC, Kaufman JM. Complications of permanent catheter drainage in spinal cord injury patients. J Urol 1978; 119:740.
24. Broecker BH, Klein FA, Hackler RH. Cancer of the bladder in spinal cord injury patients. J Urol 1981; 125:196.
25. Chai T, Chung AK, Belville WD, et al. Compliance and complications of clean intermittent catheterization in the spinal cord injured patient. Paraplegia 1995; 33:161.
26. Timoney AG, Shaw PJ. Urological outcome in female patients with spinal cord injury: the effectiveness of intermittent catheterization. Paraplegia 1990; 28:556.
27. The clinical use of urecholine in dysfunctions of the bladder. J Urol 1949; 62:300.
28. Tahagho E, Schmidt R, Orvis B. Neural stimulation for control of voiding dysfunction: a preliminary report on 22 patients with serious neuropathic voiding disorders. J Urol 1989; 142:340.
29. Schmidt RA. Advances in genitourinary neurostimulation. Neurosurgery 1986; 18:1041.
30. Rijkholl NJM, Wijkstra H, van Kerrebroeck PEV, et al. Selective detrusor activation by sacral ventral nerve-root stimulations: results of intraoperative testing in humans during implantation of a Finetech-Brindley system. World J Urol 1998; 16:337.
31. Madersbacher H, Scott FB. Twelve o'clock sphincterotomy; technique, indications, results. Urol Int 1975; 30:75.
32. Duckett JW Jr. Cutaneous vesicostomy in childhood: the Blocksom technique. Urol Clin North Am 1974; 1:485.
33. Bushman W. Spinal cord Injury. In: Gillenwater JY, Grayback JT, Howards SS, Mitchell ME, eds. Adult and Pediatric Urology. Philadelphia: Lippincott, Williams and Wilkins, 2002:1217.
34. Wyndale JJ, Michelsen D, Van Dromme S. Influence of sacral neuromodulation on electrosensation of the lower urinary tract. J Urol 2000; 163:221–224.

40

Pathophysiology and Management of Head Injury

Egon M. R. Doppenberg, M. Ross Bullock, and William C. Broaddus

INTRODUCTION

Data on multiple causes of death, as collected and provided by the National Center for Health Statistics, show that of all injury-related deaths, at least 28% involve significant injury to the brain (1). The patients at highest risk for brain injury are between 15 and 24 years of age, with males far more often affected than females.

About two million Americans are treated at hospitals in the United States every year because of a head injury, making it the most common cause of death and severe disability in adults under the age of 40 (2,3).

Although 80% to 90% of those patients who are admitted to the hospital with a head injury sustain only a mild or moderate injury, the remainder will sustain permanent disability, or die after mild/moderate injury, due to secondary brain damage, caused by ischemia and/or hematoma (4,5).

The great majority of death and disability occurs in those with severe head injury, which affects 200,000 people per year in the United States. Even in this severe head injury group, about a third of the patients who die will have spoken at some point during their clinical course after the injury, suggesting that secondary mechanisms are responsible for death (4,6,7). This indicates that there is a window of opportunity for intervention to treat the pathophysiology and try to restore normal physiology before secondary insults could potentially further develop. The quest for understanding the derangements in brain physiology after head injury has resulted in many gradual improvements in the medical and surgical treatment of the head-injured patient.

The greatest decrease in mortality due to head trauma has occurred in patients with mild to moderate injuries. In addition to better management strategies, better imaging and diagnostic tools have contributed to the improvement in outcome for these patients (8). However, despite these advances, the outcome for severe head injury patients still remains poor, with death and severe disability affecting close to 50% (6). The limited understanding of the pathophysiological mechanisms following severe head injury is a major reason for this poor outcome after severe head injury. Better strategies to monitor and treat these patients are only possible if the pathophysiology is better understood. In neurotrauma, not only the primary impact injury but also secondary and delayed mechanisms are important to understand and treat, as a means of trying to reduce the damage that results from the injury. The present chapter focuses on these considerations.

PATHOPHYSIOLOGY
General Considerations

Our current understanding of the pathophysiological events in human head injury has been developed mainly from post mortem exams, in vitro and in vivo studies in the laboratory, and studies of head-injured patients during life through imaging and monitoring. Each of these modalities has its limitations in showing the derangements in biological and structural status of the brain after head injury. For example, post mortem studies are limited due to the fact that ischemia is usually far more pronounced due to global, agonal reduction in cerebral blood flow (CBF). Therefore, more subtle and focal ischemic changes, which take place between the time of injury and the actual death, might go undetected. Also, animal models do not exactly mimic the complex mechanisms that occur in human head injury, and most often there is a combination of cascades taking place, which affect one another. Therefore, multiple trauma models are currently in use to address different aspects of trauma (9–11).

The events concerned with intracellular energy metabolism, maintenance of neuronal membrane potential, and homeostasis at synapses all have been shown to play a role in various degrees in the derangements seen after human head injury. Different insults to the brain, from intracranial hematomas/contusions, ischemia or shear injury, result in different types of disturbances of the biological homeostasis of the brain. Most often, these insults play a role simultaneously in varying severity, therefore resulting in a pathophysiological state that evolves from different mechanisms.

Intracranial Hematomas and Contusions

Intracranial hematomas (epidural and subdural hematomas, and hemorrhagic contusions) occur in about 30% to 45% of severely head-injured patients. They are by far the most important cause for preventable delayed secondary brain damage. Epidural and acute subdural hematomas are usually formed within the first hour after the injury, although they may enlarge over time (5,7). These mass lesions compromise the cerebral microcirculation, resulting in secondary ischemia and brain swelling. Subsequently, shifting of the brain occurs, and further occlusion of cerebrospinal fluid (CSF) pathways leads to increased intracranial pressure (ICP). In this way, a vicious cycle can begin with more ischemia and brain swelling.

Epidural hematomas are usually the result of focal impact to the skull with an accompanying fracture of the cranial vault in over 80% of cases (Fig. 1). The middle

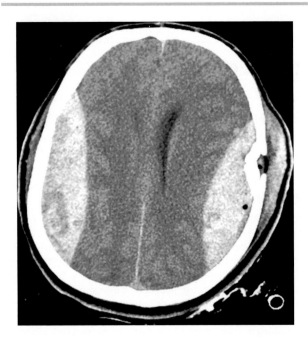

Figure 1 Head computed tomography scan demonstrating bilateral epidural (lentiform-shaped) hematomas with obvious depressed skull fracture over the left convexity.

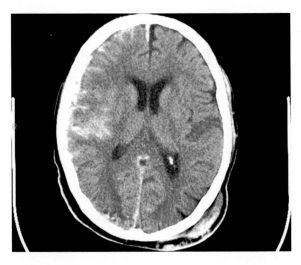

Figure 2 Traumatic subarachnoid hemorrhage over the right convexity, with associated small acute subdural hematoma.

meningeal artery is classically involved with temporal bone fractures, although venous hemorrhage can also cause or contribute to epidural hematomas. These hematomas can rapidly enlarge due to the frequent "arterial" nature of the bleeding and therefore, emergent evacuation is usually indicated. When evacuated promptly, secondary injury to the underlying brain can often be prevented, and therefore excellent outcome is frequently possible with this type of hematoma.

The *acute subdural hematoma* is usually caused by the tearing of the bridging veins that enter the sagittal sinus or by bleeding from surface vessels as a result of focal contusions and laceration of the pia (Fig. 2) (5,12). The acute subdural hematoma has a poor prognosis with a 60% rate of death or severe disability (13). Interestingly, over 50% of all patients with an acute subdural hematoma have had a period after the injury during which they were conscious, suggesting that secondary insults are taking place, resulting in further deterioration. One explanation is that in the acute subdural hematoma model in the rat, there is a zone of focal cerebral ischemia underneath the hematoma. In this zone, a sevenfold increase in glutamate was found, leading to increased metabolic activity and further ischemic insults to the brain (10,13,14).

Severe contusions may undergo delayed hemorrhage over the intermediate period from minutes to hours after impact, especially with coagulopathy (Fig. 3). Zones of ischemically damaged pyknotic shrunken neurons and swollen astrocytes are found to extend many millimeters around the margins of contusions, and this is usually associated with reduced CBF and increased metabolism leading to a flow-metabolism mismatch in the "penumbra" surrounding the contusion. This area may be potentially salvageable in the early stages before cell death and necrosis take place. However, the mechanisms involved in this process are not yet fully understood (5,15,16).

Supratentorial contusions and hematomas may induce brain shift either laterally or in a rostrocaudal direction. Lateral shift causes subfalcine herniation with consequent ischemic damage to the cingulate gyrus of the limbic system (6). Uncal transtentorial herniation is a combination of lateral and rostrocaudal shift, which pushes the medial para-hippocampal gyrus of the temporal lobe through the tentorial hiatus alongside the brain stem. This process causes, ipsilaterally, a fixed dilated pupil, as the

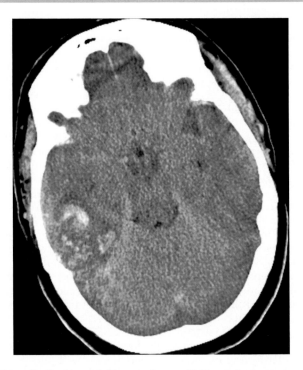

Figure 3 Head computed tomography scan. Right posterior temporal contusions. Note the hypodens surrounding edema.

(A)

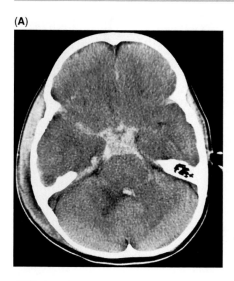

(B)

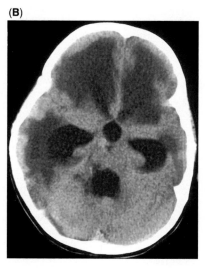

Figure 4 **(A)** Head computed tomography (CT) scan of a two-year old unrestrained female involved in a motor vehicle accident, with massive traumatic subarachnoid hemorrhage. A cerebral angiogram was performed, excluding traumatic aneurysm. **(B)** Same patient two months later. Head CT scan shows severely enlarged ventricles due to communicating hydrocephalus.

cardinal clinical sign for a mass lesion. If there is not an immediate decompression, irreversible ischemic damage occurs within the brain stem, and may be associated with the classical "flame-shaped" hemorrhage of Duret in the pons. Such brainstem hemorrhages are ominous and these patients usually die or remain in a persistent vegetative state. Herniation seldom occurs when ICP is less than 40 mmHg (normal 4–12 mmHg), but it may develop sooner in the presence of mass lesions within the temporal lobe and when there has been swelling of bilateral, frontal, and temporal lobes to cause anteroposterior shift.

Vasospasm has been shown to occur in about 30% of patients with severe head injury (17). It is more frequent in patients who have suffered an extensive subarachnoid hemorrhage (Fig. 4A).

The proximal vessels on the pial surface, or around the Circle of Willis are frequently involved. If imaging studies reveal a significant amount of blood in the subarachnoid spaces in a patient, a cerebral angiogram may be warranted to exclude a traumatic arterial aneurysm. Traumatic aneurysms typically arise at the skull base or from distal anterior or middle cerebral arteries or branches consequent to direct mural injury or to acceleration-induced shear. Once diagnosed, these aneurysms should be treated immediately either through surgical or through an endovascular approach.

Posttraumatic hydrocephalus (accumulation of CSF and dilatation of the cerebral ventricular system) due to traumatic subarachnoid hemorrhage is a frequent phenomenon that clearly worsens outcome. The blood load can cause arachnoiditis of the villi and result in communicating hydrocephalus, in which ventricular dilatation develops due to poor CSF re-absorption (CSF communication between lateral ventricles and spinal canal is retained, hence the name). This can develop as late as two to three years after the initial injury. Therefore, previously head-injured patients who arrest or regress in their recovery should always be evaluated for increased ICP due to hydrocephalus with a head computed tomography (CT) scan (Fig. 4B). A careful evaluation should be made on imaging studies to not confuse the radiographic findings with ex vacuo hydrocephalus (type of hydrocephalus in which CSF replaces

volume of tissue lost) due to brain atrophy, commonly seen in patients with diffuse axonal injury. The imaging studies should show enlargement of the ventricles, transependymal flow, and effacement of the sulci. A spinal tap may be performed to measure the ICP.

Ischemia

Ischemic brain damage is by far the dominant finding in patients who die after head injury, and its distribution is predominantly focal rather than global (6).

The interrelationship between metabolic substrate delivery and substrate demand after traumatic brain injury (TBI) has been extensively studied both in animals and in humans. It is known that in the early phase after TBI, CBF is reduced in up to one-third of the patients (18). At the same time, glutamate release is massively increased in subgroups of patients (19). This increase in glutamate then results in increased neuronal activity. This rise in excitatory activity requires an increased metabolic rate and therefore leads to an increased substrate demand. In the absence of a commensurate increase in local CBF (the source of metabolic substrates), a flow-metabolism mismatch occurs. Massive K^+ efflux has been shown to further increase aerobic metabolism, and thereby further deteriorating the already existing discrepancy between supply and demand in brain metabolism (20). Yoshino et al. showed a marked early increase in glucose utilization, followed by a hypometabolic state after animal brain injury (21). Recently, positron emission tomography (PET) studies have shown a hyperglycolytic state of the brain after severe human head injury in as many as 56% of the patients (22).

Altogether, these results clearly suggest a coupling between an increased metabolism for glucose and increased extracellular release of glutamate after TBI. Thus, the increase in lactate production seen after TBI is explained by a flow-metabolism mismatch because the increase in substrate demand cannot be met by CBF, resulting in anaerobic glycolysis and lactate generation. However, Andersen and Marmarou have shown that lactate generation is increased, following TBI in the cat, as measured by magnetic resonance (MR) spectroscopy, even when CBF was adequate to ensure substrate delivery (23). This implicates factors other than ischemia as a cause of lactate generation after TBI. This early

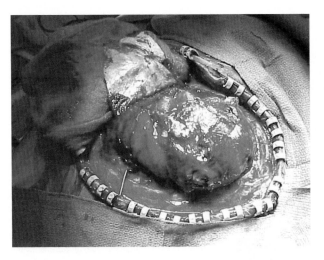

Figure 5 Intraoperative photo of a 56-year-old man who sustained a fall from a ladder. Massive brain swelling is seen, with herniation of brain tissue through the craniotomy defect.

increase in glucose utilization and lactate generation may be a consequence of the massive glutamate release, in accordance with the hypothesis of Pellerin and coworkers. They showed under physiological conditions in an in vitro study that glutamate release due to physiological stimulation results in increased lactate generation (24).

Brain Swelling

Brain swelling, as diagnosed by either cistern effacement on CT scan, or by measured raised ICP, occurs in about 70% of patients with severe head injury at some time during the clinical course (Fig. 5). Even though the cause of brain swelling is not fully understood, four pathophysiological mechanisms are thought to play a role. They are vasogenic edema, cytotoxic edema, vascular engorgement, and venous occlusion.

Delayed blood–brain barrier disruption is seen more frequently in patients with contusions, and is delayed for days after injury (5). In the early phase after injury, cytotoxic edema seems to be the most important component in the development of brain swelling. Vascular engorgement (hyperemia) is usually a reactive response to a prior focal or global ischemic event. One explanation is that the hyperemic response can only occur in relatively normal tissue, which has not undergone severe ischemic damage, sufficient to cause severe edema, and "low density" on CT (18,25). Vascular engorgement may occur in response to the release of mediators such as lactate, H^+, adenosine diphosphate, or inflammatory products, such as cytokines, and substance P.

Diffuse Axonal Injury

Brain tissue does not have the supporting structures that other organs possess, such as a collagen stroma, and it is therefore much more vulnerable to deformation and injury due to forces during trauma. Previously, diffuse axonal injury was thought to be an acute event in which widespread physical and functional disruption of axons occurred at the moment of impact. However, in severely head-injured

patients, probably a relatively small number of axons are immediately torn at the moment of impact, but varying numbers are subjected to stretching due to shear forces. The majority of axonal disruption is then a consecutive delayed event that occurs over the first 24 to 48 hours after injury in humans (26). The pathological hallmark of diffuse axonal injuries is a histological picture described as retraction balls and microglial stars, and they are not seen until 12 to 24 hours after injury.

Diffuse shearing injury causes widespread changes in neurotransmitter function and ionic homeostasis throughout the neuraxis and this results in instantaneous loss of axonal transport, disruption of energy metabolism, and coma or altered consciousness. Several animal studies using fluid percussion injury models have shown that the impact is immediately followed by massive release of neurotransmitters, including catecholamines, acetylcholine, and glutamate into the extracellular space (11,27). This may cause widespread depolarization with the influx of sodium and calcium ions into cells, and efflux of potassium into the extracellular space (20). This may then cause swelling of neurons and glia, which may proceed to cause brain edema, and high ICP.

Penetrating Head Injury

Penetrating head injury has become increasingly common due to increased availability of firearms. The pathophysiology of these injuries is at least in part distinctly different from that of the previously described closed injuries. The injuries can vary from those resulting from low velocity bullets (mostly civilian hand guns) and sharp objects to high velocity bullets and shrapnel in military injuries (Fig. 6A and B). Also, hematomas, cerebral contusions and, sometimes, significant vascular injuries to major blood vessels can occur. Arterial as well as venous injuries may be present, resulting in hematomas and/or subarachnoid hemorrhage. Delayed hemorrhage may also occur, due to development of pseudo aneurysms, arterial dissection, or direct laceration of a vessel or venous sinus. Intracerebral hematomas are the most frequent, followed by subdural hematomas and, to a lesser extent, epidural hematomas (28). High-velocity injuries, especially, may result in extensive fractures of the cranium. Penetrating injuries often cause a variety of injuries, including scalp lacerations and skull base fractures, sometimes complicated by transient or persistent CSF leak.

ICP studies have been carried out in animal models demonstrating an immediate peak in pressure after the injury. The ICP then lowers but does not return to baseline (29). At the same time, cardiac output may be impaired despite adequate fluid resuscitation. This is thought to be due, in part, to the effects on the brain stem either through direct impact or through the "shock wave" produced by the traversing projectile. This combination of increased ICP and decreased cardiac output can significantly impair cerebral perfusion, leading to secondary insults with cerebral ischemia with further brain swelling and further impairment of cerebral perfusion.

GENERAL CONSIDERATIONS IN THE CARE OF THE HEAD-INJURED PATIENT

The acutely injured brain has been shown to be vulnerable to so-called secondary insults (30). These insults include ischemia, hypoxia, and hypercarbia. The latter can result in increased cerebral blood volume and consequent increased ICP, leading in turn to further ischemia. The

(A) 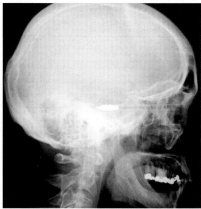   **(B)**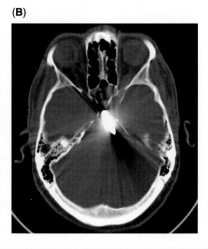

Figure 6 (**A**) and (**B**) Lateral skull X-ray and head computed tomography scan (bone window) showing a 45-year-old man with a penetrating crossbow arrow entering through the right orbit into the skull, ending just anterior of the brain stem. An emergent cerebral angiogram was performed, which was negative for vascular injury. The *arrow* was removed in the operating theatre through the entry site. This patient made a full recovery.

autoregulation of the brain to maintain its constant supply of oxygen and glucose is impaired in the head-injured patient (31). This leads to hypoperfusion of the already vulnerable brain during episodes of systemic hypotension. Several studies have shown that a large number of head-injured patients who present to a trauma center will have hypotension and/or hypoxia, resulting in a tremendous increase in morbidity and mortality from secondary injury to the brain (32–36).

Airway establishment is thus the first priority in the head-injured patient. It should also be kept in mind that approximately 7% of all patients with a Glasgow coma score (GCS) of 8 or less will have a concomitant cervical spine fracture (37). Intubation should be accomplished while the patient is in a rigid collar or preferably with in-line manual cervical immobilization. Recently, several studies have been completed in which inspired oxygen fraction (FiO_2) was increased in the head-injured patient. This improves brain biochemistry and outcome in animals. Also, this maneuver appears not to increase free-radical production in the injured brain tissue in animal models, despite concerns to the contrary (38–40).

Systemic hypotension should be treated aggressively and rapidly, with intravenous fluid (Ringers or normal saline). Hypovolemia is the most common etiology and only rarely is the hypotension caused by the primary brain injury. The choice of intravenous fluids remains a focus of debate. Hypertonic saline has been shown to redistribute extravascular fluids back into the intravascular compartment, resulting in increased cardiac output and blood pressure (41–43). However, in the injured brain where the blood–brain barrier is disrupted, the extracellular fluid may increase with the use of hypertonic solutions, possibly exacerbating the development of cerebral edema. Contrariwise, some data from animal studies show that there may be a beneficial effect on ICP in severely head-injured patients with the use of these hyperosmotic agents (44). To date, there have been no randomized clinical trials to show a clear-cut benefit (as well as risk) for their use in head-injured patients.

The main goal in the multitrauma patient is to maintain normotension and volume expansion to normal status, to ensure adequate cerebral perfusion. It is important to recognize that the fear of inducing increased ICP through aggressive fluid resuscitation to normovolemic status has been proven to be unfounded (45–47).

Furthermore, hyperglycemia may occur in diabetic and nondiabetic patients as a consequence of the physiologic stress response, which is directly related to the severity of the head injury. For this reason, hyperglycemia should be treated appropriately in the acute setting. Increased glucose levels have been linked to a worsened prognosis in animal models of brain injury, independent of the severity of the initial injury (48).

SPECIFIC MANAGEMENT OF THE HEAD-INJURED PATIENT

Historically, head-injured patients have been categorized into three main subgroups using the GCS. Mild injury is categorized as 14 or 15, moderate as 9 to 13, and severe as eight or less. The details of this scoring system are summarized in Table 1.

The neurological examination of the severely head-injured patient in the acute phase consists at a minimum of establishment of this score. Findings should be interpreted with the knowledge of concomitant injuries. These

Table 1 Glasgow Coma Score

Response	Points
Eye opening	
Spontaneous	4
To sound	3
To pain	2
None	1
Motor response	
Obeys commands	6
Localizes pain	5
Normal flexion (withdrawal)	4
Abnormal flexion (decortication)	3
Extension (decerebration)	2
None	1
Verbal response	
Oriented	5
Confused conversation	4
Inappropriate words	3
Incomprehensible sounds	2
None	1

Source: From Ref. 49.

Table 2 Admission Criteria for Patient with Mild Head Injury (GCS 14 or 15)

History of loss of consciousness
Amnesia
No reliable supervision at home
Skull fracture
CSF leak
Penetrating head injury
Abnormal CT scan
No CT scanner available
Deteriorating neurological status
Moderate/severe headache
Inability to reach medical facility quickly while at home
Alcohol/drugs intoxication

Abbreviations: CSF, cerebrospinal fluid; GCS, Glasgow coma score; CT, computed tomography.

include spinal cord injuries, which can impair motor response, as well as trauma to the orbit/globe, possibly resulting in iridoplegia. Also, intoxication by alcohol or other drugs, and the use of paralytics or other pharmacological agents such as atropine need to be taken into consideration. Unfortunately, the use of paralytic agents is very common, making a reliable neurological exam impossible at times.

Eighty percent of the total number of patients with head trauma can be categorized as minor, meaning that they have a GCS of 14 or 15. These patients will need to be admitted for observation if they show any of the findings listed in Table 2.

The moderately head-injured patient with a GCS of 9 to 13 will always require close observation, and therefore admission. These are the patients who require skillful clinical judgment and careful, close observation, usually requiring a stay in the intensive care unit (ICU). If necessary, intubation should be performed to protect the airway, with the use of continuous short-acting sedation (e.g., propofol), to ensure the possibility of intermittent neurological exams.

The severely head-injured patient, with a GCS of eight or less, is by definition comatose. He is unable to follow simple commands. This patient will always require intubation, because studies have shown that up to 30% of these patients are hypoxemic on arrival in the emergency room (35). Furthermore, these patients require continuous evaluation of their volume status and therefore require continuous blood pressure monitoring as well as central venous pressure or pulmonary artery pressure monitoring. Arterial lines and central venous lines are often placed for these reasons.

Mannitol should be given to patients who show localizing signs or who have a fixed pupil when they are hemodynamically stable, even prior to obtaining a CT scan. The osmotic effects of this agent can reduce ICP by decreasing edema in cerebral tissue and therefore decrease ICP and improve cerebral perfusion. Also, the rheological effects play a role in improving cerebral perfusion and therefore potentially might reduce secondary insults to the vulnerable brain (50,51). As soon as the patient is stable enough for transport to the CT scanner, a CT of the head without contrast is to be performed.

In general, patients who have a significant mass lesion, with brain compression and shift of normal structures, and who are not fully neurologically intact, require emergent evacuation of these lesions through a craniotomy or craniectomy. This at times can cause "conflict of interest"

between the neurosurgeon and trauma surgeon. Patients with a high suspicion of a mass lesion resulting in rapidly deteriorating neurological status and who are suspected to have significant thoracoabdominal injury should undergo a chest X-ray and abdominal CT, and, if necessary, should be taken the operating room to prevent secondary neurological deterioration due to cerebral hypoperfusion.

For cranial surgery, the main goal of intervention is to restore the supply of substrate for brain metabolism to the brain. This implies that mass lesions causing increased intracerebral pressure, and therefore decreased cerebral perfusion pressure (CPP), will need to be evacuated as soon as possible. The effects of evacuation of these lesions on brain metabolism have been described in patients recently (52). The exact surgical techniques to perform are beyond the scope of this chapter, but aggressive decompression through a generous bone flap, together with removal of clots and nonviable brain tissue, is mandatory. The neurosurgeon may also elect to leave the bone flap out (craniectomy) for reimplantation later, after subsidence of cerebral edema. In this way, the ICP in the patient will be potentially more manageable in the days after the initial impact when the effects of secondary brain injury may develop. A large bone window can ensure that the swollen brain can expand through the craniectomy site with less chance of dramatic increases in ICP.

Overall surgical treatment of gunshot wounds is similar to closed head injury with a few exceptions. First, the rule also applies that when a mass lesion is present, this should be evacuated when it causes significant compression or shift of brain structures and the patient is not fully neurologically intact. Also, bullet and skull fragments should be removed when they are readily accessible and not located in eloquent areas. Studies from Vietnam War patients have shown that less than 5% of patients developed a delayed cerebral abscess, because aggressive entry and debridement was mandatory (53). However, from these studies it became clear that the presence of retained fragments did not result in increased risk of seizures later in life. Also, obvious nonviable brain tissue in penetrating brain injury should be removed because this may help to manage ICP problems in the days after injury. Finally, dura and scalp repair or reconstruction are helpful in the prevention of CSF leak and/or infection.

The surgical management of stab wounds is grossly similar to that of gun shot wounds. Debridement and dural closure are the goals during surgery. However, removal of a penetrating object requires careful evaluation of the location of the weapon. Evaluation of vascular structures, especially, is important prior to removal. Cerebral angiography or CT-angiography is mandated, whenever major intracranial vessels maybe injured, and should be performed before removal when feasible.

Prophylactic perioperative "triple" antibiotics are frequently used, although no randomized study has shown clinical benefit.

Treatment of Increased Intracranial Pressure

There is no absolute critical threshold for ICP. However, prolonged raised ICP over 20 mmHg has been shown to correlate with worsened outcome in head injury patients, and thus should be treated promptly (54). In conjunction with this, maintenance of adequate CPP (defined as mean arterial pressure minus ICP) has been shown to improve outcome (36). Obviously, every severely head-injured patient requires close monitoring in an ICU with trained nurses who have the expertise to deal with the challenges that come with these patients. Every patient requires continuous monitoring of all "basic" vital signs, including ventilation parameters [oxygen saturation and end tidal carbon dioxide (CO_2)], arterial blood pressure, and central venous pressure. Furthermore, ICP needs to be monitored and any elevation should be aggressively treated.

Intracranial hypertension can lead to further damage through direct mechanical impact during herniation of brain tissue as well as through further decrease of blood flow, which in turn leads to ischemia. The goal of treatment is to prevent these events. Currently several devices are available commercially to monitor the ICP reliably.

Patients who should be considered for this type of monitoring are the ones with a GCS of 8 or less. Also, patients with a moderate head injury and an abnormal CT, who cannot be neurologically evaluated due to other factors, should undergo ICP monitoring. An intraventricular catheter (ventriculostomy) may be used for this purpose as previous studies and experience have validated (55). Also available are intraparenchymal transducer-tipped monitors that are more easily inserted and may be useful in patients with small ventricles. The ventriculostomy is advantageous in that it can allow treatment of elevated ICP by CSF drainage. However, the procedure to place the catheter is slightly more invasive and difficult. Both monitoring modalities are an acceptable way of following the ICP.

The treatment of increased ICP is best done by a stepwise process. First and foremost, one should ensure that any increase in ICP is not due to non-neurological causes such as inadequate ventilation, labile blood pressure, agitation, or pain. Positioning with slight elevation of the head of the bed (approximately 20 degrees) can be helpful, and the use of constricting devices, such as tight cervical collars, or tape to secure the endotracheal tube around the neck, should be avoided. Second, the possibility of an expanding mass lesion needs to be ruled out through a head CT. When a ventriculostomy is in place the next step is to drain CSF to treat raised ICP. Mannitol can be given, with monitoring of electrolytes and renal function after each dose.

One should also consider that patients with unexplained raised ICP do not have subclinical seizures, which may occur despite anticonvulsant therapy. Evaluation of intractable ICP elevation may also require evaluation of serum anticonvulsant levels, as well as an electroencephalogram (EEG) to exclude seizures.

If the above-mentioned measures do not control the ICP, sedation and paralysis are indicated. The benefit of this is twofold. These measures will decrease cerebral metabolic rate, and ventilation is more easily managed. The arterial oxygen and CO_2 partial pressures can now be more effectively controlled. For sedation, several agents can be used. First, morphine will act as both a sedative and pain reliever. However, it should not be used unless the head-injured patient is intubated and ventilated, due to the potential increase in arterial CO_2. Sedatives such as propofol or midazolam decrease the cerebral metabolic rate and therefore decrease the amount of metabolic substrate delivery that is required by the brain to maintain homeostasis. This is especially of value because there may already be a flow-metabolism mismatch present in the injured brain. Propofol has the advantage that it is very short acting and therefore can be stopped intermittently to examine the patient. Midazolam is longer acting but is currently less expensive, and

has the theoretical advantage of reducing seizure activity, which may not be clinically noticeable. Because these sedatives have no analgesic effect, a pain reliever such as morphine should always be used in conjunction with either of these agents. All of these agents may cause hypotension to some extent, and close monitoring of the blood pressure should be maintained.

Paralytic agents are also frequently used, in conjunction with sedatives and analgesia for optimal ventilation, CO_2 control, and reduction of elevated ICP. Vecuronium is one example of a short-acting nondepolarizing neuromuscular blocker that can be given by continuous intravenous administration. The use of an external nerve stimulator allows for monitoring adequate levels of paralysis.

Hyperventilation is a means of decreasing ICP. However, there is now more and more evidence that aggressive and/or prolonged hyperventilation causes cerebral vasoconstriction, decreases CBF, and therefore worsens outcome (56,57). The use of moderate hyperventilation is appropriate and can be extremely helpful to treat elevated ICP. The recommended lower threshold for arterial CO_2 is 30 to 32 mmHg (55).

Mean arterial pressure needs to be maintained to ensure adequate CPP. This is primarily done by preventing/treating hypovolemia. If there is doubt about the volume status of the patient, a Swan–Ganz catheter can be used. Usually normovolemia or slight hypervolemia will ensure adequate CPP when ICP is treated. If further increase in mean arterial blood pressure is needed to maintain CPP, pressors may be used. Dopamine and/or phenylephrine are generally effective in doing so. Dobutamine might be used in patients with decreased cardiac output. In general, based on anecdotal evidence, a CPP over 70 mmHg is accepted as adequate for the severely head-injured patient without signs of vasospasm.

Moderate hypothermia (32–33°C) has failed to show improved outcome in severely head-injured patients in a recent clinical trial (58). However, it may reduce ICP. This is at least in part due to decreasing cerebral metabolic rate and possibly subsequently reducing the release of excitatory amino acids such as glutamate (59). However, the side effects are significant; they include cardiac arrhythmias and increased risk of systemic infections due to suppression of the immune system, as well as coagulopathies. Nevertheless, the use of hypothermia remains to be more fully evaluated, as a potentially useful tool whenever the above-described measures fail to control the raised ICP.

Other Measures to Reduce ICP

Further measures to reduce ICP may be used after the above-described treatments have failed to improve the intracranial hypertension. Their efficacy is less well proven.

Decompressive craniectomies are used to give the injured brain "space to swell" as a method to reduce the ICP. A large bone flap is created and the dura is patched with a graft. The brain can now herniate out through the defect. There is some evidence that this measure improves outcome both in terms of morbidity and mortality (60).

Induced barbiturate coma is a way to minimize brain activity and therefore the need for substrate delivery, which is compromised in these patients. It requires bedside EEG monitoring to regularly evaluate brain activity. In this way, the cerebral metabolic rate is reduced and the existing flow-metabolism mismatch is positively influenced (61). Unfortunately, this comes with the risk of major complications, such as reduced cardiac output, myocardial infarction, and serious systemic infections, and is therefore reserved for situations when all other measures have failed.

There is no role for corticosteroid use in the treatment of raised ICP in the severely head-injured patient (62). It is now clear that the edema resulting from trauma to the brain is cytotoxic in nature and therefore not susceptible to the use of steroids that mainly acts on vasogenic edema (63).

Pharmacologic Intervention

As previously stated, both shearing injury and ischemic damage have been shown to result in calcium-mediated damage to intracellular structures, massive release of glutamate, and also generation of free radicals (64–66). Selective pharmacological antagonists for both presynaptic release and postsynaptic receptor binding of glutamate have been developed.

The most powerful evidence in support of glutamate-induced neurotoxicity in focal ischemia comes from many neuroprotection studies, performed with different *N*-methyl-D-aspartate (NMDA) and non-NMDA glutamate antagonists (67–69). NMDA antagonists are most effective when administered before the insult (especially competitive antagonists), but others have been effective when given up to two hours after the ischemic event. Newer glutamate antagonists, which block release of glutamate from presynaptic vesicles, may also show protection after global ischemia, which could not be demonstrated with the previous NMDA antagonists.

Unfortunately, trials in humans using free-radical scavengers and glutamate antagonists so far have not shown significant benefit. Clearly, it is now becoming accepted that mechanism-driven trials in which individual pathophysiological mechanisms are targeted may be preferable in this heterogeneous patient population. The degree of brain penetration, the safety and tolerability of the compound, and end points used for outcome assessment are major influences upon the success of these new drugs.

MONITORING THE INJURED BRAIN

In the last two decades, major advances have been made in understanding the pathophysiological mechanisms following TBI. However, the impact on clinical monitoring and management of cerebral metabolism in severely head-injured patients of this progress has been modest. The only well-established and accepted method currently available is ICP monitoring. Unfortunately, this is a relatively crude technique, and changes in ICP are only seen after major changes and derangements previously have taken place in the physiology and anatomy of the brain. As a consequence, only the final results (brain swelling) of the disturbance of the intracranial milieu are monitored. Clinically, this means that measurements that are being taken to intervene in these harmful events are by definition done relatively late, and may be too late to prevent permanent injury. This lack of sufficient monitoring for brain injury has resulted in a search for more elegant techniques, in the last decade.

Another important issue is the time course of events, following trauma. However, in humans, it remains impossible to study the first events taking place immediately after injury. New monitoring devices and imaging techniques have improved the assessment of brain physiology; they include microdialysis to study the extracellular fluid content in the brain parenchyma. In this way, one can assess the levels of metabolites, amino acids, and free-radical production in the injured brain. Measurements of brain oxygen, CO_2, and pH are also being performed more widely and this has the advantage that continuous monitoring of brain is available in the ICU (19,39,40). Also, more advanced imaging studies are now deployed to evaluate these patients. For example, PET scanning is now used to study the brain metabolism in combination with its supply of nutrients, as well as MR diffusion-weighted imaging to evaluate the water/edema seen after head injury in the parenchyma (16,22,63). However, the data and results of these new monitoring devices require careful evaluation and interpretation before their use in actual treatment of these patients will be clinically helpful.

Notwithstanding these findings, before any conclusions can be made from data obtained by means of these devices, a thorough and critical analysis is needed to better understand what exactly is measured and whether or not these labor-intensive and expensive techniques are helpful in understanding and treating the derangements in physiology seen after TBI.

SUMMARY

Traumatic brain injury is the most common cause of death and severe disability in adults under the age 40. Because a third of patients who die from this injury will have spoken at some point during their clinical course, it seems clear that a window of opportunity exists to treat the underlying pathophysiology before secondary insults develop, which irreversibly prevent restoration of normal physiology. Although much still needs to be learned about the cascade of events that are set in motion following a traumatic brain injury, our current understanding of the pathophysiologic mechanisms that previously led to death or severe disability has been effectively utilized to institute treatment strategies so that many of these patients can become productive individuals leading normal or near normal lives. Thus, adequate fluid resuscitation to ensure euvolemia, antiseizure prophylaxis, and optimization of the blood's oxygen-carrying capacity have all contributed greatly to managing these patients. Other therapeutic measures that have evolved include the prevention of hyperthermia, maintenance of cerebral perfusion pressure above 70 mmHg, and sedation. Early ventricular drainage for elevated ICP and mild hyperventilation (PCO_2 of approximately 35 mmHg) have been found to be especially beneficial in patients with a GCS of less than 8. As research continues in this important area of human disease, it is envisioned that other therapeutic alternatives will become available to salvage even more individuals in the early stages of injury when the "window of opportunity" is most advantageous.

REFERENCES

1. Collins JG. Types of injuries by selected characteristics: United States, 1985–1987. Vital Health Stat 1990; 10:175.
2. Kalsbeek WD, Mclaurin RL, Harris BS. The national head and spinal cord injury survey: major findings. J Neurosurg 1980; (Suppl 53):S19–S31.
3. Kraus JF. Epidemiology of head injury. In: Cooper PR, ed. Head Injury. Baltimore: Williams & Wilkins, 1993:1–25.
4. Blumberg PC, Jones NR, North JB. Diffuse axonal injury in head trauma. J Neurol Neurosurg Psychiatry 1989; 52:38–842.
5. Bullock R, Teasdale GM. Head injuries-surgical management: traumatic intracranial hematomas. In: Braakman R, ed. Vinken

and Bruyn's Handbook of Clinical Neurology. 24. Head Injury. Amsterdam: Elsevier Science Publishers, 1991:249–298.

6. Adams JH, Graham DI, Gennarelli TA. Head injury in man and experimental animals: neuropathology. Acta Neurochir 1983; 32:15–30.

7. Jennett B, Carlin J. Preventable mortality and morbidity after head injury. Injury 1978; 10:31–39.

8. Klauber MR, Marshall LF, Luerssen TG, Frankowski R, Tabaddor K, Eisenberg HM. Determinants of head injury mortality: importance of the low risk patient. Neurosurgery 1989; 24:31–36.

9. Kirino T, Tamura A, Sano K. Delayed neuronal death in the rat hippocampus following transient forebrain ischemia. Acta Neuropathol 1984; 64:139–147.

10. Miller JD, Bullock R, Graham DI, Chen MH, Teasdale GM. Ischemic brain damage in a model of acute subdural hematoma. Neurosurgery 1990; 27:433–439.

11. Hayes R, Jenkins LW, Lyeth BG. Neurotransmitter mediated mechanisms of traumatic brain injury: acetylcholine and excitatory amino acids. J Neurotrauma 1992;(Suppl 9):S173.

12. Stone JL, Rifai MHS, Sugar O, Lang RGA, Oldershaw JB, Moody RA. Subdural hematomas. Acute subdural hematoma: progress in definition, clinical pathology, and therapy. Surg Neurol 1983; 19:216–231.

13. Chen MH, Bullock R, Graham DI, Miller JD, Mcculloch J. Ischemic neuronal damage after acute subdural haematoma in the rat: effects of pretreatment with a glutamate antagonist. J Neurosurg 1991; 74:944–950.

14. Kuroda Y, Inglis FM, Miller JD, Mcculloch J, Graham DI, Bullock R. Transient glucose hypermetabolism after acute subdural hematoma in the rat. J Neurosurg 1992; 76:944–950.

15. Schroder ML, Muizelaar JP, Kuta AJ. Documented reversal of global ischemia immediately after removal of an acute subdural hematoma. J Neurosurg 1994; 80:324–327.

16. Hovda DA, Lee SM, Smith ML, et al. The neurochemical and metabolic cascade following brain injury: moving from animal models to man. J Neurotrauma 1995; 12:903–906.

17. Cruz J. Brain ischemia in head injury. J Neurosurg 1993; 78: 522–523 (letter).

18. Bouma GJ, Muizelaar JP, Stringer WA, Choi SC, Fatouros PP, Young HF. Ultra-early evaluation of regional cerebral blood flow in severely head-injured patients using xenon-enhanced computerized tomography. J Neurosurg 1992; 77:360–368.

19. Zauner A, Daugherty WP, Bullock MR, Warner DS. Brain oxygenation and energy metabolism: Part I. biological function and pathophysiology. Neurosurgery 2002; 51(2):289–301; discussion 302.

20. Katayama Y, Becker DP, Tamura T, Hovda DA. Massive increases in extracellular potassium and the indiscriminate release of glutamate following concussive brain injury. J Neurosurg 1990; 73:889–900.

21. Yoshino A, Hovda DA, Kawamata T, Katayama Y, Becker DP. Dynamic changes in local cerebral glucose utilization following cerebral conclusion in rats: evidence of a hyper- and subsequent hypometabolic state. Brain Res 1991; 561(1):106–119.

22. Bergsneider M, Hovda DA, Shalmon E, et al. Cerebral hyperglycolysis following severe traumatic brain injury in humans: a positron emission tomography study. J Neurosurg 1997; 86(2):241–251.

23. Andersen BJ, Marmarou A. Post-traumatic selective stimulation of glycolysis. Brain Res 1992; 585(1–2):184–189.

24. Magistretti PJ, Pellerin L, Rothman DL, Shulman RG. Energy on demand. Science 1999; 283(5401):496–497.

25. Muizelaar JP, Marmarou A, De Salles AAF, Ward JD, Zimmermann RS. Cerebral blood flow and metabolism in severely head-injured children. Part 1: relationship with GCS score, outcome, ICP and PVI. J Neurosurg 1989; 71:63–71.

26. Povlishock JT, Erb DE, Astruc J. Axonal response to traumatic brain injury: reactive axonal change, deafferentation, and neuroplasticity. J Neurotrauma 1992; 9(Suppl 1):S189–S200.

27. Faden AI, Demediuk P, Panter SS, Vink R. The role of excitatory amino acids and NMDA receptors in traumatic brain injury. Science 1989; 244:798–800.

28. Clark WC, Muhlbauer MS, Watridge CB, Ray MW. Analysis of 76 civilian craniocerebral gunshot wounds. J Neurosurg 1986; 65(1):9–14.

29. Crockard HA, Brown FD, Johns LM, Mullan S. An experimental cerebral missile injury model in primates. J Neurosurg 1977; 46(6):776–783.

30. Jenkins LW, Moszynski K, Lyeth BG, et al. Increased vulnerability of the mildly traumatized rat brain to cerebral ischemia: the use of controlled secondary ischemia as a research tool to identify common or different mechanisms contributing to mechanical and ischemic brain injury. Brain Res 1989; 477(1–2): 211–224.

31. Bruce DA, Langfitt TW, Miller JD, et al. Regional cerebral blood flow, intracranial pressure, and brain metabolism in comatose patients. J Neurosurg 1973; 38(2):131–144.

32. Shackford SR, Mackersie RC, Davis JW, Wolf PL, Hoyt DB. Epidemiology and pathology of traumatic deaths occurring at a Level I Trauma Center in a regionalized system: the importance of secondary brain injury. J Trauma 1989; 29(10):1392–1397.

33. Graham DI, Ford I, Adams JH, et al. Ischaemic brain damage is still common in fatal non-missile head injury. J Neurol Neurosurg Psychiatr 1989; 52(3):346–350.

34. Graham DI, Adams JH, Doyle D, et al. Quantification of primary and secondary lesions in severe head injury. Acta Neurochir Suppl (Wien) 1993; 57:41–48.

35. Miller JD, Sweet RC, Narayan R, Becker DP. Early insults to the injured brain. JAMA 1978; 240(5):439–442.

36. Chesnut RM, Marshall LF, Klauber MR, et al. The role of secondary brain injury in determining outcome from severe head injury. J Trauma 1993; 34(2):216–222.

37. Hills MW, Deane SA. Head injury and facial injury: is there an increased risk of cervical spine injury? J Trauma 1993; 34(4):549–553; discussion 553–554.

38. Doppenberg EM, Rice MR, Di X, Young HF, Woodward JJ, Bullock R. Increased free radical production due to subdural hematoma in the rat: effect of increased inspired oxygen fraction. J Neurotrauma 1998; 15(5):337–347.

39. Menzel M, Doppenberg EM, Zauner A, et al. Cerebral oxygenation in patients after severe head injury: monitoring and effects of arterial hyperoxia on cerebral blood flow, metabolism and intracranial pressure. J Neurosurg Anesthesiol 1999; 11(4): 240–251.

40. Menzel M, Doppenberg EM, Zauner A, Soukup J, Reinert MM, Bullock R. Increased inspired oxygen concentration as a factor in improved brain tissue oxygenation and tissue lactate levels after severe human head injury. J Neurosurg 1999; 91(1):1–10.

41. Smith GJ, Kramer GC, Perron P, Nakayama S, Gunther RA, Holcroft JW. A comparison of several hypertonic solutions for resuscitation of bled sheep. J Surg Res 1985; 39(6):517–528.

42. Auler JO Jr, Pereira MH, Gomide-Amaral RV, Stolf NG, Jatene AD, Rocha e Silva M. Hemodynamic effects of hypertonic sodium chloride during surgical treatment of aortic aneurysms. Surgery 1987; 101(5):594–601.

43. Battistella FD, Wisner DH. Combined hemorrhagic shock and head injury: effects of hypertonic saline (7.5%) resuscitation. J Trauma 1991; 31(2):182–188.

44. Gunnar W, Jonasson O, Merlotti G, Stone J, Barrett J. Head injury and hemorrhagic shock: studies of the blood brain barrier and intracranial pressure after resuscitation with normal saline solution, 3% saline solution, and dextran-40. Surgery 1988; 103(4):398–407.

45. Schmoker JD, Shackford SR, Wald SL, Pietropaoli JA. An analysis of the relationship between fluid and sodium administration and intracranial pressure after head injury. J Trauma 1992; 33(3):476–481.

46. James HE, Schneider S. Effects of acute isotonic saline administration on serum osmolality, serum electrolytes, brain water content and intracranial pressure. Acta Neurochir Suppl (Wien) 1993; 57:89–93.

47. Rosner MJ, Daughton S. Cerebral perfusion pressure management in head injury. J Trauma 1990; 30(8):933–40; discussion 940–941.

48. Lam AM, Winn HR, Cullen BF, Sundling N. Hyperglycemia and neurological outcome in patients with head injury. J Neurosurg 1991; 75(4):545–551.

49. Teasdale G, Jennett B. Assessment of coma and impaired consciousness. A practice scale. Lancet 1974; 2:81.

50. Burke AM, Quest DO, Chien S, Cerri C. The effects of mannitol on blood viscosity. J Neurosurg 1981; 55(4):550–553.

51. Muizelaar JP, Wei EP, Kontos HA, Becker DP. Mannitol causes compensatory cerebral vasoconstriction and vasodilation in response to blood viscosity changes. J Neurosurg 1983; 59(5):822–828.

52. Doppenberg EM, Watson JC, Broaddus WC, Holloway KL, Young HF, Bullock R. Intraoperative monitoring of substrate delivery during aneurysm and hematoma surgery: initial experience in 16 patients. J Neurosurg 1997; 87(6):809–816.

53. Rish BL, Dillon JD, Weiss GH. Mortality following penetrating craniocerebral injuries. An analysis of the deaths in the Vietnam Head Injury Registry population. J Neurosurg 1983; 59(5):775–780.

54. Marshall LF, Smith RW, Shapiro HM. The outcome with aggressive treatment in severe head injuries. Part I: the significance of intracranial pressure monitoring. J Neurosurg 1979; 50(1):20–25.

55. Bullock R, Chesnut RM, Clifton G, et al. Guidelines for the management of severe head injury. Brain Trauma Foundation. Eur J Emerg Med 1996; 3(2):109–127.

56. Marion DW, Bouma GJ. The use of stable xenon-enhanced computed tomographic studies of cerebral blood flow to define changes in cerebral carbon dioxide vasoresponsivity caused by a severe head injury. Neurosurgery 1991; 29(6):869–873.

57. Muizelaar JP, Marmarou A, Ward JD, et al. Adverse effects of prolonged hyperventilation in patients with severe head injury: a randomized clinical trial. J Neurosurg 1991; 75(5):731–739.

58. Marion DW. Moderate hypothermia in severe head injuries: the present and the future. Curr Opin Crit Care 2002; 8(2):111–114.

59. Busto R, Dietrich WD, Globus MY, Ginsberg MD. The importance of brain temperature in cerebral ischemic injury. Stroke 1989; 20(8):1113–1114.

60. Gaab MR, Rittierodt M, Lorenz M, Heissler HE. Traumatic brain swelling and operative decompression: a prospective investigation. Acta Neurochir Suppl (Wien) 1990; 51:326–328.

61. Eisenberg HM, Frankowski RF, Contant CF, Marshall LF, Walker MD. High-dose barbiturate control of elevated intracranial pressure in patients with severe head injury. J Neurosurg 1988; 69(1):15–23.

62. Dearden NM, Gibson JS, McDowall DG, Gibson RM, Cameron MM. Effect of high-dose dexamethasone on outcome from severe head injury. J Neurosurg 1986; 64(1):81–88.

63. Marmarou A, Portella G, Barzo P, et al. Distinguishing between cellular and vasogenic edema in head injured patients with focal lesions using magnetic resonance imaging. Acta Neurochir Suppl 2000; 76:349–351.

64. Benveniste H, Drejer J, Schousboe A, Diemer NH. Elevation of the extracellular concentrations of glutamate and aspartate in rat hippocampus during transient cerebral ischemia monitored by intracerebral microdialysis. J Neurochem 1984; 43:1369–1374.

65. Butcher SP, Bullock R, Graham DI, Mcculoch J. Correlation between amino acid release and neuropathological outcome in rat striatum and cortex following middle cerebral artery occlusion. Stroke 1990; 1:1727–1733.

66. Shimada N, Graf R, Rosner G, Heiss WD. Ischemia-induced accumulation of extracellular amino acids in cerebral cortex, white matter, and cerebrospinal fluid. J Neurochem 1993; 60:66–71.

67. Meldrum B. Protection against ischemic neuronal damage by drugs acting on excitatory neurotransmission. Cerebrovasc Brain Metab Rev 1990; 2:27–57.

68. Bullock R, Fujisawa H. The role of glutamate antagonists for the treatment of CNS injury. J Neurotrauma 1992(suppl 9): S3443–S3461.

69. Kuroda Y, Fujisawa H, Strebel S, Graham DI, Bullock R. Effect of neuroprotective N-methyl-d-aspartate antagonists on increased intracranial pressure: studies in the rat acute subdural hematoma model. Neurosurgery 1994; 35:106–112.

41

Spinal Cord Injury

Kangmin Lee and R. Scott Graham

INTRODUCTION

Spinal cord injury (SCI) is an important cause of morbidity and mortality in modern society. Injuries result in significant and permanent neurologic deficits, and the functional consequences can be devastating. Although there are a number of causes, the focus of this chapter is on traumatic cord injury. The following is a summary of the prevailing concepts in pathophysiology and treatment of traumatic SCI.

EPIDEMIOLOGY

Approximately 10,000 SCIs occur each year in the United States. Although the true incidence is unknown, the range has been estimated to be between 28 and 55 per million population (1,2). Data from the Olmsted County, Minnesota study from 1935 to 1981 reported an age- and sex-adjusted incidence rate of 54 injuries per million population. This figure was reduced to 34 per million if immediate deaths before reaching the hospital were not included (3). In comparison, the incidence rate in other developed countries ranges from 2 to 53 per million population (1,4). In the United States, injuries are due to motor vehicle accidents (36–48%), violence (5–29%), falls (17–21%) and recreational activities (7–16%) (5–7). Average age at time of injury for each cause of SCI was 30 years for motor vehicle accidents, 27 years for violence, 24 years for recreational activities, and 42 years for falls. Monetary costs are significant, and a recent study estimated total direct costs in the value of the 1995 dollar for all causes of SCI in the United States at $7.7 billion (6).

Data from the Major Trauma Outcome Study (5) showed that traumatic SCI occurred in one of every 40 injured persons presenting to trauma centers. Patients with SCI and multitrauma were more common than those with isolated spine injuries. In those with isolated SCI, 65% had cervical cord injury. In those with multiple injuries, cervical cord injury was seen in 52%. Motor vehicle accidents, pedestrian accidents, and falls were associated with the highest percentage of cervical injury, 56% to 65%. Gunshot wounds and motorcycle accidents were associated with the lowest percentage of cervical injury, 30% and 39% respectively (5).

PATHOPHYSIOLOGY

Similar to current concepts in traumatic brain injury, the pathophysiology of SCI involves a primary mechanism with initial mechanical damage and local tissue destruction and a complex cascade of secondary mechanisms. The secondary mechanisms are initiated by the primary injury and encompass systemic, cellular, and biochemical processes that lead to cellular damage and cell death. The severity of primary injury can have prognostic significance, while the severity of secondary injury can limit the potential of rehabilitative processes and contribute to the overall morbidity and mortality.

Primary Mechanisms

The primary mechanical injury occurs by way of penetration, laceration, shear, compression, and/or distraction. Depending on the mechanism of injury, duration can be either transient or persistent. Impact with transient compression is often seen with hyperextension injuries in individuals with underlying spondylosis. Burst fractures with canal compromise, fracture dislocations, and disc ruptures are examples of impact with persistent compression. The extent of the primary injury can be used to group patients into severity categories (neurologic grades). Mechanism of injury, spinal level, and neurologic grade on admission to the hospital are important prognostic indicators (8,9). The American Spinal Injury Association (ASIA) SCI grading scale is a common scale used for this purpose (Table 1).

The primary mechanical injury has a tendency to damage the central gray matter of the cord. This is probably due to its softer consistency and greater vascular requirements. Within the white matter, axons that pass through the injured segment may be physically disrupted or exhibit a decrease in myelin thickness, resulting in impaired conduction of action potentials. Mechanical disruption of venules and capillaries may result in early hemorrhage within the cord. Larger vessels such as the anterior spinal artery are relatively spared from direct mechanical injury, and the location of vascular damage is primarily in the intramedullary vascular system (8–10).

Secondary Mechanisms

The initial mechanical insult serves as the impetus for a cascade of deleterious events. Current understanding of these

---

Table 1 American Spinal Injury Association Impairment Scale

- *A = Complete*: No motor or sensory function is preserved in the sacral segments S4–S5
- *B = Incomplete*: Sensory but not motor function is preserved below the neurological level and includes the sacral segments S4–S5
- *C = Incomplete*: Motor function is preserved below the neurological level, and more than half of key muscles below the neurological level have a muscle grade less than 3
- *D = Incomplete*: Motor function is preserved below the neurological level, and at least half of key muscles below the neurological level have a muscle grade of 3 or more
- *E = Normal*: Motor and sensory function are normal

mechanisms has evolved over the past three decades, and many corollaries to recent advances in cerebral trauma and ischemia have helped to mold understanding. Numerous studies have shown that the central nervous system responds to injury in a prototypical fashion. Vascular changes, ionic derangements, neurotransmitter accumulation, free-radical production, and apoptosis as well as various other cellular and biochemical events have been shown to compromise the spinal cord after injury (Table 2). A thorough discussion of each event is beyond the scope of this chapter, but animal models point to posttraumatic ischemia as a common denominator for secondary processes following SCI. Other mechanisms such as glutamate excitotoxicity and free-radical and apoptotic mechanisms have been shown to be important sequellar posttraumatic ischemia.

Spinal Cord Ischemia

Following the initial insult, a number of systemic and local events are initiated; of primary concern is an acute reduction in blood flow to the area of the lesion. Although the precise mechanism behind this hypoperfusion is unclear, it has been shown to persist in rats and monkeys for at least 24 hours. It is speculated that vasospasm or possibly the release of a vasoactive amine is partially responsible. However, it is likely that the mechanism involves a combination

Table 2 Primary and Secondary Mechanisms of Spinal Cord Injury

Primary injury mechanisms
Compression
Impact
Missile
Stretch
Laceration
Shear
Secondary injury mechanisms
Systemic effects
    Heart rate: brief tachycardia and then prolonged bradycardia
    Blood pressure: hypertension and then prolonged hypotension
    Decreased peripheral vascular resistance
    Decreased cardiac output
    Increased catecholamine release and then decrease
    Hypoxia
    Hyperthermia
Local vascular changes
    Loss of autoregulation
    Neurogenic shock
    Hemorrhage (especially in the gray matter)
    Loss of microcirculation
    Vasospasm
    Thrombosis
Electrolyte changes
    Increased intracellular calcium
    Increased intracellular sodium
    Increased extracellular potassium
Neurotransmitter accumulation
    Catecholamines
    Glutamate
Arachidonic acid release
Free-radical production
Eicosanoid production
Lipid peroxidation
Edema
Apoptosis

Source: Modified from Ref. 11.

of processes such as hemorrhagic ischemia, thrombosis, endothelial swelling, and edema formation (8,10,12).

Normally, gray and white matter blood flow is maintained at a 3:1 ratio, reflecting the greater vascular requirements of the gray matter relative to the adjacent white matter. The metabolic requirement of spinal cord gray and white matter has important implications for understanding the response to secondary injury. Perfusion to the peripheral white matter is typically reduced within the first five minutes postinjury, with a return to normal flow within 15 minutes. In contrast, hemorrhage is often seen in the central gray matter within the first five minutes postinjury, and perfusion virtually halts within the hour. This vascular stasis has been confirmed using microangiography and fluorescent tracer studies (11,13). It is believed that the central gray matter is irreversibly damaged within the first hour after injury, and that white matter damage is irreversible beyond the first 72 hours postinjury (8).

Studies by Tator and Koyanagi using silicone rubber microangiography have elucidated some of the vascular changes in SCI. They have shown that the central area of the cord is supplied by the sulcal arteries and encompasses the anterior gray matter, the anterior half of the posterior gray matter, the inner half of the anterior and lateral white columns, and the anterior half of the posterior white columns. The peripheral white matter and the posterior portion of the posterior gray matter are supplied by the posterior spinal and pial arteries. There is also an intermediate watershed zone representing the vascular overlap between the pial and sulcal arterial systems (10). This anatomical arrangement may help to explain the hemorrhagic and ischemic changes seen in the gray matter of traumatized spinal cords. Hemorrhage in the gray matter of traumatized spinal cords has been well documented in clinical and experimental studies. Sekhon and Fehlings have proposed that it may be that obstruction or mechanical disruption of the anterior sulcal arteries leads to the hemorrhagic necrosis and subsequent central myelomalacia seen at the site of injury (11).

Impaired Autoregulation

In many cases of SCI, the primary injury is not severe enough to cause the hemorrhagic necrosis discussed above. However, vascular alterations with cord ischemia have been shown to occur in milder forms of injury as well.

Loss of autoregulatory homeostasis (i.e., a decreased ability to maintain constant blood flow over a wide range of pressures) and endothelial dysfunction are additional vascular sequelae of SCI. Endothelial dysfunction leads to increased vascular permeability with the leakage of proteinaceous fluid into the interstial space and edema at the injury site. Endothelial damage occurs early after injury, and cellular changes are observed in as early as one to two hours (12). In the setting of a markedly swollen spinal cord, ischemia may be further aggravated by the limited cross-sectional area of the bony spinal canal and rising tissue pressures. Neurologic deterioration due to spinal cord edema is well documented in SCI and may be potentially reversible in the subacute period.

Neurotransmitter Excitotoxicity

The notion of glutamate excitotoxicity is a concept that has been implicated in the pathophysiology of head trauma. As the primary excitatory neurotransmitter in the central nervous system, toxic levels are known to initiate a highly disruptive process known as glutamate excitotoxicity. This process has been implicated in SCI as well. Glutamate has been shown to flood out of injured spinal neurons, axons, and astrocytes, causing an over excitation of neighboring neurons. Glutamate acts on N-methyl-D-aspartate (NMDA) and non-NMDA receptors on neurons or glial cells, causing an influx of Ca^{2+}. This triggers a series of highly destructive events directly and indirectly through the production of numerous agents such as free-radicals. The ischemia that results from vascular changes may also be instrumental to glutamate accumulation. Hypoxia results in adenosine triphosphate depletion, which then impairs cellular uptake mechanisms. Glutamate receptor activation also appears to result in early accumulation of intracellular Na^+ and Ca^{2+} as well (8).

Free-Radical–Mediated Cell Injury

Free-radical formation is also known to be an important secondary injury mechanism in SCI. After injury, oxygen free-radicals are formed and have been shown to cause cell membrane peroxidation. Important phospholipid-dependent enzymes can be impaired disrupting ionic gradients and causing membrane lysis (8).

Apoptosis

Recent research has implicated the process of programmed cell death in a number of neurological disorders including SCI. Apoptosis can be triggered by a variety of initiating factors including cytokine release, inflammatory insults, free-radical damage, and excitotoxicity. Days or weeks after initial trauma, a wave of cell suicide or apoptosis sweeps through neurons, oligodendrocytes, microglia, and, perhaps, astrocytes. This wave can affect cells as many as four segments away from the initial trauma site (8,14,15).

Additional Pathophysiologic Considerations
Spinal Shock

The term "neurogenic" or "spinal shock" has been used in several ways. For references made in this chapter, spinal shock will refer to a sudden loss of peripheral vascular tone. This results in pooling of blood in the extremities and inadequate central venous return. The unopposed parasympathetic effects of the vagus nerve results in bradycardia, which is in marked contrast to the tachycardia associated with hemorrhagic shock. Although the pathophysiology of spinal shock is not completely understood, it is most probably due to a conduction blockade resulting from cellular K^+ ion leakage. Impulse conduction would then be dependent upon restoration of normal Na^+ and K^+ gradient (16).

EVALUATION
Neurologic Assessment

All individuals with SCI should have a thorough neurologic examination. Traumatic brain injury has been shown to coincide with nearly half of all traumatic SCIs (17). Multilevel injury to the spine is also common, and a thorough examination of the entire spine is warranted, once the diagnosis of SCI is made. The evaluation of a spinal cord–injured patient begins by determining whether the injury is complete or incomplete. This information is important for determining prognosis and often useful clinically in determining the risk and benefit ratio of early surgery

(18,19). According to the ASIA, an SCI is defined as complete when there is absence of sensory and motor function in the lowest sacral segment. In contrast, an incomplete injury is defined by the presence of sensory and/or motor function at the lowest sacral segment ("sacral sparing"). Sacral sensation includes pinprick or light touch sensation at the anal mucocutaneous junction, as well as deep anal sensation with digital exam. The test of motor function is marked by the ability to contract the external anal sphincter on digital exam. Among the SCI classification schemes, there is some disagreement regarding definition of the "level" of a SCI. ASIA criteria defines neurologic level as the most caudal segment of the spinal cord with normal sensory and, at least, antigravity strength (greater than or equal to three out of five motor strength) on both sides (20).

The severity of SCI is rated by a simple five-level (A–E) ASIA impairment scale (Table 1). The standards for neurological and functional classifications of SCI assess motor function in ten muscle groups (arms: C5-T1, legs L2-S1) and sensation (light touch and pinprick) in 28 dermatomes (C2-S4/5) on both sides of the body (Fig. 1).

CLASSIC INJURY PATTERNS

Age, level of injury, and neurologic grade have been demonstrated to be the most important premorbid factors for survival after acute SCI (21). Approximately 45% of SCIs are complete injuries (22). These injuries are more likely to be due to fracture dislocations rather than burst or compression fractures (17). It is generally accepted that thoracic injuries will more frequently produce complete SCIs than cervical or lumbar injuries. When complete injuries do occur, the greatest neurologic recovery occurs in the more rostral injuries. Cervical injuries therefore, have exhibited the greatest degree of recovery following initial complete injury (23).

Complete Spinal Cord Injuries

Complete injuries at or above the C3 level result in immediate respiratory arrest, and death will result within minutes if artificial respiration is not instituted (Fig. 2). Additionally, high cervical cord injuries are frequently accompanied by hemodynamic instability, which is the result of sudden loss of sympathetically mediated vasomotor tone, blood loss, and bradycardia from unopposed parasympathetic activity. Patients with complete injuries between the C5 and T1 levels can usually be weaned from mechanical ventilation. Prolonged ventilator support and possible tracheostomy are often necessary during the initial weeks following the injury. The reversible dysfunction of the spinal cord above the level of the injury is presumably due to effects of edema and the secondary pathways discussed earlier in this chapter.

Central Cord Syndrome

Central cord syndrome is one of the most well-recognized and common SCI injury patterns. The pattern of injury is classically characterized by disproportionate motor deficit in the upper extremities as compared to deficit in the lower extremities. Bladder dysfunction and varying degrees of sensory loss below the level of the lesion also occur. Injury typically involves hyperextension in the cervical spine,

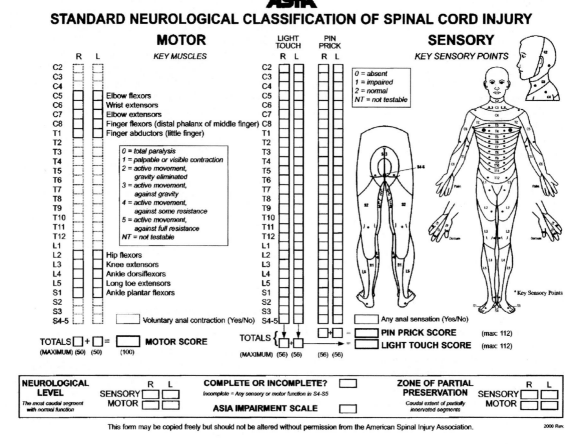

Figure 1 Standard neurological classification of spinal cord injury.

usually in association with preexisting cervical spondylosis. These injuries can occur even without apparent damage to the bony spine, but have also been described in association with vertebral body fractures or fracture-dislocation injuries. The natural history of recovery following central cord syndrome is a gradual return of neurologic function in the early stages followed by a plateau. Some patients experience late deterioration often complicated by spasticity

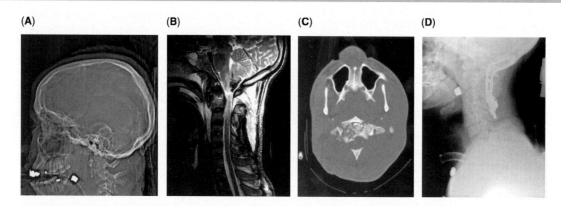

Figure 2 Radiographic findings in a case of complete spinal cord transection just below the cervicomedullary junction due to a gunshot wound. (**A**) computed tomography (CT) scout tomogram shows the bullet fragment at the angle of the mandible and a markedly comminuted C2 fracture. (**B**) Sagittal T2-weighted magnetic resonance imaging demonstrates transection of the spinal cord and thick subarachnoid hemorrhage from injury to the vertebral artery. (**C**) Axial CT shows the comminuted fractures of C1 and C2. (**D**) Postoperative lateral radiograph shows the stabilizing titanium loop and tracheostomy in place.

or pain. Although the prognosis is favorable, recovery is usually incomplete. Impaired intrinsic muscle function of the hand is a common permanent deficit with this injury pattern. Several retrospective studies have shown that increased age and poor initial motor exam are the most important predictive variables (Fig. 3) (24–29).

Conus Medullaris Syndrome

Conus medullaris syndrome is another common SCI pattern (Fig. 4). This syndrome most often results from thoracolumbar burst fractures. It involves injury to the distal portion of the spinal cord at the T12 through L2 spinal levels. The clinical presentation of this injury can occasionally be confused with cauda equina syndrome. Patients typically present with severe lower back pain at the level of the fractured vertebra. This may be accompanied by neuropathic pain in the thighs, distal lower extremities, and perineum. Motor and sensory deficits are also seen in a roughly symmetric distribution involving the distal lower extremities. Bladder and sphincter function are usually impaired with severe injuries and are the least likely deficits to regain function.

Anatomically, the injured neural elements consist of the terminal portion of the conus (central nervous system) and the cauda equina (peripheral nervous system). The prognosis is relatively good for these injuries, and many patients can regain some useful function in the lower extremities (Fig. 5). The L1 vertebra is involved in the majority of thoracolumbar fractures. At this level, many of the axons for motor neurons to the lower extremities have exited the cord. Permanent impairment is most likely to be seen in the L5 and sacral spinal cord levels, i.e., pelvis instability during gait (glutei), ankle weakness (anterior tibialis, extensor hallius longus, and gastroc), and sphincter dysfunction. Anecdotal data from case series indicate a benefit for early decompression and stabilization of these injuries (30–36).

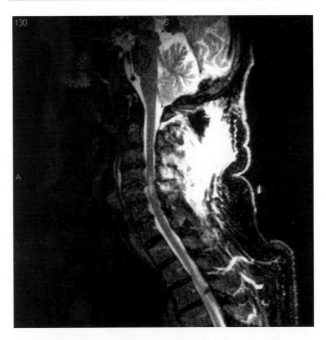

Figure 3 Sagittal T2-weighted magnetic resonance image of a typical central cord injury in a 67-year-old male. Patient presented with severe symmetric weakness of the deltoids and biceps with preservation of normal intrinsic hand and lower extremity motor function. The patient had brief paraesthsias over the upper portions of the arms, which returned to normal sensory exam shortly after the injury. Note the preexisting spondylosis and high signal within the spinal cord at the C4-5 level.

Cauda Equina Syndrome

Although cauda equina syndrome is not a SCI, it is included in this discussion because it is a relatively common

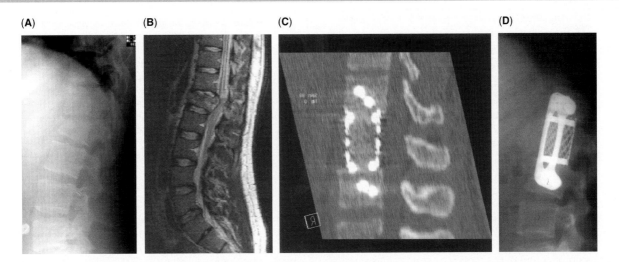

(A) **(B)** **(C)** **(D)**

Figure 4 L1 burst fracture with a complete conus medullaris syndrome; 22-year-old male who fell 30 feet from a tree. **(A)** Plain film of the lumbar spine shows an L1 burst fracture with kyphotic angulation. **(B)** The sagittal magnetic resonance imaging scan demonstrates compression of the conus and cauda equina with high signal in the distal portion of the spinal cord. **(C)** Reformated sagittal computed tomography scan shows the decompression of the spinal canal and correction of the kyphotic deformity. **(D)** The six-month postoperative X-ray shows the final alignment of the repair. The patient underwent early surgery and at six months was ambulatory with bilateral ankle braces.

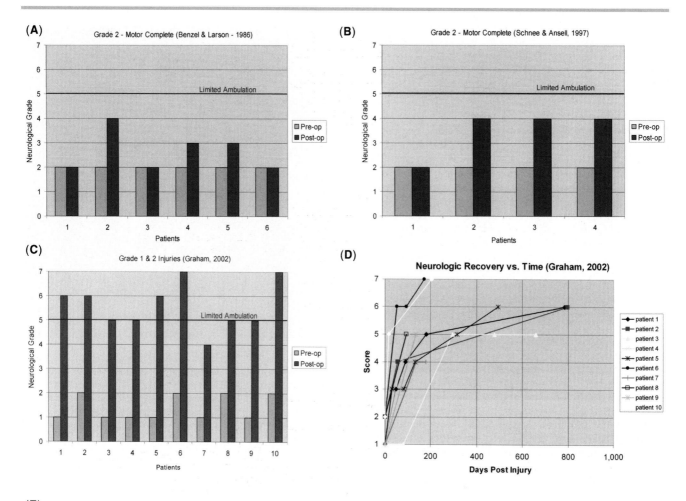

(E)

Benzel-Larson Neurological Grading System

Grade	Description
1	Complete functional neural transection: no motor or sensory function
2	Motor complete: no voluntary motor function w/ preservation of some sensation
3	Motor incomplete-nonfunctional: minimal nonfunctional voluntary motor function
4	Motor incomplete-functional (nonambulatory): some functional motor control that is useful but not sufficient for independent walking
5	Motor incomplete-functional (limited ambulation): walking w/ assistance or unassisted, but w/ significant difficulty that limits patients mobility
6	Motor incomplete-functional (unlimited ambulation): difficulty w/ micturation; significant motor radiculopathy; discoordinated gait
7	Normal: neurologically intact or minimal deficits that cause no functional difficulties

Figure 5 (**A–C**) Neurologic grade at presentation and at the final assessment for three case series of conus medullaris injuries. Data from a case series in the mid-1980s. Delayed surgery was considered the standard approach at this time. (**B**) Data from the mid-1990s in this series surgery was preformed in the first week following the injury. (**C**) The senior authors series. Surgery was completed within 24 hour of the injury unless contraindicated. (**D**) Neurologic grade for the authors' series over time. (**E**) Description of the Benzel Larson Grading scale.

compression syndrome. The pattern of neurologic deficits is similar to conus medullaris syndrome. Cauda equina syndrome usually occurs due to acute and severe midline compression of spinal nerve roots, i.e., from a massive disc rupture, most commonly at L4-5 (Fig. 6). This is often superimposed on a preexisting spinal stenosis or spondylosis. In contrast to conus medullaris lesions, pain is often the most prominent symptom and is radicular in nature. Motor and sensory deficits tend to be asymmetric. Urinary retention is the most consistent finding, and "saddle anesthesia"

is the most common sensory deficit. Studies have shown that early surgical decompression, i.e., within 24 to 48 hours of onset is particularly important in avoiding permanent neurologic deficits (37–39). This syndrome is considered a neurosurgical emergency, and recognition of patients with a possible diagnosis of cauda equina syndrome requires immediate evaluation with magnetic resonance imaging (MRI) or myelogram/computed tomography (CT) of the lumbar spine and possible urgent surgical decompression.

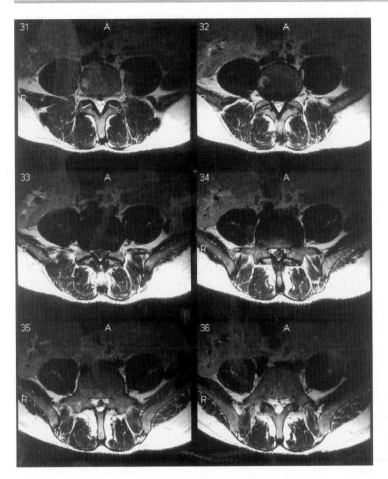

Figure 6 Axial T2-weighted magnetic resonance imaging scan in a patient presenting with cauda equina syndrome due to a large L4-5 herniated disc. Images 31 and 32 show the spinal canal with cerebrospinal fluid and nerve roots in cross section. Images 33 and 34 show the spinal canal completely obstructed with a large free fragment of disc material.

Brown-Sequard Syndrome

This syndrome occurs as a result of focal dysfunction in a hemisection of the spinal cord. Classically it was described following penetrating trauma of the cord and is reported to occur in 2% to 4% of traumatic SCIs. Although data for true incidence is lacking, it is more commonly seen in its partial form due to asymmetric distortion of the cord from compression by meningiomas, nerve sheath tumors, and disc herniations. Neurologic symptoms consist of ipsilateral loss of proprioceptive and vibratory sense as well as motor paralysis due to interruption of the posterior column and corticospinal tracts. Contralateral findings are loss of pain and temperature sensation one to two segments below the lesion. Light touch is preserved however, due to redundant ipsilateral and contralateral paths (anterior spinothalamic tracts). The prognosis for this syndrome is the best of any of the incomplete SCIs. The vast majority of patients with this syndrome will regain the ability to ambulate independently, as well as regain anal and urinary sphincter control. Sensory abnormalities are reported to persist in a higher percentage of patients with Brown-Sequard myelopathy, in comparison to other patterns of myelopathy (40–42).

Anterior Cord Syndrome

The anterior two-thirds of the spinal cord is affected by this syndrome. The lesion is typically associated with cord infarction in the territory of the anterior spinal artery. This syndrome may occur from occlusion of the anterior spinal artery or from anterior cord compression, e.g., by a dislocated bone fragment or by traumatic disc herniation. Posterior column function is typically preserved, while spinothalamic and corticospinal tract damage results in loss of pain and temperature sensation as well as paraplegia. Lesions higher than C7 can result in quadriplegia. This syndromes has the worst prognosis of the incomplete injuries. Only 10% to 20% recover functional motor control.

Posterior Cord Syndrome

This syndrome is relatively rare and is most frequently associated with isolated damage to the posterior components of the spinal cord. There is usually loss of dorsal column function producing pain and parasthesias in the neck, upper arms, and torso. There also may be mild paresis of the upper extremities.

Posttraumatic Myelopathy Associated with Syringomyelia

Posttraumatic syringomyelia is reported to develop in 0.3% to 3.2% of SCIs (43). Typically, the posttraumatic syrinx becomes symptomatic in a delayed and insidious fashion after a few years of stable neurologic functioning. Patients present with signs and symptoms of progressive neurologic dysfunction and pain. The presentation in order of frequency is local pain, loss of motor function, loss of sensory function, increased spasticity, autonomic dysreflexia, hyperhydrosis, increased sphincter dysfunction, increasing respiratory insufficiency, and Horner's syndrome. Diagnosis is confirmed by MRI or in rare cases in which an MRI cannot be obtained by delayed (1–2 hour) postmyelogram CT scanning (the delay allows time for the myelogram dye to enter the syrinx cavity). Controversy exists as to optimal management of the syrinx. Hence, many procedures have been used to treat them, including syringosubarachnoid shunting, syringopleural and syringoperitoneal shunting, fenestration of the syrinx, neurolysis of cord with duraplasty, and correction of spinal deformity. Each of these procedures has purported advantages, and specific associated risks and all of them have relatively high reoccurrence rates.

IMAGING

The diagnosis and management of SCI will often require a variety of imaging studies. If cervical injury is suspected, anteroposterior, lateral, and open-mouth radiographs can be used to define integrity and alignment of bony structures. Under these circumstances, it is important to adequately visualize the entire cervical spine from occiput to T1. Gentle traction on the patient's arms or alternatively a "swimmers view" can usually accomplish this. The negative predictive value of a normal three-view cervical spine series has been reported to range from 93% to 98% in several Class I studies (44–46). Dynamic views with flexion/extension can also be helpful and may aid in the diagnosis of ligamentous laxity. However, these views may be contraindicated, if neurologic dysfunction is noted. For suspected injuries in the thoracic or lumbar spine, anteroposterior and lateral films may be obtained.

CT is superior to plain radiography and provides better resolution of bony structures. These films may be obtained when a fracture is suggested by plain film or full visualization of the cervical spine to T1 is not attainable. Sagittal and coronal reconstructions may be done if further anatomic information is required or the patient is a surgical candidate. Ideally, scan thickness in the cervical spine is 1.5 mm and 3 mm in the lumbar and thoracic spine. High-quality images can diagnose cord hemorrhages, mass effects, and disc herniations. Although invasive, the combination of myleography and CT remains the gold standard for visualization of cord or nerve root compression. This combination is especially useful when MRI is contraindicated or spinal instrumentation distorts imaging with artifact.

If it is crucial to visualize the spinal cord, MRI remains the best available study. MRI would also be indicted, if evidence of SCI is evident without skeletal abnormality. Each examination should include at least one T1-weighted sagittal sequence, a sagittal sequence with water displayed bright (T2 spin echo, fast spin echo, or gradient refocused images), and a series of axial images. There has been a recent interest in diffusion weighted imaging of the spinal cord, given its significant value in detecting early brain injury.

MANAGEMENT OF ACUTE SCI
Initial Management

The major causes of immediate death in SCI are aspiration and shock (47). Therefore, the basic tenets of advanced trauma life support procedure are critical in the management of SCI. It is also important to be aware that SCI may mask other injuries, i.e., abdominal injuries below the level of the SCI.

Immobilization prior to and during extrication in the fields is important to prevent passive or active movements of the spine. However, if cardiopulmonary resuscitation is necessary, resuscitation takes precedence. The patient should be placed on a backboard with sandbags placed on both sides of the head. A 3-in. strip of adhesives tape from one side of the backboard to the other across the forehead and allows movement of the jaw and provides access to the airway. The backboard may be maintained to facilitate transfer, i.e., to the CT table. However, once urgent studies are completed, the backboard should be removed as soon as possible. Early removal will improve patient comfort and reduce the risk of decubitus ulcers.

It is important to avoid hypotension in SCI patients, and systolic blood pressure should be maintained above 90 mmHg. Therapeutic measures may include the use of pressors, fluids, and military antishock trousers (MAST). MAST immbolizes the spine and can also compensate for decreased or lost muscle tone in the patient and prevent venous pooling. Dopamine may be used if necessary and is the pressor of choice. Vasomotor collapse may also contribute loss of temperature control, and the patient should be provided with cooling or warming blankets.

Adequate oxygenation is also vital, and oxygen via nasal cannula or face mask should be delivered if intubation is not indicated. If intubation is required, then chin lift (not jaw thrust), without neck extension should be performed. If at all possible, tracheostomy or cricothyroidotomy should be avoided, because it may compromise later anterior cervical surgical approaches.

Nasogastric tube suctioning is also often implemented in order to prevent vomiting and aspiration, as well as provide decompression of the stomach. Placement of a Foley catheter is also advised in order to prevent bladder distension from urinary retention.

Critical Care and Management of Complications

Assuming survival after initial injury, it was commonly believed that renal failure and urinary tract infections were the leading causes of death in SCI patients. However, more recent studies show that pulmonary complications such as pneumonia are the leading cause of death (48). Cardiac dysfunction is also known to be common sequelae of SCI. These life-threatening events may occur episodically despite early resuscitation and initial restoration of cardiopulmonary function. Early detection through cardiopulmonary monitoring in the intensive care unit (ICU) setting can result in improved neurologic recovery. This is especially true for the patient with cervical cord injury above C5. The muscles of the diaphragm are innervated by the phrenic nerve (C3–C5). Injury at or above this level can thus result in apnea and require ventilator support for the patient. However, even for injuries below C5, respiratory function is often quite compromised. A flaccid paralysis of the intercostal muscles initially occurs—as the diaphragm contracts and descends, the chest wall contracts rather than expands. Forced vital capacity and maximal inspiratory force are reduced by 70%. Eventually, the intercostal muscles become spastic, and respiratory function improves. Approximately five months after injury, the forced vital capacity and the maximal inspiratory force are about 60% of predicted preinjury levels. Perhaps the most significant respiratory complication associated with SCI is ventilator-associated pneumonia. Common organisms include *Streptococcus pneumoniae, Haemophilus influenzae, Pseudomonas aeruginosa,* and *Staphylococcus aureus.* Cardiovascular irregularities such as hypotension, arrhythmias, and even cardiac arrest can also occur. Therapy involves resuscitation with pressors as well as hemodynamic monitoring with a pulmonary artery catheter. Unfortunately, there is no clear consensus on the appropriate end point for volume resuscitation (49).

Patients with SCI have a threefold increase in risk for thromboembolic disease (50). Given this risk, it is important to initiate prophylaxis in the ICU setting. Methods available include pneumatic compression devices, stockings, anticoagulants, and inferior vena cava (IVC) filters. Mechanical devices are clearly advisable but insufficient for prophylaxis. Low-molecular-weight-heparin can be added unless contraindicated, in which case an IVC filter may be a consideration. Studies of patients with spinal injuries have shown that the risk of deep venous thrombosis is quite low in the first 72 hours after SCI (51). Anticoagulation may then be held for this initial period. Thereafter it is advisable that anticoagulation be started. Although the optimum length of stay in the ICU is unknown, the available studies show that cardiac and respiratory events often occur within the first week or two after injury. This time frame may be dependent upon the severity of SCI (52).

Management of Instability

Clinical stability can be defined as the ability of the spine to resist displacement, under physiologic loads and prevent irritation or injury to the spinal cord or nerve roots. In general, the spine can be viewed as being composed of three columns. Injury to any two of these columns may be regarded as sufficient to raise suspicion for clinical instability. The anterior column is composed of the anterior longitudinal ligament, the anterior half of the vertebral body, and the anterior half of the annulus fibrosis. The middle column includes the posterior half of the vertebral body, the posterior half of the annulus fibrosis, and the posterior longitudinal ligament. The posterior column consists of the spinous processes, laminae, articular processes, and the ligamentum flavum. After SCI, the objective of management is to mechanically limit displacement and pharmacologically prevent the progression of secondary damage. Mechanical stabilization can be provided by bed rest, external orthoses, or immediately through internal fixation.

Cervical traction/reduction restores and maintains normal alignment immobilizing the spine to prevent further injury. Reduction may decompress the spinal cord or roots. The timing of reduction is controversial, and it is contraindicated in atlanto-occipital dislocation as well as type IIA or III Hangman's fractures. A number of cranial tongs are available, and Gardner-Wells tongs are probably the most common tongs in use. The tongs are placed in the temporal ridge (above the temporalis muscle) 3 to 4 cm above the pinna. Traction weight is 5 lbs for the upper C-spine and 10 lbs for lower levels. Halo rings can be used initially for traction or later as a postoperative measure for immobilization.

The indications and timing of surgical decompression for acute SCI have been controversial for many years. Considering the steady improvement in surgical technology and widespread capability to quickly complete the trauma evaluation and obtain necessary studies and radiographic evaluations, early surgery for SCI is becoming increasingly feasible. Therefore, we will briefly consider the knowledge base regarding the timing of decompression of acute SCIs.

There have been multiple animal studies providing persuasive evidence that SCI has a reversible component. Studies in primates, cats, dogs, and rodents have convincingly shown that early decompressive intervention enhances neurologic recovery in SCI. A study by Dimar et al., using a weight drop model, showed that neurologic recovery in rats was significantly dependent on time to decompression after injury (53).

Unfortunately, clinical studies in humans have been less compelling. Basic definitions such as the time frame for "early surgery" have yet to be established. Due to the lack of Class I data, the clinical benefits of surgery for fracture dislocations are difficult to determine. However, there have been several reports of cervical cases receiving significant benefit after decompression with early traction. Overall, the data is lacking and is insufficient to produce practice guidelines or standards.

Posttraumatic Deformity

The vast majority of unstable spinal injuries are recognized in the acute setting. However, posttraumatic kyphosis may develop in a delayed fashion. Most cases occur in patients initially managed "nonoperatively" with spinal bracing. Additionally, it is also seen in operatively managed cases that fail to fuse properly or at levels not incorporated into the fusion. The most common presenting symptom is spinal pain, followed by postural changes, increasing neurologic deficits, and, rarely, the development of a syrinx. Treatment is indicated for cases that demonstrate progression over time and for those associated with new or progressive neurologic deficits. A localized kyphotic deformity greater than 30 degrees is associated with an increased risk of chronic pain (54).

Pharmacologic Management

There has been a significant evolution of thought in the pathophysiology of SCI within the past two decades. This has led to further progress in the surgical and medical treatment of SCI. The primary strategy has focused on limitation of secondary injury mechanisms.

The first positive clinical trial [National Acute Spinal Cord Injury Study (NASCIS II)] for pharmacological treatment for SCI was reported in 1990 (55,56). In a multicenter clinical study, high-dose methylprednisolone was reported to reduce disability when given within eight hours of trauma. Although the mechanism of action has yet to be fully elucidated, it is thought to act in part to reduce swelling, inflammation, glutamate release, and free-radical accumulation. Results of the latest NASCIS III (57,58) showed that high-dose methylprednisolone, started between three and eight hours after injury and continued for 48 hours, was reported to preserve more motor function than treatment for 24 hours. It has become common practice in the United States to administer methylprednisolone (30 mg/kg) within the first eight hours after injury. Treatment started within the first three hours is continued (5.4 mg/kg/hr) for 24 hours. Treatment initiated between three and eight hours is continued for 48 hours.

However, the use of methylprednisolone remains a topic of heated debate and is a controversial issue in many countries. Treatment with high-dose methylprednisolone is associated with a number of complications, including gastric bleeding and wound infection. The NASCIS studies have opened the door for investigation of other pharmacologic agents such as monosialoganglioside sodium (GM1 ganglioside), naloxone, and tirilazad.

REHABILITATION

Early and aggressive rehabilitation is an important key to prevention of medical complications after SCI and for the psychological adjustment of the patient. Following intensive inpatient rehabilitation, most individuals with SCI continue their rehab work in an outpatient setting with physical, occupational, and vocational therapist. However, yearly follow-ups with functional assessments by physiatrists or other specialists with knowledge of SCI are recommended.

Urinary and sexual dysfunction are areas of great concern for the SCI patients. Urinary tract infections are common and more often result in serious complications of sepsis and chronic renal insufficiency. Some patients will require chronic suppressive antibiotics. Many males with SCI struggle with erectile and ejaculatory dysfunction. Semen quality and motility can be reduced secondary to recurrent urinary tract infections, drugs, prostatic fluid stasis, retrograde ejaculation, and changes in seminal fluid. Treatment for these issues can be medical or surgical and are beyond the scope of this chapter. However, pregnancy rates for individuals with SCI have improved over the past decade and are between 10% and 60%.

ADVANCED THERAPIES

There have been a number of advancements in the management of the very severe disabilities encountered by individuals with SCI. These therapies attempt to limit the effect of SCI on everyday life and maximize existing functional ability. Common options include tendon transfer, functional electrical stimulation, and the use of adaptive equipment and environmental control devices.

Tendon transfer is an underused treatment for restoration of limited but useful motor function. Muscle groups that serve redundant roles (e.g., elbow flexion is done by both biceps brachii and brachioradialis) may be used for transfer. The muscles need to be sufficiently strong (at least four out of five) and should be trained to take over lost movements. The most frequent tendon transfers are used for elbow/wrist extension and thumb flexion.

Transcutaneous or direct electrical stimulation of muscle can be achieved, but is only useful when lower motor neurons and peripheral nerves are still intact. Denervated muscle cannot be used because the currents necessary would be injurious to the muscle. Transcutaneous electrical activation of leg muscles has been used for strength training and cardiovascular conditioning. Bowel and bladder control is perhaps the function that is the most distressing to individuals with SCI, and functional electrical stimulation is an available therapy for this issue.

RESTORATION OF FUNCTION

Fortunately, the damaged spinal cord does not require complete restoration in order to improve quality of life. Small anatomical gains are known to produce a disproportionate improvement in function. Fewer than 10% of functional long-tract connections are required to allow locomotion. This level of connectivity often remains in the doughnut-like outer rim of white matter following trauma. However, axons in this outer rim may be nonfunctional as a result of demyelination. Therefore, remyelination of intact connections is one reasonable approach to improvement of function.

Spinal Cord Regeneration

With the increase in understanding of the pathologic processes involved in SCI and neurobiology of the developing spinal cord obtained over the past two decades, research efforts have begun to focus on strategies to promote regeneration of the injured spinal cord. Clinically useful drugs and techniques are still many years into the future, and a complete discussion of the topic is beyond the scope of this chapter. However, we will highlight some of the hurdles to be overcome. Effective neuroprotection to limit the degree of secondary injury, preserve intact axonal fibers crossing the injured segment, and the neuronal cell bodies at the level of the cord injury is a prerequisite for spinal cord regeneration therapies. The NASCIS II and NASCIS III were positive clinical trials for the use of methylprednisolone and tirilazad as neuroprotectants, following SCI (55–58). However, more effective drugs and timing of decompressive surgery have yet to be established.

The regenerative capacity of the central nervous system poses additional substantial hurdles: (i) injured neurons have a limited intrinsic ability to regenerate, and (ii) the area of the injury into which they must send axons is not permissive to regeneration. Intense research efforts are underway focusing on the development of neurotrophic agents and delivery mechanisms to enhance the regenerative capacity of the injured neurons. Stem cell, Schwann cell, and olfactory-ensheathing cell transplantation are under investigation as potential means of bridging the gliotic barrier at the site of the injury (59). Complicating the matter further, animal studies demonstrate that the regenerative responses to both neurotrophic factors and tissue grafting decline precipitously within a few weeks to months following the initial injury (11,59–61).

SUMMARY

The pathophysiology of SCI involves a sequence of primary and secondary mechanisms. Although the primary injury is fated by the mechanism of the trauma, the progression of secondary injury may be amenable to therapy. Secondary mechanisms of injury encompass an array of interwoven biochemical and cellular processes. Our continued understanding of these mechanisms will provide a framework for future medical and surgical treatment paradigms.

REFERENCES

1. Burke DA, Linden RD, Zhang YP, Maiste AC, Shields CB. Incidence rates and populations at risk for spinal cord injury: a regional study. Spinal Cord 2001:274–278.
2. Kraus JF, Franti CE, Riggins RS, Richards D, Borhani NO. Incidence of traumatic spinal cord lesions. J Chronic Dis 1975:471–492.
3. Griffin MR, O'Fallon WM, Opitz JL, Kurland LT. Mortality, survival and prevalence: traumatic spinal cord injury in Olmsted County, Minnesota, 1935–1981. J Chronic Dis 1985:643–653.
4. Botterell EH, Jousse AT, Kraus AS, Thompson MG, Wynne-Jones M, Geisler WO. A model for the future care of acute spinal cord injuries. Can J Neurol Sci 1975:361–380.
5. Burney RE, Maio RF, Maynard F, Karunas R. Incidence, characteristics, and outcome of spinal cord injury at trauma centers in North America. Arch Surg 1993:596–599.
6. DeVivo MJ. Causes and costs of spinal cord injury in the United States. Spinal Cord 1997:809–813.

7. McDonald JW, Sadowsky C. Spinal-cord injury. Lancet 2002: 417–425.

8. Dumont RJ, Okonkwo DO, Verma S, et al. Acute spinal cord injury, part I: pathophysiologic mechanisms. Clin Neuropharmacol 2001:254–264.

9. Marino RJ, Ditunno JF, Donovan WH, Maynard F. Neurologic recovery after traumatic spinal cord injury: data from the model spinal cord injury systems. Arch Phys Med Rehabil 1999:1391–1396.

10. Tator CH, Koyanagi I. Vascular mechanisms in the pathophysiology of human spinal cord injury. J Neurosurg 1997:483–492.

11. Sekhon LH, Fehlings MG. Epidemiology, demographics, and pathophysiology of acute spinal cord injury. Spine 2001:S2–S12.

12. Sandler AN, Tator CH. Effect of acute spinal cord compression injury on regional spinal cord blood flow in primates. J Neurosurg 1976:660–676.

13. Rivlin AS, Tator CH. Regional spinal cord blood flow in rats after severe cord trauma. J Neurosurg 1978:844–853.

14. Abe Y, Yamamoto T, Sugiyama Y, et al. Apoptotic cells associated with Wallerian degeneration after experimental spinal cord injury: a possible mechanism of oligodendroglial death. J Neurotrauma 1999:945–952.

15. Shuman SL, Bresnahan JC, Beattie MS. Apoptosis of microglia and oligodendrocytes after spinal cord contusion in rats. J Neurosci Res 1997:798–808.

16. Tator CH. Biology of neurological recovery and functional restoration after spinal cord injury. Neurosurgery 1998: 696–707.

17. Tator CH. Epidemiology and general characteristics of the spinal cord-injured patient. In: Tator C, Benzel EC, eds. Contemporary Management of Spinal Cord Injury: From Impact to Rehabilitation. Park Ridge, IL: American Association of Neurological Surgeons, 2000:9–15.

18. Clinical assessment after acute cervical spinal cord injury. Neurosurgery 2002:S21–S29.

19. Silber JS, Vaccaro AR. Summary statement: the role and timing of decompression in acute spinal cord injury: evidence-based guidelines. Spine 2001:S110.

20. Burns AS, Ditunno JF. Establishing prognosis and maximizing functional outcomes after spinal cord injury: a review of current and future directions in rehabilitation management. Spine 2001:S137–S145.

21. Claxton AR, Wong DT, Chung F, Fehlings MG. Predictors of hospital mortality and mechanical ventilation in patients with cervical spinal cord injury. Can J Anaesth 1998:144–149.

22. Tator CH, Duncan EG, Edmonds VE, Lapczak LI, Andrews DF. Changes in epidemiology of acute spinal cord injury from 1947 to 1981. Surg Neurol 1993:207–25.

23. Tator CH. Spine-spinal cord relationships in spinal cord trauma. Clin Neurosurg 1983:479–494.

24. Guest J, Eleraky MA, Apostolides PJ, Dickman CA, Sonntag VK. Traumatic central cord syndrome: results of surgical management. J Neurosurg 2002:25–32.

25. Newey ML, Sen PK, Fraser RD. The long-term outcome after central cord syndrome: a study of the natural history. J Bone Joint Surg Br 2000:851–855.

26. Tow AM, Kong KH. Central cord syndrome: functional outcome after rehabilitation. Spinal Cord 1998:156–160.

27. Chen TY, Lee ST, Lui TN, et al. Efficacy of surgical treatment in traumatic central cord syndrome. Surg Neurol 1997:435–440.

28. Penrod LE, Hegde SK, Ditunno JF Jr. Age effect on prognosis for functional recovery in acute, traumatic central cord syndrome. Arch Phys Med Rehabil 1990:963–968.

29. Roth EJ, Lawler MH, Yarkony GM. Traumatic central cord syndrome: clinical features and functional outcomes. Arch Phys Med Rehabil 1990:18–23.

30. Aebi M, Mohler J, Zach G, Morscher E. Analysis of 75 operated thoracolumbar fractures and fracture dislocations with and without neurological deficit. Arch Orthop Trauma Surg 1986:100–112.

31. Benzel EC, Larson SJ. Operative stabilization of the posttraumatic thoracic and lumbar a comparative analysis of the Harrington distraction rod and the modified Weiss spring. Neurosurgery 1986:378–385.

32. Jacobs RR, Asher MA, Snider RK. Thoracolumbar spinal injuries. A comparative study of recumbent and operative treatment in 100 patients. Spine 1980:463–477.

33. Jiang JM, Jin DD, Chen JT, et al. Decompression and internal fixation in the treatment of thoracolumbar spine and spinal cord injury: report of 166 cases. Di Yi Jun Yi Da Xue Xue Bao 2002:82–83.

34. McEvoy RD, Bradford DS. The management of burst fractures of the thoracic and lumbar spine. Experience in 53 patients. Spine 1985:631–637.

35. Schnee CL, Ansell LV. Selection criteria and outcome of operative approaches for thoracolumbar burst fractures with and without neurological deficit. J Neurosurg 1997:48–55.

36. Wiberg J, Hauge HN. Neurological outcome after surgery for thoracic and lumbar spine injuries. Acta Neurochir (Wien) 1988:106–112.

37. Kennedy JG, Soffe KE, McGrath A, Stephens MM, Walsh MG, McManus F. Predictors of outcome in cauda equina syndrome. Eur Spine J 1999:317–322.

38. Ahn UM, Ahn NU, Buchowski JM, Garrett ES, Sieber AN, Kostuik JP. Cauda equina syndrome secondary to lumbar disc herniation: a meta-analysis of surgical outcomes. Spine 2000:1515–1522.

39. Shapiro S. Medical realities of cauda equina syndrome secondary to lumbar disc herniation. Spine 2000:348–351.

40. Kobayashi N, Asamoto S, Doi H, Sugiyama H. Brown-Sequard syndrome produced by cervical disc herniation: report of two cases and review of the literature. Spine J 2003:530–533.

41. Kohno M, Takahashi H, Yamakawa K, Ide K, Segawa H. Postoperative prognosis of Brown-Sequard-type myelopathy in patients with cervical lesions. Surg Neurol 1999:241–246.

42. Little JW, Halar E. Temporal course of motor recovery after Brown-Sequard spinal cord injuries. Paraplegia 1985:39–46.

43. Lee TT, Alameda GJ, Camilo E, Green BA. Surgical treatment of post-traumatic myelopathy associated with syringomyelia. Spine 2001:S119–S127.

44. Ajani AE, Cooper DJ, Scheinkestel CD, Laidlaw J, Tuxen DV. Optimal assessment of cervical spine trauma in critically ill patients: a prospective evaluation. Anaesth Intensive Care 1998:487–491.

45. Berne JD, Velmahos GC, El Tawil Q, et al. Value of complete cervical helical computed tomographic scanning in identifying cervical spine injury in the unevaluable blunt trauma patient with multiple injuries: a prospective study. J Trauma 1999: 896–902.

46. MacDonald RL, Schwartz ML, Mirich D, Sharkey PW, Nelson WR. Diagnosis of cervical spine injury in motor vehicle crash victims: how many X-rays are enough? J Trauma 1990:392–397.

47. Chesnut RM. Emergency management of spinal cord injury. In: Narayan RK, Wilberger JE, Povlishock JT, eds. Neurotrauma. New York: McGraw-Hill, 1996:1121–1138.

48. DeVivo MJ, Kartus PL, Stover SL, Rutt RD, Fine PR. Cause of death for patients with spinal cord injuries. Arch Intern Med 1989:1761–1766.

49. Ball PA. Critical care of spinal cord injury. Spine 2001: S27–S30.

50. Velmahos GC, Oh Y, McCombs J, Oder D. An evidence-based cost-effectiveness model on methods of prevention of posttraumatic venous thromboembolism. J Trauma 2000:1059–1064.

51. Green D, Rossi EC, Yao JS, Flinn WR, Spies SM. Deep vein thrombosis in spinal cord injury: effect of prophylaxis with calf compression, aspirin, and dipyridamole. Paraplegia 1982: 227–234.

52. Management of acute spinal cord injuries in an intensive care unit or other monitored setting. Neurosurgery 2002:S51–S57.

53. Dimar JR, Glassman SD, Raque GH, Zhang YP, Shields CB. The influence of spinal canal narrowing and timing of decompression on neurologic recovery after spinal cord contusion in a rat model. Spine 1999:1623–1633.

54. Vaccaro AR, Silber JS. Post-traumatic spinal deformity. Spine 2001:S111–S118.

55. Bracken MB, Shepard MJ, Collins WF, et al. A randomized, controlled trial of methylprednisolone or naloxone in the treatment of acute spinal-cord injury. Results of the Second National Acute Spinal Cord Injury Study. N Engl J Med 1990:1405–1411.

56. Bracken MB, Shepard MJ, Collins WF Jr, et al. Methylprednisolone or naloxone treatment after acute spinal cord injury: 1-year follow-up data. Results of the Second National Acute Spinal Cord Injury Study. J Neurosurg 1992:23–31.

57. Bracken MB, Shepard MJ, Holford TR, et al. Administration Of methylprednisolone for 24 or 48 hours or tirilazad mesylate for 48 hours in the treatment of acute spinal cord injury. Results of the Third National Acute Spinal Cord Injury. Randomized Controlled Trial. National Acute Spinal Cord Injury Study. JAMA 1997:1597–1604.

58. Bracken MB, Shepard MJ, Holford TR, et al. Methylprednisolone or tirilazad mesylate administration after acute spinal cord injury: 1-year follow up. Results of the third National Acute Spinal Cord Injury. Randomized Controlled Trial. J Neurosurg 1998:699–706.

59. Kwon BK, Tetzlaff W. Spinal cord regeneration: from gene to transplants. Spine 2001:S13–S22.

60. Decherchi P, Gauthier P. Regrowth of acute and chronic injured spinal pathways within supra-lesional post-traumatic nerve grafts. Neuroscience 2000:197–210.

61. Houle JD, Ye JH. Changes occur in the ability to promote axonal regeneration as the post-injury period increases. Neuroreport 1997:751–755.

42

Injuries to Peripheral Nerves

Irvine G. McQuarrie, Thomas C. Chelimsky, and Karen Bitzer

INTRODUCTION

The management of nerve injuries poses special difficulties for the surgeon. Although the majority heal satisfactorily without surgical intervention, a year may pass before it is evident that a particular injured nerve will not heal on its own. By then, it is too late to do a nerve repair ("neurorrhaphy") and have this followed by a satisfactory motor recovery. To obtain a good result from neurorrhaphy, it must be performed within six months after injury. On the other hand, the result obtained from carrying out a timely neurorrhaphy is not as good as the result from spontaneous recovery. Neurorrhaphy is to be avoided unless clearly indicated; often this decision must be made before a spontaneous recovery is evident from changes in the neurologic examination. This chapter addresses the pathophysiology of nerve injury and the physiologic basis of nerve repair. It also provides a strategy for the timely identification of nerve lesions that require operative intervention. To accomplish these goals, we only consider mechanical trauma to large mixed (motor and sensory) nerves.

ANATOMY AND PHYSIOLOGY

Fascicular Anatomy

Although physicians agree that the safe and effective treatment of injuries is based on a knowledge of the relevant anatomy and physiology, this is especially true for nerve injuries. Here, the most important consideration is the intraneural anatomy. Each mixed nerve contains 4 to 20 bundles ("fascicles") of nerve fibers (axons within myelin sheaths) that combine, divide, and rotate within the nerve while moving distally to assemble into motor and cutaneous branches. As shown in Figure 1, an unbranched 3 cm length of a mixed nerve contains 5 to 10 fascicles that interconnect to such an extent that most axons come to lie in a different quadrant and have different neighbors after traveling that distance (1). Because of this anatomic circumstance, it is impossible for the surgeon who performs a neurorrhaphy to perfectly match the fascicles in a proximal nerve stump to those in a distal nerve stump. Even if neurorrhaphy appears necessary, the surgeon may want to carry out an electrophysiologic investigation at the operating table before deciding to resect an incomplete nerve lesion.

The incomplete lesion of greatest concern is the "neuroma-in-continuity," a fusiform enlargement of the nerve, which often occurs within weeks following a nontransecting nerve injury. Although a variable fraction of axons may have been broken ("axonotmesis") at the time of injury, the mass effect is less a result of the axonal sprout formation than of a proliferation of Schwann cells, fibroblasts, and collagen, which has been evoked by the force of injury (Fig. 2).

If the "perineurium" enclosing the fascicles has been breached, misdirected axonal sprouts grow for short distances in the "epineurium" (connective tissue that separates fascicles) before rounding up into small neuromas. If the perineurium remains intact, sprouts remain within the fascicle, and there is more than a 90% chance of spontaneous recovery after approximately one year (2). However, there is less than a 60% chance of a good result from excising a neuroma-in-continuity and performing a neurorrhaphy (2) because regenerating axons have a reduced chance of entering the correct fascicle in the distal nerve stump (3–5).

When a neuroma-in-continuity contains broken fascicles (perineurial rupture in addition to axonotmesis—an injury termed "neurotmesis"), most axon sprouts enter the epineurium and are unable to traverse the lesion. In that event, the only possibility for recovery lies in neurorrhaphy. Because the majority of civilian nerve injuries produce a neuroma-in-continuity that is initially associated with a complete loss of nerve function, the decisions of whether and when to operate assume paramount importance (2).

Homeostasis and Microvasculature

The special environment of the central nervous system (CNS) tissues is maintained by the blood–brain barrier, which is physically enforced by tight junctions between capillary endothelial cells. Thus, protein is excluded from the extracellular fluid of the CNS. Active transport mechanisms within the endothelial cells permit the transfer of

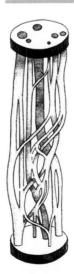

Figure 1 Intraneural fascicular anatomy of a 3-cm segment from the musculocutaneous nerve of a human cadaver. *Source*: From Ref. 1.

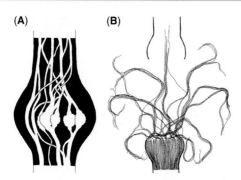

Figure 2 Schematic representation of a neuroma-in-continuity. **(A)** Intraneural fascicular anatomy is depicted in contrast with a dark background representing the proliferation of Schwann cells, fibroblasts, and collagen, which occurs at any site of nerve contusion; five of the fascicles have sustained perineurial rupture, producing a neurotmesis-type lesion (1). **(B)** Intrafascicular axonal anatomy is depicted at a site of perineurial rupture (distal fascicle stump is at the top of the figure); a number of "minifascicles" have formed in response to a complete axotomizing lesion, and one of these has found its way to the distal fascicle stump.

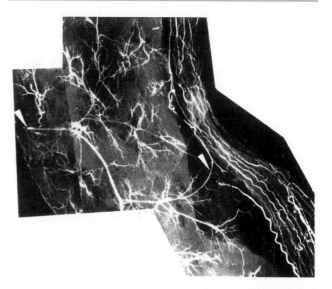

Figure 3 Microradiograph of the rat sciatic nerve (*right*) and the caudofemoralis muscle (*left*) after infra-arterial injection of 25% micropaque. The two arrowheads mark the course of the anastomotic artery as it arises in the muscle, emerges from the anterior muscle border, and joins the arteria comitans along the posterior surface of the nerve (×9). *Source*: From Ref. 6.

specific substances into the extracellular fluid of the brain. Similar mechanisms remove metabolic waste products and toxic substances from the extracellular fluid, because the CNS has no lymphatic vessels. In the peripheral nervous system, each fiber (axon with its supporting Schwann cells) is bathed in endoneurial fluid, which has a composition similar to that of cerebrospinal fluid. As in the CNS, there are no lymphatic vessels, capillaries are nonfenestrated, and endothelial cells are joined by tight junctions (6). The perineurial cells that enclose the endoneurial space are also joined by tight junctions. A breakdown of this "blood–nerve barrier" causes a loss of function in the nerve fibers of the affected fascicle. This pathophysiologic event may not be associated with any change in the ultrastructure of the fibers, and function is restored on restitution of the perineurium (7).

The intraneural blood supply is from longitudinally directed arterioles and venules, located in both the epineurium and endoneurium, which connect with intrafascicular capillaries (Fig. 3). These lie between nerve fibers, and the mean distance between capillaries is only 0.15 mm (1). Although the largest nerves (median and sciatic) have nutrient vessels that are larger than arterioles, more than 90% of the intraneural vessels are less than 10 μm in diameter. Because of the length of the arterioles and venules, and the collateralization of intraneural vessels, blood flow rates are little affected by mobilization of the nerve or nerve transection. Experimental studies in cats show that the flow returns to the normal range of 40 to 50 mL/100 g/min in both stumps by one hour after transection (1,8). The surgeon can safely mobilize 20 to 30 cm lengths of nerve without being concerned about blood supply (1), a maneuver that makes it possible to bridge a 5 cm gap if the extremity is splinted in a position of functional flexion.

Impulse Conduction

Nerve impulses (action potentials) are conducted over the axon surface to the axon terminal through a propagated reversal of charge that maintains the impulse at a constant amplitude and velocity. Although the rate of conduction may exceed 100 m/sec (because of myelin insulation, which forces the impulse to jump from one node of Ranvier to the next), it is much slower than electric conduction over a copper wire. Axons are actually poor electric conductors: a 30 V stimulus could not produce a potential of 1 V at the end of an axon 1 m long without the energy-requiring process that mediates the reversal of charge at the axon surface.

Following axonotmesis, the nerve action potential (NAP) cannot propagate across the point of injury. However, the axons of the distal nerve stump retain the ability to propagate an impulse for up to four days after injury. Thereafter, the axon surface loses its functional integrity as a result of the segmentation of the axon into myelin-bound "ovoids" or "digestion chambers," where the axon is phagocytosed—a process termed "wallerian degeneration" (9).

Nerve Cell Body Reaction to Axonotmesis

The possibility of axonal regeneration depends on the survival of the neuron. Because 95% to 99% of the cytoplasm in peripherally projecting neurons is located in the axon and a large fraction of the axonal volume is in the terminal arborization (10,11), axonotmesis removes most of the neuronal cytoplasm. This often results in the death of a small percentage of neurons. The main reason neurons survive the loss of such a large amount of cytoplasm is that the protein synthesis machinery of the neuron is spared (12,13). In response to axonotmesis, the nerve cell body undergoes a series of biochemical, physiologic, and anatomic changes that have been termed "chromatolysis" because of the reduction in cytoplasmic basophilia. This tinctorial change is attributable to the diffusion of cytoplasmic RNA (located mainly within polyribosomes), secondary to the disruption of the rough endoplasmic reticulum and an increase in the cell volume (12). Biochemical changes include an early and sharp reduction in the synthesis of proteins used for neurotransmitter production. This decrease is roughly balanced by an increase in the synthesis of proteins used for regrowing an axon, which include tubulin, actin, and "growth-associated proteins" (12–15). Physiologic changes include a prompt internalization and degradation of cell-surface receptors, a marked reduction in the amplitude of excitatory postsynaptic potentials (EPSPs), and a reduction in the velocity of impulse conduction in the surviving or "parent" axon (12). Anatomic changes vary with the type of neuron but commonly include a withdrawal of axon terminals from the cell body and dendrites of the injured neuron (accounting for the reduced amplitude of EPSPs), atrophy of dendrites, enlargement of the nucleolus, eccentric positioning of the nucleus, an increase in peri-karyal volume, and a thinning of the parent axon (accounting for the reduced rate of impulse propagation) (12).

There is abundant evidence that the nerve cell body reaction plays a prominent role in axonal regeneration (12). In addition, the "environment" of the newly formed "daughter" axon is important to the success of regeneration (13,16). Two recent developments support the primacy of neuronal events. First, studies over the past decade have shown that axonal outgrowth can be accelerated by the use of a conditioning lesion. This axonotmesis initiates a "crop" of regenerating axons, which is removed days later by a second (testing) lesion. The second crop forms sooner and advances faster than the first (13,17,18). This acceleration appears to be based on the increased synthesis and axonal transport of tubulin, actin, and certain growth-associated proteins (13). The environment faced by the second crop of axons, an environment of wallerian degeneration, is not the primary cause for accelerated outgrowth (13,17,18). The neuronal control of outgrowth is also evident from its rapid response to changes in the status of the axon tip. The nerve cell body receives information quickly by means of "retrograde axonal transport" and makes appropriate changes in its protein synthesis and axonal transport priorities (14). It is by this process, for example, that the nerve cell body comes to know within a few hours that it has sustained an axotomy (19).

Axonal Transport During Axonal Regeneration

The motive force for axonal outgrowth appears to be the axonal transport system, which is responsible for supplying all the protein needs of the axon (11,13,20). Membranous organelles are carried "by fast transport;" structural proteins and the enzymes of intermediary metabolism are carried by the two subcomponents of "slow transport" (10). The proteins that are used for synaptic transmission and renewal of the axolemma are conveyed in tubulovesicular form by fast transport at approximately 400 mm/day. During regeneration, fast transport provides the glycoproteins that form the new axon membrane. In experimental studies, fast transport is labeled with radioactive glycoproteins (which are enriched fivefold in growth cones) to measure axonal outgrowth distances (17).

The principal cytoskeletal proteins are tubulin, actin, and the neurofilament triplet. These are conveyed through the axon by slow transport as both monomers and polymers (microtubules, actin microfilaments, and neurofilaments). The 30 to 40 proteins that associate with actin microfilaments move in a group at 2 to 6 mm/day as slow component b (SCb) of slow transport. The protein triplet composing neurofilaments is transported 1 to 2 mm/day as slow component a,

in association with most of the microtubules. During axonal outgrowth, there are changes in the relative amounts of several proteins moving with both fast and slow transport, but proteins are neither added nor deleted (11). However, both the average rate and the overall amount of protein transport via SCb increases (11,13,20). This correlates with the evidence indicating that the rate of outgrowth cannot exceed the rate of SCb (11,13,20). The governing role of SCb may relate to (i) the dependence of growth cone function on the polymerization of actin into microfilaments and (ii) the dependence of axonal elongation on the assembly of tubulin into microtubules (11,13).

Examination of these two hypotheses in laboratory animals favors the former: radiolabeling of axonal proteins following nerve injury shows that polymerization of both actin and tubulin upregulates, and radiolabeling prior to injury shows that only actin upregulates (21).

Stages of Axonal Regeneration

Four stages of axonal regeneration precede the onset of voluntary motor activity: (i) the "initial delay," consisting of sprout formation and the advance of sprouts to the lesion site; (ii) the "scar delay," during which the sprouts cross the lesion; (iii) the "outgrowth period," during which the axons elongate within fascicles of the distal nerve; and (iv) the "maturation delay," during which the axons that contact an appropriate end organ initiate a series of recovery events. These include the reversal of end-organ atrophy, radial growth of the axon, and myelination.

In experimental studies on sciatic nerves of the rat, sprouts begin to form within a few hours of injury and many acquire a cytoskeleton by 27 hours (18). The zone of "traumatic degeneration" (same pathology as wallerian degeneration but located at the proximal nerve stump) must be traversed before sprouts can attempt to reach the distal nerve stump (22). The average initial delay in rats is 36 hours, and the scar delay at a neurorrhaphy is approximately 48 hours (23). In monkeys, the combined initial and scar delay is one to three weeks (24,25). This is much shorter than the five to seven weeks required by chimpanzees, suggesting that the evolutionary step from monkeys to anthropoid apes involves a major change in neuronal growth potential (24).

The outgrowth period terminates with the arrival of axons at an end organ. If an incompatible end organ is encountered, as in the case of a sensory axon reaching a motor end plate, the maturation phase is not initiated, and the axon remains small in caliber (26). If the contact is appropriate, the axon undergoes radial growth (through the addition of neurofilaments), which triggers the formation of myelin by Schwann cells (27,28). The axon initiates myelin formation through both a chemical signal to the Schwann cell and the physical influence of its radial growth (23,28). After the nerve fiber has matured and end-organ atrophy has been reversed through the resumption of neurotrophic activity, function is recovered. The mismatches between motor axons and muscle fibers (e.g., when a motor axon that had originally projected to a flexor muscle reinnervates an extensor muscle) are partially compensated by changes in the sensory connections within the CNS (5) and the neurotrophic induction of changes in muscle fiber type (29).

The pathophysiology that we have gleaned from these animal studies can be related to nerve injuries in humans. If the times of onset for voluntary movements (in a proximal-to-distal series of muscles served by an injured nerve) and the distances from the lesion to the motor point (where each muscle is innervated) are noted (1), a regression function of distance on time can be plotted. When this is extrapolated to zero distance, the number of days indicated on the x-axis represents the "latent period" (Fig. 4). This is a combination of the initial delay, the scar delay, and the maturation delay. In a classic study that applies this method to a number of patients following neurorrhaphy, the latent period is estimated to be about 13 weeks (30). These patients were compared to others having closed crush injuries (axonotmesis) and therefore a negligible scar delay, where the latent period is about nine weeks. Thus, the average scar delay is four weeks. Because most of the nerve repairs (in this study of World War II injuries) were carried out more than six months after injury, the maturation delay would not have been the optimal four weeks but rather six to eight weeks (25,31). Subtracting that six- to eight-week interval from the nine-week latent period (seen after axonotmesis) leaves an initial delay of one to three weeks. With the four-week scar delay after neurorrhaphy added, there is a five- to

seven-week delay before axons begin to elongate within the distal nerve stump, as in chimpanzees (24). Experience with testing the NAP across the lesion site during surgery has validated this estimate (2). Accordingly, an operation that is partly done for the purpose of recording NAPs from axons that have crossed a suspected neuroma-in-continuity must be delayed until 8 to 10 weeks after injury (2).

PATHOLOGY

With acute nerve compression of mild degree and short duration, the local pathology is limited to "paranodal demyelination" (a retraction and thinning of myelin at the nodes of Ranvier) (32). Greater compression causes a loss of myelin between nodes of Ranvier ("segmental demyelination"). These forms of demyelination block the transmission of action potentials without interrupting the axon, producing a "neurapraxia" (Fig. 5A) (22). Greater compression breaks the axon without disrupting the basement membrane of the Schwann cell (endoneurial tube) or the perineurium (33). This is termed "axonotmesis," meaning "a break in the axon" (Fig. 5B). Finally, cutting objects, shearing forces, and percussive forces produce additional connective tissue disruption and break the perineurium and/or the nerve. This is termed "neurotmesis," meaning "a break in the nerve."

Myelin is readily displaced and thinned by pressure, especially at paranodes. When this occurs, impulse transmission is interrupted even though the axon remains intact. The susceptibility of axons to pressure increases with the degree of myelination. This is best illustrated in a pure neurapraxia, such as "Saturday night palsy," where an intoxicated person develops paralysis and loss of sensation in the upper extremity because of sleeping for prolonged periods in a position that either stretches or compresses a nerve (usually the radial) or the brachial plexus. Examination often shows total paralysis associated with an absence

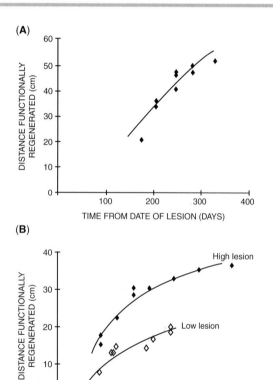

(A)

(B)

Figure 4   Functional motor recovery in patients sustaining radial nerve injuries, illustrating the progress seen after an axonotmesis-type injury within a neuroma-in-continuity (**A**) versus a neurotmesis-type injury repaired by nerve suture (**B**). Distances from the lesion site to the muscle nerve entry point are plotted on the ordinate, and the time from injury (or nerve suture) to the onset of recovery (voluntary contractions) is plotted on the abscissa. Latent period is estimated by extrapolating the regression function of distance on time to zero distance. (**A**) Radial nerve axonotmesis: high lesion; the regression function indicates that the motor axon outgrowth rate is approximately 3 mm/day. (**B**) Radial nerve sutures: low versus high lesion; regression functions indicate that the axon outgrowth rate is approximately 1 mm/day. *Source*: From Ref. 30.

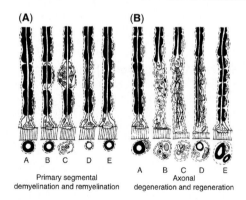

Figure 5   Sequence of changes in a myelinated fiber sustaining a neurapraxia-type injury (**A**) versus an axonotmesis-type injury (**B**) as a result of nerve compression. (**A**) Neurapraxia-type injuries produce segmental demyelination and remyelination. A, Normal fiber; B, retraction of paranodal myelin with widening of nodal gap; C, destruction of myelin sheath and Schwann cell mitoses; D and E, remyelination through the intercalation of short internodes. (**B**) Axonotmesis-type injuries produce axonal degeneration and regeneration. A, Normal fiber; B, by one week after axotomy, Schwann cells containing axon and myelin debris have divided to form "bands of Büngner"; C, during the second week, axon sprouts extend from the enlarged terminus of the proximal axon stump; D, one of the newly formed sprouts becomes myelinated; E, end-organ reconnection occurs. *Source*: From Ref. 22.

of proprioception and touch sensation in the distribution of one or more nerves. However, a pin sensation can be perceived as a dull ache, and a normal density of sweat droplets can be discerned (by examining the skin with an ophthalmoscope set at +20 D). Thus, the functions served by myelinated axons have been lost, but those served by unmyelinated axons have been retained. These patients begin to recover within two weeks and are fully recovered by three months. When the force of compression is greater, there is a break in the axon (axonotmesis). Axonal transport is blocked at the point of breakage, and the axon distal to that point undergoes wallerian degeneration. This process occurs simultaneously at all levels, and all axons show degeneration by the fifth day after injury (9).

The most straightforward classification of acute nerve injuries is open versus closed, depending on whether there has been a break in the skin. If closed, the lesion is either an "acute compression injury" (closed crush) or a "traction injury." Acute compression injuries are usually secondary to fractures, with the radial nerve being involved most often (34). The pathology is paranodal demyelination secondary to increased endoneurial fluid pressure (35). A traction component occurs if the nerve is stretched over a bone fragment. Pure traction injuries because of motorcycle accidents are commonly seen in emergency rooms. In these accidents, the nerve injury occurs because the rider tries to maintain a grip on the handlebars in an attempt to stay with the motorcycle. The upper brachial plexus is involved if the motorcycle stops suddenly, throwing the rider over the handlebars; the lower plexus is involved if the rider is thrown off and dragged while the motorcycle keeps moving.

Of the open injuries, there are two types—those caused by bullet wounds and those caused by cutting objects such as glass. A bullet that misses a nerve may still block function. This is because a "percussion injury" is caused as the bullet passes near the nerve and a pressure wave creates a temporary cavity in the tissues. The pathology is usually a combination of segmental demyelination and wallerian degeneration, producing a combination of neurapraxia and axonotmesis (32,36). The extent of nerve damage depends on the proximity of the bullet to the nerve and the amount of kinetic energy that is transferred to the nerve. With a high-velocity bullet (moving at more than 2500 ft/sec), nerve fascicles can be ruptured even though the bullet misses the nerve. This is because the kinetic energy of the bullet is proportional to its weight and the "square" of its velocity. A small bullet moving at several thousand feet per second is going to cause more damage than a large bullet moving at several hundred feet per second. A military assault rifle (e.g., the M-16 used by the U.S. Forces) produces the former condition, whereas a pistol produces the latter condition. A high-velocity bullet causes a prolonged initial delay because the zone of traumatic degeneration is longer than it would be with a simple laceration (the length of this zone being proportional to the kinetic energy of the bullet) (1). For a low-velocity bullet wound, it is appropriate to wait for 8 to 10 weeks before exploring the nerve to test whether a NAP can be transmitted across the lesion, but a wait of 12 to 16 weeks is necessary for a high-velocity bullet wound (1).

ASSESSMENT OF THE DEFICIT

Assessment should (i) name the injured nerve, (ii) locate the injury along its course, (iii) differentiate neurapraxia from a complete lesion (axonotmesis or neurotmesis), and (iv) list both negative changes (motor and sensory losses) and positive changes (paresthesias, dysesthesias, pain, and altered autonomic activity). A careful neurologic examination is the most important part of the assessment. In addition, certain neurophysiologic tests are useful. These include nerve conduction studies (NCSs) that are done together with electromyography (EMG). In addition, autonomic testing may be appropriate when pain is present.

Neurologic Examination

It is important to assess sensory disturbances, focusing on any loss of sensation that may have occurred in the autonomous cutaneous zone of the injured nerve. Experience has shown that these zones are only innervated by a particular mixed nerve. Neither congenital anomaly nor collateral sprouting from adjacent nerves can provide innervation of these zones; so anesthesia denotes a complete nerve lesion (1). With incomplete nerve lesions, sensation is retained in the autonomous zones, and abnormal spontaneous sensations (paresthesias) or abnormal responses to stimuli (dysesthesias) commonly occur. Dysesthesias can include decreased or increased sensitivity of a normal type (hypoesthesia and hyperesthesia). All sensory changes, including anesthesia, can have a painful component. When a non-noxious stimulus produces pain, the term "allodynia" is used.

The pathophysiology of pain after nerve injury has been studied in great detail, and an excellent review has been published by Wall (37). The most important pain syndrome is "causalgia," which is a severe burning pain that follows nerve injury and may extend beyond the distribution of the injured nerve; both allodynia and abnormalities of autonomic function are typical findings (38,39). It occurs after approximately 2% of incomplete transections (40) but is rarely seen when complete transections are promptly repaired. Causalgia is diagnosed when there is constant burning pain within the distribution of an injured nerve and examination shows allodynia in association with autonomic changes. These changes may include skin that is smooth and glossy, an increase or decrease in the rate of hair growth, tapered digits, thickened nails, periarticular fibrosis, and osteoporosis (41).

The pathophysiology of causalgia has been thought to involve an excess of activity in sympathetic motor axons and the transmission of this activity to somatic sensory axons by means of synapse-like connections in the proximal stump neuroma (42,43). Accordingly, there have been many attempts to treat causalgia pharmacologically (by systemic or local administration of agents that block sympathetic activity) and surgically (by sympathectomy) (44). More recently, however, this teaching has come under criticism (39).

Following nerve injury, autonomic function is lost in the areas of cutaneous anesthesia. Sweat secretion is undetectable when the skin is examined with the +20 D lens of an ophthalmoscope. The ninhydrin sweat test can also be used to document both the absence of sweat formation and any recovery caused by collateral sprouting or axonal regeneration. The "erectores pillae" muscles at the base of each hair follicle do not erect the hair in response to cooling, and the skin is warm because of the absence of innervation to arterial smooth muscle. Later, as the β-adrenergic receptors on these muscle cells proliferate in response to the absence of normal innervation, the cells become supersensitive to congeners of the missing neurotransmitter. This may be manifested by the extremity becoming cool in response to the epinephrine released from the adrenal medulla during environmental or emotional stress.

Assessment of the response of muscles to voluntary effort is achieved through manual testing techniques that are specific to the nerve injury in question. For these to be diagnostic, the examiner must be aware of trick movements or substitution patterns. The distribution and extent of muscle atrophy is recorded as mild to severe and is quantified by measuring the circumference of extremities at fixed distances from the bony landmarks. Deformities of posture must be described and interpreted. For example, a "claw hand" deformity denotes an ulnar nerve lesion. The extent of muscle contractures in the hand is determined by applying standard tests for intrinsic and extrinsic tightness (45). Joint contractures are measured with a goniometer and judged to be either reducible or fixed (46).

For motor disturbances, the principal problem is muscle atrophy. Both disuse and the lack of neurotrophic influences contribute to this problem. If the muscle is not reinnervated within two to three years, all the muscle cells are replaced by connective tissue. If the muscle is not maintained in dynamic activity (by passive range-of-motion exercises) while it is denervated, much of the rehabilitative potential is lost because of muscle fiber atrophy occurring in concert with endomysial fibrosis. Immobilization and paralysis also cause venous and lymphatic stasis, which further reduce blood flow and cause edema. Finally, joint contractures often occur because of decreased muscular support, edema, fibrosis, and the unopposed action of normally innervated muscles. Although it is clear that passive range-of-motion exercises are worthwhile, the presence of pain may be a limitation. In that event, the regular use of regional anesthesia may be necessary to allow an exercise program to occur.

Examination of Specific Nerves

For the "median nerve," the autonomous zone of skin innervation includes the digital pads of the thumb and index finger, and the dorsum of the terminal phalanx of the index finger. An absence of pin sensation and sweat formation in these areas indicates a complete nerve lesion. The equivalent loss in terms of motor function is an absence of voluntary contraction of the abductor pollicis brevis muscle; without this muscle, it is impossible to elevate the thumb from the palm and rotate it into a position of grasp. If the median nerve injury is near the elbow, other movements are impossible after a complete lesion. These include pronation of the forearm and flexion of the thumb and index finger joints, which results in the "benediction sign" when the patient is asked to make a fist.

For the "radial nerve," there is no autonomous sensory zone. In most individuals, however, a total nerve lesion causes loss of sensation over the radiodorsal forearm and the dorsum of the thumb. On motor examination, the fingers cannot be extended at the metacarpophalangeal joints, the thumb cannot be extended at any joint, and the hand cannot be extended at the wrist.

For the "ulnar nerve," the autonomous zone is over the terminal phalanx of the fifth finger. None of the fingers can be adducted or abducted, and the metacarpophalangeal joints cannot be flexed without first flexing the interphalangeal joints. A claw hand deformity is common. This involves hyperextension of the metacarpophalangeal joints and flexion of the interphalangeal joints.

In the lower extremity, the "common peroneal nerve" does not have an autonomous zone of skin sensation.

However, a complete lesion commonly causes a loss of sensation over part of the mid-dorsum of the foot and the web space between the great and second toes. On motor examination, there is an inability to evert the foot, dorsiflex the ankle, or extend the toes. For the "tibial nerve," the autonomous zone is the entire sole of the foot. The motor deficit is a loss of plantar flexion at the ankle and metatarsophalangeal joints. Complete lesions of the "sciatic nerve" produce combinations of the patterns of loss for the tibial and common peroneal nerves.

Nerve blocks may be needed to be certain of which nerves have been injured and whether those injuries are complete or incomplete in terms of the loss in function. After a thorough neurologic examination, it may appear that an incomplete nerve injury has occurred because there are strong voluntary contractions of one or two muscles served by the injured nerve while all others are unresponsive. In that event, it is important to block conduction in the uninjured nerves that could be providing anomalous innervation to the myotome traditionally served by the injured nerve. For example, function can be retained in median-innervated muscles of the hand (abductor pollicis brevis and opponens pollicis) in 15% of patients following a complete transection of the median nerve at the wrist because of the Martin–Gruber anastomosis between the median and ulnar nerves in the forearm (1). A "procaine block" of the ulnar nerve at the wrist would demonstrate this.

Neurophysiologic Tests

Electrophysiologic tests (NCS and EMG) are of great value after nerve injuries. There are two types of NCS, motor and sensory. For motor, the stimulus is a supramaximal electric discharge delivered by a surface (skin) electrode to an underlying nerve (e.g., the median nerve at the wrist). The motor response is the electric potential recorded over a muscle subserved by the nerve (e.g., the abductor pollicis brevis). This consists of the summed motor unit action potentials (MUAPs), each of which represents the response of muscle fibers innervated by a single motor axon. These responses act to amplify the NAP. In contrast, detection of the sensory response requires recording a NAP directly (e.g., from the median nerve at the wrist after stimulating the digital nerves of the index finger). Accordingly, MUAPs have a large amplitude, in the range of 3 to 15 mV, whereas sensory NAPs have a small amplitude, in the range of 5 to 50 μV.

NCS yields two values: an amplitude of response (in microvolts or millivolts) and a latency of response (in milliseconds). The conduction velocity, normally 40 to 60 m/sec, is calculated by dividing the latency into the length of the nerve segment over which the study is performed. Nerve conduction is readily examined following nerve injuries, usually by stimulating distally with digital cuff electrodes and recording sensory NAPs proximally with needle or skin electrodes. By five days after axonotmesis, motor axons distal to the lesion are unable to conduct NAPs because of wallerian degeneration (9). Thus, motor NCS can be used to differentiate neurapraxia from axonotmesis within a week after injury.

In general, the findings on NCS depend on the type of injury (whether a neurapraxia or complete lesion), the interval since injury, the severity of negative neurologic changes (motor and sensory loss), and the severity of positive neurologic changes (paresthesia, pain, and autonomic changes). The most useful information is obtained if electrophysiologic tests are carried out both immediately and at three weeks after the nerve injury. The first study, if done within two to three days, localizes the lesion by NCS because conduction is absent across the site of injury but intact above and below. (A slowing of conduction velocity is characteristic of a demyelinating lesion, but a total loss of myelin results in a "conduction block," which is indistinguishable from a complete lesion.) The second study determines whether there is a complete lesion, in which case conduction is lost below the lesion and fibrillations are present in denervated muscles.

In axonal injury, the degeneration of nerve fibers becomes complete in five days for motor responses and in seven days for sensory responses. (The difference is due to the sensitivity of the neuromuscular junction to blocked axonal transport.) With the demyelinating lesion of neurapraxia, the distal response is never affected.

By one week after injury, nerve conduction changes reach their nadir and the character of the lesion can be fully discerned. With a pure neurapraxia, only the myelin must be reconstituted, and this usually occurs in three to six weeks. With a pure axonal lesion, the axon must grow back to an end organ similar to the original. This occurs at approximately 1 mm/day, as previously described, and depends on daughter axons entering a vacated endoneurial tube distal to the lesion, which then directs the outgrowing axon to an appropriate end organ. With neurorrhaphy, the choice of endoneurial tube is essentially random. Recovery usually takes many months. Motor recovery sometimes begins in weeks because of collateral sprouting, which provides motor axons from nearby uninjured nerves to reinnervate muscles denervated by the injury.

EMG examines the pattern of individual MUAPs seen after inserting a bipolar (concentric) needle electrode into a muscle. Complete lesions produce two types of abnormalities (Fig. 6). First, spontaneous discharges are the most important, including positive deflections that occur

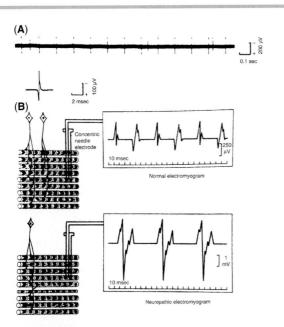

Figure 6 (A) Fibrillation potentials recorded at slow and fast sweep speeds. (B) EMG responses during weak voluntary contractions: normal EMG contrasted with neuropathic EMG seen following axonal regeneration. *Abbreviation*: EMG, electromyogram. *Source*: From Refs 47,48.

with needle insertion and, later, fibrillation potentials. Both are regular discharges, which represent denervation supersensitivity of the muscle cell. Second, with the onset of motor recovery, there is an alteration in the shape and amplitude of voluntary MUAPs. EMG is of particular value whenever there is a total loss of nerve function as a result of injuries that are unlikely to have divided the nerve. These include nerve compression resulting from a compartment syndrome, nerve traction resulting from a fracture, and nerve percussion resulting from a bullet. The most useful information is obtained when the test is carried out as early as possible after injury and again at three weeks. By this time, wallerian degeneration has eliminated any neurotrophic influence of axonal transport on the denervated muscle, and sufficient time has passed for muscle fibers to become supersensitive to the missing neurotransmitter by producing extrajunctional acetylcholine receptors. Fibrillations depend on these.

The EMG method of electrophysiologic testing uses a concentric needle electrode to record from muscles in the distribution of the lesioned nerve. After the needle is placed in a muscle, the patient is asked to attempt a movement using that muscle. If no MUAPs are recorded, the nerve is stimulated by inserting a needle electrode near the nerve between the muscle and the lesion site. When the lesion is a neurapraxia, nerve stimulation elicits MUAPs without difficulty—even though none can be elicited by voluntary effort and the muscle is electrically silent when the nerve is not being stimulated. By one week after axonotmesis or neurotmesis, MUAPs cannot be elicited by stimulation of the distal nerve; by three weeks, the muscle exhibits fibrillations at rest and stimulation does not alter that activity. Fibrillation potentials (Fig. 6A) are never seen in normally innervated muscles and differ from MUAPs by having a regular firing pattern. Fibrillations occur at a frequency of 5 to 15 per second, arise from single muscle fibers, and are thought to be the result of supersensitivity of the muscle fiber membrane to acetylcholine-like molecules that enter extracellular fluid from the blood stream. The EMG is very helpful for detecting axonal reconnection at motor end plates: fibrillations disappear and are replaced by nascent MUAPs that mature into large polyphasic potentials (Fig. 6B). The use of NCS and EMG for differential diagnosis is summarized in Table 1.

Imaging techniques have advanced to the point of detecting that a muscle has been denervated. A magnetic resonance imaging technique termed "short time to inversion recovery" reveals a specific increase in signal intensity (49). Further study in a rat model has shown that gadolinium enhancement augments the sensitivity enough to detect denervation 24 to 48 hours after nerve transection (50).

Autonomic testing is important when causalgia is suspected. The general principle of testing is to compare the unaffected and affected extremities for measures of autonomic function. Different laboratories may employ different methods. When resting sweat output and axon reflex sweat output are tested, and both results are abnormal, there is a 98% chance of "reflex sympathetic dystrophy" (RSD), a syndrome that differs from causalgia by not requiring a prior nerve injury. RSD and causalgia may or may not be associated with "sympathetically maintained pain" (39). The finding of warmer skin over the affected limb when compared to its normal counterpart suggests a positive response to sympathetic block. If bilateral axon reflex abnormalities are present, the prognosis for response to a sympathetic block is poor. In our laboratory, at this time, we use the combination of six tests of autonomic function: resting and

Table 1 Uses of NCSs and EMG for Differential Diagnosis

Time	Axonal injury (axonotmesis)		Demyelinating injury (neurapraxia)	
	NCS	EMG	NCS	EMG
0 days	Amplitudes drop proximal to point of injury	Reduced recruitment; no fibrillations; normal MUAPs	Amplitudes drop proximal to point of injury; slowing may be present	Reduced recruitment; no fibrillations; normal MUAPs
5 days	Distal motor amplitude reaches nadir	No change	No change	No change
7 days	Distal sensory amplitude reaches nadir	No change	No change	No change
10 days	No change	Insertional activity appears	No change	No change
21 days	No change	Insertional activity appears	Amplitude and slowing begin to improve	Recruitment may improve
6 wks	Slight motor amplitude improvement by collateral sprouting	Polyphasic MUAPs (nascent units); fibrillations decrease	Further improvement	Further improvement
3 mos	Sensory amplitude may improve	Increased "duration" of MUAPs, less polyphasic	Maximal recovery	Maximal recovery
6 mos	Maximal motor improvement; continued sensory amplitude improvement	Increased "amplitude" of MUAPs	No change	No change
1 yr	EMG: collateral sprouts are replaced by regenerating axons ("remodeling"); MUAP amplitudes may drop, and recruitment may be normalized	No change	No change	No change

Abbreviations: NCS, nerve conduction study; EMG, electromyography; MUAP, motor unit action potentials.

axon reflex sweat output (by direct sudorometry), blood flow in both skin (by laser Doppler) and muscle (by plethysmography), limb volume (by water-volume displacement), and skin temperature (by infrared probe). All but sweat output are done both before and after a quantitated exercise load to the extremity. Thus, autonomic testing after nerve injury can determine whether sympathetically maintained pain is present and whether the pain is likely to respond to sympathetic block.

TREATMENT APPROACH
Principles of Nonsurgical Treatment

Initially, the potential for rehabilitation is evaluated. This must include a careful assessment of the cause for dysfunction. Otherwise, patients may be treated with a pain management program, for example, when partial paralysis is the main obstacle to progress but goes undetected. Dysfunction may arise from any one or combination of the following, and each should be considered by history, examination, and appropriate neurophysiologic tests: (i) loss of nerve function to produce hypoesthesia and weakness; (ii) excess nerve function to produce pain and hypersensitivity to touch, pressure, temperature change, or movement; (iii) tissue changes, such as edema, loss of hair, loss of skin turgor, or loss of joint mobility; (iv) CNS abnormalities, as may occur with sympathetically maintained pain, which create a "pain cycle" and sometimes adventitial movements (spasms and dystonias); (v) psychologic factors, including adjustment abnormalities, anxiety disorders, and even major depression; and (vi) issues of secondary gain, such as litigation, manipulation of family members, or lack of desire to be in the workforce. A psychologist is needed to help in the assessment of the last two factors.

The presence of sympathetically maintained pain requires a multidisciplinary rehabilitation approach. The team includes a neurologist who adjusts oral medications and coordinates treatment, a surgeon who decides on the appropriateness and timing of operative intervention, an anesthesiologist who carries out nerve blocks, a psychologist who evaluates the patient's motivation and provides treatment with biofeedback and other modalities, and, most importantly, experienced physical and occupational therapists who provide exercise programs and physical treatments designed to improve function. The patient should be told from the outset that the goal is to increase function rather than reduce pain. Medications are selected according to the requirements for treating the patient's greatest source of limitation. Tricyclic antidepressants have great utility in addressing several frequent problems: loss of sleep, depressed mood, and deep or burning pain. Anticonvulsants and mexiletene are effective with lancinating pain. Baclofen, metho-carbomol, and clonazepam are useful in reducing spontaneous movements and postures, including spasms and dystonias. Capsaicin ointment is helpful for the treatment of superficial burning pain. Nonsteroidal anti-inflammatory drugs help control deep aching pain. The use of narcotics is controversial. These may be safe and beneficial when used in a patient with whom the physician has a solid and long-term relationship, provided that a clear-cut contract is arrived at, giving both an exact duration of the trial and the end point. The selection of a nerve block method depends primarily on what is effective. Bier blocks provide regional anesthesia to the involved limb and are least invasive. Sympathetic blocks are traditionally used in the diagnosis and treatment of sympathetically maintained pain. Longer lasting analgesia may be obtained from epidural, plexus, and axillary blocks.

Psychologic techniques include biofeedback, relaxation training, behavior modification, and psychologic investigation of the basic conflicts that may be exacerbating the pain (e.g., reliving an emotionally traumatic event that caused the injury in the first place). Other techniques that may also be useful, but remain unproved, include self-hypnosis and acupuncture. The occupational and physical therapists' roles are most crucial, and the approach depends on the exact type of limitation. All patients require a combination of limb loading and unloading, usually accomplished by the combination of stress loading and water aerobics. For allodynia, desensitization is used with gradually less abrasive materials. Limitations in range-of-motion can be addressed by a continuous passive range-of-motion machine, used during the night, and set at an ever-increasing range.

Principles of Surgical Treatment

The main goals are to preserve fascicular anatomy (1) and ensure that the end organs become reinnervated within eight months after injury (1,31). To achieve these goals, axonotmesis must be differentiated from neurotmesis with certainty by three months after injury. This is not difficult if there is a skin laceration directly over the course of a nerve that has lost all function below the level of the laceration. The wound should be explored immediately; if the nerve has been transected, it should be repaired. Any delay results in scar formation that necessitates trimming 1 to 2 cm off each nerve stump when the delayed neurorrhaphy is performed. However, if the soft tissues show evidence of contusion (petechial hemorrhages and discoloration) or if a bacterial infection is likely because the wound was not closed within 12 to 24 hours of injury, delayed neurorrhaphy (two to three weeks) is preferable. When there is a high-velocity bullet wound and the initial debridement does not reveal a nerve lesion, any loss of nerve function must be attributed to the percussive force of the bullet. During the Vietnam War, 69% of the casualties recovered spontaneously after three to nine months (51). Nerve injuries caused by acute compression, traction, or the percussive force of a low-velocity bullet often recover spontaneously (34). An element of neurapraxia is usually present, so that NCS is often effective in identifying the patients with a favorable prognosis. When NCS shows no conduction below the level of injury after two to three months and EMG shows only denervation, the nerve should be explored for intraoperative NAP testing (12,25,52). Most patients who are going to recover spontaneously have EMG evidence of recovery in the most proximal denervated muscles within three months. This includes the disappearance of fibrillation potentials and the appearance of nascent MUAPs. These changes occur one to two months before voluntary contractions can be elicited (2,25).

Hoffmann's sign of sensory axon regeneration may mislead the surgeon into delaying the exploration for NAP testing. This crude test was described by military surgeons during World War I. It is elicited by light percussion of the distal nerve stump, beginning distally and proceeding proximally. When the leading sensory axons are percussed, the patient feels a tingling sensation in the normal cutaneous distribution of the injured nerve. There are two possible causes of false-positive findings. One is that percussion of the nerve within 10 cm of the lesion may produce traction on the lesion. This stimulates regenerating sensory axons that are arrested within a neuroma-in-continuity. The other problem is that the sign is positive even if only a few axons have bridged a neurotmesis to enter the distal nerve stump (53). The sign must be easily elicited at progressively more distal points along the nerve before it can be interpreted as presumptive evidence of sensory axon regeneration, and the rate of progression must be appropriate—at least 1.5 mm/day at points proximal to the wrist or ankle (1,54). Following

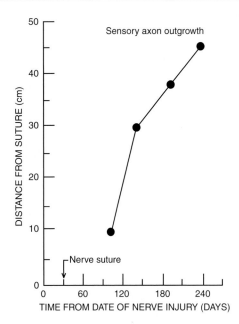

Figure 7 Progress of Hoffmann's sign of sensory axon outgrowth in a patient sustaining a neurotmesis injury of the ulnar nerve at the elbow. By extrapolating the regression function to zero distance, the latent period can be estimated to be seven to eight weeks after nerve suture. With this test of nerve function, there is no maturation delay; the axon terminal is continuously and exquisitely sensitive to mechanical stimuli (31,55–57). Thus, the latent period simply represents the sum of the initial delay and the scar delay. *Source*: From Ref. 54.

neurorrhaphy, the sign should be elicited at 10 cm below the repair within 9 to 12 weeks, assuming an initial delay of two weeks and a scar delay of four weeks (Fig. 7) (1).

Treatment of Neuroma-in-Continuity

From the point of view of pathology, a neuroma-in-continuity (fusiform enlargement of the nerve) involves a proliferation of connective tissue elements that may, if a fascicle has been ruptured, include thin axons that lack linear organization. Ruptured fascicles must be identified and repaired within three months if the patient is to have a reasonable chance of satisfactory motor recovery (2,31,52). Ruptured fascicles are identified by intraoperative NAP testing (52), done after a period of time that allows the neuroma to be crossed by any axon within the unruptured fascicles. An appropriate interval is two months after injuries caused by acute compression or low-velocity missiles and three months after injuries caused by traction or high-velocity missiles.

It is not reasonable to carry out nerve exploration earlier than two months after injury unless there is reason to think that the diagnosis is neurotmesis. Even if all fascicles are intact, one cannot expect to demonstrate NAPs across the lesion site if testing is carried out before seven to eight weeks (2). For high-velocity missile wounds and most traction injuries, there should be a 12-week wait because of the greater extent of traumatic degeneration in the proximal stump. However, delaying definitive diagnosis and treatment any longer only serves to increase the likelihood of a poor result should neurorrhaphy prove necessary.

This is because axonal regeneration proceeds slowly, at an overall rate of 1 mm/day, and distances of over 250 mm often must be overcome before end-organ atrophy can be reversed by the arrival of regenerating axons. After one year, the effects of atrophy and endomysial fibrosis on striated muscle fibers reach a stage that is not compatible with good motor recovery (1,31). When nerve lesions that are caused by a bullet or fracture are explored, a great amount of scarring is encountered in the region. In these cases, the nerve is initially identified in the normal tissues above or below the site of injury. These operations can be facilitated by consulting a useful guide that has been written by Henry (58).

Treatment of Nerve Gap

When a nerve gap is discovered at surgery and the nerve stumps have been trimmed back to the point at which endoneurial tissue bulges beyond the cut edge, and microscopic examination shows no endoneurial fibrosis, the gap between stumps can be measured. When the extremity is flexed to a position of function, and the residual gap is more than 3 to 5 cm, it is unreasonable to expect that a tension-free neurorrhaphy can be achieved with extensive mobilization of the nerve. In this situation, it is preferable to reconnect the fascicles with several free autogenous nerve grafts of small caliber taken from a long cutaneous nerve serving a small skin area (59,60). The sural nerve is most commonly used for this purpose. To restore fascicular anatomy most effectively, it is important to make a map of the location and size of fascicles in the proximal and distal stumps (and the position of blood vessels on the surface of the nerve) as a guide for reconnecting appropriate quadrants of the nerve and matching major fascicles (60).

REHABILITATION AFTER NEURORRHAPHY
Principles of Rehabilitation

Current rehabilitation programs are effective in addressing most of the sensory, autonomic, and motor disturbances that result from denervation (55). Although we recognize that most nerve lesions consist of a neuroma-in-continuity and that many of these have a neurapraxic element that does not involve denervation, we focus here on the rehabilitation of patients after neurorrhaphy. Three phases of rehabilitation can be recognized: the denervation phase that precedes end-organ reconnection, the recovery phase during which end-organ atrophy is reversed, and the adaptation phase during which the CNS makes adjustments to altered connectivity. In each of these phases, rehabilitation methods are aimed at preventing unnecessary disability. This is accomplished by using the existing motor and sensory capability and by preserving denervated structures in a state that is optimal for reinnervation.

Throughout the rehabilitation program, the outlook of the injured person is an important element in recovery. Beginning with that first moment of despair, patients see their skills destroyed, their careers ruined, and their family life jeopardized. Self-esteem and identity invariably suffer. During the slow and tedious recovery process, the personality of the patient is truly tested. Some patients devote considerable time and effort to assist in the recovery process, whereas others remain indifferent and apathetic. To some, the injured part remains useless despite reinnervation; to others, a permanently disabled part is seen as serving in a useful capacity. Still other patients exploit their injury for monetary and secondary gains.

The rehabilitation program must respect the importance of human interactions between the patient and the health professional (especially the occupational therapist). These play a vital role in rebuilding the patient's feelings of confidence and trust, feelings that are indispensable to the success of the rehabilitation program. However, even the most devoted professional attention can be rendered ineffectual if the patient does not receive the interest and support of friends and family. At every stage, both the patient and these key people must be advised together about the problems and expectations of the rehabilitation effort. In the end, however, the success of the rehabilitation outcome largely depends on the trust, courage, and determination of the patient (45).

Retraining in the activities of daily living is promoted throughout the rehabilitation program, regardless of the extent of motor and sensory recovery or the degree to which the patient has made a psychologic adjustment to the injury. Emphasis is placed on the patient's existing strengths, with the use of adaptive techniques and devices that encourage the patient to achieve the highest level of performance possible. The activities that are important for self-care, homemaking, recreation, school, and work are broken down into their key components, and a graded program is created to facilitate maximal independent function at each stage of recovery.

Denervation Phase

The denervation phase begins at the onset of injury and continues until there is evidence of reconnection. Emphasis is placed on keeping denervated tissues in optimal condition pending reinnervation. Absence of sensation, decreased sweating and circulation, and the presence of edema are impairments that must be addressed swiftly and aggressively to minimize their negative effects. The first part of the sensory reeducation process, protective sensory reeducation, starts when wound closure has been achieved and dressings are no longer necessary. Patients must be educated to appreciate the degree and extent of their sensory deficit, learn to compensate for it, and adopt appropriate safety precautions. They must learn to rely more heavily on their vision while performing activities, and avoid applying excessive pressure to denervated skin by looking for signs of trauma—redness, edema, and warmth (45). Skin that is dry and smooth because of the absence of sweat formation should be treated to prevent cracking. Daily warm water soaks followed by the application of oils help to retain moisture and improve circulation. Blood flow through denervated muscles can also be improved by actively contracting nonparalyzed muscles, thereby exerting a pull on paralyzed muscles through the interconnecting fascial sheaths. Retrograde massage, avoidance of extremes of temperature, and passive range-of-motion exercises are also helpful in this regard.

Scar massage and gentle soft-tissue mobilization techniques are used to minimize scar hypertrophy and to prevent adherence of the skin to underlying tissues. Ultimately, this serves to minimize loss of motion as a result of restricted soft-tissue mobility and assists in managing hyperesthesias, which may develop as sensation returns. Passive range-of-motion exercises and active use of uninvolved muscles are essential for improving circulation and maintaining musculotendinous excursion, preventing stiffness and adhesion formation, and decreasing edema (45). This program can minimize the trophic changes that otherwise occur in denervated skin by improving blood flow and reducing the frequency and severity of minor trauma.

Denervated muscles must be maintained with dynamic activity to slow the process of myofibrillar atrophy and endomysial fibrosis. Immobilization (beyond that which is needed to prevent tension on the neurorrhaphy) must be avoided because it promotes tissue edema, reduces blood flow, and encourages the development of muscle contractures. Nonetheless, splinting may be indicated for several purposes: (i) to prevent the overstretching of paralyzed muscles, (ii) to support joints, (iii) to balance the forces on joints and tendons, and (iv) to facilitate the active contraction of uninvolved muscles in a manner that substitutes for paralyzed muscles. The type and design of these splints must be individualized to the patient's needs, and relief from the splint must be provided several times daily to combat the adverse effects of immobilization once the repair has undergone adequate healing.

The application of heat in the form of warm water or oil increases circulation without harming sensitive, denervated tissues. Joint stiffness and ankylosis can occur as a result of decreased muscular support, edema, contractures, and the unopposed action of normally innervated muscles. Joint mobility and the ranges of tendon excursion can be preserved by daily passive exercises. Edema, which is caused largely by the inactivity of muscle masses, is combated by elevation, active contraction of uninvolved muscles, massage, use of Jobst intermittent pressure pump, and the application of compression wraps.

The use of electric stimulation to prevent denervation atrophy of affected muscles remains controversial because there are no controlled studies in human subjects (55). Although muscle stimulation cannot prevent denervation atrophy, there is considerable experimental evidence suggesting that its use reduces the rate and degree of atrophy and that the electric properties of the stimulated muscle more closely resemble those of the normal muscle (56). However, there is no benefit in terms of final twitch tension or tetanic tension after reinnervation. To reduce the degree of atrophy, treatment must begin soon after injury. The stimulus strength must be sufficient to cause long contractions without pain or discomfort; 15 to 20 contractions per session, with low-frequency stimulation in the range of 10 to 12 Hz, are applied three to four times a day. Treatment is abandoned in favor of active contraction after reinnervation has been documented (1).

Recovery Phase

The recovery phase begins with axonal reconnection at an appropriate end organ. During this phase, the therapist plays an important role, monitoring the progress of nerve regeneration through the use of manual muscle testing, sensibility testing, and clinical observation. At each visit, the therapist carefully observes the posture of the involved limb, looking for subtle changes that may indicate the early return of motor function (61). In addition, specific tests of innervation density and sensory threshold are performed. These test the responses to pinprick, temperature, vibration, moving touch/pressure, and static touch/pressure. The Semmes–Weinstein Monofilament Test (North Coast Medical), a standardized threshold test, provides the therapist with an accurate measure of sensibility to graded point pressures throughout the reinnervation period: from unresponsiveness to the return of deep pressure sensation, to the return of protective sensation, to the return of light touch sensation, and to the return of normal sensation (62). Test results are recorded in a color-coded diagram of the limb, providing a clear, simple visual representation of the reinnervation process, which can be forwarded to the surgeon. Early signs of sensory recovery include feelings that "something is happening," tenderness to pressure exerted on muscles, and an advancing Hoffmann's sign (55). The reinnervation of sensory receptors results in altered sensation. Normal tactile stimuli may be perceived as noxious, leading patients to complain of pain, paresthesias, or hyperesthesias. A desensitization program can be quite effective in reducing these symptoms. Patients are taught to expose the sensitive skin to graded textures (e.g., cotton progressing to sandpaper), vibratory stimuli (of increasing frequencies), and solid particles (45). Treatment begins with the exposure to the least aversive stimuli, and the patient is taught to increase the intensity and duration of stimulation each day. This progression continues until normal stimulation is tolerated. The Three-Phase Desensitization Test (originally, the Downey Community Hospital hand sensitivity test) is a readily available (North Coast Medical), standardized test for hypersensitivity that provides a systematic, reliable method for performing and documenting a desensitization protocol with the items described above (62). Other methods of providing sensory input that have been shown to decrease hyperesthesias include massage, application of heat, and percussion or tapping of the sensitive area (62,63).

The principles of pain treatment following nerve injury include measures directed at the pain itself and use of the involved part. The latter is of value because pain is largely a result of the combined effects of vasomotor dysfunction, scar tissue near the proximal nerve stump, and traction on this scar from movement of the limb. To address the pain directly, transcutaneous electric nerve stimulation (TENS) provides relief in almost half the patients. TENS uses an electric device to emit a pulsed current to skin electrodes in a biphasic asymmetric wave. TENS is so effective in treating pain from peripheral nerve injuries that mild transcutaneous stimulation using surface electrodes may be sufficient even for the treatment of sympathetically maintained pain (64,57). Different forms of stimulation are achieved by adjusting the amplitude, frequency, and duration of the pulse. Constant stimulation of the large-diameter afferent fibers reduces the perception of pain, which depends on slowly conducting nonmyelinated fibers. TENS is not a cure for pain but rather an adjunct to the specific treatment of the nerve injury. Its purpose is to decrease pain to a degree that allows patients to participate in the rehabilitation program and perform functional activities.

The pattern of sensory recovery begins with the return of pain and temperature appreciation. This is followed by awareness of vibration at 30 Hz, moving touch stimuli, and then vibration at 256 Hz. The last modalities to recover are the localization of tactile stimuli and two-point discrimination (65). Modality tests include pinprick, temperature discrimination, vibration, moving touch/pressure, and constant touch/pressure. The return of function is assessed from tests of moving and static two-point discrimination, the response to a ridge-shaped sensitometer, and tactile gnosis (the ability to feel the shape, weight, and texture of objects well enough to identify these) (45). The Moberg pickup test is particularly useful because the ability to pick up a series of 10 to 12 small objects of various sizes and then place them into a small container is readily timed and compared to results for the normal hand (45). Qualitative differences in prehension patterns may also become apparent during testing. An effort must be made to standardize the conditions for these tests at follow-up examination, because there are many uncontrollable factors affecting the transmission of sensory impulses from the periphery to the CNS.

Muscle atrophy is reversed by reinnervation of the motor end plate, provided that endomysial fibrosis is not advanced. Rehabilitative efforts are aimed at maximizing voluntary motion, motor control, and strength. The therapist must be familiar with the expected order of reinnervation following repair of the particular nerve lesion being treated, information that is readily obtained from standard texts (1). Treatment methods during the recovery phase include muscle reeducation, biofeedback, resistive exercises (initially resisting gravity alone), proprioceptive facilitation techniques (to maximize the stimulation of muscle afferents), and the use of patterns of movement that recruit the maximal number of muscle fibers (46).

Adaptive Phase

Once end-organ function has been restored, central changes occur, which reflect adaptation to a new pattern of connectivity. An important part of this phase, which can be influenced by the rehabilitation program, is the reeducation of integrative mechanisms in the CNS. This facilitates new patterns for acquiring sensory information and distributing commands to muscle groups. Sensory recovery may slowly progress for more than three years before it is complete. Improvement occurs both through the maturation of reunited axon-receptor systems and the subliminal reeducation of integrative mechanisms. Because the CNS acquires sensory information differently after neurorrhaphy (because end-organ reinnervation is a random event), the sensations that occur early in the recovery phase may be somewhat foreign to those normally perceived in a particular part of the CNS (5,58).

Sensory reeducation involves a graded series of specific sensory exercises that are instituted at appropriate times in the recovery process. An attempt is made to facilitate central reorganization so that patients can interpret the altered profile of neural impulses reaching consciousness. In the early stages of recovery, patients relearn modality-specific perceptions (e.g., moving vs. constant touch). In the later stages, patients progress to the second phase of sensory reeducation: discriminative sensation. Readiness for progression to this phase is determined by the patient's results on the Semmes–Weinstein monofilament test. The patient must be able to perceive filament number 4.31 (2.35 g) before discriminative training proves useful (66). At that time, various structured activities are performed with the ultimate goal of the return of tactile gnosis (name recognition of objects in the hand; two-point discrimination). Various stimuli are applied to the patient's hand with the patient's vision occluded. The patient attempts to identify the stimulus, and if unsuccessful, the stimulus is applied while the patient watches. The patient continues this training method, alternating eye occlusion and then using direct visualization in an effort to reorganize and integrate the cortical processing of sensory information from the altered periphery. The patient is challenged with the task of first identifying specific characteristics of the object (e.g., metallic vs. wooden and round vs. square). Ultimately, the patient attempts to name the object itself (e.g., key, coin, and paperclip). Graphesthesia activities and puzzles or mazes that are performed with vision occluded are higher-level tasks that also facilitate the return of discriminative sensation (66). This program is continued until the patient assumes responsibility for self-education and returns to work, avocations, and self-care. With sensory reeducation, maximal recovery may occur within two years (65), shortening the adaptive phase by a year or more.

Surgical procedures for the relief of pain caused by peripheral nerve injuries include the excision of any neuromas and sympathectomy. However, the former is rarely effective (67) and the latter has largely been replaced by TENS, ganglion blocks, and phenoxybenzamine (57,68). Muscle mass is regained through repeated exercises and the use of the injured part in activities of daily living.

Permanent Denervation

Specific adaptive techniques, support personnel, or appliances may be required when functional impairment is substantial and permanent (63). Sufficient time should be allowed to elapse before evaluating the extent and significance of recovery. Although reconstructive procedures may be effective if performed in a timely manner, the patient will realize that the hoped-for recovery cannot occur. These procedures include arthrodesis, tendon transfers, tendon translocation, tenodesis, nerve transfers (69), microsurgical free muscle transplants, muscle transfers using an intact neurovascular island pedicle, and amputation with prosthetic fitting. These procedures require specific rehabilitation methods and goals.

SUMMARY

Peripheral nerve injuries are rarely followed by a full recovery of function and often leave patients with a significant disability. Most nerve injuries involve an upper extremity and therefore threaten hand function. To minimize the extent and incidence of permanent disability, it is important to preserve as much of the microanatomy of the injured nerve as possible. This may mean "leaving well enough alone." To know when to intervene surgically and, more importantly, when not to intervene requires an in-depth understanding of the anatomy and physiology of normal nerves. Diagnostic tools such as NCS and EMG are critical in sorting out the nature of the injury. To maintain what has been obtained by successful initial management requires the use of active rehabilitation measures that take account of any residual limb pain. Therapy must begin soon after injury, continue during the phases of recovery, and maximize the patient's independence in the performance of daily activities.

REFERENCES

1. Sunderland S. Nerves and Nerve Injuries. Edinburgh: Churchill Livingstone, 1978.
2. Kline DG, Hackett ER. Reappraisal of timing for exploration of civilian peripheral nerve injuries. Surgery 1975; 78:545.
3. Brushart TM, Mesulam MM. Alteration in connections between muscle and anterior horn motoneurons after peripheral nerve repair. Science 1980; 208:603.
4. Lisney SJW. Changes in the somatotopic organization of the cat lumbar spinal cord following peripheral nerve transection and regeneration. Brain Res 1983; 259:31.
5. Wall JT, Felleman DJ, Kaas JH. Recovery of normal topography in the somatosensory cortex of monkeys after nerve crush and regeneration. Science 1983; 221:771.
6. Bell MA, Weddell AGM. A descriptive study of the blood vessels of the sciatic nerve in the rat, man, and other mammals. Brain 1985; 107:871.

7. Hudson A, Kline D. Progression of partial experimental injury to peripheral nerve. II. Light and electron microscopic studies. J Neurosurg 1975; 42:15.

8. Smith DR, Kobrine AI, Rizzoli HV. Blood flow in peripheral nerves. Normal and post severance rates. J Neurol Sci 1977; 33:341.

9. Donat JR, Wisniewski HM. The spatio-temporal pattern of wallerian degeneration in mammalian peripheral nerves. Brain Res 1973; 53:41.

10. Grafstein B, McQuarrie IG. Role of the nerve cell body in axonal regeneration. In: Cotman CW, ed. Neuronal Plasticity. New York: Raven Press, 1978.

11. McQuarrie IG. Role of the axonal cytoskeleton in the regenerating nervous system. In: Seil FJ, ed. Nerve, Organ, and Tissue Regeneration: Research Perspectives. New York: Academic Press, 1983.

12. Grafitein B, Forman DS. Intracellular transport in neurons. Physiol Rev 1980; 60:1167.

13. McQuarrie IG. Effect of a conditioning lesion on axonal transport during regeneration: the role of slow transport. In: Elam J, Cancalon P, eds. Advances in Neurochemistry. Vol. 6. New York: Plenum Press, 1984.

14. Benowitz LI, Yoon MG, Lewis ER. Transported proteins in the regenerating optic nerve: regulation by interactions with the optic rectum. Science 1983; 222:185.

15. Skene HHP, Willard M. Axonally transported proteins associated with axon growth in rabbit central and peripheral nervous systems. J Cell Biol 1981; 89:96.

16. Bray GM, Rasminsky M, Aguayo AJ. Interactions between axons and their sheath cells. Annu Rev Neurosci 1981; 4:127.

17. McQuarrie IG. Accelerated axonal sprouting after nerve transection. Brain Res 1979; 167:185.

18. McQuarrie IG. Effect-of a conditioning lesion on axonal sprout formation at nodes of Ranvier. J Comp Neurol 1985; 231:239.

19. Singer PA, Mehler S, Fernandez HL. Blockade of retrograde axonal transport delays the onset of metabolic and morphologic changes induced by axotomy. J Neurosci 1982; 2:1299.

20. Wujek JR, Lasek RJ. Correlation of axonal regeneration and slow component B in two branches of a single axon. J Neurosci 1983; 3:243.

21. Lund LM, Machado VM, McQuarrie IG. Increased Beta-actin and tublin polymerization in regrowing axons: relationship to the conditioning lesion effect. Exper Neurol 2002; 178:306.

22. Weller RO, Cervos-Navarro J. Pathology of Peripheral Nerves. London-Boston: Butterworth Publishers, 1977.

23. Forman DS, Wood DK, DeSilva S. Rate of regeneration of sensory axons in transected rat sciatic nerve repaired with epineurial sutures. J Neurol Sci 1979; 44:55.

24. Kline DG, Hayes GJ, Morse AS. A comparative study of response to species to peripheral nerve injury. J Neurosurg 1964; 21:980.

25. Kline DG, Hackett ER, May PR. Evaluation of nerve injuries by evoked potentials and electromyography. J Neurosurg 1969; 31:128.

26. Sanders FK, Young JZ. The influence of peripheral connexion on the diameter of regenerating nerve fibers. J Exp Biol 1946; 22:203.

27. Friede RL. Control of myelin formation by axon caliber (with a model of the control mechanism). J Comp Neurol 1972; 144:233.

28. Politis MJ et al. Studies on the control of myelinogenesis. IV. Neuronal induction of Schwann cell myelin-specific protein synthesis during nerve fiber regeneration. J Neurosci 1982; 2:1252.

29. Gordon T, Stein RB. Reorganization of motor-unit properties in reinnervated muscles of the cat. J Neurophysiol 1982; 48:1175.

30. Bowden REM, Sholl DA. The advance of functional recovery after radial nerve lesions in man. Brain 1950; 73:17.

31. Richter HP. Impairment of motor recovery after late nerve suture: experimental study in the rabbit. I. Functional and electromyographic findings. Neurosurgery 1982; 10:70.

32. Gilliatt RW. Physical injury to peripheral nerves. Physiologic and electrodiagnostic aspects. Mayo Clin Proc 1981; 56:361.

33. Dyck PJ et al. Structural alterations of nerve during cuff compression. Proc Nad Acad Sci USA 1990; 87:9828.

34. Pollock FH et al. Treatment of radial neuropathy associated with fractures of the humerus. J Bone Joint Surg 1981; 63A:239.

35. Lundborg G, Myers R, Powell H. Nerve compression injury and increased endoneurial fluid pressure: a "miniature compartment syndrome." J Neurol Neursurg Psychiatry 1983; 46:1119.

36. Richardson PM, Thomas PK. Percussive injury to peripheral nerve in rats. J Neurosurg 1979; 51:178.

37. Wall PD. The painful consequences of peripheral injury. J Hand Surg 1984; 9B:37.

38. Treede RD et al. Peripheral and central mechanisms of cutaneous hyperalgesia. Prog Neurobio 1992; 38:397.

39. Verdugo RJ, Ochoa JL. Sympathetically maintained pain. Neurology 1994; 44:1003.

40. Rothberg JM, Tahmoush AJ, Oldakowski R. The epidemiology of causalgia among soldiers wounded in Vietnam. Milit Med 1983; 148:347.

41. Merskey H. Classification of chronic pain. Pain 1986(suppl 3):1.

42. Devor M, Janig W. Activation of myelinated afferents ending in a neuroma by stimulation of the sympathetic supply in the rat. Neu Rosci Lett 1981; 24:43.

43. Roberts WJ. A hypothesis on the physiological basis for causalgia and related pains. Pain 1986; 24:297.

44. Shir Y, Seltzer Z. Effects of sympathectomy in a model of causalgiform pain produced by partial sciatic nerve injury in rats. Pain 1991; 45:309.

45. Hunter JM et al. Rehabilitation of the Hand: Surgery and Therapy. 3rd ed. St. Louis: Mosby, 1990.

46. Nickel VL. Orthopedic Rehabilitation. Edinburgh: Churchill Livingstone, 1982.

47. Goodgold J, Eberstein A. Electrodiagnosis of Neuromuscular Diseases. Baltimore: Williams & Wilkins, 1978.

48. Bradley WG. Disorders of Peripheral Nerves. Oxford: Blackwell Scientific Publications, 1974.

49. Mcdonald CM et al. Magnetic resonance imaging of denervated muscle: comparison to electromyography. Muscle Nerve 2000; 23:1431.

50. Bendszus M, Koltzenburg M. Visualization of denervated muscle by gadolinium-enhanced MRI. Neurology 2001; 57:1709.

51. Omer GE. Injuries of nerves of the upper extremity. J Bone Joint Surg 1974; 56A:1615.

52. Terzis JK, Dykes RW, Hakstian RW. Electrophysiological recordings in peripheral nerve surgery: a review. J Hand Surg 1976; 1:52.

53. Napier JR. The significance of Tinel's sign in peripheral nerve in juries. Brain 1949; 72:63.

54. McQuarrie IG. Nerve regeneration and thyroid hormone treatment. J Neurol Sci 1975; 26:499.

55. Wynn Parry CB. Rehabilitation of the Hand. 3rd ed. London: Butterworth Publishers, 1978.

56. Nix WA. The effect of low-frequency electrical stimulation on the denervated extensor digitorum longus muscle of the rabbit. Acta Neurol Scand 1982; 66:521.

57. Meyer GA, Fields HL. Causalgia treated by selective large fibre stimulation of peripheral nerve. Brain 1972; 95:163.

58. Henry AK. Extensile Exposure. 2nd ed. Edinburgh: Churchill Livingstone, 1973.

59. Haase J, Bjerre P, Simensen K. Median and ulnar nerve transections treated with microsurgical interfascicular cable grafting with auto genoussural nerve. J Neurosurg 1980; 53:73.

60. Millesi H. Interfascicular grafts for repair of peripheral nerves of the upper extremity. Orthop Clin North Am 1977; 8:387.

61. Hallin RG, Wiesenfeld Z, Lindblom U. Neurophysiological studies on patients with sutured median nerves: faulty sensory localization after nerve regeneration and its physiological correlates. Exp Neurol 1981; 73:90.

62. Waylett-Rendall J. Desensitization of the traumatized hand. In: Hunter JM, Mackin EJ, Callahan AD, eds. Rehabilitation of the Hand: Surgery and Therapy. 4th ed. St. Louis: Mosby, 1995:693.

63. Trombly CA, Scott AD. Occupational Therapy for Physical Dysfunction. Baltimore: Williams & Wilkins, 1977.

64. Campbell JN, Long DM. Peripheral nerve stimulation in the treatment of intractable pain. J Neurosurg 1976; 45:692.

65. Dellon AL. Evaluation of Sensibility and Reeducation of Sensation in the Hand. Baltimore: Williams & Wilkins, 1981.

66. Callahan AD. Methods of compensation and reeducation for sensory dysfunction. In: Hunter JM, Mackin EJ, Callahan AD, eds. Rehabilitation of the Hand: Surgery and Therapy. 4th ed. St. Louis: Mosby, 1995:701.

67. Noordenbos W, Wall PD. Implications of the failure of nerve re section and graft to cure chronic pain produced by nerve lesions. J Neurol Neurosurg Psychiatr 1981; 44:1068.

68. Ghostine SY et al. Phenoxybenzamine in the treatment of causalgia: report of 40 cases. J Neurosurg 1984; 60:1263.

69. Chacha PB, Krishnamurti A, Soin K. Experimental sensory reinnervation of the median nerve by nerve transfer in monkeys. J Bone Joint Surg 1977; 59A:386.

43

Physiology of Arterial, Venous, and Lymphatic Flow

Dennis F. Bandyk and Paul A. Armstrong

INTRODUCTION

Clinical evaluation of patients with vascular disease requires a thorough understanding of the anatomy and hemodynamics of the arterial, venous, and lymphatic circulations. The continued improvement of noninvasive ultrasound techniques that produce high-resolution vascular imaging and depict system hemodynamics has resulted in improved understanding of arterial and venous disease pathophysiology, and has better defined the physiologic significance of anatomic disease. The ability to monitor the hemodynamics of arterial and venous flow and vessel anatomy serially has allowed detection of disease progression, resulting in a more cost-effective and timely intervention. In this chapter, the functional anatomy and hemodynamics of the arterial, venous, and lymphatic components of the circulatory system will be discussed. Special emphasis will be placed on how the biophysical properties of the circulation (e.g., pressure, flow velocity, and turbulence) can be measured in man, and how such measurements are used in the evaluation of patients with vascular disease. The discussion will focus primarily on the principles of arterial, venous, and lymphatic flow in the lower extremity; however, the concepts are equally germane and applicable to the upper extremity and cerebrovascular circulation.

PERIPHERAL ARTERIAL SYSTEM

The purpose of the arterial system is to deliver blood and its various components to tissue capillaries in amounts sufficient to maintain normal cellular function. Metabolic demands of body tissues and organs vary widely, in normal (resting), exercising, and diseased states. The ability of the arterial circulation to respond to a variable demand is reflected in the anatomic and physical properties of the cardiovascular system and is mediated through two regulatory mechanisms: local control of blood flow through the tissue according to its metabolic state (autoregulation) and neural control of peripheral vascular resistance. These factors, acting in concert, control tissue blood flow and consequently regulate cardiac output. Control of blood flow is also strongly influenced by factors such as those involved in the regulation of extracellular fluid volume and urinary output.

The functional elements of the arterial system include the "heart," which generates the energy necessary to maintain arterial pressure and blood flow at an appropriate level, "arteries," which transport blood to the periphery, "arterioles," which regulate flow of blood into the microcirculation, and "capillaries," which are the site of nutrient and metabolic exchange to the tissues. Depending on their position in the arterial system, arteries can act as "storers" of

pressure energy produced in the heart, by cushioning vessels that convert the pulsatile flow of the blood into smooth flow, and acting as resistance vessels involved in the microcirculation. Arterial wall structure and neural innervations accordingly reflect the specialized function(s) of the various arterial system elements.

As blood proceeds through the arterial system, the network of conducting vessels undergoes repeated branching accompanied by a decrease in caliber, resulting in many parallel distributing vessels that terminate in the capillary beds. In the arterial system of the lower extremity, branching produces potential collateral networks that can bypass blood around a hemodynamically significant, i.e., pressure-reducing, obstruction in a conduit artery (Fig. 1). The total cross-sectional area progressively increases each time branching occurs, with a concomitant decrease in mean flow

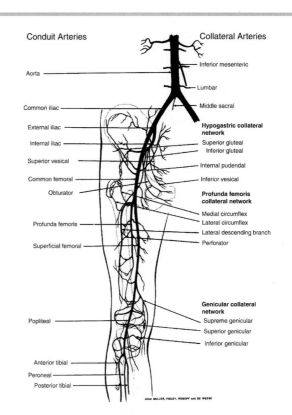

Figure 1 Diagram of the arterial circulation to the lower extremity, indicating the main conduit arteries and corresponding potential collateral arteries.

Table 1 Physical and Hemodynamic Characteristics of the Human Arterial System

	Total blood volume (%)	Cross-sectional area (cm^2)	Mean flow velocity (cm/s)	Pressure (mmHg)	Resistance (%)
Aorta	8	2.5	14–18	100	4
Branching arteries	5	20	12	90	21
Arterioles	2	40		55	41
Capillaries	5	2500	0.07	25	27

velocity (Table 1). At the capillary level, the cross-sectional area is approximately 1000 times that of the aorta. Each red blood cell remains in the microcirculation for only one to three seconds, an exceedingly short time during which all nutrient diffusion and fluid exchange occur.

Approximately 20% of the entire blood volume of the body is in the arterial system, in contrast to the 64% in the venous system. The heart contains 7% of the blood, and the pulmonary vessels 9%. Surprisingly, only 5% of the total blood volume resides in the capillaries. Although total capillary volume is small, surface and cross-sectional areas are immense to facilitate the transfer of oxygen, carbon dioxide, water, nutrients, and electrolytes through the capillary walls. In the resting state, the lower limbs receive about 300 to 400 mL/min, two to three times of that in the upper limbs, primarily because of differences in muscle mass.

The heart, through cyclic muscle wall contraction, generates a complex pressure pulse and provides the energy for blood flow. The ability of the heart to vary its output is based on its three fundamental properties: the capacity to vary the rate of contraction (chronotropism), the rate of isometric tension development, which is a function of cardiac muscle fiber length (Frank–Starling mechanism), and the ability to alter the velocity of muscle fiber shortening (inotropism). From these properties, four factors that are independent determinants of cardiac output can be defined. These are commonly referred to as ventricular preload, ventricular contractility, ventricular afterload, and heart rate. The output of the heart mainly reflects the demands of the peripheral circulation. The frequency of contraction is determined by the interplay of neural and humeral adrenergic and neural cholinergic activity on the sinoatrial node. The velocity and force of ventricular–muscular contraction are influenced by both circulating and neuron-released catecholamines acting on the muscle fibers themselves. The work output of the heart is the amount of energy that the heart transfers to the blood. This energy, which is in the form of potential energy of pressure and the kinetic energy of blood flow, is used to accelerate blood to its ejection velocity through the aortic valve. In the distribution of blood to the various capillary beds, the viscoelastic properties of the artery walls and the tapered, converging vessel caliber are important physical characteristics maintaining blood pressure and minimizing pressure and kinetic fluid energy losses.

Arterial Wall: Structural Features

The composition and structure of the arterial wall in the different segments of the arterial system reflect the local wall mechanics and its functional role. With the exception of the capillaries, the artery wall consists of three concentric layers: tunica intima, tunica media, and tunica adventitia.

The tunica intima is the innermost layer and consists of monolayer endothelium lining the lumen, a thin basal lamina, and a subendothelial layer (present in the large elastic arteries of the thorax and abdomen), composed of collagenous bundles, elastic fibrils, and smooth cell muscles. The tunica media is in the middle layer and is made up of predominantly smooth muscle cells in a varied number of elastic sheets (laminae), bundles of collagenous fibrils, and a network of elastic fibrils. The tunica adventitia consists of dense fibroelastic tissue without smooth muscle cells. The adventitia also contains the nutrient vessels of the arterial wall (vaso vasorum) and both vasomotor and sensory nerves of the vascular wall.

Arteries can be classified by the respective amounts of elastin, smooth muscle, and collagen in their walls. The distensibility of an artery wall generally correlates with the elastin content. The large arteries of the thorax and abdomen, such as the aorta, innominate, iliac, subclavian, and common iliacs, are referred to as elastic or "pressure storer" arteries because their walls contain a predominance of elastin and few smooth muscle cells. The large elastic arteries instantaneously accommodate each stroke volume of the heart, storing a portion during systole and draining this volume during diastole (windkessel effect). This helps to propel the blood toward the periphery during diastole and promotes continuous flow to the capillaries. The internal systole pressure in the large arteries is normally about 120 to 160 mmHg.

Proceeding distally, the muscular or branching arteries such as brachial, radial, femoral, and popliteal have a media with a predominance of smooth muscle and collagen, but little elastic tissue. The varying arterial wall properties distant from the heart are related to the proportions of collagen and elastin in the media, the linkage between these two elements, the insertions of elastin and muscle on collagen fibers, and the contractile state of the vascular smooth muscle. Proceeding from the thoracic aorta distally, there is a gradual decline in the elastin–collagen ratio. Thus, the initial segment of the arterial tree has a lower vascular impedance, and oscillatory component of work required distally to maintain cardiac output is reduced. The increased relative stiffness of the distal muscular arteries is important to ensure that undamped transmission of the pressure pulse to the baroreceptors (e.g., at the carotid bifurcation) occurs. At the level of the arterioles, the arterial wall is composed almost entirely of smooth muscle. These vessels provide the major site of resistance to the arterial system, and provide for the regulation of blood flow to the microcirculation (Table 1). Mean pressure in the arterioles ranges from 40 to 60 mmHg. The smooth muscle of the media is well innervated by sympathetic nerves. At the cutaneous level, these nerve fibers are involved with temperature regulation, vasoconstriction in cool weather to conserve heat and vasodilatation in warm conditions to dissipate heat. Exceptions to this can occur in the septic states, severe emotional distress, or profound shock, where vasodilatation predominates secondary to sympathetic innervation. Additionally, metabolites at a local level also cause vasodilatation, as does exercise. This autoregulation disappears at pressures below 30 mmHg, where flow occurs secondary to perfusion pressure alone.

The collagen content of the arterial wall correlates with its tensile strength, with the adventitia collagen responsible for the majority of wall stability. This is evident from the maintenance of vessel integrity by the adventitia following surgical endarterectomy, which removes the intima and large portion of the media. In naturally occurring aneurysms, the collagen content of the adventitia is decreased and failure of wall integrity occurs. Degradation of collagen results in arterial wall rupture. The circumferential tension (*T*) in the arterial wall is calculated as the product of the transmural pressure, P_t (inside pressure minus outside pressure), and the radius (*R*). This relationship, known as the Law of Laplace, can be expanded to include the factor of wall thickness (µm):

$$T = P_t R / \mu m \ (dynes/cm)$$

In arteries with a radius and wall thickness of equal proportions, wall tension varies with transmural pressure. For example, the small radius and low pressure of a capillary requires only a thin wall to support the wall tension, whereas the aorta with its greater pressure and radius requires a thicker wall to prevent rupture.

The elastic properties of any blood vessel can be described by Young's modules (*E*), which is stress divided by strain. Because arteries are subject to pulsatile pressure, measurements of elasticity are determined from the strain that accompanies a period of time in which stress is varied, producing what is called dynamic modules (Edyn). The most important component of stress in arteries is the first harmonic of the pressure pulse, i.e., heart rate. The dynamic elastic modules of an artery are also a determinant of pulse wave velocity. In vivo arterial wall motion occurs predominantly in the circumferential direction. The variation of vessel diameter with each cardiac cycle closely resembles the pressure waveform. Intrathoracic arteries vary 12% to 18% in diameter with each pressure pulse, whereas peripheral arteries change 8% to 10% in diameter. The distensibility characteristic of arteries also depends on the extent of stretch (transmural pressure). At low pressure and small diameters, arteries are very distensible, whereas they become gradually stiffer with increasing pressure and diameter.

The viscoelastic properties of arteries are altered not only in diseased states but also change with age. With age, artery diameter and length increase, and so do the wall thickness and collagen-to-elastin ratios. These changes result in tortuosity, increased arterial stiffness, and an increase in vascular impedance. Although an increase in the thickness of the intima, which initially occurs in atherosclerosis, has little effect on the elastic properties of the artery, the accompanying changes within the media and adventitia, particularly if the wall nutrition through vaso vasorum is involved, may have marked effects of hemodynamic characteristics and further disease progression.

Viscous Properties of Blood Flow

Blood is a viscous fluid composed of cells and plasma. When blood flows, frictional forces develop between the cellular components of blood, causing it to exhibit the property of viscosity. Because the red blood cells comprise the majority of the cellular component, the hematocrit is a major determinant of blood viscosity, as illustrated in Figure 2. If measured with reference to water, the relative viscosity of blood having a hematocrit of 40 is approximately 3.6. This means that three to four times as much pressure is required to force blood than water through the same tube. Blood viscosity is not constant in the arterial system but exhibits a non-Newtonian fluid property: the faster it flows, the lower is its viscosity. The chief determinants of this property are the red cell concentrations and plasma concentration of fibrinogen and globulins. Blood viscosity decreases in small caliber

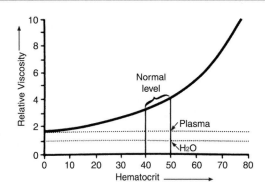

Figure 2 Effect of hematocrit on relative velocity of blood. Note that as the hematocrit increases, the relative viscosity increases disproportionately. *Source*: From Ref. 1.

tubes (less than 200 µm) such as the arterioles, capillaries, and venules. This phenomenon is known as Fahraeus–Lindqvist effect and is related to red cell orientation and lower hematocrit in small vessels. The rheology of blood in the capillary circulation is poorly understood, although the deformability of the red cell membrane and erythrocyte velocity are important factors. Rheologic agents focus on increasing the membrane flexibility of the red blood cells and therefore decrease the overall viscosity of blood. They also promote decreased platelet aggregation.

The viscosity of blood is important not only for its effect on the resistance to blood flow, but also in producing impairment of tissue perfusion. Increased blood viscosity can potentiate the low flow states seen in pathologic conditions such as polycythemia, trauma, and other hyperviscosity syndromes. Increased blood viscosity combined with a low flow promotes erythrocytes to aggregate into stocks or "rouleaux," with resultant tissue ischemia.

Essentials of Arterial Hemodynamics

Hemodynamics is a discipline concerned with the interrelationships of the physical characteristics of blood and pulsatile flow conditions in the visoelastic arterial and venous circulations. As a first step toward understanding the complexity of arterial flow, it is useful to discuss the energy principles involved in arterial circulation and the interrelationships between pressure, flow, and resistance under steady flow conditions.

Fluid Energy

In general, blood flows from a point of high pressure to one of lower pressure, but the true driving force is the differential in total fluid energy. "Total fluid energy" associated with blood flow is of three types: intravascular pressure, gravitational, and kinetic. The intravascular pressure (*P*) has three components: (i) the dynamic pressure produced by the contraction of the heart, (ii) the hydrostatic pressure, and (iii) the static filling pressure. Both the gravitational energy and the hydrostatic pressure are determined by the product of the specific gravity of blood (ρ), the acceleration of gravity (980 cm/sec)(g), and the distance (h) above the right atrium. Gravitational energy (+ρgh) is the ability of the blood to do work on the basis of its height and is of the opposite value of the hydrostatic pressure (-ρgh). The static filling pressure is the residual pressure that exists in the absence of arterial flow. This pressure is determined by the volume of blood and the compliance of the arterial system, and is in the range of 5 to 10 mmHg. Because the hydrostatic pressure and the gravitational potential energy cancel each other out and the static filling pressure is relatively low, the dynamic pressure produced by the heart is the major source of potential energy used in moving blood.

Kinetic energy (Ek) is the ability of blood to do work on the basis of its motion. It is proportional to the specific gravity of blood (p) and the square of the blood velocity (v):

$$Ek = \tfrac{1}{2}pv^2$$

Omitting the term for gravitational energy (i.e., $+pgh$), the total fluid energy per volume of blood (E) can be expressed as:

$$Ek = P + \tfrac{1}{2}pv^2$$

where P is intravascular pressure. In an idealized fluid system of steady flow and/or frictional energy losses, total fluid energy along a streamline remains constant with the relationship between the different energy forms described by Bernoulli's principle of the conservation of energy:

$$P + \tfrac{1}{2}\,pv_1{}^2 = P2 + \tfrac{1}{2}\,pv_2{}^2 + \text{heat}$$

In the horizontal diverging tube shown in Figure 3, steady flow between two points is accomplished by an increase in cross-sectional area and a decrease in flow velocity. Although fluid energy moves against a pressure gradient ($p_2 - p_1$) of 2.4 mmHg and gains potential energy, total fluid energy remains constant because of a lower velocity and a proportional loss of kinetic energy. In the normal arterial system in which ideal flow conditions are absent and vessels change diameter only gradually, the pressure gradients caused by viscous losses as predicted by Poiseuille's law far outweigh the extremely small interconversions to kinetic energy and pressure. In certain disease states, however, such as sudden vessel widening into an aneurysm or narrowing

as a result of an atherosclerotic plaque, the Bernouille effect and the production of turbulence with the associated changes in kinetic energy explain the pressure and flow changes that develop under these conditions.

It is important to emphasize that the pressure–flow relationship described in Poiseuille's law is based on assumptions involving idealized fluid mechanics that significantly underestimate the energy losses present in the viscoelastic pulsatile flow conditions of the human circulation. Poiseuille's law represents the minimum pressure gradient produced by viscous losses that may be expected in arterial flow. In addition to energy loss caused by friction, inertial energy losses related to changes in the velocity and the direction flow occur. In the arterial system, particularly in the presence of disease, energy losses caused by inertial effects usually exceed viscous energy loss.

Energy losses related to inertia are proportional to the specific gravity of blood and the square of the blood velocity. Because the density of blood is constant, inertial losses result when blood accelerates, decelerates, or changes direction. In the arterial system, inertial energy losses occur at points of curvature, variations of lumen diameter, and at bifurcations of the vasculature. Blood velocity usually increases from large luminal size to smaller luminal size. The acceleration and deceleration of blood in pulsatile flow add inertial forces to the constant kinetic energy of steady flow.

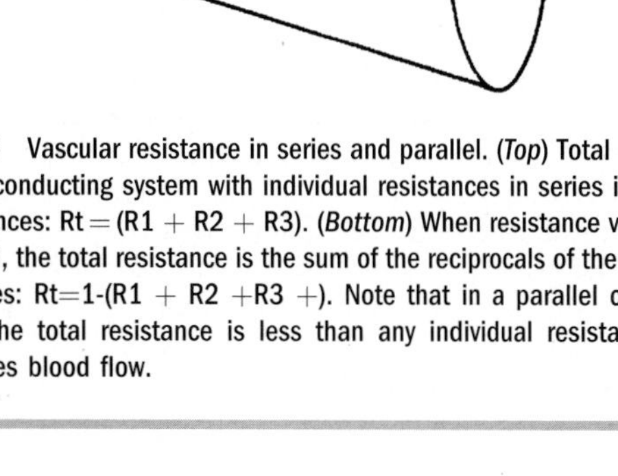

Resistance to Flow

The relations between flow and pressure in cylindrical tubes were first accurately described by the French physician, Poiseuille, in 1846. Under the conditions of his experiments, the volume flow (Q) through a vessel is determined by:

$$Q = \frac{P\pi r^4}{8l\mu}\,\text{ml/min}$$

where P is perfusion pressure, or the pressure gradient between the ends of the vessel, r is the vessel radius, l is the vessel length, and μ is viscosity of the fluid. Poiseuille's law describes the viscous energy losses that occur in a steady-flow, idealized fluid model. The theoretic derivation rests in the assumptions that each particle of the fluid moves at a constant velocity parallel to the vessel wall, that the force opposing this motion is proportional to fluid viscosity, and that the velocity gradient is perpendicular to the direction of flow. This means that in a cylindrical tube, the fluid moves in a series of concentric lamina and flow is laminar. Steady laminar flow results in a parabolic velocity profile in the tube. As predicted by this law, the resistance to flow is most dependent on vessel radius. Resistance is proportional to vessel length and viscosity, but inversely proportional to the fourth power of the radius. Assuming a constant blood viscosity, a doubling of conduit length will double the resistance, whereas halving the radius increases the resistance 16 times. In the human peripheral arterial system, flow is primarily determined by active changes in the arteriole, arteries less than 200 μm in diameter, and the capillary. Artery caliber varies according to the state of contraction of the vascular smooth muscle, which depends on perfusion pressure, activity of the sympathetic nervous system, and local mechanisms involving metabolic, humeral, and physiologic factors.

In a flow model governed by Poiseuille's law, the physical properties of the system (tube dimensions and fluid viscosity) determine the magnitude of pressure gradient required to produce a given flow. The ratio of mean pressure gradient

$A_1 = 1\ \text{cm}^2$
$V_1 = 80\ \text{cm/sec}$
$P_1 = 100\ \text{mm Hg}$

$A_2 = 16\ \text{cm}^2$
$V_2 = 5\ \text{cm/sec}$
$P_2 = 102.5\ \text{mm Hg}$

Figure 3   Vascular resistance in series and parallel. (*Top*) Total resistance (Rt) of a conducting system with individual resistances in series is the sum of resistances: Rt = (R1 + R2 + R3). (*Bottom*) When resistance vessels are in parallel, the total resistance is the sum of the reciprocals of the individual resistances: Rt=1-(R1 + R2 +R3 +). Note that in a parallel conducting system, the total resistance is less than any individual resistance level. Q indicates blood flow.

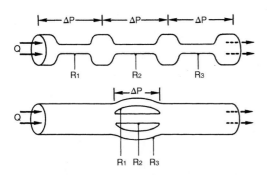

Figure 4 Effect of increasing cross-sectional area on pressure in friction-less fluid system. Although pressure increases, total fluid energy remains constant because of a decrease in velocity. *Abbreviations*: A, area; V, velocity; P, pressure. *Source*: From Ref. 2.

to mean flow is thus a measure of the opposition to flow, commonly termed "vascular resistance." When Poiseuille's law is simplified to an expression, pressure = flow times resistance, it is exactly analogous to Ohm's law of electric circuits, $V = 1 \times Re$, when Poiseuille's equation is rearranged to:

$$P = Q \frac{8l\mu}{\prod r^4} \, mmHg$$

where the term $(8l\mu)/\prod r^4$ expresses electrical resistance (Re), P is voltage (V), and Q is flow of current (I). Vascular and electrical resistances both express the dissipation of energy per unit flow within a system. In the arterial system, resistance is expressed as peripheral resistance units (PRU), where 1 PRU equals the resistance to flow encountered when there is a pressure difference between two points of 1 mmHg and flow is 1 m/sec. The resistance of the entire systemic circulation is approximately 1 PRU, calculated using a 100-mmHg pressure gradient between the left ventricle and the right atrium and an average blood flow of 100 mL/sec.

The total resistance of a conducting system depends on whether the vessels are in series or in parallel (Fig. 4). When vessels are in series, total resistance is equal to the sum of the individual resistances. On the other hand, if the conducting vessels are in parallel, total resistance is the reciprocal of the total conductance. This means that in a parallel conducting system, total resistance is less than any of the individual resistance vessels. Also resistance usually tends to increase as velocity increases along a fixed diameter artery.

Arterial Flow Patterns

The combination of viscous (frictional) and inertial forces acting on blood determines whether flow is laminar or turbulent (i.e., disturbed flow). The transition to turbulent flow is physiologically important because a greater pressure gradient is needed to maintain flow. Frictional interactions at the inner wall of an artery can also produce flow pattern variations, referred to as boundary layer separation. The clinical importance of local flow patterns in arteries resides in their role in the pathogenesis of atherosclerosis, and the ability of duplex ultrasound systems to detect and grade the severity of disease through the disturbed flow produced.

Laminar and Turbulent Flow

As previously discussed, the blood flow follows streamlines or is laminar in the steady flow conditions specified by Poiseuille's law. The velocity profile is parabolic in shape (Fig. 5). In contrast to the concentric laminae of laminar flow, turbulence is a condition in which the flow velocity vectors are moving in a random fashion with respect to space and time. The point at which flow changes from laminar to turbulent, termed the "critical velocity," depends on the ratio of inertial forces to viscous forces and is best defined in terms of a dimensionless entity known as Reynolds number:

$$Re = \rho d v / \mu$$

where ρ is the blood density, d is the vessel diameter, v is the mean velocity, and μ is the viscosity. Below a Reynolds number of 2000, flow is laminar because viscous forces predominate and damping of random inertial forces on the flow stream occurs. At a Reynolds number above 2000, the inertial forces may disrupt the laminar flow pattern, the result being increased energy dissipation as sound and heat. Energy dissipation in laminar flow is proportional to flow velocity, whereas losses in turbulent flow occur with the velocity squared. Flow conditions that predispose to the development of turbulence include an increased flow velocity (ascending aorta), a decreased vessel diameter (diseased), or a reduced blood viscosity (anemia, over hydration). An important clinical sign of turbulence is the presence of a bruit. Streamline (laminar) flow is silent, but turbulence produces wall vibrations that can often be heard with a stethoscope, termed a "bruit." Bruits produced by stenoses are loudest over the stenotic segment and are transmitted in a distal direction.

Under conditions of turbulent, viscoelastic flow, the arterial velocity profile changes from the parabolic shape of laminar flow to a blunt or rectangular shape. Although turbulent flow is uncommon in arteries, a condition of disturbed flow commonly occurs. Disturbed flow is a transient perturbation in the laminar streamlines that disappears with time or as the flow proceeds downstream. Sites of focal disturbed flow can be identified in the thoracic aorta during the flow deceleration phase of each heart cycle, in regions of

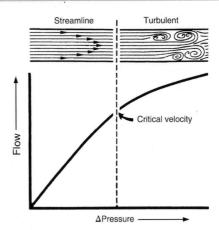

Figure 5 Relationship between velocity of flow and turbulence. *Source*: From Ref. 3.

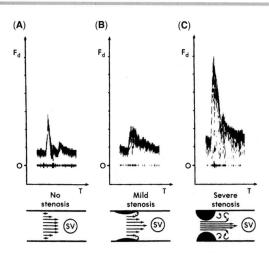

Figure 6 Center stream flow from a normal artery is laminar and is demonstrated on the spectrum (**A**) as a narrow band of frequencies during systole, with a clear window beneath the frequency envelope. Disturbed flow caused by mild stenosis appears as spectral broadening on the frequency spectrum (**B**) without producing changes in the park systolic velocity. Highly disturbed flow (turbulence) is characterized by high peak velocities and spectral broadening throught the cardiac cycle. Also note the increase in end-diastolic velocity associated with severe stenosis (**C**). *Abbreviations*: SV, systolic velocity; T, time. *Source*: From Ref. 4.

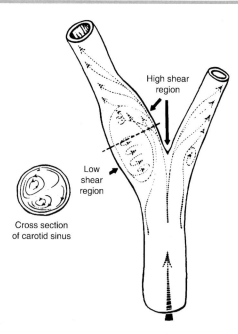

Figure 7 Flow patterns at model carotid bifurcation. Adjacent to the outer wall of the bulb, flow is stagnant (a region of flow separation), may reverse, or may be diverted across the vessel lumen. Rapid flow is associated with high shear stress, whereas the slow flow in the separation zone produces a region of low shear. *Source*: From Ref. 5.

arterial branching, and in the carotid bulb. Disturbed flow, however, can represent the initial hemodynamic abnormality produced by atherosclerotic plaque formation seen in occlusive disease. Plaque formation alters wall compliance and reduces cross-sectional lumen area, resulting in disturbed flow and an increase in blood flow velocity. The recognition that the kinetic energy losses associated with disturbed flow conditions helps to explain the gross underestimation of energy loss when Poiseuille's law is used alone to evaluate flow changes produced by arterial stenosis.

The magnitude of disturbed flow can be divided into three categories on the basis of the Doppler velocity spectra pattern: undisturbed (laminar), disturbed, and highly disturbed (turbulent). As shown in Figure 6, the velocity spectra of blood flow through a stenosis demonstrates the focal disruption of laminar flow at and distal to the lesion. Highly disturbed velocity spectra associated with pressure–flow– reducing stenosis exhibit high-frequency Doppler shifts and spectral broadening throughout the pulse cycle. Turbulent flow can initiate platelet aggregation, which may lead to thrombus formation. Disturbed velocity waveforms contain high-frequency components only during peak systole and typically indicate a transitional flow condition detected under normal flow conditions in the ascending aorta and at arterial bifurcations. Undisturbed velocity waveforms exhibit negligible high-frequency content and are representative of laminar flow.

Boundary Layer Separation

The outer layer of fluid in a flow stream adjacent to the vessel wall is referred to as the boundary layer. Radial-directed velocity gradients exist as a result of the fractional interactions of fluid with the vessel wall and the more rapidly moving fluid in the center of the vessel. When vessel geometry changes suddenly, such as at points of curvature and

bifurcations, small pressure gradients are created, causing the boundary layer to stop or reverse direction. This results in a complex, localized flow pattern known as an area of flow separation. Areas of flow separation have been observed in models of arterial anastomoses and the carotid bifurcation depicted in Figure 7; an area of flow separation is seen to have formed along the outer wall as a result of the diverging carotid bulb diameter. The complex flow patterns identified in normal human carotid bifurcation include vortex flow as well as regions of flow separation and reversal along the lateral, posterior wall of the bulb. Shear rate is the variation of velocity of flow changes between concentric laminae of blood. Shear stress at the vessel wall (Dw) can be characterized by the following formula:

$$Dw = 4\frac{V}{r} = 4\frac{Q}{\pi r^3}$$

$$\Gamma w = 4\eta \frac{V}{r} = 4\eta \frac{Q}{\pi r^3}$$

where Γw is the shear stress at the wall, V, the mean velocity, r, radius, Q, mean flow, and η, the blood viscosity. Therefore shear rate and stress are directly proportional to mean velocity, turbulence, and viscosity and inversely proportional to the inner radius of the vessel. At bifurcations and vessel curves, shear is highest at the wall where the velocity of flow is also highest. It has been shown that arterial vasoconstriction and vasodilatation occur with shear rate changes, most likely via production of endothelium-derived relaxing factor, now known to be nitric oxide (NO). Production of NO in the wall in response to increased shear causes relaxation of the media smooth muscle, resulting in vasodilatation.

Chapter 43: Physiology of Arterial, Venous, and Lymphatic Flow   **837**

The disturbed flow and low shear stress in regions of boundary layer separation may contribute to the formation of atherosclerotic plaques. Examination of carotid and iliac bifurcations, both at autopsy and during surgery, indicate that intimal thickening and plaque formation tend to occur in the regions of flow separation. Within these zones, there is an opportunity for a synergistic effect for rheologic and contact activation of blood elements with the intima. The role of localized flow disturbances as an initiator or promoter of atherosclerosis is speculative and awaits further analysis and research.

Principles of Pulsatile Flow

In the arterial system, pressure and flow vary continuously with time, and the velocity profile changes throughout the cardiac cycle. The addition of a pulsatile component on steady flow increases fluid energy expenditure. As much as 30% of the energy in cardiac output is dissipated as a result of pulsatile flow. With increasing heart rate, energy losses caused by pulsatile flow decrease exponentially up to a heart rate of approximately 150 beats/min. The remainder of cardiac output energy is used for tissue perfusion, and therefore primarily dissipates in the arteriolar and capillary bed. Although the true nature of pulsatile energy loss remains poorly defined, contributing factors include inertia energy loss with acceleration, geometric vessel tapering, vessel curvature, and bifurcation, production of disturbed flow, and the non-Newtonian character of blood. It is apparent that Poiseuille's law cannot accurately predict all the hemodynamic characteristics of flow through the artery.

Of importance to the surgeon is that, with pulsatile flow, the energy losses produced by arterial reconstructions, which commonly have anatomic and physical characteristics much different from the normal arterial system, are likely to be much greater than predicted by the equations governing steady flow. Although pulsatile flow appears less efficient than steady laminar flow, studies indicate that individual organs require pulsatile flow for optimum function. Perfusion of a kidney with a steady flow instead of pulsatile flow results in a reduction of urine volume and sodium excretion. Pulsatile flow and pressure probably exert their effect at the microvascular level. Although the exact mechanism is unknown, transcapillary exchange, arteriolar and venular tone, and lymphatic flow are all responsive to pulsatile pressure.

With each stroke volume of the heart, blood is pumped into the distensible arterial tree, which acts as an elastic reservoir or *windkessel* absorbing the cardiac energy that is later released during ventricular diastole. The physiologic effect is to damp the flow/no-flow effect of the heart so that the pressure and flow are maintained during diastole. As blood is forced into the aorta, the instantaneous increase in volume is transmitted along the artery as a pressure and flow wave. As shown in Figure 8, the increase in flow starts almost synchronously with the rise in pressure, but the peak flow velocity precedes peak pressure. The instantaneous flow rate is not determined by the magnitude of the pressure pulse but by the pressure gradient developed along the artery. The pressure gradient is determined by recording the pressure at two points, a short distance apart, and subtracting the downstream pressure from the upstream pressure during the cardiac cycle. The effect of the traveling pressure wave is to produce a oscillatory pressure gradient. The magnitude of the pressure gradient determines both instantaneous flow velocity and the

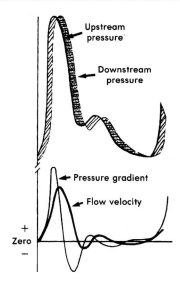

Figure 8 Generation of flow velocity waveform by traveling pressure pulse wave. Simultaneous pressure pulse and flow velocity pulse recordings from an arterial segment. Although similar in configuration, peak flow occurs before the systolic pressure peak, indicating a complex relationship between these hemodynamic parameters. Flow is determined by the pressure gradient that develops along the arterial segment.

direction of flow. Unless there is a marked decrease in the mean pressure along the artery, there will always be a period during the pulse cycle when the pressure gradient is reversed. This reversal of gradient causes a rapid deceleration of flow, and, if it continues after the forward flow has been brought to a halt, flow reversal can occur. Indeed, flow reversal during diastole is a normal pattern of blood flow in peripheral limb arteries.

As the pressure-pulse wave travels from the aorta to the periphery, its speed, magnitude, and configuration are altered. The pressure wave is produced by the sudden ejection of blood into the aorta. The pressure wave velocity increases from 4 to 6 cm/sec to approximately 13 cm/sec in the muscular arteries of the lower limb. The velocity of the pressure wave is 20 times greater than the mean velocity imparted to the blood in the aorta (20–40 cm/sec), illustrating that the pressure wave has no direct relationship to flow and can be recorded under "no flow" conditions of acute arterial occlusion. The acceleration of the pressure wave in the peripheral arteries is caused primarily by increasing wall stiffness. Because of this relationship, the transmission velocity of the pressure wave has been used as an index of arterial distensibility. The amplitude of the pressure wave, otherwise known as the pulse pressure, increases, as wave configuration changes with propagation to the periphery (Fig. 9). With increasing distance from the heart, the rate of systolic pressure rise increases, and the sharp inflection of the downslope known as the "dicrotic notch" becomes rounded and disappears in the abdominal aorta, where dicrotic waves appear. In the arteries of the lower limb, systolic pressure is higher, and diastolic pressure is lower than that in the aorta. This is the result of the viscoelastic characteristics of the arterial conduits, the effect of pressure waves being reflected from sites of increased peripheral resistance (i.e., from sites of tapering and branching), and the abrupt increase in resistance at the level of the arterioles.

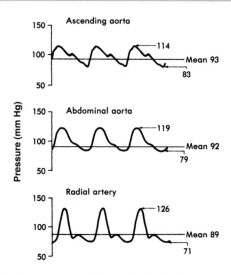

Figure 9 Pressure waves at different sites in the arterial tress. With pressure wave transmission into the distal aorta and large arteries, the systolic pressure increases, and the diastolic pressure decreases with a resultant increase in pulse pressure. Note that mean arterial pressure declines steadily.

It is important to note that the mean pressure decreases with the distance from the heart, but the pressure loss in the large arteries of the thorax and abdomen is small because of their large radius. As shown in Table 2, systolic and diastolic pressures recorded from large arteries are influenced by various hemodynamic factors. Careful analysis of the pressure wave configuration and its transmission can provide useful clues to important cardiac and peripheral arterial physiology.

The pulsatile characteristics of the pressure wave are dampened considerably at the level of arterioles at which mean pressure reaches values up to 40 to 60 mmHg. In general, perfusion pressure in the capillaries is nonpulsatile, and pressure waves in the venous system are caused primarily by pressure changes in the right heart and not the left. Exercise increases total leg blood flow 5X to 10X in the normal patient. In the diseased extremity seen during treadmill duplex evaluation, ankle pressure drops severely and requires prolonged periods of time to recover.

Measurement of Arterial Pressure

A major advance in the understanding of and approach to patients with arterial occlusive disease came with the recognition that the physiologic disturbance responsible for symptoms is predominantly related to development of a pressure gradient in the proximal arterial segment. Pressure measurement is a more sensitive index of an occlusive process than is the measurement of flow, because in the presence of moderate arterial disease blood flow is essentially normal,

Table 2 Main Determinants of Aortic Systolic and Diastolic Pressures

Systolic pressure	Diastolic pressure
Stroke volume	Systolic pressure
Aortic distensibility	Aortic distensibility
Ejection velocity	Heart rate
	Peripheral resistance

owing to the reduction of resting arteriolar resistance compensating for the increased resistance of the proximal arterial system. Although flow measurement techniques (i.e., indicator dilution methods and impedance flowmeter) have clinical value in the determination of cardiac output, flow volume measurement in the limbs is of limited value as a clinical or diagnostic tool. For these reasons, a variety of direct and indirect arterial pressure measurement techniques are available using noninvasive instrumentation.

Direct pressure measurement involves placing a needle or catheter into the artery and recording the pressure waveform with the aid of manometer or strain-gauge transducers. From a continuous recording of the pressure waveform, systolic pressure is the peak pressure during the pulse cycle, and diastolic pressure is the lowest pressure. The difference between these two pressures is the pulse pressure. Mean pressure, the force responsible for the mean flow of blood to an organ, can be determined electronically by calculating the area of the pulsatile waveform or estimated from systolic and diastolic pressure measurements (mean pressure = diastolic pressure + 1/3 pulse pressure). Although direct pressure measurements provide the most accurate data, their routine clinical use is not warranted, because the technique is invasive and requires sterile conditions, and pressure data obtained indirectly are sufficiently accurate for diagnostic purposes.

Indirect pressure measurements depend on (i) the production of Korotkoff sounds, which are the result of turbulence in the flow stream, (ii) the appearance and disappearance of the pressure pulse, or (iii) the reappearance of flow when a proximally located pneumatic cuff has been inflated and slowly deflated above the regional perfusion pressure. Auscultatory (Riva–Ricci method) and palpatory techniques to measure upper limb arterial pressure are the most common hemodynamic assessments of the arterial circulation. To avoid measurement errors, the occluding cuff should be 20% wider than the limb diameter. If it is too narrow, the pressure will be erroneously high; if it is too wide, the reading may be erroneously low.

Several techniques are used clinically to measure systolic pressure in the limbs, including plethysmography (mercury strain gauge, air, and photocell) and the ultrasonic velocity detector (continuous-wave Doppler). These instruments are used as sensors to indicate return of flow with cuff deflation. Plethysmography operates on the principle that changes in the circulation of the blood to a body part (e.g., leg) will result in corresponding changes in the size of that part that are measurable. Such changes in size can be measured by displacement of air or mercury in a strain gauge or emission of light in a photoelectric cell, as is done in photoplethysmography. In general, devices with ultrasound are most commonly used because instruments are inexpensive and simple to use, and the Doppler-derived pressure measurements have been thoroughly evaluated and have been noted to be as accurate as plethysmographic measurements. Even when an ultrasonic signal is difficult to obtain, it is almost always possible to record a pressure with the photoplethysmograph. Digital volume changes are then amplified and can be recorded. This allows pressures to be recorded in digits in the presence of severe obstructive arterial disease, when flow velocities are too low to be picked up by a Doppler transducer.

The assessment of arterial flow with ultrasound is made on the basis of the Doppler effect, which refers to the shift in frequency that occurs when sound is reflected from a moving object. Moving red blood cells reflect the ultrasound beam and shift the frequency proportional to the flow velocity. The Doppler signal can be (i) amplified to provide an audible sound, with the pitch directly proportional to blood velocity, (ii) converted into an analog waveform using a zero-crossing frequency meter, or (iii) analyzed for its frequency–amplitude content. Failure to obtain a Doppler signal from an artery usually indicates occlusion; however, an extremely low flow rate (under 2 cm/sec) may not produce detectable Doppler frequency shift.

The systolic pressure at any level of an extremity can be measured by applying a pneumatic cuff and positioning the Doppler probe over a patent artery distal to the cuff (Fig. 10). The arterial signal is distinguished from the adjacent venous signal by its characteristic high pitch that corresponds to the cardiac cycle. When the cuff is inflated above systolic pressure, the arterial flow signal disappears. As cuff pressure is gradually lowered, the point at which flow resumes is recorded as the systolic pressure. In the lower limb, the use of multiple cuffs placed at the high-thigh, above and below the knee, ankle, and digital levels permits the measurement of segmental pressures. The level of pressure measurement is determined by cuff placement and not the site of Doppler flow detection. The difference in systolic pressure between any two adjacent cuffs or between corresponding segments in the opposite limb is less than 20 mmHg in normal individuals. Because of cuff artifact, proximal thigh systolic pressure normally exceeds brachial pressure by 30 to 40 mmHg.

As the distance increases from the heart, an amplification of the pressure wave produces a higher systolic pressure to be measured at the ankle than in the brachial artery, which, in the absence of disease, is nearly equal to central aortic pressure. To compensate for variation in central perfusion pressure and to permit comparisons of serial measurements, the ankle systolic pressure is expressed as a ratio of brachial pressure, termed the ankle-brachial systolic pressure index (ABI). The normal ABI is equal or greater than 1 (mean value of 1.1 ± 0.1), and reductions correlate with the degree of arterial insufficiency. In limbs with intermittent claudication, the ABI (mean + S.D.) is 0.58 ± 0.15, in limbs with ischemic rest pain, 0.26 ± 0.13, and in limbs with gangrene, 0.05 ± 0.08.

The measure of toe pressures can be used to identify obstructive disease distal to the ankle and to measure pressure in diabetic patients in whom ankle pressure measurement by the cuff method is artifactually high because of the incompressibility of calcified arteries. Normal systolic toe pressure is approximately 80% of the brachial systolic pressure. Photoplethysmographic techniques are better suited than the ultrasonic methods of flow determination at the digital level, because of vessel caliber and a low flow velocity in the digital arteries.

Real-Time Ultrasound Arterial Imaging and Flow Analysis

Since the 1970s, ultrasound technology has developed instrumentation to both image vascular anatomy and display blood flow patterns within the lumen in real time. The technique referred to as color duplex ultrasonography, which combines real-time imaging (B-mode) with pulsed Doppler flow detection, is most versatile and permits the arterial and venous circulations to be mapped analogous to arteriography or venography in body regions accessible to interrogation by ultrasonic energy. Duplex scanning can be used to address specific queries concerning location and extent of vascular disease and disease morphology (stenosis, occlusion, or aneurysm), to measure vessel diameter and grade stenosis severity, and to measure occlusion length based on visualization or exit and reentry collateral vessels. In atherosclerotic lesions, B-mode imaging with high (10–15 MHz) frequency transducers can demonstrate features such as ulceration, calcification, acoustic heterogeneity, and intraplaque hemorrhage.

Blood flow velocity within visualized vessels is characterized with the use of a Doppler velocity detector. Accurate characterization of blood flow patterns requires the use of a pulsed Doppler whose sample volume (the point in space from which blood flow is detected) is small in relation to the vessel diameter. The Doppler signal is processed by a real-time spectrum analyzer to determine the velocity of blood, the direction of flow, and the velocity distribution of the RBCs in the sample volume. When the pulsed Doppler sample volume is positioned in the midstream of nondisturbed (laminar) arterial flow, the Doppler signal will contain a narrow range of frequencies (spectral width) of similar amplitude corresponding to streamline movement of RBCs during the pulse cycle. Undisturbed flow produces a "clear window" in the spectra beneath the frequency envelope and is characteristic of normal peripheral arterial hemodynamics.

Calculation of blood flow velocity requires estimation and assignment of the angle between the incident Doppler beam and the blood velocity vector. An operator-controlled line on the B-mode image indicates the direction of the sound beam from the pulsed Doppler probe. In general, the Doppler beam is adjusted to intersect the flow stream at an angle of approximately 60. A "cursor" on the Doppler beam indicator locates the position of the sample volume and can be placed at any point in the vessel. The Doppler angle is calculated electronically by the operator positioning

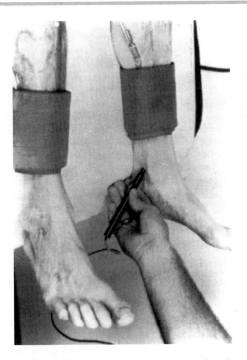

Figure 10 Measurement of ankle systolic pressure. Doppler probe is positioned over the posterior tibial artery.

a cursor parallel to the longitudinal axis of the vessel. Blood flow velocity is calculated from the frequency spectra waveform measurements using the Doppler equation:

$$\text{Flow velocity} = \frac{C\,Fs}{2\,Fo}\cos\Theta\,(\text{cm/sec})$$

where C is the average speed of sound in tissue [$1.54 \times 10^6\,\text{cm/sec}$], Fs is the shift in frequency between the transmitted and reflected Doppler beam, Fo is the frequency of the transmitted Doppler beam, and Θ is the Doppler beam angle.

If the mean frequency shift can be electronically extracted from the Doppler spectrum, the spatial average velocity (Vsa) as a function of time can be calculated. Volumetric blood flow (Q) can then be determined from a measurement of lumen diameter (D) by the equation:

$$Q = \frac{Vsa\,\prod D^2}{4}\,(\text{mL/min})$$

Although the determination of volumetric flow is attractive, the accurate calculation of Vsa can be quite difficult, because it requires complete insonation of the flow stream across the vessel lumen, knowledge of the velocity profile configuration, and a correction for both the forward and reverse components of pulsatile flow.

Duplex scanning provides both anatomic and physiologic informations regarding arterial flow. Tables 3 and 4 provide normal arterial lower limb mean and peak velocities and velocity waveform configurations seen with duplex scanning. This information has been applied clinically to the evaluation and classification of the atherosclerotic occlusive disease involving the carotid bifurcation, visceral arteries (renal, celiac, and superior mesenteric), the abdominal aorta, and the arteries of the lower limb. Under normal conditions, the flow in peripheral and carotid arteries is undisturbed (Figs. 11 and 12). As discussed previously, turbulence is responsible for most of the fluid energy loss associated with arterial disease. Because turbulence occurs at lesser degrees of stenosis than that causing detectable changes in mean flow and pressure, assessment of arterial flow by duplex scanning permits a more accurate diagnosis of altered hemodynamics than is possible by using techniques that monitor pressure and flow. Distal to a site of stenosis, turbulence is evident in the Doppler signal by an increase in peak systolic velocity, an alteration in the velocity waveform, and the presence of spectral broadening corresponding to the disordered, random movement of red blood cells in the flow stream. Accurate characterization of vessel anatomy and

Table 4 Normal Blood Flow Velocity Waveform Configurations in Peripheral Arteries

Arterial location	Biphasic	Triphasic
Cerebrovascular		
Internal, common carotid	X	
External carotid		X
Vertebral	X	
Visceral		
Celiac	X	
Superior mesenteric		
Fasting		X
Post-prandial	X	
Renal	X	
Peripheral (upper/lower limbs)		
Resting		X
After exercise	X	

flow in both normal and diseased states is possible by duplex mapping of the peripheral arterial system. Accuracy approximates that of contrast and magnetic resonance imaging and can also estimate whether lesions seen on angiogram are hemodynamically significant. Risks, cost, and discomfort are less than that of contrast and magnetic resonance imaging studies, although it is operator dependent and well-trained experienced technologists are required. Natural history studies of atherosclerosis using duplex scanning have demonstrated anatomic and hemodynamic features associated the initiation and progression of vascular disease. Compared with arteriography, diagnostic accuracy of duplex scanning is in excess of 80% in detection of greater than 50% diameter–reduction arterial stenosis or occlusion. Clinical applications include preintervention testing of peripheral, cerebrovascular, and visceral arterial disease, venous testing for acute/chronic venous thrombosis and venous insufficiency, intraoperative assessment of surgical and endovascular therapies, and postoperative graft surveillance and vascular disease.

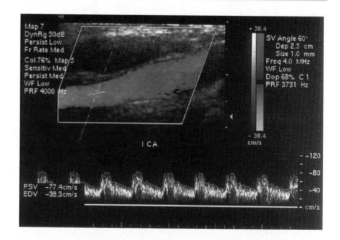

Figure 11 Color duplex scan imaging of the internal carotid artery. Sample volume of the pulsed Doppler probe is positioned in the proximal internal carotid artery. Narrow band of frequencies during the pulse cycle and the clear area beneath the waveform are characteristics of laminar flow in a normal carotid artery.

Table 3 Duplex-Derived Flow, Diameter, and Mean/Peak Systolic Flow Velocity Measurements from Lower Limb Artery Segments

	Artery segment			
Duplex	Common femoral	Popliteal	Anterior tibial	Posterior tibial
Flow (mL/min)	371	140	11	16
Diameter (mm)	8.6	6.6	2.2	2.3
Mean velocity (cm/s)	11	7	4	5
Peak velocity (cm/s)	89	66	58	57

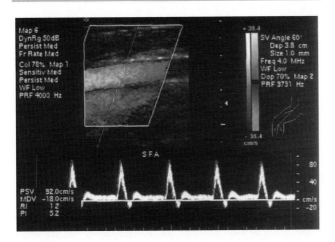

Figure 12 Color duplex examination of normal superficial femoral artery flow. Velocity spectra and waveform configuration are typical of normal flow in a limb artery.

THE VENOUS SYSTEM

The most important role of the venous system is probably that of a return conduit for blood from the peripheral tissues back to the heart and lungs for oxygenation. Veins also serve as a fluid reservoir for the vascular system, with up to 75% of the circulating blood volume being found in the venous system at any one time. In addition to these functions, the venous system is capable of augmenting ventricular filling pressure, thereby increasing cardiac output and stroke volume by sympathetic stimulated vasoconstriction. The mechanisms responsible are best addressed by considering first the anatomic configuration and unique structure of the venous channels, and then the interaction of the structural characteristics with the forces responsible for normal venous return.

Venous Anatomy

The venous system of the lower extremities is divided into superficial and deep systems. There is great variability in the anatomy of the deep and superficial veins, including segmental and complete duplicated systems. In the lower limbs, the common femoral vein is medial to the common femoral artery. The greater saphenous vein joins the common femoral vein at the saphenofemoral junction. The deep and superficial femoral veins generally join 3 to 5 cm cephalad to this point. The greater saphenous venous system begins anterior to the medial malleolus and travels subcutaneously on the anteriomedial aspect of the lower leg, 1 to 2 cm posterior to the tibia. It joins the femoral vein 2 to 4 cm lateral to the pubic tubercle and inferior to the inguinal ligament in the fossa ovalis. The superficial circumflex iliac vein and superficial inferior epigastric vein join the greater saphenous vein also in this area.

The venous system is more complex than the arterial system because veins are collapsible, affected by gravity and a low pressure system, contain valves, and are affected by the right side of the heart. The superficial system of the legs consists of the greater and lesser saphenous veins that are located in the subcutaneous tissue superficial to the deep fascia (Fig. 13). The veins are usually three times the size of their accompanying arteries and are composed of intima, media, and adventitia layers. Generally as one proceeds down the lower extremity, they encounter more valves. These superficial channels are responsible for collection of venous blood from the skin and subcutaneous tissues, and terminate by penetrating the deep fascia at the groin and popliteal fossa, respectively, to enter the deep venous channels. The superficial veins are subject to increased hydrostatic pressure and are therefore relatively thick walled. The superficial veins contain numerous bicuspid valves that facilitate flow from the periphery of the limb to the central portion of the limb and prevent flow in a retrograde direction. Competency of the valves in the lower extremities is more critical as compared to the upper extremity, where a malfunction more often leads to deep vein thrombosis, venous insufficiency, and venous stasis ulcers.

The deep system veins accompany the major muscular arteries and are similarly named. In the periphery of the limb, these channels are frequently present in duplicate and, because they are protected from the force of gravity by the muscles in the lower extremity, are relatively thin walled. Bicuspid valves are also present in these veins, with the greatest density occurring peripherally, and relatively few valves being located in the more central larger channels. For example, the superior and inferior vena cava, as well as the common iliac veins are devoid of valves, whereas the external iliac vein infrequently has a single bicuspid valve present. The popliteal vein has one to two valves, while the greater and lesser saphenous systems have about 8 to 10 valves each.

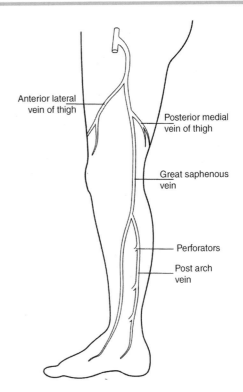

Figure 13 Diagrammatic representation of the major anatomic features of the greater and lesser saphenous veins and their tributaries.

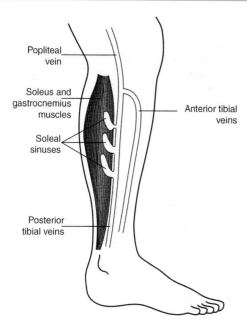

Figure 14 Schematic representation of the soleal sinuses and their relationship to the calf muscles and deep venous system. It should be noted that these empty directly into the deep venous system and also on occasion receive communications from the superficial system.

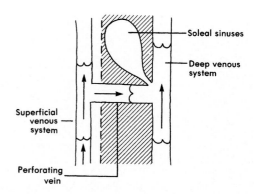

Figure 15 Schematic representation of the valvular relationships in the superficial veins, the connecting veins or perforators, and the deep venous system. It can be seen that under normal circumstances flow only occurs from the superficial to deep channels.

A second major component of the deep venous system is the soleal sinuses, a group of endothelium-lined venous reservoirs or "lakes" located within the substance of the gastrocnemius and soleus muscles (Fig. 14). These venous lakes are compressed by the calf muscles and are emptied during contraction, thereby facilitating venous emptying of the lower limb. These vein segments are also devoid of valves, and are a common site of early thrombus formation. Distally, they coalesce to join the peroneal and posterior tibial vessels.

The superficial and deep venous systems of the lower extremity are united by a series of perforating veins that pass from the superficial venous system through the deep fascia to the deep venous channels. These perforators range in number from 100 to 200, and are also most frequently located below the level of the knee. Bicuspid valves are also located in these channels so that, under normal circumstances, the flow occurs only from the superficial to the deep venous system (Fig. 15). Venous flow in the lower extremity, therefore, always travels in centripetal direction from peripheral to central channels. The presence of valves prevents reflux in the superficial, deep, and connecting systems. The necessity for valves is greatest at the most peripheral locations, where the gravitational force is greatest, and is least important in the central venous channels, where the pressure changes generated by respiration are sufficient to overcome the effects of gravity. In addition to blood traveling from the peripheral to central regions, it also moves preferentially from the superficial to the deep system, with only 10% of the venous outflow being conducted by the superficial veins and 90% by the deep veins.

Venous Structural Features

Vein wall thickness varies from one-third to one-tenth the thickness of the artery wall. Elastin wall content is considerably less than in the arterial wall, but like arteries, the amount of smooth muscle in the media is variable. The major factor influencing the smooth muscle content is not the necessity for control of regional blood flow as in arteries, but rather the gravitational force from blood the wall must withstand. The great saphenous vein has the highest percentage of smooth muscle, because it is located in the subcutaneous tissue in the lower limbs where it is exposed to maximum gravitational force with standing. At the foot and ankle, the smooth muscle may account for as much as 80% of the total wall thickness, whereas in the axillary vein, it composes only 5% of the vein wall.

The smooth muscle fibers are arranged in helical bundles united by strands of connective tissue, with a tough outer layer of predominately collagen fibers constituting the adventitia. Luminal to the smooth muscle layer is the intima, the most important component of which is the single layer of endothelial cells responsible for the blood and vessel wall interface. Perhaps because of the relatively low velocity in the venous system, these cells contain abundant quantities of fibrinolytic agents, with the veins in the lower extremity having higher concentrations than the intimal cells of the upper extremity. The lowest concentration of fibrinolytic active substances is found in the deep veins of the calf region and may in part explain the predisposition for thrombi to form in this location.

Because the deep veins are surrounded by skeletal muscles, which protect them from the adverse effects of gravity, they contain smaller amounts of smooth muscle and larger amounts of collagen. Increased collagen is the major factor responsible for the relative stiffness of these veins. In the large central veins such as the vena cava and iliac veins, this property is of major importance in determining shape changes induced by alterations in pressure–volume characteristics. Reductions in the volume of blood in these vessels result in collapse of the wall and assumption of an elliptical shape (Fig. 16). Restoration of volume to normal is associated with a resumption of the normal resting circular cross section. This shape change can also be demonstrated with more minimal external forces such as that generated by the respiratory cycle. However, the most common factor influencing the central veins is the overall circulatory blood volume.

These changes in the venous volume are accomplished with minimal changes in pressure because most

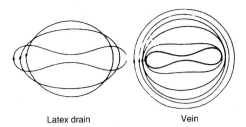

Latex drain   Vein

Figure 16 Capacitance of collapsible tubes. Effect of volume change on the cross-sectional area of veins showing the small cross-sectional ellipsoid state and the significant increase in cross-sectional area associated with filling. This change occurs without a change in circumference; because the wall is not stretched, the change can occur with the application of relatively minor force.

veins are partially collapsed during resting conditions. The importance of this is appreciated when it is realized that 40% of the total blood volume may be found in these large central veins at a pressure of 5 mmHg, whereas a reduction to 5% is accompanied by a fall in pressure of only a few millimeters of mercury. This is an example of how the central veins are able to collapse and auto-transfuse their volume into the arterial system, in order to maintain adequate blood flow. Thus the central venous system may be classified as a high-compliance, high-capacitance system as compared to the low-compliance, low-capacitance arterial system. Then, of practical clinical importance is the fact that the pressure measured in the central veins may be used as an index of the moment-to-moment blood volume, i.e., high pressure represents an expanded blood volume, and low pressure represents a volume deficiency.

Unlike arterioles, which are very sensitive to local mediators, veins and venules are controlled exclusively by sympathetic adrenergic activity except for the vein in skeletal muscle, which are without sympathetic influence, and the cutaneous veins, which are primarily thermoregulatory. Venous constriction may occur secondary to Valsalva maneuvers, muscular exercise, pain, hyperventilation, emotional stress, or with vasoconstrictive medications. Venous dilation can occur in conditions of shock, general anesthesia, or with vasodilator medications.

Pressure–Flow Relationships

In contrast to the arterial system, blood flow throughout the venous system is not mediated by a central pumping mechanism. The forces affecting pressure and therefore flow in the venous system are generated by respiration and exercise. The relative importance and interaction of these forces is best understood by considering the independent effects of each one and how they impact on the gravitational forces that must be overcome in the erect position.

Gravitational Effects

Gravitational forces have a negative effect on venous flow from the lower extremity, and are best appreciated by considering the pressure relationships first in the supine position when gravity is not a factor. In the supine position, the venular end of the capillaries has a pressure of approximately 15 mmHg, and the pressure in the right atrium is 5 mmHg. There is a point in the venous system located in the inferior vena cava close to the diaphragm, termed the hydrostatic indifference point where the pressure is always zero, regardless of attitude (Fig. 17). These pressure gradients are adequate to sustain normal venous return in the supine position, but are augmented by respiratory-induced pressure changes.

Assumption of the erect position results in profound changes in these pressure relationships. The system can then be likened to a vertical column of fluid, approximately 180 cm in height, in a hypothetic six-foot "dead man," although certain modifications of this model are required to parallel the real circumstances (Fig. 17). As noted earlier, the pressure at the hydrostatic indifference point is unchanged by the erect position, and right atrial pressure is normally 0 mmHg. The veins above this point will either fill or collapse, depending on the degree of filling in the system and the effects of respiration. This is best seen in the external jugular vein clinically, where intermittent filling and decompression are readily apparent. The skull acts as a protective barrier against these collapsing forces and maintains the intracerebral venous channels distended even in the erect position. Below the hydrostatic indifference point, the pressure gradually increases so that at the foot level a hydrostatic pressure of 80 mmHg is produced. This has two profound effects, the first of which is cessation of flow from the lower extremities and progressive pooling

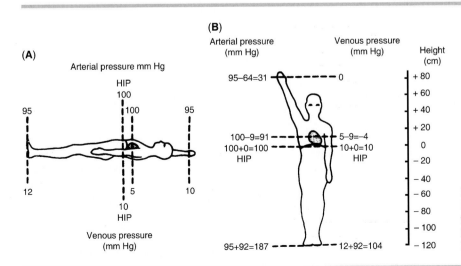

Figure 17 Pressure relationships in the various levels of the arterial and venous system shown in the supine (**A**) and the erect positions (**B**). HIP is located just below the diaphragm. *Abbreviation:* HIP, hydrostatic indifference point.

in the leg veins. This associated reduction in venous return secondarily produces a major decrease in cardiac output and, if the stimulus is long enough, may activate the syncope reflex. This pressure is also apparent in a change of the fluid dynamics at the tissue level, and, again, if it persists for any prolonged period, massive extravascular fluid extravasation may occur, further depleting venous return. This negative effort on venous circulation by gravity is overcome by the combined effects of respiration and exercise.

Effects of Respiration

The effects of respiration on venous flow are, again, most easily understood by first considering the pressure characteristics and changes that occur with the subjects in the supine position. During inspiration, negative pressure is generated in the thoracic cavity, which facilitates flow into the superior mediastinum from the venous channels in the head, neck, and upper extremity. Descent of the diaphragm produces an increase in intra-abdominal pressure that compresses the inferior vena cava and is associated with a marked reduction in flow from the lower extremities. The pressure changes produced by respiration are insufficient to overcome the gradient that exists between the peripheral venules and the right atrium, and therefore, even during inspiration, there is some venous outflow from the lower extremities. However, cessation of flow may be produced by increasing the pressure a few millimeters of mercury, as occurs with a Valsalva maneuver. Conversely, during expiration, venous return from the upper extremities and head and neck is interrupted, and flow from the lower extremities is augmented (Fig. 18).

Assumption of the erect position, however, introduces the force of gravity that drastically alters the pressure–flow relationships. Without the pulsatile pump of the arterial system, the venous circulation does not contain an intrinsic mechanism capable of overcoming this effect. Clearly the relatively small changes induced by respiration are inadequate for normal venous return, and additional forces must be activated. Prolonged assumption of the erect position without activation of other mechanisms results in a serious disturbance of the hydrostatic forces at the tissue level, with

the development of both peripheral edema and venous pooling in the lower extremities. A major force responsible for maintenance of normal venous return in the erect position is contraction of the calf muscles of the lower extremities.

Pressure Changes with Exercise

The calf muscle pump is to the venous system what the left ventricle is to the arterial system. The changes produced by calf muscle contraction are best considered by reviewing (i) the overall net effect after multiple muscle contractions and (ii) the step-by-step pressure relationships. Calf muscle contractions exert a force in excess of 80 mmHg on the walls of the calf veins, thus exceeding that exerted by gravity and resulting in a net efflux of blood out of the limb. With each contraction, the venous pressure is progressively lowered until the mean pressure at the ankle level falls to approximately 15 mmHg, similar to that in the resting supine state. These pressure changes are responsible for an overall reduction in the resistance of the peripheral vascular system and an associated increase in arterial inflow to the extremity, as required with exercise. Although this is the mean effect of exercise, the moment-to-moment pressure changes are more complex.

During the phase of calf muscle relaxation or diastole, the large venous channels are distended, and the pressure in the deep veins falls below that in the superficial veins. During calf muscle contraction, however, the pressure in the deep veins increases dramatically to exceed the pressure in the superficial veins, with a pumping effect being generated and forcing venous blood out of the extremities in an antegrade direction. During calf muscle relaxation, therefore, flow occurs from the superficial venous system to the deep venous system through the perforating veins; this flow is facilitated by the unidirectional valves contained in the perforating veins. During calf muscle contraction, the unidirectional valves in the deep venous system lead to the blood being forced to flow in a centripetal direction, with the valves in the perforating veins preventing reflux of blood into the superficial system. At the completion of calf muscle contraction, the cycle is again repeated (Fig. 19). Therefore, peripheral muscle pump resembles the working heart as it promotes the circulation of blood out of the lower extremities and empties the deep vein system, decreasing edema and venous congestion in the extremities, both of which result in an increased central blood volume. The increase in frequency and depth of respiration associated with exercise acts to facilitate overall venous return as well, although to a somewhat smaller degree.

Venous Endothelium

The endothelium is involved in the apperception of changes in blood flow and can influence vessel luminal size by changing the degree of contraction of the smooth muscle present in the vessel wall. Both natural and pharmaceutical grade compounds have been shown to alter vessel size by either vasodilatation or vasoconstriction, depending on the presence of an intact endothelium. Vessels devoid of endothelium, however, most often react with vasoconstriction alone. The endothelial cell–dependant dilation is related to the production of a nonprostanoid endothelial factor that results in a rise in cyclic guanosine monophosphate. NO, which is derived from L-arginine present in high concentrations in small resistant vessels also promotes vasodilatation. Intact endothelium has been shown to reduce platelet-induced spasms of the vessel wall. If the endothelial lining is

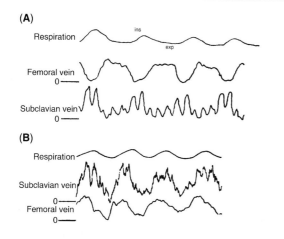

Figure 18 Relationship between respiration and flow in the femoral and subclavian veins in the supine (**A**) and in the erect positions (**B**). *Abbreviations*: Ins, inspiration; Exp, expiration.

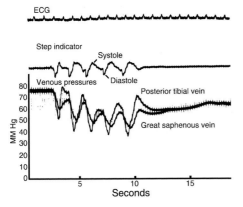

Figure 19 Pressure relationship between the superficial and deep venous system during walking. It should be noted that during calf muscle contraction or systole, the pressure in the deep system exceeds that in the superficial; whereas during calf muscle relaxation, pressure in the deep system is less than in the superficial. Filling of the calf muscle pump therefore occurs as with the heart during diastole. Posterior tibial veins are deep veins and great saphenous veins are superficial veins.

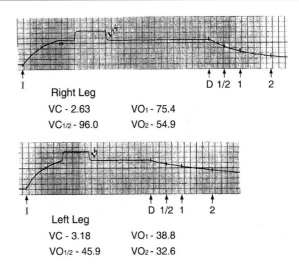

Figure 20 Plethysmographic recordings from a 60-year-old man four months after left iliofemoral deep vein thrombasis. Recordings were obtained from the right leg with no deep vein thrombosis and left leg with superficial femoral vein thrombosis. Recordings are obtained by inflating a pressure cuff above venous pressure followed by instantaneous release of the pressure. Rate of emptying is significantly less in right leg compared to left leg, a fact that can be used in a diagnostic investigation. *Abbreviations*: I, inflate; D, deflate; VC, venous capacitance; VO, venous exit flow.

undiminished, the complete absence of blood flow for a prolonged period of time does not result in clotting. Furthermore, the endothelium produces several antithrombotic substances as well as a number of procoagulants such as heparin sulfate and thrombomodulin prostaglandin I2 (prostacyclin), Factor 8, and von Willebrand Factor (vWF).

Changes Induced by Disease
Acute Venous Thrombosis
The development of deep venous thrombosis (DVT) in the major axial veins of the venous system will obviously have an effect of preventing normal venous outflow from the extremities (Fig. 20). This effect can be used as a diagnostic test with plethysmographic methods, to identify this condition. In veins with acute thrombosis, the venous pressure initially stays the same, but as obstruction increases, there is steady rise in the venous pressure as well. This results in accompanying increased edema and inflammation seen in this condition. This effect, however, can be quite variable and depends not only on the location and extent of the venous thrombosis, but also on the availability of collateral venous channels to compensate for the obstruction. It is, therefore, not infrequent to observe that venous thrombosis may not be associated with significant edema, especially in the setting of a well-functioning collateral venous network.

A secondary effect of an occlusive thrombus and the development of peripheral venous hypertension is that the minor pressure changes produced by respiration are not transmitted beyond the area of obstruction. Duplex venous ultrasound is now the gold standard for the diagnosis of this condition and demonstrates nicely the flow disturbances associated with DVT. With acute DVT, the flow distal to the obstruction loses its normal phasic relationship to respiration and becomes continuous (Fig. 21). Flow now does not augment well with manual compression distal to the obstruction. Visualizing thrombus is possible with duplex, which carries a 96% specificity and a 94% sensitivity with an overall accuracy of 96%.

Air plethysmography has been used to quantitate venous reflux and calf muscle pump ejection volume

(Fig. 22). The instrument uses an air-filled chamber wrapped around the lower leg to determine absolute volume changes in the leg as a result of exercise. Baseline limb volume is measured with the patient supine and the leg elevated 45°, to empty the veins. Volume measurements are then made during non–weight-bearing standing, and with single and repetitive calf muscle contractions. Calculations are then made to determine venous filling index, ejection fraction, and residual volume fraction. Plethysmography is usually used to evaluate the venous system in preparation for venous surgery, to correct severe venous valve reflux.

Chronic Post-thrombotic Venous Insufficiency
The adverse long-term sequelae of venous thrombosis are produced by the residual venous obstruction and the destruction of valves in both the deep axial veins and the perforating

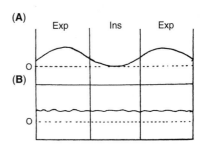

Figure 21 Venous flow patterns in the normal state (**A**) and in the presence of venous obstruction (**B**). It should be noted that in the latter there is a loss of the oscillatory pattern produced by respiration. *Abbreviations*: Exp, expiration; Ins, inspiration.

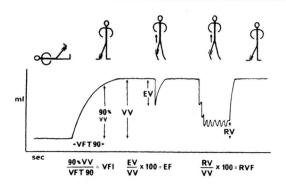

Figure 22   Methods of deriving air plethysmography values. *Abbreviations*: EV, evoked potential; RV, residual volume; RVF, residual volume fraction; VFI, venous filling index; VFT, venous filling time; VV, venous volume. *Source*: From Ref. 6.

veins. This latter effect, in particular, produces profound changes in the dynamics of the venous circulation during exercise, which at least, in part, is responsible for the clinical changes of edema, hyperpigmentation, and ulceration.

The most significant changes are demonstrated during exercise. Valve destruction adversely affects the flow patterns produced by the pressure changes seen with exercise, and, instead of flowing in a centripetal direction and from superficial to deep, blood may be forced under high pressure from the deep system, during calf muscle contraction, through incompetent perforating veins, into the superficial system producing severe superficial hypertension. In the deep system, the normal antegrade flow pattern is completely interrupted and venous return from the leg is significantly reduced.

Instead of a gradual reduction in venous pressure in the lower extremity produced by exercise, in severe cases, exercise may actually be associated with an increase in the venous pressure in both the deep and superficial systems, as depicted in Figure 23. The likelihood of developing severe complications such as venous ulceration is closely related to the degree of ambulatory venous hypertension that occurs in such patients as shown in Table 5.

LYMPHATIC SYSTEM

The lymphatic system consists of: (i) lymphatic vessels or plexuses, which consist of a network of closed endothelial tubes that function to recover fluid and macromolecules (e.g., albumin and other proteins) that have diffused into the interstitium at the capillary level; (ii) lymph nodes, which

Table 5   Relation of Ambulatory Venous Hypertension to Incidence of Ulceration

Ambulatory venous pressure (mmHg)	Incidence of ulceration (%)
45	0
45–50	5
50–59	15
60–69	50
70–79	75
80	80

are small aggregates of lymph tissue that filter the lymph circulation as it moves more centrally; and (iii) lymphoid tissues, which are responsible for fat absorption in the form of chylomicrons, when found in the gastrointestinal tract (e.g., lactiles), and are involved in the humeral mechanism of the immune reaction, when found elsewhere (e.g., spleen, tonsils, and thymus). Although the lymphatic system is involved with gastrointestinal and immune function, it is its role in protein and interstitial fluid reabsorption that is of significant importance to circulatory pathophysiology. Disruption of the balance of arteriovenous hydrostatic or oncotic pressures can produce an imbalance in lymphatic transport capacity and lead to the development of lymphedema.

Anatomy

Similar to the venous system of the extremities, the lymphatic system is composed of superficial and deep lymphatic systems. The basic unit of the superficial lymphatic vasculature is an initial lymphatic sinus. These terminal sinuses are lined by a single layer of lymphoid endothelial cells. They coalesce to form lymphphatic aerola, which serve as collection stations for lymph drainage from the skin and subcutaneous tissues. Lymphatic aerola are connected by precollector lymph channels and eventually empty into larger collector lymph channels. One way valves are spaced every several millimeters (mm) throughout the precollector and collector lymph channels and provide with one way lymph flow. The superficial lymphatics are estimated to handle 90% to 95% of the lymphatic effluent from the extremities. The deeper system of the lymphatic vasculature serves to drain the subfascial structures of the musculoskeletal system and the deep circulatory vessels. These two systems seem to run parallel in the extremities, joining in the regions of the pelvis or axilla.

In the lower extremities, the lymphatic channels approximate 1 to 2 mm in diameter. The major superficial lymph channels begin in the dorsum of the foot and course primarily along the medial aspect of the leg in the distribution of the saphenous vein. In the upper thigh, these channels terminate in the superficial inguinal lymph nodes and in turn empty into the deep nodal basins. Usually five to eight major lymphatic channels are located at this level. The deep lymphatic channels are less numerous and course in close proximity to the deep muscular arteries of the extremities. In the high thigh, they empty into the deep inguinal lymph nodes as well. In the lower extremities, the lymph circulation then flows from the deep nodal basins into the lymph nodes/channels along the pelvic brim. Again these channels course intimately with the major pelvic vessels. At the level of the lumbosacral joints, these channels form the para-aortic lymph channels that course along the aorta and through the central retroperitoneum. At this level, the lymph from the lower extremities now joins chyle from the intestinal lymphatics in the cisterna chyle, which is eventually transported via the thoracic duct through the thorax, terminating in the posterior triangle on the left side at the junction of the internal jugular and subclavian veins. In the upper extremities, the superficial and deep systems coalesce in the axillary regions and the travel in larger lymph channel to the venous circulation. The thoracic duct drains lymph from the entire body except that of the right arm, neck, head, and thorax. The lymphatics on this side of the body use a lymphatic pathway that empties lymph into the right lymphatic duct that in turn empties in the junction of the right subclavian and internal jugular veins.

Physiology

Bicuspid valves are located every few centimeters along the course of the lymphatic channels and enable lymph flow to occur from peripheral to more central regions. The lymphatic adventitia contains smooth muscle fibers and is capable of exhibiting vasomotion and self-propagation of fluid. Independent contractions, also called propulsor lymphaticum, can produce pressures in the vicinity of 50 mmHg every four to five minutes. These contractions mimic venous and arterial vasomotion and are mediated by sympathomimetic agents (alpha- and beta-adrenergic agents), arachidonic acid metabolism (thromboxanes and prostaglandins), and neurogenic stimuli. Contraction of adjacent muscle groups as well as the respiratory cycle also serves to assist in the return of lymph flow to the venous system. Intrinsic lymphatic contractility increases in response to tissue edema, temperature change, exercise, and hydrostatic pressure.

The understanding of the exchange dynamics at the capillary level is paramount in defining the role of the lymphatics in recovering interstitial proteins and fluids. Capillary filtration and diffusion are the two main processes that drive this exchange and recovery process. The movement of fluid across the capillary membrane is known as filtration. This process is governed by the principles of the Starling hypothesis. Basically, intravascular hydrostatic pressure and osmotic pressure oppose interstitial hydrostatic and osmotic pressure at the capillary level (Fig. 23). A relative increase in the intravascular hydrostatic pressure or a decrease in oncotic pressure favors an increased filtration of fluid out of the capillary membrane. Under normal circumstances, there is a slight excess of fluid filtered at the arterial capillary end over that reabsorbed at the venous end. It is this excess fluid, which approximates 0.003 mL/min/g of tissue in the moving lower limb, that is transported in the lymphatics.

Diffusion also plays a major role in the exchange of molecules across the capillary membrane. The semipermeable capillary membrane and the size of the pores govern the diffusion process of micro- and macroprotiens. The lymphatic sinuses of the terminal lymphatics are highly permeable to these proteins and act as suction pumps to facilitate the recovery of these lost proteins. Contraction of the lymphatic wall may result in the generation of a positive pressure proximal to the area of contraction and a negative pressure at the bulbous terminal portion of the lymphatic that facilitates entry of the protein rich interstitial fluid. As much as 50% (150–200 g) of circulating albumin is lost into the interstitial space every 24 hours. The lymphatic system allows for the return of two to four liters of this protein-rich lymph to the venous circulation.

Lymphatics in Disease

Disruption in lymphatic flow from occlusion, trauma, infection, or other illness can interfere with the lymphatic system's role in fluid dynamics, homeostasis, and immune function, termed as secondary lymphedema. Primary lymphedema reflects heritable defects in lymphatic development and function and is classified by the age of onset. Congenital lymphedema is apparent within the first two years of life, represents 15% of clinical cases, and is caused by aplasia or hypoplasia of lymphatic channels. Lymphedema prascox comprises 75% of clinical cases and is first detected at puberty. Lymphedema tarda, which typically appears after the age of 35, can result from either hypo- or hyperplastic lymphatic vasculature. Skin and limb changes with lymphatic obstruction or inefficient lymphatic outflow are different from those seen with arterial or venous obstruction. Obstructed lymphatic vessels have been known to have pressures as high as 50 to 60 mmHg, and unlike the vascular system, a collateral network does not exist. If flow in the vascular system becomes impaired or obstructed, the supply of essential nutrients to tissues is impaired and tissue ischemia results.

Because valves are absent in the terminal sinuses of the minute lymphatic capillaries of the dermal plexuses, disruption or obstruction in the larger lymph channels results in a significant increase in extracellular fluid retention and resultant edema. This edema, also called "lymphedema," appears gradually with lymphatic obstruction. An accumulation of large protein molecules in the tissue results in increased oncotic pressure and a net accumulation of extracellular fluid. The delivery of nutrients is typically only minimally impaired, and tissue viability is generally maintained. Eventually a steady state will be reached at which the hydrostatic pressure exerted by the fluid in the tissues will balance that of the oncotic pressure, and essentially normal fluid exchange will continue. Despite what seems like a restoration of fluid homeostasis, the edema will remain, unless additional therapy is instituted.

Treatment programs, also known as lymphedema clinics, institute a multidiscipline team approach toward dealing with this condition. Medical management and dietary counseling is undertaken. Physical therapy and exercise programs are initiated. These programs typically use a combination of compression garments and massage therapies to reduce the peripheral edema. Occasionally, lymphatic pumps can also be employed. The role of surgery for the condition of lymphedema continues to decline due in part to the success of these programs.

SUMMARY

The circulatory system as a whole serves to maintain normal tissue nutrition under conditions of rest and exercise, with both the arterial and venous systems, like many other body systems, having a sizeable functional reserve capacity. The arterial and venous systems are primarily involved in the maintenance of a favorable tissue milieu for normal

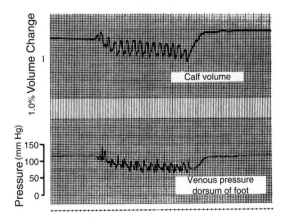

Figure 23 Effect of calf muscle exercise on ankle pressure in patients with the postthrombotic syndrome. There is no significant decrease in venous pressure associated with exercise as is seen in the normal state.

metabolism, with the lymphatics functioning as a scavenger system to remove macromolecules and any excess of fluid that is extravasated from the capillary mechanism. Whereas the arterial system is dynamic with the energy being provided intrinsically by contraction of the left ventricle, both the venous and lymphatic systems are uniquely designed to facilitate movement of fluid under relatively low pressures and rely predominately on extrinsic forces such as respiration and skeletal muscle contraction to offset the "edema-producing" effects of gravity.

REFERENCES

1. Smith JJ, Kampine JP. Circulatory Physiology. 2nd ed. Baltimore: Williams & Wilkins, 1984.
2. Zierler RE, Strandness DE. In: Moore WS, ed. Vascular Surgery–A Comprehensive Review. New York: Grune & Stratton, 1983.
3. Ruch TC, Patton HD. Physiology and Biophysics. Philadelphia: WB Saunders, 1974.
4. Roederer G, Langlois Y, Strandness DE Jr, et al. Comprehensive noninvasive evaluation of extracranial cerebrovascular disease. In: Hershey FB, Barnes RW, Sumner DS, eds. Noninvasive Diagnosis of Vascular Disease. Pasadena, Calif: Appeleton-Davies, 1984.
5. Summer DS. Pitfalls on noninvasive cerebrovascular testing and angiography. In: Bernhard VM, Towne JB, eds. Complications in Vascular Surgery. 2d ed. New York: Grune & Stratton, 1985.
6. Belcaro G, Laurora G, Christopoulos S, et al. Noninvasive tests in venous insufficiency. J Cardiovasc Surg 34; 3:1993. Reprinted with permission.

FURTHER READINGS

Burton AC. Physiology and Biophysics of the Circulation. Chicago: Year Book Medical Publishers, 1972.
Cockett FB, Dodd H, eds. The Pathology and Surgery of the Veins of the Lower Limb. Edinburgh: Churchill Livingstone, 1976.
Folkow B, Neil E. Circulation. Oxford: Oxford University Press, 1971.
Guyton AC. Human Physiology and Mechanism of Disease. 2d ed. Phildelphia: WB Saunders, 1982.
Milnor WR. Hemodynamics. Baltimore: Williams & Wilkins, 1982.
Strandness DE, Sumner DS. Hemodynamics for Surgeons. New York: Grune & Stratton, 1975.
Szuba A, Rockson S. Lymphedema anatomy, physiology, and pathogenesis. Vasc Med 1977; 2:321–326.

44

Aorta and Arterial Disease of the Lower Extremity

Christopher K. Zarins and Sheila M. Coogan

INTRODUCTION

Degenerative changes in the aorta and atherosclerosis of lower extremity arteries account for the majority of vascular complications in elderly patients (1). Aging of the baby boom population will result in rapid growth of the elderly population. By the year 2040, people older than 65 will comprise 22% of the U.S. population, or 67 million people. The most striking aspect of this trend is the increased rate of survival of those older than 75 (2). Obviously, the management of atherosclerotic complications of the aorta and its branches will play an increasingly significant role in the primary health care of a major portion of the adult American population.

Atherosclerotic arterial disease is characterized by the formation of intimal plaques. These plaques may obstruct the lumen, ulcerate and embolize, cause thrombosis, or contribute to aneurysmal degeneration of the arterial wall. Each of these processes may result in a spectrum of clinical presentations requiring different diagnostic and therapeutic approaches. In this chapter, we consider some of the general features of the atherosclerosis, along with its pathologic and clinical manifestations in the lower extremity, and discuss diagnostic methods and current treatment alternatives.

ATHEROSCLEROSIS

Risk Factors

The risk factors for atherosclerosis may be divided into two major categories, reversible and irreversible. Major reversible factors include cigarette smoking, diabetes mellitus, hyperglycemia, hypertension, abnormalities of lipid metabolism, obesity, and low levels of physical activity. Nonreversible factors are primarily sex, age, and genetic influences of family history.

It has been generally assumed that the factors associated with plaque formation and development in the extracoronary arteries are the same as those in the coronary arteries (2). However, there have been few population-based studies of risk factors associated with atherosclerosis of the aorta or the lower extremity branches. Several early studies considered only the symptomatic form of the disease (3,4). More recently, noninvasive methods have been used to identify and include asymptomatic subjects in these investigations (5,6). These findings are summarized in Table 1. The most significant risk factors apparently have independent effects (i.e., not cumulative) on the vasculature of the abdomen, pelvis, and lower extremity.

Control of certain risk factors may have a beneficial effect on the expression, of the disease. Cessation of tobacco use has a beneficial effect on peripheral occlusive disease, and limb loss rates and arterial graft patency rates are improved in patients who can successfully abstain from tobacco (7,8). Optimization of serum lipid profiles and control of hypertension have less certain impact on the progression of lower extremity arterial disease, but are known to be beneficial in preventing progression of coronary atherosclerosis (2). Physical exercise may ameliorate the symptoms, of aortic and peripheral occlusive disease, and may play a role in preventing progression of disease. Weight reduction and control of environmental stress also play important roles. Recent data from the Diabetes Control and Complication Trial suggest that close control of serum glucose does not prevent progression or complications of peripheral vascular occlusive disease as measured by limb salvage in the setting of insulin-dependent diabetes mellitus (9).

Configuration and Composition of Atherosclerotic Plaque

Although atherosclerotic plaques contain varying amounts of lipids, it is unclear whether all lesions containing lipids are necessarily precursors of clinically significant atherosclerotic plaques. A prime example of this uncertainty is demonstrated by the questionable significance of the so-called fatty streak lesion. This term describes a flat, yellow, focal luminal patch or streak, representing an accumulation of lipid-laden foam cells in the intima, evident in most people older than three years. They are identified with increasing frequency between the ages of 8 and 18, after which many apparently resolve. Fatty streaks exist at any age, often adjacent to or even superimposed on advanced atherosclerotic plaques. Fatty streaks and atheromata, however, do not have identical patterns of localization, and fatty streaks do not compromise the lumen or ulcerate (10). Although this subject remains controversial, the link and

Table 1 Risk Factors Associated with the Development of Lower Extremity Arterial Disease, Disease Progression, and Mortality

Risk factor	Development of disease	Progression	Mortality
Smoking	Yes	Yes	Yes
Diabetes	Yes	NAI	Yes
Hyperlipidemia	Yes	NAI	NAI
Hypertension	Yes	NAI	Yes
Physical activity	Yes	NAI	Yes
Hemorheologic factors	NAI	NAI	NAI
Obesity	No; however, may be a weak risk factor in men	NAI	NAI
Genetic factors	NAI	NAI	Yes

Abbreviation: NAI, not adequately investigated.

transition between fatty streak and fibrous plaque formation remain to be clarified.

The term *fibrous plaque* identifies the characteristic and unequivocal atherosclerotic lesion. These intimal deposits appear in the second decade of life, becoming predominant or clinically significant only during or after the fourth decade. Fibrous plaques usually are eccentric and are covered by an intact endothelial surface. Although considerable variation exists in plaque composition and configuration, a characteristic architecture prevails. The immediate subendothelial region of the plaque consists of a compact and well-organized stratified layer of smooth muscle cells and connective tissue fibers known as the fibrous cap. This structure may mimic medial architecture, including the formation of a subendothelial elastic lamina, which may function to sequester the underlying necrotic and thrombogenic plaque core from the luminal surface. This surface usually is regular, with a concave contour corresponding to the circular or oval cross-sectional lumen of the uninvolved vessel wall segment. The stable necrotic core occupies the deeper plaque (Fig. 1). The core contains amorphous, crystalline, and droplet forms of lipid. Cells of undetermined origin, with morphologic, functional, and cell surface receptor characteristics of smooth muscles or macrophages are noted beneath the core. These cells also may contain lipid vacuoles. Calcium and myxoid deposits, collagen and elastin matrix fibers, basal lamina, and amorphous ground substance are also evident. Atherosclerotic plaques grow in an episodic fashion, demonstrating dense fibrocellular regions adjacent to organizing thrombus and atheromatous debris. Intermittent ulceration and healing occur, with thrombi being incorporated into the lesion.

Vasa vasorum may nourish the plaque, facilitating the organization of thrombotic deposits and the remodeling of the plaque and artery wall (11). Attenuation of the subadjacent media promotes outward bulging of the plaque toward the adventitia. Although this attenuation sequesters plaque, enlarges the artery, and stabilizes the wall, a predominant lytic reaction may result in excessive arterial dilation or aneurysmal degeneration. Experimental evidence suggesting such a mechanism for aneurysm formation has been obtained in nonhuman primates in our laboratory (12) and by other investigators (13).

Tissues between the necrotic core and the media, however, usually are densely fibrotic. Arterial wall support may thus be maintained by the integrity of the fibrous cap or thickened adventitia. Advanced lesions, particularly those associated with aneurysms, may appear to be atrophic and relatively acellular, consisting of dense fibrous tissue and a minimal necrotic center. Calcification is a prominent feature, involving the superficial and deeper layers. Terms such as *fibrocalcific*, *lipid-rich*, *necrotic*, and *myxomatous* describe various predominant aspects of advanced plaques. Calcific deposits are most prominent in plaques in older people and in the abdominal aorta or coronary arteries, where the earliest plaques form in animal models and in humans (14). The usual eccentric plaque bulges outward from the lumen; the external cross-sectional contour of an atherosclerotic artery becomes oval while retaining a circular lumen (Fig. 1) (15,16).

Localizing Factors in the Development of Atherosclerotic Lesions

Adaptive changes in arterial luminal diameter are determined by changes in blood flow. During embryologic growth and development, lumen diameter is determined by the volume of blood flow. After birth, increases in artery diameter continue as a response to increases in blood flow (17). This phenomenon is also demonstrated in mature arteries after cessation of growth, with enlargement of arteries proximal to arteriovenous fistulas and a decrease in the size of arteries proximal to amputated limbs (18).

Luminal diameter adaptation is responsive to wall shear stress, as determined by the effective velocity gradient at the endothelial-blood interface (19). In mammals, wall shear stress normally ranges between 10 and 20 dynes/cm^2 at all locations throughout the arterial vasculature. In arteriovenous fistulas, the afferent artery enlarges enough to restore shear stress to this physiologic range (20). This response depends on the presence of an intact endothelial surface (21) and may be mediated by the release of endothelium-derived relaxant factors, including nitric oxide or other vasoactive agents (22). Near-wall properties of arterial flow fields and the distribution of mural wall shear stress correspond closely to atherosclerotic plaque localization (23–30). Plaques develop where shear stress is reduced (25,26), not elevated, with an intact endothelial surface, even in the absence of platelet deposition (31). The revised response to injury hypothesis now stresses on metabolic or functional changes sustained by intact endothelial cells that alter binding or metabolism of lipid molecules or modify transendothelial transport, rather than denudation of the endothelium itself (32).

Atherosclerosis tends to occur principally in three locations within the arterial vasculature: the carotid-cerebral, coronary, and aortic-peripheral system. Within these predisposed regions, lesions form in predictable geometric configurations, demonstrating the influence of shear stress and flow patterns. Size as well as localization closely correlates with low wall shear stress and departures from unidirectional

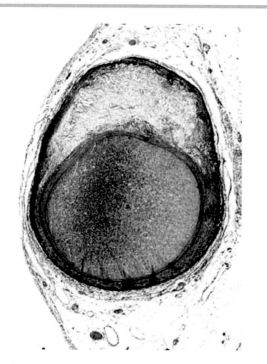

Figure 1 Atherosclerotic plaque demonstrating the fibrous cap over a necrotic center. Note the oval external contour with the round lumen typical of these plaques.

flow (25,26). Plaque initiation and localization are the result of low rather than high shear stress, low flow velocity, flow separation, and oscillation in wall shear direction (33).

Regions of increased mural tensile stress about branches (23), pulsatile wall motion (34), and wall thickness and density (35,36) are also associated with selective plaque localization. Conversely, regions of relatively elevated wall shear stress or reduced tensile stress, at flow dividers and along the outer or convex aspects of curved arterial segments, generally are spared (37). Hemodynamics and tensile influences are also important in plaque progression and evolution (38,39) and influence potential plaque regression (40). As an example of this influence on regression, hypertension was found to sustain experimental plaque progression in a hypercholesterolemic cynomolgus monkey model, despite a reduction in serum cholesterol level (41). Reduced flow and consequent reduction in wall shear stress also tend to induce intimal thickening. An increase in wall volume, including cell enlargement, cell proliferation, and net matrix accumulation, is demonstrated in long-term reactions (42).

A sieving effect related to these changes in wall composition (43,44) and porosity (35) has been proposed. Wall thickening, including intimal thickening, may retard transmural mass transport, providing the basis for intimal lipid deposition (45). The accumulation of matrix fibers with affinity for lipid molecules (46–50) and the fusion or accretion of lipid particles on these components may also be responsible.

PATHOPHYSIOLOGIC PROCESSES AFFECTING THE AORTA AND LOWER EXTREMITY ARTERIES

The processes affecting the arteries to the lower extremity include plaque formation with obstruction of the lumen and subsequent limitation of flow, thrombosis resulting in acute ischemia, ulceration of the plaque with distal embolization, and weakening of the arterial wall with aneurysmal formation resulting in rupture or thrombosis.

Stenosis

Progressive intimal plaque deposition may result in narrowing of the lumen, or stenosis. Mild degrees of stenosis producing less than 50% reduction in lumen diameter usually do not obstruct blood flow. It is not until lumen diameter falls below a critical point that resistance to blood flow increases. This is referred to as *critical arterial stenosis*, or the percentage by which the lumen diameter must be reduced to produce a measurable drop in blood flow. Under experimental conditions, there is no significant pressure drop and no reduction in flow until there is more than 80% reduction in lumen cross-sectional area (equivalent to 55% diameter reduction) (51). However, pressure drops across stenoses are critically dependent on flow, and noncritical stenoses at rest may develop significant pressure gradients when flow is increased with exercise. This can account for the clinical observation of disappearing pedal pulses after exercise and symptoms of claudication in patients with palpable pedal pulses.

The extent of disability from an obstruction is related to the location of the lesion, the degree of obstruction, the length and number of obstructions, the metabolic needs of the tissues distal to the obstruction, and the ability of collateral vessels to provide the necessary flow. *Collateral blood flow* may be quite extensive in occlusive disease. Collateral

vessels are naturally existing branches of large- and medium-sized arteries that enlarge to carry blood flow around an obstruction. They do not represent neovascularization but adaptation of existing vessels to an increased demand of blood flow. The collateral blood flow that develops in the face of a developing, progressive obstruction usually can supply the demands of resting tissue. However, it often is unable to supply the flow necessary for an exercising muscle group.

There are a number of well-recognized collateral beds that develop in the presence of atherosclerosis of the aorta and distal tree:

1. Intercostal and lumbar arteries
2. Superior and inferior mesenteric arteries
3. Hypogastric artery
4. Profunda-genicular arteries
5. Peroneal-tibial arteries

Patients may have a totally occluded abdominal aorta for several years, with relatively mild symptoms of hip and buttock claudication. Under these circumstances, the intercostal arteries, superior epigastric arteries, and visceral arteries become important sources of collateral flow to the lower extremity (Fig. 2). For example, blood supply to the distal aorta may be through the inferior mesenteric artery, which derives collateral supply from the superior mesenteric artery. In addition, the inferior mesenteric artery

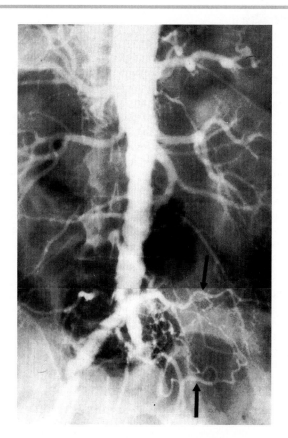

Figure 2 Angiogram revealing severe aortoiliac disease. Note the large collateral vessels (*arrows*) that have developed in response to occlusion of the left iliac artery.

can be an important source of collateral flow to the lower extremity through the superior hemorrhoidal network.

Thrombosis

The causes of *acute arterial obstruction* can be divided into two categories: embolism and thrombosis. Emboli arise from a proximal source, either the heart or proximal great vessels, and obstruct the tapering arterial tree at a branch point or at the point where the embolus is larger than the lumen diameter. Mural thrombus that forms in a fibrillating atrium is the most common source of arterial emboli (52), but emboli can also arise from areas of recent transmural infarction, ventricular aneurysms, and diseased valves. Spontaneous thrombosis usually occurs in arteriosclerotic arteries as a result of slow flow caused by severe stenotic lesions or as a result of sudden dissection or hemorrhage under a previously nonstenotic plaque.

Acute thrombosis usually results in very sudden and severe symptoms of arterial ischemia. The severity of clinical symptoms is related to the site of the obstruction, the size and extent of the thrombus, and the adequacy of the collateral vessels. In severe ischemia, one or more of the often-described five Ps may be present: pulselessness, pallor, paresthesia, pain, and paralysis. The loss of motor power and sensation in the toes and foot indicates very severe ischemia and limb loss unless the ischemia is relieved promptly. Acute thrombosis of a previously stenosed artery that has excellent collateral vessels about it may occur with only mild symptoms and little risk of limb loss.

Ulceration

Ulceration occurs when breakdown of the fibrous cap over a lesion exposes the necrotic core of the plaque to the circulation. This may be the site for platelet deposition (1) and thrombus formation or may result in embolization of the plaque contents itself, producing cholesterol emboli in the distal arterial tree.

The most common clinical syndrome in the peripheral circulation associated with distal embolization from a proximal ulcerated plaque is the *blue toe syndrome.* Patients may have normal pedal pulses but suddenly develop one or more cold, blue, painful toes—a condition that resolves in three to four days. These symptoms may be caused by cholesterol emboli in the digital arteries of the feet. The source of the emboli usually is a proximal ulcerated lesion in the aorta, iliac, or femoral vessels. Unrecognized and untreated repeated embolization to the foot results in obstruction of the small arteries of the foot, gangrene, and limb loss.

Aneurysm Formation

An aneurysm is a localized arterial dilation. A *true aneurysm* is one in which there is thinning or atrophy of all layers of the artery wall, with enlargement of the lumen. This should be distinguished from *a false aneurysm,* which results from a rupture of the artery wall, usually caused by trauma, with containment of the blood stream by fibrous tissue surrounding the vessel. Thus in a true aneurysm there is an inadequate artery wall, whereas in a false aneurysm there is absence of the artery wall.

As the lumen radius of an aneurysm enlarges, there is an increase in *tension* on the vessel wall (T), according to the law of Laplace ($T = Pr$), where P is pressure and r is radius. The larger the radius, the greater is the tension and the greater is the tendency for further enlargement of the lumen.

This explains why larger aneurysms have a greater tendency to expand and rupture than do smaller aneurysms. Blood flow in the dilated aneurysmal sac is slower than normal, producing an increased tendency to thrombosis. Most large abdominal aortic aneurysms are lined by laminated mural thrombus. Mural thrombus may be so thick that the lumen caliber on angiography does not appear enlarged. However, mural thrombus provides little, if any, support for the artery wall and no protection from aneurysm rupture.

ARTERIAL OCCLUSIVE DISEASE OF THE AORTA AND PERIPHERAL ARTERIES

The manifestations of atherosclerosis in the aorta and peripheral arteries are either occlusive disease or aneurysm formation. The arteries of importance in the circulation to the lower extremities are diagrammed on Figure 3. Obstructive plaques may occur in each of the vessels shown but are most common in the infrarenal abdominal aorta, iliac arteries, and superficial femoral arteries. The profunda femoris artery is relatively spared, and diabetic patients are more prone to develop lesions in the tibial arteries.

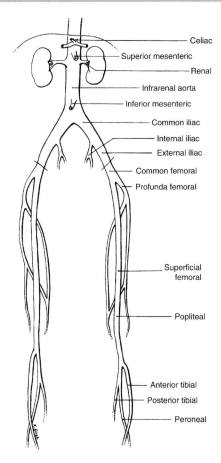

Figure 3　Arterial supply to the viscera and lower extremity. Obstructive or aneurysmal changes can occur in each of these vessels. The clinical signs and symptoms vary depending on the location and blood supply distribution of a given artery. Full angiographic evaluation of the aorta and lower extremity vessels should demonstrate flow through each of these arteries.

Clinical Manifestations of Peripheral Occlusive Disease

The clinical manifestations and physical findings of peripheral occlusive disease are as follows:

Clinical manifestation	Physical findings
Claudication	Absent or diminished pulses
Rest pain	Bruits
Ulceration	Skin pallor
Gangrene	Hair loss
Impotence	Dependent rubor
	Skin and muscle atrophy
	Trophic changes of the nails
	Tissue necrosis

Claudication

Claudication arises from the term *claudicatio*, which means to limp. It is a clinical syndrome of pain on exercise, which is relieved by rest and results from a fixed obstruction or stenosis in arteries to the lower extremity. Although circulation may be adequate at rest, with exercise there is an increasing demand for flow. When such flow is obstructed by a stenosis, the muscle served by that vessel becomes ischemic and begins to function with anaerobic metabolism. This results in pain and symptoms of fatigue, causing the patient to stop and rest. Typically, the patient rests for one to two minutes, allowing the circulation to again restore aerobic conditions, after which the patient can again exercise. Patients with aortoiliac occlusive disease have symptoms of claudication in the hips and buttocks, whereas patients with superficial femoral artery obstruction have symptoms of claudication in the calf. The level of claudication is always below the level of the arterial obstruction.

Most patients with claudication, although symptomatic, are at low risk for developing gangrene. Only 33% of patients with proven arterial stenosis report symptoms of claudication. It is a stable disease in 70% to 80% of patients, and it is generally clinically accepted that only 25% of claudicants deteriorate (53–57). Thus patients with stable, nonlimiting claudication may be safely followed, and revascularization should be reserved for those with disabling symptoms. Reconstructive surgery to improve blood flow is done in less than 10% of all patients with claudication. Amputation may be required in 1% to 5% (58). The benign nature of this symptom should be carefully considered when planning any type of intervention, either catheter based or via traditional open arterial surgery.

Rest Pain

Patients with worsening ischemia develop a clinical syndrome called rest pain. The condition of rest pain indicates a much more severe degree of ischemia than claudication and, unlike claudication, indicates that the patient is at high risk for developing gangrene and limb loss. Typically, the patient experiences pain in the toes and forefoot during the night, which causes him or her to awaken from sleep. The patient usually sits up in bed, dangles the legs over the side of the bed, and frequently relieves the symptoms by getting up and walking. After a short period of time, the patient's symptoms have disappeared and the patient can return to sleep. The symptoms of rest pain occur because of severe ischemia in the forefoot and toes, brought about by two conditions: (i) the patient is recumbent and thereby eliminates the hydrostatic pressure gradient that assists the arteriolar perfusion pressure when erect; and (ii) during sleep there is a diminution of cardiac output that correspondingly diminishes the volume of peripheral blood flow. When the patient dangles the feet, he or she restores the hydrostatic gradient; when the patient gets up to walk, he or she increases cardiac output and thereby improves the perfusion of the lower extremities. Sometimes patients complain of nocturnal cramps in the calf muscles. Such cramps are usually not related to vascular ischemia and should be differentiated from nocturnal rest pain, which typically is in the toes and forefoot rather than in the calf.

Ulceration

Cutaneous ulcers may be the first evidence of peripheral vascular disease. These ulcers are caused by severe ischemia from proximal arterial occlusions and often are initiated by minor skin trauma. However, there are many causes of skin ulceration, which must be differentiated from ischemic ulcers:

- Venous stasis
- Infection
- Neoplasm
- Neurotropism
- Hematologic abnormalities
- Allergic reactions
- Insect bites
- Injections

Each type of ulcer has certain clinical and physical characteristics. The ischemic ulcer is most commonly found on the toes, heel, dorsum of the foot, or lower third of the leg. The pain is usually severe and persistent, and worsens at night. The ulcer itself is generally irregular, with a pale or necrotic base.

At times, patients have ulcerations that are attributed to venous disease that may in fact be the result of a combination of arterial ischemia and venous stasis. Ulcerations not in the classic position for venous disease (at the medial malleolus) should be considered as potentially being of an arterial origin. Even if a component of venous disease is present, the arterial component must be evaluated if effective therapy is to be instituted.

Gangrene

Progressive ischemia caused by atherosclerosis can result in gangrenous changes of the tissues. Most commonly the digits are affected initially, but progression to the forefoot is not unusual. Small amounts of infection superimposed on a severe chronic ischemic state can progress very rapidly to gangrene. Clinically, dry and wet gangrene should be differentiated. *Dry gangrene* represents mummification of tissue, and active purulent tissue and cellulitis are absent. *Wet gangrene* is characterized by active infection with cellulitis and purulent tissue planes and is an indication for urgent amputation to prevent ascending infection.

Impotence

Penile erection requires a threefold increase in blood flow through the penile arteries, which is shunted into the vascular spaces of the corpora cavernosa. Arterial obstruction that prevents this increase in blood flow can result in erectile impotence in much the same way that symptoms of claudication are brought about by exercise when there is an unmet demand for increased blood flow. Rene Leriche in 1923 first noted the association among atherosclerotic occlusion of the aorta, hip claudication, buttock atrophy, and erectile impotence. This is now known as the *Leriche syndrome.*

Obstruction can occur at any level from the abdominal aorta, the common iliac arteries, the internal iliac arteries, the internal pudendal arteries, or the penile arteries, resulting in erectile impotence. Although the majority of cases of impotence have psychogenic or urologic causes or are the result of the side effects of medication, the importance of an adequate vascular supply is becoming increasingly recognized and can be objectively assessed, as is discussed below.

EVALUATION OF PERIPHERAL VASCULAR OCCLUSIVE DISEASE

Peripheral vascular occlusive disease is evaluated on the basis of a thorough medical history and clinical examination, noninvasive vascular testing, continuous acquisition ("spiral") computed tomography (CT) scanning, magnetic resonance (MR) angiography, and intra-arterial contrast angiography.

Clinical Examination

Peripheral oscular occlusive disease may be accurately diagnosed with a careful history and thorough physical examination of the patient. In addition to the important determination of symptoms of claudication or rest pain, the patient's level of activity and walking distance should be noted. Often patients with very severe disease do not walk enough to develop symptoms. A careful evaluation of all pulses should be made, although the presence of a palpable pulse does not rule out the possibility of significant arterial occlusive disease. A bruit may be appreciated during the physical examination. Bruits are produced by the turbulence of blood just distal to a stenosis but may also be produced by angulations and bends in arteries. Bruits may be audible with a stethoscope over and distal to an area of stenosis. A high-pitched bruit may be indicative of a severe stenosis. Finally, the temperature, quality, and color of the skin, hair, and nails should be noted, including the presence of skin ulcerations or gangrenous changes.

Noninvasive tests are used after the clinical examination to confirm the presence of occlusive disease, identify the level and severity of the disease, and assess whether angiography is required to further evaluate these patients.

Objective Assessment with Vascular Laboratory Techniques

Doppler Ankle Pressure

The ready availability of the handheld Doppler ultrasound has made measurement of lower extremity blood pressure simple and convenient and has permitted the development of objective means of assessing lower extremity perfusion. The Doppler ultrasound probe emits high-frequency sound waves in the range of 2 to 10 MHz. The sound is reflected by the movement of red blood cells in the vessel, which produces a frequency shift that is picked up by the receiving crystal of the Doppler probe. This frequency shift is proportional to the blood flow velocity. This *Doppler shift* can be expressed by the following formula:

$$\Delta f = \frac{2fV\cos\theta}{C}$$

where V is velocity, f is frequency of the incident sound beam, C is velocity of sound in tissue, and θ is the angle of the incident sound beam to the vessel examined. Because V, C, and θ can be constant, the shift in frequency is proportional to the velocity of the blood flow.

To measure the blood pressure in the legs, a blood pressure cuff is placed at the ankle just above the malleoli and inflated while a handheld Doppler is used to listen to the flow in the dorsalis pedis and posterior tibial artery. Inflation of the cuff above systolic pressure causes obliteration of the Doppler signal, and systolic blood pressure can be recorded as the cuff is deflated and flow resumes in the measured vessel. Because a patient's blood pressure may fluctuate, more precision can be gained by comparing the ankle pressure to the brachial pressure. Usually, the ankle systolic pressure is divided by the brachial systolic pressure to produce an *ankle-brachial index* (*ABI*). Such an index is quite useful in assessing the severity of peripheral occlusive disease. Patients without occlusive disease have an ABI of 1, whereas patients with claudication have an ABI of 0.5 to 0.6. Patients with rest pain, gangrene, and ulceration have an ABI of 0.4 and less (Fig. 4). Despite these ranges, considerable overlap can be present, especially around an ABI of 0.5. This measurement is useful for differentiating patients with lower extremity pain caused by spinal stenosis, arthritis, or other nonvascular conditions. Patients with diabetes frequently have calcified vessels that cannot be compressed by the blood pressure cuff. This may lead to a false elevation of the ABI. In the setting of incompressible ankle vessels, toe pressure or waveforms may be more accurate.

It is important to note that the pressure measured is determined by the location of the cuff rather than the location of the listening probe. Thus an ankle pressure can be recorded by placing a cuff at the level of the malleoli, and a below-knee or above-knee pressure can be recorded by appropriate blood pressure cuff placement. Patients with superficial femoral artery occlusion have a normal pressure reading in the upper thigh but an abnormal pressure reading below the knee and at the level of the ankle. The resting ankle index is the most accurate of the noninvasive techniques for objectively assessing the presence or absence of occlusive disease. It is reproducible, and hence the index can be followed to identify the progression of disease.

It should also be recognized that listening for and hearing flow in the dorsalis pedis and posterior tibial arteries does not represent a pulse. A pulse is palpated with the fingers. Flow can be heard at very low levels of circulation in the dorsalis pedis and the posterior tibial arteries, and patients may have frank gangrene of their foot even though audible Doppler signals are heard. One should not be lulled into a false sense of security of good perfusion of the foot if Doppler flow signals in the foot are heard but pulses cannot be palpated.

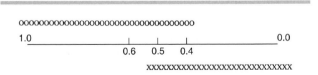

Figure 4 Ankle-brachial index is used to determine severity of lower extremity ischemia. *Circles* denote range consistent with claudication; *Xs* denote area of limb-threatening ischemia. Note area of considerable overlap around 0.5.

Stress Testing

Because patients with claudication develop their symptoms only with exercise, stress testing is a useful means for documenting the degree of walking impairment. Treadmill exercise can be performed at a standard pace of 1.5 miles/hr at a 7-degree grade. Normally, one has no diminution of the ankle pressure following exercise. On walking to the point of claudication, there is a substantial drop in ABI because blood flow is shunted to the proximal thigh muscle and cannot pass through the obstruction to the distal vascular bed. There is return of ankle pressure to normal with rest. The symptom of reduction in ankle pressure is similar to the finding of disappearing pulses with exercise, seen on clinical examination.

Doppler Waveform Analysis

Doppler detectors can provide an analog signal that is proportional to the velocity of the blood in vessels studied. The shape of the waveform reflects the status of the vessel. Normally, a *triphasic* waveform is seen, indicative of reversal of flow in early diastole. Stenosis proximal to the vessel examined first eliminates this reversed flow. As the stenosis becomes more severe, the peak of the waveform is blunted, and the waveform widens (Fig. 5). Qualitative analysis of these waveforms at different levels of the extremity can identify the level and severity of occlusive lesions.

Analysis of the Doppler waveforms in conjunction with systolic pressures at several levels in the leg can allow the clinician to make an accurate diagnosis of the location and extent of peripheral vascular occlusive disease. For example, Figure 6 illustrates the decrease in the waveform and systolic pressures across an obstructed superficial femoral artery. A decrease in systolic blood pressure of 30 mmHg or more between any two levels in the leg usually indicates total occlusion of the intervening artery.

Doppler Ultrasound Imaging and Duplex Scanning

B-mode ultrasound imaging of arteries and plaques combined with pulsed Doppler ultrasound flow determination and sound spectral analysis is now a routine method evaluating the common femoral, superficial femoral, and popliteal arteries. This technique provides the ability to noninvasively image arteries and to assess flow. This technology has also been used to image autogenous vein grafts to prevent vein graft thrombosis and failure. Routine postoperative vein graft surveillance using duplex ultrasound imaging every six months can detect elevated flow velocities (peak systolic velocity >200 cm/sec) within the vein graft or at the anastomotic sites (59,60). Early detection

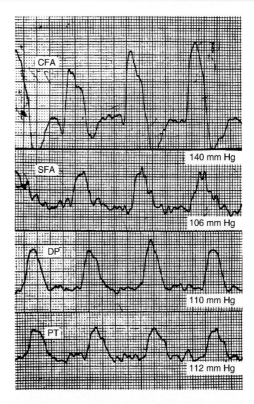

Figure 6 Doppler flow velocity waveforms recorded at four places in an extremity with SFA occlusion demonstrated by angiography. Recordings were made at the CFA, SFA, DP artery, and PT artery. Associated systolic blood pressures were measured to be 140 mmHg in the thigh and 106 mmHg below the knee. This 34 mmHg drop in pressure indicates occlusion of the intervening artery (in this case, the SFA). Distal arteries fill through collateral vessels. Note the change in Doppler velocity waveforms. *Abbreviations*: CFA, common femoral artery; SFA, superficial femoral artery; DP, dorsalis pedis; PT, posterior tibial.

of vein graft stenoses allows localized treatment with surgical revision or endovascular treatment and thus may prevent graft occlusion and prolong graft patency (61,62). Duplex ultrasound scanning may also be used to identify aneurysms and stenotic and ulcerated lesions in the aortoiliac and femoropopliteal arteries, which may be potential sources for distal emboli.

Penile Brachial Pressure Index

The simplest and most reliable assessment of the adequacy of penile perfusion is the measurement of arterial pressure in the corpora cavernosa supplied by the penile arteries. A Doppler velocity probe is positioned directly over one of the six penile arteries, and a small pneumatic cuff is placed around the penis proximal to the probe. The cuff is inflated until arterial flow is abolished and is then allowed to slowly deflate until flow returns, which indicates the systolic blood pressure. The penile systolic pressure is divided by the brachial systolic pressure to provide a penile-brachial index (PBI). A PBI greater than 0.9 is normal. A PBI less than 0.7 is consistent with a vascular occlusive cause of impotence.

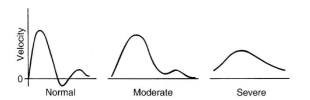

Figure 5 Doppler ultrasound velocity waveforms indicating the normal triphasic waveform, the loss of the reverse flow component seen in moderately stenotic vessels, and the blunted waveform of a severely stenotic vessel.

Catheter-Based Angiography

Catheter-based angiography provides the most definitive anatomic assessment of obstructing vascular lesions and is performed before vascular reconstruction. This includes visualization of the abdominal and infrarenal aorta, the iliac arteries, and the femoral, popliteal, tibial, and pedal vessels throughout their length (Fig. 3). Angiography is usually performed through a transfemoral approach, which has the advantage of allowing selective catheterization and the study of individual arteries as needed. Transbrachial and translumbar aortography can also be used successfully. Newer techniques of digital subtraction and computer enhancement of images permit the use of smaller volumes of iodinated contrast materials. Patients should be well hydrated before and after angiography to minimize the possibility of renal failure caused by the osmotic diuresis produced by the hypertonic contrast medium (63).

CT and MR Angiography

Advances in computer technology have resulted in significant advances in CT and MR imaging. Timed bolus injection of a contrast agent allows vascular imaging, which rivals the resolution that can be obtained with contrast arteriography. Continuous acquisition of data using helical or spiral CT techniques allows three-dimensional (3-D) image reconstruction with image rotation, shaded-surface display, and curved planar reformation of images. CT angiographic techniques allow imaging not only of the lumen contour but also of the artery wall and extravascular structures. Thus CT angiographic imaging is the imaging procedure of choice for thoracic and abdominal aortic aneurysms and is used to plan endovascular treatments, as well as to follow patients who have undergone treatment of aneurysms (64,65). CT angiography can also be used to study the carotid artery (66) and peripheral vessels. Multislice spiral CT scans with 16-row detectors can precisely image the aortoiliac and femoral vessels as well as infrageniculate arteries in 13 seconds using as little as 130 mL of iodinated contrast (67).

MR angiography using gadolinium contrast agent, which is not nephrotoxic, is currently being used to supplant catheter-based, contrast angiography in some centers (68): In addition to anatomic data, however, MR sequences can encode for flow volume (69) and the oxygen saturation of hemoglobin (70,71). Although still limited in quality and the field of view available compared to a traditional aortogram with bilateral runoff, MR anatomic and flow imaging may ultimately replace catheter-based, invasive arterial diagnostic methods.

TREATMENT OF PERIPHERAL VASCULAR OCCLUSIVE DISEASE

The treatment of peripheral vascular occlusive disease is determined by the severity of the patient's symptoms and the anatomic location and extent of obstructing lesions. Treatment options include nonoperative measures, minimally invasive procedures such as transluminal angioplasty and stenting, and operative revascularization.

Nonoperative Measures

Patients with peripheral occlusive disease usually have one or several risk factors for the development of vascular disease, including cigarette smoking, hyperlipidemia, hypertension, and diabetes mellitus. Every effort should be made to control these factors to prevent progression of obstructive disease. Patients with symptoms of claudication, which are not physically limiting have a low risk for limb loss (72) and usually respond well to a program of cessation of smoking and walking exercise to stimulate enlargement of collateral circulation and to condition the muscles to function at a higher level with the available blood supply. Exercise programs are effective in improving walking distance. In a meta-analysis of randomized trials of supervised exercise trials for intermittent claudication, exercise therapy improved pain-free walking time by 180% and maximal walking time by 150% at six months. However, exercise programs must be maintained in order to remain effective. Cessation of the exercise program usually returns the patient to the same level of claudication as present originally. Patients often adjust their levels of activity and coexist well with occlusive disease for many years. Those who continue to smoke have the poorest outlook.

Risk Factor Modification

A comprehensive program of risk factor modification should be undertaken in patients with peripheral artery disease, including smoking cessation, increased physical activity, blood pressure control, reduction of elevated total and low-density lipoprotein (LDL) cholesterol levels, antiplatelet therapy, angiotensin-converting enzyme–inhibitor therapy, weight reduction, and glycemic control in patients with diabetes mellitus. Tobacco use is the single most important modifiable risk factor for peripheral occlusive disease. Smoking increased the risk of intermittent claudication by a factor of 8 to 10 and smoking cessation resulted in a 50% reduction in intermittent claudication over a 20-year period among Icelandic men (73). Rest pain developed in 16% of smokers, with intermittent claudication, but there was no disease progression in nonsmoking patients, with intermittent claudication (74). Long-term graft patency is significantly better in patients who quit smoking than in those who continue to smoke (75). Lowering of cholesterol with statin drugs has been shown to reduce the incidence of new or worsening intermittent claudication by 38% (76). Several studies have confirmed an increase in pain-free and total walking distances, as well as improvement in overall physical function in patients treated with statin drugs. Dietary modifications to reduce cholesterol and statin therapy with a target LDL of less than 100 mg/dL is recommended. Antiplatelet therapy with aspirin has been shown to reduce overall cardiovascular morbidity and mortality in patients with peripheral occlusive disease. Ticlid has benefits similar to aspirin but is associated with a risk of thrombocytopenia and neutropenia and is therefore not routinely recommended. Clopidogrel has been shown to be superior to aspirin but is considerably more expensive than aspirin. There is evidence to suggest that the combined use of clopidogrel and aspirin may provide added benefit. Strict glycemic control with a target hemoglobin A1c of less than 7.0 is recommended for diabetic patients with peripheral occlusive disease (77). Reduction in hemoglobin A1c by 1% has been shown to result in an 18% reduction in myocardial infarction, a 15% reduction in stroke and, a 42% reduction in symptomatic peripheral occlusive disease in the prospective U.K. diabetes study (78).

Medical Therapy

A number of vasodilating drugs have been used in an attempt to diminish vasospasm and improve peripheral perfusion in patients with peripheral occlusive disease. These, in general, have been found to be ineffective and most have been removed from the market. Nifedipine has been found to be useful in the treatment of vasospasm as seen in Raynaud's disease (79), but has no beneficial effect in peripheral occlusive disease.

Pentoxifylline was the first medication approved by the Food and Drug Administration (FDA) for the treatment of intermittent claudication. Pentoxyfylline is a xanthine derivative that is believed to exert its effect by decreasing the rigidity of erythrocytes so that they can more readily deform and pass through the small capillary beds, thereby increasing tissue perfusion. A multicenter trial of patients with claudication demonstrated a 30% increase in walking distance in patients treated with pentoxyfylline as compared to placebo (80). However, more recent studies suggest that improvement in walking distance with pentoxyfylline is unpredictable and may offer little benefit over placebo. There is no evidence for a beneficial effect from pentoxyfylline for patients with rest pain, ulceration, or gangrene.

Cilostazol is a phosphodiesterase inhibitor with antiplatelet and antiproliferative activity. It is the second FDA-approved drug for the treatment of intermittent claudication and appears to provide significant benefit compared to placebo. In a meta-analysis of eight randomized, placebo-controlled trials of cilostazol in patients with intermittent claudication, after 12 to 24 weeks of therapy, patients on cilostazol had an increase in pain-free walking of 40% to 70% and an increase in maximum walking distance of 65% to 83% compared to placebo controls (81). Cilostazol is contraindicated in patients with congestive heart failure because of a proarrhythmic effect. However, it may be considered as initial medical therapy in addition to smoking cessation and walking exercise in patients with mild-to-moderate claudication.

Although metabolism-enhancing drugs such as 6-propionyl carnitine, agents such as L-arginine, dietary supplements such as gingko biloba, and pneumatic compression stockings may hold promise for patients with intermittent claudication, they have yet to demonstrate clinical efficacy in prospective, controlled clinical trials. Intravenous prostaglandin infusion, which has a significant vasodilator and platelet inhibitory effect, has been proposed for the treatment of ischemic ulcers, but no significant improvement in rest pain of ischemic ulcer healing has been demonstrated in controlled clinical trials.

Endovascular Treatment

Endovascular catheter-based therapy of stenotic lesions and short-segment occlusions has gained acceptance as an effective treatment modality for peripheral occlusive disease. While the overall long-term results are not as durable as surgical reconstruction and bypass procedures, the procedures are minimally invasive and well tolerated by patients. Endovascular treatment is usually percutaneous and is performed in the angiography suite under fluoroscopic image guidance. Proper patient selection is important and clinical criteria for treatment, similar to those used to select patients for surgical treatment, should be used. Treatment consists of transluminal balloon dilation of lesions with or without stenting. Dilation of lesions that appear to be significant on angiographic images but, which produce minimal or no symptoms, should be avoided. The best candidate for transluminal angioplasty is a patient with severe claudication, with an isolated hemodynamically significant common iliac artery stenosis.

Transluminal Angioplasty

Transluminal balloon angioplasty is accomplished by first performing a diagnostic arteriogram to localize the occlusive lesion. A catheter with a balloon that has a predetermined maximal diameter at its tip is then passed over a guide wire under X-ray control through the obstructing lesion. Inflation of the balloon disrupts the plaque and stretches the arterial wall, resulting in enlargement of the lumen. This enlargement of the lumen cross-sectional area occurs by separating the plaque from the underlying tunica media and stretching the artery wall (Fig. 7). At times, the media is stretched and thinned to the point of media rupture, in which case vessel integrity is maintained by the adventitia (82). There is no plaque compression or removal of the lesion, and long-term patency depends on the vessel wall remaining in the overstretched state. When the vessel contracts to its predilated state, restenosis occurs. This occurs in a substantial number of patients and is a significant limitation of the procedure. Intra-arterial stents have been introduced as a method, of maintaining lumenal patency after angioplasty. Stents have improved the long-term effectiveness of angioplasty by preventing recoil, intimal flaps, and dissections, such as seen in Figure 8.

Intraluminal Stenting

Stenting of recanalized or dilated arterial segments prevents lumen collapse and recoil and maintains lumen caliber. Stents also tack down dissected and separated intimal flaps, preventing lumen obstruction and occlusion (Fig. 8A–C). Stents are either balloon expandable or self-expanding and are widely used for coronary artery stenoses and occlusions. They are FDA approved for use in iliac artery lesions and recently have been approved for high-risk patients with carotid stenosis. Balloon-expandable stents provide maximal radial strength and allow precise positioning. They, however,

(A)   **(B)**

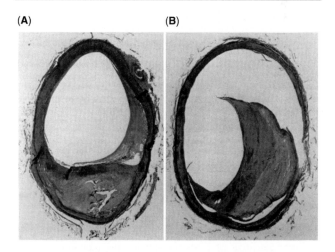

Figure 7 Mechanism of balloon dilation of arteries. **(A)** Human superficial femoral artery that has been fixed with an intraluminal pressure of 100 mmHg and cut in cross section. Note the eccentric plaque and round lumen. **(B)** Segment of the same artery after balloon dilation. Note the separation of plaque from the media and protrusion of the plaque into the lumen. The media is thinner and has ruptured, and lumen integrity is maintained by the adventitia. Disruption and stretching of the artery wall results in a larger lumen area. There is no plaque compression. *Source:* From Ref. 82.

(A)   **(B)**   **(C)**

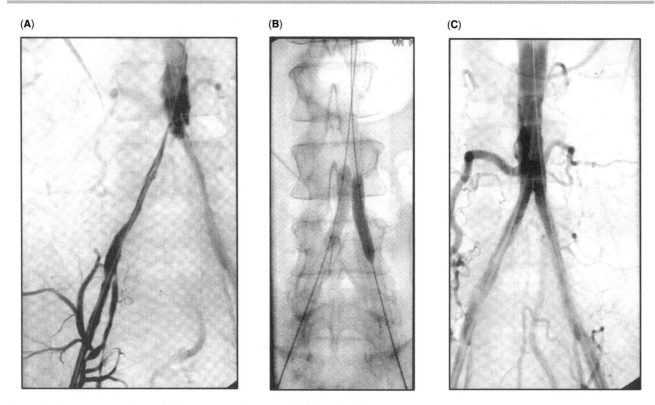

Figure 8   Endovascular treatment of bilateral common iliac stenoses: **(A)** following balloon angioplasty, dissection flaps and residual stenoses are seen; **(B)** Balloon expandible stents are deployed in the common iliac arteries; **(C)** completion angiogram demonstrating no residual stenosis and smooth lumen caliber.

may be compressed by extrinsic force. Self-expending stents are commonly oversized to create a continual outward force resisting recoil. The hoop strength of self-expanding stents is less than for balloon-expandable stents but they are useful in vessels at risk for external compression, such as the carotid artery or the superficial femoral artery.

While stenting has largely eliminated intimal flaps and early recoil following balloon angioplasty, restenosis and intimal hyperplasia remain a problem, particularly for smaller-caliber arteries. Promising results in controlling restensosis of the coronary circulation has been achieved with drug-eluting stents. Drug-eluting stents are bare-metal stents that are coated with a drug that acts locally to inhibit or prevent cellular proliferation and restenosis. Restenosis is a significant problem for superficial femoral artery stenting as well as popliteal and tibial artery stenting, and drug-eluting stents are not yet available for these vessels.

Adjunctive Endovascular Treatments

Laser angioplasty of peripheral artery lesions has fallen into disfavor because of high restenosis and recurrence rates. Transcatheter atherectomy devices that shave or debulk plaque are currently being investigated but there is no evidence that these will be more successful in avoiding restenosis. Secondary treatments of restenotic lesions can be carried out with cutting balloon techniques and cold thermal energy application, but the effectiveness of these therapies are unproved. Medical therapy aimed at inhibiting platelet aggregation with glycoprotein IIb/IIIa complex inhibition has been shown to decrease in-stent restenosis (83) and treatment with the antiplatelet agent cilostazol has been

shown to have a beneficial effect in preventing coronary stent restenosis (84). New and improved methods to control and treat in-stent restenosis can be expected to expand the role of endovascular therapy in the near future.

Results of Endovascular Therapy

The results of transluminal balloon angioplasty and stenting are to a large degree determined by the location and character of the lesion being treated. The predictors of success include the location and length of the target lesion, whether the lesion is a stenosis or an occlusion, and the adequacy of the outflow vascular bed. In general, the larger the artery being treated and the shorter the lesion being treated, the better the results. Thus, in the lower extremity vessels, the best results are achieved with short-segment stenoses in the common iliac artery. Long-term patency of angioplasty of selected common iliac lesions is comparable to open surgical bypass. The long-term patency of common iliac balloon angioplasty of common iliac stenoses at one year is 90%, at three years is 80%, and at five years is 70% (85). The results for iliac occlusions with stenting is somewhat less favorable, but considering the minimally invasive nature of the endovascular treatment, iliac angioplasty and stenting should be considered for isolated iliac artery lesions. Results for external iliac stenoses are not as favorable as for common iliac lesions and surgical bypass should probably be considered for patients with diffuse aortoiliac disease, which involves the external iliac artery. Results for angioplasty and stenting below the inguinal ligament are distinctly inferior to those for iliac stenting. Bypass surgery for superficial femoral artery occlusions, particularly with autogenous saphenous vein bypass, is the procedure of choice for such patients. However, even though long-term patency rates may not be high, significant benefit can be achieved in some patients who are facing limb loss and who have no satisfactory options for bypass. An example is shown in Figure 9. This elderly diabetic patient with gangrene of the toes had occlusion of anterior tibial, posterior tibial, and peroneal arteries and no saphenous or upper extremity veins. A balloon angioplasty of the diffusely diseased and occluded anterior tibial artery was successful in restoring flow to the foot and allowed a transmetatarsal amputation to heal. Even though the anterior tibial artery restenosed eight months later, the transmetatarsal amputation remained fully healed and the patient was able to ambulate. The recent codification of reporting standards for endovascular procedures including angioplasty should facilitate future comparisons with existing surgical standards, and help clarify the relative indications for angioplasty (86). Despite technical issues, cost, and ongoing problems with restenosis, interest in non–angioplasty-related endovascular procedures such as rotational arthrectomy, laser-mediated plaque obligation, and thermal- or laser-assisted angioplasty continues (87).

Surgical Revascularization
Endarterectomy
Endarterectomy is a surgical procedure in which the obstructing intimal plaque is removed from an artery to restore flow. The cleavage plane for endarterectomy is usually just below the internal elastic lamina, although the media below extensive plaque is often degenerated and is removed along with the intimal plaque. In these circumstances, the cleavage plane is at the external elastic lamina, and thus only the adventitial layer contains the blood stream. The adventitial layer alone provides sufficient structural support, and aneurysmal dilation of endarterectomized arterial segments does not occur.

Although endarterectomy is the standard mode of treatment for carotid bifurcation atherosclerosis, it has a more limited usefulness in the treatment of peripheral vascular occlusive disease. This is because carotid plaques are

localized in the carotid bifurcation, whereas lower extremity atherosclerosis usually is extensive, with no discrete starting or end points. Some patients with localized aortoiliac disease and no distal occlusive disease are candidates for local aortoiliac endarterectomy, but bypass procedures are more commonly performed. If a local endarterectomy is to be considered, these patients must not have aneurysmal disease or fibrotic small-caliber vessels. Results of *local* aortoiliac endarterectomy compare favorably to aortobifemoral bypass grafts.

Most surgeons occasionally use local endarterectomy as an adjunctive procedure to aortobifemoral bypass grafting. Such local endarterectomies are frequently performed in the common and profunda femoris arteries at the time of anastomosis of bypass grafts; but primary endarterectomies have limited usefulness in the peripheral circulation.

Bypass Procedures
Procedures to bypass occlusive lesions are the standard surgical methods for treatment of lower extremity peripheral occlusive disease. Procedures are usually considered as inflow or outflow procedures, depending on the level of obstruction. Inflow procedures refer to those used for aortoiliac obstructions, and outflow procedures are those used for superficial femoral and popliteal artery obstructions, with the level of the inguinal ligament usually being the dividing line. Angiographic, vascular, laboratory, and clinical criteria are used to determine the primary level of obstruction. If a patient has both inflow and outflow disease, the proximal, or inflow, obstruction is treated first and usually is sufficient to relieve symptoms.

Aortofemoral Bypass
The indications for surgical intervention in patients with aortoiliac occlusive lesions are severe claudication and limb-threatening ischemia as defined by rest pain, ulcerations, and gangrene. The standard surgical treatment for bypass of aortoiliac obstructions is the aortofemoral bypass graft (88). In this procedure, a knitted or woven Dacron bifurcation graft is sutured from the infrarenal aorta, which is usually free of disease, to the common femoral arteries. This graft bypasses the entire aortoiliac segment, which includes the inferior mesenteric artery and internal iliac arteries. The proximal anastomosis is placed just below the level of the renal arteries and may be performed in either an end-to-end or an end-to-side fashion (Fig. 10). When an *end-to-end anastomosis* is used, the distal aorta is ligated, and the entire aortic outflow passes through the graft. Blood is supplied to the distal aorta and the inferior mesenteric and internal iliac arteries by retrograde flow from the common femoral artery through the external iliac artery. With an *end-to-side proximal anastomosis*, blood flows in parallel in the bypass graft and in the distal aorta. This anastomosis is preferred when the external iliac arteries are occluded and would prevent retrograde fill of the aorta from the groin. The distal anastomosis is usually placed on the common femoral artery, with outflow through the superficial femoral and profunda femoris vessels. If there is associated superficial femoral artery occlusion, the profunda femoris artery alone can serve as the outflow bed, with relief of symptoms. Concomitant endarterectomy of the orifices of the superficial femoral and profunda femoris arteries can be undertaken to improve the distal anastomosis. *Profundaplasty* is performed by extending the opening of the common femoral artery onto the profunda femoris artery and suturing the Dacron graft onto the profunda femoris

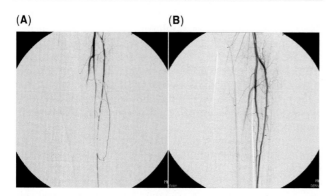

(A)   **(B)**

Figure 9 Angiogram of infrapopliteal arteries in a diabetic patient with gangrene of toe. **(A)** The posterior tibial and peroneal arteries are occluded in mid calf and the anterior tibial artery is diffusely narrowed with a focal occlusion. The distal anterior tibial artery reconstitutes by a large collateral vessel. **(B)** Following balloon angioplasty, the anterior tibial artery is patent with restoration of a normal dorsalis pedis pulse. The patient successfully healed a toe amputation.

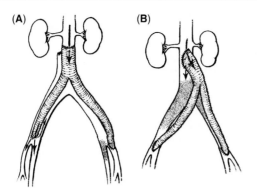

Figure 10 Aortofemoral bypass for aortoiliac obstruction. Proximal anastomosis may be performed end-to-end **(A)** or end-to-side of the aorta **(B)**. With an end-to-end anastomosis, perfusion of the internal iliac arteries and distal aorta is retrograde from the common femoral artery in the groin.

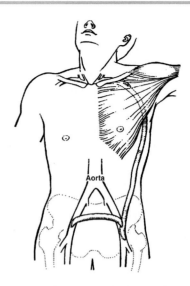

Figure 11 Illustration of extra-anatomic bypasses for aortoiliac obstruction. Axillofemoral bypass graft courses in the subcutaneous space in the midaxillary line and brings blood from the subclavian artery to the femoral artery to bypass an aortic obstruction. Femorofemoral bypass graft brings blood from one femoral artery across to the other. "Steal" phenomenon does not occur if there is no obstruction to the inflow of the donor artery.

artery. This results in enlargement of the lumen of the proximal profunda femoris artery and is useful when there is a stenosis at that site.

Aortofemoral bypass graft is a stable and durable operation that effectively eliminates the inflow obstruction. Surgical mortality rate is less than 2%, and the five-year graft patency rate is greater than 90% (89). Should these operations fail, they generally do so because of progression of disease in the arteries at or distal to the groin anastomosis rather than because of failure of the Dacron graft itself.

Early complications of aortobifemoral grafts are caused mainly by technical misadventures. These include postoperative hemorrhage, early graft thrombosis, distal embolization, groin hematomas, and lymph leaks. Long-term complications include graft infection, pseudoaneurysm formation, and aortoduodenal fistula. Details of these problems are expanded on below.

Extra-Anatomic Bypass

Patients who require bypass of aortoiliac lesions but are too ill to withstand an intra-abdominal operation for placement of an aortobifemoral graft may be revascularized with an axillofemoral or femorofemoral bypass graft (Fig. 11). These operations are effective in relieving aortoiliac, or inflow, obstruction but do not require that the abdominal cavity be entered. The bypass is tunneled in the subcutaneous space, and incisions to expose the axillary and femoral vessels can be performed while the patient is under local anesthesia. Thus they are safer and more amenable to use in high-risk patients. *Axillofemoral bypass grafts* are also useful to bypass the aorta in situations of infection within the abdominal cavity. There is no steal of blood from the upper extremity when an axillofemoral bypass is placed because there is an increase in flow in the feeding subclavian artery. This increase is sufficient to supply the arm and both legs. However, the great length of the axillofemoral graft makes it prone to thrombosis. Recent reports suggest that the long-term patency of axillofemoral bypass grafting supports its use in highly selected cases when in-line anatomic reconstruction is less desirable (90). However, proximal anastomotic disruption remains a serious though infrequent complication (91).

Afemorofemoml bypass graft can be used to bypass an iliac artery occlusion if the opposite patent iliac artery is disease free. In this situation, one iliac artery is able to deliver enough flow to supply both legs. Five-year patency rates for femorofemoral grafts vary from 44% to 74%. Axillofemoral bypass grafts have a poorer patency rate than aortofemoral grafts, with five-year patency rates reported near 75% (92). These grafts fail more commonly than an aortobifemoral graft because of their longer course and the risk of external compression in the subcutaneous tunnel. Thus extra-anatomic grafts should be considered only when endovascular treatments, aortobifemoral grafts, or local aortoiliac endarterectomies are not feasible.

Femoropopliteal and Femoral Distal Bypass Grafts

Claudication or severe ischemia of the legs despite a good aortoiliac segment is usually the result of obstruction of the superficial femoral or popliteal artery and its branches. A preoperative angiogram demonstrates which distal vessels are patent and of adequate caliber to accept a bypass graft. If the popliteal artery is patent with runoff through at least one of the tibial vessels, a *femoropopliteal bypass graft* is the procedure of choice. If the popliteal artery is occluded, bypass should be performed to the tibial artery that best fills the plantar arch.

The saphenous vein is the most suitable conduit for bypasses below the inguinal ligament. It may be used as a reversed or in situ vein bypass (Fig. 12). In a *reversed saphenous vein femoropopliteal bypass graft*, the saphenous vein is excised, and all branches are ligated and divided. The vein position is reversed so that the distal end of the vein is sewn to the common femoral artery, whereas the proximal portion of the vein is sewn to the popliteal artery. This permits arterial flow to course in the vein in the direction of the valves. An *in situ vein bypass graft* is left in its normal position (93).

The proximal vein is sewn to the common femoral artery, and the distal portion is sewn to the popliteal (or

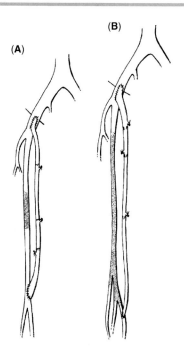

Figure 12 Saphenous vein bypass grafts in the lower extremity for treatment of femoropopliteal occlusions. These may be performed as a reversed saphenous vein bypass graft **(A)** or an in situ saphenous vein bypass graft **(B)**. In the in situ bypass graft, the saphenous vein valves must be cut to render them incompetent. Selection of the site of distal anastomosis depends on angiographic demonstration of the patency of distal arteries.

tibial) artery. To permit blood to flow in the vein against the direction of the valves, the valve leaflets must be cut to render them incompetent. The in situ graft avoids extensive dissection of the vein, provides a better size match between the smaller distal artery and vein, and allows the use of smaller veins that might not be suitable for reversed vein bypass. Autogenous vein is far superior to prosthetic materials in all infrainguinal positions, and every effort should be made to use the vein, even if the arm veins or lesser saphenous veins are employed.

Limb salvage rate for patients undergoing femoropopliteal bypass grafting with autogenous tissue is 73% at four years; for femoral distal bypass grafts, limb salvage is 80% at four years (94). The limb salvage rates are usually 15% higher than the actual graft patency rates. The patency of each individual graft depends on the adequacy of inflow, the type of graft material used, the quality of the outflow vessels, and the technical aspects of the procedure (94).

The complications of femoropopliteal and femoral distal bypass grafts are similar to those associated with an aortobifemoral procedure. Early thrombosis is the most serious early problem and usually represents technical error or inadequate runoff vessels. Prompt thrombectomy and recognition of the technical problem returns function to the graft but usually results in reduction of long-term patency (95).

Sympathectomy

Lumbar sympathectomy produces vasomotor paralysis, which increases blood flow by decreasing peripheral resistance. Before the advent of direct arterial surgery,

sympathectomy was the chief surgical therapeutic approach for peripheral occlusive disease. With progressive improvement in the ability to directly revascularize ischemic tissue, lumbar sympathectomy has fallen into disfavor. It has no beneficial effect in the treatment of claudication but has been reported to improve rest pain in approximately 50% of patients. It has been shown to increase cutaneous, but not muscle, blood flow and thus has been recommended for the treatment of ischemic ulcers. Some surgeons use sympathectomy as an adjunct to arterial reconstruction, believing that sympathectomy adds to the total improvement of blood flow to the extremity by causing vasodilation in the small vessels of the foot. However, there is little evidence that there is improved flow over and above the benefit derived from arterial reconstruction alone. In addition, there are potential complications of lumbar sympathectomy, including postsympathectomy neuralgia and failure of ejaculation. Although sympathectomy has limited usefulness in the treatment of arteriosclerosis obliterans, it is effective in the treatment of causalgia and hyperhidrosis.

Embolectomy/Thrombectomy

Acute arterial occlusion with severe ischemia may be caused by emboli, which usually arise from the heart, or by thrombosis of a diseased artery. In addition to the ischemia caused by the embolus, the limb is threatened by propagation of thrombus in the arteries distal to the embolus where blood flow is slow. Therefore patients with acute arterial occlusion should be immediately anticoagulated with heparin. In addition to preventing clot propagation, anticoagulation helps prevent recurrent embolization from the heart.

Removal of the obstructing embolus is readily accomplished using the *Fogarty balloon catheter* (Fig. 13). An incision is made in the femoral artery, and the catheter with the balloon deflated is passed through the thrombus. The balloon is then inflated, and the clot extracted. This procedure is very effective in removing fresh thrombus and restoring blood flow in patients with embolism. However, bypass may be required to restore flow in patients who have thrombosis induced by severe stenotic plaques.

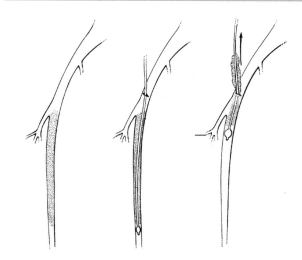

Figure 13 Fogarty balloon catheter embolectomy. Deflated balloon is passed through the thromboembolus. Balloon is inflated and withdrawn, and the embolus is extracted from the artery.

Percutaneous catheter-directed *thrombolysis* may be used as initial therapy for patients with acute arterial ischemia due to embolization or thrombosis and intact neuromuscular function. Thrombolytic agents such as streptokinase, urokinase, and recombinant tissue plasminogen activators (alteplase and recombinant plasminogen activator-reteplase) induce a systemic fibrinolytic state and carry a risk of inducing hemorrhage. However, the risk of hemorrhage may be reduced by direct infusion of the thrombolytic agent into the clot, using an infusion catheter. Such catheter-directed thrombolysis has been shown to be effective in removing thrombus, reducing the need for subsequent surgery and improving limb salvage in three prospective randomized clinical trials (96).

ANEURYSMAL DISEASE OF THE AORTA

The abdominal aorta is particularly vulnerable to aneurysm formation and contains 90% of all aneurysms. Aneurysms are usually located in the infrarenal abdominal aortic segment, with sparing of the first 1 to 2 cm below the level of the renal arteries. Aneurysms are usually clinically silent but may enlarge, cause symptoms, and rupture.

Cause of Aortic Aneurysms

Special anatomic features of the infrarenal abdominal aorta may make it vulnerable to the development of aneurysms.

The aortic media is composed of groups of smooth muscle cells surrounded by layers of elastin in a network of collagen fibers. The elastin layers serve to allow distensibility of the aortic wall in pulse propagation, whereas the collagen fibers provide tensile strength and prevent overdistention and rupture. The number of medial lamellar units increases proportionally with the aortic diameter to support the tensile stress. The aortic media is nourished by diffusion from the lumen to a depth of approximately 29 medial lamellar units (97). However, if the aorta is thicker than 29 layers, adventitial vasa vasorum penetrate the media to supply nutrition. The relationship between the number of medial layers and the depth of penetration of vasa vasorum in the aortic media applies to both the thoracic aorta and abdominal aortic segment in most mammals. However, the human abdominal aorta is a noticeable exception in that it contains fewer lamellar units than would be expected for its diameter and the media is devoid of vasa vasorum (98). Thus each layer is thicker than expected and sustains an increased tension per lamellar unit. This may make the aorta vulnerable to relative ischemic injury of the medial smooth muscle cells, leading to medial atrophy in aneurysm formation (99).

Atherosclerotic plaques are also prone to develop in the infrarenal abdominal aorta and may be a factor in aneurysm formation. Intimal plaques may obstruct diffusion of nutrients from the lumen to the media. Usually there is ingrowth of new medial vasa vasorum to supply the media and plaque under these circumstances. When this does not occur, aneurysmal degeneration may take place because of inadequate medial nutrition. Vasa vasorum usually arise from the renal arteries, and the immediate infrarenal aortic segment may have a better vasa vasorum supply than the rest of the aorta. This may explain the relative protection from aneurysm formation in this area.

Other etiologic factors in aneurysm formation have been proposed, including increased elastase or collagenase activity, hemodynamic factors in the infrarenal aorta, and genetic predisposition.

Aneurysms are also found in the femoral and popliteal arteries, although much less commonly. Patients with peripheral aneurysms usually have coexistent abdominal aortic aneurysms, suggesting a more general aneurysmal diathesis.

Clinical Manifestations

The biologic fate of an aneurysm of the abdominal aorta is to increase in size with eventual rupture. When first detected in a patient, aneurysms may be asymptomatic, symptomatic, or ruptured. In addition, slow flow within the dilated aneurysm may result in thrombus formation along the wall, which occasionally may totally occlude the lumen, causing acute ischemia, or may embolize to the distal arterial vasculature. The prevalence of aneurysms increases with age. Aneurysms are more common in men than in women and approximately 1 in 10 men over the age of 75 will have an aneurysm.

Asymptomatic Aneurysms

Aneurysms are remarkable by their clinical silence in the majority of cases. Asymptomatic aneurysms are frequently discovered by palpating a pulsatile mass during physical examination of the abdomen. Because the aortic bifurcation is located at the level of the umbilicus, the pulsatile mass is usually in the epigastrium. However, aneurysms less than 5 cm in diameter are difficult to palpate, especially in corpulent people; most aneurysms are discovered incidentally during ultrasound X ray or CT examination for gastrointestinal, genitourinary, orthopedic, or other lesions. The best screening test for abdominal aortic aneurysms is an abdominal ultrasound examination (100).

The single most important prognostic feature of asymptomatic abdominal aortic aneurysms is the size, or transverse diameter. The absolute risk of rupture related to size is unknown. Best estimates suggest that small abdominal aortic aneurysms less than 4 cm in diameter have a low risk of rupture whereas aneurysms greater than 8 cm in diameter have a 75% risk of rupture within five years (Fig. 14).

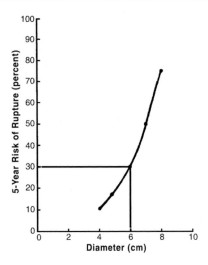

Figure 14 Relationship between the five-year risk of rupture and the diameter of infrarenal abdominal aortic aneurysms. A 6-cm abdominal aneurysm has a 30% risk of rupturing within five years.

Enlarging and Symptomatic Aneurysms

Aneurysms tend to progressively enlarge because of the increased tension on and thinning of the artery wall. If this process is slow, symptoms do not appear or are very late in appearing. If, however, enlargement is relatively rapid, symptoms of pain may arise as a result of pressure on the somatic sensory nerve elements of the retroperitoneal soft tissue in the vicinity of the aneurysmal sac. The pain is usually severe, constant, unrelated to posture, and boring in character; it is most commonly located in the lumbar spine region, in the midabdomen, or in the pelvis. Such symptoms indicate the impending rupture of the aneurysm and require immediate clinical attention.

Serial follow-up examinations using clinical and radiologic methods identify the patient with an aneurysm that is expanding and yet asymptomatic. The rate of enlargement can be variable and unpredictable. The mean rate of expansion of infrarenal abdominal aortic aneurysms is 0.4 cm/yr (101); however, some do not change at all, whereas others enlarge at twice that rate.

Ruptured Aneurysms

Aneurysms may rupture into the retroperitoneal space, with the development of severe back pain and sudden hypotension. If the rupture occurs anteriorly, free intraperitoneal hemorrhage results, with rapid exsanguination and death. Rupture can also occur into the inferior vena cava, resulting in the development of an *aortocaval fistula* with hypotension and an elevated central venous pressure. Approximately 50% of patients who sustain aneurysm rupture die suddenly, before medical help can arrive. Of those who survive to reach the hospital, mortality rates range from 50% to 80%. For patients who are stable with normal blood pressure, operative mortality may be as low as 10%. However, patients who are in shock and have required cardiopulmonary resuscitation have mortality rates approaching 90%. Thus, overall mortality rates for ruptured aortic aneurysms are in the range of 80% to 90%. On physical examination, ruptured aneurysms, even large ones, may be difficult to palpate because of hypotension and because the aortic aneurysm is often diffuse and ill defined as a result of obliteration of the margins of the aneurysm by retroperitoneal hematoma.

Diagnosis

The diagnosis of abdominal aortic aneurysm may be made on physical examination. However, physical examination commonly overestimates the true size of the aneurysm by 1 to 2 cm when compared to ultrasound or CT examination. A *cross table lateral X-ray* may demonstrate a rim of calcium outlining the anterior wall of the abdominal aorta and indicate the presence of an aneurysm. This X-ray film is taken with the patient lying supine, with the X-ray beam running horizontally, allowing intestinal gas to rise superiorly and the retroperitoneum to be visualized. Physical examination and a lateral X-ray film were in the past the predominant methods of evaluation for an abdominal aortic aneurysm. However, in view of the new development of ultrasound, the lateral abdominal X-ray film is currently used infrequently.

B-mode ultrasound is the most commonly used method of diagnosing an abdominal aortic aneurysm. It is simple, safe, noninvasive, and accurate and can be readily repeated for serial evaluation of aneurysms. It provides information on the presence or absence of an aneurysm and on the transverse diameter, length, and presence or absence of mural thrombus. It is the procedure of choice for routine evaluation for aneurysm.

CT scan provides better resolution and imaging of aneurysms than does ultrasound, especially when intravenous contrast enhancement is used. It provides the most detailed evaluation of the aortic wall and mural thrombus and the most accurate assessment of aneurysm size and characteristics of the infrarenal aortic neck. It also allows the evaluation of retroperitoneal extravasation and rupture. The CT scan offers significant advantages over ultrasound in assessing the thoracoabdominal aorta, because ultrasound does not pass through the air in the lung and cannot visualize the thoracic aorta. Thus it is particularly helpful in assessing thoracoabdominal aneurysms. In addition, CT is very useful in evaluating the pelvis for the presence of internal iliac aneurysms. CT scanning is essential for preoperative planning for endovascular aneurysm repair.

Angiography is useful in the evaluation of abdominal aortic aneurysms but provides little information on aneurysm size because only the aortic lumen is visualized. Aneurysms frequently contain mural thrombus, which may result in a normal or relatively normal lumen contour and diameter. This mural thrombus provides no structural strength to the aortic wall, and such aneurysms are just as likely to rupture as those without extensive mural thrombosis. CT scanning has largely replaced angiography in the evaluation of aortic aneurysms and provides, other important information regarding (i) accurate assessment of the proximal extent of the aneurysm in relation to the renal arteries, (ii) the status of the renal arteries and the presence of accessory renal arteries arising from the aneurysm itself, (iii) the inferior mesenteric artery and its collateral blood supply to the left colon, (iv) coexistent occlusive disease of the iliac and femoral vessels, and (v) identification of congenital abnormalities of the kidneys such as horseshoe kidney.

Treatment

Indications for Surgery

Indications for surgical repair of abdominal aortic aneurysms depend on the presence or absence of symptoms, the size of the aneurysm, and the general medical condition of the patient. If a patient has a ruptured aortic aneurysm, immediate surgical treatment is imperative. No diagnostic tests should be performed, and resuscitation should be carried out in the operating room. Fluid resuscitation may be useful during transport.

Patients with symptoms attributable to an aneurysm but without hypotension or signs of rupture should undergo confirmatory CT examination and urgent operative repair of the aneurysm. Similarly, if there is evidence of rapid enlargement of the aneurysm on routine physical examination or imaging follow-up such as B-mode ultrasound, urgent repair of the aneurysm is advised.

The absolute size of the aneurysm also determines whether repair should be undertaken. Studies of the natural history of aneurysms reveal that the risk of rupture of untreated aneurysms is directly proportional to their size (102,103). Aneurysms greater than 5 cm in transverse diameter as measured by ultrasound or CT scan or aneurysms that have more than twice the diameter of the adjacent, non-aneurysmal aorta should be surgically repaired if the patient has no medical contraindications to surgery, such as severe cardiac, pulmonary, renal, or neoplastic disease. However, it must be realized that aneurysms smaller than 5 cm can also rupture and must be carefully observed.

Surgical Repair

The surgical treatment of an abdominal aortic aneurysm consists of excluding the aneurysm from the circulation and replacing it with a Dacron prosthetic bypass graft. The aorta is clamped proximal to the aneurysm, below the level of the renal arteries, and distal to the aneurysm. The aneurysm sac is opened, and the graft is sutured to the normal, nonaneurysmal aorta from within the aneurysm. The graft may be a straight "tube" graft confined to the abdominal aorta or a bifurcation graft to the iliac arteries if the aortic bifurcation and iliac arteries are involved (Fig. 15). The aneurysm sac is not excised but closed over the graft after it is in place to isolate the graft from the bowel. This prevents possible erosion of the bowel, aortoduodenal fistula formation, and graft infection. The inferior mesenteric artery, which always arises from the aneurysm, is usually ligated. Collateral circulation from the celiac and superior mesenteric arteries and internal iliac arteries maintains flow to the sigmoid colon. Occasionally, when collateral flow is insufficient, the inferior mesenteric artery must be reimplanted into the bypass graft to avoid colonic ischemia.

Endovascular Aneurysm Repair

During the past decade a new less invasive strategy for treating aortic aneurysms has been introduced. This strategy involves the transfemoral placement of self-expanding endoluminal devices to exclude the aneurysm from the circulation. The first FDA-approved devices appeared in 1999 and favorable long-term results extending to six years and longer have been reported (104). All current FDA-approved devices are self-expanding, bifurcated, modular stent grafts that are introduced through the femoral arteries and deployed under fluoroscopic image guidance. Endovascular aneurysm repair requires a suitable infrarenal aortic neck and iliac arteries to allow secure fixation and sealing of the endovascular device (Fig. 16). Precise preoperative imaging with high-quality CT scanning and 3-D image reconstruction is required to select appropriate candidates for endovascular repair. Because endovascular aneurysm repair requires only groin exposure of the femoral arteries, the procedure can be performed in elderly, high-risk patients who are not suitable candidates for open surgical repair. However, not all patients with infrarenal aortic aneurysms are suitable candidates for endovascular repair because of adverse morphologic features such as a short (<15 mm long) or severely angulated infrarenal aortic neck, absent infrarenal aortic neck, large diameter (>28 mm) aortic neck, iliac aneurysms, or iliac stenosis. Thus, careful preoperative

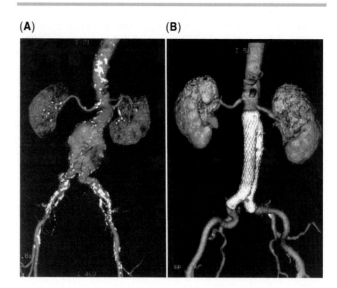

(A)   **(B)**

Figure 16 **(A)** Three-dimensional reconstruction of spiral computed tomography (CT) scan demonstrating a 5.8 cm-abdominal aortic aneurysm. **(B)** CT scan following endovascular aneurysm repair using a stent graft.

patient evaluation and planning are required to obtain satisfactory results.

Results: Open vs. Endovascular Repair

Both open and endovascular aneurysm repair are highly effective in achieving the primary objective of aneurysm repair, namely prevention of aneurysm rupture. Operative mortality for elective open surgical repair is approximately 5% to 6% (105,106) although elective operative mortality rates of less than 2% are reported from high-volume specialized centers (107–109). Operative mortality for endovascular aneurysm repair is 1% to 2% even though most series include high-risk patients who would not be candidates for open surgical repair (106). Two recent prospective randomized trials comparing open to endovascular repair in good-risk patients revealed a statistically significant reduction in operative mortality in patients undergoing endovascular repair (1–2%) compared to patients undergoing elective open repair (4–5%) (110,111). In addition to reduced operative mortality, there is a significant reduction in morbidity following endovascular repair, with a reduction in blood loss and transfusion requirements, shorter intensive care unit and hospital stay, and earlier return to function. Thus, endovascular repair has significant short-term advantages over open surgical repair and is favored for most patients who have suitable anatomy (112). However, the long-term outcome of endovascular repair is uncertain, because long-term outcome data is limited. Adverse outcomes of endovascular aneurysm repair include continued blood flow in the aneurysm sac (endoleak), device migration over time, aneurysm enlargement, and possible late rupture. These adverse events may require secondary procedures, including possible conversion to standard open repair in the future. Although open surgical repair appears to be needed in no more than 5% of patients at five years, more complete long-term outcome analysis will be required to fully define the role of endovascular aneurysm repair.

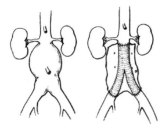

Figure 15 Repair of abdominal aortic aneurysm. Aneurysm sac is opened, and a Dacron graft is sutured to the normal, nonaneurysmal artery. Aneurysm is not excised, but it is excluded from the circulation.

Regardless of the mode of therapy, elective aortic aneurysm repair has far better results than emergent repair of ruptured aortic aneurysms. Operations for ruptured abdominal aortic aneurysms have a mortality rate of 50% to 80% or higher (105,109,113). Thus, every effort should be made to repair abdominal aortic aneurysms before rupture. Improved operative techniques with better preoperative and perioperative care, including central hemodynamic monitoring, earlier diagnosis, improvements in fluid management, and refinements in anesthesia techniques, have allowed elective aneurysm repair to be carried out with a similar low mortality rate even in octogenarians (114). Thus, age alone is not a contraindication to aneurysm repair.

The long-term survival of patients who have undergone abdominal aortic aneurysm repair is approximately 60% at five years (106). Associated coronary artery disease is responsible for the majority of deaths in the long-term follow-up of these patients. In a matched group, the expected five-year survival is 80% (108). It is possible that with more aggressive treatment of coexistent coronary disease this mortality rate can be decreased. The overall survival and long-term outlook with elective repair of abdominal aortic aneurysms is significantly better than that for nonsurgical treatment.

PERIPHERAL ARTERY ANEURYSMS

Although it is not common, aneurysms can form in arteries other than the aorta. The most commonly involved peripheral arteries are the common femoral and popliteal arteries, which together account for 90% of all peripheral aneurysms. The popliteal artery accounts for 70% of these aneurysms. *Popliteal aneurysms* are unique in that they are found almost exclusively in males, and the vast majority are atherosclerotic in origin. Approximately two-thirds of the patients have bilateral aneurysms, with one-half of these patients having associated abdominal aortic aneurysms.

Popliteal aneurysms are usually symptomatic when discovered, and over 50% have complications at the first medical visit (114). The most common complication is thrombosis of the aneurysm, which is associated with a 33% amputation rate. Embolization of mural thrombus from within the aneurysm to the distal arterial tree also occurs and is associated with a high amputation rate. Rupture of popliteal aneurysms is unusual but can occur. Compression of the popliteal vein with lower extremity edema and neurologic pain syndromes from nerve compression are also possible.

Treatment of popliteal aneurysms consists of ligation of the aneurysm to exclude it from the circulation, followed by bypass grafting from the femoral artery to either the popliteal or tibial vessels. Results of surgery are influenced by the status of the leg at the time of presentation and the extent of coexistent occlusive disease in the tibial vessels and vessels of the foot. If these are obstructed because of prior and repeated embolization from the aneurysm, prospects for revascularization are poor. There is minimal risk for limb loss in patients with asymptomatic aneurysms, but 34% of limbs are lost if the patient initially has symptoms (114). Therefore, popliteal aneurysms should be repaired electively when found, before symptoms of embolization or thrombosis occur.

Femoral artery aneurysms are similarly found in elderly men and are caused by atherosclerosis. Associated hypertension is extremely common. Associated abdominal aortic aneurysms are present in 51% to 85% of patients (115,116) and associated popliteal aneurysms are present in 17% to 44%

of patients (116,117), suggesting an aneurysmal diathesis. As in the popliteal artery, symptoms may be caused by local pressure from the expanding aneurysm on the adjacent femoral vein or nerve, distal embolization, acute or chronic thrombosis, or rupture of the aneurysm. Because of the risk for limb loss from acute thrombosis and distal embolization, surgical management of these aneurysms is advised in all patients who are reasonable medical risks. Surgical techniques include replacement of the aneurysm with an interposition graft (118).

COMPLICATIONS OF VASCULAR PROCEDURES

Complications following vascular procedures fall into two categories: those involving the generalized disease process of atherosclerosis and those involving local factors related to the vascular procedure or bypass graft.

The generalized process of atherosclerosis involves not only the peripheral arteries but also the carotid and coronary arteries. The risk factors of hypertension, hyperlipidemia, diabetes mellitus, and cigarette smoking are important in determining whether there is disease progression, stabilization, or regression, and control of these factors is important. The major cause of morbidity and mortality in the vascular surgical patient is disease progression in the coronary arteries, with myocardial infarctions accounting for the majority of deaths in these patients despite successful peripheral vascular procedures. Stroke from progression of cerebrovascular disease is also a major problem. These same risk factors play a major role in the progression of distal disease following bypass grafts and are a common reason for restenosis and subsequent graft occlusion and its related morbidity.

Local factors related to vascular procedures may produce a number of complications following vascular procedures. Graft thrombosis in the early postoperative period may be the result of a technical error in the graft-to-artery anastomosis or caused by an obstructed outflow bed with slow flow in the graft. Late graft occlusion is usually caused by progression of atherosclerotic occlusive disease in the inflow or outflow vessels or by a hypertrophic proliferative response of intima at the anastomosis and can usually be corrected by reoperation.

Pseudoaneurysms may form at the sites of vascular anastomoses and must be distinguished from true aneurysms that involve dilation of all layers of the artery wall. In a pseudoaneurysm, there is separation of the vascular graft from the artery wall, and the blood stream is contained by surrounding fibrous tissue. The integrity of an anastomosis of prosthetic graft to artery is forever dependent on the integrity of the suture line. Failure of the suture or excess tension on the suture line can result in the disruption of the anastomosis with pseudoaneurysm formation. In addition, anastomotic breakdown with pseudoaneurysm formation may be a harbinger or sign that infection of the prosthetic bypass graft has occurred. Treatment of a pseudoaneurysm mandates replacement of that segment with a prosthetic graft if it is not infected. However, infected grafts must be totally removed because prosthetic grafts are foreign bodies and infection cannot be eradicated until all foreign material is excised.

Revascularization under these circumstances is complex and usually involves the use of an "extra-anatomic" bypass in a clean, noninfected area. An example of such a bypass is an axillofemoral bypass to bypass an infected intra-abdominal aortoiliac bypass graft.

SUMMARY

Atherosclerosis is a degenerative disease process that affects the aorta and peripheral arteries, as well as coronary and carotid arteries. It can result in occlusive disease, obstructing the lumen, or aneurysmal disease, with dilation of the lumen. Occlusive disease can result in stenosis and diminished blood flow or embolization with occlusion of distal arteries. Obstruction of blood flow can result in ischemia of the lower extremities, producing symptoms of claudication, rest pain, ulceration, or gangrene. Obstructions can be detected with the use of clinical, noninvasive, and angiographic diagnostic techniques. Revascularization of the lower extremities with a bypass or with transluminal balloon angioplasty can restore circulation and help avoid limb loss.

Aneurysmal disease results in progressive arterial enlargement and weakening of the aortic wall, with eventual rupture unless the patient dies of intercurrent disease. The larger the aneurysm, the higher the risk of rupture. Most aneurysms are asymptomatic and are detectable by noninvasive techniques. Operative replacement of aneurysmal segments of artery with a Dacron graft or endovascular aneurysm repair prevents further degeneration and aneurysm rupture.

REFERENCES

1. Fann JI, Dalman RL. Genetic and metabolic causes of arterial disease. Ann Vasc Surg 1993; 7:594.
2. Vogt MT, Wolfion SK, Kullen LN. Lower extremity arterial disease and the aging process. J Clin Epidemiol 1992; 45:529.
3. Reunanen A, Takkunen H, Aromaa A. Prevalence of intermittent claudication and its effect on mortality. Acta Med Scand 1982; 211:249.
4. Kannel WB, Mcbee DL. Update on some epidemiological features of intermittent claudication. The Framingham Study. J Am Geriatr Soc 1985; 33:13.
5. Scheoll M, Murck O. Estimation of peripheral arteriosclerotic disease by ankle pressure measurements in a population study of 60 year old men and women. J Chron Dis 1981; 34:261.
6. Criqui MH, Browner D, Fronek A, et al. Peripheral arterial disease in large vessels is epidemiologically distinct from small vessel disease. An analysis of risk factors. Am J Epidemiol 1989; 129:1110.
7. Knipski WC. The peripheral vascular consequences of smoking. Ann Vasc Surg 1991; 5:291.
8. Powell JT, Greenhalgh RM. Arterial bypass surgery and smokers. Br Med J 1994; 308:607.
9. Diabetes Control and Complications Trial Research Group. The effect of intensive treatment of diabetes on the development and progression of long-term complications in insulin-dependent diabetes mellitus. N Engl J Med 1993; 329:977.
10. Wissler RW, Hiltscher l, Oinuma T, et al. Pathogenesis of atherosclerosis—the lesions of atherosclerosis in the young: from fatty streaks to intermediate lesions. In: Fuster V, Ross R, Topol E, eds. Atherosclerosis and Coronary Artery Disease. New York: Lippincott-Raven Press, 1995:475–489.
11. Paterson JC. Vascularization and haemorrhage of the intima of arteriosclerotic arteries. Arch Pathol 1936; 22:312.
12. Zarins CK, Glagov S, Vesselinovitch D, Wissler RW. Aneurysm formation in experimental atherosclerosis: relationship to plaque formation. J Vasc Surg 1990; 12(3):246–256.
13. Strickland HL, Bond MG. Aneurysms in a large colony of squirrel monkeys (*Saimiri sriures*). Lab Anim Sci 1983; 33:589.
14. Riflin RD, Parisis HF, Follard E. Coronary calcification in the diagnosis of coronary artery disease. Am J Cardiol 1979; 44:141.
15. Glagov S, Eckner FAO, Lev M. Controlled pressure fixation apparatus for hearts. Arch Pathol 1963; 76:640.
16. Zarins CK, Zatina MA, Glagov S. Correlation of postmortem angiography with pathologic anatomy: quantitation of atherosclerotic lesions. In: Bond MG, et al., ed. Clinical Diagnosis of Atherosclerosis. New York: Springer-Verlag, 1983:283.
17. Mulvihill DA, Harvey SC. The mechanism of the development of collateral circulation. N Engl J Med 1931; 104:1032.
18. Holman E. Problems in the dynamics of blood flow. I. Condition controlling collateral circulation in the presence of an ateriovenous fistula following ligation of an artery. Surgery 1949; 26:889.
19. Kamiya A, Tbgawa T. Adaptive regulation of wall shear stress to flow change in the canine carotid artery. Am J Physiol 1980; 239:H14.
20. Furchgott RF. Role of endothelium in responses of vascular smooth muscle. Circ Res 1983; 53:557.
21. Langille BL, O'Donnel F. Reductions in arterial diameter produced by chronic decreases in blood flow are endothelium dependent. Science 1986; 231:405.
22. Ying H, Harris EJ, Dalman RL. Unpublished observations, 1992–1993.
23. Thubrikar M, Maker J, Nolan S. Inhibition of atherosclerosis associated with reduction of arterial intramural stenosis in rabbits. Arteriosclerosis 1988; 8:410.
24. Friedman MH. Some atherosclerosis may be a consequence of the normal adaptive vascular response to shear. Atherosclerosis 1990; 82:193.
25. Zarins CK, et al. Carotid bifurcation atherosclerosis: quantitative correlation of plaque localization with flow velocity profiles and wall shear stress. Circ Res 1983; 53:502.
26. Ku DN, et al. Pulsatile flow and atherosclerosis in the human carotid bifurcation: positive correlation between plaque localization and low oscillating shear stress. Arteriosclerosis 1985; 5:292.
27. Karino T. Microscopic structure of disturbed flows in the arterial and venous systems and its implication in the localization of vascular disease. Int Angiol 1986; 5:297.
28. Glagov S, Rowley DA, Kohut R. Atherosclerosis of human aorta and its coronary and renal arteries. Arch Pathol 1961; 72:558.
29. Svindland A. The localization of sudanophilic and fibrous plaques in the main left coronary arteries. Atherosclerosis 1983; 48:139.
30. Giddens DP, Zarins CK, Glagov S. The role of fluid mechanics in the localization and detection of atherosclerosis. J Biomech Eng 1993; 115:588.
31. Fingerle J, Johnson R, Clowes AW. Role of platelets in smooth muscle cell proliferation and migration after vascular injury in rat carotid artery. Proc Natl Acad Sci USA 1989; 86:8412.
32. Falcone DJ, Haijar DP, Minick CR. Lipoprotein and albumin accumulation in re-endothelialized and de-endothelialized aorta. Am J Pathol 1984; 114:112.
33. Bassinouny HS, et al. Quantitative inverse correlation of wall shear stress with experimental intima thickening. Surg Forum 1988; 39:328.
34. Lyon RT, Hass A, Davis HR. Protection from atherosclerotic lesion formation by reduction of artery wall motion. J Vasc Surg 1987; 5:59.
35. Caro GG, et al. Influence of vasoreactive agents on arterial hemodynamics: possible relevance to atherogenesis. Biorheology 1986; 23:197.
36. Glagov S. Microarchitecture of arteries and veins. In: Abrahson D, Dobrin P, eds. Blood Vessels and Lymphatics. Orlando, Florida: Academic Press, 1984:3.
37. Glagov S, et al. Hemodynamics and atherosclerosis: insights and perspectives gained from studies of human arteries. Arch Pathol Lab Med 1988; 112:1018.
38. Glagov S, et al. Establishing the hemodynamic determinants of human plaque configuration, composition and complication. In: Yoshida Y, et al., ed. Role of Blood Flow in Atherogenesis. New York: Springer-Verlag, 1988:3.
39. Born VRG, Richardson PD. Mechanical properties of human atherosclerotic lesions. In: Glagov S, Newman WP, Schaffer SA,

eds. Pathobiology of the Human Atherosclerotic Plaque. New York: Springer-Verlag, 1990:413.

40. Zarins CK, et al. Artery stenosis inhibits regression of diet-induced atherosclerosis. Surgery 1980; 88:86.

41. Xu Chengpei, Glagov S, Zatina M. Hypertension sustains plaque progression despite reduction of hypercholesterolemia. Hypertension 1991; 18:123.

42. Zarins CK, et al. Shear stress regulation of artery lumen diameter in experimental atherogenesis. J Vasc Surg 1987; 5:413.

43. Fry DL. Problems and progress in understanding "endothelial permeability" and mass transport in human arteries. In: Glagov S, Newman WP, Schaffer SA, eds. Pathobiology of the Human Atherosclerotic Plaque. New York: Springer-Verlag, 1990:271.

44. Smith EB. Accumulating evidence from human artery studies of what is transported and what accumulates relative to atherogenesis. In: Glagov S, Newman WP, Schaffer SA, eds. Pathobiology of the Human Atherosclerotic Plaque. New York: Springer-Verlag, 1990.

45. Tracy RE, Kissling GE. Comparisons of human populations for histologic features of atherosclerosis. Arch Pathol Lab Med 1988; 112:156.

46. Frank JS, Fogelman AM. Ultrastructure of the intima in WHHL and cholesterol-fed rabbit aortas prepared by ultrarapid freezing and freeze-etching. J Lipid Res 1989; 30:967.

47. Berenson GS, et al. In: Glagov S, Newman WP, Schaffer SA, eds. Pathobiology of the Human Atherosclerotic Plaque. New York: Springer-Verlag, 1990:189.

48. Kramsh DM, Hollander W. The interaction of serum and arterial lipoproteins with elastin of the arterial intima and its role in the Kpid accumulation in atherosclerotic plaque. J Clin Invest 1973; 52:236.

49. Wagner WD, et al. Low density lipoprotein interaction with artery derived proteoglycan: the influence of LDL particle size and the relationship to atherosclerosis susceptibility. Atherosclerosis 1989; 75:49.

50. Grande J, et al. Effect of an elastin growth substrate on cholesteryl ester synthesis and foam cell formation by cultured aortic smooth muscle cells. Atherosclerosis 1987; 68:87.

51. May AG, De Weese JA, Rob CG. Hemodynamic effects of arterial stenosis. Surgery 1963; 53:513.

52. Thompson JE, et al. Arterial embolectomy: a 20 year experience with 163 cases. Surgery 1970; 67:212.

53. Coffinan JD. Intermittent claudication-be conservative. N Engl J Med 1991; 325:557.

54. Jelnes R, et al. Fate in intermittent claudication: outcome and risk factors. Br Med J 1986; 293:1137.

55. Sibert S, Zazeela H. Prognosis in arteriosclerotic peripheral vascular disease. JAMA 1958; 156:1816.

56. Kallero KS. Mortality and morbidity in patients with intermittent claudication as defined by venous occlusion plethysmography. A ten year follow-up study. J Chron Dis 1981; 34:455.

57. Croneneitt JL, et al. Intermittent claudication. Current results at non-operative management. Arch Surg 1984; 119:430.

58. Dormandy J, et al. Fate of the patient with chronic leg ischemia. J Cardiovasc Surg 1989; 30:50.

59. Bandyk DF. Essentials of graft surveillance. Semin Vasc Surg 1993; 6:92.

60. Mills JL, et al. The origin of infrainguinal vein graft stenosis. A prospective study based on duplex surveillance. J Vasc Surg 1995; 21:16.

61. Bandyk DF, et al. Intraoperative duplex scanning of arterial reconstructions: rate of repaired and unrepaired defects. J Vasc Surg 1994; 20:426.

62. Ferris BL, Mills JL Sr, Hughes JD, Durrani T, Knox R. Is early postoperative duplex scan surveillance of leg bypass grafts clinically important? J Vasc Surg 2003; 37(3):495–500.

63. Shehadi WH, Tbnielo G. Adverse reactions to contrast media. Radiology 1980; 137:299.

64. Rubin GD, et al. Three dimensional spiral computed tomographic angiography: an alternative imaging modality for the abdominal aorta and its branches. J Vasc Surg 1993; 18:656.

65. Napel S, Rubin GD, Jeffiey RB Jr. STS-MIP: a new reconstruction technique for CT of the chest. J Comput Assist Tomogr 1993; 17:832.

66. Marks MP, et al. Diagnosis of carotid artery diseases: preliminary experience with maximum intensity projection spiral CT angiography. Am J Roentgenol 1993; 160:1267.

67. Boll DT, Lewin JS, Fleiter TR, Duerk JL, Merkle EM. Multidetector CT angiography of arterial inflow and runoff in the lower extremities: a challenge in data acquisition and evaluation. J Endovasc Ther: Official J Int Soc Endovasc Specialists 2004; 11(2):144–151.

68. Carpenter JP, et al. Peripheral vascular surgery with magnetic resonance angiography as the sole preoperative imaging modality. J Vasc Surg 1994; 20:861.

69. Debatin JE, et al. Phase contrast MRI assessment of pedal blood flow. Eur Radiol 1995; 194:321.

70. Li KCP, et al. Oxygen saturation of blood in the superior mesenteric vein: in vivo verification of MR imaging measurements in a canine model. Radiology 1995; 194:321.

71. Li KCP, et al. Simultaneous measurement of flow in the superior mesenteric vein and artery with cine phase-contrast MR imaging: value in diagnosis of chronic mesenteric ischemia. Radiology 1995; 194:327.

72. Peabody CN, Kannel WB, McNamara PM. Intermittent claudication: surgical significance. Arch Surg 1974; 109:693.

73. Ingolfsson IO, Sigurdsson G, Sigvaldason H, Thorgeirsson G, Sigfusson N. A marked decline in the prevalence and incidence of intermittent claudication in Icelandic men 1968–1986: a strong relationship to smoking and serum cholesterol—the Reykjavik Study. J Clin Epidemiol 1994; 47(11):1237–1243.

74. Jonason T, Bergstrom R. Cessation of smoking in patients with intermittent claudication. Effects on the risk of peripheral vascular complications, myocardial infarction and mortality. Acta Med Scand 1987; 221(3):253–260.

75. Ameli FM, Stein M, Provan JL, Prosser R. The effect of postoperative smoking on femoropopliteal bypass grafts. Ann Vasc Surg 1989; 3(1):20–25.

76. Pedersen TR, Kjekshus J, Pyorala K, et al. Effect of simvastatin on ischemic signs and symptoms in the Scandinavian simvastatin survival study (4S). Am J Cardiol 1998; 81(3):333–335.

77. Stoyioglou A, Jaff MR. Medical treatment of peripheral arterial disease: a comprehensive review. J Vasc Interv Radiol 2004; 15(11):1197–1207.

78. Group UPDSU. Intensive blood-glucose control with sulphonylureas or insulin compared with conventional treatment and risk of complications in patients with type 2 diabetes (UKPDS 33). UK Prospective Diabetes Study (UKPDS) Group [see comment] [erratum appears in Lancet 1999 Aug 14; 354(9178):602]. Lancet 1998; 352(9131):837–853.

79. Smith CD, McKendry RJ. Controlled trial of nifedipine in the treatment of Raynaud's phenomenon. Lancet 1982; 2:1299.

80. Porter JM, et al. Pentoxifylline efficacy in the treatment of intermittent claudication. Am Heart J 1982; 104:66.

81. Thompson PD, Zimet R, Forbes WP, Zhang P. Meta-analysis of results from eight randomized, placebo-controlled trials on the effect of cilostazol on patients with intermittent claudication. Am J Cardiol 2002; 90(12):1314–1319.

82. Zarins CK, et al. Arterial disruption and remodeling following dilatation. Surgery 1982; 92:1086.

83. Yalcin R, Erkan A, Ergun MA, Yurtcu E. The effect of clopidogrel on apoptosis an in vivo study. Cell Biol Int 2004; 28(6):477–481.

84. Douglas JS, Weintraub WS, Holmes D. Rationale and design f the randomized, multicenter, cilostazol for RESTenosis (CREST) trial. Clin Cardiol 2003; 26(10):451–454.

85. (TASC) TI-SC. Treatment of intermittent claudication in Management of Peripheral Arterial Disease (PAD). J Vasc Surg 2000; 31(1):S77.

86. Ahn SS, et al. Reporting standards for lower extremity arterial endovascular procedures. J Vasc Surg 1993; 17:1103.

87. Dalman RL, Taylor LM, Porter JM. Current status of extracoronary endovascular procedures. Ann Vasc Surg 1990; 3:1.

88. Rutherford RB. Aortofemoral bypass: the gold standard. Technical considerations. Semin Vasc Surg 1994; 7:11.

89. Brewster DC, Darling RC. Optimal methods of aortoiliac reconstruction. Surgery 1978; 84:739.

90. Taylor CM, et al. Axillofemoral grafting with externally supported PTFE. Arch Surg 1994; 129:588.

91. Taylor CM, et al. Acute disruption of polytetrafluoroethylene grafts adjacent to axillary anastomosis: A complication of axillofemoral grafting. J Vasc Surg 1994; 20:520.

92. Farm JI, Harris EJ, Dalman RL. Extra-anatomic bypass. Ann Vasc Surg 1993; 7:378.

93. Corson JD, et al. In situ vein bypasses to distal tibial and limited outflow tracts for limb salvage. Surgery 1984; 96:756.

94. Dalman RL, Taylor CM. Basic data regarding intrainguinal revascularization procedures. Ann Vasc Surg 1990; 4:309.

95. Craver JM, et al. Hemorrage and thrombosis as early complications of femoropopliteal bypass grafts: causes, treatment, and prognostic implications. Surgery 1971; 74:839.

96. Giannini D, Balbarini A. Thrombolytic therapy in peripheral arterial disease. Curr Drug Targets Cardiovasc Haematol Disord 2004; 4(3):249–258.

97. Wolinsky H, Glagov S. Nature of species differences in the medial—distribution of aortic vasa vasorum in mammals. Circ Res 1967; 20:409.

98. Wolinsky H, Glagov S. Comparison of abdominal and thoracic aortic medial structure in mammals: deviation of man from the usual pattern. Circ Res 1969; 25:677.

99. Zarins CK, Glagov S. Aneurysms and obstructive plaques: differing local response to atherosclerosis. In: Bergan JJ, Yao JST, eds. Aneurysms: Diagnosis and Treatment. New York: Grune & Stratton, 1982.

100. Lederle FA. Ultrasonographic screening for abdominal aortic aneurysms.[see comment][erratum appears in Ann Intern Med. 2003 Nov 18;139(10):873]. Ann Intern Med 2003; 139(6): 516–522.

101. Bernstein EF, et al Growth rates of small abdominal aortic aneurysms. Surgery 1976; 80:765.

102. Bernstein EF. The natural history of abdominal aortic aneurysms. In: Najarian JS, Delaney JP, eds. Vascular Surgery. Miami, Florida: Symposia Specialists, 1978.

103. Szilagyi DE, Elliott JP, Smith RE. Clinical fate of patients with asymptomatic abdominal aortic aneurysm and unfit for special treatment. Arch Surg 1972; 104:600.

104. Zarins CK. Aneu Rx Clinical I. The US AneuRx Clinical Trial: 6-year clinical update 2002. J Vasc Surg 2003; 37(4):904–908.

105. Zarins CK, Harris EJ Jr. Operative repair for aortic aneurysms: the gold standard. J Endovasc Surg 1997; 4(3):232–241.

106. Zarins CK, Heikkinen MA, Lee ES, Alsac JM, Arko FR. Short- and long-term outcome following endovascular aneurysm repair. How does it compare to open surgery? J Cardiovasc Surg (Torino) 2004; 45(4):321–333.

107. DeBakcy MD, et al. Aneurysms of the abdominal aorta: analysis of results of graft replacement therapy one to eleven years after operation. Ann Surg 1964; 160:622.

108. Thompson JE, et al. Surgical management of abdominal aortic aneurysms: factors influencing mortality and morbidity—a 20 year experience. Ann Surg 1975; 188:654.

109. Brewster DC, Cronenwett JL, Hallett JW Jr, Johnston KW, Krupski WC, Matsumura JS, Joint Council of the American Association for Vascular S, and Society for Vascular S. Guidelines for the treatment of abdominal aortic aneurysms. Report of a subcommittee of the Joint Council of the American Association for Vascular Surgery and Society for Vascular Surgery. J Vasc Surg 2003; 37(5):1106–1117.

110. Prinssen M, Verhoeven EL, Buth J, et al. Dutch Randomized Endovascular Aneurysm Management Trial G. A randomized trial comparing conventional and endovascular repair of abdominal aortic aneurysms. [see comment]. N Eng J Med 2004; 351(16):1607–1618.

111. Greenhalgh RM, Brown LC, Kwong GP, Powell JT, Thompson SG, participants Et. Comparison of endovascular aneurysm repair with open repair in patients with abdominal aortic aneurysm (EVAR trial 1), 30-day operative mortality results: randomised controlled trial. [see comment]. Lancet 2004; 364(9437):843–848.

112. Lee WA, Carter JW, Upchurch G, Seeger JM, Huber TS. Perioperative outcomes after open and endovascular repair of intact abdominal aortic aneurysms in the United States during 2001. J Vasc Surg 2004; 39(3):491–496.

113. Garrett HE, Ilabaca PA. The ruptured abdominal aortic aneurysm. In: Bergan JJ, Yao JST, eds. Aneurysms: Diagnosis and Treatment. New York: Grune & Stratton, 1982.

114. Evans WE, Conley JE, Bernhard V. Popliteal aneurysms. Surgery 1971; 70:762.

115. O'Donnel TF Jr, Darling RC, Linton RR. Is 80 years too old for aneurysmectomy? Arch Surg 1976; 111:1250.

116. Cutler BS, Darling RC. Surgical management of arteriosclerotic femoral aneurysms. Surgery 1973; 74:764.

117. Graham L, et al. Clinical significance of arteriosclerotic femoral artery aneurysms. Arch Surg 1973; 115:502.

118. Baud RJ, et al. Arteriosclerotic femoral artery aneurysms. Can Med Assoc J 1977; 117:1306.

45

Cerebrovascular Disease and Upper-Extremity Vascular Disease

Bruce L. Gewertz and James F. McKinsey

INTRODUCTION

In each calendar year, nearly 500,000 people in the United States suffer cerebral infarctions; in 175,000 patients, the strokes are fatal, and the remaining patients experience variable disability. The emotional and economic consequences of advanced cerebrovascular disease are staggering; the cost of care and loss of earnings secondary to permanent disability or death have been estimated at more than $10 billion annually.

In contrast to these depressing statistics, there has been a persistent 10-year decline in the death rate from stroke, which has exceeded the general decline in cardiovascular mortality observed over the same time period (1). It is difficult to explain this phenomenon. Although surgery for extracranial occlusive disease has become much more common in the last 15 years, improved medical and surgical care can account for only a small fraction of the change in death rate. It is most likely that the decline in cardiovascular mortality reflects better control of arterial hypertension, changes in lifestyle, and the general reduction in cigarette smoking (2,3).

Although the natural history of stroke in the United States was defined in an earlier era, studies performed from 1950 to 1975 provide useful information regarding the indications and timing of cerebrovascular surgery (4,5). The following are now accepted facts.

1. Patients who have survived one cerebral infarction have a high incidence of *recurrent strokes* (approximately 25%). More than half of these recurrent strokes are fatal.
2. Prodromal symptoms of stroke, such as *transient cerebral ischemic attacks*, identify the patients at greatest risk of suffering later completed strokes. The cumulative stroke rate approaches 50% at five years and is highest in the first year after the transient ischemic episode (6,7).
3. Patients suffering transient ischemic attacks (TIA) or strokes from *atheromatous stenotic lesions* of the carotid bifurcation are significantly benefited by carotid endarterectomy if the complications of the procedure are equal to or less than current norms.

In this chapter, the anatomy and physiology of cerebral blood flow will be reviewed, the variable clinical presentations of cerebral ischemia characterized, and the diagnostic and therapeutic options considered. In addition, clinically relevant upper-extremity vascular disease will also be reviewed. It has become clear that only through better understanding of cerebrovascular physiology and upper-extremity vascular pathology can the care of patients with advanced vascular disease be improved.

CEREBRAL BLOOD FLOW

Anatomy

The brain is perfused by paired carotid and vertebral arteries that communicate with each other through the circle of Willis at the base of the skull. Although there is substantial variation in the effectiveness of this collateral network (less than 20% of patients have "complete" circles), occlusion of one vessel is frequently compensated for without neurologic deficit. In general terms a carotid artery supplies only the ipsilateral cerebral hemisphere through the middle, anterior, and posterior cerebral vessels. The vertebral arteries join to form a single basilar artery that supplies the brainstem and cerebellum with additional contributions to the posterior aspect of the circle of Willis (Fig. 1).

Boundary zones or "watershed" areas between the primary perfusion territories of the middle, anterior, and posterior cerebral arteries can be demonstrated by anatomic studies. These areas are most at risk for ischemia and infarction during hypotension or vascular occlusion. Perhaps because of the lower basal vascular tone of these vessels, boundary zones are frequently the site of intracerebral hemorrhages associated with acute hypertension.

The subclavian origin of both vertebral arteries makes possible the unique subclavian steal syndrome that will be discussed in greater detail in the section on "Vertebrobasilar Disease" (Fig. 2). This syndrome occurs when an occlusive lesion proximal to the origin of the vertebral vessels decreases perfusion pressure in the distal subclavian artery. The vertebral artery then functions as a collateral pathway for the arm, and reversal of flow (away from the cranium) can be demonstrated angiographically. This flow pattern "steals" blood from the basilar system and may result in cerebellar ischemia or infarction.

Characteristics of Flow

The cerebral circulation is supplied with nearly 15% of cardiac output. Resting total blood flows range from 50 to 60 mL/min/100 g of tissue, with higher values in the cellular gray matter (100 mL/min/100 g) and lower flows in the cell-poor white matter (20 mL/min/100 g) (8,9). Cerebral blood flow is regulated by both metabolic and myogenic mechanisms that tend to maintain or "autoregulate" perfusion to avoid cerebral infarction during hypotension and cerebral hemorrhage during hypertension (10,11). Cerebral infarcts may result when regional blood flows decline below 15 mL/min/100 g, although the metabolic state of the brain strongly influences the likelihood of cell death (12). Barbiturate coma has been shown to decrease the ischemic limit to as low as 5 mL/min/100 g (13).

The cerebral circulation is further distinguished by a *blood–brain barrier* that effectively isolates brain tissue from

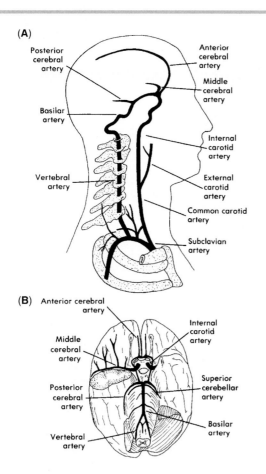

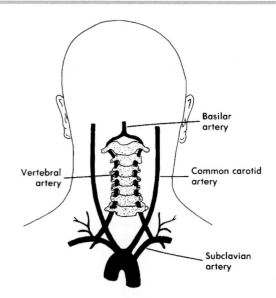

Figure 1   **(A)** Carotid artery supplies middle cerebral and anterior cerebral arteries predominantly, with major contributions to posterior cerebral artery. **(B)** Vertebral arteries form the basilar artery that supplies cerebellar vessels and posterior cerebral arteries.

Figure 2   Subclavian origin of vertebral arteries allows these vessels to function as collateral pathways for upper extremity. Cerebellar ischemia may result from the "steal" of blood flow.

serum ionic changes and humoral factors (14). The barrier is both a physical and biochemical impediment to the transport of protein and polar substances into cerebral extracellular fluid. Anatomic features include very tight junctions between endothelial cells, with only a few scattered pores and minimal transport by pinocytotic vesicles. A membrane-bound enzyme system, primarily composed of monoamine oxidase, effectively degrades circulating catecholamines and limits cerebral extraction to less than 5%. It is noteworthy that the areas of the brain responsible for hormone regulation, such as the hypothalamus, pituitary gland, and pineal gland, do *not* demonstrate the anatomic or functional characteristics of the blood–brain barrier.

The blood–brain barrier is disrupted in areas of tissue infarction and during periods of severe hypertension (15). These observations are clinically important because breakdown of the blood–brain barrier (i) facilitates the diagnosis of cerebral infarcts by radionuclide scanning, and (ii) explains the occurrence of late hemorrhage in previously "bland" infarcts when patients become severely hypertensive.

Measurement Techniques

Diverse methods have been used to measure cerebral blood flow in experimental settings, including venous outflow

collections, radioactive microspheres, autoradiography, and heat or hydrogen clearance (16). In clinical practice, most measurements of total and regional cerebral blood flow are made on the basis of the clearance of inhaled inert gases including xenon-133. Using the modified Kety–Schmidt technique, xenon-133 washout is monitored by external gamma scintillation counters and subjected to "curve stripping" to remove any component of extracranial blood flow (17). This technique is most accurate in the middle cerebral distribution and least helpful in evaluating the posterior cerebral or cerebellar circulations.

The recent introduction of positron emission tomography allows repeated imaging of radionuclide concentration in any transverse section of the brain (18). Depending on the labeled element, regional blood flow $H_2^{15}O$ or substrate use (C^{11}-glucose) can be measured (19). Although this technology was once only regarded as a research tool, now it provides the most precise metabolic and flow data available in a wide range of clinical settings.

Flow Regulatory Mechanisms

Pressure-flow autoregulation is the ability of an organ to maintain normal blood flow despite variations in blood pressure. This protective mechanism is well documented in the cerebral circulation. Most physiologists agree that the process is an intrinsic property of blood vessels, involving a continuous readjustment of the myogenic activity of vascular smooth muscle, which depends on changes in transmural pressure and the local (extracellular) chemical environment. Increased intravascular pressure (hypertension) predictably results in compensatory vasoconstriction, whereas decreased pressure (hypotension) elicits vasodilation (20). Although early experiments suggested that pCO_2 was the primary chemical regulator of vascular tone, it has become well accepted that the hydrogen ion concentration in the extracellular space provides the vasodilatory influence (21,22).

Decreasing pCO_2 results in lower hydrogen ion concentration and vasoconstriction. An elevated pCO_2 leads to higher hydrogen ion concentration and vasodilation. This relationship is applied clinically in the management of severe head injuries; hyperventilation with resultant hypocarbia and decreased hydrogen ion concentration decreases cerebral blood flow and attenuates posttraumatic cerebral edema. Responses to changes in pCO_2 are less vigorous, although hypoxia does result in moderate cerebral vasodilation.

Sympathetic stimulation and other neural stimuli have only a small influence on cerebrovascular resistance and blood flow autoregulation (23). In fact, there is minimal histologic evidence of adrenergic vasoconstrictive fibers on cortical vessels (18). Neurally mediated vasoconstriction is limited to large vessels outside the brain proper and, as such, does not represent a primary regulatory mechanism (24).

CLINICAL PRESENTATION OF CEREBROVASCULAR DISEASE

Definitions

For purposes of discussion, clinicians have grouped neurologic deficits into four categories. *TIA* are classically defined as short-lived, often repetitive alterations of mentation, vision, motor, or sensory function that are completely reversed within 24 hours. Although TIA often involve the middle cerebral artery distribution and present with contralateral arm, leg, and facial weakness, perhaps the most well-recognized episodes involve transient monocular blindness (*amaurosis fugax* or "fleeting blindness"). TIA that last only a few minutes may be prognostically different from those deficits that persist for longer than two hours. For this reason, longer-lasting episodes (2–72 hours) that still result in no permanent neurologic deficit or radiologic evidence of brain infarction are usually designated *reversible ischemic neurologic deficits*.

A documented cerebral infarction (*stroke* or *cerebrovascular accident*) implies a permanent neurologic deficit that is usually associated with computed tomography scan evidence. Neurologic recovery is quite variable and may be complete, but the time course of recovery (weeks or months) clearly distinguishes infarcts from TIA or reversible ischemic neurologic deficits. A "stuttering stroke" in which the neurologic deficit "waxes and wanes" has been termed *stroke-in-evolution*. This type of presentation is not as common but has received much recent attention because of the potential that therapeutic maneuvers could improve the eventual outcome (25,26).

Although the above definitions have aided communication, they can be criticized for arbitrarily grouping diverse mechanisms with quite variable prognoses. For example, TIA can be caused by migraines, seizure disorders, and intracranial aneurysms, as well as carotid artery lesions. This "lumping" phenomenon is most confusing when large multicenter studies attempt to characterize the natural history of a clinical presentation without rigorous preselection on the basis of cause.

Mechanisms

Symptoms of cerebrovascular disease reflect both the mechanism of ischemia and the specific areas affected. In general, ischemia and infarction result from either *low flow* in large- or medium-sized vessels associated with obstructive lesions or hypotension, or *emboli* in smaller vessels from proximal ulcerative lesions or turbulent flow. Hemodynamic derangements predisposing to the low flow are manifest clinically by neurologic deficits corresponding to the "watershed areas" between the main cerebral artery perfusion territories.

Symptoms of embolic occlusion depend on the site of distal impaction. Predictably, the size of the embolus determines the vessel it will occlude. Both mechanisms can result in permanent and reversible deficits (27). In particular, repetitive short-lived neurologic deficits (i.e., TIA) are compatible with either (i) recurrent ischemia of watershed areas, or (ii) impaction and lysis of intermittent platelet emboli following a consistent route mandated by hemodynamics and anatomy.

Arterial Pathology

The most common disease process involving the cerebral and extracranial vessels is atherosclerosis (28). Although the disease is most prevalent in patients over the age of 50, presentations of younger patients are not rare. In roughly half of the cases, the atheroma is localized to the extracranial bifurcation of the common carotid into the internal and external carotid arteries. Such atherosclerotic plaques may slowly encroach on the arterial lumen or suddenly occlude following intraplaque hemorrhage (29).

Other pathologic processes are less common and may more frequently involve younger patients. These include spontaneous subintimal dissections of the internal carotid and fibromuscular dysplasia.

Although it is generally accepted that the majority of emboli arise from ulcerated atherosclerotic lesions in the common or internal carotid artery, the intracranial carotid siphon near the origin of the ophthalmic artery can also harbor symptomatic ulcerative lesions. Stenoses and occlusions can involve either the extracranial or the intracranial carotid arteries, both areas simultaneously (tandem lesions), or any portion of a specific cerebral artery (30,31).

The mechanisms that underlie plaque instability may involve *biologic factors* that are intrinsic to plaque structure and *biomechanical factors* that induce structural breakdown or specific cellular responses. Ongoing histopathologic studies at the University of Chicago have found that large symptomatic and asymptomatic plaques, often highly stenotic, possess remarkably similar histopathologic features with regard to the presence of necrosis, calcification, fibrous-cap ulceration, hemorrhage, and surface thrombosis (32,33). Although intraplaque hemorrhage, hematoma, and surface thrombosis have been regarded by other investigators as cardinal features of symptomatic plaques, such a finding was not substantiated in these studies. It was consistently observed, however, that proximity of the necrotic core to the overlying fibrous cap and lumen was associated with embolic symptoms. In symptomatic plaques, the necrotic core was twice as close to the lumen when compared with asymptomatic plaques, whereas the degree or location of calcification had little effect. Symptomatic plaques also exhibited a greater degree of macrophage infiltration in and about the fibrous cap and were associated with fibrous-cap thinning and erosion. This implicated an ongoing inflammatory or immune-mediated response as a factor in plaque instability.

The potential role of biomechanical forces in inducing structural fatigue of plaque constituents and the localization of plaque neoformation and inflammatory cell response is also of interest. Marked elevation of wall shear stress occurs within stenoses that are associated with large plaques. Although high shear may inhibit plaque formation (34), changes in flow dynamics associated with marked stenoses, including wall vibration, flutter, and cyclical collapse (35), could induce disruptions within plaques, lumen ulcer formation, and associated surface irregularities.

TYPES OF CEREBROVASCULAR DISEASE

Extracranial Carotid Artery Disease

Clinical Presentation

The symptoms of extracranial carotid disease can be described by the timing of impairment (permanent, transient, or relapsing) and the type of neurologic deficit (motor, sensory, cognitive, or communicative). As discussed earlier in this chapter, both decreases in cerebral blood flow and embolic occlusions can produce the entire clinical spectrum. The persistence of any neurologic deficit is synonymous with death of brain tissue. Transient and relapsing episodes unassociated with infarctions are distinguished by the return of the neurologic examination to normal.

The exact nature of a deficit can be directly correlated with the area of brain rendered ischemic. The most commonly involved area is the perfusion territory of the middle cerebral artery (the parietal lobe), which is the main outflow vessel of the carotid artery. The patient with middle cerebral ischemia presents with contralateral hemiparesis or hemiplegia, usually more severe in the arm, and paralysis of the contralateral lower part of the face ("central seventh nerve paralysis"). Associated findings include some degree of hypesthesia (decreased sensation) on the paralyzed side and a contralateral homonymous hemianopsia (visual-field deficit). Aphasia (difficulty with speech) is noted if the dominant hemisphere is involved. The left hemisphere is dominant in nearly all right-handed people and roughly 50% of left-handed people. Such defects can be expressive (Broca's aphasia), receptive (Wernicke's aphasia), or complete. If the nondominant hemisphere is affected, a curious "neglect response" is noted in which the paralyzed extremity is essentially ignored by the patient.

Ischemia of the anterior cerebral artery most commonly presents with contralateral monoplegia involving only the lower extremity; visual–spatial problems and cortical sensory loss are also common.

Posterior cerebral artery ischemia may result from carotid occlusive disease, but is also closely related to vertebral–basilar lesions. Presentations often include visual-field defects and may overlap with symptoms of ischemia of the posterior portion of the middle cerebral distribution, such as language disturbances and contralateral hemiparesis. Other neurologic signs consistent with posterior cerebral artery ischemia include ipsilateral third–cranial nerve palsy and contralateral complete sensory loss (thalamic syndrome).

Diagnosis

Symptomatic carotid artery disease is commonly associated with the above neurologic presentations. However, it is essential to exclude other causes for such syndromes, including migraines, brain tumors, intracranial hemorrhage, and vascular malformations.

The physical finding most consistent with extracranial carotid disease is a demonstration of a *bruit* on auscultation of the upper cervical region, reflecting turbulent blood flow at a stenosis. Classic carotid bruits have the following characteristics: they are (i) high pitched and fade into diastole, (ii) localized to the angle of the jaw, and (iii) best heard with the bell rather than the diaphragm of the stethoscope. Unfortunately, even experienced examiners frequently cannot distinguish internal or common carotid bruits from clinically irrelevant turbulence in the distal external carotid artery or other cervical blood vessels. As many as 50% of symptomatic ulcerations may be unassociated with stenoses and hence may not present with bruits. Finally, when a stenosis exceeds 90% of vascular cross-sectional area, the intensity of the bruit often decreases because of lower volume flow. This lack of specificity of cervical bruits is most disturbing in asymptomatic patients with bruits, because physical examination alone does not allow assessment of the degree, or even the presence, of carotid disease.

Many noninvasive tests have been developed to better characterize extracranial carotid disease without the risk of angiographic procedures. They are most widely used in asymptomatic patients with cervical bruits and in the long-term follow-up of patients already treated with carotid endarterectomy.

Imaging Techniques

Direct noninvasive tests using ultrasound techniques to visualize the extracranial vessels have largely replaced the indirect methods previously used to detect and quantitate disease (e.g., oculoplethysmography). When combined with sophisticated range-gated pulsed Doppler instruments (duplex scanning), the velocity and volume flow can be determined (1). The resolution of duplex scanning has improved recently such that ulcerative nonstenotic lesions can be detected in most patients.

Arteriography for cerebrovascular disease commonly includes imaging of the aortic arch and selective injections of the common carotid arteries, with delineation of the carotid siphon and intracranial vessels (Figs. 3 and 4). The common carotid artery and its bifurcation are readily visualized along with any associated stenoses or ulcerated plaques. Perhaps the most significant advantage of cerebral arteriograms is their ability to demonstrate intracranial lesions and aortic arch disease. Relevant intracranial lesions include tumors, aneurysms, arteriovenous malformations, and arterial occlusive disease, particularly of the carotid siphon. Indeed, ulcerative or occlusive lesions of the aortic arch or intracranial vessels may produce symptoms identical to those associated with carotid artery disease such as TIA or amaurosis fugax. When associated with carotid bifurcation disease, such proximal or distal occlusive lesions are termed "tandem" lesions.

Due to its invasive nature, contrast angiography has associated morbidity and mortality (36). These adverse reactions can be grouped into three major categories: local, systemic, and neurologic. Local complication rates (ranging from 5% to 15%) include hemorrhage, hematomas, pseudoaneurysms, and formation of thrombi or emboli at the arterial puncture site.

Systemic complications include allergic reactions to the contrast agent, as well as renal and cardiovascular manifestations. While the incidence of serious allergic reactions to radiographic contrast agents is less than 2% in most reported series, in patients with a history of contrast allergy, the incidence of anaphylactic reactions may be as high as 20% (37). Allergic reactions range from minor sequelae such as nausea, vomiting, hives, and chills, to major life-threatening reactions such as hypotension, bronchospasm, laryngospasm, and pulmonary edema. Radiographic contrast agents can also produce a deterioration in renal function, especially in patients with preexisting kidney disease. One series reported that nonazotemic patients experienced a 2% incidence of acute renal failure following all types of angiography, while patients with chronic azotemia suffered a 33% incidence (38). However, the same study revealed that the occurrence of acute renal failure was less in patients undergoing carotid–vertebral studies than in patients undergoing visceral angiograms with more direct delivery of dye to the kidneys. Cardiac complications of cerebral

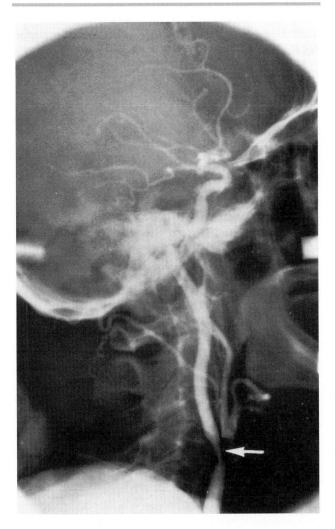

Figure 3 Preoperative angiogram of patient presenting with repeated episodes of contralateral hemiparesis demonstrates severe stenosis of both internal (*arrow*) and external carotid arteries.

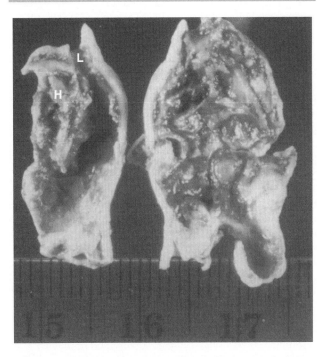

Figure 4 Operative specimen (bivalved) reveals narrow lumen (*L*) with fresh hemorrhage (*H*) within atherosclerotic plaque. Extensive ulcerations are noted.

angiography include hypotension, arrhythmias, myocardial ischemia or infarction, and even cardiac arrest.

Neurologic complications are the most important risk of cerebral angiography (39). Events range from TIA (lasting less than 24 hours) to completed strokes. Hankey et al. reviewed eight prospective studies consisting of 2227 patients with mild ischemic cerebrovascular disease (40). A 4% incidence of postangiographic neurologic complications was observed, of which 1% were permanent. As would be expected, the incidence was higher in patients with active symptoms or bilateral severe carotid artery stenoses.

Magnetic resonance arteriography (MRA) is another noninvasive method of imaging the extracranial carotid arteries. It has an advantage over conventional angiography in that there is no risk of stroke, arterial injury, or systemic complications such as contrast reactions. Rigorous correlation between magnetic resonance angiography and carotid endarterectomy specimens has yet to be reported. In our early experience with this technique, the degree of stenosis is often factitiously overestimated. Even modest degrees of turbulence at the carotid bifurcation or siphon (such as 50% stenoses) may appear to be critical lesions.

Operative Indications

The indications for carotid endarterectomy are constantly being reevaluated and redefined. In a recent multicenter randomized trial, it has been shown that carotid endarterectomy will significantly decrease the risk of stroke in symptomatic patients with carotid stenoses of 70% to 99% of diameter (41). Symptoms referable to carotid stenosis included hemispheric TIA with resultant loss of motor and/or sensory function on one side of the body, monocular ipsilateral blindness (amaurosis fugax), or a nondisabling stroke. In this study, there was a reduction in risk of major or fatal stroke from 13.1% in the medical therapy group to 2.5% in the surgical group over two years.

The timing of carotid endarterectomy after a completed stroke due to an ipsilateral carotid lesion is somewhat controversial. Most would agree that endarterectomy should be considered unless the patient has sustained a severely disabling stroke such that there is minimal salvageable function in the affected carotid artery distribution. The procedure should be delayed until the patient's neurologic status has stabilized, usually three to six weeks after the stroke (42). The risk of recurrent stroke after carotid endarterectomy is approximately 1.6% per year (15% at nine years), as compared to a recurrent stroke rate of 50% at five years in those patients not undergoing carotid endarterectomy (9). Nevertheless, many surgeons will not operate if severe intracranial disease or cardiac risk factors would decrease the effectiveness or increase the morbidity of the procedure.

The prognosis of asymptomatic patients with highly stenotic carotid lesions remains difficult to characterize (25,43). Long-term follow-up of patients with persistent disease of the contralateral carotid artery following unilateral carotid endarterectomy documents a 20% incidence of cerebrovascular symptoms; the incidence of stroke without antecedent TIA is approximately 3% to 5% (44). The recent Veterans Affairs Cooperative Study found a benefit for endarterectomy if the stenosis was greater than 50%, but the endpoints included all neurologic events, not just stroke (45). Because experienced surgeons document a perioperative stroke rate of less than 2%, operative intervention may be appropriate in asymptomatic patients with limited anesthetic risk factors and those undergoing major surgical procedures that may predispose to hypotension (36).

Nonoperative Treatment

The most significant risk factor for stroke is hypertension. Hence, the control of hypertension is most important in the medical management of patients with cerebrovascular disease (46). Evaluation of serum lipoproteins will likely assume a greater role in the prevention and retardation of atherosclerosis as dietary and drug therapies for specific abnormalities become more clear.

Direct medical therapy for cerebrovascular disease has focused on anticoagulation (heparin and warfarin) and antiplatelet drugs (aspirin, dipyridamole, and sulfinpyrazone) (47,48). Mechanisms of action differ considerably, but the common rationale includes prevention of sudden thrombosis of stenotic lesions and inhibition of platelet activation on ulcerative lesions. Although many studies have suggested a benefit of long-term anticoagulation, the methodologies of these investigations have been seriously questioned, especially regarding their lack of randomization and precise patient selection. Furthermore, the statistically significant reduction in stroke rate (from 19% to 12% in one series) does not compare to better results achieved by carotid endarterectomy (49,50).

Many clinicians believe that antiplatelet agents are most appropriate in patients with minimal ulcerative non-stenotic lesions and only one episode or one closely spaced series of TIA (7). If symptoms recur in such patients, endarterectomy remains an option. Other candidates for anticoagulation include patients with very high operative risk or those with severe associated intracranial disease.

Operative Techniques and Results

Carotid endarterectomy is the surgical procedure of choice for disease of the common carotid artery or the extracranial portion of the internal carotid artery (51). The procedure can be performed under general or local anesthesia. Patients at greatest risk for a perioperative ischemic stroke include patients with previous infarcts, those with contralateral carotid occlusions, and those with unstable neurologic deficits (52). Some surgeons routinely use an indwelling vascular shunt to maintain carotid cerebral perfusion during endarterectomy, whereas others use shunts selectively or not at all. Intraoperative monitoring of electroencephalograms or retrograde carotid perfusion pressure ("stump pressure") has been used to assess the need for shunt placement. Because it is likely that embolic events account for the majority of perioperative strokes, precise dissection technique is crucial in patients with thrombotic or ulcerative plaques (53).

Exposure of the vessels must be carried out in an unhurried and gentle manner, mindful of surrounding cranial nerves, especially the vagus, hypoglossal, superior laryngeal, and glossopharyngeal nerves. We administer heparin and clamp the distal internal carotid prior to any manipulation of the bifurcation. Only then is the lateral carotid bulb sharply dissected free and rotated anteromedially. The arteriotomy is made in this lateral aspect and usually extended past the distal edge of the plaque. Unhindered visualization of the end point is essential. It is also important that the proximal extent of the endarterectomy achieves a suitable nondiseased segment of the vessel. If there is any question of the distal "feather" of the endarterectomy, fine tacking sutures are placed; such sutures should not be tied too tightly or puckering of the luminal surface may result. It has also been our practice to tack the edges of the proximal end point if a thickened intimal layer has separated from the medial layer. Intraoperatively, Doppler signals are evaluated in both the internal and the external carotid arteries. Completion duplex ultrasonography or arteriography is not used routinely; however, both are employed if deemed necessary.

Recently we have applied more liberal indications for placement of prosthetic or vein patch (extensive arteriotomy into the internal carotid artery, vessels smaller than 3 mm, female sex, or active smoking). For example, patching was performed in about 10% of our patients during 1981 through 1987, and nearly half of patients in the more recent period. The type of patch does not seem to strongly influence early or late outcomes, but care must be taken to avoid excessively enlarging the artery and altering flow dynamics.

The incidence of perioperative stroke varies with operative indication. Most large series report stroke rates of 1% to 2% in patients with TIA and 3% to 5% in patients with previous strokes or contralateral carotid occlusion (54). Other postoperative complications include cranial nerve injury (especially the hypoglossal and recurrent laryngeal nerves) and myocardial infarction. Because the carotid sinus regulates blood pressure homeostasis, postoperative hypotension or hypertension is noted in many patients during the 24 hours required for baroreceptor reacclimation (55).

Death following carotid endarterectomy is infrequent and is more commonly due to myocardial infarction than stroke. In our series of 367 consecutive carotid endarterectomies, two of the three deaths were attributable to acute myocardial infarction, while none of the four patients suffering perioperative neurologic deficits died (56). This experience is not unique. In 1981, Lees and Hertzer (57) reported a total of 10 postoperative deaths in 335 patients, many of whom underwent other major surgical procedures during the same hospitalization. Myocardial infarction was the cause of 6 of the 10 deaths, and only two deaths were due to stroke. In the multicenter Asymptomatic Carotid Atherosclerosis Study (58), only one patient in the 825-patient surgical group died following surgery; the cause of death was myocardial infarction. In the North American Symptomatic Carotid Endarterectomy Trial report (41) in 1991, of the 328 patients undergoing surgical treatment of severe carotid stenoses, two deaths were noted (0.7%), one from stroke and one from myocardial infarction or arrhythmia. In the multicenter Veterans Medical Centers study of asymptomatic stenoses described by Hobson et al. (45), all four surgical deaths (1.9%) resulted from myocardial infarction.

The occurrence of myocardial ischemia and infarction has been linked to hypertension. Riles et al. (59) specifically linked the overzealous use of α-adrenergic agents to increase carotid artery "stump" pressure intraoperatively with both myocardial ischemia and infarction. In their view, the incidence of myocardial infarction was 4.9% in 284 patients with hypertension as compared with zero in 207 normotensive patients. The well-described fluctuations in systemic blood pressure in the postoperative period (including hypertension and hypotension) also contribute to cardiac morbidity (55,60). The risk for myocardial complications and death appears to increase slightly with age. Meyer et al. (61) reported an overall mortality of 1.3% in 749 carotid endarterectomies performed on patients 70 years of age or older, between 1971 and 1989; 6 of 10 deaths were due to myocardial infarction. A more recent series of 63 endarterectomies in patients 75 years or older, from Perler and Williams (62), included five major cardiac complications but no deaths.

It has been well accepted that the indications for surgery and the neurologic status strongly influence outcome. For example, in a large series of more than 1700 carotid endarterectomies, Thompson (63) reported an operative mortality rate of 3.4% for patients with previous stroke, 1.1% for patients with TIA, and 0% for asymptomatic patients. Taken as a whole, it seems clear that mortality reflects cardiac status and management, while neurologic morbidity reflects patient selection and technical aspects of the operation.

Recurrent stenoses occur in approximately 8% to 10% of patients, if followed closely, although the incidence of symptomatic recurrence is much lower (3%). Restenosis within 24 months usually represents exuberant intimal regeneration, whereas later presentations reflect recurrent atherosclerosis (64).

Carotid Angioplasty and Stenting

The recent and remarkable improvements in interventional devices and skills offer nonsurgical options for treatment of carotid and vertebral lesions. The advantages of angioplasty and stenting include extending the definitive treatment of carotid lesions to higher-risk patients as well as those with special considerations mitigating against operative repair. This population would include patients with previous endarterectomies, in whom cranial nerve injury might be a concern, and patients with cervical radiation (65,66).

Initial experience in angioplasty and stenting was limited to patients with severe comorbidities, which precluded safe operative repair (67). Technical success was observed in more than 95% of patients treated in a number of recognized centers, although the incidence of neurologic complications exceeded the best operative endarterectomy series (68). Increasing experience in endovascular techniques and the introduction of various types of "cerebral protection devices" (which filter or trap atheroembolic debris downstream from the dilated lesion) have both contributed to lower complication rates in the current literature (69). More widespread use of this endovascular approach is occurring, although the proper assessments of the safety and durability of these procedures await the completion of a number of ongoing randomized clinical trials.

Vertebrobasilar Disease

Clinical Presentation

As noted earlier, the paired vertebral vessels join to form the basilar artery. For this reason, proximal occlusion or ligation of only one vertebral vessel will not cause symptoms unless the contralateral vessel is diseased or hypoplastic. More distal disease of one vertebral vessel with occlusion of the small branches supplying the lateral medulla can result in neurologic deficits.

The most frequent symptoms of basilar insufficiency include nausea, vertigo, ipsilateral facial numbness, ipsilateral Horner's syndrome, and limb ataxia (70). Although ischemic symptoms are generally mild, true posterior fossa infarction can be progressive and lethal, as a result of extensive edema and midbrain compression. Emboli can contribute to posterior cerebral and cerebellar ischemia, but occlusive disease of the vertebral arteries or the basilar artery is the most common mechanism. The thrombotic process may involve the basilar artery proper or the basilar branch vessels that penetrate into the brain stem (49).

A classic syndrome of vertebrobasilar insufficiency (subclavian steal syndrome) is associated with subclavian or innominate arterial occlusive disease (71). The subclavian origins of the vertebral arteries allow the vessels to function as collaterals for the upper extremity. During arm exercise, flow is reversed in the vertebral artery, and basilar arterial blood flow and perfusion pressure are decreased. Symptoms of posterior cerebral and cerebellar ischemia can result, especially if any flow-limiting carotid lesions are present. The anatomic relationship favors left-sided involvement, approximately in the ratio of 4:1 (72).

The diagnosis of subclavian steal syndrome is supported by complaints of intermittent vertigo, lightheadedness, and nausea and vomiting intensified by arm exercise. Physical findings include supraclavicular bruits and 40- to 60-mmHg blood pressure discrepancies between the arms.

Diagnosis

Measuring blood pressure in both upper extremities is essential in any patient with cerebral symptoms. More sophisticated tests include B-mode imaging of the subclavian and vertebral vessels and the use of directional dopplers to document reversal of vertebral-artery blood flow.

The primary diagnostic test remains arteriography (70). It is important to obtain delayed films to adequately demonstrate retrograde flow through the vertebral into the distal subclavian (Figs. 5 and 6). The origin of the contralateral vertebral artery and the status of the basilar artery should also be evaluated with oblique films if necessary. The incidental demonstration of subclavian steal during arteriography for some other reasons is, in itself, not cause for concern or surgical therapy.

Operative Indications and Techniques

Symptomatic patients with multiple vertebral occlusive lesions or subclavian steal syndrome should be considered for elective surgery. Procedures include endarterectomy of the proximal vertebral artery or carotid subclavian bypass to restore antegrade vertebral flow (73). The latter can be accomplished by bypass graft or division of the cervical subclavian artery with reimplantation into the common carotid artery. These procedures can be performed through a cervical incision (Figs. 7 and 8).

In patients with associated carotid artery disease, carotid endarterectomy alone may relieve symptoms of vertebrobasilar insufficieny, by increasing collateral flow to the posterior cerebral artery and cerebellum (28). This is most appropriate in symptomatic patients with severe carotid stenoses and those with more distal vertebral or basilar occlusion.

Results and Complications

Patency of vertebral endarterectomies and carotid subclavian bypass grafts exceeds 90%. In most cases, symptoms are completely relieved by successful bypass. Failure to

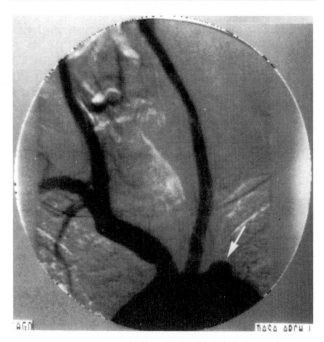

Figure 5   Preoperative angiogram in patient presenting with stroke in basilar distribution (superior cerebellar) demonstrates complete occlusion of left subclavian artery (*arrow*).

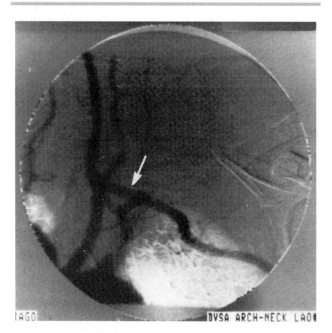

Figure 7   Postoperative intravenous digital angiogram demonstrates patent carotid–subclavian bypass (*arrow*) with return of cephalad flow in left vertebral artery.

achieve symptomatic improvement may be caused by continued carotid disease or intracranial lesions (75).

Perioperative complications include injuries to the phrenic nerve, cervical sympathetic ganglia (with Horner's

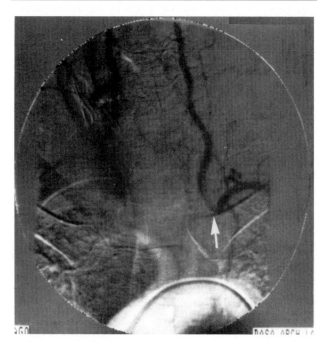

Figure 6   Delayed films document reversed flow in large left vertebral artery (*arrow*) with reconstitution of distal subclavian artery (subclavian steal syndrome).

syndrome), or the thoracic duct. Basilar territory infarction after carotid subclavian bypass is very rare; even early graft failure should not further compromise vertebral flow.

UPPER-EXTREMITY VASCULAR DISEASE

Symptomatic arterial insufficiency of the upper extremity is relatively uncommon, accounting for approximately 2% of all peripheral vascular reconstructive procedures. Although atherosclerosis is the predominant cause of arterial ischemia of the upper extremity, there are other etiologies including extrinsic compression, vasospasm, arteritis, connective tissue disorders, trauma, Buerger's disease, previous radiation therapy, and occupational injury.

Nonatherosclerotic Disease

Extrinsic compression of the subclavian artery usually occurs at the thoracic outlet and may result in distal extremity ischemia or emboli. While impingement on the subclavian artery is commonly positional and temporary, long-standing external compression can lead to fibrosis and permanent arterial stenoses. If arteriography with positional maneuvers confirms a persistent and significant stenotic or ulcerative lesion, simple excision of the local soft tissue, primarily the medial scalene muscle and first rib, will not be sufficient treatment. Exclusion and bypass of the involved portion of the subclavian artery should be performed.

In some patients, upper-extremity arterioles are exceptionally sensitive to sympathetic stimuli, resulting in *vasospasm* with intermittent ischemia and even gangrene. Vasospasm of the hands presents with a characteristic progression of color changes in the fingers: digits first become pallorous, secondary to decreases in the flow of oxygenated blood, then cyanotic, and finally ruborous as the vasospasm decreases and reperfusion occurs. This clinical syndrome is

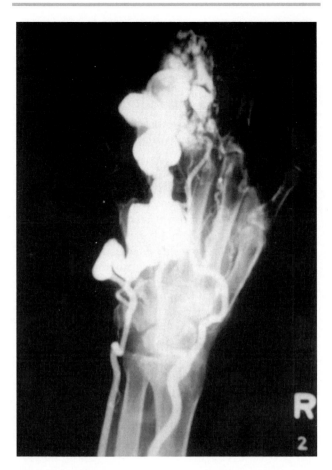

Figure 8 Aneurysms of palmar vessels secondary to repetitive hand trauma in a meat packer.

termed "Raynaud's phenomenon," after the French physician who first described it. Patients with Raynaud's phenomenon should be screened for collagen-vascular diseases such as lupus erythematosis, rheumatoid arthritis, and scleroderma. In approximately 50% of patients with manifestations of severe digital ischemia, the phenomenon predates or is associated with these disorders.

The most critical therapy of Raynaud's phenomenon is avoidance of the cold, wind, and moisture, which classically trigger each episode; in some patients, stress also is a major factor. Vasoactive drugs including sympatholytics, which reduce the uptake and subsequent release of local norepinephrine, and calcium-channel blocking agents can be helpful. Finally, cervical dorsal sympathectomy can be employed if tissue loss is threatened or if symptoms are intolerable; unfortunately, the benefits of this procedure are not uniform or particularly durable.

Two other causes for digital ischemia are *vibratory injury* to the palmar and digital vessels and *Buerger's disease.* Vibratory injury results from repetitive blunt trauma to the hands, which are associated with certain occupations (construction work, especially with jack-hammers, meat packing, etc.) (76). The cumulative force of the injuries results in medium-vessel occlusions as well as true aneurysms due to medial and adventitial necrosis (Fig. 9). Patients may present with distal ulcers from ischemia and embolization. If aneurysms are demonstrated, direct microvascular

repair is indicated to prevent enlargement and continued embolization.

Buerger's disease is a progressive medium- and small-vessel obliterative disease associated with nicotine abuse. Patients present with distal ischemia of both upper and lower extremities; recurrent venous thrombophlebitis is a frequent comorbidity. Local treatments of ischemic lesions and sympathectomy may be successful, but *only* if smoking cessation is *complete.* Unfortunately, this goal is almost never attained at this level of addiction to smoking.

Takayasu's Disease is an example of an inflammatory large vessel arteritis resulting in fibrosis and scarring of the aorta and its primary branches. Symptoms start as fever, myalgias, and anorexia, but then progress to upper-extremity arterial insufficiency (77). The progression of arterial stenosis leads to the loss of the upper-extremity pulses, hence the name "pulseless disease." Takayasu's disease primarily affects people of Asian descent, with a strong predominance for females (8:1) less than 40 years of age. The etiology is still uncertain, although infection and autoimmune processes have been implicated; the disease is associated with rheumatoid arthritis, ankylosing spondylitis, and ulcerative colitis. Laboratory evaluation may reflect a generalized inflammatory process with an elevation of the erythrocyte sedimentation rate and a mild hypochromic anemia.

Takayasu's arteritis can be divided into four types based on the distribution of lesions (77,78). Type I is limited to the aortic arch and its primary branches, Type II includes lesions of the descending thoracic and abdominal aorta, Type III extends from the aortic valve to the abdominal aorta, and Type IV includes pulmonary artery involvement and/or associated aneurysms (77,78).

The majority of patients present during the "pulseless" stage, and symptoms reflect the organ or extremity that is rendered ischemic. Complaints can include headache, light-headedness, hemiparesis, blurring of vision, diplopia, and blindness. The classic ocular findings include optic atrophy and retinal vein or artery thrombosis (79). Extremity symptoms can be limited to exercise-related complaints or progress to rest pain and tissue loss.

Initial therapy, especially in the prepulseless stage, is centered upon the administration of corticosteroids. If a patient with symptomatic lesions has failed corticosteroid therapy, operative therapy is directed toward bypass of the involved or occluded vessels (80). If at all possible, operative intervention should be delayed until the acute phase of the disease has resolved. This may not be possible in patients presenting with active cerebrovascular symptoms. Endarterectomy has not proven effective, due to the transmural inflammatory response and the tendency toward aneurysmal degeneration. Bypass grafts are the preferred treatment and should originate and terminate in arteries known to be free of disease by both angiography and inspection (81); often, grafts must originate from the ascending aorta. Distal anastomotic stenoses occur in 20% to 30% of cases and may require reoperation.

Atherosclerotic Upper-Extremity Arterial Disease
Clinical Presentation
Atherosclerosis of the subclavian or innominate arteries is the most common cause of upper-extremity ischemia; symptoms may be due to low flow or emboli. Lesions involving the *innominate artery* can result in thrombotic atherosclerotic emboli to either the right vertebral artery or the right

(A)

(B)

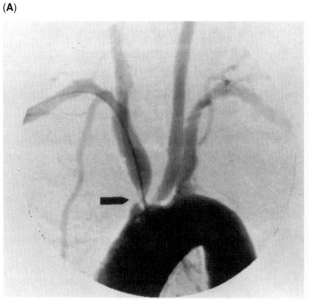

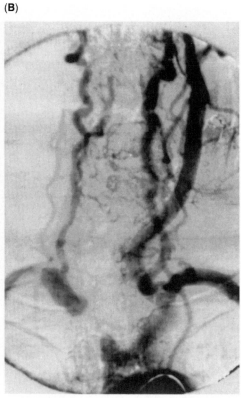

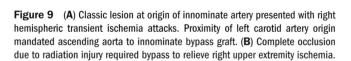

Figure 9 (A) Classic lesion at origin of innominate artery presented with right hemispheric transient ischemia attacks. Proximity of left carotid artery origin mandated ascending aorta to innominate bypass graft. (B) Complete occlusion due to radiation injury required bypass to relieve right upper extremity ischemia.

common carotid artery, with resulting TIA or strokes (Fig. 10). Emboli to the left cerebral hemisphere can also originate from the innominate artery lesions, due to the proximity of the origin of the left common carotid artery to the innominate artery. In one large series, 77% of the patients with symptomatic innominate artery lesions presented with neurologic symptoms, not upper-extremity problems (82).

Stenosis or occlusion of the *subclavian artery* occurs three to four times more commonly on the left than the right subclavian artery. As noted earlier, a proximal subclavian artery occlusion or stenosis can result in reversal of flow in the left vertebral artery. The clinical presentation of unilateral upper-extremity weakness or coolness, vertigo with upper-extremity exercise (subclavian "steal" syndrome), or ischemic lesions of the hand should raise a suspicion of subclavian artery stenosis or occlusion. The diagnosis is suspected by comparing upper-extremity arterial pressures, and is confirmed by arteriography. Arteriograms will not only define the extent of disease of the subclavian artery, but will also evaluate the thoracic aorta, carotid arteries, and the vertebral arteries.

Treatment

Symptomatic patients should be considered for arterial revascularization (83). Innominate lesions are usually approached directly through a median sternotomy (Fig. 11) (74). Both endarterectomy and bypass from the aortic arch are durable procedures. The selection of the specific procedure is based on the nature of the lesion and the location of origin of the left carotid artery. If it originates close to the innominate, clamping of the latter vessel for endarterectomy is inadvisable and bypass is preferred (82).

Bypass procedures for subclavian disease include transposition of the subclavian artery to the adjacent non-diseased carotid artery or carotid artery to subclavian artery bypass with a prosthetic graft (Fig. 8) (74). Transposition entails the complete mobilization of the subclavian artery proximal to the origin of the vertebral artery. The subclavian artery is divided and the proximal arterial stump oversewn. An anastomosis is created between the side of the proximal carotid artery and the end of the subclavian artery. If the subclavian cannot be mobilized enough for a tension-free apposition to the proximal carotid artery, a carotid–subclavian bypass can be performed. In these instances, the preferred bypass graft conduit is a synthetic graft, due to its decreased tendency to kink. Both subclavian artery transposition and carotid–subclavian artery bypass have similar long-term patencies of greater than 95% (84).

Thoracic Outlet Syndrome
Clinical Presentation

Thoracic outlet syndrome is best described as an intermittent but reproducible compression irritation of the brachial plexus caused by congenital fibromuscular bands, cervical ribs, or the anterior scalene muscle (Fig. 12) (85,86). Classic symptoms include shoulder pain with radiation to the occiput and down the arm along the C8 to T1 distribution. Numbness and tingling frequently accompany the pain. In advanced cases, weakness of the hands and forearm may be noted. Although the subclavian artery may also be compressed by the same anatomic configuration, most symptoms of thoracic outlet syndrome relate directly to neurologic rather than vascular compromise.

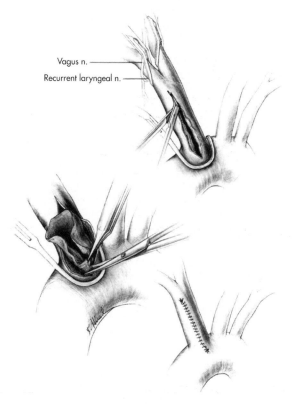

Figure 10 Innominate endarterectomy can be performed if a vascular clamp can be applied proximal to the lesion without also obstructing the left carotid artery origin. *Source*: From Ref. 74.

A history of neck or shoulder trauma can be elicited in many patients, which some clinicians consider to be suggestive of scalene muscle spasm being an initiating event. Whiplash injuries are frequently implicated, but documentation of a

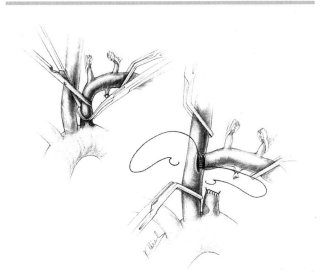

Figure 11 Subclavian reconstructions include both carotid–subclavian bypass and transposition of the distal subclavian into the carotid artery (illustrated here). *Source*: From Ref. 74.

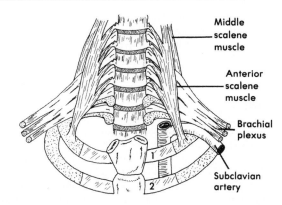

Figure 12 Brachial plexus compression occurs at triangular outlet between scalene muscles and first rib.

cause-and-effect relationship is nearly impossible. The differential diagnosis includes carpal tunnel syndrome, cervical disk compression, arthritis, tendonitis, and angina pectoris.

Diagnosis

The chronicity and lack of specificity of the clinical presentation is paralleled by a lack of definitive diagnostic tests other than chest x-ray film demonstration of an abnormal cervical rib. The Adson maneuver is a positional test long associated with thoracic outlet syndrome. The test is considered positive if the radial pulse disappears during abduction and external rotation of the arm. Unfortunately, the Adson maneuver is frequently positive in asymptomatic patients and negative in patients with classic symptoms of thoracic outlet syndrome, again emphasizing the neurologic as opposed to vascular origin of the pain syndrome. Angiographic demonstration of subclavian artery compression in extreme abduction also does not contribute significantly to the diagnosis unless there is evidence of a persistent blood pressure gradient in the involved arm (5).

Electromyograms and nerve conduction velocities have been suggested as objective measures of thoracic outlet nerve compression. Unfortunately, enthusiasm for these studies has decreased recently because of the difficulty of electrically stimulating nerves proximal to the presumed site of compression and the intermittent nature of the syndrome. Furthermore, clinical correlations between positive nerve conduction studies and symptomatic relief following surgery have not been very convincing.

Operative Indications and Techniques

Initial therapy should include shoulder girdle exercises and avoidance of extreme posturing. If pain remains and symptoms are fully consistent and reproducible, surgical therapy is appropriate. Unfortunately, even experienced surgeons report complete relief in only 80% to 85% of patients.

The most common operation is transcervical or transaxillary resection of the first rib or a cervical rib, if present. In some patients, merely transecting the insertion of the anterior scalene muscle onto the first rib may suffice (87). Although there has been some enthusiasm for concurrent cervical sympathectomy, this is usually unnecessary unless symptoms of posttraumatic sympathetic dystrophy (causalgia) are evident.

Complications

The failure rate from all procedures remains relatively high in thoracic outlet syndrome (88). Complications of surgery include Horner's syndrome, direct injury to the brachial plexus, lymphatic leaks, and pneumothorax.

SUMMARY

Although cerebrovascular disease remains a major cause of morbidity and mortality in our population, improved understanding of the mechanisms and pathologic processes involved has allowed a wider application of preventive medical and surgical therapies. Appropriate selection of noninvasive tests to evaluate asymptomatic patients with signs of extracranial cerebrovascular disease has further characterized the natural history of these disorders. Although specific recommendations for medical or surgical therapy will continually be modified, it is generally accepted that patients with repetitive neurologic deficits (TIA) associated with extracranial atherosclerotic disease benefit significantly from surgical intervention. In patients with upper-extremity ischemia, extensive medical evaluation and careful assessments of the brachial–cephalic arterial system are mandatory.

REFERENCES

1. Lees RS, Kistler JP, Sanders D. Duplex Doppler scanning and spectral bruit analysis for diagnosing carotid stenosis. Circulation 1982; 66(2 Pt 2):I102–I105.
2. Levy RI. Stroke decline: implications and prospects. N Engl J Med 1979; 300(9):490–491.
3. Whisnant JP. Epidemiology of stroke: emphasis on transient cerebral ischemia attacks and hypertension. Stroke 1974; 5(1): 68–70.
4. Wolf PA, Kannel WB, Sorlie P, McNamara P. Asymptomatic carotid bruit and risk of stroke. The Framingham study. JAMA 1981; 245(14):1442–1445.
5. Judy KL, Heymann RL. Vascular complications of thoracic outlet syndrome. Am J Surg 1972; 123(5):521–531.
6. West H, Burton R, Roon AJ, Malone JM, Goldstone J, Moore WS. Comparative risk of operation and expectant management for carotid artery disease. Stroke 1979; 10(2):117–121.
7. Goldner J, Wisnant JP, Taylor WF. Long-term prognosis of transient cerebral ischemic attacks. Stroke 1971; 2(2):160–167.
8. Diaz FG, Ausman JI, de los Reyes RA, et al. Combined reconstruction of the vertebral and carotid artery in one single procedure. Neurosurgery 1983; 12(6):629–635.
9. Mani RL, Eisenberg RL. Complications of catheter cerebral arteriography: analysis of 5,000 procedures. III. Assessment of arteries injected, contrast medium used, duration of procedure, and age of patient. Am J Roentgenol 1978; 131(5):871–874.
10. Dinsdale HB, Robertson DM, Haas RA. Cerebral blood flow in acute hypertension. Arch Neurol 1974; 31(2):80–87.
11. Gregory PC, McGeorge AP, Fitch W, Graham DI, MacKenzie ET, Harper AM. Effects of hemorrhagic hypotension on the cerebral circulation. II. Electrocortical function. Stroke 1979; 10(6): 719–723.
12. Lassen NA, Henriksen L, Paulson O. Regional cerebral blood flow in stroke by 133Xenon inhalation and emission tomography. Stroke 1981; 12(3):284–288.
13. Wechsler RL, Drips PO, Kety SS. Blood flow and oxygen consumption of the human brain during anesthesia produced by thiopental. Anesthesia 1951; 12:308.
14. Abboud FM. Special characteristics of the cerebral circulation. Fed Proc 1981; 40(8):2296–2300.
15. Johansson B, Li CL, Olsson Y, Klatzo I. The effect of acute arterial hypertension on the blood-brain barrier to protein tracers. Acta Neuropathol (Berl) 1970; 16(2):117–124.
16. Busija DW, Heistad DD, Marcus ML. Continuous measurement of cerebral blood flow in anesthetized cats and dogs. Am J Physiol 1981; 241(2):H228–H234.
17. Marcus ML, Bischof CJ, Heistad DD. Comparison of microsphere and Xenon-133 clearance method in measuring skeletal muscle and cerebral blood flow. Circ Res 1981; 48(5):748–761.
18. Raichle ME, Hartman BK, Eichling JO, Sharpe LG. Central noradrenergic regulation of cerebral blood flow and vascular permeability. Proc Natl Acad Sci USA 1975; 72(9):3726–3730.
19. Raichle ME, Welch MJ, Grubb RL Jr, Higgins CS, Ter-Pogossian MM, Larson KB. Measurement of regional substrate utilization rates by emission tomography. Science 1978; 199(4332):986–987.
20. Ekstrom-Jodal B. On the relation between blood pressure and blood flow in the canine brain with particular regard to the mechanism responsible for cerebral blood flow autoregulation. Acta Physiol Scand Suppl 1970; 350:1–61.
21. Borgstrom L, Johannsson H, Siesjo BK. The relationship between arterial po2 and cerebral blood flow in hypoxic hypoxia. Acta Physiol Scand 1975; 93(3):423–432.
22. Greenberg JH, Alavi A, Reivich M, Kuhl D, Uzzell B. Local cerebral blood volume response to carbon dioxide in man. Circ Res 1978; 43(2):324–331.
23. D'Alecy LG, Feigl EO. Sympathetic control of cerebral blood flow in dogs. Circ Res 1972; 31(2):267–283.
24. Heistad DD, Marcus ML. Evidence that neural mechanisms do not have important effects on cerebral blood flow. Circ Res 1978; 42(3):295–302.
25. Humphries AW, Young JR, Santilli PH, Beven EG, deWolfe VG. Unoperated, asymptomatic significant internal carotid artery stenosis: a review of 182 instances. Surgery 1976; 80(6):695–698.
26. Mentzer RM Jr, Finkelmeier BA, Crosby IK, Wellons HA Jr. Emergency carotid endarterectomy for fluctuating neurologic deficits. Surgery 1981; 89(1):60–66.
27. Pessin MS, Hinton RC, Davis KR, et al. Mechanisms of acute carotid stroke. Ann Neurol 1979; 6(3):245–252.
28. Solberg LA, Eggen DA. Localization and sequence of development of atherosclerotic lesions in the carotid and vertebral arteries. Circulation 1971; 43(5):711–724.
29. Javid H, Ostermiller WE Jr, Hengesh JW, Dye WS, Najafi H, Julian OC. Natural history of carotid bifurcation atheroma. Surgery 1970; 67(1):80–86.
30. Craig DR, Meguro K, Watridge C, Robertson JT, Barnett HJ, Fox AJ. Intracranial internal carotid artery stenosis. Stroke 1982; 13(6):825–828.
31. Eisenberg RL, Nemzek WR, Moore WS, Mani RL. Relationship of transient ischemic attacks and angiographically demonstrable lesions of carotid artery. Stroke 1977; 8(4):483–486.
32. Bassiouny HS, Davis H, Massawa N, Gewertz BL, Glagov S, Zarins CK. Critical carotid stenoses: morphologic and chemical similarity between symptomatic and asymptomatic plaques. J Vasc Surg 1989; 9(2):202–212.
33. Bassiouny HS, Sakaguchi Y, Mikucki SA, et al. Juxtalumenal location of plaque necrosis and neoformation in symptomatic carotid stenosis. J Vasc Surg 1997; 26(4):585–594.
34. Zarins CK, Bomberger RA, Glagov S. Local effects of stenoses: increased flow velocity inhibits atherogenesis. Circulation 1981; 64(2 Pt 2):221–227.
35. Cancelli C, Pedley TJ. A separated flow model for collapsible rube oscillations. J Fluid Mech 1985; 157:375–404.
36. Makhoul RG, Moore WS, Colburn MD, Quinones-Baldrich WJ, Vescera CL. Benefit of carotid endarterectomy after prior stroke. J Vasc Surg 1993; 18(4):666–670; discussion 670–671.
37. Witten DM, Hirsch FD, Hartman GW. Acute reactions to urographic contrast medium: incidence, clinical characteristics and relationship to history of hypersensitivity states. Am J Roentgenol Radium Ther Nucl Med 1973; 119(4):832–840.
38. D'Elia JA, Gleason RE, Alday M, et al. Nephrotoxicity from angiographic contrast material. A prospective study. Am J Med 1982; 72(5):719–725.

39. Faught E, Trader SD, Hanna GR. Cerebral complications of angiography for transient ischemia and stroke: prediction of risk. Neurology 1979; 29(1):4–15.

40. Hankey GJ, Warlow CP, Sellar RJ. Cerebral angiographic risk in mild cerebrovascular disease. Stroke 1990; 21(2):209–222.

41. Beneficial effect of carotid endarterectomy in symptomatic patients with high-grade carotid stenosis. North American Symptomatic Carotid Endarterectomy Trial Collaborators. N Engl J Med 1991; 325(7):445–453.

42. Whittemore AD, Mannick JA. Surgical treatment of carotid disease in patients with neurologic deficits. J Vasc Surg 1987; 5(6):910–913.

43. Busuttil RW, Baker JD, Davidson RK, Machleder HI. Carotid artery stenosis—hemodynamic significance and clinical course. JAMA 1981; 245(14):1438–1441.

44. Podore PC, DeWeese JA, May AG, Rob CG. Asymptomatic contralateral carotid artery stenosis: a five-year follow-up study following carotid endarterectomy. Surgery 1980; 88(6): 748–752.

45. Hobson RW II, Weiss DG, Fields WS. The Veterans Affairs Cooperative Study Group. Efficacy of carotid endarterectomy for asymptomatic carotid stenosis. N Engl J Med 1993; 328(4):221–227.

46. Kannel WB, Dawber TR, Sorlie P, Wolf PA. Components of blood pressure and risk of atherothrombotic brain infarction: the Framingham study. Stroke 1976; 7(4):327–331.

47. Brust JC. Transient ischemic attacks: natural history and anti-coagulation. Neurology 1977; 27(8):701–707.

48. Olsson JE, Brechter C, Backlund H, et al. Anticoagulant versus anti-platelet therapy as prophylactic against cerebral infarction in transient ischemic attacks. Stroke 1980; 11(1):4–9.

49. A randomized trial of aspirin and sulfinpyrazone in threatened stroke. The Canadian Cooperative Study Group. N Engl J Med 1978; 299(2):53–59.

50. Fields WS, Lemak NA, Frankowski RF, Hardy RJ. Controlled trial of aspirin in cerebral ischemia. Stroke 1977; 8(3):301–314.

51. Thompson JE, Talkington CM. Carotid surgery for cerebral ischemia. Surg Clin North Am 1979; 59(4):539–553.

52. Goldstone J, Moore WS. A new look at emergency carotid artery operations for the treatment of cerebrovascular insufficiency. Stroke 1978; 9:599.

53. Steed DL, Peitzman AB, Grundy BL, Webster MW. Causes of stroke in carotid endarterectomy. Surgery 1982; 92(4): 634–641.

54. DeWeese JA, Rob CG, Satran R, et al. Results of carotid endarterectomies for transient ischemic attacks-five years later. Ann Surg 1973; 178(3):258–264.

55. Bove EL, Fry WJ, Gross WS, Stanley JC. Hypotension and hypertension as consequences of baroreceptor dysfunction following carotid endarterectomy. Surgery 1979; 85(6):633–637.

56. McKinsey JF, Desai TR, Bassiouny HS, et al. Mechanisms of neurologic deficits and mortality with carotid endarterectomy. Arch Surg 1996; 131(5):526–531; discussion 531–532.

57. Lees CD, Hertzer NR. Postoperative stroke and late neurologic complications after carotid endarterectomy. Arch Surg 1981; 116(12):1561–1568.

58. Executive Committee for the Asymptomatic Carotid Atherosclerosis Study. Endarterectomy for asymptomatic carotid artery stenosis. JAMA 1995; 273(18):1421–1428.

59. Riles TS, Kopelman I, Imparato AM. Myocardial infarction following carotid endarterectomy: a review of 683 operations. Surgery 1979; 85(3):249–252.

60. Towne JB, Bernhard VM. The relationship of postoperative hypertension to complications following carotid endarterectomy. Surgery 1980; 88(4):575–580.

61. Meyer FB, Meissner I, Fode NC, Losasso TJ. Carotid endarterectomy in elderly patients. Mayo Clin Proc 1991; 66(5): 464–469.

62. Perler BA, Williams GM. Carotid endarterectomy in the very elderly: Is it worthwhile? Surgery 1994; 116(3):479–483.

63. Thompson JE. Carotid endarterectomy, 1982—the state of the art. Br J Surg 1983; 70(6):371–376.

64. Cossman D, Callow AD, Stein A, Matsumoto G. Early restenosis after carotid endarterectomy. Arch Surg 1978; 113(3):275–278.

65. Jordan WD Jr, Voellinger DC, Fisher WS, Redden D, McDowell HA. A comparison of carotid angioplasty with stenting versus endarterectomy with regional anesthesia. J Vasc Surg 1998; 28(3):397–402; discussion 402–403.

66. New G, Roubin GS, Iyer SS, et al. Safety, efficacy, and durability of carotid artery stenting for restenosis following carotid endarterectomy: a multicenter study. J Endovasc Ther 2000; 7(5):345–352.

67. Roubin GS, New G, Iyer SS, et al. Immediate and late clinical outcomes of carotid artery stenting in patients with symptomatic and asymptomatic carotid artery stenosis: a 5-year prospective analysis. Circulation 2001; 103(4):532–537.

68. Hertzer NR, Ouriel K. Results of carotid endarterectomy: the gold standard for carotid repair. Semin Vasc Surg 2000; 13(2): 95–102.

69. Al-Mubarak N, Colombo A, Gaines PA, et al. Multicenter evaluation of carotid artery stenting with a filter protection system. J Am Coll Cardiol 2002; 39(5):841–846.

70. Caplan LR, Rosenbaum AE. Role of cerebral angiography in vertebrobasilar occlusive disease. J Neurol Neurosurg Psychiatry 1975; 38(6):601–612.

71. Fisher CM. A new vascular syndrome: "the subclavian steal". N Engl J Med 1961; 265:912.

72. Fields WS, Lemak NA. Joint Study of extracranial arterial occlusion. VII. Subclavian steal—a review of 168 cases. JAMA 1972; 222(9):1139–1143.

73. Clark K, Perry MO. Carotid vertebral anastomosis: an alternate technic for repair of the subclavian steal syndrome. Ann Surg 1966; 163(3):414–416.

74. Zarins CK, Gewertz BL. Atlas of Vascular Surgery. New York: Churchill Livingstone, Inc., 1989.

75. Allen GS, Cohen RJ, Preziosi TJ. Microsurgical endarterectomy of the intracranial vertebral artery for vertebrobasilar transient ischemic attacks. Neurosurgery 1981; 8(1):56–59.

76. Clark ET, Mass DP, Bassiouny HS, Zarins CK, Gewertz BL. True aneurysmal disease in the hand and upper extremity. Ann Vasc Surg 1991; 5(3):276–281.

77. Ishikawa K. Natural history and classification of occlusive thromboaortopathy (Takayasu's disease). Circulation 1978; 57(1):27–35.

78. Lupi E, Sanchez G, Horwitz S, Gutierrez E. Pulmonary artery involvement in Takayasu's arteritis. Chest 1975; 67(1):69–74.

79. Takayasu M. Case with unusual change of the vessels in the retina. Acta Soc Ophthalmol 1908; 12:554.

80. Alpert HJ. The use of immunosuppressive agents in Takayasu's arteritis. Med Ann Dist Columbia 1974; 43(2):69–71.

81. Weaver FA, Yellin AE, Campen DH, et al. Surgical procedures in the management of Takayasu's arteritis. J Vasc Surg 1990; 12(4):429–437; discussion 438–439.

82. Cherry KJ Jr, McCullough JL, Hallett JW Jr, Pairolero PC, Gloviczki P. Technical principles of direct innominate artery revascularization: a comparison of endarterectomy and bypass grafts. J Vasc Surg 1989; 9(5):718–723; discussion 723–724.

83. Whitehouse WM Jr, Zelenock GB, Wakefield TW, Graham LM, Lindenauer SM, Stanley JC. Arterial bypass grafts for upper extremity ischemia. J Vasc Surg 1986; 3(3):569–573.

84. Salam TA, Lumsden AB, Smith RB III. Subclavian artery revascularization: a decade of experience with extrathoracic bypass procedures. J Surg Res 1994; 56(5):387–392.

85. Kirgis HD, Reed AF. Significant anatomic relations in the syndrome of the scalene muscles. Ann Surg 1948; 127:1182.

86. Roos DB. Congenital anomalies associated with thoracic outlet syndrome. Anatomy, symptoms, diagnosis, and treatment. Am J Surg 1976; 132(6):771–778.

87. Sanders RJ, Monsour JW, Gerber WF, Adams WR, Thompson N. Scalenectomy versus first rib resection for treatment of the thoracic outlet syndrome. Surgery 1979; 85(1):109–121.

88. Urschel HC Jr, Razzuk MA, Albers JE, Wood RE, Paulson DL. Reoperation for recurrent thoracic outlet syndrome. Ann Thorac Surg 1976; 21(1):19–25.

46

Venous and Lymphatic Abnormalities of the Limbs

Jose R. Parra and Julie A. Freischlag

INTRODUCTION

William Harvey's monumental work nearly four centuries ago on the circulation of blood first emphasized the important role that the extremity veins play in this process. The impact of derangements in venous and lymphatic function of the limbs is staggering and contributes substantially to human disease. This chapter discusses our current understanding of these disorders and the physiologic rationale underlying their management.

ANATOMY

Veins of the lower extremity can be classified as deep, superficial, or perforating venous systems. The superficial veins run in the subcutaneous tissue external to the deep fascia. The two major tributaries in the superficial venous system are the greater and lesser saphenous veins. The greater saphenous vein, formed by the confluence of the medial veins of the dorsum and plantar aspect of the foot, is found anterior to the medial malleolus and travels along the medial aspect of the leg until it crosses laterally at the proximal thigh to join the common femoral vein (Fig. 1). This junction is commonly 2 to 4 cm lateral to the pubic tubercle and inferior to the inguinal ligament. Cutaneous sensation to the medial aspect of the lower leg is provided by the saphenous branch of the femoral nerve, which runs adjacent to or crosses the greater saphenous vein in the lower leg. This is an important anatomic finding in that saphenous nerve injury can result in a troublesome neuropathy. The lesser saphenous vein, arising behind the lateral malleolus, takes its origin from the veins draining the lateral aspect of the foot and travels through the midline of the posterior calf to join the popliteal vein behind the knee (Fig. 1). Both of these major veins are commonly used as bypass conduits and are also the main sites of superficial venous reflux.

The deep veins of the calf include the peroneal, posterior tibial, and anterior tibial vein, which ascend along the course of their corresponding artery (Fig. 2). In addition, there is a complex of veins within the soleal and gastrocnemius muscles often referred to as venous lakes, which are important physiologically because of their propensity to generate thrombus. These venous lakes coalesce and join the posterior tibial and peroneal veins. The aforementioned veins then merge with the anterior tibial vein to form the popliteal vein at the knee. This vein continues proximally as the superficial femoral vein and joins the deep femoral vein below the inguinal ligament to become the common femoral vein. The common femoral vein, traveling medial to the femoral artery, passes beneath the inguinal ligament and continues as the external iliac vein. As a rule, deep veins are duplicated below the knee and are the first structures identified when dissecting out the arteries.

Perforating veins traverse the deep fascia and connect the superficial and deep venous systems. These veins play a critical role in the pathophysiology of chronic venous insufficiency insofar as they can transmit elevated pressures from the deep venous system into the superficial system.

Superficial and deep venous systems are present within the upper extremity (Fig. 3). The major superficial veins are the cephalic vein, which runs from the anatomic snuffbox along the lateral aspect of the arm to empty into the axillary vein at the deltopectoral groove, and the basilic vein, which travels along the medial aspect to empty into the brachial vein in the upper arm. These veins are commonly used as outflow tracts for arteriovenous fistulas created for hemodialysis. The deep veins parallel the radial

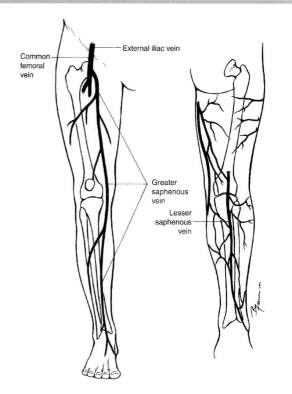

Figure 1 Diagram depicting the two main superficial tributaries of the venous system: the greater saphenous vein and lesser saphenous vein.

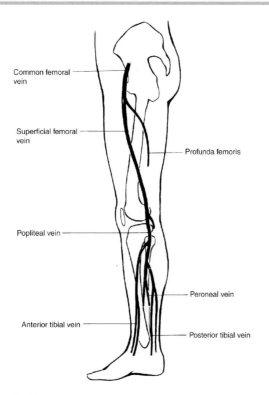

Figure 2   Diagram depicting the deep venous system of the lower extremity.

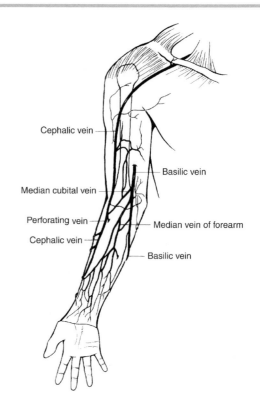

Figure 3   Diagram depicting the upper-extremity venous anatomy.

and ulnar arteries below the elbow and then coalescence to form the brachial vein. The brachial vein merges with the basilic vein to become the axillary vein followed by the subclavian vein at the lateral border of the first rib. The subclavian vein then drains into the innominate vein ultimately ending up in the superior vena cava.

VENOUS PHYSIOLOGY

The venous system is a low-pressure capacitance system with significant redundancy, which depends upon external compression and compartmentalization to return blood to the heart. The veins have an intima, media, and adventitia but lack a significant muscular and elastic layer in all but the most central veins. A feature unique to the venous circulation is the presence of bicuspid valves in all veins distal to the common iliac vein. These one-way valves are oriented so to maintain a unidirectional flow of blood toward the heart. Upon standing, the column of venous blood is arrested as the valves slam shut and reflux is prevented. The valves of the perforating veins are crucial in preventing reflux of blood from the deep to the superficial systems, which prevents superficial venous hypertension.

In the supine position at rest, the foot vein has a pressure of approximately 15 mmHg. On standing, the gravitational hydrostatic forces are added increasing the measured foot vein pressure to approximately 115 mmHg. Assuming the standing position also increases venous volume with an increase in the capacitance by about 500 cm^3. Ambulation produces contraction of the calf muscles that serve as an external "pump" to squeeze the venous blood in a cephalad direction and lower the venous

pressure. With competent valves and a functioning calf pump during exercise, venous blood in these capacitance vessels is returned to the heart. A clinical application of this action is the use of pneumatic compression devices in patients at bed rest. These devices rhythmically inflate to mimic the function of the calf muscles and reduce stasis and the risk for venous thrombosis.

VENOUS DISORDERS OF THE LOWER EXTREMITY
Deep Venous Thrombosis

Deep venous thrombosis (DVT) is the most serious and potentially life-threatening disorder of the venous system. The most lethal complication, pulmonary embolism (PE), is the cause of approximately 200,000 deaths each year in the United States (1). More than half of the patients surviving DVT suffer from the postphlebitic syndrome notable for disabling edema and potential stasis ulcers. Much of the pathophysiology of DVTs was first postulated by Virchow. He described three conditions (Virchow's triad) that permit the development of a venous thrombus: stasis, hypercoagulability, and vessel wall damage. Stasis is the most important predisposing factor in the surgical patient. With the induction of general anesthesia, there is a considerable reduction in the venous flow because of the loss of the ability to contract the muscles of the lower extremity and a generalized peripheral dilation that is present throughout the procedure. Furthermore, a hospitalized patient frequently remains at bed rest, which also induces stasis and subsequent DVT. It is this consequence that provides the stimulus for early ambulation in most surgical patients. Other risk factors for DVT include age, obesity, malignancy, oral contraceptive use, hypercoagulability syndromes, and pregnancy (2). Each of these factors alters venous stasis or coagulopathy.

Clinical Presentation

Clinical signs of venous thrombosis are found in only 40% of the patients. When symptoms are present, they initially include edema and calf pain. The level at which swelling occurs is determined by the site of venous obstruction. If the swelling is confined to the calf or foot, obstruction is at the femoropopliteal level, whereas swelling at the thigh level implies iliofemoral obstruction. Physical examination reveals calf tenderness on palpation and occasionally a palpable cord representing the thrombosed vein. Homans' sign, tenderness or tightness in the back of the calf with forcible dorsiflexion of the foot, may be present but is nonspecific and unreliable. There is a higher incidence of DVTs in the left leg compared to the right.

Most DVTs involve the popliteal vein and its tributaries. However, if the thrombus extends proximally to involve the iliofemoral system, there may be massive swelling from the toes to the inguinal ligament. The clinical picture of pain, extensive pitting edema, and blanching is referred to as *phlegmasia alba dolens* or "milk leg." With the progression of the thrombus, venous return becomes compromised and produces a painful, cyanotic leg known as *phlegmasia cerulea dolens* (3). If left unchecked, venous congestion and swelling can eventually limit arterial flow leading to gangrene of the extremity (Fig. 4). However, as previously mentioned, most patients are asymptomatic, and these dramatic presentations represent a very small percentage of the patients with venous thrombosis.

Diagnosis

Diagnostic tests are critical in establishing the diagnosis because false-positive clinical signs have been found to occur in up to 45% of the patients evaluated (4). Duplex ultrasonography scanning is noninvasive and can be conveniently used at the bedside to detect venous thrombi with an accuracy of approximately 90%. Flow abnormalities such as a loss of phasicity or augmentation with distal compression are suggestive of thrombi. The most sensitive test, however, is a loss of compressibility of the normally compliant vein (Fig. 5). In the femoral vein, duplex scanning has a specificity of 100% and sensitivity of 95% (5). Diagnostic accuracy is lower in the calf. Nevertheless, it has been suggested that duplex scanning replaces venography as the standard method of diagnosing femoropopliteal DVT.

Venography is the most accurate means of establishing the diagnosis of venous thrombosis and its extent of involvement. This test requires injection of a contrast medium into a foot vein while the superficial veins are occluded by a tourniquet to promote filling of the deep venous system. Filling defects and nonvisualization of the deep veins identify the thrombus. This invasive test carries the risk of producing venous thrombosis secondary to the thrombogenicity of the injected contrast medium. Other rare complications include cellulitis or skin necrosis secondary to extravasation of contrast and gangrene (6). This test remains the gold standard.

Venography can also be performed with isotope injection and thus eliminate some of these complications. A gamma scintillation counter is then used to record the flow of the isotope. The image with this technique is not as well defined, but this method may be valuable for the sequential study of patients. A similar technique involves radioactive-labeled fibrinogen scanning. This technique involves intravenous injection of ^{125}I-labeled fibrinogen. A developing thrombus incorporates fibrinogen with an increase in radioactivity that represents an organizing thrombus. This test is primarily used in clinical research studies given its oversensitivity to clot formation.

Impedance plethysmography is another alternative to venography. This method measures the rate of volume changes in the extremity following rapid deflation of a blood pressure cuff. A prolongation of the outflow following deflation is indicative of occlusive thrombus. This technique has largely been supplanted by duplex ultrasonography.

Prophylaxis

Several prophylactic measures can be used in the hospitalized patient. The goals of these measures are to reduce stasis or alter blood coagulability. Early ambulation has become a routine part of a patient's postoperative course in an attempt to prevent stasis. Other options to reduce stasis include graded compression stockings and intermittent pneumatic compression devices, both of which augment venous flow. These devices are placed on the patient just prior to surgery and remain in place until the patient is actively ambulating.

Anticoagulation therapy using heparinoids is commonplace. Heparin and its derivative low-molecular-weight heparin (LMWH) bind to anti–thrombin III, which causes an increased inhibition of factors IIa, Xa, IXa, XIIa, and thrombin. Unfractionated heparin (5000 U subcutaneously) can be given two hours preoperatively and then every 8 to 12 hours postoperatively until the patient is ambulating. Although controversy exists over its efficacy, a large randomized series of surgical patients showed protection against DVT and a markedly decreased incidence of PE (7). LMWH is composed entirely of lower-molecular-weight heparin moieties and has the benefit of lowering the risk of bleeding complications. Other advantages include a lower incidence of the heparin-induced thrombocytopenia (HIT) syndrome and lower risks of osteopenia with long-term use. Several different brands of LMWH are available and the dosing for prophylaxis varies among the brands (8).

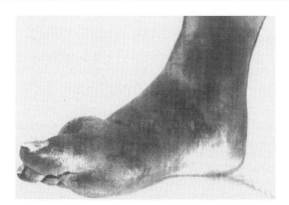

Figure 4 Venous gangrene following iliofemoral deep venous thrombosis associated with malignancy.

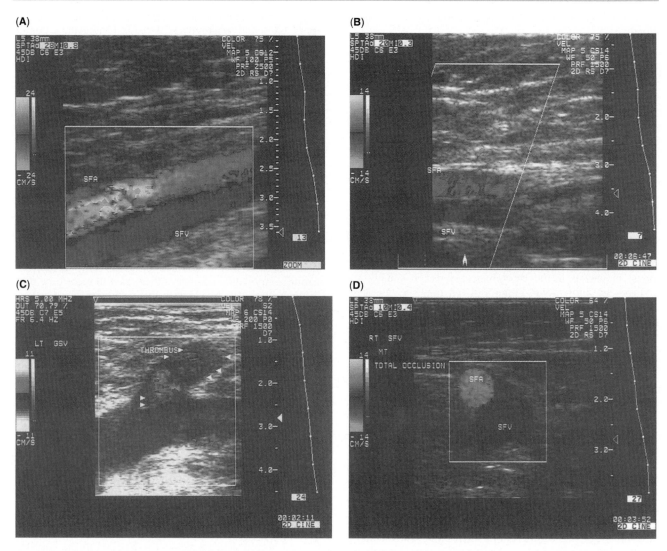

Figure 5   (A) Longitudinal view using the duplex scan to identify normal flow in the superficial femoral artery (SFA) and superficial femoral vein (SFV). (B) Longitudinal view using the duplex scan demonstrating normal SFA and loss of venous flow in the SFV caused by thrombus. (C) Duplex scan of the greater saphenous vein showing nonoccluding thrombus identified by *arrows*. (D) Transverse view of the SFA and SFV demonstrating no flow in a completely thrombosed SFV.

Colditz et al. (9) evaluated general surgery patients using a variety of different types of prophylaxis. The incidence of DVT using the fibrinogen uptake test or venography was estimated to be 27% without any therapy, while those treated with subcutaneous heparin had an incidence of 9.6%, those with compression stockings 6.3%, and those with pneumatic compression devices 17.6%. A combination of heparin and stockings revealed an incidence of DVT of 6.3%, and stockings with intermittent pneumatic compression revealed an incidence of 4.5% (9).

Indications for prophylaxis depend upon the type of surgery as well as associated risk factors. There are three levels of risk ranging from negligible risk not warranting treatment to high risk requiring multi-modality treatment. Patients undergoing outpatient surgery with no risk factors do not require prophylaxis, while patients undergoing major general surgery and/or having multiple risk factors need one of the prophylactic measures described above. Trauma, orthopedic and neurosurgical procedures, and/or

several risk factors require therapy with two of the above measures (e.g., compression devices and LMWH).

Treatment

The goal of DVT management is to halt the propagation of thrombus, prevent PE, and promote resolution of existing clot to minimize the risk for postphlebitic syndrome. The mainstay of initial therapy for DVT is anticoagulation with heparin. This can take the form of an adjusted dose heparin drip or LMWH. Traditional dosing of a heparin drip consists of a 80 U/kg intravenous bolus followed by 18 U/kg/hr as a continuous infusion. The adequacy of anticoagulation is monitored by serial partial thromboplastin time levels, which are maintained between 60 and 80 seconds. Adjusted dose heparin therapy requires inpatient treatment. In contradistinction, LMWH is administered as subcutaneous injections and can be given in the outpatient setting. Treatment with LMWH has been shown to have a lower rate of major and minor bleeding as well as lower rates of PE than adjusted dose heparin (10). A predictable pharmacokinetic profile obviates the need for any type of monitoring except in obese and renal failure patients. However, an anti-Xa assay can be obtained to verify efficacy with a target goal of between 0.6 and 1.0 IU/mL (11). Heparin limits any further propagation of the thrombus and prevents the formation of new thrombi. It does not break up the original thrombus. The affected extremity should be elevated when the patient is not ambulatory to reduce swelling and tenderness. Compression stockings should be used to prevent edema formation.

Once the patient is anticoagulated, oral warfarin (Coumadin) therapy is begun. Warfarin acts by inhibiting the synthesis of the vitamin K–dependent clotting factors, II, VII, IX, and X. The prothrombin time (PT) or international normalized ratio (INR) is used to monitor warfarin therapy. The PT is brought to within 1.3 to 1.5 times the control value or an INR of 2 to 3 to maintain sufficient anticoagulation. Warfarin therapy should be continued for at least three months when identifiable risk factors are present, six months for an idiopathic thromboembolism, and 12 months to lifetime in patients with a hypercoagulable condition (12). Recently, a randomized trial demonstrated that lower INRs in the 1.5 to 2.0 range were as efficacious as higher doses with lower bleeding complications (13).

Both heparin and warfarin therapy have serious potential side effects. Side effects associated with heparin treatment include bleeding, thrombocytopenia, hypersensitivity reaction, arterial thromboembolism, and osteoporosis in patients receiving long-term therapy (14). HIT syndrome is an antibody-mediated reaction to heparin leading to venous and arterial thromboses (15). A drop in the platelet count by 50% or skin lesions at the site of injection are highly suggestive of HIT syndrome. Laboratory assays that can detect HIT antibodies exist. Treatment of this syndrome involves cessation of heparin use and administration of direct thrombin inhibitors such as lepirudin or argatroban. Coumadin should be avoided in these patients because there are multiple reports of warfarin-induced venous limb gangrene. Arterial thromboembolism caused by HIT is the most severe complication.

Complications associated with warfarin therapy include bleeding, skin necrosis, dermatitis, and a painful blue toe syndrome. Skin necrosis occurs in areas with significant adipose tissue such as thighs, breasts, and buttocks. It has been found that thrombosis of venules and capillaries supplying this region occurs as a result of an underlying protein C deficiency. Protein C and protein S are the first factors to decrease following the administration of Coumadin, which results in a transient hypercoagulable state amplified in patients with a preexisting protein C deficiency. A blue toe syndrome can occur secondary to bleeding into an arterial plaque, which results in distal embolization and ischemia. Warfarin is also teratogenic and should not be used during pregnancy. Heparin is the drug of choice during pregnancy and is given subcutaneously for long-term treatment.

Fibrinolytic therapy for the management of DVT has been an area of great interest. Bleeding is the major complication associated with this course of treatment and is therefore contraindicated in patients who have had recent surgery, trauma, or hemorrhagic stroke. This technique is most effective when performed within 72 hours of the event and involves placement of a catheter directly into the thrombus and providing a local infusion of the lytic agent. Urokinase has been found to be more effective than streptokinase with fewer hemorrhagic and allergic complications (16).

Objectives of this form of therapy include reduction of lower-extremity edema and pain and preservation of venous valve function. The presence of an iliofemoral DVT resulting in phlegmasia cerulea dolens or venous gangrene is a situation where thrombolysis or surgical thrombectomy is indicated to prevent limb loss. A more controversial indication for thrombolysis has been to preserve venous valve integrity by rapid resolution of the thrombus so as to protect against the development of valvular incompetence and subsequent postphlebitic syndrome (17). Early recanalization is important in preserving valve integrity; however, it is not clear that postphlebitic syndrome can be prevented by early lytic therapy (18,19). Quality-of-life assessments have shown a benefit to the use of lysis in patients with iliofemoral DVTs (20).

Complications of DVT

Pulmonary Embolism

The most fatal complication of DVT is a PE. PEs occur most frequently between 7 and 10 days postoperatively; if the symptoms remain unrecognized and untreated, the mortality is approximately 30%.

Pathophysiology. A patient with a DVT of the lower extremity has a 50% chance of PE if the thrombus reaches the iliofemoral system. Even though thrombi may develop in the smaller veins of the calf, the risk of PE is less until the thrombus extends to the level of the femoral and iliac veins. Once embolization occurs and pulmonary blood flow is interrupted, a regional ventilation–perfusion mismatch and a bronchoconstrictive response are produced. Occlusion of more than 30% of the pulmonary vascular bed leads to a rise in pulmonary artery pressures, while a 50% occlusion leads to a fall in systemic pressures. The classic presentation is that of sudden pleuritic chest pain, dyspnea, and tachypnea. Other findings can include cough, tachycardia, and hemoptysis; hemoptysis is an uncommon finding indicative of pulmonary infarction. Physical examination reveals tachycardia, a prominent second heart sound, and cyanosis.

Diagnosis. The clinical presentation of a PE mimics several other life-threatening conditions. An electrocardiogram is essential to exclude a myocardial infarction. Nonspecific ST and T wave changes are a nonspecific finding with PE. Chest X rays demonstrate enlargement of the central vasculature, a lack of the vascular markings with segmental or lobar ischemia (Westermark's sign), or pleural effusion. A wedge-shaped infiltrate is occasionally seen. Arterial blood gas analysis shows hypoxemia coupled with alkalosis. Central venous pressure is elevated or normal if hemodynamic compensation has occurred, with a low central venous pressure essentially excluding PE.

Definitive diagnosis of PE requires a computed tomography (CT) scan, ventilation–perfusion scan, or pulmonary arteriography. The ventilation–perfusion scan involves intravenous infusion of labeled albumin, to demonstrate perfusion abnormalities, combined with xenon gas inhalation, to demonstrate ventilation abnormalities. The combination of a poorly perfused area that shows excellent ventilation has the highest probability of representing a PE. Lesser concordances are given lower probabilities. With this technique, there is a high false-positive rate, because other diseases such as pneumonia or atelectasis can lead to similar results. Spiral CT scans of the chest with intravenous contrast have sufficient resolution to allow discrimination of thrombosis in the segmental pulmonary arteries (21). The sensitivity of this test varies widely (63–94%), but it has a high specificity (22). Pulmonary angiography remains the gold standard for identification of PE, but it is best reserved for situations where there is disagreement or uncertainty with the other imaging techniques.

Treatment. Anticoagulation with heparin is the mainstay of treatment, and the technique of administration is the same as that described for DVT. Again, heparin therapy is initiated and is converted to oral anticoagulation for three to six months. Those patients in whom anticoagulation is contraindicated are candidates for inferior vena caval interruption to prevent further DVTs.

Surgical thrombectomy is another procedure for treating iliofemoral DVTs. The indications for this treatment include phlegmasia, venous gangrene, and the inability of patients to be treated by anticoagulation or thrombolysis. A longitudinal venotomy is made in the distal common femoral vein and an Esmarch bandage (i.e., a wide, thick rubber band) is used to squeeze thrombus from the distal veins, while balloon catheters are used to extract clot from the proximal veins. A temporary arteriovenous fistula is often created to increase venous patency. This procedure is associated with an early patency rate of 87% and a significant decrease in the incidence of reflux following treatment (23). This procedure is somewhat morbid with potential for significant intraoperative blood loss and high rates of postoperative hematomas and groin infections.

Although anticoagulation remains the mainstay of treatment for DVT, this therapy is contraindicated in some patients leaving them at high risk for the development of pulmonary emboli. To treat patients in this situation, several techniques to "filter" the vena cava have been explored. Inferior vena cava filters are made by several manufacturers but basically consist of a metallic screen that filters the vena cava of thrombi. These filters can be placed percutaneously and are usually deployed in the vena cava between the caval bifurcation and the lowest renal vein. Complications of inferior vena cava filters include misplacement, insertion-site DVT, migration of the filter, erosion of the device into the inferior vena cava wall and inferior vena cava obstruction, and PE (24,25). Although this procedure has a relatively low morbidity and mortality, the complications can be severe, and placement should be reserved for those patients who have absolute contraindications to traditional anticoagulation. Temporary filters are currently under investigation.

For patients with a massive PE with refractory hypotension, an emergent pulmonary embolectomy may be required. A thoracotomy is performed to surgically remove the thrombus. Given the high mortality rate associated with this procedure, alternative approaches using interventional techniques have been developed although the only Food and Drug Administration–improved device is the Greenfield aspiration (26). Other devices and techniques use mechanical means to break up the thrombus.

Thrombolytic therapy has also been used as an alternative treatment for those patients not in shock. Urokinase and tissue plasminogen activator are available lytic agents proven to be effective. The patient's symptoms often improve quickly with the dissolution of the clot; however, no improvement has been seen in early mortality in patients with pulmonary emboli, who have been treated with thrombolytic therapy (27). In addition, there are significant complications secondary to bleeding, which have limited the use of this therapy.

Postphlebitic Syndrome

Chronic venous insufficiency is a disabling venous disorder characterized by chronic lower-extremity edema, skin changes, and a propensity for ischemic ulcer formation. *Postphlebitic syndrome* is the chronic venous insufficiency that occurs following a DVT; 74% of patients with DVTs involving the femoral or iliac vein develop this condition (28).

Clinical Presentation. Hyperpigmentation and edema of the lower extremity are the earliest signs of chronic venous insufficiency (Fig. 6). The swelling has been described as brawny and nonpitting. The hyperpigmentation is associated with a dermatitis (venous eczema) that leads to severe pruritus, frequently the initial complaint. In addition to the skin changes, the patient experiences an aching discomfort or night cramps that are aggravated by dependency and relieved with elevation. Venous claudication or a throbbing pain throughout the leg may occur with ambulation.

These changes occur because valves in the deep venous system are compromised by the inflammation associated with a DVT. Blood is diverted into the communicating veins and into the superficial venous system with the development of venous hypertension and varicosities. Chronic venous hypertension leads to increased hydrostatic pressure at the capillary level, causing transudation of fluid and proteins as well as hemosiderin-laden red blood cells. The latter is responsible for the typical brownish skin pigmentation seen in these patients. From a histologic perspective, there is fat necrosis and fibrosis of the skin and subcutaneous tissue, a condition commonly referred to as *lipodermatosclerosis*. All these factors promote an inflammatory reaction conducive to skin breakdown and ulceration (29). Ultimately, patients can develop ulcerations in the region of the medial or lateral malleolus (Fig. 7).

Diagnosis. The diagnosis is generally made on history and physical examination alone. In an attempt to distinguish chronic venous insufficiency from lymphedema, one can focus on the extent of edema. Edema secondary to venous insufficiency begins at the ankle and extends to involve primarily the lower leg, whereas lymphedema begins in the toes and foot and involves the entire extremity. Also, those patients with lymphedema do not have pigmentation of the skin. Diagnostic studies such as duplex scanning or

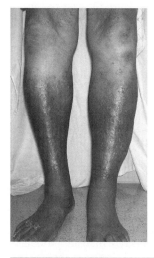

Figure 6 Chronic venous insufficiency with a small amount of stasis dermatitis around the right toes.

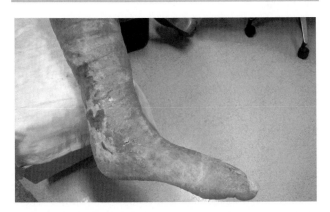

Figure 7 Venous stasis ulcer in a patient with chronic venous insufficiency.

venography are infrequently performed. However, these tests can be used to locate areas of valvular incompetence if surgery is contemplated.

Treatment. Ideally, the best treatment is prevention, and this is accomplished by applying the prophylactic measures against DVT previously described. Unfortunately, those who develop postphlebitic syndrome often require a lengthy and frustrating treatment course. It is essential that patients avoid prolonged standing and elevate their legs when sitting and sleeping. Graded compression stockings are also required to increase venous return. The skin is extremely fragile, and all efforts must be taken to avoid trauma. The skin is frequently dry, flaky, and itchy; therefore liberal use of skin emollients to prevent cracking and subsequent ulceration is necessary. When venous ulcers are present, an occlusive protective paste dressing such as Unna's boot is used. This dressing allows for ambulation while providing compression and protection from trauma. Healing of venous ulcers is slow, and it is not uncommon to require many months of vigilant wound care. Erickson et al. examined 99 limbs with venous stasis ulcers. They found that those patients with low venous refill times ($\leq$10 seconds), indicative of severe venous insufficiency, took significantly longer to completely heal. Although 91% of the ulcers healed at a median of three months, 56% of the healed ulcers recurred (20).

Antibiotics should be reserved for the presence of frank cellulitis. If the ulcer is slow to heal, split thickness skin grafting can be employed if there is a viable granulation bed. A plethora of other wound care treatments have been suggested for use in venous stasis ulcers.

Incompetent perforating veins contribute to elevated lower-extremity pressures and are often associated with recalcitrant ulcer healing. Ligation of these veins can be performed via an open approach or an endoscopic approach. Endoscopic perforating vein ligation results in healing of 88% of ulcers at one year, although approximately 28% of the ulcers will reoccur after two years (30). Overall, 50% of patients with postthrombotic deep venous involvement will remain ulcer-free at three years. Transplantation of competent valves from the axillary vein to the popliteal vein has also been employed to assist in the healing of ulcers. This technique results in ulcer healing rates of 79% with 50% to 65% remaining ulcer-free at six years (31). Other procedures that attempt to reduce reflux by surgically reconstructing incompetent valves have been investigated.

Varicose Veins

Varicose veins are superficial veins that have become dilated and tortuous (Fig. 8). The development of varicose veins is thought to result from venous valve incompetence and defects in the elastic properties of the vein wall. This venous valve incompetence can arise secondary to local trauma, thrombophlebitis, familial weakness in the valve structure, increased blood volume as seen after DVT, and hormonal changes especially during pregnancy (32–34). Incompetence leads to the unimpeded reflux of blood into the lower veins, which results in a significant rise in resting venous pressure. This chronic elevation of pressure contributes to the dilation and elongation of the veins and formation of varicosities. In addition, enzymatic abnormalities in the vein segments distant from the varicosities have been identified suggesting that additional biochemical defects may be present as well (35).

Varicosities of the lower extremity can be classified as primary varicose veins or secondary varicose veins depending on the cause. Primary varicose veins have an unclear etiology and occur in individuals with no previous history of DVT. Studies of select populations have found that 20% to 40% of patients with primary varicosities have a family history of this disease (36). Women have a threefold greater risk of developing varicose veins compared to men. Female hormones are thought to contribute to this increased risk. Specifically, progesterone, a hormone whose levels are elevated during the second phase of the menstrual cycle and during pregnancy, causes passive dilation of varicosities (37). This distention renders the valves incompetent and initiates the formation of varicose veins or makes existing varicosities more symptomatic. Advancing age, obesity, and increased intra-abdominal pressure are other factors associated with primary varicose veins.

Secondary varicose veins arise subsequent to the consequences of DVTs or as a result of venous obstruction. Venous obstruction may be caused by compression of the proximal venous system or by an intra-abdominal or pelvic tumor. The underlying increased venous pressure and vascular incompetence caused by these conditions result in reflux of blood from the deep to the superficial veins and the development of varicosities.

Clinical Presentation

Varicose veins may or may not produce symptoms. In fact, many women have asymptomatic varicosities; however, they seek medical attention because of the unsightly blue, dilated, and tortuous veins. Those with symptoms usually complain of pain, fatigue, and aching, most noticeable in the calves

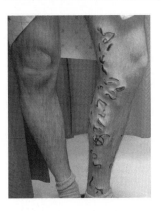

Figure 8 Varicose veins marked prior to vein stripping.

and ankles especially at the end of the day. A feeling of heaviness is often described by the patient, particularly if the day has been spent standing or sitting without much walking. These symptoms are relieved by lying down, elevating the leg, or wearing elastic support stockings. The symptoms are exacerbated in women during their menstrual cycle because of venous valve dilation and worsening incompetence. Physical examination must include the abdomen and pelvis to access the possibility of venous obstruction secondary to a tumor. Examination of the legs should be performed in the standing and supine position. Varicose veins should be examined and palpated. Palpation can detect hidden varicosities in obese legs where they may not be visualized. Arterial pulses should be palpated as well.

Preoperative Testing

There are several clinical tests that are applied to evaluate deep venous patency and valvular competence. The Perthes test is performed by placing a tourniquet around the proximal thigh snug enough to compress the superficial veins. The patient is then asked to walk, and attention is paid to the superficial ankle veins. If the veins become less prominent, the perforator and deep vein valves are intact; however, if the veins remain the same size, the perforator valves are incompetent. If the veins should become more prominent with exercise and the patient complains of pain, it can be assumed that there is significant deep venous insufficiency along with incompetent perforators.

The retrograde filling test or Trendelenburg test aids in distinguishing between superficial valvular incompetence and perforator valvular incompetence. This procedure is done by elevating the leg initially to empty the veins and then placing a tourniquet over the saphenofemoral junction. The patient is then asked to stand, and the pattern of superficial venous refill is noted. If the varicosities do not fill on standing but do so immediately after releasing the tourniquet, the perforating veins are competent and the varicosities are secondary to superficial venous valve incompetence. If the patient stands and there is rapid filling of the varicosities with the tourniquet still in place, the perforator veins are incompetent secondary to deep venous disease.

Duplex scanning can be performed to document venous valvular reflux as well. The test is important if there are clinical findings or a history suggestive of DVT. A hand-held Doppler probe can also give the information needed to demonstrate deep venous patency and venous reflux especially at the saphenofemoral junction and at the level of the perforators (38). With the patient sitting on the examining table with the legs hanging over the edge of the table, the popliteal and posterior tibial veins can be examined for venous valvular insufficiency using compression above and below the Doppler probe. A delayed response with augmentation can indicate poor outflow secondary to obstruction. This is quite rare unless the patient has a history of DVT. Reflux heard during proximal compression confirms the diagnosis of venous valvular insufficiency. Venous reflux can be determined in a similar manner in the perforator veins. Saphenofemoral junction incompetence can be ascertained with the Doppler probe by placing it over the site and having the patient perform a Valsalva maneuver. This should be repeated with a tourniquet placed around the proximal thigh area. The reflux should disappear when the Valsalva maneuver is performed again with the tourniquet in place.

Treatment

Conservative therapy is recommended for those with minimal varicosities or for those who desire to avoid invasive measures to cure the disease. Graded compression stockings can relieve the symptoms. The stockings are put on in the morning and removed at night. Patients are encouraged to avoid long periods of standing and to elevate the legs while sitting. Patients are also encouraged to walk as much as possible, which helps facilitate venous outflow by using the calf muscle pump.

For those patients with symptomatic varicosities or for those who do not like the unsightly nature of their varicose veins, there are several treatment options for cure. Sclerotherapy has become a popular treatment option given its success and availability in an outpatient setting. Venous sclerotherapy is an ablative procedure that actually causes thrombosis in the affected vein, preferably without blood in the lumen (27). The procedure is performed by having the patient stand to mark the varicose veins and perforating veins. With the patient remaining standing, 23-gauge butterfly needles are placed approximately 1 cm apart along the course of the varicose veins (Fig. 9). One proceeds from distal to proximal until all veins have been cannulated. The patient is then placed in the supine position, and each site is injected with 0.5% to 1% of the sclerosing agent. The preferred sclerosing agent is sodium tetradecyl sulfate. Up to 60 sites and 30 mL of this solution can be used during venous sclerotherapy of one limb without sequelae. Immediately after the injection, the butterfly needle is removed, and a gauze and foam rubber pad are placed over the injection site. A stockinette and compression stocking are then placed over the gauze and pad. These should remain in place for

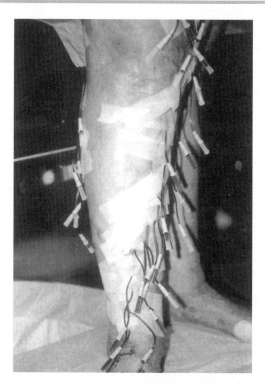

Figure 9 Multiple butterfly needles seen placed along the course of symptomatic varicose veins prior to injection of a sclerosing agent.

three weeks without being removed. The patient is encouraged to walk and remain active. When stocking, gauze, and pad are removed after three weeks, inspection and palpation can document the obliteration of the varicose vein. Those patients with saphenofemoral junction incompetence have high recurrence rates with venous sclerotherapy alone; therefore high ligation of the saphenofemoral junction should be performed in these patients either prior to or in conjunction with venous sclerotherapy.

The main complication resulting after venous sclerotherapy is localized phlebitis, which occurs approximately 10% of the time (39,40). It is usually self-limiting and requires little intervention. Other uncommon complications include skin necrosis and ulceration secondary to extravasation of the sclerosing agent, intraluminal hematomas, and pigmentation of the surrounding skin.

Vein stripping is an alternative method of treating varicose veins. This procedure requires a general or regional anesthetic and potential overnight stay in the hospital, even though most patients do go home the same day of the procedure. After marking all varicosities, the patient is given a general anesthetic, and attention is given to ligation of the saphenous vein and all other tributaries at the saphenofemoral junction. The vein stripper, a flexible rod, is then passed up the length of the vein from a distal venotomy at the level of the medial malleolus. The divided vein at the saphenofemoral junction is tied to the stripper, and the vein is removed with the instrument. Prior to stripping the vein, the other varicosities that are located away from the course of the stripper are treated. This is accomplished by making very small incisions by stabbing the skin over the vein with a No. 11 blade scalpel. The vein is grasped with fine forceps and divided. Each end is then avulsed by direct traction and removed through the incision. Bleeding is controlled with pressure; no ligatures are used. After removal of the stripper and therefore avulsion of the main venous channel from the perforators, the leg is wrapped firmly from the toes to the groin to allow the perforators to thrombose. The patient may resume daily activities but is encouraged to sit with the leg elevated and avoid prolonged standing.

Complications after vein stripping are infrequent. They may include bleeding, with ecchymosis being the most common complication appearing three to five days postoperatively. This usually resolves within three to four weeks. Leg edema is common but is relieved by the use of the elastic support stockings. Hypoesthesia of the skin particularly at the level of the ankle may occur because of trauma to the saphenous and sural nerves (39).

Other options for the treatment of varicosities include radio frequency and laser ablation of the saphenous vein. These techniques can be performed as outpatient procedures and, when combined with high ligation techniques, have reasonable success rates.

Superficial Thrombophlebitis

Thrombophlebitis is a local inflammatory process that is restricted to the superficial veins. This condition most commonly occurs in varicose veins of the lower extremity below the level of the knee. Thrombophlebitis can also occur in association with intravenous cannulation, local trauma, and parenteral drug abuse. The typical clinical finding is an indurated, painful, and erythematous venous cord as a result of the thrombosed superficial vein.

When thrombophlebitis involves the distal aspect of the greater saphenous venous system, therapy is managed in the outpatient setting. Treatment consists of symptomatic relief with bed rest, leg elevation, and warm compresses to the affected vein. Anticoagulation therapy is not warranted, because embolization virtually never occurs. However, if the thrombophlebitis extends above the knee, the risk of embolization exists. These patients require close observation in the hospital setting; if they remain refractory to symptomatic therapy, anticoagulation is initiated. If the thrombophlebitis worsens despite these interventions, excision of the affected vein may become necessary. Formation of an abscess in the thrombosed segment—septic thrombophlebitis—also mandates surgical excision.

VENOUS DISORDERS OF THE UPPER EXTREMITY
Axillary/Subclavian Vein Thrombosis

DVT of the upper extremity is now more common than previously reported. Earlier studies have cited a 1% to 2% incidence; however, with the increasing use of subclavian venous access, the incidence has risen (41). In fact, subclavian catheters are the number one cause of axillary and subclavian venous thrombosis (42,43). The presence of an upper-extremity DVT is not an innocuous event. Studies indicate that 12% of patients with an upper-extremity DVT have had a documented pulmonary embolization (43).

The most common causes of axillary/subclavian vein thrombosis are (i) central venous lines or pacemakers; (ii) malignancy secondary to tumor compression of the vein or the hypercoagulable state associated with the malignancy; (iii) effort thrombosis or primary thrombosis, frequently referred to as *Paget–Schroetter syndrome* (42). Several factors are involved in the pathophysiology of effort thrombosis. First, there is compression of the axillary/subclavian vein resulting in stasis. This may be due to an anomalous subclavius or anterior scalene muscle or the presence of a cervical rib. Second, repetitive movement at the level of the arm and shoulder may cause intimal tears in the vessel. Third, the stress of exercise may temporarily produce a hypercoagulable state. All these factors are conductive to the development of a thrombus. Primary or effort thrombosis develops clinically as an acute swelling of the involved extremity. It is frequently found in young otherwise healthy men with a recent history of trauma or heavy exertion. It is often noted after activities requiring the arm to be hyperabducted and externally rotated such as painting, throwing a baseball or football, or chopping wood. The involved extremity is usually the patient's dominant arm.

Clinical Presentation

The diagnosis of an upper-extremity DVT can be clinically difficult, especially in the case of iatrogenic injury from a central venous catheter. Often, it has a relatively indolent course that is infrequently associated with symptoms. The subtlety of this injury may be a result of the well-developed venous collateral system of the upper extremity and its ability to compensate in the case of obstruction of a major vein (44).

With increased activity of the involved arm, arterial flow increases in the face of venous outflow obstruction resulting in venous hypertension. This promotes effusion of edema fluid into the tissues and distention of the superficial veins. This venous congestion may make the arm feel heavy or achy. In addition, a dusky cyanosis may develop especially with exertion and dependency of the arm. Physical examination discloses an obvious size and color discrepancy in the upper extremity. Frequently, the superficial veins of the hand and forearm are distended. This can be accentuated with the arm in the dependent position; the veins remain paradoxically distended when the arm is elevated.

Diagnosis

Duplex scanning can often diagnose the problem by revealing the presence of the thrombus in the subclavian or axillary vein. Venography is used to locate the thrombus anatomically and provide access for thrombolytic therapy. Venographic demonstration of prominent collateral veins bypassing an obstructed axillary/subclavian vein provides the definitive diagnosis of thrombotic obstruction (Fig. 10).

Treatment

The traditional treatment of axillary/subclavian vein thrombosis has been bed rest with limb elevation and anticoagulation. With this conservative approach, resolution without recurrence of symptoms has been reported in only 25% of patients (45). Other studies have shown that 50% to 70% of those with an upper-extremity DVT proceed to develop significant postphlebitic sequelae. The recent development of thrombolytic therapy has improved results dramatically. Most patients with primary or effort thrombosis are young and healthy and excellent candidates for thrombolysis. A successful protocol for effort thrombosis described by Machleder (46) recommends continuing the anticoagulation for three months. This is followed by transaxillary first rib resection and decompression with subsequent balloon angioplasty in cases of residual stenosis. Surgical decompression by first rib resection is advocated to correct the anatomic abnormality that caused the thrombosis and prevent recurrent thrombosis. Subsequent angioplasty or stenting of residual venous stenoses may be required.

In cases of secondary thrombosis or catheter-related thrombosis, removal or correction of the offending cause is important. Thrombolytics and anticoagulation are the mainstay of therapy, and surgical intervention is usually not warranted.

The most significant complication of upper-extremity DVT is pulmonary embolization. This was formerly thought to be almost nonexistent; however, rising numbers of upper-extremity thrombosis studies have found a 12% incidence of pulmonary embolization (43). Other complications include postphlebitic changes and long-term disability, septic thrombophlebitis, and loss of central venous access. A rare but morbid complication is venous gangrene. Severe edema of the fingers from venous hypertension can occlude arterial inflow and produce ischemia. This rare condition is best treated with thrombectomy or thrombolysis.

Superficial Thrombophlebitis

The cause of superficial thrombophlebitis of the upper extremity is usually secondary to prolonged intravenous cannulation or infusion of an acidic fluid. The incidence has risen in the recent years, secondary to intravenous drug abuse. Treatment involves elevation, warm compresses, and pain control with nonsteroidal anti-inflammatory drugs. Surgical excision is reserved for septic thrombophlebitis.

LYMPHEDEMA
Clinical Presentation

The embryonic development of the lymphatic system begins with paired jugular and iliac sacs, the cisterna chyli, and a second retroperitoneal sac. It is from these sacs that the lymph vessels sprout and course throughout the body following the major venous pathways (Fig. 11). The cisterna chyli within the abdomen communicates with the paired jugular sacs by two lymphatic channels. The more predominant channel connecting the cisterna chyli to the left jugular bud is known as the thoracic duct. The elaborate network of lymphatic channels and regional nodes of the upper and lower extremities drain lymph into the thoracic duct and cisterna chyli, respectively, which then return the lymph to the venous system. The lymphatics are formed by a layer of endothelial cells with a discontinuous basement membrane in contrast to the continuous basement membrane found in blood capillaries (47). The lymphatic capillaries are a valved system that allows for unidirectional flow of lymph back to the venous system.

The functions of the lymphatic system include resorption of interstitial fluid, particularly macromolecular proteins such as albumin; lymph node filtering of bacteria and other antigenic particles; and transport of certain substances (vitamin K and long-chain fatty acids) from the gastrointestinal tract to the venous system (48). During a 24-hour period, approximately 4 L of lymph flow containing 100 g of plasma protein is returned to the venous circulation.

(A)   **(B)**

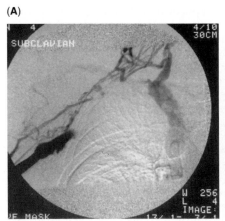
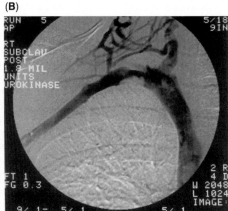

Figure 10 **(A)** Venogram revealing a thrombosed right subclavian vein in a patient with effort thrombosis. **(B)** Following urokinase infusion, venous outflow is restored. However, an irregular proximal subclavian vein remains.

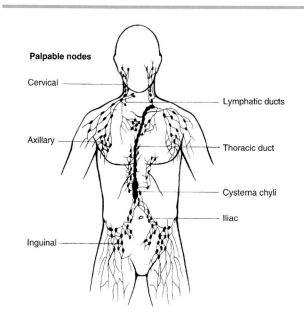

Palpable nodes

Cervical

Axillary

Inguinal

Lymphatic ducts

Thoracic duct

Cysterna chyli

Iliac

Figure 11 Normal anatomy of the lymphatic system.

If the lymphatics fail to return this considerable volume of protein-rich fluid, lymphedema results.

Lymphedema can be categorized as either primary (congenital) or secondary depending on its cause. Primary lymphedema is subdivided according to the age of onset; however, all forms are a result of the congenial abnormalities in the development of the lymphatic system. Congenital lymphedema is present from birth. *Milroy's disease* is a hereditary form of congenital lymphedema with a sex-linked dominant pattern and characteristic hypoplasia of the lymphatic trunks. *Lymphedema praecox* becomes apparent from the adolescent years to age 35 and accounts for approximately 80% of the patients with congenital lymphedema. *Lymphedema tarda* occurs after age 35. The anatomic anomalies seen in these three forms of primary lymphedema include hypoplasia (the most common), aplasia, and hyperplasia (varicose pattern) of the lymphatic system. Primary lymphedema is found to affect women three times more frequently than it is found to affect men. The left leg is more often involved than the right, and the upper extremity is rarely involved. There is no single identifiable precipitating factor that can account for these findings.

Secondary or acquired lymphedema is the most common form of lymphedema. Worldwide, the most common cause is filariasis, resulting in the obstruction of lymph nodes by the parasite *Filaria bancrofti*. In the United States, a common cause is surgical excision of lymph nodes and irradiation for malignant disease. For those who undergo mastectomy with axillary node dissection and radiation therapy, the incidence of lymphedema in the ipsilateral arm can be as high as 38% (49). Prostate carcinoma or other pelvic carcinomas can also cause lymphatic obstruction. Other causes of secondary lymphedema include trauma or infection.

Diagnosis

The diagnosis of lymphedema can frequently be made on clinical grounds alone. Because the most common cause of unilateral extremity swelling is venous disease, one must be able to distinguish between this and lymphedema. Edema secondary to venous disease presents with decreased capillary perfusion, a brawny discoloration of the involved skin, and ulceration. These findings are not indicative of lymphedema. Venous edema also improves after several hours of limb elevation, whereas lymphedema may require several days of extremity elevation to see a decrease in swelling. If there is any question in the differentiation, noninvasive evaluation is required. Duplex examination is the preferred test to rule out DVT. Lymphangiography is rarely used, because it is invasive and hazardous. Complications include dye allergy, oil embolism, and worsening lymphedema.

Lymphoscintigraphy is now becoming the diagnostic procedure of choice for lymphedema. This test is noninvasive, without side effects, and has an overall diagnostic accuracy of 93% (50). The procedure involves a subcutaneous injection of a radiolabeled tracer particle specific for the lymphatics. The diagnosis of lymphedema is made when no radioactivity can be detected in the regional lymph nodes one hour after injection. A CT scan of the pelvis should also be considered in those patients with lymphatic obstruction to rule out malignancy.

Treatment

Palliative therapy is the only treatment option for lymphedema, because there is no medical or surgical cure. The goal of therapy is to reduce the limb volume and prevent infectious complications. Medical treatment begins with the treatment of the inciting event if the lymphedema is acquired as in the case of filariasis. Concomitantly, all patients must be fitted with compressive stockings. For those who are refractory to stocking compression, the use of pneumatic compression has been shown to be effective in reducing the swelling. Compression therapy and skin care alone has resulted in an 80% improvement rate in patients with lymphedema of the lower extremity (51). It is imperative that patients understand the chronicity of this disease and the need to maintain the use of compressive stockings. In addition, it must be stressed to these individuals that meticulous foot care is also necessary to avoid fungal infections.

Pharmacotherapy has consisted of diuretics and benzopyrones. Diuretics are not recommended for routine use. They do remove excess fluid but do not change the high interstitial protein concentration and therefore do not alter the underlying pathology. Diuretics can provide short-term relief of the painfully swollen limb, when used on an intermittent basis. Benzopyrones have been demonstrated to reduce lymphedema by enhancing proteolysis via increased macrophage phagocytic activity (52). These drugs are used to provide slow relief of chronic lymphedema but have yet to be approved for use in the United States.

Only a small percentage of the patients with lymphedema require surgical intervention. Indications for operation include an extremely edematous limb, resulting in loss of function, and recurrent infections that are refractory to medical management. The operations for lymphedema are divided into two categories—excisional and physiologic procedures. Excisional operations remove the lymphedematous subcutaneous tissue and skin. This is preferably accomplished by staged subcutaneous excisions with preservation of a viable skin flap for primary closure. If this is not possible, the wound can be covered with split-thickness skin grafts; however, breakdown and ulceration of the skin graft is common, and therefore primary closure is preferred.

Physiologic procedures are geared toward reconstruction of lymphatic drainage. Microlymphatic venous anastomosis has been used for the treatment of obstructive lymphedema. This procedure is not applicable to those with primary lymphedema caused by hypoplastic lymphatics. The patient must have patent lymphatic vessels distal to the site of obstruction. The microsurgical lymph vessel-to-vein anastomosis is constructed to bypass the obstructed lymphatics. Long-term subjective improvement and limb volume reduction have been reported (53).

Complications

Episodes of lymphangitis occur several times a year in patients with lymphedema. This accounts for a significant amount of morbidity and accelerates the process of fibrosis. When infection occurs, systemic antibiotics and bed rest with leg elevation are required. *Streptococcus* is the most common inciting organism. In patients with recurrent infections, prophylactic antibiotic therapy is recommended.

A rare but deadly complication of lymphedema is lymphangiosarcoma. This malignant lesion is most frequently associated with postmastectomy lymphedema. It presents as a reddish purple lesion of the skin and subcutaneous tissue, usually appearing approximately 10 years after the onset of lymphedema. Treatment consists of radical amputation; however, prognosis remains dismal with an average survival of less than two years.

SUMMARY

Of all the venous disorders, DVT is the most serious and potentially life threatening. More than 50% of those with DVT progress to develop postphlebitic syndrome with its disabling consequences. Prophylactic measures in the hospitalized surgical patient are essential. Heparin therapy remains the mainstay of care for the patient diagnosed with DVT, and the inferior vena cava filter is an effective alternative for those with contraindications to anticoagulation.

Of the lymphatic disorders, lymphedema is the most important. This disorder may result from a congenital cause or may be the result of lymphatic obstruction from malignancy and radiation therapy. Therapy is based on external compression and avoidance of infection. A select group of patients with severe disease may benefit from operative intervention. All treatment is palliative, because there is no known cure for lymphedema.

REFERENCES

1. Dalen JE, Alpert JS. Natural history of pulmonary embolism. Prog Cardiovasc Dis 1975; 17:259–270.
2. Rosendaal FR. Risk factors for venous thrombotic disease. Thromb Haemost 1999; 82:610–619.
3. Bertelsen S, Anker W. Phlegmasia cerulea dolens: pathophysiology, clinical features, treatment, and prognosis. Acta Chir Scand 1968; 134:107–114.
4. Haeger K. Problems of acute deep venous thrombosis. I. The interpretation of signs and symptoms. Angiology 1969; 20:219–223.
5. Mitchell DC, Grasty MS, Stebbings WS, et al. Comparison of duplex ultrasonography and venography in the diagnosis of deep venous thrombosis. Br J Surg 1991; 78:611–613.
6. Thomas LM, MacDonald LM. Complications of phlebography of the leg. Br Med J 1978; 2:317–318.
7. Kakkar VV, Corrigan T, Spindler J, et al. Efficacy of low doses of heparin in prevention of deep vein thrombosis after major surgery: a double-blind, randomised trial. Lancet 1972; 2(7768):101–106.
8. Hirsh J, Warkentin TE, Shaughnessy SG, et al. Heparin and low-molecular-weight heparin. Chest 2001; 119:64S–94S.
9. Colditz GA, Tuden RL, Oster G. Rates of venous thrombosis after general surgery: combined results of randomized clinical trials. Lancet 1986; 2(8499):143–146.
10. Anderson DR, O'Brien BJ, Levine MN, et al. Efficacy and cost of low-molecular-weight heparin compared with standard heparin for the prevention of deep vein thrombosis after total hip arthroplasty. Ann Intern Med 1993; 119:1105–1112.
11. Abbate R, Gori AM, Fari A, et al. Monitoring of low-molecular weight heparins. Am J Cardiol 1998; 82:33L–36L.
12. Hyers TM, Agnelli G, Hull RD, et al. Antithrombotic therapy for venous thromboembolic disease. Chest 2001; 119:176S–193S.
13. Ridker PM, Goldhaber SZ, Danielson E, et al. Low-intensity warfarin for prevention of venous thromboembolism. NEJM 2003; 348:1425–1434.
14. Greenfield LJ. Deep vein thrombosis: prevention and management. In: Veith FJ, et al., eds. Vascular Surgery. Principles and Practice. 2d ed. New York: McGraw-Hill, 1994.
15. Warkentin TE. Heparin-induced thrombocytopenia: a clinico-pathologic syndrome. Thromb Haemost 1999; 82(suppl):439–447.
16. Semba C, Dake M. Iliofemoral deep venous thrombosis: aggressive therapy with catheter-directed thrombolysis. Radiology 1994; 191:487.
17. Killewich LA, et al. Spontaneous lysis of deep venous thrombi: rate and outcome. J Vasc Surg 1989; 9:89.
18. Kakkar VV, Lawrence D. Hemodynamic and clinical assessment after therapy for acute deep vein thrombosis. A prospective study. Am J Surg 1985; 150:54–63.
19. Meissner MH, et al. Deep venous insufficiency: the relationship between lysis and subsequent reflux. J Vasc Surg 1993; 18: 596–605.
20. Comerota AJ, Throm RC, Mathias SD, Haughton S, Mewissen M. J Vasc Surg 2000; 32:130–137.
21. Drucker EA, Rivitz SM, Shepard JA, et al. Acute pulmonary embolism: assessment of helical CT for diagnosis. Radiology 1998; 209:235–241.
22. Mullins MD, Becker DM, Hagspiel KD, Philbrick JT. The role of spiral volumetric computed tomography in the diagnosis of pulmonary embolism. Arch Intern Med 2000; 160:293–298.
23. Plate G, Einarsson E, Ohlin P, Jensen R, Qvarfordt P, Eklof B. Thrombectomy with temporary arteriovenous fistula: the treatment of choice in acute iliofemoral venous thrombosis. J Vasc Surg 1984; 1:867–876.
24. Greenfield LJ, Michna BA. Twelve-year experience with the Greenfield vena cava filter. Surgery 1988; 104:706–712.
25. Becker DM, Philbrick JT, Selby BJ. Inferior vena cava filters. Indications, safety, effectiveness. Arch Intern Med 1992; 152:1985–1994.
26. Greenfield LJ et al. Transvenous management of pulmonary embolic disease. Ann Surg 1974; 180:461–468.
27. Urokinase Pulmonary Embolism Trial Study Group. Urokinase pulmonary embolism trial. Phase I results. A cooperative study. JAMA 1970; 214:2163–2172.
28. Browse NL, Clemenson G, Thomas MI. Is the postphlebitic leg always postphlebitic? Relation between phlebographic appearances of deep-vein thrombosis and late sequelae. Br Med J 1980; 281:1167–1170.
29. Pappas PJ, Duran WN, Hobson RW. The pathology and cellular physiology of chronic venous insufficiency. In: Gloviczki P, Yao J, eds. Handbook of Venous Disorders. 2d ed. New York: Oxford University Press, Inc., 2001:58–67.
30. Gloviczki P, Bergan JJ, Rhodes JM, Canton LG, Harmsen S, Ilstrup DM, and the North American Study Group. Mid-term results of endoscopic perforator vein interruption for chronic venous insufficiency: lessons learned from the North American Subfascial Endoscopic Perforator Surgery (NASEPS) registry. J Vasc Surg 1999; 29:489–502.

31. O'Donnell TF. Venous valve transplantation and vein transposition for valvular incompetence of deep veins. In: Gloviczki P, Yao J, eds. Handbook of Venous Disorders. 2d ed. New York: Oxford University Press, Inc., 2001:336–346.

32. Burnand KG, Whimster I, Clemenson G, Thomas ML, Browse NL. The relationship between the number of capillaries in the skin of the venous ulcer-bearing area of the lower leg and the fall in foot vein pressure during exercise. Br J Surg 1981; 68:297.

33. Duffy DM. Small vessel sclerotherapy: an overview. Adv Dermatol 1988; 3:221–242.

34. Greene GL. Estrogen and progesterone receptor measurements with monoclonal antibodies. Int J Biol Markers 1988; 3:57–59.

35. Parra JR, Cambria RA, Hower CD, et al. Tissue inhibitor of metalloproteinase-1 is increased in the saphenofemoral junction of patients with varices in the leg. J Vasc Surg 1998; 28:669–675.

36. Hobbs JJ, ed. The Treatment of Venous Disorders. Philadelphia: JB Lippincott, 1977.

37. Bergan JJ. Varicose veins: chronic venous insufficiency. In: Moore WS, ed. Vascular Surgery. A Comprehensive Review. 3d ed. Philadelphia: WB Saunders, 1991.

38. O'Donnell TF Jr, et al. Doppler examination vs clinical and phlebographic detection of the location of incompetent perforating veins—a prospective study. Arch Surg 1977; 112:31.

39. Keith LM Jr, Smead WI. Saphenous vein stripping and its complications. Surg Clin North Am 1983; 63:1303–1312.

40. Sadick NS. Treatment of varicose and telangiectatic leg veins with hypertonic saline: a comparative study of heparin and saline. J Dermatol Surg Oncol 1990; 16:24–28.

41. Monreal M, Lafoz E, Ruiz J, Valls R, Alastrue A. Upper extremity deep venous thrombosis and pulmonary embolism: a prospective study. Chest 1991; 99:280–283.

42. Aburahma AF, Sadler DL, Robinson PA. Axillary-subclavian vein thrombosis. Changing patterns of etiology, diagnostic, and therapeutic modalities. Am Surg 1991; 57:101–107.

43. Horattas MC, Wright DJ, Fenton AH, et al. Changing concepts of deep venous thrombosis of the upper extremity—report of a series and review of the literature. Surgery 1988; 104: 561–567.

44. Erickson CA, Lanza DJ, Karp DL, et al. Healing of venous ulcers in an ambulatory care program: the roles of chronic venous insufficiency and patient compliance. J Vasc Surg 1995; 22(5):629–636.

45. Tilney NL, Griffiths HJG, Edwards EA. Natural history of major venous thrombosis of the upper extremity. Arch Surg 1970; 101:792–796.

46. Machleder HI. Evaluation of a new treatment strategy for Paget-Schroetter syndrome: spontaneous thrombosis of the axillary-subclavian vein. J Vasc Surg 1993; 17:305–315.

47. Leak LV. Electron microscopic observations on lymphatic capillaries and the structural components of the connective tissue-lymph interface. Microvasc Res 1970; 2:361–391.

48. Turk AE, Miller TA. Lymphedema and tumors of the lymphatics. In: Moore WS, ed. Vascular Surgery. A Comprehensive Review. 3d ed. Philadelphia: WB Saunders, 1991.

49. Kissin MW, Querci della Rovere G, Easton D, Westbury G. Risk of lymphoedema following the treatment of breast cancer. Br J Surg 1986; 73:580–584.

50. Gloviczki P, Calcagno D, Schirger A, et al. Noninvasive evaluation of the swollen extremity: experiences with 190 lymphoscintigraphic examinations. J Vasc Surg 1989; 9:683–689.

51. Pappas CJ, O'Donnell TF. Long-term results of compression treatment for lymphedema. J Vasc Surg 1992; 16:555–562.

52. Piller NB. Lymphedema, macrophages, and benzopyrones. Lymphology 1980; 13:109–119.

53. O'Brien BM, Mellow CG, Khazanchi RK, Dvir E, Kumar V, Pederson WC. Long-term results after microlymphaticovenous anastomoses for the treatment of obstructive lymphedema. Plast Reconstr Surg 1990; 85:562–572.

54. Sladen JG. Compression sclerotherapy: preparation, technique, complications, and results. Am J Surg 1983; 146:228–232.

47

Diseases of the Thoracic Aorta

Michael P. Macris and O. Howard Frazier

INTRODUCTION

With the advent of cardiopulmonary bypass, improved anesthetic techniques, and synthetic grafts, diseases of the thoracic aorta have become amenable to surgical treatment. However, despite these advances, surgical repair of aortic lesions remains one of the greatest challenges in cardiovascular surgery. These procedures are associated with substantial postoperative morbidity; for example, patients undergoing surgical repair of descending or thoracoabdominal aortic aneurysms have a 3.6% to 16% rate of postoperative paraplegia or paraparesis (1,2). Therefore, many surgeons do not perform thoracic aortic repairs, and others will do so only as a last resort.

Lesions of the thoracic aorta that may necessitate surgery include aneurysms, dissections, and traumatic pseudoaneurysms. In the past, syphilitic aneurysms were common; now, however, most thoracic aortic diseases result from atherosclerotic and degenerative processes. Early recognition and diagnosis, along with timely surgical intervention and improved preoperative and postoperative care, have resulted in long-term survival for patients with these lesions.

This chapter discusses the factors responsible for the development of thoracic aneurysms, aortic dissections, and traumatic pseudoaneurysms. It also discusses the physiologic principles that underlie the management of these conditions.

INTRINSIC THORACIC AORTIC DISEASE
Thoracic Aneurysms
Classification

Aneurysms of the thoracic aorta are classified according to type, shape, and location. Classification allows the surgeon to use a systematic approach in the treatment of these challenging vascular lesions. Thoracic aortic aneurysms involving all three layers of the arterial wall are called true aneurysms, whereas those involving only the tunica adventitia are called false aneurysms or pulsating hematomas. False aneurysms usually result from traumatic rupture, most commonly seen in decelerating blunt chest trauma.

Fusiform aneurysms, in which the vessel assumes a spindle shape, result in circumferential dilation of all layers of the aorta. These aneurysms may affect a localized portion or an extensive segment of the aorta, and they are usually related to degenerative diseases such as arteriosclerosis and cystic medial necrosis (3). Saccular aneurysms are localized spherical dilations that affect one segment of the vessel wall and are connected to the lumen by a mouth. The aneurysmal sac is usually filled with thrombus. These lesions typically form after an episode of bacterial endocarditis.

Aneurysms involving the aortic arch are classified into four categories, according to their location (4). Type A lesions are localized and saccular, involving only the transverse arch. Type B lesions are fusiform and involve the ascending aorta and arch. Type C lesions extend into the proximal descending aorta, and type D lesions are more extensive, involving the entire descending aorta (Fig. 1). Although type D lesions are the least common of the four types, they are the most challenging in terms of surgical therapy.

Aneurysmal disease of the aorta is often multifocal. In a review of 1510 patients with aortic aneurysms, Crawford and Cohen (5) found 191 patients (12.6%) with multifocal disease. Abdominal aortic aneurysms commonly accompany thoracic aneurysms. For this reason, the entire aorta should be evaluated when a patient is being considered for surgical treatment of an aortic aneurysm, because better results are obtained when both lesions are corrected at the same time.

Traumatic rupture of the aorta produces a false aneurysm, usually distal to the left subclavian artery at the level of the ligamentum arteriosum. This type of lesion is generally saccular and constitutes a surgical emergency, so it is most commonly seen in major trauma centers. These aneurysms are discussed below in the section on Traumatic Pseudoaneurysms.

Pathophysiology

Saccular and fusiform aneurysms of the aorta result from loss of structural integrity of the aortic wall and its individual components (6). Alterations in the tunica adventitia (7) and loss of lamellar units in the tunica media (8) have been cited as the major causes of aneurysmal dilation of the aorta. Unusual hemodynamic stresses and impaired blood flow may cause these pathologic changes as a result of deficient delivery of nutrients and ischemia of the vessel wall related to involvement of vasa vasorum by various degenerative, inflammatory, and infectious disease states. This assumption is supported by the following facts: (i) aneurysms are more common in the abdominal aorta than in the thoracic aorta and (ii) compared with the abdominal aorta, which has single lumbar vessels, the thoracic aorta has more vasa vasorum originating from a system of paired intercostal arteries (9).

Currently, most aneurysms of the ascending aorta exhibit the histologic characteristics of cystic medial necrosis (10), as originally described by Erdhiem (11). This type of pathologic lesion is found in patients with Marfan's syndrome (MFS) (12,13) and usually affects the aortic root, which is subject to high stress because of the velocity and

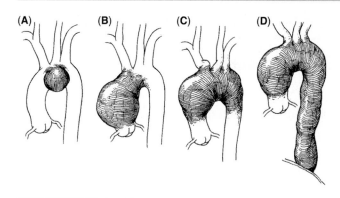

Figure 1 Cooley classification of aortic arch aneurysms. **(A)** Type A lesions are saccular lesions, confined to the arch. **(B)** Type B lesions are fusiform, involving the ascending aorta and proximal arch. **(C)** Type C lesions extend into the proximal descending aorta. **(D)** Type D lesions involve the entire descending aorta. *Source*: From Ref. 4.

turbulence of blood flow in this region.[a] The histologic pattern reveals necrosis and disappearance of muscle cells in the middle third of the tunica media, with disintegration of elastic laminae and collagen. A mucinoid material fills the cystic spaces. The primary lesion is accompanied by secondary tears caused by the underlying focal weakness (12–14). Annuloaortic ectasia represents a severe form of cystic medial necrosis in which electron-microscopic changes occur that are similar to those found in patients with MFS or forme fruste annuloaortic ectasia (15). This ectatic condition affects the entire ascending aorta, extending from the aortic annulus to the innominate artery. It may cause severe congestive heart failure related to aortic insufficiency, with a high risk of aortic rupture or dissection (16).

The concept of cystic medial necrosis as an intrinsic disease of the tunica media that causes aneurysms of the aorta has been challenged by Schlatmann and Becker (17). In histologic studies of the aortic media in 100 patients of different ages with normal aortas, these investigators found changes attributable to cystic medial necrosis, the frequency of which increased with age. They proposed that these changes result from hemodynamic stress on the vessel wall and represent a process of injury and repair in the normal aging aorta. Therefore, the ascending aorta, which is subject to relatively high hemodynamic stress, is the most common site of histologic changes caused by cystic medial necrosis.

Because of a steady increase in both the elderly population and clinicians' ability to control the late complications of syphilis, arteriosclerosis has become a more common cause of aortic aneurysmal disease. Arteriosclerotic aneurysms, which are confined mainly to the descending and distal thoracic aorta, are fusiform. Once the tunica media and tunica adventitia have been weakened by arteriosclerosis, the disease progresses steadily. It is aggravated by hypertension, progression of the dilation, and further ischemia of the aneurysmal wall. The primary factors that contribute to the formation of arteriosclerotic aneurysms are alterations in flow to the vasa vasorum of the vessel wall and disturbances in intraluminal flow patterns (7). Moreover, flow across stenotic plaques creates high lateral pressures, and turbulent,

reversed flow likewise strikes against the vessel wall. These stresses, which result in structural fatigue and subsequent dilation (18), may be of etiologic importance.

Through suppurative or granulomatous processes, infections of the vessel wall cause the formation of mycotic aneurysms (19). These aneurysms are usually saccular and can develop in any part of the aorta. Previously damaged vessels are most likely to be affected, and the resultant symptoms depend on the size and location of the lesion. Aortitis of unknown cause or associated with different autoimmune disorders is also characterized by aortic dilation and the formation of aneurysms. The exception is Takayasu's arteritis, which is primarily an inflammatory disease associated with severe stenotic lesions of the aorta and other large- and medium-sized vessels (19). Nonspecific aortitis may also result in multiple saccular aneurysms of the aorta, leading to death attributed to rupture (20).

Inflammatory aneurysms of the aorta are usually located in the terminal aorta and are accompanied by a severe retroperitoneal inflammatory process that encases the ureters and, sometimes, the vena cava. Histologic analysis reveals destruction of both the tunica media and the tunica adventitia, with replacement of these structures by a thick, fibrotic wall. Both layers are infiltrated with lymphocytes, plasma cells, lymphoid follicles, and multinucleated giant cells (21). When these aneurysms occur in the thoracic aorta, however, they usually do not involve the surrounding mediastinum and pleura.

Diagnosis

Clinical Presentation

The clinical presentation and symptomatology of thoracic aneurysms are related to the location of the lesion and the compression of adjacent structures. Erosion of large masses through the ribs and sternum is a late finding that is, fortunately, rarely seen these days. Symptoms include pain, stridor, and coughing caused by aneurysmal compression of the vagus nerves, trachea, and bronchi. With ascending aortic aneurysms that involve the aortic annulus, congestive heart failure commonly occurs as a result of aortic insufficiency. Free rupture into the pericardial sac or pleura is catastrophic and is usually diagnosed postmortem.

Occasionally, the diagnosis is suspected in a patient without symptoms, in whom routine chest roentgenography shows an upper mediastinal mass contiguous with the aortic shadow. In such cases, further studies are indicated to confirm the diagnosis.

---

[a] These conditions make aneurysms of the ascending aorta particularly dangerous to repair. Surgeons at Grady Hospital in Atlanta in the 1940s sometimes referred to these lesions as "four-poster" aneurysms; patients afflicted with them would be placed in four-poster beds with sheets hung over the posts to protect the ceiling from being spattered with blood when the aneurysm ruptured.

Special Diagnostic Techniques

The patient with thoracic aortic aneurysmal disease requires a thorough multidisciplinary evaluation to provide the surgeon with all the information necessary to plan the surgical procedure. Routine chest roentgenography and arteriography remain the standard evaluative techniques to which newer ones are compared. However, because the invasiveness of arteriography entails specific risks for critically ill patients, there is a trend toward use of less invasive diagnostic techniques. In particular, computed axial tomography is useful in clarifying certain characteristics of thoracic aneurysms, including their configuration and location, the extent of the disease process, and tissue modifications (Fig. 2).

Another method, magnetic resonance imaging (MRI), can produce images of mediastinal vessels along their axes and create sagittal and coronal views without degradation of spatial resolution (22). This technique is especially helpful in the recognition of annuloaortic ectasia and the serial evaluation of postoperative results or disease progression. Furthermore, recent advances in cardiovascular MRI technology allow the detection and even quantification of aortic valve insufficiency (23). Although MRI is not currently a primary method of assessing the condition of the coronary arteries, advances are being made in this area (24,25).

Since the early 1980s, two-dimensional (2-D) transesophageal echocardiography (TEE) has emerged as an important technique for visualizing the thoracic aorta (26–29). This method is highly sensitive and specific, particularly in the diagnosis of aortic dissection (30). It also seems well suited to detecting thoracic aortic aneurysms, especially in patients with unstable hemodynamics and a risk of aneurysmal rupture (26). Major advantages include safety, reproducibility, cost-effectiveness, and portability (because TEE can be performed at any location).

Although these newer techniques are attractive in the diagnosis of aneurysmal disease of the thoracic aorta, aortography is still usually preferred, because it provides a detailed image of the aortic lesion, the coronary arteries, and the branches of the aortic arch (27). Nevertheless, the newer techniques provide important information that, combined with the aortographic results, gives the surgeon a more complete anatomic picture of the diseased aorta and its branches.

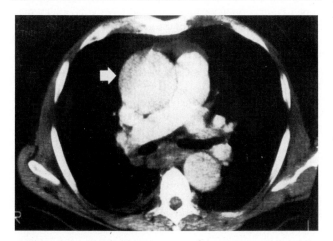

Figure 2 Computed axial tomogram showing an aneurysm of the ascending aorta (*arrow*).

Treatment

With the introduction of cardiopulmonary bypass, modern techniques of hypothermic circulatory arrest, and improved synthetic vascular grafts, surgical treatment of thoracic aortic aneurysms has become the standard approach to these difficult lesions. Most patients who do not undergo surgery for the treatment of these aneurysms die of rupture. Overall survival after emergency surgery is also dismal. Elective intervention, on the other hand, clearly results in lower mortality and morbidity rates (31). For these reasons, elective surgical repair is recommended if the patient has symptoms related to the aneurysm, if the diameter of the lesion is greater than 10 cm, or, in cases involving smaller lesions, if enlargement has been documented (32). Elective repair is also recommended for the patient with MFS, whose ascending aorta is more than 5.5 to 6.0 cm in diameter (32). Early and late risks of death are related to advanced age, the need for emergency surgery, and the presence of congestive heart failure and arterial hypertension.

The best surgical approach varies according to the aneurysm's location and specific anatomic characteristics. Unique surgical techniques and complications associated with aneurysms of the different segments of the thoracic aorta are discussed below.

Ascending Aorta

The treatment of choice for most ascending aortic aneurysms is surgical resection and graft replacement. Cardiopulmonary bypass with cannulation of the right atrium and femoral artery is instituted, when cannulation of the ascending aorta or proximal transverse aorta is not possible; otherwise, the ascending aorta is the preferred site. Once full cardiopulmonary bypass flow has been established, the patient is cooled to 18–22°C, after which the circulation is arrested. The distal ascending aorta is then transected, and an open distal anastomosis is performed (33,34). This technique allows better visualization of the distal aorta and is technically easier, because it allows better handling of the distal aorta. The flow is slowly restarted, and air is evacuated from the aorta. The graft is clamped, full flow is re-established, and the patient is rewarmed as the proximal anastomosis is performed.

A modified technique is used in the presence of associated aortic valve insufficiency and coronary ostial involvement. When the sinuses of Valsalva are not grossly dilated, supracoronary grafting and conventional aortic valve replacement is the procedure of choice, but care must be taken to prevent hemorrhage, damage to the coronary ostia, or the formation of pseudoaneurysms. If the sinuses of Valsalva are involved in the aneurysmal dilation and the coronary ostia are displaced 2 cm or more cephalad, one should use a valved conduit and reimplant the coronary ostia into the graft (Fig. 3) (4).

Normally, we prefer the classic technique of Bentall and De Bono (35) for repairing annuloaortic ectasia. Still, this approach can result in postoperative bleeding and false aneurysm formation at the anastomotic site between the coronary orifices and the valve-containing graft. To minimize the risk of these complications, we routinely create a fistula between the perigraft space and the right atrium, as recommended by Cabrol et al. (36). This step is accomplished by sewing the proximal apex of the aortotomy to a 2-cm slit in the medial aspect of the right atrial appendage. The rest of the aorta is wrapped snugly around the graft (37).

(A)

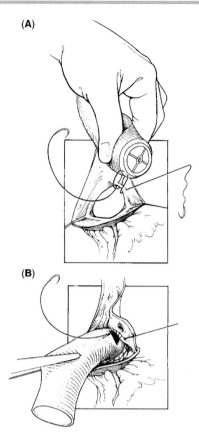

(B)

Figure 3 **(A)** Graft replacement of the ascending aorta with a valved conduit. **(B)** Reimplantation of the coronary ostia into the conduit. *Source*: From Ref. 4.

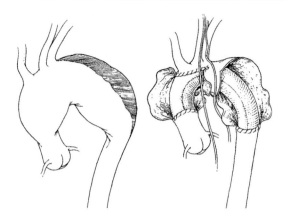

Figure 4 Graft replacement of a type C aortic arch aneurysm, with reimplantation of the great vessels into the graft. *Source*: From Ref. 4.

Transverse Arch

The treatment of transverse aortic arch aneurysms presents a special challenge to the cardiovascular surgeon. The most serious surgical complications are (i) cerebral damage resulting from cerebral ischemia and (ii) air or particulate embolization during graft replacement. Because of these risks, indications for surgery should be evaluated on an individual basis; elective surgical intervention should be reserved for lesions that approach 6 to 8 cm in diameter and cause symptoms related to the compression of vital structures.

Strategies for treating these lesions have included insertion of a temporary tube bypass, placement of temporary and permanent bypass grafts, cardiopulmonary bypass with separate perfusion of the brachiocephalic vessels, and cardiopulmonary bypass with profound hypothermia and circulatory arrest (4,38–40). Bypass techniques are complicated, however, as is separate perfusion of the brachiocephalic vessels, and the results are inconsistent.

Surgeons at the Texas Heart Institute in Houston have used hypothermic circulatory arrest, which provides adequate cerebral protection during arch replacement and eliminates the need for perfusion cannulas and excessive clamps, thereby offering a simplified operative field (41). The patient's core temperature is lowered to between 18°C and 22°C with a pump oxygenator and heat exchanger. The circulation is arrested, and the aneurysm is then repaired with a low-porosity woven polyethylene terephthalate

fiber (Dacron) graft, which is impregnated with collagen (Hemashield; Meadox Medicals, Oakland, New Jersey, U.S.A.) and does not require preclotting with autologous plasma and autoclaving (42). The proximal and distal anastomoses are created with a running, nonabsorbable monofilament suture (Fig. 4). Circulation is resumed gradually, with care to allow the air–fluid level of the blood to increase slowly, thus minimizing the risk of gross air embolization. The patient is gradually rewarmed at a rate of 1°C every three minutes, to minimize the production of gaseous microemboli.

This simplified technique of moderate hypothermia satisfactorily protects the cerebrum and myocardium for 20 to 30 minutes during circulatory arrest. Most of the neurologic deficits that result from this technique are transient; however, most fixed deficits appear to be caused by emboli; so special precautions should be taken to avoid particulate embolization from atherosclerotic aneurysms during graft replacement.

In recent years, further attempts at reducing neurologic injuries have included various forms of limited cerebral perfusion during the period of circulatory arrest. These techniques involve several approaches to perfusion: retrograde perfusion, which can be accomplished through the superior vena caval cannula; various antegrade methods, which may include direct cannulation of the great vessels; or cannulation of the right axillary artery, which perfuses the brain through the right vertebral and carotid arteries.

Descending Aorta

Most cardiovascular surgeons consider graft replacement the best surgical treatment for descending aortic aneurysms. They disagree, however, as to which approach should be used to avoid the complications related to this procedure.

Since the early days, when Carrel (43) found postoperative paraplegia in animals, this problem has been the most dreaded complication associated with operations on the descending thoracic aorta. The mechanism that causes spinal cord injury after cross-clamping of the proximal descending thoracic aorta is poorly understood. Several factors are probably responsible, but the primary ones appear to be interruption of blood flow and distal ischemia of the spinal cord, in addition to elevation of the cerebrospinal fluid pressure as a result of proximal hypertension (44,45). Accordingly, special attention has been devoted to understanding how blood is supplied to the distal spinal cord. The arteria radicularis magna anterior, also known as the artery of Adamkiewicz, originates between T9 and T12 and is responsible for supplying most of the blood to this segment of the spinal cord. Isolated ligation of this vessel in animals, without proximal cross-clamping or other hemodynamic alterations, results in a paraplegia rate of 71.4% (46), thereby establishing this artery's importance.

During the early days of aortic surgery, the value of systemic hypothermia as an adjunct for preventing ischemic spinal cord injury was demonstrated experimentally and clinically by Cooley et al. (4), DeBakey et al. (47), and by Pontius et al. (48). Nevertheless, the risk of cardiac arrhythmias and coagulopathies resulting from systemic hypothermia remained a problem (49). Other researchers have recommended the use of various shunts and partial bypass techniques (50–53), but the results have been inconsistent. Furthermore, these techniques are relatively complicated, so the operation is prolonged and made more difficult for surgeons who do not use these techniques routinely. Because the problem of perioperative paraplegia remains so serious, investigations have continued. Among the more commonly reported are techniques in serial clamping, selective cannulation and perfusion of the mesenteric and renal vessels, more extensive reimplantation of the intercostal arteries, and drainage of cerebrospinal fluid (54–59).

On the basis of their experience with these complex lesions, experts at two major vascular surgical centers advocate a simple cross-clamping technique without the use of adjuncts to prevent ischemia (40,60–62). They also recommend preventing hypotension, expeditiously removing the aneurysm and restoring distal flow, and avoiding cross-clamp times longer than 30 minutes, which are associated with a higher risk of postoperative paraplegia (63). We favor an "open" distal anastomosis technique, in which a single cross-clamp is placed proximal to the aneurysm to exsanguinate the lower body. The exsanguinated blood is collected by an autotransfusion device and returned to the patient. This approach minimizes the risk of spinal cord injury and renal insufficiency yet allows the distal anastomosis to be completed efficiently, with a short ischemic time (33,34).

Aortic Dissection

Pathophysiology

Dissection of the thoracic aorta is a unique entity characterized by a spontaneous tear of the tunica intima and part of the tunica media of the aortic wall. Blood escapes under pressure into the aortic laminae, causing a pathologic separation of the tunica media along the longitudinal axis of the aorta, parallel to the blood flow. This "false" dissecting channel in the middle of the aortic wall spreads downstream for a variable distance. It usually starts 2 cm distal to the aortic valve cusps (4,64). In most cases, a transverse intimal tear marks the beginning of the dissection, but this finding can vary. A tear in the ascending aorta is usually located in the right lateral aortic wall, and the dissection progresses along the greater curvature of the aorta. A reentry tear occurs much less frequently and may be difficult to identify. Dissections may also begin in the transverse arch or the proximal descending thoracic aorta, usually at the level of the isthmus, distal to the origin of the left subclavian artery. Once the dissecting process has begun, it progresses rapidly, depending mainly on the systemic blood pressure and the velocity of blood flow. The extent of the dissection appears

to be influenced by intrinsic characteristics of the vessel wall itself, but medial scarring related to atherosclerotic plaque formation seems to be the factor that usually limits the dissection (64).

A working classification of aortic dissections according to site of origin and extension provides a practical approach to these lesions and aids in their management (64). Type A dissections originate from a tear in the ascending aorta and may extend distally into the descending aorta. These dissections carry the greatest risk of rupture and are associated with acute aortic regurgitation and myocardial infarction related to dissection and obstruction of the coronary arteries. Type B dissections originate in the descending aorta, distal to the arch (Fig. 5). The dissecting process usually extends distally, but proximal dissection is also possible.

The cause of aortic dissection is still a subject of debate. This lesion was previously called a dissecting aneurysm, but the term "acute aortic dissection" is more appropriate, because the pathologic process is different from that of a true aneurysm, and aneurysmal expansion is seldom a particularly prominent feature. Although dissection was formerly attributed to cystic medial necrosis, Schlatmann and Becker (17) showed that the morphologic changes of aortic dissection may result from injury and repair within the aortic wall. Such changes alter the structural properties of the vessel wall, leading to dilation. The local hemodynamic circumstances determine whether further dilation, dissection, or rupture occurs. Patients with MFS, who most frequently have aortic dissections, have an underlying connective tissue disorder that makes them susceptible to aortic complications at an early age (65). Arterial hypertension is present in approximately 70% of patients with aortic dissection and is the most common predisposing factor for this condition. Other associated findings include trauma, a bicuspid aortic valve, aortic isthmic coarctation, and a previous aortotomy for cannulation in cardiopulmonary bypass.

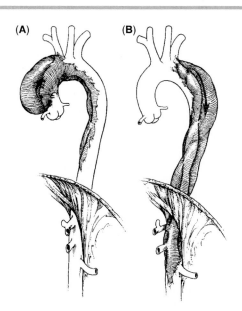

Figure 5 Classification of aortic dissections. **(A)** Type A lesions comprise the ascending aorta and may extend into the aortic arch. **(B)** Type B lesions originate in the proximal descending aorta, extending distally. *Source*: From Ref. 4.

Diagnosis

Clinical Presentation

The presenting symptoms of aortic dissection vary according to the location of the tear, the associated complications, and the degree of ischemia of vital organs in the presence of a blood supply that has been compromised by the dissecting process. The most common symptom is acute, severe chest pain that radiates to the back and abdomen. When the dissection extends into the innominate artery, compromising the right subclavian artery, the patient may also report numbness or pain in the right arm. Proximal dissections may result in aortic valve insufficiency, in which case, a diastolic murmur can be heard. In severe cases, the clinical presentation may involve signs and symptoms compatible with congestive heart failure.

Complications of acute aortic dissection are varied. Rupture of the aorta is the most devastating complication, leading to immediate exsanguination. Rupture may occur anywhere between the pericardial sac and the abdominal cavity. Obstruction of blood flow to vital organs by a medial hematoma of the wall vessel that supplies those particular organs may result in ischemia, producing myriad symptoms, depending on which organs are involved. Myocardial infarction, cerebrovascular insufficiency, stroke, transient ischemic attacks, renal failure, mesenteric ischemia, and even paraplegia may be the presenting manifestation of aortic dissection. As noted earlier, proximal dissection can result in dilation of the aortic annulus, causing acute aortic regurgitation and congestive heart failure.

Special Diagnostic Techniques

As with thoracic aneurysmal disease, aortography remains the gold standard for establishing the diagnosis of aortic dissection. The most common angiographic findings are opacification of the false lumen, visualization of the intimal flap, and deformity of the true lumen (Fig. 6).

Other, less invasive techniques are being used with increasing frequency. Two-dimensional echocardiography, particularly TEE, is useful in diagnosing dissection of the ascending aorta. In fact, many experts now consider TEE the method of choice in this setting (26,28,29,66). It has the advantage of being a bedside procedure, and it provides other useful information regarding the differential diagnosis. Moreover, it is faster and more accurate than aortography or computed tomography (CT) (67). The criteria for aortic dissection are (i) an aortic root measuring at least 42 mm, (ii) an intraluminal structure within the proximal aorta consistent with an intimal flap, and (iii) a high frequency of intimal flap oscillations, which is the most specific sign (68). Although computed axial tomography may be useful in elucidating various features of aortic dissection, 2-D echocardiography, especially TEE, offers better resolution, because it can more easily identify the intimal flap in cases of dissection (69).

Ultimately, MRI may prove the most useful of the new techniques. Currently, it is limited by high cost, long image-acquisition time, nonportability, and unsuitability for patients in a hemodynamically unstable condition. When further refined, however, MRI could rival TEE for diagnosing aortic dissection (70).

Treatment

Treatment of aortic dissection depends on location and associated complications. Type A dissections should undergo immediate surgical intervention and repair.

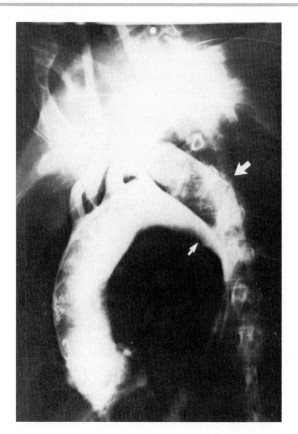

Figure 6 Arteriogram of a type B aortic dissection. Notice the opacification of the false lumen (*large arrow*) and compression of the true lumen (*small arrow*).

Uncomplicated type B lesions may be managed medically with close observation, intravenous administration of peripheral vasodilators to lower the systemic blood pressure, and β-adrenergic blockers to reduce the cardiac ejection velocity (71). Nevertheless, patients must be watched carefully to prevent associated complications, and not all authorities agree that medical management is the best approach. After analyzing results of surgical treatment of type B lesions, Reul et al. (72) recommended that patients with acute and chronic descending aortic aneurysms undergo early surgical repair before extension, rupture, or massive enlargement occurs.

Prophylactic surgery for aortic dissection is indicated in cases of MFS, in which the ascending aorta reaches a diameter of 6 cm, or twice the diameter of the normal aorta, as measured by echocardiography or CT scan. These patients are candidates for a composite graft repair, and early intervention has proved highly beneficial (73).

TRAUMATIC PSEUDOANEURYSMS

The present-day ubiquity of motor vehicles has produced a high incidence of blunt deceleration injuries. Traumatic rupture of the thoracic aorta occurs in approximately 10% to 21% of fatal traffic accidents (74,75). When traumatic aortic pseudoaneurysm occurs, only 20% of patients survive the initial injury. For this small group, mortality rate increases with time, with 49% dying within the first 48 hours, and only 2% surviving for more than four months if left untreated (76). Death results from rupture with immediate exsanguination.

Disruption is a result of shearing stresses at the junction of the fixed and mobile parts of the aorta (74), usually distal to the left subclavian artery at the ligamentum arteriosum. If the tear is complete, exsanguination is immediate, resulting in death at the scene. If the tunica intima and tunica media are disrupted but the tunica adventitia remains intact, a false aneurysm forms. The tunica adventitia, which contains the pulsating hematoma, cannot withstand the bursting pressure that an intact aorta could. Moreover, the tunica adventitia is susceptible to rupture during aggressive fluid resuscitation in the emergency department or at induction of anesthesia, when measures to counteract hypotension are taken (77). For this reason, if aortic rupture is suspected, careful monitoring of the systemic blood pressure to avoid extremes and rapid changes is mandatory.

Aortic transection should be suspected in any patient with blunt chest trauma. Chest roentgenography is the initial step in making the diagnosis. Loss of the aortic knob contour appears to be the most consistent and reliable sign of aortic laceration. Other findings include (i) a mediastinal-width/chest-width ratio greater than 0.25 on a supine chest radiograph, (ii) a left apical cap, (iii) rightward displacement of the nasogastric tube, the trachea, or both, (iv) displacement of the right paraspinous interface, and (v) depression of the left main stem bronchus (Fig. 7) (78). If the chest roentgenogram appears suspect, immediate aortography is indicated to confirm the diagnosis and localize the tear in order to plan a surgical approach (Fig. 8). Alternatively, TEE or CT may be used to screen patients for aortography (25).

Acute aortic transection and false aneurysm formation should be treated with immediate surgical repair through a left thoracotomy. Most of these lesions can be repaired primarily or with an interposition graft. Whether adjunctive measures to prevent spinal cord ischemia and renal failure are necessary, or even useful, remains controversial. As a rule, during operation for aortic transection, one should make sure that the left ventricle is not subjected to excessive

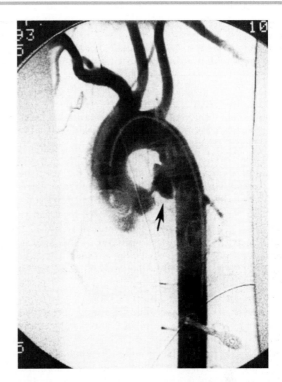

Figure 8 Digital-subtraction angiogram of the thoracic aorta in a patient with traumatic aortic transection and development of a false aneurysm distal to the left subclavian artery at the level of the ligamentum arteriosum (*arrow*).

stress as a result of proximal cross-clamping and that the total distal ischemic time is minimized. To accomplish these goals, surgeons have used numerous adjuncts, including partial bypass techniques and different types of shunts. Bypass techniques entail a higher mortality rate than do shunting and simple cross-clamping (79), probably because bypass necessitates the use of heparin (with its attendant complications) in the presence of multiple injuries. Simple aortic cross-clamping and use of an expeditious surgical technique to keep the ischemic time to less than 30 minutes form the procedure of choice for repairing acute traumatic rupture of the aorta (79,80).

SUMMARY

Because of the increasing size of the elderly population, aneurysmal disease of the thoracic aorta is usually related to chronic degenerative processes involving the different layers of the vessel wall. The concept of cystic medial necrosis as a primary disease of the ascending aorta has been challenged. Aneurysms are now believed to be a response to local hemodynamic factors that stress the aortic wall. Distal to the ascending aorta, arteriosclerosis is usually responsible for aneurysmal dilation of the aorta. The cause of arteriosclerosis is still uncertain, and preventive measures are controversial.

In addition, the genetic basis of aortic aneurysms is being currently investigated, in particular for Marfan kindreds, such that screening may be offered to the relatives and descendants of these patients (81–83). Ascending aortic

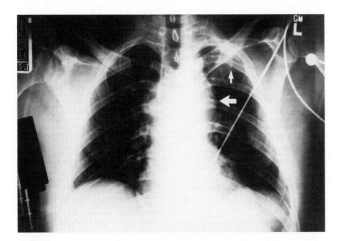

Figure 7 Chest X-ray of a patient with aortic transection. Note the widened mediastinum (*large arrow*), which indicates a mediastinal hematoma. Other findings include a left apical cap, loss of the aortic knob contour, and fracture of the left second and third ribs (*small arrow*).

aneurysms leading to type A dissections [thoracic aortic aneurysms and dissections (TAAD)] are the major cardiovascular complications of MFS, a pleiotropic disorder with involvement of the cardiovascular, ocular, and skeletal systems (84). MFS is inherited in an autosomal-dominant manner, and is caused by mutations in the fibrillin gene (FBN) 1 on chromosome 15q. FBN1 encodes fibrillin-1, a large glycoprotein that is a component of extracellular matrix structures called microfibrils. Clinical studies have indicated that up to 19% of nonsyndromic TAAD patients referred for surgery have affected first-degree relatives, supporting the hypothesis that genetic factors influence the formation of TAAD in individuals who do not have MFS. Aortic imaging of individuals at risk and analysis of the pedigrees determined that the condition is inherited primarily as an autosomal-dominant disorder with decreased penetrance and variable expression. Mapping studies using families with TAAD have identified three loci for the condition, TAAD1 on 5ql3-14, TAAD2 on 3p24–25, and FAA1 on 11q (85). Therefore, it is possible that, someday, gene therapy may even be available for some patients with aortic aneurysms.

The clinical presentations of thoracic aneurysms and dissections have been well described, and aortography has generally been the procedure of choice in confirming the diagnosis. Recently, however, there has been a trend toward the use of less invasive techniques. In some cases, particularly those involving thoracic aortic dissection, TEE has begun to supplant aortography. MRI, magnetic resonance angiography, and 3–D CT scan reconstruction are also very useful imaging methods.

Surgical repair is the treatment of choice for thoracic aneurysms and dissections. Because of the availability of cardiopulmonary bypass, improved anesthesia, advanced hypothermic techniques, and better prosthetic grafts, patients with these difficult lesions now have a greater chance of survival. Nonetheless, surgical repair retains a considerable amount of risk. As a result, the development of endovascular methods of excluding abdominal aortic aneurysms (86) has inspired several groups of investigators to attempt endovascular exclusion of thoracic and thoracoabdominal aneurysms. Reports of these studies describe mortality and paraplegia rates similar to or lower than those of surgery, but still less than optimal (87–90). Additionally, the long-term outcomes of these procedures are still being evaluated.

Combined surgical and endovascular approaches are also being tried. In these "hybrid" techniques, the endoluminal insertion of a stent graft to exclude the aneurysm may be preceded by surgical revascularization of adjacent arteries or followed by surgical fixation of the graft to the aorta (91–93). These techniques have only been tried in a small number of patients, however, and their long-term sequelae are not yet known. In conclusion, judging from the greatest improvements of the last 50 years, the management of thoracic aortic disease will continue to inspire surgeons for generations to come.

REFERENCES

1. Safi HJ, Miller CC, Huynh TTT, et al. Distal aortic perfusion and cerebrospinal fluid drainage for thoracoabdominal and descending thoracic aortic repair: ten years of organ protection. Ann Surg 2003; 238:372–381.
2. Svensson L, Crawford E, Hess K, Coselli J, Safi H. Experience with 1509 patients undergoing thoracoabdominal aortic operations. J Vasc Surg 1993; 17:357–370.
3. Richards MA. Medionecrosis aortae idiopathica cystica. Am J Pathol 1932; 8:717.
4. Cooley DA, Kneipp M, Lawrence EP. Surgical Treatment of Aortic Aneurysms. Philadelphia: Saunders, 1986.
5. Crawford ES, Cohen ES. Aortic aneurysm: a multifocal disease. Arch Surg 1982; 117:1393–1400.
6. Robicsek F, Tam W, Daugherty HK, Mullen DC. The applicability of Bernoulli's law in the process of enlargement and rupture of aortic aneurysms. J Thorac Cardiovasc Surg 1971; 61:472–475.
7. De Takats G, Pirani CL. Aneurysms: general considerations. Angiology 1954; 5:173–208.
8. Pomerance A, Yacoub MH, Gula G. The surgical pathology of thoracic aortic aneurysms. Histopathology 1977; 1:257–276.
9. Benjamin HB, Becker AB. Etiologic incidence of thoracic and abdominal aneurysms. Surg Gynecol Obstet 1967; 125: 1307–1310.
10. Klima T, Spjut HJ, Coelho A, et al. The morphology of ascending aortic aneurysms. Hum Pathol 1983; 14:810–817.
11. Erdheim J. Medionecrosis aortae idiopathica. Virchows Arch Pathol Anat 1929; 273:454.
12. Baer RW, Taussig HB, Oppenheimer EH. Congenital aneurysmal dilatation of the aorta associated with arachnodactyly. Bull Johns Hopkins Hosp 1943; 72:309–331.
13. Bahnson HT, Nelson AR. Cystic medial necrosis as a cause of localized aortic aneurysms amenable to surgical treatment. Ann Surg 1956; 144:519–529.
14. Rotino A. Medial degeneration, cystic variety in unruptured aortas. Am Heart J 1940; 19:330.
15. Savunen T, Aho HJ. Annulo-aortic ectasia: light and electron microscopic changes in aortic media. Virchows Arch A Pathol Anat Histopathol 1985; 407:279–288.
16. Chapman DW, Beazley HL, Peterson PK, Webb JA, Cooley DA. Annulo-aortic ectasia with cystic medial necrosis: diagnosis and surgical treatment. Am J Cardiol 1965; 16:679–687.
17. Schlatmann TJ, Becker AE. Histologic changes in the normal aging aorta: implications for dissecting aortic aneurysm. Am J Cardiol 1977; 39:13–20.
18. Holman E, Peniston W. Hydrodynamic factors in the production of aneurysms. Am J Surg 1955; 90:200–209.
19. Lande A, Berkmen YM. Aortitis: pathologic, clinical and arteriographic review. Radiol Clin North Am 1976; 14:219–240.
20. Henochowicz SI, Lindsay J Jr, Furlong MJ, Fulenwider AK, Greenfield DI, Ross EM. Multiple saccular aortic aneurysms in nonspecific aortitis. Am J Cardiol 1986; 57:377–378.
21. Crawford JL, Stowe CL, Safi HJ, Hallman CH, Crawford ES. Inflammatory aneurysms of the aorta. J Vasc Surg 1985; 2:113–124.
22. Moore EH, Webb WR, Verrier ED, et al. MRI of chronic posttraumatic false aneurysms of the thoracic aorta. AJR Am J Roentgenol 1984; 143:1195–1196.
23. Hoffmann U, Frank H, Stefenelli T, Kaiser B, Klaar U, Globits S. Afterload reduction in severe aortic regurgitation. J Magn Reson Imaging 2001; 14:693–697.
24. Kim WY, Danias PG, Stuber M, et al. Coronary magnetic resonance angiography for the detection of coronary stenoses. N Engl J Med 2001; 345:1863–1869.
25. Earls JP, Ho VB, Foo TK, Castillo E, Flamm SD. Cardiac MRI: recent progress and continued challenges. J Magn Reson Imaging 2002; 16:111–127.
26. Blanchard DG, Kimura BJ, Dittrich HC, DeMaria AN. Transesophageal echocardiography of the aorta. JAMA 1994; 272:546–551.
27. Earnest FT, Muhm JR, Sheedy PF II. Roentgenographic findings in thoracic aortic dissection. Mayo Clin Proc 1979; 54:43–50.
28. Goldstein SA, Mintz GS, Lindsay J Jr. Aorta: comprehensive evaluation by echocardiography and transesophageal echocardiography. J Am Soc Echocardiogr 1993; 6:634–659.
29. Wiet SP, Pearce WH, McCarthy WJ, Joob AW, Yao JS, McPherson DD. Utility of transesophageal echocardiography in the diagnosis of disease of the thoracic aorta. J Vasc Surg 1994; 20:613–620.
30. Ballal RS, Nanda NC, Gatewood R, et al. Usefulness of transesophageal echocardiography in assessment of aortic dissection. Circulation 1991; 84:1903–1914.

31. Pressler V, McNamara JJ. Aneurysm of the thoracic aorta: review of 260 cases. J Thorac Cardiovasc Surg 1985; 89:50–54.

32. Moreno-Cabral CE, Miller DC, Mitchell RS, et al. Degenerative and atherosclerotic aneurysms of the thoracic aorta: determinants of early and late surgical outcome. J Thorac Cardiovasc Surg 1984; 88:1020–1032.

33. Cooley DA, Baldwin RT. Technique of open distal anastomosis for repair of descending thoracic aortic aneurysms. Ann Thorac Surg 1992; 54:932–936.

34. Scheinin SA, Cooley DA. Graft replacement of the descending thoracic aorta: results of "open" distal anastomosis. Ann Thorac Surg 1994; 58:19–22.

35. Bentall H, De Bono A. A technique for complete replacement of the ascending aorta. Thorax 1968; 23:338–339.

36. Cabrol C, Pavie A, Mesnildrey P, et al. Long-term results with total replacement of the ascending aorta and reimplantation of the coronary arteries. J Thorac Cardiovasc Surg 1986; 91:17–25.

37. Lewis CT, Cooley DA, Murphy MC, Talledo O, Vega D. Surgical repair of aortic root aneurysms in 280 patients. Ann Thorac Surg 1992; 53:38–45.

38. Cooley DA. Aneurysms of the ascending aorta: surgical treatment using hypothermic arrest. Cardiology 1990; 77:373–387.

39. Crawford ES, Saleh SA, Schuessler JS. Treatment of aneurysm of transverse aortic arch. J Thorac Cardiovasc Surg 1979; 78:383–393.

40. Kay GL, Cooley DA, Livesay JJ, Reardon MJ, Duncan JM. Surgical repair of aneurysms involving the distal aortic arch. J Thorac Cardiovasc Surg 1986; 91:397–404.

41. Livesay JJ, Cooley DA, Reul GJ, et al. Resection of aortic arch aneurysms: a comparison of hypothermic techniques in 60 patients. Ann Thorac Surg 1983; 36:19–28.

42. Cooley DA, Romagnoli A, Milam JD, Bossart MI. A method of preparing woven DACRON aortic grafts to prevent interstitial hemorrhage. Cardiovasc Dis 1981; 8:48–52.

43. Carrel A. Experimental surgery of the aorta and heart. Ann Surg 1910; 52:83–95.

44. Blaisdell FW, Cooley DA. The mechanism of paraplegia after temporary thoracic aortic occlusion and its relationship to spinal fluid pressure. Surgery 1962; 51:351–355.

45. Oka Y, Miyamoto T. Prevention of spinal cord injury after cross-clamping of the thoracic aorta. Jpn J Surg 1984; 14:159–162.

46. Wadouh F, Lindemann EM, Arndt CF, Hetzer R, Borst HG. The arteria radicularis magna anterior as a decisive factor influencing spinal cord damage during aortic occlusion. J Thorac Cardiovasc Surg 1984; 88:1–10.

47. DeBakey ME, Cooley DA, Creech O Jr. Resection of the aorta for aneurysms and occlusive disease with particular reference to the use of hypothermia; analysis of 240 cases. Trans Am Coll Cardiol 1955; 5:153–157.

48. Pontius RG, Brockman HL, Hardy EG, Cooley DA, Debakey ME. The use of hypothermia in the prevention of paraplegia following temporary aortic occlusion: experimental observations. Surgery 1954; 36:33–38.

49. Cooley DA, Ott DA, Frazier OH, Walker WE. Surgical treatment of aneurysms of the transverse aortic arch: experience with 25 patients using hypothermic techniques. Ann Thorac Surg 1981; 32:260–272.

50. Donahoo JS, Brawley RK, Gott VL. The heparin-coated vascular shunt for thoracic aortic and great vessel procedures: a ten-year experience. Ann Thorac Surg 1977; 23:507–513.

51. Laschinger JC, Cunningham JN Jr, Nathan IM, Knopp EA, Cooper MM, Spencer FC. Experimental and clinical assessment of the adequacy of partial bypass in maintenance of spinal cord blood flow during operations on the thoracic aorta. Ann Thorac Surg 1983; 36:417–426.

52. Lawrence GH, Hessel EA, Sauvage LR, Krause AH. Results of the use of the TDMAC-heparin shung in the surgery of aneurysms of the descending thoracic aorta. J Thorac Cardiovasc Surg 1977; 73:393–398.

53. Zacharopoulos L, Symbas PN. Internal temporary aortic shunt for managing lesions of the descending thoracic aorta. Ann Thorac Surg 1983; 35:240–242.

54. Coselli JS, Conklin LD, LeMaire SA. Thoracoabdominal aortic aneurysm repair: review and update of current strategies. Ann Thorac Surg 2002; 74:S1881–1884.

55. Koksoy C, LeMaire SA, Curling PE, et al. Renal perfusion during thoracoabdominal aortic operations: cold crystalloid is superior to normothermic blood. Ann Thorac Surg 2002; 73:730–738.

56. Coselli JS. The use of left heart bypass in the repair of thoracoabdominal aortic aneurysms: current techniques and results. Semin Thorac Cardiovasc Surg 2003; 15:326–332.

57. LeMaire SA, Miller CC III, Conklin LD, Schmittling ZC, Koksoy C, Coselli JS. A new predictive model for adverse outcomes after elective thoracoabdominal aortic aneurysm repair. Ann Thorac Surg 2001; 71:1233–1238.

58. Coselli JS, Lemaire SA, Koksoy C, Schmittling ZC, Curling PE. Cerebrospinal fluid drainage reduces paraplegia after thoracoabdominal aortic aneurysm repair: results of a randomized clinical trial. J Vasc Surg 2002; 35:631–639.

59. Coselli JS, LeMaire SA, Conklin LD, Koksoy C, Schmittling ZC. Morbidity and mortality after extent II thoracoabdominal aortic aneurysm repair. Ann Thorac Surg 2002; 73:1107–1115.

60. Crawford ES, Rubio PA. Reappraisal of adjuncts to avoid ischemia in the treatment of aneurysms of descending thoracic aorta. J Thorac Cardiovasc Surg 1973; 66:693–704.

61. Crawford ES, Walker HS III, Saleh SA, Normann NA. Graft replacement of aneurysm in descending thoracic aorta: results without bypass or shunting. Surgery 1981; 89:73–85.

62. Livesay JJ, Cooley DA, Ventemiglia RA, et al. Surgical experience in descending thoracic aneurysmectomy with and without adjuncts to avoid ischemia. Ann Thorac Surg 1985; 39:37–46.

63. Safi HJ, Winnerkvist A, Miller CC III, et al. Effect of extended cross-clamp time during thoracoabdominal aortic aneurysm repair. Ann Thorac Surg 1998; 66:1204–1209.

64. Roberts WC. Aortic dissection: anatomy, consequences, and causes. Am Heart J 1981; 101:195–214.

65. Schlatmann TJ, Becker AE. Pathogenesis of dissecting aneurysm of aorta: comparative histopathologic study of significance of medial changes. Am J Cardiol 1977; 39:21–26.

66. Borner N, Erbel R, Braun B, Henkel B, Meyer J, Rumpelt J. Diagnosis of aortic dissection by transesophageal echocardiography. Am J Cardiol 1984; 54:1157–1158.

67. Erbel R, Engberding R, Daniel W, Roelandt J, Visser C, Rennollet H. Echocardiography in diagnosis of aortic dissection. Lancet 1989; 1:457–461.

68. Granato JE, Dee P, Gibson RS. Utility of two-dimensional echocardiography in suspected ascending aortic dissection. Am J Cardiol 1985; 56:123–129.

69. Iliceto S, Ettorre G, Francioso G, Antonelli G, Biasco G, Rizzon P. Diagnosis of aneurysm of the thoracic aorta: comparison between two noninvasive techniques: two-dimensional echocardiography and computed tomography. Eur Heart J 1984; 5:545–555.

70. Amparo EG, Higgins CB, Hoddick W, et al. Magnetic resonance imaging of aortic disease: preliminary results. AJR Am J Roentgenol 1984; 143:1203–1209.

71. Doroghazi RM, Slater EE, DeSanctis RW. Medical therapy for aortic dissections. J Cardiovasc Med 1981; 6:187.

72. Reul GJ, Cooley DA, Hallman GL, Reddy SB, Kyger ER III, Wukasch DC. Dissecting aneurysm of the descending aorta: improved surgical results in 91 patients. Arch Surg 1975; 110:632–640.

73. Gott VL, Pyeritz RE, Magovern GJ Jr, Cameron DE, McKusick VA. Surgical treatment of aneurysms of the ascending aorta in the Marfan syndrome: results of composite-graft repair in 50 patients. N Engl J Med 1986; 314:1070–1074.

74. Greendyke RM. Traumatic rupture of aorta; special reference to automobile accidents. JAMA 1966; 195:527–530.

75. Richens D, Kotidis K, Neale M, Oakley C, Fails A. Rupture of the aorta following road traffic accidents in the United Kingdom 1992–1999: the results of the co-operative crash injury study. Eur J Cardiothorac Surg 2003; 23:143–148.

76. Parmley LF, Mattingly TW, Manion WC, Jahnke EJ Jr. Nonpenetrating traumatic injury of the aorta. Circulation 1958; 17:1086–1101.

77. Stiles QR, Cohlmia GS, Smith JH, Dunn JT, Yellin AE. Management of injuries of the thoracic and abdominal aorta. Am J Surg 1985; 150:132–140.

78. Sefczek DM, Sefczek RJ, Deeb ZL. Radiographic signs of acute traumatic rupture of the thoracic aorta. AJR Am J Roentgenol 1983; 141:1259–1262.

79. Mattox KL, Holzman M, Pickard LR, Beall AC Jr, DeBakey ME. Clamp/repair: a safe technique for treatment of blunt injury to the descending thoracic aorta. Ann Thorac Surg 1985; 40:456–463.

80. Svensson LG, Antunes MD, Kinsley RH. Traumatic rupture of the thoracic aorta: a report of 14 cases and a review of the literature. S Afr Med J 1985; 67:853–857.

81. Khau Van Kien P, Wolf JE, Mathieu F, et al. Familial thoracic aortic aneurysm/dissection with patent ductus arteriosus: genetic arguments for a particular pathophysiological entity. Eur J Hum Genet 2004; 12:173–180.

82. Hasham SN, Willing MC, Guo DC, et al. Mapping a locus for familial thoracic aortic aneurysms and dissections (TAAD2) to 3p24–25. Circulation 2003; 107:3184–3190.

83. Kakko S, Raisanen T, Tamminen M, et al. Candidate locus analysis of familial ascending aortic aneurysms and dissections confirms the linkage to the chromosome 5ql3–14 in Finnish families. J Thorac Cardiovasc Surg 2003; 126:106–113.

84. Milewicz DM, Urban Z, Boyd C. Genetic disorders of the elastic fiber system. Matrix Biol 2000; 19:471–480.

85. Hasham SN, Guo DC, Milewicz DM. Genetic basis of thoracic aortic aneurysms and dissections. Curr Opin Cardiol 2002; 17:677–683.

86. Howell MH, Strickman N, Mortazavi A, Hallman CH, Krajcer Z. Preliminary results of endovascular abdominal aortic aneurysm exclusion with the AneuRx stent-graft. J Am Coll Cardiol 2001; 38:1040–1046.

87. Dake MD, Miller DC, Mitchell RS, Semba CP, Moore KA, Sakai T. The "first generation" of endovascular stent-grafts for patients with aneurysms of the descending thoracic aorta. J Thorac Cardiovasc Surg 1998; 116:689–703.

88. Fattori R, Napoli G, Lovato L, et al. Descending thoracic aortic diseases: stent-graft repair. Radiology 2003; 229:176–183.

89. Czerny M, Cejna M, Hutschala D, et al. Stent-graft placement in atherosclerotic descending thoracic aortic aneurysms: midterm results. J Endovasc Ther 2004; 11:26–32.

90. Scheinert D, Krankenberg H, Schmidt A, et al. Endoluminal stent-graft placement for acute rupture of the descending thoracic aorta. Eur Heart J 2004; 25:694–700.

91. Lawrence-Brown M, Sieunarine K, van Schie G, et al. Hybrid open-endoluminal technique for repair of thoracoabdominal aneurysm involving the celiac axis. J Endovasc Ther 2000; 7:513–519.

92. Kotsis T, Scharrer-Pamler R, Kapfer X, et al. Treatment of thoracoabdominal aortic aneurysms with a combined endovascular and surgical approach. Int Angiol 2003; 22:125–133.

93. Flye MW, Choi ET, Sanchez LA, et al. Retrograde visceral vessel revascularization followed by endovascular aneurysm exclusion as an alternative to open surgical repair of thoracoabdominal aortic aneurysm. J Vasc Surg 2004; 39:454–458.

48

Secondary Hypertension: Pathophysiology and Operative Treatment

James C. Stanley and Gerard M. Doherty

INTRODUCTION

Hypertension is a common clinical abnormality in the Western world. Even though its precise etiology remains to be elucidated, it can be effectively managed in most patients with lifestyle changes, such as exercise and weight control, either alone or in conjunction with a variety of pharmacological agents, including diuretics, angiotensin-converting enzyme (ACE) inhibitors, calcium channel blockers, and beta-adrenergic antagonists. In contrast, surgically correctable forms of hypertension are infrequently encountered in clinical practice. Two diseases of the adrenal gland exhibiting abnormal aldosterone and catecholamine production and a number of renal artery occlusive lesions associated with excess renin–angiotensin activity, often present clinically with blood pressure elevations. Several other endocrine diseases, including hyperthyroidism, pituitary-dependent Cushing's disease, ectopic adrenocorticotropin (ACTH) production by pancreatic tumors, and reninomas can all cause hypertension, however, they are very rare. Similarly, renal artery occlusions and secondary hypertension due to emboli and dissections are quite uncommon. Contemporary practice requires a thorough understanding of the more common correctable forms of hypertension associated with adrenal and renal diseases. An understanding of these abnormalities is the focus of this chapter. For a more comprehensive discussion of adrenal gland physiology and pathophysiology, the reader is referred to the chapter on that subject.

ADRENAL DISEASE AND HYPERTENSION
Normal Adrenal Anatomy and Mineral Corticoid Production

The adrenal glands are paired organs with a normal combined weight of 7 to 12 g (1). They can expand 100-fold in the setting of adrenal hyperplasia or tumors. The right adrenal gland is located superior to the right kidney and directly posterior to the inferior vena cava along the right crus of the diaphragm. The left adrenal gland resides atop the left renal vein, medial to the superior pole of the left kidney, just lateral to the aorta, and posterior to the tail of the pancreas.

The adrenal gland arterial blood supply varies, with each gland often supplied by numerous, small branches from the aorta, inferior phrenic artery, renal artery, gonadal artery, and intercostal arteries. The venous drainage is more constant, with a single, main adrenal vein. The right adrenal vein is several millimeters in both width and length, draining directly from the anterior surface of the gland into the posterolateral aspect of the inferior vena cava. The left adrenal vein drains from the mid-portion of the posterior gland into the left renal vein. It is often joined by the left inferior phrenic vein. The majority of the lymphatic drainage from the adrenal glands is to the para-aortic, paracaval, and perirenal lymph nodes. The adrenal gland is divided into an outer cortex and inner medulla. The zona glomerulosa of the cortex, where aldosterone is produced, and the medulla, which produces catecholamines, are the two important functional areas of the gland.

Aldosterone

Aldosterone is the principal mineralocorticoid, secreted by zona glomerulosa cells, and regulated by the renin–angiotensin system, by plasma potassium concentration, and, to a lesser degree, by ACTH and plasma sodium concentration. Physiologic states that stimulate the renin–angiotensin system and aldosterone release include dehydration, hemorrhage, and upright posture. Postural effects are mediated by the sympathetic nervous system. Volume repletion decreases the activity of the renin–angiotensin system.

Normal daily aldosterone production is 100 to 150 mg. This hormone binds to albumin and transcortin, with only a small percentage of free aldosterone remaining available to target tissues. Plasma aldosterone half-life is 15 minutes. Aldosterone is metabolized in the liver and conjugated to glucuronidase, leading to its excretion in the urine. In liver failure, metabolism of aldosterone is impaired, leading to its elevated levels with subsequent fluid retention.

Aldosterone is the major regulator of extracellular fluid volume and potassium homeostasis. Its receptors are expressed on cells of the distal renal tubule, which is the major site of its action. Aldosterone binds to these receptors with high affinity. This results in retention of sodium and excretion of potassium. Sodium retention then leads to passive reabsorption of water and an increase in extracellular fluid volume. To balance aldosterone-mediated retention of positively charged sodium ions, the kidney epithelium releases intracellular potassium into the distal convoluted tubule for excretion in the urine. Hydrogen ion is also released, acidifying the urine (2).

Hyperaldosteronism

Hyperaldosteronism is a syndrome manifest by hypertension and hypokalemia, due to the autonomous adrenal secretion of aldosterone. It may result from an adrenal neoplasm with suppressed plasma renin, or it may be secondary, as a result of elevated plasma renin.

Primary hyperaldosteronism is twice as common in women as in men, and usually occurs between the ages of 30 and 50. Screening of hypertensive patients with plasma aldosterone and plasma renin activity (PRA) has revealed that primary hyperaldosteronism may be the underlying cause of up to 10% of cases of essential hypertension (3). Primary hyperaldosteronism is due to an aldosterone-producing adrenal adenoma in approximately a third of cases. This is responsible for Conn's syndrome. Idiopathic bilateral adrenal hyperplasia is responsible for the remaining cases. Adrenocortical carcinoma is a rare cause of primary hyperaldosteronism, as is an autosomal-dominant glucocorticoid-suppressible hyperaldosteronism resulting from the fusion of the ACTH-responsive 11-beta-hydroxylase gene promoter to the aldosterone synthase gene.

Secondary hyperaldosteronism is a physiologic response to the activated renin–angiotensin system, in cases of renal artery stenosis, cirrhosis, congestive heart failure, and normal pregnancy. In these situations, the adrenal cortex functions normally and secretes aldosterone in response to an elevated plasma renin and angiotensin. Secondary hyperaldosteronism is responsive to treatment of the underlying cause (3).

Clinical manifestations of primary hyperaldosteronism are attributable to aldosterone-mediated retention of sodium and excretion of potassium and hydrogen ion by the kidney, causing moderate diastolic hypertension. Edema is absent. Hypokalemia affects 80% to 90% of patients with primary hyperaldosteronism and can be easily provoked in the remaining patients. Potassium depletion in this setting frequently causes symptoms of muscle weakness and fatigue, polyuria and polydipsia, as well as impaired insulin secretion and fasting hyperglycemia. Primary hyperaldosteronism should be suspected in hypertensive patients with spontaneous hypokalemia (serum potassium concentration $< 3.5 \, \text{mEq/L}$), moderate hypokalemia (serum potassium concentration < 3.0) during diuretic therapy despite supplementation with oral potassium or use of potassium-sparing diuretics, or refractory hypertension without explanation. Because as many as 50% of hypertensive patients with hyperaldosteronism are normokalemic, it is advocated that all newly diagnosed hypertensive patients be screened by determining the aldosterone to renin ratio. A ratio of greater than 30 on two separate occasions in a normokalemic patient warrants further investigation (4,5). The essential hallmarks of primary hyperaldosteronism are (i) diastolic hypertension without edema; (ii) suppression of plasma renin in the face of volume depletion; and (iii) hypersecretion of aldosterone, which fails to suppress with intravascular volume expansion. Diagnostic evaluation must establish primary hyperaldosteronism, differentiate a surgically correctable adrenal adenoma from medically treatable idiopathic hyperplasia, and localize an adrenal tumor, if present.

Demonstration of an elevated plasma aldosterone concentration (PAC) in the setting of suppressed PRA is the best test to establish a diagnosis of primary hyperaldosteronism. The ratio of PAC to PRA in normal subjects and patients with essential hypertension is 4 to 10, compared to more than 30 in most patients with primary aldosteronism. A PAC $>20 \, \text{ng/dL}$ and a PAC/PRA ratio greater than 30 are diagnostic of an aldosteronoma, with almost 90% sensitivity. A serum potassium value less than $3.5 \, \text{mEq/L}$ and urinary potassium excretion greater than $30 \, \text{mEq/dL}$ also support the diagnosis of primary hyperaldosteronism. Hypokalemia and inappropriate kaliuresis may be present as well. It is important to recognize that before biochemical evaluation, patients need to be potassium repleted, have an adequate sodium intake, and medications including ACE inhibitors and spironolactone should be withheld for at least four weeks before testing.

An elevated PAC/PRA ratio alone does not establish the diagnosis of primary hyperaldosteronism, which must be confirmed by demonstrating inappropriate aldosterone secretion of less than $14 \, \mu\text{g}/24 \, \text{hr}$ in the urine with salt loading. This involves a 24-hour urine collection for sodium and aldosterone after three days of a high-sodium diet. An intravenous saline infusion test, fludrocortisone suppression test, and captopril challenge test are also reliable methods to confirm the diagnosis of primary hyperaldosteronism, although these tests are not usually required (3).

Once the diagnosis of primary hyperaldosteronism is established, distinction must be made between an aldosteronoma and idiopathic adrenal hyperplasia. Postural testing can give some indication of the source of hyperaldosteronism; however, a more definitive diagnosis depends on radiographic imaging and functional localization (6,7).

High-resolution computed tomography (CT) of the adrenal gland is adequate for localization of aldosterone-producing adenomas in more than 90% of cases (Fig. 1). The presence of a unilateral mass greater than 1 cm on CT and supportive biochemical evidence of an aldosteronoma are generally all that is needed to make the diagnosis in patients less than 40 years of age. The contralateral adrenal gland must be examined in patients presumed to have an aldosterone-producing adenoma, to ensure that bilateral hyperplasia is not present. Magnetic resonance imaging (MRI) may be useful during pregnancy or in situations in which administration of intravenous contrast medium is undesirable. NP-59 scintigraphy may also identify functional tumors but requires a tumor size greater than 1 cm for the imaging to be dependable (8).

Adrenal vein sampling to lateralize the source of aldosterone production is useful in patients with hyperaldosteronism when there is no adrenal abnormality on cross-sectional imaging, or when both adrenal glands are abnormal but asymmetric. Further, patients over 40 years of age, in whom the possibility of a nonfunctioning adenoma is statistically higher, may benefit from routine sampling. Percutaneous transfemoral cannulation of both

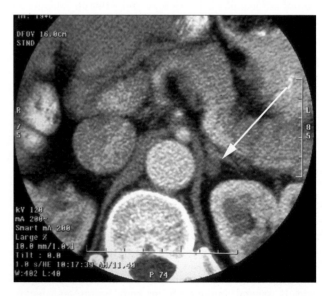

Figure 1 Computed tomography evidence of typical small, benign-appearing adrenal aldosterone-producing adenoma.

adrenal veins is performed and simultaneous blood samples for aldosterone and cortisol are taken before and after ACTH injection, and their ratios are determined. The aldosterone concentration should be at least fourfold higher on the side of an adenoma, whereas there is little or no gradient in patients with bilateral adrenal hyperplasia. A tenfold gradient of cortisol in adrenal veins to a peripheral sample ensures adequacy of adrenal vein cannulation. The former study is greater than 90% accurate and alters management in 30% to 50% of patients, even in those with an apparent unilateral adenoma. The test is technically difficult and may be unsuccessful in 25% of patients. Emerging data suggest that adrenal vein sampling may be superior to CT in differentiating the source of aldosterone production in patients with hyperaldosteronism (5,9).

Surgical removal of an aldosterone-secreting adenoma results in a durable improvement regarding hypertension and hypokalemia in 70% to 90% of patients. Laparoscopic adrenalectomy is the preferred approach to remove these tumors. Morbidity and mortality following these procedures are negligible. Preoperative spironolactone and potassium are given to replenish potassium stores and correct any existing alkalosis. A good response to spironolactone predicts a successful outcome after adrenalectomy. Response to adrenalectomy is also influenced by the duration and severity of hypertension. Age greater than 50 years, male gender, and the presence of multiple nodules within the adrenal are associated with a poor response to surgery.

Management of idiopathic adrenal hyperplasia is medical. In fact fewer than 20% of patients with this particular disease are cured by adrenalectomy. Idiopathic adrenal hyperplasia is treated with spironolactone or with the newer aldosterone antagonist eplerenone. Other potassium-sparing diuretics may be used, including triamterene and amiloride. Treatment of glucocorticoid-suppressible hyperaldosteronism includes dexamethasone 0.5 to 1.0 mg daily. Glucocorticoids are used in small doses to avoid Cushing's syndrome (5).

Normal Adrenal Catecholamine Production

Catecholamines of the adrenal medulla include epinephrine, norepinephrine, and dopamine. These vasoactive hormones are derivatives of the amino acid tyrosine. The biosynthetic pathway that converts tyrosine to active catecholamines involves four sequential enzymatic reactions: (i) tyrosine is converted to l-dihydroxyphenylalanine (dopa) by tyrosine hydroxylase; (ii) dopa is converted to dopamine by aromatic-l-amino acid decarboxylase; (iii) dopamine is converted to norepinephrine by dopamine beta-hydroxylase; and (iv) norepinephrine is converted to epinephrine by phenylethanolamine-*N*-methyltransferase(PNMT).Epinephrine is the major (80%) catecholamine stored in the adrenal medulla, followed by norepinephrine (20%) and dopamine (<1%). Tissue expression of the enzyme PNMT is limited to cells of either the adrenal medulla or the organ of Zuckerkandl, located near the aortic bifurcation; thus, most extra-adrenal pheochromocytomas produce norepinephrine, rather than epinephrine (10).

A complex regulatory network governs synthesis and secretion of catecholamines. Catecholamines are stored and secreted from granules within cells of the medulla, in association with the matrix protein chromogranin. Chromogranin A is measurable in the blood and its quantitation may support the biochemical testing for pheochromocytoma, as well as other functional neuroendocrine tumors.

Catecholamines act upon target tissues through membrane-bound adrenergic receptors. Pharmacologic distinction of adrenergic receptors is made based on their relative responsiveness to natural and artificial bioamines. The affinity of alpha-adrenergic receptors is highest for norepinephrine, less for epinephrine, and least for isoproterenol. Beta-adrenergic receptors are most responsive to isoproterenol and least responsive to norepinephrine. In addition, specific antagonists recognize each receptor class: alpha receptors are antagonized by phentolamine and phenoxybenzamine, and beta receptors are blocked by propranolol and related compounds. Beta-adrenergic receptor subtypes include beta-1 receptors, present in cardiac muscle, adipose tissue, and small intestine, and beta-2 receptors that occur in vascular, tracheal, and uterine smooth muscle, skeletal muscle, and liver. Alpha-adrenergic receptors are similarly subdivided: α-1 receptors mediate vasoconstriction, whereas α-2 receptors modulate presynaptic norepinephrine release and platelet aggregation (10).

Metabolism of Catecholamines

Metabolism of catecholamines occurs through three mechanisms: (i) specific uptake by sympathetic neurons, (ii) nonspecific uptake and degradation by peripheral tissues, and (iii) excretion in the urine. Catecholamines are metabolized in liver and kidney by two enzymes, monoamine oxidase (MAO) and catechol-O-methyltransferase (COMT). MAO and COMT convert epinephrine or norepinephrine to normetanephrine, and metanephrine, 3,4-dihydroxy-mandelic acid, and 3-methoxy-4-hydroxy-mandelic acid. These inactive metabolites are excreted by the kidney and are measurable in the plasma and the urine, either as free compounds or as conjugates of glucuronide or sulfate (10).

Adrenal Medullary Hyperfunction: Pheochromocytoma

Pheochromocytomas are rare adrenal tumors that are usually benign. However, primary tumors can occur outside of the adrenal gland, and tumors that arise either within or outside the adrenal gland can be malignant. This tumor is often described by the rule of ten's, that is, 10% familial, 10% bilateral, 10% extra-adrenal, 10% malignant, and 10% occurring in children. However, these figures underestimate the incidence of both malignancy and extra-adrenal primary tumors, each of which probably occur in closer to 20% of patients with pheochromocytoma (11).

Unilateral pheochromocytoma that occurs without evidence of familial tendency, based on family history, is still associated, in 25% of patients, with a germline abnormality predisposing to these tumors. This significant frequency mandates direct genetic testing in patients with apparently sporadic pheochromocytoma, to assess for multiple endocrine neoplasia type 2 syndromes, von Hippel–Lindau syndrome, and familial paraganglioma syndromes (12).

Clinical Presentation

Clinical presentation of a pheochromocytoma includes baseline hypertension, "spells," which classically include exacerbation of hypertension, and a variety of signs and symptoms that may include paroxysmal headache, dizziness, anxiety, tachycardia, nausea, or visual changes. The spells may occur seemingly spontaneously, or may predictably follow certain activities. This can be particularly true for some of the ectopic sites, where spells can be caused by local mechanical changes, such as micturition, sexual intercourse, or defecation, with tumors adjacent to the bladder (13). Patients may occasionally present with severe systemic illness, or death from hormone release from a previously occult tumor (10).

Diagnosis

Biochemical assessments should be performed before adrenal imaging in patients suspected of pheochromocytomas. The best test for the assessment of adrenal medullary hyperfunction is measurement of plasma free-metanephrine levels. This diagnostic test has supplanted the measurement of urine catecholamines and their metabolites. It is accurate and sensitive, and is marred only by some false-positive results with borderline elevated values. Measurements are interfered by use of a variety of drugs and dietary habits. In particular, patients should be withdrawn from adrenergic-blocking agents, and should refrain from consumption of grapefruit. Once the biochemical diagnosis is assured, then diagnostic imaging is appropriate.

Imaging, once the biochemical diagnosis of pheochromocytoma has been made, will localize the tumor. Because most pheochromocytomas reside in the adrenal gland, the initial localizing test should be a cross-sectional study of the adrenals, either by a high-resolution CT scan or by an MRI (Fig. 2). If the study shows a unilateral adrenal mass, without suggestion of malignancy or other extra-adrenal findings, then no further testing is necessary. In a consecutive series from the University of Michigan, of the 48 patients with a biochemical diagnosis of pheochromocytoma and a unilateral adrenal mass on CT or MRI, none had additional disease defined by the ^{123}I-metaiodobenzylguanidine (MIBG) scan. Of the 48 patients, 47 had a single unilateral focus of uptake defined on MIBG scan, and the remaining patient had a false-negative MIBG scan. Thus, the MIBG scan can be reserved for either patients whose disease is not apparent on the cross-sectional imaging, or those who have additional abnormalities, such as bilateral adrenal masses or extra-adrenal lesions (14). In the latter group of patients,[123]I-MIBG scans or somatostatin-receptor scintigraphy can identify other sites of disease (15).

Extra-Adrenal Primary Pheochromocytoma

Although most pheochromocytomas are unilateral adrenal-based lesions, occasional patients have tumors elsewhere in the body. Patients with disease at ectopic sites typically present with the same symptoms as those with adrenal gland tumors. Extra-adrenal tumors occur along the sympathetic chain, at any site from the skull base to the pelvis. The most common site for extra-adrenal pheochromocytomas, which are also sometimes called paragangliomas, particularly when they do not make appreciable amounts of catecholamines, is

the organ of Zuckerkandl. They may occur in the neck, posterior chest, atrium, renal hilum, and bladder. A common location of extra-adrenal tumors is between the aorta and vena cava at the level of the left renal vein, cephalad to the organ of Zuckerkandl tumors arising on either side of the superior mesenteric artery or more distally to the aortic bifurcation, where such may be mistaken for a lymph node metastasis. Middle mediastinal tumors, which may involve the heart, occur more frequently than was previously recognized. Extra-adrenal tumors have a higher reported malignancy rate of 25% to 40%, although not all reports agree on the differential aggressiveness of the extra-adrenal lesions (16,17).

Increased recognition of ectopic sites of primary pheochromocytomas is due a variety of newer diagnostic options. First, it is the improved accuracy of biochemical testing for pheochromocytoma with the current testing methods, particularly with the widespread availability of plasma metanephrine testing, and then, with the subsequent increased level of diagnostic certainty, improved imaging can be selectively and diligently applied. Current imaging, including high-resolution CT scan, MRI, and nuclear imaging with ^{123}I-MIBG or somatostatin-receptor scintigraphy, can localize tumors in many sites, which were simply not practical in the past, particularly if the biochemical diagnosis was equivocal (Fig. 3) (15,18).

Pheochromocytomas can also produce hormones other than catecholamines, including ACTH, calcitonin, somatostatin, vasoactive intestinal peptide (VIP), or serotonin. The production of these unusual hormones and their syndromes can lead to an extensive work-up to identify the responsible tumor.

Surgical Management

The best therapy for a localized pheochromocytoma at any site is resection, because this is the only potentially curative treatment. Regardless of site or number of tumors, all patients should be prepared with an α-adrenergic antagonist for one to two weeks preoperatively. One proven agent is phenoxybenzamine (Dibenzyline), which can be administered three times a day. Starting with a dose of 30 mg/day, the dose is increased every third day by 30 mg. The endpoint of therapy is orthostatic hypotension, although a clinical sign that the dose is adequate is the development of nasal congestion. This may be achieved with the starting dose, although some patients have required as much as 360 mg/day. An experienced and prepared

(A)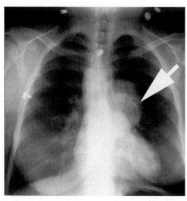

(B)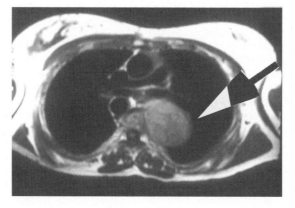

Figure 2 Ectopic pheochromocytoma during pregnancy. Worsening hypertension led to a biochemical evaluation that diagnosed pheochromocytoma. Initial imaging with ultrasound and abdominal magnetic resonance imaging (MRI) showed no evidence of the site of disease. **(A)** Chest x-ray revealed a left thoracic mass (*arrow*), and a **(B)** subsequent MRI provided improved anatomic delineation (*arrow*) facilitating second-trimester resection of the tumor.

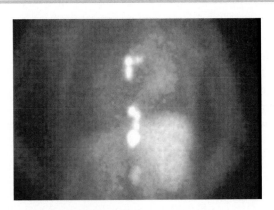

Figure 3 Metaiodobenzylguanidine scan demonstration of systemic malignant pheochromocytoma disease, with diffuse intra-abdominal and intrathoracic nodal disease.

anesthesiologist should be considered essential in managing the patient during surgery. Central venous and arterial pressure lines are placed for monitoring during induction of anesthesia and throughout the operative procedure (10).

A wide variety of operative approaches to the adrenal gland have evolved during the last eight decades. Each approach has its utility, and all belong in the repertoire of any surgeon operating on the adrenal gland. The initial approach to the adrenal glands was anterior, through bilateral subcostal or vertical midline incision. This allows wide exposure and the opportunity to explore both adrenal beds. A right thoracoabdominal incision allows access to the right chest and abdomen, to permit resection of large right adrenal tumors. It has the added advantage of facilitating vena cava and right atrium control for adrenal tumors with significant vascular invasion. The retroperitoneal approach uses posterior incisions in a prone patient. This offers the least morbidity to the patient, but is inadequate for resection of large adrenal tumors. However, the posterior approach offers advantages after extensive prior abdominal or retroperitoneal surgery. It has otherwise been superseded by laparoscopic adrenalectomy (19).

Minimally invasive approaches to the adrenal gland include anterior or lateral transabdominal laparoscopy (1,20, 21). Further, endoscopic retroperitoneal adrenalectomy can use either traditional laparoscopic instruments or 2 mm needlescopic instruments (22,23). Several authors have demonstrated the technical feasibility of a laparoscopic resection of lesions up to 15 cm. Because most hormonally active tumors are benign, and are identified at less than 5 cm diameter, the laparoscopic approach has proved ideal for most resections (24–28).

Numerous high-quality studies have compared traditional, open adrenalectomy to laparoscopic adrenalectomy (29–38). These have consistently demonstrated that patients who have the laparoscopic approach have decreased intraoperative blood loss, decreased length of hospital stay, decreased use of postoperative analgesics, increased rate of return to normal activities, improved cosmesis, and decreased late morbidity. Laparoscopic adrenalectomy has reduced overall costs, compared with open surgery (34,39). In spite of these advances, the traditional open approach retains utility for management of very large tumors, tumors with local invasion, and patients with extensive prior

surgery precluding insufflation. Extra-adrenal lesions, like those confined to the adrenal gland itself, now can be approached with minimally invasive resection techniques.

Malignant Pheochromocytoma

Malignant pheochromocytomas account for 10% to 15% of all cases, although various authors have reported an incidence ranging from 5% to as high as 46%. Extra-adrenal pheochromocytomas have been associated with a higher incidence of malignancy in most series reported, ranging from 20% to 40%, but this is not uniform (16). When collected series of pheochromocytomas are evaluated, and taking into account for selective referral bias, an overall malignancy incidence of 15% appears to be a reasonable estimate (11).

There are no certain histologic criteria that distinguish benign from malignant tumors. Even upon retrospective review, the distinction is often impossible because vascular and capsular invasion as well as mitotic figures can be readily identified in both benign and malignant lesions. Tumors without evidence of capsular or vascular invasion may have metastasized to distant sites, while other tumors with local capsular or even major venous invasion have apparently been cured by surgical excision. Malignancy can be positively diagnosed only when there is local invasion of tumor into surrounding soft tissue, or when the presence of tumor in nonchromaffin-bearing tissue outside the region of the sympathetic chain is identified. Tumors, also at increased risk for malignancy, are those pheochromocytomas that secrete only dopamine (10).

The median time of recurrence or identification of metastases is five to six years. Long-term follow-up is therefore advised, which should include regular blood pressure monitoring as well as annual biochemical studies for catecholamines and their metabolites. The current approach is to evaluate using plasma metanephrine measurements at least annually, except in those tumors that make only dopamine or ACTH, in which case, the specific biochemical follow-up depends upon the initial biochemical presentation (40–43).

The most common site for metastatic lesions is bone, where they present as lytic lesions of the spine, skull, or ribs. Other sites include liver, lung, and retroperitoneal or mediastinal lymph nodes. Malignant pheochromocytomas usually are slow-growing tumors, and long-term survival, although rare, has been reported, provided that control of symptoms caused by increased catecholamines is possible (10).

Once the diagnosis of malignant pheochromocytoma is established or suspected, ^{123}I-MIBG scintiscanning has proven effective in detecting the extent of the disease in most patients. CT and MRI may give additional anatomic information that may be helpful in determining resectability in patients whose disease is limited to soft tissue. Octreotide scanning and technetium bone scans have also proved useful in some cases (15).

Therapy

Therapy of malignant pheochromocytomas should initially be with an α-adrenergic-blocking drug, with the exception of those rare tumors secreting only dopamine. Most prefer phenoxybenzamine, gradually increasing the dose, to control hypertension. Small doses of a β-blocking drug, even when epinephrine levels are not excessively high, may also prove beneficial. In patients whose symptoms or blood pressure cannot be readily controlled with an α-blockade, additional antihypertensive therapy may be required. For patients with unresectable metastatic disease, alpha-methyltyrosine should be considered. This drug inhibits the

Table 1 Clinical Reports of Therapy for Pheochromocytoma with Cyclophosphamide, Dacarbazine, and Vincristine

Institution	Patients	Biochemical responses	Tumor responses
National Cancer Institute, USUHS (47)	14	11	8
University of Tsukuba, Japan (46)	3	3	Not reported
University of Michigan (45)	6	3	3

synthesis of catecholamines and may, in conjunction with an adrenergic blockade, offer long-term control of catecholamine-related symptoms.

After appropriate blockade, management of metastatic disease or recurrences includes wide local excision of surgically resectable disease as a first line of treatment. Unfortunately, this may only be palliative because of the presence of bone metastases. However, when tumor is limited to soft tissue, surgical excision may offer long-term palliation and even cure. Complete resection may require retroperitoneal lymph node dissection, liver resection, or soft tissue resection that includes other organs (e.g., kidney, bowel, and distal pancreas). Careful preoperative planning and imaging can help to "draw the dotted lines" sufficiently widely around the tumor to give the best opportunity for cure (16).

Until the past decade, no effective chemotherapeutic regimen had been reported. No single agent such as adriamycin or streptozotocin has ever been shown to be beneficial. However, a combination of cyclophosphamide, vincristine, and dacarbazine has resulted in a high incidence of both biochemical improvement (decrease in catecholamines) and tumor growth inhibition (Table 1) (44–47). This combination is currently considered the drug regimen of choice when chemotherapy is indicated.

External beam radiation treatment is effective for the palliation of bone pain. Therapeutic ^{131}I-MIBG has been used to treat patients with functioning metastases with encouraging results in selected patients with respect to decrease in both tumor size and circulating catecholamines (46,48–50). Less than a third of patients are candidates for treatment, which is based on the tumor's ability to concentrate sufficient ^{131}I-MIBG to be irradiated effectively. Although regression of tumor has been well documented

in some cases, the duration of effect has been limited to approximately two years and no patient has been cured.

RENAL ARTERY OCCLUSIVE DISEASE AND HYPERTENSION
Normal Physiology of the Renin–Angiotensin System

The renin–angiotensin system is of paramount importance in renovascular hypertension. Elements of this system that contribute to blood pressure control include (i) renin, produced in the kidney; (ii) angiotensinogen, produced in the liver; (iii) ACE, which is most active in the endothelium of the lung; (iv) angiotensin II, produced from angiotensin I by ACE; and (v) aldosterone, produced in the adrenal gland (Fig. 4).

Renin

Renin is produced by the juxtaglomerular apparatus of the kidney (Fig. 5). Major components of this anatomic region include (i) myoepithelioid cells or granular cells, located on the wall of the afferent arterioles; (ii) the macula densa, which is a specialized region of tubular epithelial cells, located in the glomerular hilus at the transition of Henle's loop to the distal convoluted tubule; and (iii) lacis cells, located in the region of the efferent glomerular arteriole and the macula densa. The lacis cells are intimately associated with the glomerulus and are anatomically similar to mesangial cells. An interrelationship clearly exists between these structures, with the function of the juxtaglomerular apparatus being translation of various signals into altered glomerular filtration and secretion of renin.

Mechanisms controlling renin production and its release from the kidney are very complex. Renal baroreceptors appear responsible for release of renin from juxtaglomerular cells, with these cells specifically acting as stretch receptors. The cellular basis for activation of these receptors seems to involve the calcium ion, with experimental evidence documenting an inverse relationship between renin release and intracellular calcium levels. Stimuli for renin release also include pressure changes at the afferent renal arteriole level, and renal interstitial volume and pressure changes. The importance of the tubular fluid milieu and the macula densa has been well established, with

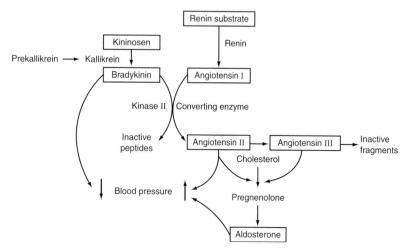

Figure 4 Renin–angiotensin system interrelation with aldosterone and bradykinin in the regulation of blood pressure. *Source*: From Ref. 51.

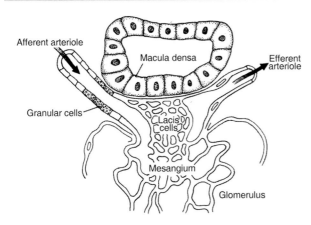

Figure 5 Anatomic components of the juxtaglomerular apparatus.

changes in sodium and chloride content of tubular fluid altering renin release. However, the relative importance of macula densa receptors in activation of the renin–angiotensin system in renovascular hypertension is uncertain. Stimulation of postganglionic sympathetic neurons to renal arterioles, many of which end in the region of the juxtaglomerular apparatus, also causes increased renin release. This may be due to afferent arteriolar constriction with decreased stretch of intrarenal vascular receptors and decreased sodium load to the macula densa, but it is more likely a direct result of catecholamine action on β-adrenergic receptors of the juxtaglomerular cells.

Renin, a proteolytic enzyme, is active at a neutral pH on its only known substrate, angiotensinogen. The renin gene in humans is located on chromosome 1 (Figs. 6 and 7).

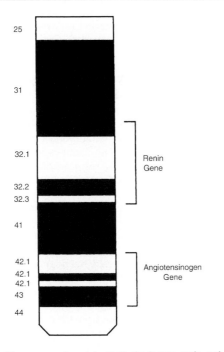

Figure 6 Chromosome 1 contains both the human renin and angiotensinogen genes.

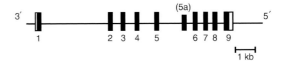

Figure 7 Human renin gene, consisting of nine exons and eight introns, with a 9bp miniexon (5a) of unknown function located between exon five and six. This gene is approximately 12.18 kb in length. The coding sequence (*black boxes*) is contained in the second to eighth exons and portions of the first and ninth exons.

It consists of nine exons and an additional miniexon, interrupted by eight introns. The renin gene is transcribed into renin mRNA and translated into a pre-prorenin molecule with a molecular weight of 45,000. Following cleavage and glycosylation in the rough endoplasmic reticulum, prorenin is produced with a molecular weight of 47,000. It is transferred into the Golgi complex, where it is rapidly secreted and processed to active renin, a single-chain polypeptide with a molecular weight of approximately 38,000. Extrarenal renin or renin-like enzymes (isorenins) have been found in the submaxillary salivary gland, uterus, placenta, and brain. No documentation exists that these latter substances are functionally important in elevating blood pressure.

Renin, once synthesized, is stored as granules within the juxtaglomerular cells, and, in some instances, as granules within the arteriolar wall. The release of both protein and renin into the extracellular space occurs by exocytosis. Renin has a half-life of approximately 20 to 30 minutes. Peripheral levels of circulating renin appear to be in a steady state, the sum of renin activity from both renal veins being approximately 48% greater than that in the infrarenal vena cava or arterial circulation (52). The major site for removal and clearance of renin is the liver (53).

Biochemical events related to the renin–angiotensin system have been relatively well defined (Fig. 8). The primary and perhaps only function of renin is the hydrolysis of the circulating renin substrate, angiotensinogen, to form angiotensin I. Angiotensinogen is an α_2-globulin with a molecular weight of 60,000, produced in the liver. The human gene for angiotensinogen is located on chromosome 1 (Figs. 6 and 9). It is composed of five exons interrupted by four introns. Gene expression is subject to a variety of physiologic and pathophysiologic stimuli, including steroid

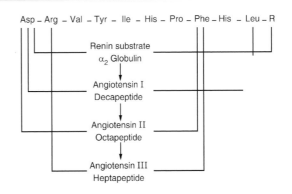

Figure 8 Biochemical composition of renin substrate and the angiotensins.

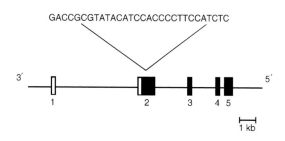

Figure 9 Human angiotensinogen gene, consisting of five exons and four introns. This gene is approximately 14.55 kb in length. The coding sequence (*black boxes*) for angiotensinogen is contained in the second to fifth exon. The second exon contains the coding sequence for angiotensin I.

hormones, angiotensin II, salt loading, and various drugs. Angiotensinogen itself is not vasoactive.

Angiotensin I

Angiotensin I, the decapeptide produced by the renin substrate–renin reaction, is relatively inactive. It does exert some effect on the adrenal medulla, the sympathetic and central nervous systems, and the renal arterioles. Quantitation of this intermediary is the basis for many radioimmunoassays of renin activity.

Angiotensin II

Angiotensin II is produced when two C-terminal peptides are cleaved from angiotensin I by a carboxypeptidase known as ACE. The resulting octapeptide is the major contributor to the vasoactive element of renovascular hypertension. Angiotensin II stimulates liver production of angiotensinogen, but in normal individuals, it provides a continuous negative feedback on the renal release of renin. Angiotensin II has a half-life of approximately four minutes.

Angiotensin III

Angiotensin III, which is a heptapeptide, is derived by aminopeptidase cleavage of angiotensin II to 1-des-aspartyl angiotensin II. Angiotensin III has biologic activity, although its levels are so low that its physiologic importance is questioned. Angiotensin III inhibits angiotensin II. Perhaps, its most relevant effect is stimulation of aldosterone synthesis.

Aldosterone

Aldosterone, a mineralocorticoid, is secreted from the zona glomerulosa of the adrenal cortex. The biosynthesis of this substance initially involves cleavage of the side of cholesterol to form pregnenolone. This step is facilitated by both angiotensin II and III. Aldosterone increases renal conservation of sodium and water, with a resultant expansion of the extracellular fluid volume and an eventual increase in blood pressure.

Angiotensin Converting Enzyme

ACE is a zinc metallopeptidase responsible for the generation of angiotensin II from angiotensin I by removing C-terminal peptides. The enzyme has a molecular weight of 150,000 to 180,000. Its gene has been mapped to chromosome 17 in humans. ACE has its highest concentration in the lung on the surface of endothelial cells. It also can be found at lower levels in the blood and kidney, as well as in other vascular beds. Conversion of angiotensin I to angiotensin II, at

physiologic concentrations, has been shown to occur in a single passage through the lungs.

ACE also plays an important role in the metabolism of the vasodepressor bradykinin. At least two enzymes appear to be responsible for the inactivation of bradykinin. The first is kinase I, which cleaves the carboxyl-terminal arginine of bradykinin. The second enzyme, kinase II, cleaves the carboxyl-terminal dipeptide group, Phe–Arg. Kinase II and ACE are considered the same, in that they have nearly identical substrate specificities, cofactor requirements, and antigenic specificities.

The most common technique for determination of PRA involves measurement of angiotensin I generation using a radioimmunoassay. PRA is expressed as the hourly rate of angiotensin I generation per unit of volume assayed. The assay involves two phases: (i) incubation of plasma to generate angiotensin I and (ii) measurement of generated angiotensin by the radioimmunoassay. Actual renin secretion is calculated as the renal arteriovenous difference in renin activity multiplied by renal plasma flow, and it is usually expressed as ng/mL/hr. Assay methods may vary among laboratories, often making interlaboratory comparisons difficult.

Angiotensins have actions on the cardiovascular system, central nervous system, adrenal gland, and kidneys (Fig. 10). The effects on cardiac activity, vascular smooth muscle reactivity, and salt and water metabolism are profound, and all contribute to increased arterial pressure. The most important consequence of renal artery occlusive disease is the production of angiotensin II, which by weight is one of the most potent pressor substances known. Angiotensin II acts directly on the arteriolar smooth muscle of nearly all vascular beds. The splanchnic, renal, and cutaneous circulations are most sensitive to its effects. Despite an acceptance of the central importance of angiotensin in the generation of renovascular hypertension, the relevance of absolute plasma levels remains unknown. The end-organ sensitivity to these vasoactive substances is often impossible to predict, because it is different in various physiologic and pathologic settings. In addition, the exact role in renovascular hypertension of locally secreted renin and locally generated angiotensin remains poorly defined.

Renal Blood Flow–Mediated Changes in the Renin–Angiotensin System

Hemodynamic responses to activation of the renin–angiotensin system by changes in renal artery blood flow depend on the rate at which renal blood flow is decreased, as well as whether one or both kidneys are at risk. Acute reductions in renal blood flow result in prompt blood pressure increases and increased plasma renin levels. Experimental animal models of renovascular hypertension are defined as two kidney–one clip (2K–1C), two kidney–two clip (2K–2C), or one kidney–one clip (1K–1C), depending on whether one or both renal arteries are constricted.

In instances of 2K–1C renovascular hypertension, where the total renal mass is not affected, the hypertension is characterized by renin hypersecretion from the affected kidney and contralateral suppression of kidney renin production (55,56). Sodium avidity within the affected kidney is counterbalanced by continuous sodium excretion from the contralateral kidney, resulting in relative intravascular volume depletion. This form of hypertension is angiotensin II dependent and responds to angiotensin antagonists and ACE inhibitors.

When the entire renal mass is at risk with 2K–2C or 1K–1C renovascular hypertension, pathophysiologic

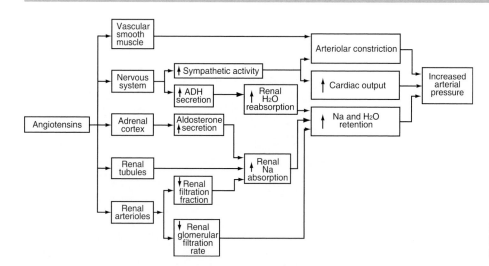

Figure 10 Effects of angiotensins contributing to increased arterial pressure. *Source*: From Ref. 54.

alterations are quite different and undoubtedly relate to changes other than vasoconstriction. Angiotensin II is known to be involved with sodium retention, decreases in glomerular filtration, stimulation of aldosterone production, and stimulation of norepinephrine release from the adrenergic nervous system. These effects may occur acutely, but in chronic 2K–2C or 1K–1C renovascular hypertension, it appears that sodium retention accounts for late reductions in renin secretion, although the absolute renin activity may be abnormal in relation to the existing state of sodium balance. Studies have been unable to demonstrate that blood pressure elevations depend on the renin–angiotensin system in sodium-replete chronic renovascular hypertension. In fact, angiotensin receptor antagonists or ACE inhibitors are effective in reducing elevated blood pressures only when the subjects are depleted of sodium.

Pathologic Types of Renal Artery Occlusive Disease

Various occlusive diseases affect the renal arterial circulation, ranging from common macrovascular narrowings to unusual microvascular arteriopathies associated with connective tissue diseases. Although relatively uncommon, renal artery emboli, spontaneous dissections, and traumatic occlusions are occasionally associated with acute forms of renin-mediated hypertension. The most often encountered causes of hypertension, secondary to renal artery occlusive disease, are those associated with atherosclerosis, arterial fibrodysplasia, and developmental renal artery stenoses (57–63).

Atherosclerosis

Atherosclerosis is the most common renal artery occlusive disease, accounting for approximately 95% of reported cases of renovascular hypertension. Atherosclerotic renovascular lesions are usually recognized in the sixth decade of life. Men are twice as likely as women to exhibit this disease. It is important to note that some degree of atherosclerotic renal artery stenotic disease affects nearly half the elderly population and that this is not always associated with elevated blood pressures.

Atherosclerotic renal artery occlusive disease typically involves the proximal third of the vessel with eccentric or concentric stenoses. In nearly 80% of patients, these lesions represent a "spill-over" stenosis associated with aortic

atherosclerosis (Fig. 11). Such lesions are bilateral in three-quarters of patients. When unilateral, the lesions seemingly affect the right and left sides with equal frequency, although the left renal artery often appears more severely diseased. Subendothelial and medial accumulation of cholesterol-laden foam cells and fibrosis are present in these lesions. Necrosis, hemorrhage, deposition of cholesterol crystals, calcification, and luminal thrombus formation are characteristic of complicated atherosclerotic plaques associated with advanced disease.

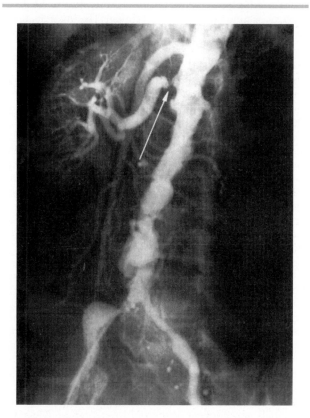

Figure 11 Characteristic proximal aortic spillover plaque of an arteriosclerotic renal artery stenosis.

Arterial Fibrodysplasia

Arterial fibrodysplasia is the second most common type of renal artery disease, affecting nearly 5% of patients with renovascular hypertension. Renal artery stenoses caused by dysplastic disease are a heterogeneous group of lesions classified by the specific pathologic process and the region of the vessel wall most affected. These lesions include intimal fibroplasia, medial fibrodysplasia, and perimedial dysplasia. The latter two entities appear to be a continuum of the same disease process. Each category has certain characteristic features that deserve mention.

Intimal Fibroplasia

Intimal fibroplasia accounts for approximately 5% of all dysplastic renal artery lesions. It affects infants and young adults more often than the elderly, and occurs with equal frequency in female and male patients. The cause of primary intimal fibroplasia is unknown, although some of these lesions may represent persistent myointimal cushions, originally occurring during fetal development. Secondary intimal fibroplasia has been attributed to trauma and the sequela of an earlier arteritis. Progression of intimal fibroplasia may cause an accelerated proliferation of fibrous tissue and rapid compromise of the arterial lumen.

Intimal fibroplasia usually appears as long, tubular stenoses of the main renal artery or web-like segmental renal artery lesions in young patients and as smooth, focal stenoses in adults. Proximal intimal stenoses are, most often, secondary lesions associated with aortic hypoplasia or coarctations, frequently in patients with neurofibromatosis. Subendothelial accumulations of irregularly arranged mesenchymal cells surrounded by loose fibrous connective tissue are typical of these intimal lesions that protrude as hillocks of tissue into the vessel lumen. The internal elastic lamina is usually intact, but partial fragmentation may occur.

Medial Fibrodysplasia

Medial fibrodysplasia is the most common dysplastic renal artery disease, accounting for 85% of such stenoses. It invariably affects women. Clinical presentation occurs most often during the fourth decade of life. This disease in its classic form has not been encountered before menarche. Medial fibrodysplasia appears to be a systemic arteriopathy in certain patients, with the internal carotid, superior mesenteric, and external iliac arteries being the extrarenal vessels most often affected. The cause of medial fibrodysplasia remains poorly defined, but appears to be associated with estrogenic effects on smooth muscle in women during their reproductive years, unusual stretch forces on affected vessels, and mural ischemia resulting from a paucity of vasa vasorum blood flow.

Morphologic changes of medial fibrodysplasia range from solitary stenoses in the middle and distal main renal artery to multiple constrictions with intervening mural dilations. The latter produce the lesion's classic string-of-beads appearance (Fig. 12). Actual macrovascular aneurysms, usually occurring at branchings, affect a little more than 10% of patients with arterial fibrodysplasia, but are rarely a cause of hypertension. Extension of medial fibrodysplasia into segmental branches occurs in approximately 25% of cases. Bilateral disease affects nearly 60% of patients and is usually most severe in the right renal artery. Unilateral lesions more commonly involve the right renal artery, with isolated disease of the right and left renal arteries existing in 30% and 10% of patients, respectively. Progression has

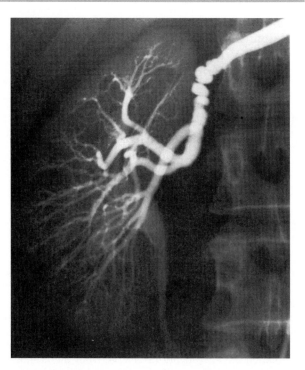

Figure 12 Characteristic string-of-beads appearance of renal artery medial fibrodysplasia.

been recognized in approximately 20% of patients, occurring more frequently in premenopausal women.

Diffuse medial fibrodysplasia is typified by severe disorganization of smooth muscle and the predominance of myofibroblasts, which appear responsible for excessive accumulations of ground substance encroaching on the vessel lumen. These stenoses occur adjacent to areas of atrophic smooth muscle and medial thinning, which are responsible for the mural dilations. Peripheral medial fibrodysplasia is a second form of this disease. It is characterized by fibroproliferative changes and loss of normal smooth muscle limited to the outer portion of the media. The latter findings are usually associated with less severe stenoses than with diffuse disease. Both the diffuse and peripheral forms of this disease may be observed in the same vessel.

Perimedial Dysplasia

Perimedial dysplasia accounts for nearly 10% of dysplastic renal artery disease. It invariably affects women, with its recognition usually occurring during the fifth decade of life. This particular dysplastic lesion appears to be more progressive than medial fibrodysplasia. Only 20% of patients have bilateral disease. Perimedial disease appears as solitary or multiple constrictions without intervening mural dilations. These stenoses involve distal portions of the main renal artery, usually without branch involvement. Excessive accumulation of elastic tissue in inner adventitial regions is characteristic of perimedial dysplasia. Abnormal increases in medial ground substances may also accompany this type of renal artery dysplasia. Certain histologic and ultrastructural features are common to both perimedial dysplasia and medial fibrodysplasia. Although perimedial dysplasia is classified as a separate pathologic entity, this may not be an appropriate distinction.

Developmental Renal Artery Stenoses

Developmental renal artery stenoses represent a third category of renal artery occlusive disease. Most are ostial in location, and many are associated with abdominal aortic narrowings. There is no gender predilection for any of the developmental lesions. Most are encountered in late childhood. Nearly 80% of patients with these stenoses have multiple renal arteries. It is believed that most of these lesions evolve because of faulty union of the metanephric vessels to the aorta during fetal development; at the same time, the two embryonic aortas fuse to become a single vessel. Other developmental stenoses are seen in association with neurofibromatosis, in which case, a growth disturbance of mesenchymal tissue is likely to underlie the hypoplastic character of these renal arteries. Fragmentation of the internal elastic lamina, incomplete formation of the media, and excesses of perimedial elastic tissue typify the stenoses of these diminutive vessels.

Renovascular Hypertension

The exact prevalence of renovascular hypertension among all patients with elevated diastolic blood pressures is unknown, but is probably close to 1%. It clearly occurs much more often in individuals having moderate or severe diastolic blood pressure elevations, with as many as 5% of such patients exhibiting underlying renovascular hypertension.

Clinical findings suggestive of renovascular hypertension include (i) systolic–diastolic upper abdominal bruits, (ii) initial diastolic blood pressures greater than 115 mmHg or sudden worsening of mild preexisting essential hypertension, (iii) development of hypertension during childhood, or (iv) sudden development of high blood pressure after the age of 50. Drug-resistant hypertension and malignant hypertension are also more likely to be associated with renovascular hypertension. Patients whose renal function deteriorates while receiving multiple antihypertensive drugs, especially ACE inhibitors, must also be tested for renal artery stenotic disease and renovascular hypertension. Clinical screening of patients is important before undertaking diagnostic studies for suspected renovascular hypertension. Otherwise, the costs of indiscriminate evaluations for this type of hypertension would be prohibitive. Many diagnostic and prognostic tests for renovascular hypertension represent methods of defining the anatomic presence of renal artery disease or pathophysiologic derangements of renal function due to the stenotic disease.

Contrast Arteriography

In the past, conventional contrast arteriography has been a standard study for the evaluation of all patients with suspected renovascular hypertension. Oblique aortography and multiple-plane selective renal arteriography can precisely define the morphologic character and extent of a stenotic lesion. Collateral vessels circumventing a stenosis are evidence of a lesion's hemodynamic and functional importance. Pressure gradients of approximately 10 mmHg are necessary for development of collateral circulation, and the same degree of pressure change is associated with activation of the renin system. Accordingly, collateral vessels circumventing a renal artery stenosis are invariably associated with increased renin release. Thus the importance of an otherwise benign-appearing stenosis may be established when collateral vessels are present (Fig. 13), or when dilution defects representing noncontrast-containing blood from collateral vessels entering the poststenotic portion of the vessel are identified with selective renal arteriography.

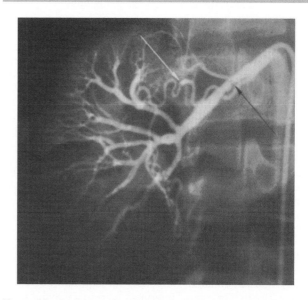

Figure 13 Arteriogram of a benign-appearing renal artery stenosis (*black arrow*) associated with a large collateral vessel (*white arrow*) circumventing the lesion, defining hemodynamic significance of the stenosis and implicating its functional importance. *Source*: From Ref. 64.

Digital subtraction arteriography following intra-arterial contrast injection has become commonplace. This technique allows the use of smaller amounts of contrast agents as compared to conventional arteriography, lessening potential nephrotoxicity. This is especially relevant in patients with preexisting impairment of renal function. The use CO_2 or gadolinium in the latter circumstances is also appealing, but may not always provide sufficient anatomic detail for clinical decision-making in patients with segmental arterial disease. Arteriography evidence of arterial nephrosclerosis should not be considered an indication that renal revascularization or angioplasty will not have a beneficial effect on blood pressure. This is in keeping with previous reports that biopsy evidence of nephrosclerosis is of limited prognostic value (65).

Computed Tomographic Arteriography

Computed tomographic arteriography (CTA) is another frequently used means of assessing coexistent renal artery and aortic disease. It allows computer generated visualization of the vessels from many different angles not possible with conventional biplanar studies. Newer 64-slice CTA images are likely to replace catheter-based angiographic studies. However, CTA does carry a similar risk of contrast-induced nephrotoxicity, which accompanies conventional iodine-related angiography.

Magnetic Resonance Angiography

Application of magnetic resonance technology to vascular imaging, especially with gadolinium enhancement, has evolved to a sufficient extent that it often provides high-resolution images of the renal arteries (66). Magnetic resonance angiography is not available at all institutions, and recent advances require further evaluation before it becomes widely used in assessing patients suspected of renovascular disease. Nevertheless, its noninvasiveness and lack of nephrotoxicity make it an attractive diagnostic test.

Deep Abdominal Renal Artery Ultrasonography

Hemodynamically significant renal artery narrowings and, in many instances, functionally important narrowings may often be identified by imaging the renal arteries and characterizing renal resistive indices and flow-velocity patterns with abdominal duplex ultrasonography (67–69). Such studies have been advocated in screening for renovascular disease and are useful in establishing the existence of a stenosis when peak systolic velocities are in the range of 180 to 200 cm/sec and the ratio of these velocities to those in the aorta approaches 3.5. Unfortunately, this technology does not provide discrimination of renal artery lesions exceeding 60% cross-sectional narrowing. Failure to identify a main renal artery in cases where no parenchymal flow signal exists suggests existence of a main renal artery occlusion. However, occluded accessory or segmental renal arteries may go unrecognized and thus contribute to false-negative assessments.

Renin Activity of Peripheral and Renal Venous Blood

Renin activity in peripheral and renal venous blood provides information about the functional importance of renal artery disease. To reduce interpretive errors evolving from minor fluctuations in basal renin activity, the renin–angiotensin system should be stimulated before sampling blood for renin assays. Blood samples for renin assays in the peripheral and renal circulations should be obtained simultaneously, or nearly simultaneously, with the patient tilted to a semi-upright position. Sodium intake should be limited to 20 mEq/day and a diuretic administered for three days before testing. Renin-suppressing drugs are discontinued when possible. Blood pressure elevations in such circumstances should be controlled with renin-stimulating agents such as hydralazine. The effect of ACE inhibitors in stimulating renin release and thus improving renin-assay results has not been achieved in general practice.

Renal Vein Renin Ratios

Renal vein renin ratios (RVRRs) are calculated by dividing the renin activity in venous blood from the affected kidney by that from the contralateral kidney. An RVRR >1.48 indicates functionally important renovascular disease (55,56). Because this test compares one kidney to another, it is not helpful in the presence of bilateral disease when both kidneys exhibit equal elevations of renin secretion. In fact, approximately 15% of patients benefiting from surgery have an RVRR <1.48.

Renal:Systemic Renin Index

Renal:systemic renin index (RSRI) is an expression of a single kidney's renin secretion. It is calculated by subtracting systemic renin activity from an individual kidney's venous renin activity and dividing the remainder by the systemic renin activity (55). In nonrenovascular hypertension, renal venous activity from each kidney is usually 24% higher than systemic activity (52). Thus the total of both kidneys' activity is usually 48% higher than systemic levels, balancing hepatic degradation and establishing a steady state.

In renovascular hypertension, the RSRI of the affected kidney becomes greater than 0.24. This is normally accompanied by suppression of contralateral kidney renin production with a drop in its RSRI <0.24. In the case of bilateral renal artery disease, this servomechanism may be lost, and autonomous release of renin from both kidneys may cause the sum of the individual RSRIs to be greater than 0.48. Renin production then exceeds normal hepatic degradation, and a hyperreninemic state evolves (Fig. 14).

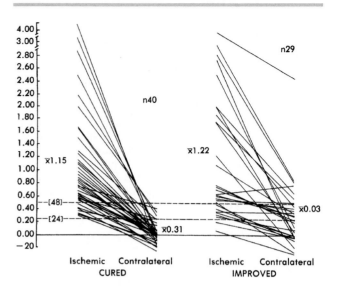

Figure 14 Renal:systemic renin indices, depicting their prognostic usefulness. *Source*: From Ref. 70.

RSRI documentation of renin hypersecretion and suppression allows the differentiation of patients most likely to be cured or improved following treatment (Fig. 9). The validity of ischemic renin hypersecretion (RSRI >0.48) from the kidney being revascularized and the contralateral renin suppression (RSRI <0.24, approaching 0) in identifying patients who will be cured has been well documented (55,56,60). However, the prognostic accuracy of RSRI may be limited in that approximately 10% of patients who are cured do not exhibit contralateral renin suppression.

Hypertensive Urography

It is a poor diagnostic test for renovascular hypertension, because of its limited sensitivity (71). Bilateral or segmental disease often precludes recognition of gross differences in contrast excretion between the two kidneys. In a large series of patients with proven renovascular hypertension, urograms were abnormal in only 27% of pediatric patients, 48% of patients with arterial fibrodysplastic disease, and approximately 72% of patients with atherosclerotic lesions (72). Nevertheless, rapid-sequence urography may contribute to the diagnosis of renovascular hypertension when (i) at least a two-minute delay in contrast appearance occurs within the collecting system of the affected kidney compared to that of the contralateral kidney; (ii) a length discrepancy is found, with the right kidney being 2 cm shorter than the left, or the left being 1.5 cm shorter than the right; and (iii) hyperconcentration of contrast in the collecting system of the affected kidney is observed on late urograms. Ureteral or pelvic irregularities caused by large collateral vessels may also accompany these urographic features.

Isotopic Renography

It has been used with both imaging and analysis of the washout curve of several tracers, the most common being ^{99m}Tc-DTPA (diethylenetriamine penta acetic acid),^{123}I or ^{131}iorthoiodohippurate,^{99m}Tc-MAG$_3$ (mercaptoacetylglycyl glycylglycine),^{99m}Tc-DMSA (dimercaptosuccinic acid), and ^{99m}glucoheptonate. These compounds provide an assessment of both renal blood flow and excretory function. Unfortunately, different states of hydration and intrarenal vascular resistance often result in flow abnormalities with false-positive studies in nonrenovascular hypertensive patients. The specificity and sensitivity of current studies are both approximately 75%. However, the sensitivity may be improved by administration of an ACE inhibitor to block the compensatory change in glomerular filtration, causing it to fall on the side of a stenosis. The sensitivity of the renogram increases to more than 80%, and the specificity of such a modified study approaches 85%. Renal perfusion–excretion ratios and more sophisticated computer programs offer a potential means of increasing the predictive value of radionuclide screening for renovascular hypertension, but they are not yet in widespread use.

Treatment

Treatment outcomes following interventions for renovascular hypertension relate to an accurate diagnosis and proper execution of an appropriate intervention, whether the intervention is arterial reconstructive surgery, ablative surgery, transcatheter renal infarction, percutaneous transluminal angioplasty, or institution of drug therapy. The specific type of renovascular disease being treated is also relevant to the expected therapeutic outcome. Although prospective randomized studies comparing medical and surgical therapy have yet to be published, long-term drug therapy has not been favored by most physicians responsible for the care of these patients.

Antihypertensive Drugs

Antihypertensive drugs developed during the past two decades have resulted in major improvements in the medical management of patients with renovascular hypertension. Vasoconstriction assumes greatest importance with a unilateral stenosis in patients having a normal contralateral kidney (2K–1C). Excessive sodium retention and hypervolemia become important factors in patients with bilateral renal artery stenoses (21C–2C), in those with unilateral stenoses affecting a solitary kidney (1K–1C), or in patients with contralateral parenchymal disease. Blood pressure elevations in most, if not all, patients with renovascular hypertension may be reduced by appropriate drug interventions. However, side effects, compliance, and effects on renal function must be considered before pursuing drug treatment.

Beta-blocking agents are usually the first drugs administered in known cases of renovascular hypertension, with subsequent reductions in renin release causing a lowering of the blood pressure (73). Propranolol and atenolol are most frequently used, although other β-blockers are also effective in treating renovascular hypertension. High doses of these drugs may be required to control the blood pressure, although in most cases, suppression of renin release may be accomplished with very small doses. In instances of more refractory hypertension, especially that caused by bilateral renal artery stenoses or unilateral lesions with contralateral parenchymal disease, addition of a standard diuretic such as a thiazide, a hydrogenated thiazide, or substituted compound is recommended. In cases of impaired renal function secondary to decreased blood flow, a loop diuretic such as furosemide provides a more effective diuretic action.

ACE inhibitors, such as captopril and enalapril, are used for treating hypertension in general. Antihypertensive effects other than decreased angiotensin II generation, such as those involving bradykinin, probably occur with the use of these agents. ACE inhibitors may be supplemented with β-blockers or diuretics in resistant hypertension. In more severe hypertension, vasodilators such as minoxidil may be required. It is important to recognize the deleterious

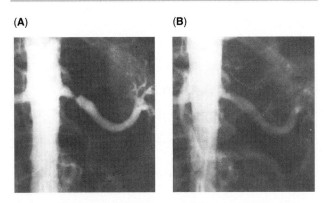

Figure 15 Percutaneous transluminal angioplasty. Renal artery stenosis: **(A)** before dilation and **(B)** after dilation.

effects of ACE inhibitors on renal function. This becomes especially evident in patients with bilateral renal artery stenoses, in cases of unilateral stenosis together with contralateral parenchymal disease, or when stenosis occurs in a solitary kidney (74). In these instances, severe deterioration of glomerular filtration may occur, and use of these agents is contraindicated.

Percutaneous Transluminal Renal Angioplasty

Percutaneous transluminal angioplasty (PTA) of renal arteries for the management of renovascular hypertension has important patient safety and cost benefits (Fig. 15). However, certain issues must be considered, including (i) differences in treating various types of renal artery disease, (ii) the frequency of being unable to catheterize or dilate a given type of stenosis, (iii) the long-term effects of angioplasty on the vessel wall, (iv) the incidence of renal and extrarenal complications, and (v) the durability of a successfully performed dilation.

Renal Artery Fibrodysplasia PTA provides the most benefits and fewest complications compared to PTA for other forms of renovascular disease. Medial dysplastic stenoses are most amenable to PTA and this is considered primary therapy for those lesions limited to the main renal artery. Excellent early technical and clinical results usually follow renal artery PTA in these patients (75–80). Similarly, these patients have experienced excellent long-term clinical results, with a primary patency rate of 87% after more than three years of follow-up (Table 2).

Table 2 Percutaneous Transluminal Angioplasty for Fibrodysplastic Renovascular Hypertension

Institution	Patients	Follow-up mean (mo)	Postprocedural blood pressure response (%)		
			Cured	Improved	Failed
Mayo Clinic	105	43	22	41	37
University of Virginia	66	39	39	59	2
University Hospital, Zurich, Switzerland	28	15	50	39	11
University of Florida	23	6	52	22	26
University Hospitals, Leuven, Belgium	22	26	95	–	5
Hospital Broussais, Paris	20	19	68	16	15

Source: From Ref. 81.

Table 3 Percutaneous Transluminal Angioplasty with Stent Placement for Arteriosclerotic Renovascular Disease

| Institution | Patients | Indication | | Follow-up mean (mo) | Post procedural blood pressure response (%)[a] | | |
		Hypertension	Renal insufficiency		Cured	Improved	Failed
Dorros-Feuer Foundation	76	76	48	6	6	46	48
University Hospital, Freiburg, Germany	68	68	29	27	16	62	22
Ochsner Clinic	66	66	Unknown	19	2	64	34
Polyclinique D'Essey	59	59	10	14	19	57	24
Hotel-Dieu de Montreal	33	33	17	13	6	61	33
University of Texas Health Center (Multicenter Study)	28	28	14	7	11	54	36

[a]Outcomes defined in reports from individual institutions.

Developmental renal artery narrowings represent true hypoplastic vessels that are less likely to be successfully dilated (82). In a like fashion, less common causes of renovascular hypertension in children, including arteritis, William's syndrome, and neurofibromatosis, do not respond well to renal artery PTA.

Aortic spill-over arteriosclerosis and isolated renal artery arteriosclerosis are quite different in regard to long-term clinical results (83–92). Historically, PTA alone, without stent placement, has resulted in a technical success rate of only 70% to 80%. Ostial spill-over lesions treated by PTA alone have a technical success rate of only 30% to 50%. These latter stenoses often manifest excessive recoil and many exhibit acute dissections. As a result of high early post-PTA restenosis rates, stenting of atherosclerotic lesions is considered appropriate in most patients. Results following renal artery stenting for atherosclerotic disease vary depending on outcome definitions and the indication for intervention, yet many studies have good long-term technical results (Table 3). In treating patients for hypertension, long-term benefits have been reported in 50% to 75% of cases. PTA with stenting for progressive ischemic nephropathy is not as effective at reversing renal failure. In these cases, benefits appear related to the degree and duration of ischemic nephropathy prior to PTA, with those having a serum creatinine of less than 2 mg/dL demonstrating the best response.

Complications accompanying renal artery PTA, for either atherosclerotic or fibrodysplastic disease, are uncommon, with severe complications occurring in less than a few percent of cases. Intimal disruption occurs more often with proximal renal artery dilation, where the vessel elasticity is greater and medial disruption is less likely. Medial tears are more common with distal renal artery dilation where vessel elasticity is less. Surgery following failed renal artery PTA is much more hazardous than primary surgery alone. PTA failures are associated with a much higher incidence of emergent repair and nephrectomy, and blood pressure benefits are significantly lower, being 57% after reoperation versus 89% for a primary operation (93).

Bypass Procedures

These are the most frequently used means of open renal revascularization for both atherosclerotic and fibrodysplastic stenoses (Fig. 16). Autogenous saphenous vein is the graft employed most often (59). Autogenous internal iliac arteries are the preferred graft when undertaking bypasses in pediatric patients (63), in that vein grafts placed in younger patients are often associated with late aneurysmal changes (94). Prosthetic grafts of knitted Dacron or expanded Teflon are used when autogenous conduits are not available. Limitations of prosthetic grafts relate to their potential for infection and technical difficulties in anastomosing them to small arteries. Although most bypass procedures are fashioned as aortorenal reconstructions, the aorta may be an inappropriate site for the graft to originate. In these latter circumstances, nonanatomic reconstructions with grafts originating from the hepatic or splenic arteries may be best for

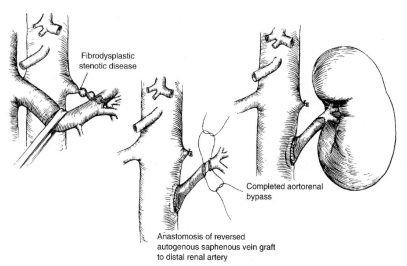

Fibrodysplastic stenotic disease

Completed aortorenal bypass

Anastomosis of reversed autogenous saphenous vein graft to distal renal artery

Figure 16 Renal revascularization. Bypass procedure with autogenous saphenous vein.

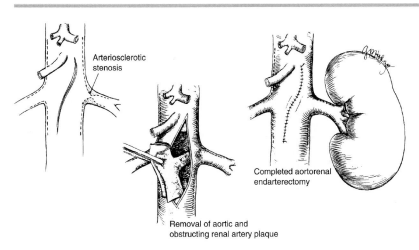

Figure 17 Renal revascularization by performance of an endarterectomy.

the patient (95,96). In some patients with ostial disease, especially in the pediatric-aged group (63), aortic reimplantation of the normal renal artery beyond its stenosis may be better than a conventional bypass.

Ex Vivo Renal Artery Reconstruction
It is an alternative to in situ repair for treating select cases of complex renovascular hypertension (97–99). This technique allows temporary removal of the kidney for precise microsurgical repair of the diseased vessel. Disruption of preexisting collateral channels, the need to cool the kidney, and the longer duration of such procedures are disadvantages of ex vivo reconstructions. This form of reconstruction is most applicable when treating multiple stenoses and aneurysms of segmental vessels.

Endarterectomy
Endarterectomy has been advocated in the treatment of most atherosclerotic renal artery stenoses (59,100–105). A transaortic approach with an aortotomy, extending along the lateral aorta from the level of the superior mesenteric artery to below the renal orifices anteriorly, is usually preferable to a direct longitudinal renal arteriotomy and local endarterectomy (Fig. 17). Endarterectomy through the transected infrarenal aorta during aortic reconstructive procedures has gained favor over bypass reconstructions in certain patients.

Conventional Surgical Therapy
Results of conventional surgical therapy for renovascular hypertension have been documented from many centers.

Loss of life during renovascular surgery occurs infrequently today, with overall operative mortality in most large series usually being less than 0.5%. Renal preservation and maintenance of renal function is clearly very important in assessing clinical experiences. Cumulative primary and secondary nephrectomy rates should not exceed 10%. Nephrectomy may provide good early results but obviously leaves the patient at considerable risk if contralateral disease evolves later. The incidence of nephrectomy during second surgery, for failed primary procedures, approaches 50% and emphasizes the importance of an appropriately performed primary revascularization (106).

Contemporary surgical treatment differences among the various series usually reflect the most prevalent renal artery disease entity causing the secondary hypertension (Table 4) (59). Pediatric patients with renovascular hypertension are most likely to be cured after restoration of renal blood flow, with a beneficial response expected in approximately 95% of such cases (Table 5). Adults with arterial fibrodysplasia benefit from surgery more often than those with atherosclerotic disease, which probably reflects the fact that coexisting essential hypertension and nephrosclerosis is quite uncommon in younger patients with arterial fibrodysplasia, compared to those with atherosclerosis (Tables 6 and 7). Atherosclerotic renovascular hypertension has often been considered a homogenous disease entity. However, at least two clinical subgroups of patients with atherosclerotic lesions exist: (i) those having focal renal artery disease, whose only clinical manifestation of their atherosclerosis is secondary renovascular hypertension,

Table 4 Comparative Results of Surgical Treatment of Renovascular Hypertension in Specific Patient Subgroups, University of Michigan Experience

Subgroup	Patients	Postoperative status[a]			Operative mortality rate (%)
		Cure rate (%)	Improvement rate (%)	Failure rate (%)	
Pediatric disease	34	85	12	3	0
Arterial fibrodysplasia	144	55	39	6	0
Arteriosclerosis					
Focal renal artery disease	64	33	58	9	0
Overt extrarenal disease	71	25	47	28	8.5

[a]Represents outcome of 405 operations (346 primary, 59 secondary), including initial nephrectomy in 17 patients.
Cure: Blood pressures were 150/90 mmHg or less for a minimum of six months postoperatively, during which no antihypertensive medications were administered. *Improvement*: Normotensive while on drug therapy, or if diastolic, blood pressures ranged between 90 and 100 mmHg, but were at least 15% lower than preoperative levels. *Failure*: Diastolic blood pressures greater than 90 mmHg but less than 15% lower than preoperative levels or greater than 110 mmHg. Lower pressure standards were used in evaluating children.
Source: From Ref. 72.

Table 5 Renovascular Hypertension in Children

Institution	Patients	Operative outcome (%)			Surgical mortality rate (%)
		Cured	Improved	Failed	
University of Michigan	57	79	19	2	0
Cleveland Clinic	27	59	18.5	18.5	4
University of California, Los Angeles	26	84.5	7.5	4	4
Vanderbilt University	21	68	24	8	0
University of Pennsylvania	17	76.5	23.5	0	0
Argentinean Institute, Buenos Aires	15	53	13	27	7
University of California, San Francisco	14	86	7	0	7

Source: From Ref. 59.

and (ii) those with clinically overt extrarenal atherosclerosis. The severity and duration of hypertension, age, and sex distribution in these two subgroups are often similar, but the surgical outcomes are very different. Improved renal function following revascularization is a well-recognized event, occurring most often among patients with profound preoperative impairment in renal function.

SUMMARY

Although most forms of hypertension can be effectively managed nonoperatively, three abnormalities fall under the umbrella of surgically correctable hypertension. These include two diseases of the adrenal gland exhibiting abnormal aldosterone and catecholamine production and a number of renal artery occlusive lesions associated with excessive renin–angiotensin activity. Of the three, renovascular hypertension is the most common cause of surgically

Table 6 Fibrodysplastic Renovascular Hypertension in Adults

Institution	Patients	Operative outcome (%)			Surgical mortality rate (%)
		Cured	Improved	Failed	
University of Michigan	144	55	39	6	0
Baylor College of Medicine	113	43	24	33	0
Cleveland Clinic	92	58	31	11	Unstated
University of California, San Francisco	77	66	32	1.3	0
Mayo Clinic	63	66	24	10	Unstated
University Hospital Leiden, The Netherlands	53	53	34	13	2
Vanderbilt University	44	72	24	4	2.3
Columbia University	42	76	14	10	Unstated
Bowman Gray	40	33	57	10	0
University of Lund, Malmo, Sweden	40	66	24	10	0

Source: From Ref. 59.

Table 7 Arteriosclerotic Renovascular Hypertension in Adults

Institution	Patients	Operative outcome (%)			Surgical mortality rate (%)
		Cured	Improved	Failed	
Wake Forrest University	500	12	73	15	4.6
University of Michigan	135	29	52	19	4.4
University of California, San Francisco	84	39	23	38	2.4
Cleveland Clinic	78	40	51	9	2
Columbia University	67	58	21	21	Unstated
University of Lund, Malmo, Sweden	66	49	24	27	0.9
Hospital Aiguelongue, Montpellier, France	65	45	40	15	1.1
Vanderbilt University	63	50	45	5	9

Source: From Ref. 59

correctable high blood pressure and results from altered renal circulatory hemodynamics causing the release of renin. This form of hypertension can be altered by several drug interventions, including those that diminish the release of renin, block the conversion of angiotensin I to angiotensin II. However, derangements of renovascular hypertension are best reversed by correction of the altered renal hemodynamics that usually result from renal artery stenosis. Surgical intervention with renal revascularization and PTA are presently the most appropriate means to this end. With respect to aldosterone or catecholamine-secreting tumors of the adrenal gland, surgical removal of the affected gland usually results in permanent cure of the hypertension. In most situations, this can be accomplished laparoscopically.

REFERENCES

1. Lal G, Duh QY. Laparoscopic adrenalectomy—indications and technique. Surg Oncol 2003; 12:105–123.
2. Linos D, van Heerden JA, eds. Adrenal glands: diagnostic aspects and surgical therapy. Berlin: Springer, 2005.
3. Gordon RD, Stomacher M. Overview of mineralocorticoid excess syndromes. In: Linos D, van Heerden JA, eds. Adrenal Glands: Diagnostic Aspects and Surgical Therapy. Berlin: Springer, 2005:115–126.
4. Stomacher M, Gordon RD, Gunasegaram TG, et al. High rate of detection of primary aldosteronism, including surgically treatable forms, after 'non-selective' screening of hypertensive patients [see comment]. J Hypertens 2003; 21:2149–2157.
5. Stowasser M, Gordon RD. Primary aldosteronism. Best Pract Res Clin Endocrinol Metabol 2003; 17:591–605.
6. Radin DR, Manoogian C, Nadler JL. Diagnosis of primary hyperaldosteronism: importance of correlating CT findings with endocrinologic studies. AJR 1992; 158:553–557.
7. Doppman JL, Gill J, John R, et al. Distinction between hyperaldosteronism due to bilateral hyperplasia and unilateral aldosteronoma: reliability of CT. Radiology 1992; 184:677–682.
8. Dunnick NR, Leight J, George G, et al. CT in the diagnosis of primary aldosteronism: sensitivity in 29 patients. AJR 1993; 160:321–324.

9. Stowasser M, Gordon RD. Primary aldosteronism—careful investigation is essential and rewarding. Mol Cell Endocrinol 2004; 217:33–39.

10. Gray DK, Thompson NW. Pheochromocytoma. In: Doherty GM, Skogseid BS, eds. Surgical Endocrinology. Philadelphia: Lippincott Williams & Wilkins, 2001:247–262.

11. Stenstrom G, Svardsudd K. Pheochromocytoma in Sweden 1958–1981. An analysis of the National Cancer Registry Data. Acta Med Scand 1986; 220:225–232.

12. Neumann HP, Bausch B, McWhinney SR, et al. Germ-line mutations in nonsyndromic pheochromocytoma [see comment]. NEJM 2002; 346:1459–1466.

13. Thrasher JB, Rajan RR, Perez LM, Humphrey PA, Anderson EE. Pheochromocytoma of urinary bladder: contemporary methods of diagnosis and treatment options. Urology 1993; 41:435–439.

14. Miskulin J, Shulkin BL, Doherty GM, Sisson JC, Burney RE, Gauger PG. Is preoperative iodine 123 meta-iodobenzylguanidine scintigraphy routinely necessary before initial adrenalectomy for pheochromocytoma? Surgery 2003; 134: 918–922.

15. Kaltsas G, Korbonits M, Heintz E, et al. Comparison of somatostatin analog and meta-iodobenzylguanidine radionuclides in the diagnosis and localization of advanced neuroendocrine tumors. J Clin Endcrinol Metabol 2001; 86:895–902.

16. Pommier RF, Vetto JT, Billingsly K, Woltering EA, Brennan MF. Comparison of adrenal and extraadrenal pheochromocytomas. Surgery 1993; 114:1160–1165; discussion 1165–1166.

17. Lumachi F, Polistina F, Favia G, D'Amico DR. Extraadrenal and multiple pheochromocytomas. Are there really any differences in pathophysiology and outcome? J Exp Clin Cancer Res 1998; 17:303–305.

18. Velchik MG, Alavi A, Kressel HY, Engelman K. Localization of pheochromocytoma: MIBG, CT and MRI correlation. J Nucl Med 1989; 30:328–336.

19. Kebebew E, Duh QY. Operative strategies for adrenalectomy. In: Doherty GM, Skogseid BS, eds. Surgical Endocrinology. Philadelphia: Lippincott Williams & Wilkins, 2001:273–290.

20. Kumar U, Albala DM. Laparoscopic approach to adrenal carcinoma. J Endourol 2001; 15:339–342; discussion 342–333.

21. Heniford BT, Arca MJ, Walsh MR, Gill IS. Laparoscopic adrenalectomy for cancer. Semin Surg Oncol 1999; 16:293–306.

22. Walz MK, Peitgen K, Hoermann R, Giebler RM, Mann K, Eigler FW. Posterior retroperitoneoscopy as a new minimally invasive approach for adrenalectomy: results of 30 adrenalectomies in 27 patients. World J Surg 1996; 20:769–774.

23. Gagner M, Garcia-Ruiz A. Technical aspects of minimally invasive abdominal surgery performed with needlescopic instruments. Surg Laparosc Endosc 1998; 8:171–179.

24. Gagner M, Pomp A, Heniford BT, Pharand D, Lacroix A. Laparoscopic adrenalectomy: lessons learned from 100 consecutive procedures. Ann Surg 1997; 226:238–246; discussion 246–237.

25. Hobart MG, Gill LS, Schweizer D, Sung GT, Bravo EL. Laparoscopic adrenalectomy for large-volume (> or = 5 cm) adrenal masses. J Endourol 2000; 14:149–154.

26. Brunt LM, Moley JF, Doherty GM, Lairmore TC, DeBendetti MK, Quasebarth MA. Outcomes analysis in patients undergoing laparoscopic adrenalectomy for hormonally active adrenal tumors. Surgery 2001; 130:629–634.

27. Wells SA, Merke DP, Cutler GB Jr, Norton JA, Lacroix A. Therapeutic controversy: the role of laparoscopic surgery in adrenal disease. J Clin Endocrinol Metabol 1998; 83:3041–3049.

28. Kebebew E, Siperstein AE, Duh QY. Laparoscopic adrenalectomy: the optimal surgical approach. J Laparoendosc Adv Surg Tech A 2001; 11:409–413.

29. Bonjer HJ, Lange KF, Kazemoer G, De Herder WW, Steyerberg EW, Bruining HA. Comparison of three techniques for adrenalectomy. Br J Surg 1997; 84:679–682.

30. Duh QY, Siperstein AE, Clark OH, et al. Laparoscopic adrenalectomy. Comparison of the lateral and posterior approaches. Arch Surg 1996; 131:870–875; discussion 875–876.

31. Dudley NE, Harrison BJ. Comparison of open posterior versus transperitoneal laparoscopic adrenalectomy. Br J Surg 1999; 86:656–660.

32. Thompson GB, Grant CS, vanHeerden JA, et al. Laparoscopic versus open posterior adrenalectomy: a case-control study of 100 patients. Surgery 1997; 122:1132–1136.

33. Imai T, Kikumori T, Ohiwa M, Mase T, Funahashi H. A case-controlled study of laparoscopic compared with open lateral adrenalectomy. Am J Surg 1999; 178:50–53; discussion 54.

34. Jacobs JK, Goldstein RE, Geer RJ. Laparoscopic adrenalectomy. A new standard of care. Ann Surg 1997; 225: 495–501; discussion 501–492.

35. Smith CD, Weber CJ, Anderson JR. Laparoscopic adrenalectomy: new gold standard. World J Surg 1999; 23:389–396.

36. Prinz RA. A comparison of laparoscopic and open adrenalectomies. Arch Surg 1995; 130:489–494.

37. Barreca M, Presenti L, Renzi C, et al. Expectations and outcomes when moving from open to laparoscopic adrenalectomy: multivariate analysis. World J Surg 2003; 27: 223–228.

38. Brunt LM, Doherty GM, Norton JA, Soper NJ, Quasebarth MA, Moley JF. Laparoscopic adrenalectomy compared to open adrenalectomy for benign adrenal neoplasms. J Am Coll Surg 1996; 183:1–10.

39. Hobart MG, Gill IS, Schweizer D, Bravo EL. Financial analysis of needlescopic versus open adrenalectomy. J Urol 1999; 162:1264–1267.

40. Eisenhofer G, Lenders JW, Linehan WM, Walther MM, Goldstein DS, Kesier HR. Plasma normetanephrine and metanephrine for detecting pheochromocytoma in von Hippel-Lindau disease and multiple endocrine neoplasia type 2. NEJM 1999; 340:1872–1879.

41. Sawka AM, Jaeschke R, Singh RJ, Young WF Jr. A comparison of biochemical tests for pheochromocytoma: measurement of fractionated plasma metanephrines compared with the combination of 24-hour urinary metanephrines and catecholamines [comment]. J Clin Endocrinol Metabol 2003; 88: 553–558.

42. Eisenhofer G. Editorial: biochemical diagnosis of pheochromocytoma—is it time to switch to plasma-free metanephrines? [comment]. J Clin Endocrinol Metabol 2003; 88:550–552.

43. Eisenhofer G, Keiser H, Friberg P, et al. Plasma metanephrines are markers of pheochromocytoma produced by catechol-O-methyltransferase within tumors. J Clin Endocrinol Metabol 1998; 83:2175–2185.

44. Averbuch SD, Steakley CS, Young RC, et al. Malignant pheochromocytoma: effective treatment with a combination of cyclophosphamide, vincristine, and dacarbazine. Ann Intern Med 1988; 109:267–273.

45. Tada K, Okuda Y, Yamashita K. Three cases of malignant pheochromocytoma treated with cyclophosphamide, vincristine, and dacarbazine combination chemotherapy and alpha-methyl-p-tyrosine to control hypercatecholaminemia. Hormone Res 1998; 49:295–297.

46. Sisson JC, Shapiro B, Shulkin BL, Urba S, Zempel S, Spaulding S. Treatment of malignant pheochromocytomas with 131-I metaiodobenzylguanidine and chemotherapy. Am J Clin Oncol 1999; 22:364–370.

47. Rao F, Keiser HR, O'Connor DT. Malignant and benign pheochromocytoma: chromaffin granule transmitters and the response to medical and surgical treatment. Ann NY Acad Sci 2002; 971:530–532.

48. Loh KC, Fitzgerald PA, Matthay KK, Yeo PP, Price DC. The treatment of malignant pheochromocytoma with iodine-131 metaiodobenzylguanidine (131I-MIBG): a comprehensive review of 116 reported patients. J Endocrin Invest 1997; 20:648–658.

49. Pujol P, Bunger J, Faurous P, Jaffiol C. Metastatic pheochromocytoma with a long-term response after iodine-131 metarodobenzylguanidine therapy. Eur J Nucl Med 1995; 22:382–384.

50. Nakabeppu Y, Nakajo M. Radionuclide therapy of malignant pheochromocytoma with 131I-MIBG. Ann Nucl Med 1994; 8:259–268.

51. Stanley JC, Graham LM, Whitehouse WM Jr. Renovascular hypertension. In: Miller TA, Rowland BJ, eds. Physiologic Basis of Modern Surgical Care. St Louis: CV Mosby, 1988: 734–739.

52. Sealey JE, Buhler FR, Laragh JH, Vaughan ED Jr. The physiology of renin secretion in essential hypertension: estimation of renin secretion rate and renal plasma flow from peripheral and renal vein renin levels. Am J Med 1973; 55:391–401.

53. Schneider EG, Davis JO, Baumber JS, Johnson JA. The hepatic metabolism of renin and aldosterone: a review with new observations on the hepatic clearance of renin. Circ Res 1970; 175:26–27.

54. Stanley JC, Graham LM. Renovascular hypertension. In: Miller TA, ed. Physiologic Basis of Modern Surgical Care. 2nd. St Louis: Quality Medical Publishing, 1998:918–934.

55. Stanley JC, Gewertz BL, Fry WJ. Renal:systemic renin indices and renal vein renin ratios as prognostic indicators in remedial renovascular hypertension. J Surg Res 1976; 20:149–155.

56. Vaughan ED Jr, Buhler FR, Laragh JH, Sealey JE, Baer L, Bard RH. Renovascular hypertension: renin measurements to indicate hypersecretion and contralateral suppression, estimate renal plasma flow, and score for surgical curability. Am J Med 1973; 55:402–414.

57. Graham LM, Zelenock GB, Erlandson EE, Lindenauer SM, Coran AG, Stanley JC. Abdominal aortic coarctation and segmental hypoplasia. Surgery 1979; 86:519–529.

58. Cherr GS, Hansen KJ, Craven TE, et al. Surgical management of atherosclerotic renovascular disease. J Vasc Surg 2002; 35:236–245.

59. Stanley JC. The evolution of surgery for renovascular occlusive disease. Cardiovasc Surg 1994; 2:195–202.

60. Stanley JC, Fry WJ. Renovascular hypertension secondary to arterial fibrodysplasia in adults: criteria for operation and results of surgical therapy. Arch Surg 1975; 110:922–928.

61. Stanley JC, Gewertz BL, Bove EL, Sottiurai VS, Fry WJ. Arterial fibrodysplasia: histopathologic character and current etiologic concepts. Arch Surg 1975; 110:561–566.

62. Stanley JC, Graham LM, Whitehouse WM Jr, et al. Developmental occlusive disease of the abdominal aorta and the splanchnic and renal arteries. Am J Surg 1981; 142:190–196.

63. Stanley JC, Zelenock GB, Messina LM, Wakefield TW. Pediatric renovascular hypertension: a thirty-year experience of operative treatment. J Vasc Surg 1995; 21:212–227.

64. Stanley JC, Graham LM, Whitehouse WM Jr. Limitations and errors of diagnostic and prognostic investigations in renovascular hypertension. In: Bernhard VM, Towne JM, eds. Complications in Vascular Surgery. Orlando: Grune & Stratton, 1985: 213–222.

65. Vidt DG, Yutani FM, McCormack LJ, et al. Surgical treatment of unilateral renal vascular disease: prognostic role of vascular changes in bilateral renal biopsies. Am J Cardiol 1972; 30:827–831.

66. Prince MR, Narasimham DL, Stanley JC, et al. Gadolinium-enhanced magnetic resonance angiography of abdominal aortic aneurysms. J Vasc Surg 1995; 21:656–669.

67. Hansen KJ, Tribble RW, Reavis SW, et al. Renal duplex sonography: evaluation of clinical utility. J Vascular Surg 1990; 12:227–236.

68. Hoffman U, Edwards JM, Carter S, et al. Role of duplex scanning for the detection of atherosclerotic renal artery disease. Kidney Int 1991; 39:1231–1239.

69. Motew SJ, Cherr GS, Craven TE, et al. Renal duplex sonography: main renal artery versus hilar analysis. J Vasc Surg 2000; 32:462–471.

70. Stanley JC, Fry WJ. Surgical treatment of renovascular hypertension. Arch Surg 1977; 112:1291.

71. Thornbury JR, Stanley JC, Fryback DC. Hypertensive urogram: a nondiscriminatory test for renovascular hypertension. AJR 1992; 138:43–49.

72. Stanley JC, Whitehouse WM Jr, Graham LM, Cronenwett JL, Zelenock GB, Lindenauer SM. Operative therapy of renovascular hypertension. Br J Surg 1982; 69:S63–S66.

73. Buhler FR, Laragh JH, Baer L, Vaughan ED Jr, Brunner HR. Propranolol inhibition of renin secretion. NEJM 1972; 287: 1209–1214.

74. Hricik DE, Browning PJ, Kopelman R, Goorno WE, Madias NE, Dzau VJ. Captopril-induced renal insufficiency in patients with bilateral renal artery stenosis or renal artery stenosis in a solitary kidney. NEJM 1983; 308:373–376.

75. Bonelli FS, Mckusick MA, Textor SC, et al. Renal artery angioplasty: technical results and clinical outcome in 320 patients. Mayo Clin Proc 1995; 70:1041–1052.

76. Cluzel P, Raynaud B, Beyssen B, Pagny JY, Gaux JC. Stenoses of renal branch arteries in fibromuscular dysplasia: results of percutaneous transluminal angioplasty. Radiology 1994; 193: 227–232.

77. Davidson R, Barri Y, Wilcox CS. Predictors of cure of hypertension in fibromuscular renovascular disease. Am J Kidney Dis 1996; 28:334–338.

78. Luscher TF, Keller HM, Imhoff HG, et al. Fibromuscular hyperplasia: extension of the disease and therapeutic outcome. Results of the University Hospital Zurich Cooperative Study on Fibromuscular Hyperplasia. Nephron 1986; 44:109–114.

79. Sos TA, Pickering TG, Sniderman K, et al. Percutaneous transluminal renal angioplasty in renovascular hypertension due to atheroma or fibromuscular dysplasia. NEJM 1983; 309: 274–279.

80. Tegtmeyer CJ, Selby JB, Hartwell GD, Ayers C, Tegtmeyer V. Results and complications of angioplasty in fibromuscular disease. Circulation 1991; 83:1155–1161.

81. Stanley JC, Upchurch GR Jr. Renal artery occlusive disease. In: Greenfield LJ, Mulholland MW, Oldham KT, Zelenock GB, Lillimoe KD, eds. Surgery, Scientific Principals and Practice. 3rd ed. Philadelphia: Lippincott Williams & Wilkins, 2001: 1708–1724.

82. Martin EC, Diamond NC, Casarella WJ. Percutaneous transluminal angioplasty in nonatherosclerotic disease. Radiology 1980; 135:27–33.

83. Ayerdi J, Hodgson KJ. Balloon angioplasty and stenting for renovascular occlusive disease. Pers Vasc Surg Endovasc Ther 2004; 16:25–42.

84. Blum U, Krumme B, Flugel P, et al. Treatment of ostial renal artery stenoses with vascular endoprostheses after unsuccessful balloon angioplasty. NEJM 1997; 336:459–465.

85. Boisclair C, Therasse E, Oliva VL, et al. Treatment of renal angioplasty failure by percutaneous renal artery stenting with Palmaz stents: midterm technical and clinical results. AJR 1997; 168:245–251.

86. Dorros G, Jaff M, Mathiak L, et al. Four-year follow-up of Palmaz-Schatz stent revascularization as treatment for renal artery stenosis. Circulation 1998; 98:642–647.

87. Harjai K, Khosla S, Shaw D, et al. Effect of gender on outcomes following renal artery stent placement for renovascular hypertension. Cathet Cardiovasc Diagn 1997; 42:381–386.

88. Henry M, Amor M, Henry I, et al. Stent placement in the renal artery: three-year experience with the Palmaz stent. J Vasc Intervent Radiol 1996; 7:343–350.

89. Knipp BS, Dimick JB, Eliason JL, et al. Diffusion of new technology for the treatment of renovascular hypertension in the United States: surgical revascularization versus catheter-based therapy, 1998–2001. J Vasc Surg 2004; 40:717–723.

90. Leertouwer TC, Gussenhoven EJ, Bosch JL, et al. Stent placement for renal arterial stenosis: where do we stand? A meta-analysis. Radiology 2002; 216:78–85.

91. Rees CR, Palmaz JC, Becker GJ, et al. Palmaz stent in atherosclerotic stenoses involving the ostia of the renal arteries: preliminary report of a multicenter study. Radiology 1991; 181:507–514.

92. Weibull H, Bergqvist D, Bergentz SE, Jonsson K, Hulthen L, Manhem P. Percutaneous transluminal renal angioplasty versus surgical reconstruction of atherosclerotic renal artery

stenosis: a prospective randomized study. J Vasc Surg 1993; 18:841–852.

93. Wong JM, Hansen KJ, Oskin TC, et al. Surgery after failed percutaneous renal artery angioplasty. J Vasc Surg 1999; 30: 468–482.

94. Stanley JC, Ernst CB, Fry WJ. Fate of 100 aortorenal vein grafts: characteristics of late graft expansion, aneurysmal dilatation, and stenosis. Surgery 1973; 74:931–944.

95. Khauli RB, Novick AC, Ziegelbaum M. Splenorenal bypass in the treatment of renal artery stenosis: experience with sixty-nine cases. J Vasc Surg 1985; 2:547–551.

96. Moncure AC, Brewster DC, Darling RC, Atnip RG, Newton WD, Abbott WM. Use of the splenic and hepatic arteries for renal revascularization. J Vasc Surg 1986; 3:196–203.

97. Belzer PO, Raczkowski A. Ex vivo renal artery reconstruction with autotransplantation. Surgery 1982; 92:642–645.

98. Brekke IB, Sodal G, Jakobsen A, et al. Fibromuscular renal artery disease treated by extracorporeal vascular reconstruction and renal autotransplantation: short- and long-term results. Eur J Vasc Surg 1992; 6:471–476.

99. van Bockel JH, van den Akker PJ, Chang PC, Aarts JC, Hermans J, Terpstra JL. Extracorporeal renal artery reconstruction for renovascular hypertension. J Vasc Surg 1991; 13:101–110.

100. Cambria RP, Brewster DC, L'Italien G, et al. Simultaneous aortic and renal artery reconstruction: evolution of an eighteen-year experience. J Vasc Surg 1994; 21:916–925.

101. Clair DG, Belkin M, Whittemore AD, Mannick JA, Donaldson MC. Safety and efficacy of transaortic renal endarterectomy as an adjunct to aortic surgery. J Vasc Surg 1995; 21:926–933.

102. Dougherty MJ, Hallett JW Jr, Naessens J, et al. Renal endarterectomy versus bypass for combined aortic and renal reconstruction: is there a difference in clinical outcome? Ann Vasc Surg 1995; 9:87–94.

103. Hansen KJ, Starr SM, Sands RE, Burkart JM, Plonk GW Jr, Dean RH. Contemporary surgical management of renovascular disease. J Vasc Surg 1992; 16:319–331.

104. McNeil JW, String ST, Pfeiffer RB Jr. Concomitant renal endarterectomy and aortic reconstruction. J Vasc Surg 1994; 20: 331–336.

105. Stoney RJ, Messina LM, Goldstone J, Reilly LM. Renal endarterectomy through the transected aorta: a new technique for combined aortorenal arteriosclerosis—a preliminary report. J Vasc Surg 1989; 9:224–233.

106. Stanley JC, Whitehouse WM Jr, Zelenock GB, Graham LM, Cronenwett JL, Lindenauer SM. Reoperation for complications of renal artery reconstructive surgery undertaken for treatment of renovascular hypertension. J Vasc Surg 1985; 2:133–144.

49

Calcium and Phosphorus Metabolism and the Parathyroid Gland

Fiemu E. Nwariaku

INTRODUCTION

The parathyroid glands comprise a group of endocrine structures (usually 4 in number) that either hug the posterior surface of the thyroid gland or are in close proximity to it. Although exceedingly small in size, they play crucial roles in the maintenance of calcium and phosphorus balance. Their function spans a range of activities, including blood coagulation, modulation of membrane permeability, muscle contraction, neuromuscular excitability, and the regulation of various signal transduction processes within cells. Their importance to the surgeon is usually related to states of overactivity in which hypercalcemia may ensue. Occasionally, these glands also become important in surgical practices when a state of hypocalcemia results, as may occur after total thyroidectomy for goiter or neoplasia. The intricate control systems regulated by the parathyroid glands to maintain calcium and phosphorus balance are the subject of this chapter.

CALCIUM HOMEOSTASIS

Intracellular signaling systems are exquisitely sensitive to the intracellular calcium concentration. Increased intracellular calcium concentrations generate further release of calcium stores in the sarcoplasmic reticulum, triggering the desired cellular response. Calcium-dependent intracellular signaling systems are affected by serum and extracellular fluid calcium concentration, necessitating tight control of serum calcium levels. This is especially true for neuromuscular and secretory cells whose functions are disrupted by small alterations in extracellular calcium concentrations. Serum calcium concentration is tightly regulated by the intestinal tract (absorption), bone (calcium stores), and kidney (excretion). Regulation of these processes occurs through the actions of several hormones, including parathyroid hormone (PTH) and vitamin D 1,25-dihydroxy vitamin D (1,25-$(OH)_2D$), calcitonin, estradiol, glucocorticoids, and the growth hormone. Of these, PTH and (1,25-$(OH)_2D$) appear to be the main regulators of calcium homeostasis in humans. Both hormones stimulate bone-resorbing osteoclasts, promoting calcium release into the extracellular fluid. PTH also stimulates renal hydroxylation of 25-$(OH)D_3$ to 1,25-$(OH)_2D_1$ and distal renal tubular calcium reabsorption.

More than 98% of the total body calcium is present in bone and about 1% appears to be freely exchangeable with the extracellular fluid through both physicochemical and cell-mediated mechanisms. Figure 1 illustrates the exchangeable calcium compartments. Calcium circulates in the extracellular fluid in three distinct fractions: about 50% comprises the biologically important "free" or "ionized" fraction, 40% is protein-bound and not filterable by the kidney, and 10% is complexed to anions such as bicarbonate, citrate, sulphate, phosphate, and lactate. Most of the protein-bound calcium is bound to albumin, the remainder being complexed to globulins. Disorders that lower serum albumin also lower total concentration of serum calcium, but have a lesser effect on the free "ionized" calcium level. In general, 1 g/dL of albumin binds about 0.2 mmol/L (0.8 mg/dL) of calcium, allowing for a simple estimate of an acceptable value for serum calcium when patients have hypoalbuminemia. If one begins with a normal serum value of 4.0 g/dL and subtracts 0.2 mmol/L from the total calcium concentration for each 1 g/dL decrease in albumin concentration, an expected value for serum calcium will be obtained, which can be compared to the patient's actual value to determine the presence of hypercalcemia or hypocalcemia. Figure 2 illustrates this relationship.

Binding of calcium to albumin is also affected by the extracellular fluid pH. Acidemia decreases protein binding and increases the ionized calcium fraction. For each 0.1 decrease in pH, ionized calcium rises by about 0.05 mmol/L. Extracellular calcium compartments are of interest to the clinician because multiple factors may influence the metabolically active, ionized fraction. During venipuncture, the prolonged use of a tourniquet that causes ischemia and acidosis could artificially elevate ionized calcium. Similarly, inappropriate specimen collection could cause an elevation in pH and subsequent artificial lowering of ionized calcium measurement. Electrodes used to measure ionized calcium are sensitive to temperature, calcium-chelating anticoagulants, and loss of carbon dioxide; thus, these methods generally underestimate the ionized calcium fraction.

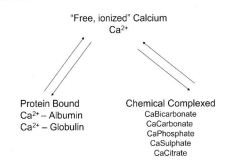

Figure 1 Physicochemical state of calcium in serum.

$$[\text{Expected Ca}^{2+}] = 4.0 \text{ g/Dl} - ([\text{Albumin}]_N - [\text{Albumin}]_O) * 0.8 \text{ g/Dl}$$

and

$$[\text{Expected Ca}^{2+}] = 4.0 \text{ g/Dl} - (\text{pH}_N - \text{pH}_O) * 0.5 \text{ g/unit pH}$$

where:
4.0 g/Dl is the normal serum concentration of Ca^{2+}
$[\text{Albumin}]_N$ = normal serum albumin concentration
$[\text{Albumin}]_O$ = measured serum albumin in the patient
pH_N = normal pH
pH_O = measured pH in the patients

Figure 2 Alterations of serum calcium due to changes in albumin concentration and pH.

Intestine

Calcium absorption varies by location in the gastrointestinal (GI) tract. The stomach does not absorb calcium, but facilitates its absorption by solubilizing the mineral in acid. The rate of calcium absorption is greatest at the duodenum and progressively decreases in the jejunum and ileum. Although the duodenum has the greatest ability to absorb calcium, it is relatively short. Because the jejunal length and transit time are greater than that of the duodenum, quantitatively greater amounts of calcium are absorbed in the jejunum. The colon is also capable of absorbing calcium, but sequestration of calcium within stool prevents contact with the colonic epithelial surface.

Calcium absorption may be active or passive. Active absorption is very efficient, but of limited magnitude. Calcium active transport systems are mediated by saturable protein carriers that transport up to a maximal rate and not beyond it. These systems are important when calcium must be transported against steep concentration gradients. Calcium absorption also occurs across steep gradients by passive transport. Because passive transport is not saturable, when there is a large concentration gradient, large quantities of calcium can be absorbed. This is what occurs when the dietary calcium content is high. When there is little calcium in the diet, calcium absorption is facilitated by active transport systems.

The small intestine demonstrates two levels of control, immediate and long term. The fraction of calcium absorbed will differ according to the quantity delivered to the GI tract. During ingestion of small quantities of calcium, most of the ingested calcium (80–100%) is absorbed. With larger amounts (100–500 mg), less calcium (20–60%) is absorbed. With long-term dietary changes in the intake of calcium, adaptation is regulated by changes in calciotropic hormones. For example, poor calcium intake will lead to lower blood calcium and, in turn, higher serum PTH and 1,25-(OH)$_2$D, which then boosts intestinal calcium absorption. The opposite occurs when dietary calcium intake is excessive. Soluble fiber and phosphate may inhibit calcium absorption by binding it within the intestinal lumen. PTH indirectly increases both active and passive calcium absorption by increasing vitamin D synthesis and release.

Bone

Bone is a dynamic structure that is in constant flux by a process known as remodeling. Cortical bone which constitutes 80% of bone mass is commonly found in the appendicular skeleton (arms and legs) and accounts for only 4% of remodeling compared to trabecular bone which accounts for 20%

of bone mass, but 80% of bone surface area. Because most calcium stores are in bone, it may act as a "calcium sink" storing excess calcium or providing additional calcium in times of need. Many derangements of calcium metabolism, such as hyperparathyroidism, result in changes in bone density.

Kidneys

The kidneys are critically important for the maintenance of calcium homeostasis. Amongst the most common causes of abnormal calcium metabolism are the renal failure syndromes. The kidney filters very large amounts of calcium, 10 g daily and must resorb almost all of it to maintain normal calcium levels. Consequently, only 100 to 200 mg of calcium is excreted into the urine daily. Because of the large amount of calcium passing through the kidney, relative minor alterations in renal function can have a large impact on calcium homeostasis.

Sixty to seventy percent of calcium reabsorption occurs in the proximal tubule. Another 20% is reabsorbed in the thick ascending loop of Henle, 5% to 10% in the distal tubule, and the remainder is reabsorbed in the collecting ducts. If renal filtration decreases due to volume depletion or declining renal function, less calcium is lost in the urine. Alternatively, if renal filtration increases due to volume overload, more calcium is excreted into the urine. This observation explains the efficacy of forced diuresis as a treatment for hypercalcemia.

PTH regulates the degree of renal tubular calcium resorption. During hypocalcemia, PTH secretion from the parathyroid glands is increased resulting in an enhanced calcium resorption from the renal tubules. In contrast, when serum calcium increases with a resultant decrease in serum PTH levels, there is less renal tubular resorption of calcium. Dumping calcium into the urine is one of the mechanisms utilized to lower serum calcium levels.

Acidosis and dietary acid loads impair renal calcium reabsorption; alkalosis and dietary alkali loads produce the opposite effect. Excess dietary intake of salt enhances calcium excretion by increasing extracellular fluid volume and by impairing renal calcium reabsorption. Finally, loop diuretics such as furosemide increase renal calcium losses, while thiazide diuretics and lithium act on the distal tubule to reduce urinary calcium resorption.

HORMONAL REGULATION OF EXTRACELLULAR CALCIUM CONCENTRATION

Parathyroid Hormone

PTH is produced by the parathyroid glands, located adjacent to the thyroid gland in the neck. While most humans have four parathyroid glands, in some there may be as few as two glands or up to eight glands. PTH is initially synthesized as part of a larger (112 amino acid) molecule, pre-pro-PTH, which is immediately shortened to pro-PTH. Enzymatic cleavage of the nonbiologically active pro-PTH frees the 84–amino acid peptide, PTH, for release into the circulation, where it is broken into two fragments, principally in the liver and kidney. The parathyroid gland also releases hormone fragments. There are three forms of circulating PTH: the 84–amino acid molecule (intact PTH), an amino-terminal fragment with a short half-life, and a carboxylterminal fragment with a longer half-life. Only the whole molecule and the amino-terminal fragment are biologically active. These are rapidly cleaved within the circulation resulting in a serum half-life of less than five minutes.

The short half-life is indicative of the importance in maintaining tight control of calcium levels. Rapid degradation of parathyroid hormone facilitates the rapid response to changes in calcium levels, enabling the body to keep serum calcium levels at nearly constant levels. When serum calcium levels fall, PTH secretion immediately increases with the opposite occurring when serum calcium rises, facilitating the minute-by-minute control of serum calcium concentration. The immediate response to changes in serum calcium levels by PTH secretion is mediated by a calcium-sensing receptor (CaSR) on the surface of the parathyroid cells. PTH secretion is 50% of the maximal level at a serum ionized calcium level of 4 mg/dL (1 mmol/L), which is the calcium set point for PTH secretion. Exploitation of the short half-life of PTH has been useful during intraoperative monitoring of PTH and has improved our ability to ensure that all hypersecreting parathyroid tissue has been resected during parathyroidectomy in patients with primary hyperparathyroidism (pHPT).

In addition, serum phosphate concentration indirectly affects PTH secretion. Hyperphosphatemia directly raises serum PTH, and phosphorus binds calcium leading to low serum calcium concentrations, which in turn stimulate PTH secretion. This has important implications for the management of patients with severe renal insufficiency, which leads to hyperphosphatemia and secondary to hyperparathyroidism from chronic parathyroid stimulation. Phosphate-reduction therapy (phosphate-binding agents, etc.) is frequently required to reduce the high PTH levels in such patients.

PTH maintains the serum calcium level by several mechanisms and by acting on several organ systems to raise serum calcium and lower serum phosphate concentrations. It directly and indirectly promotes calcium entry into the blood at the three sites of calcium exchange: gut, bone, and kidney. PTH indirectly contributes to the net GI absorption of calcium by inducing the renal synthesis of calcitriol. PTH directly inhibits the synthetic function of osteoblasts, indirectly stimulates osteoclast differentiation, stimulates tubular calcium reabsorption, enhances phosphate clearance, and stimulates the enzyme that completes the synthesis of calcitriol in the kidney. Under physiologic conditions, PTH feedback loops prevent serious derangements of calcium concentrations, such as hypercalcemia or hypocalcemia. The net effects of PTH are enhancement of bone resorption, decreased loss of urinary calcium, and increased intestinal calcium absorption. Although it is well known that pHPT is caused by the overproduction of PTH, the cause of this overproduction and the development of sporadic pHPT are unknown. Clearly, the normal negative feedback loop is altered and the abnormal parathyroid gland(s) continue to secrete excessive amounts of PTH despite high serum calcium levels.

Circulating PTH is now measured using antibodies that detect intact PTH. This sandwich technique uses two antibodies, one for the amino-terminus and another for the carboxy-terminus. These double-antibody immunoassays are highly sensitive and specific and have replaced other assays due to their improved accuracy in detecting the intact (biologically active) hormone. In patients with pHPT, there is an inappropriate and excessive secretion of PTH, relative to the serum calcium level, from the abnormal parathyroid gland(s) allowing the clinician to specifically establish pHPT as the cause of hypercalcemia.

Vitamin D (1,25-(OH)$_2$D)

The active form of vitamin D, 1,25-(OH)$_2$D, is produced by a complicated pathway involving the skin, liver, and kidneys. First, 7-dehydrocholesterol in the skin is converted to previtamin D$_3$ by ultraviolet light, and this product is converted to vitamin D$_3$ by isomerization, a process that is impaired in the elderly. At northern latitudes in the winter, the lack of sufficient ultraviolet light prevents adequate synthesis of vitamin D$_3$. Patients with highly pigmented skin require greater duration of exposure to ultraviolet light to synthesize adequate amounts of vitamin D$_3$, because melanin also absorbs these ultraviolet spectrum wavelengths. Vitamin D$_3$ is transported in the blood by the vitamin D–binding protein (VDBP) to the liver, where it is 25-hydroxylated to 25-hydroxyvitamin D (25-(OH)D) or calcifediol. Vitamin D$_2$ (plant sources) and vitamin D$_3$ (animal sources) may also reach the liver after dietary ingestion via the portal circulation. 25-(OH)D is then transported to the kidney also by VDBP. Most of the 25-(OH)D in the kidneys is shunted to the first step of a degradation pathway by 24-hydroxylase (CYP24) and is converted into 24,25-dihydroxyvitamin D in the kidneys, but a small amount of 25-(OH)$_2$D is converted to the active hormone, 1,25-(OH)$_2$D or calcitriol by the 1-α-hydroxylase (or CYP1α) in a tightly regulated process. Calcitriol appears to be the major active form of vitamin D in humans. Although its plasma level of 25 to 40 pg/mL is much lower than that of calcifediol, it is over 100 times as potent on a weight basis.

An understanding of vitamin D metabolism allows the clinician to understand the derangements in calcium metabolism that occur with liver and kidney diseases. Liver disease impairs 25-hydroxylation of 7-dehydrocholesterol in the liver and decreases the concentration of precursors of active vitamin D needed in the kidney. Renal disease suppresses the 1α-hydroxylation resulting in low levels of the most active form of vitamin D. Both diseases thus result in low vitamin D levels and subsequent aberrations in calcium metabolism.

Hypophosphatemia and high serum PTH stimulate production of active vitamin D. In addition, active vitamin D inhibits its own production by suppressing PTH and the 1-α-hydroxylase and enhances its own degradation by upregulating transcription of 24-hydroxylase through negative feedback loops. Similar to PTH, 1,25-(OH)$_2$D raises serum calcium primarily by increasing intestinal calcium absorption, but it also increases bone resorption and serum phosphate concentrations. Although 1,25-(OH)$_2$D directly increases intestinal phosphate absorption and renal phosphate reabsorption to a modest degree, its main effect on serum phosphate is probably better explained by its direct suppression of PTH secretion. The normal range for calcitriol varies with the season (lower in winter), age (lower in older persons), and serum calcium level. Although, calcitriol production is autoregulated, other hormones such as prolactin, growth hormone, and sex steroids may also modulate its production. Receptors for calcitriol are present in many tissues other than bone, kidney, and intestine, including the parathyroid glands, pancreatic islets, mammary glands, and fibroblasts, indicating that it has effects that reach beyond the three organs that are primarily involved in calcium metabolism.

Calcitonin

The role of calcitonin in humans is unclear, but in fish, the hormone plays an important role in calcium metabolism.

The 32–amino acid polypeptide is derived from the C-cells of the thyroid glands. Secretion of calcitonin is stimulated by hypercalcemia and the GI hormone, gastrin. Because gastrin secretion is also increased by calcium, calcitonin has been postulated to prevent postprandial hypercalcemia. Binding of calcitonin to its receptor on the surface of osteoclasts is responsible for the hormone's main action, to decrease bone resorption. In humans, calcitonin seems to play a minor role in calcium metabolism. Calcitonin insufficiency (postthyroidectomy) or excess (medullary thyroid carcinoma) both have no effect on bone mineral density. However, pharmacologic doses of calcitonin effectively decrease bone turnover in humans, and parenteral or intranasal formulations are approved to treat osteoporosis, hypercalcemia and Paget's disease of the bone, a disease characterized by high bone turnover, bone pain, and bone deformities. At pharmacologic doses in humans, calcitonin may also increase renal calcium excretion, though the effects of calcitonin on hypercalcemia are modest. As such, the role of calcitonin in managing hypercalcemia is as an adjuvant.

Other Hormones

Estradiol

Estradiol prevents bone resorption, increases renal calcium reabsorption, and augments intestinal calcium absorption. After menopause, rapid bone loss occurs transiently for three to seven years, after which the rate of bone loss returns to baseline. Estradiol has been used to prevent bone loss due to hyperparathyroidism with mixed results. This effect is discussed below.

Glucocorticoids

Steroids act via a vitamin D–independent mechanism to decrease intestinal calcium absorption. In the short term, high-dose glucocorticoids increase renal calcium loss by reducing renal calcium reabsorption. The combined effects on the kidney and the intestine may cause compensatory secondary hyperparathyroidism in some patients. However, the main effect of glucocorticoids is on bone, where glucocorticoids increase bone resorption, decrease bone formation, and cause apoptosis of osteoblasts and osteocytes. Of these mechanisms, the latter two appear to be most important. When a patient is treated with glucocorticoids, rapid bone loss occurs within the first six months, and then continues at a slower rate.

Growth Hormone and Thyroid Hormone

Growth hormone increases both bone resorption and bone formation, but greater stimulation of bone formation generally leads to gain in bone mass. Patients with growth hormone deficiency have a low bone mass, and their bone mineral density increases with growth hormone treatment. In contrast, acromegalic patients who have excessive secretion patterns of growth hormone tend to have low bone mass probably because of concomitant changes caused by the pituitary tumor such as hypogonadism. Thyroid hormone increases bone resorption and bone loss. The resulting higher ionized calcium suppresses PTH, 1,25-$(OH)_2$D, and intestinal calcium absorption. Modest hypercalcemia may occur in up to 20% of patients with Graves' disease.

Parathyroid Hormone-Related Protein

The precise role of parathyroid hormone-related protein (PTHrP) has not been determined. First found to be the cause of humoral hypercalcemia of malignancy, PTH-related protein, or its messenger RNA, has been identified in many tissues, including the placenta, fetal parathyroid, and adult keratinocytes, neurons, pancreatic islets, kidney, and bone. This molecule closely resembles PTH at its amino-terminal end, but it is longer and more complex than PTH. The first 13 amino acids of PTHrP are almost identical to those of PTH, but there is no homology in the remainder of the 141–amino acid structure. There are two important aspects of PTH-related protein. First, it shares a single receptor with PTH. Second, PTH-related protein appears to have a second biologically active domain in addition to the PTH-like region. This second active site plays a role in calcium transport in the placenta, thereby making PTH-related protein the important hormone regulating calcium metabolism in the fetus. One clinically relevant effect of PTHrP is the excess secretion by tumors thus producing the humoral hypercalcemia of malignancy.

The CaSR and Calcium Regulation

Since the CaSR was cloned in 1993, much investigation has focused on its function and the effect of receptor mutations in human disease. Inactivating mutations have been shown to cause hypercalcemic disorders [familial hypocalciuric hypercalcemia (FHH), neonatal severe hyperparathyroidism, etc.] while activating mutations cause hypocalcemia (autosomal dominant hypoparathyroidism) (1,2). The calcium sensing receptor is located in the parathyroid glands, C-cells of the thyroid, kidney, intestine, and focal areas of the brain. In the parathyroid gland, a rise in serum calcium activates the CaSR and results in suppression of PTH secretion. On the other hand, hypocalcemia results in higher serum PTH because the CaSR provides less inhibition. Thus, a CaSR may act as a short-feedback loop to avoid hypercalcemia. CaSR has also been shown to bind gadolinium, neomycin, and magnesium. Several clinical scenarios may be explained by these observations. First, hypermagnesemia often accompanies hypercalcemia in patients who have inactivating mutations of the CaSR; and hypomagnesemia and hypocalcemia arise in patients with activating mutations. Second, in patients without CaSR mutations, either high serum calcium or magnesium induces renal wasting of both calcium and magnesium. Finally, magnesium excess decreases the secretion of PTH. The receptor is potentially an important therapeutic target for disorders in which the receptor is inappropriately overactive or underactive. Clinical trials are currently underway to assess the efficacy of calcimimetic CaSR agonists in the treatment of primary and uremic HPT. In these trials, calcimimetics decrease the circulating PTH level more than 50% within minutes in patients with pHPT. In patients with HPT, calcimimetics reset the elevated calcium set point, which controls the response of pathological parathyroid glands to the serum calcium level. It is also likely that a CaSR antagonist would be very useful in the treatment of calcium-containing renal stones. A kidney-selective CaSR antagonist would produce, in effect, benign FHH, without altering the set point of the parathyroid to calcium therefore, producing hypercalcemia (3). In fact, a recent study demonstrated marked improvement in serum PTH levels in patients with secondary hyperparathyroidism given a calcimimetic (4).

Physicochemical Effect

At very high levels of blood calcium or phosphate, metastatic calcification (deposition of calcium phosphate) occurs in the soft tissues. The location of the involved tissues varies. With hypercalcemia, metastatic calcification occurs in lung, conjunctiva, lining of stomach, and/or endothelium of arteries. The distribution is different in the setting of hyperphosphatemia. It may occur in cerebral basal ganglia and lens thus causing cataracts, or in the dermis. Either hypercalcemia or hyperphosphatemia may calcify the kidneys or periarticular tissues. This can sometimes be manifested by the clinical condition of calciphylaxis, which is associated with tissue ischemia and necrosis. High urinary calcium concentrations are a major cause of calcium-containing stones in nephrolithiasis. This clinical presentation occurs most frequently in patients with hypercalciuria due to pHPT.

DISORDERS OF CALCIUM METABOLISM

Hypercalcemia

Calcium regulatory mechanisms are highly effective under physiologic circumstances. For example, when dietary calcium suddenly increases, a smaller fraction of each dose is absorbed. If this adjustment is not sufficient, ionized calcium rises and, via the CaSR, suppresses serum PTH and, in turn, 1,25-(OH)$_2$D secretion. Moreover, calcitonin secretion is stimulated by activation of calcium sensors within the C-cells of the thyroid. These hormonal changes correct serum calcium by reducing intestinal calcium absorption, bone resorption, and renal calcium reabsorption. The CaSR further corrects hypercalcemia by augmenting urinary calcium excretion. Despite these safeguards, hypercalcemia occurs when calcium influx into the extracellular fluid from the intestine and/or bone exceeds the efflux to bone and/or excretion by the kidney. For example, an influx of calcium from bone often occurs in patients with malignancy or increased PTH (pHPT), while increased influx from the intestine occurs in patients with hypervitaminosis D. Hypercalcemia occurs when these influxes exceed the capacity of the kidney to excrete the excess calcium presented to it. Symptoms due to hypercalcemia vary depending on duration and severity of hypercalcemia. For example, a normal volunteer infused with calcium would become lethargic or even comatose once serum calcium exceeds 14 mg/dL. In contrast, individuals with chronic hypercalcemia (i.e., slow-growing parathyroid carcinoma) present with minimal changes in mental status even when calcium exceeds 19 mg/dL. Because a variety of common disorders are responsible for abnormalities in serum calcium, the treatment of both hypercalcemia and hypocalcemia depends on the underlying disorder, the magnitude of the deviation of the serum calcium, and the severity of symptoms.

Differential Diagnosis of Hypercalcemia

With routine biochemical screening, hypercalcemia is detected with a prevalence of 1 per 600 to 1 per 1000 people, depending on the population screened. The upper limit of normal for serum calcium is about 10.5 mg/dL (2.6 mmol/L) and severe, potentially life-threatening hypercalcemia occurs when levels exceed 14 mg/dL (3.5 mmol/L). The most common cause of hypercalcemia in hospitalized patients is malignancy, while pHPT is most commonly the cause in non-hospitalized patients. Table 1 lists the other causes of hypercalcemia. Hypercalcemia may be the most common metabolic complication of cancer and, overall, 10% to 20% of cancer patients develop hypercalcemia at some time during their disease. Less commonly, granulomatous

Table 1 Nonparathyroid Nonmalignant Causes of Hypercalcemia

Benign FHH
Granulomatous disease (sarcoidosis, berylliosis, and tuberculosis)
Hyperthyroidism
Hypothyroidism
Vipoma
Addison's disease
Pheochromocytoma
Excessive vitamin A and D intake
Calcium intoxication
Milk-alkali syndrome
Immobilization
Thiazides
Lithium

Abbreviation: FHH, familial hypocalciuric hypercalcemia.

disease (e.g., tuberculosis, and sarcoidosis) and hyperthyroidism cause hypercalcemia. Macrophages activated by the granulomas metabolize 25(OH) vitamin D to the more active calcitriol, and the resulting endogenous hypervitaminosis D increases the intestinal absorption of calcium, thus leading to hypercalciuria, hypercalcemia, and suppression of PTH. Hypercalcemia due to hyperthyroidism is caused by a direct stimulation of osteoclastic bone resorption by thyroxine; however, this rarely causes hypercalcemic crisis because the marked symptoms of hyperthyroidism manifest earlier and are usually controlled before the hypercalcemia becomes apparent. When hypercalcemia does complicate hyperthyroidism, it may mask the hypermetabolic symptoms and signs of thyrotoxicosis, which may then become more difficult to diagnose. In the hypercalcemia of hyperthyroidism, PTH secretion is suppressed. Locally produced cytokines that stimulate osteoclastic bone resorption may also be the most important cause of hypercalcemia associated with metastases. However, local skeletal destruction may also occur without stimulation of osteoclasts; furthermore, many skeletal metastases secrete PTH-related polypeptide, which is the most common cause of hypercalcemia of malignancy. Table 2 lists the common mechanisms of hypercalcemia.

Hypercalcemia of Malignancy

The three main mechanisms of hypercalcemia of malignancy [PTHrP, local factors, and 1,25-(OH)$_2$D] are discussed below. The most common malignancies associated with hypercalcemia include lung or breast carcinoma (60%), renal cell carcinoma (10–15%), head and neck squamous cell carcinoma

Table 2 Mechanisms of Hypercalcemia

Mechanism	Cause
Increased bone resorption	Hyperparathyroidism, malignancy, granulomatous disease, immobilization, hyperthyroidism, hypervitaminosis A or D
Increased intestinal calcium absorption	Hyperparathyroidism, granulomatous disorders, hypervitaminosis D, milk-alkali syndrome
Decreased renal calcium excretion	Renal failure, volume depletion, hyperparathyroidism, FHH, milk-alkali syndrome, thiazides, lithium
Decreased bone formation	Immobilization

Abbreviation: FHH, familial hypocalciuric hypercalcemia.

(10%), and myeloma or lymphoma (10%). Patients with humoral hypercalcemia of malignancy have manifestations similar to those seen in hyperparathyroid patients, including mild hypophosphatemia and an elevated urinary cyclic adenosine monophosphate (cAMP) level. However, the patients with humoral hypercalcemia of malignancy are more likely to be anemic and less likely to be hyperchloremic compared to patients with pHPT. Perhaps the most valuable difference between humoral hypercalcemia of malignancy (HHM) and pHPT is that both the PTH and the calcitriol levels are in the low or lower normal range in patients with humoral hypercalcemia of malignancy.

Role of PTHrP

PTHrP-induced hypercalcemia, also known as HHM, is the most common cause of hypercalcemia of malignancy (80%). PTHrP is expressed only in neoplasms associated with HHM, such as squamous carcinomas, carcinomas of the breast, kidney, and bladder, and some lymphomas. Local implantation of such tumors in animal models results in hypercalcemia before metastases occur, and antibodies to PTHrP reverse this effect. Finally, the majority of patients with HHM have elevated PTHrP. Although the actions of PTHrP share similarities to those of PTH, there are several differences worthy of discussion. Similar to patients with pHPT, those with HHM have elevated serum calcium, low-normal or low serum phosphate, and elevated urinary calcium, phosphate and cAMP. Both PTH and PTHrP raise serum $1,25\text{-}(OH)_2D$ by stimulating the renal 1-α-hydroxylase. However, serum $1,25\text{-}(OH)_2D$ in patients with HHM is generally low, for unclear reasons. Further, patients with HHM tend to have more hypercalciuria, more bone resorption, but less bone formation compared to those with pHPT.

Local Osteolytic Hypercalcemia

In about 20% of patients with hypercalcemia of malignancy, elaboration of paracrine factors by the tumor in the skeleton causes hypercalcemia. These factors, which include interleukin (IL)-1, IL-6, tumor necrosis factor, and prostaglandin E_2 (PGE_2), drive osteoclastogenic bone resorption and bone loss. If coupled with impaired renal calcium excretion, hypercalcemia may result. Tumors believed to cause local osteolytic hypercalcemia (LOH) include multiple myeloma, breast carcinoma, and lymphoma.

Vitamin D–Mediated Hypercalcemia of Malignancy

Rarely, lymphomas contain 1-α-hydroxylase, which may produce $1,25\text{-}(OH)_2D$ in quantities high enough to cause hypercalcemia. This hormone drives intestinal calcium absorption and bone resorption. The body compensates by increasing renal calcium excretion. With renal impairment or severe calcium overload, hypercalcemia may result.

Nonparathyroid, Nonmalignant Causes of Hypercalcemia

Vitamin D–mediated hypercalcemia, either by excess intake or by excess production, is the most common cause of nonparathyroid, nonmalignant hypercalcemia. Hypercalcemia is mediated by increased intestinal calcium absorption, and to a lesser degree, increased bone resorption. Hypercalcemia occurs only after the kidney's excretory reserve is overwhelmed. Vitamin D, either ingested from the diet or supplements or that produced in the skin, is converted to

25-(OH)D. However, the renal 1-α-hydroxylase is normally so tightly regulated that $1,25\text{-}(OH)_2D$ should not increase in hypercalcemic patients despite excess substrate. Because 25-(OH)D is much less potent at the vitamin D receptor (VDR), hypercalcemia requires very high concentrations in 25-(OH)D-driven disease. This only occurs after pharmacologically excess intake of 25-(OH)D or vitamin D, which is readily converted to 25-(OH)D in the liver. In contrast, $1,25\text{-}(OH)_2D$ may be produced in granulomatous tissue in multiple disorders (most commonly sarcoidosis and tuberculosis) or prescribed by a physician. In these cases, serum 25-(OH)D would be low or normal, but $1,25\text{-}(OH)_2D$ would be elevated. Patients with hypercalcemia from granulomatous disease tend to have other symptoms related to their disease to suggest the diagnosis.

Other causes of hypercalcemia include vitamin A intoxication and hyperthyroidism. Both of these increase bone resorption, and hypercalcemia results when renal calcium excretion is overwhelmed. Alkali, thiazides, and lithium decrease renal calcium excretion. When coupled with excess calcium intake or bone resorption, hypercalcemia ensues. Long-term therapy with lithium is also associated with pHPT. This effect is believed to be due to elevation of the set point for PTH secretion by effects on the CaSR. Withdrawal of lithium therapy usually resolves the condition; however, parathyroidectomy may be required for patients with severe hypercalcemia who are unable to avoid lithium therapy. The milk-alkali syndrome results from huge intake of calcium and alkali (often from milk and antacids). Over time, the high delivery of calcium and alkali to the kidney additionally causes renal insufficiency. Again, hypercalcemia only develops when the mechanisms of renal calcium excretion are overwhelmed. In addition, it has been noted that hypercalcemia of immobilization is more common in conditions with very high bone turnover, such as childhood (active bone modeling and remodeling), or metabolic bone diseases, such as Paget's (osteitis deformans).

The differential diagnosis of hypercalcemia is further refined by excluding pseudoelevation of serum calcium and by obtaining a serum PTH level. Conditions that potentially affect the measured serum calcium level include the following: (i) serum albumin level changes greater than $1\,g/dL$ (alters the protein-bound serum calcium by $0.8\,mg/dL$ in the same direction), (ii) serum globulin concentration changes greater than $1\,g/dL$ (alters protein-bound calcium by $0.16\,mg/dL$ in the same direction), (iii) a change in the serum pH of greater than 0.1 (alters the protein-bound calcium level by $0.17\,mg/dL$ in the same direction), and (iv) dehydration (volume depletion) falsely increases in serum protein-bound calcium concentration. The serum level of intact PTH is elevated in patients with pHPT and suppressed in patients with nonparathyroid causes of hypercalcemia except the following three conditions: lithium intake, FHH, and, rarely, secretion of true PTH by a tumor. The intact PTH immunoradiometric assay as well as the mid-region–specific radioimmunoassay of PTH demonstrate equivalent sensitivity in differentiating between malignancy associated with hypercalcemia and pHPT. However, most laboratories now perform intact (1-84) PTH measurements using the chemiluminescent assay. This intact PTH assay is highly sensitive. Mallette and associates observed that the intact PTH assay is much more accurate for identifying the cause of hypercalcemia in patients with renal insufficiency, because the results of the mid-region–specific assay are sensitive to changes in renal function and biologically inactive fragments of PTH

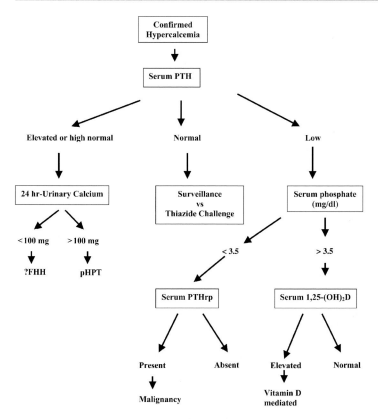

Figure 3 Algorithm to work-up confirmed hypercalcemia.

are mainly cleared by the kidneys (5,6). Our preferred algorithm for evaluation and management of hypercalcemia is shown in Figure 3. If the serum PTH level is high in the presence of hypercalcemia, then pHPT is very likely. Normal or low PTH levels should trigger additional evaluation. The serum phosphate level is useful in identifying patients with vitamin D abnormalities. Numerous studies have documented the high sensitivity of inappropriately elevated serum PTH levels in patients with pHPT. Figure 4 illustrates the separation of serum calcium and PTH levels in normal and hyperparathyroid patients.

Urinary cAMP levels may be of distinguishing value in patients with pHPT. Because cAMP levels are often elevated in primary HPT and only variably elevated in hypercalcemia of malignancy, the detection of low levels of urinary cAMP would make the possibility of coexisting HPT less likely in a patient with malignancy. While serum 1,25-$(OH)_2D$ levels are elevated in primary HPT, they are rarely elevated in hypercalcemia of malignancy, which typically shows decreased measurable, 1,25-$(OH)_2D$ metabolites. Patients with lymphoma can have elevated levels of 1,25-$(OH)_2D$, but they represent a minority of patients with hypercalcemia of malignancy. In 1974, Palmer and associates suggested using the serum chloride–phosphate ratio to differentiate hypercalcemia caused by primary HPT from other causes of hypercalcemia. They found that 96% of patients with pHPT had a serum chloride–phosphate ratio greater than 33, whereas 92% of patients with hypercalcemia due to other causes had a serum chloride–phosphate ratio of less than 30 (7). In pHPT, serum levels of phosphate and bicarbonate are commonly decreased, and the serum chloride level usually exceeds 102 mg/L.

Clinical Manifestations of Hypercalcemia

Intravascular volume contraction is present in almost all patients with severe hypercalcemia and this forms the basis for volume repletion as first line therapy for severe hypercalcemia. Other features depend on the severity of the hypercalcemia and the rapidity of the rise in serum calcium. Anorexia, nausea, vomiting, and mental obtundation are concerning clinical findings in hypercalcemic crisis. The dehydration that is invariably present should result in hypotension, but hypercalcemia increases vascular tone, so the blood pressure may be an inaccurate reflection of the severity of volume contraction. Malignancy is the most common cause of hypercalcemic crisis, and it is important to establish whether the patient has humoral hypercalcemia of malignancy or skeletal metastases. Reliable assays for PTH-related polypeptide are now available, but the results of PTH and calcitriol assays may not be available for several days; therefore, blood studies have a limited role in establishing an early diagnosis of the cause of hypercalcemic crisis. With new-onset localized skeletal pain, radiographs of the affected area should confirm a diagnosis of skeletal metastases. A complete blood count provides clues to the presence of multiple myeloma or other hematologic malignancy, with confirmatory bone marrow examination when indicated. Bradyarrhythmias, bundle-branch blocks, complete heart block, and even cardiac arrest are all well documented complications of acute hypercalcemia. Hypercalcemia potentiates the action of digoxin on the heart, such that any cardiac side effects of this drug may become clinically more significant during hypercalcemic crisis.

Clinical manifestations of hypercalcemia present mainly in the kidney, bone, GI tract, and nervous system.

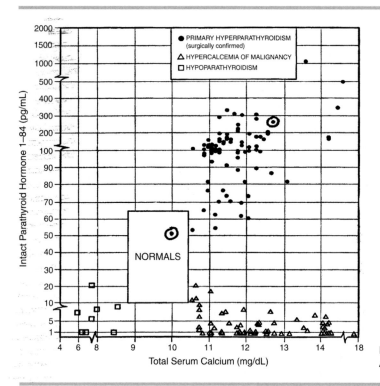

Figure 4 Relationship between PTH values and serum calcium. *Abbreviation*: PTH, parathyroid hormone.

These conditions include nephrolithiasis, nephrocalcinosis, and renal insufficiency. Bone manifestations reflect increased bone turnover (bone pain, pathologic fractures, and osteitis fibrosa cystica). Peptic ulcer disease and pancreatitis reflect GI involvement, whereas neuromuscular derangements are reflected by proximal muscle weakness, atrophy, tongue fasciculations, depression, anxiety, confusion, and in extreme stages, lethargy and coma.

Severe Hypercalcemia

Although severe hypercalcemia is often treated as a medical emergency, it is rarely fatal; therefore cautious, methodical management is recommended. Hypercalcemia of malignant origin is, however, a grave complication, with a survival rate of 45% at three months. Hypercalcemia due to malignant tumors usually develops rapidly and is associated with weight loss. It is also associated with a serum calcium level often exceeding 14 mg/dL, low serum chloride level, elevated or normal serum phosphate and bicarbonate, elevated alkaline phosphatase level, and erythrocyte sedimentation rate. Only 25% of patients with pHPT have a serum calcium level exceeding 14 mg/dL. The acute clinical findings during hypercalcemic crisis invariably include evidence of volume depletion, metabolic encephalopathy, and GI symptoms. There may be associated renal and cardiovascular manifestations beyond those attributable to volume contraction. As with most metabolic emergencies, the clinical presentation depends on acuity of onset and absolute level of hypercalcemia.

Treatment of Severe Hypercalcemia

General Measures. Two chief mechanisms causing hypercalcemic crisis include increased bone resorption and inability of the kidneys to excrete the huge increased filtered load of calcium. Therefore the treatment of hypercalcemia should include efforts to decrease bone resorption and increase urinary calcium excretion. Prompt treatment of severe hypercalcemia should be targeted toward a specific etiology. However, the general treatment measures outlined in Table 3 should begin prior to determination of etiology. Severe hypercalcemia is always associated with water and sodium depletion; therefore, volume expansion with isotonic saline solution is the essential first step of any therapeutic regimen. In addition to providing the necessary fluid, there is an obligatory calcium diuresis with a sodium-induced diuresis. This maneuver dilutes extracellular fluid calcium, expands extracellular volume, and increases urinary calcium excretion. Volume expansion (2–4 L/day) for the first 48 hours improves the glomerular filtration rate and enhances renal excretion of calcium, and lowers the serum calcium level by 1.5 to 2.0 mg/dL during the first 24 to 48 hours. Although volume expansion rarely returns serum calcium levels to normal in patients with severe hypercalcemia, a loop diuretic (e.g., furosemide or ethacrynic acid) enhances the calciuric effects of volume expansion by

Table 3 Acute Management of Severe Hypercalcemia

Encourage saline-induced diuresis (Infuse NaCl 2–4 L daily)

After appropriate diuresis, add loop diuretic (furosemide), 40–80 mg, q 2–4 hourly

Add calcitonin 4 IU/kg subcutaneously or intramuscularly q 12 hourly

Monitor serum sodium, potassium, calcium, and magnesium, q 2–4 hourly

Obtain serum phosphate, chloride, and parathyroid hormone levels

Consider bisphosphonates (Pamidronate 90 mg IV over 24 hr, Alendronate)

Consider steroids if malignancy is confirmed or highly suspected

Consider dialysis for patients with renal insufficiency or unresponsive to prior interventions

Urgent parathyroidectomy may be necessary for patients with parathyroid carcinoma

Abbreviation: IV, intravenous.

inhibiting calcium reabsorption in the thick ascending limb of the loop of Henle. However diuretics should not be administered until there is clear evidence of adequate intravascular volume expansion documented by brisk diuresis or vascular monitoring. If signs of fluid overload develop, the saline infusion is slowed, and a loop diuretic such as furosemide can be given to control volume overload and promote both a sodium and calcium diuresis. However, loop diuretics increase sodium excretion more profoundly than calcium excretion, and if the sodium excretion exceeds the intravenous saline replacement, renal sodium-conserving mechanisms are activated, thus limiting calcium excretion and probably aggravating hypercalcemia.

Volume repletion is clearly ineffective in hypercalcemic crisis patients with severely impaired renal function for reasons other than volume contraction. In such patients, first-line therapy must be hemodialysis, which can be administered with any available dialysate, until a low- or zero-calcium dialysate fluid is available, because the calcium concentration in all dialysis fluids is less than the plasma level in patients with hypercalcemic crisis. Thiazide diuretics are contraindicated because they enhance distal tubular calcium reabsorption. A review of medications and nutritional status is prudent to identify and discontinue drugs such as calcium supplements, vitamin D preparations, and other agents known to increase the serum calcium level or inhibit calcium excretion. Ongoing efforts at identifying the etiology of hypercalcemia should not be interrupted during the management of acute hypercalcemia.

Specific Therapy. The administration of inhibitors of osteoclast-mediated bone resorption (e.g., bisphosphonates, plicamycin, and calcitonin) is the next step in the treatment of hypercalcemia. Recently, the Food and Drug Administration approved gallium nitrate, which blocks PTH-induced calcium resorption of bone, for parenteral treatment of hypercalcemia. Ideally, if the cause of the hypercalcemia is known, specific therapy is preferable, e.g., glucocorticoids for hypercalcemic crisis due to granulomatous disease. The bisphosphonates directly inhibit osteoclast function, and the first-line bisphosphonate for hypercalcemic crisis is pamidronate (Aredia®). These agents are poorly absorbed from the GI tract, but when given intravenously, the bisphosphonates reduce serum calcium levels to normal in most patients with hypercalcemia of malignancy.

Pamidronate is more potent and possibly less toxic than etidronate. In clinical trials using 24-hour infusions of pamidronate, 70% to 100% of patients had lower serum calcium levels within 24 hours of initiation of treatment. Thus, pamidronate, in conjunction with vigorous saline hydration, is indicated for moderate or severe hypercalcemia due to malignancy. If normocalcemia is not achieved with an initial infusion, a second infusion will certainly decrease serum calcium levels. One disadvantage of bisphosphonates is that plasma calcium levels typically do not become normal for three to six days after their administration. This may be unduly long for critically ill patients in hypercalcemic crisis. The more common adverse reactions to pamidronate include transient mild temperature elevation soon after the drug is given, local infusion site reactions, mild GI symptoms, mild hypophosphatemia, hypokalemia, and hypomagnesemia. The first-generation bisphosphonate, Etidronate (Didronel®), is also FDA-approved for treating acute hypercalcemia, but it is considered less effective compared to pamidronate, because pamidronate lowers the calcium level more rapidly and predictably than etidronate. Because excretion of etidronate occurs mainly in the kidneys, it is important to adjust the dose for impaired renal function. Possible adverse reactions to Etidronate include elevations of BUN or serum creatinine, metallic or altered taste in up to 5% of patients, and transient elevations of serum phosphate levels.

Calcitonin inhibits osteoclastic bone resorption and thereby decreases serum calcium concentrations. It is a naturally occurring peptide produced by the C-cells of the thyroid gland. In addition to its osteoclast inhibiting effect, it has a moderate calciuric effect and an analgesic effect as well. The greatest advantage of this particular antiresorptive agent is that it has a fairly rapid onset of action. Serum calcium concentrations may begin to decline within several hours of the initiation of administration. At a dosage of 4 to 8 units/kg every 6 to 12 hours subcutaneously or intravenously, some degree of calcium lowering is seen in approximately 75% of patients. The disadvantage of this medication is that, in general, it is not as potent as either of the bisphosphonates, gallium nitrate, or plicamycin (mithramycin), and the hypocalcemic effect of calcitonin is fairly short-lived. Thus, for the treatment of hypercalcemic crisis, calcitonin should be considered an adjunctive rather than a primary therapy. The most common adverse reactions to calcitonin are nausea, with or without vomiting. Local inflammatory reactions at the site of calcitonin injection also occurs in about 10% of patients receiving this agent, and flushing of the face or hands occurs in a small percentage of patients.

Plicamycin (mithramycin) is produced by a *Streptomyces* microorganism and is effective for treating hypercalcemia. It acts by inhibiting cellular RNA synthesis and reduces the serum calcium level more quickly than do the bisphosphonates. With a plicamycin dose of 25 mg/kg of body weight administered intravenously in 5% dextrose in water over a period of four to six hours, most patients achieve normocalcemia within one to three days. If necessary, it may be readministered for three or four consecutive days. Plicamycin is more potent than calcitonin, but its effectiveness is often limited by hepatotoxicity, nephrotoxicity, and thrombocytopenia.

Gallium nitrate can be used in the management of severe hypercalcemia of malignancy. It inhibits bone resorption, although the precise mechanism of action is not clear. It may be administered as a continuous intravenous infusion of 200 mg/m^2 body surface area for five consecutive days. In clinical trials, this dose of gallium nitrate reduces the serum calcium level to normal in 75% to 82% of treated patients, but its maximum effect may require five to six days of treatment. Gallium nitrate is indicated for the treatment of clearly symptomatic cancer-related hypercalcemia that has not responded to general measures (i.e., volume repletion with or without loop diuretics). A serious adverse effect of gallium nitrate is nephrotoxicity. For this reason, it is generally recommended that gallium nitrate not be administered to patients with baseline serum creatinine levels greater than 2.5 mg/dL. Transient hypophosphatemia, mild respiratory alkalosis, anemia, nausea, vomiting, and hypotension have also been reported with gallium nitrate. However, the lack of familiarity with gallium combined with the availability of other effective and less toxic hypocalcemic agents limit the widespread use of gallium nitrate for hypercalcemia.

Glucocorticoids are the treatment of choice for hypercalcemia caused by vitamin D toxicity, certain malignancies (such as multiple myeloma and lymphoma), sarcoidosis, or other granulomatous diseases in which the production of

1,25-(OH)$_2$D is the known mechanism for causing hypercalcemia. Typically a 200 to 300 mg dose of hydrocortisone is administered intravenously daily for three to five days. However, the maximal calcium-lowering effect does not occur for at least several days after initiating therapy. Glucocorticoids act by inhibiting the inflammatory cell proliferation within granulomatous tissue and hematologic malignancies and thereby decreasing the 1,25-(OH)$_2$D levels that cause hypercalcemia. In most patients with hypercalcemic crisis, the glucocorticoids are of limited utility because, although they decrease intestinal calcium absorption and increase urinary calcium excretion, their onset of action is relatively slow. They are best reserved as an adjunctive therapy for hypercalcemic crisis.

Phosphate Therapy. Although phosphate therapy was initially proposed for the treatment of hypercalcemia, concerns regarding the precipitation of calcium-phosphate salts in soft tissue have limited the enthusiasm for intravenous phosphate administration in patients with hypercalcemia.

Hypocalcemia

Hypocalcemia, which results when calcium excretion exceeds intake, may result in several clinical manifestations. The most common symptoms relate to neuromuscular excitability. The first symptoms, paresthesias, occur particularly in perioral and acral (hands and feet) positions. Numbness and tingling also occur with hyperventilation in normal individuals, because ionized calcium falls when respiratory alkalosis shifts free calcium to the albumin-bound fraction. Muscular cramping usually starts at the hands and feet (carpopedal spasm) but may occur elsewhere. Tetany may become generalized across the body during severe hypocalcemia. Smooth muscle spasm may lead to abdominal pain, bronchospasm, and laryngospasm. The latter two conditions could result in wheezing and shortness of breath. Severe hypocalcemia may also result in confusion or even psychosis. Conduction abnormalities may result in seizures. Hypocalcemia also may affect cardiac function resulting in palpitations, due to arrhythmia or shortness of breath and other symptoms of congestive heart failure. Physical findings of neuromuscular excitability may be induced at the bedside in patients with hypocalcemia. *Chvostek's sign* is a contraction of facial muscles on the side of the face on tapping the facial nerve 1 to 2 cm anterior to the external auditory meatus. When floridly positive, the facial muscles on the same side contract at the eye, nose, and lips. Chvostek's sign is not pathognomonic for hypocalcemia because 10% of normal subjects may demonstrate a mild response such as twitching of the lips toward the side of the tapping. Unlike hypocalcemic patients, the response in normal individuals is usually blunted with repeated stimulation, i.e., repeated tapping progressively extinguishes the response. *Trousseau's sign*, a carpal spasm elicited by inflating a blood pressure cuff on the arm 20 mm above systolic blood pressure for three minutes, is more specific for hypocalcemia. Adduction of the thumb, extension of the phalanges, and flexion of the metacarpophalangeal joints and the wrist characterize the spasm.

Mechanisms of Hypocalcemia

The causes of hypocalcemia are grouped according to the main mechanisms: lack of PTH effect, lack of vitamin D effect, and calcium binding or redistribution. These are described below.

Lack of PTH Effect

The most common cause in this category is postsurgical hypoparathyroidism, in which the parathyroid glands are removed or injured during surgical procedures in the neck. Autoimmune destruction is the second most common cause of lack of PTH effect. Although the latter patients may have isolated hypoparathyroidism, they often have multiple accompanying abnormalities such as moniliasis, hypoadrenalism, diabetes mellitus, Hashimoto's thyroiditis, hypogonadism, autoimmune hepatitis, vitiligo, etc. The parathyroid glands may be congenitally absent in the 22q11.2 deletion syndrome (DiGeorge, velocardiofacial, and conotruncal anomaly face syndromes). Infiltration of the parathyroid glands with iron (hemachromatosis), copper (Wilson's disease), amyloid, or tumor also decreases their function. A recently discovered familial cause of hypoparathyroidism involves activating mutations of the CaSR. In these patients, serum PTH is suppressed even when serum calcium is relatively low. Hypomagnesemia causes resistance to and, with increasing severity, decreased secretion of PTH. Finally, patients suffer PTH resistance. Apart from its functions to raise serum calcium, PTH also lowers serum phosphorus by enhancing renal phosphorus excretion. Therefore patients with lack of PTH effect, have both hypocalcemia and hyperphosphatemia. The hyperphosphatemia may result in additional clinical manifestations due to soft tissue calcium deposition. Patients with hypoparathyroidism may have cataracts, calcification of the basal ganglia in the brain, and even moderate-to-severe cerebral calcification and mental retardation. Basal ganglia calcification may result in Parkinson's disease.

Lack of Vitamin D Effect

The effects of vitamin D may be a result of inadequate intake, impaired production, increased destruction, or resistance to vitamin D.

Inadequate Nutrition/Sunlight. Vitamin D$_3$ is present in only few foods such as vitamin D–fortified milk (100 IU/cup), cod liver oil, and fatty fish such as salmon. Thus, it is difficult to achieve sufficient intake (600–800 IU/day) by dietary sources alone. Vitamin D may also be produced in the skin with adequate ultraviolet light exposure. However, conditions that limit ultraviolet light exposure impair vitamin D synthesis in the skin. These include dwelling in northern latitudes and temperate climates with poor sunlight, and individuals with darker skin. Finally, the ability of the skin of older individuals to produce vitamin D is impaired.

Impaired Production. Rarely, inadequate 25-hydroxylation of vitamin D may occur due to a lack of the hydroxylase enzyme or severe liver disease. Impaired production of 1,25-(OH)$_2$D due to deficiency of the renal 1-α-hydroxylase or a phosphate-wasting disorder is a clinical rarity. In patients with hypocalcemia from hypoparathyroidism, 1,25-(OH)$_2$D production is suppressed due to low serum PTH and high serum phosphate, thus the need for concurrent vitamin D and calcium replacement in patients with postoperative hypoparathyroidism.

Catabolism or Loss. This is a poorly recognized but common cause of vitamin D insufficiency. Drugs such as phenobarbital and phenytoin increase catabolism of 25-(OH)D, or vitamin D substrates may be lost in the stool or urine. Fat malabsorption impairs the absorption of vitamin D, a fat-soluble vitamin, because vitamin D is normally secreted into the bile and reabsorbed in the ileum. Diarrhea may interrupt this enterohepatic loop by increasing bowel motility. In proteinuric states, vitamin D insufficiency results because VDBP with its bound vitamin D and 25-(OH)D is expelled into the urine.

Resistance. The key effects of vitamin D are mediated via its nuclear receptor, the VDR. Mutations in VDR result in a resistant state characterized by low serum calcium and phosphate, but elevated serum PTH and 1,25-(OH)$_2$D.

Binding/Redistribution of Calcium. A common cause of hypocalcemia is binding of calcium by phosphates, citrate, or other substances in blood or tissue. Phosphate binds calcium avidly, and if both calcium and phosphate concentrations are sufficiently high, calcium phosphate may precipitate in soft tissues. Elevated serum phosphate occurs due to reduced urinary excretion in renal failure or by shift out of other compartments such as massive lysis of tumor cells or necrosis of muscle with tissue injury (rhabdomyolysis). Citrate, a preservative in blood to prevent clotting by binding calcium, may cause symptomatic hypocalcemia by lowering ionized calcium even though total calcium remains in the normal range. Similarly, alkalosis reduces ionized, but not total calcium, by increased albumin binding. In patients with pancreatitis, one postulated cause of hypocalcemia is calcium saponification of the fatty acids within the pancreas and intra-abdominal tissues.

Assessment and Management of Patients with Hypocalcemia

Prior to beginning an extensive evaluation in patients with hypocalcemia, pseudohypocalcemia caused by hypoalbuminemia should be excluded. Moreover, patients with alkalosis and normal serum total calcium may have true symptoms of hypocalcemia, due to the shift of ionized calcium to the protein-bound fraction. It is sometimes necessary to directly measure ionized calcium and avoid these confounding variables. Once true hypocalcemia is confirmed, history and physical may provide helpful clues to its underlying cause. A specific congenital defect is suggested by onset of hypocalcemic symptoms early in life and by a positive family history. Vitamin D deficiency presents in patients with poor vitamin D intake, low sunlight exposure, diarrhea, and hyperpigmented skin, in old age, or in patients residing in northern latitudes. A history of neck surgery, cancer, or recent trauma points to decreased PTH secretion.

The most clinically useful initial test in patients with normal renal function is the serum phosphate. An elevated serum phosphate (>3.5 mg/dL) indicates a diminished PTH effect, and serum PTH should be measured. If PTH is low, deficient vitamin D production or severe hypomagnesemia is likely. On the contrary, if PTH is elevated, PTH resistance should be suspected. In contrast, low serum phosphate (<3.5 mg/dL) implicates diminished action of vitamin D. Such patients should have a compensatory increase in serum PTH. Vitamin D insufficiency is confirmed by low serum 25-(OH)D. If serum 25-(OH)D is normal, then serum 1,25-(OH)$_2$D should be measured. Low levels of 1,25-(OH)$_2$D establish the diagnosis of 1-α-hydroxylase deficiency, whereas high 1,25-(OH)$_2$D levels suggest vitamin D resistance. Figure 5 illustrates our preferred algorithm for evaluating patients with hypocalcemia. Patients with low serum phosphate should be treated with calcium and vitamin D. Serum calcium less than 7.0 mg/dL in a newly

diagnosed patient with moderately symptomatic hypocalcemia should be treated with intravenous calcium. Dairy intake, an excellent source of calcium and phosphate, should be encouraged in these patients. Moreover, calcium supplementation should be ingested separate from meals to avoid binding phosphate. In contrast, dairy should be avoided and calcium supplementation should be given with all meals to control serum phosphate in patients with hyperphosphatemia. Intravenous calcium, when necessary, should be given with extreme caution, if at all, in patients with hyperphosphatemia because of the previously mentioned risk of soft tissue deposition of calcium phosphate.

PHOSPHATE METABOLISM

Inorganic phosphate (Pi) is an important regulator of bone formation, acid–base regulation, and cellular metabolism. Numerous intracellular signaling activities require the high-energy phosphate bonds present in adenosine triphosphate. The bulk of phosphate resides in bone (600–700 g) with the remainder in soft tissues. In contrast to serum calcium, the regulation of phosphate metabolism depends less on hormonal effects but primarily on GI absorption and renal excretion. Most phosphate absorption occurs in the jejunum and ileum, and in normal individuals correlates linearly with dietary phosphate intake. The cellular process of phosphate uptake is by diffusional flux and active transport, with most of the uptake occurring by the former process. Phosphate deficiency due to inadequate oral intake is rare because most diets contain abundant amounts of phosphate. In contrast, hyperphosphatemia can occur due to inadequate renal excretion. Normally, phosphate concentration in the glomerular ultrafiltrate is 90% of plasma concentrations. However approximately 70% of this amount is reabsorbed in the proximal convoluted tubule. The proximal convoluted tubules, proximal straight tubule, and distal tubule all contain a PTH-sensitive adenylate cyclase. There is evidence suggesting that PTH decreases phosphate reabsorption by cAMP-dependent and independent mechanisms. cAMP-dependent protein kinase A and phospholipase C-protein kinase C both modulate PTH effects on the renal tubular phosphate reabsorption.

Disorders of Phosphate Metabolism
Hyperphosphatemia
Hyperphosphatemia is the result of increased intake (intravenous administration or phosphate enemas), decreased renal excretion (renal failure, hypoparathyroidism and PTH resistance, acromegaly, etidronate, and tumoral calcinosis), increased production from tissue injury (rhabdomyolysis, tumor lysis, hemolytic anemia, leukemia, acidosis, fulminant hepatitis, and hyperthermia), or a combination of these causes. Hyperphosphatemia due to excessive intestinal phosphate is seen mainly in children receiving phosphate-containing laxatives. In adult clinical practice, hyperphosphatemia is most commonly observed as a consequence of renal insufficiency. Management of mild to moderate hyperphosphatemia is by dietary phosphate reduction. This strategy is rarely successful because low-phosphate diets tend to be unpalatable. The use of aluminum hydroxide antacids or similar compounds to bind intestinal phosphate, thus preventing its absorption, is effective in patients with renal insufficiency. Hemodialysis is also effective for acute severe hyperphospatemia.

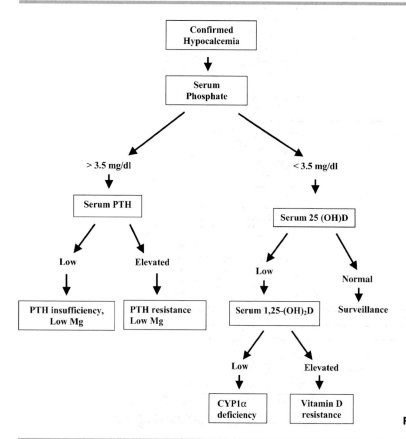

Figure 5 Algorithm to evaluate patients with hypocalcemia.

Hypophosphatemia

Hypophospatemia most frequently results from inadequate intake or increased renal excretion of phosphate. Because western diets contain abundant phosphate, inadequate absorption is usually the result of phosphate binding in the GI tract. This can be caused by aluminum or calcium, both of which avidly bind intraluminal phosphate. Renal phosphate excretion can be increased during pHPT, Fanconi's syndrome, hypophosphatemic rickets, or oncogenic osteomalacia. Potassium deficiency may also cause phosphate wasting. The initial management of hypophosphatemia is oral phosphate administration.

Oral administration of phosphate is usually well tolerated. Because oral phosphate also binds calcium in the GI tract, the preferred method of oral phosphate administration is in divided doses. Phosphate is also better tolerated when administered with food. Oral phosphate is administered as a total of 1 to 2 g of elemental phosphate daily in divided doses. Diarrhea limits the total amount of oral phosphate that can be administered. Intravenous phosphate administration may be necessary in patients with acute severe hypophosphatemia, however it should be given very cautiously, especially when serum calcium levels are elevated. This is to avoid the risk of precipitation of calcium/phosphate salts in soft tissues. Intravenous phosphate should be considered only for severe hypophosphatemia (<1.0 mg/dL) or symptomatic hypophosphatemia. Rates of administration should be less than 2 to 8 mmol/hr over four to eight hours and serum calcium and phosphate levels should be monitored every 6 to 12 hours.

THE PARATHYROID GLANDS
Anatomy of the Parathyroid Glands

During the end of the first month in utero, the inferior parathyroids (parathyroid III) proliferate from the third pharyngeal pouch along with the thymus, while the superior parathyroids (parathyroid IV) proliferate from the fourth branchial pouches in association with the lateral anlage of the thyroid. Parathyroid III (the inferior parathyroids) descends with the thymus usually to the lower border of the thyroid. Because parathyroid III migrates further than parathyroid IV (the superior parathyroids) during embryogenesis, the *lower parathyroid glands are more likely to be situated in abnormal locations.* Parathyroid IV (the superior parathyroids) migrates with the thyroid gland and usually comes to rest on the posterolateral aspect of the thyroid where the recurrent laryngeal nerve enters posterior to the cricothyroid muscle. Supernumerary (>4) parathyroid glands can occur in up to 22% of patients and up to eight glands have been reported. In contrast, fewer than four glands are present in 3% to 5% of individuals. The superior parathyroid glands are usually located on the posteromedial aspect of the thyroid gland, within a 2 cm circumference and 1 cm above the point of intersection of the recurrent laryngeal nerve and inferior thyroid artery. The inferior parathyroids usually lie on the posterolateral aspect of the lower pole of the thyroid gland, below (inferior to) the inferior thyroid artery and anterior to the recurrent laryngeal nerve but may be found within the thymus, carotid sheath, thyroid gland, or in an undescended position. Lower parathyroid glands can also be located at the level of the carotid bulb, (parathymus) or in the aortopulmonary window. This information is helpful when one parathyroid gland cannot be identified intraoperatively. It allows a directed search for missing parathyroid glands in the neck. The most common ectopic site for the inferior parathyroid glands is in or near the thymus, whereas the most common ectopic site for the superior glands is deep in the neck, in the tracheoesophageal groove, or posterior superior mediastinum posterior to the inferior thyroid artery. The inferior thyroid artery usually supplies the superior and the inferior parathyroid glands, although some parathyroids receive their blood supply from the superior thyroid artery and from anastomoses between the inferior and superior thyroid artery.

Primary Hyperparathyroidism

pHPT is the most common cause of hypercalcemia in the ambulatory setting. In hospitalized patients, pHPT is second in frequency to cancer as a cause of hypercalcemia; thus pHPT and cancer together account for 90% of all cases of hypercalcemia. Until the early 1970s, when routine serum electrolyte tests became widely available using multichannel laboratory analyzing machines, renal colic and kidney stones were the main presenting features of pHPT. Currently, most patients with pHPT are identified during routine biochemical screening (8,9).

The estimated incidence of pHPT in the United States is one new case each year per 2000 to 4000 persons in the general population (80,000–100,000 new cases annually) (10–12). pHPT occurs in 0.1% to 0.3% of the general population and is more common in women (1/500 women) than in men (1/2000 men). Primary HPT is also common in peri- or postmenopausal women and is rare in children. Approximately 87% of patients with pHPT have parathyroid adenomas, 12% have multigland hyperplasia, while 0.1% harbor a parathyroid cancer (5). This distribution is illustrated in Table 4.

Pathology of pHPT

Normal parathyroid glands in adults are usually ovoid shaped, yellow–brown, encapsulated, weighing about 35 to 40 mg, and measuring $5 \times 3 \times 1$ mm. The color varies with the amount of stromal fat present. Early in life, the glands are composed of sheets of chief cells lacking stromal fat and appear reddish brown. With increasing age, stromal fat increases to approximately 30% to 40% of the gland volume. The stromal fat also depends on body size and composition, thus overweight individuals tend to develop fatty parathyroid glands. The normal parathyroid glands tend to be soft and flabby, often taking the shape of the surrounding structures. Histologically, the normal gland has a thin fibrous capsule. Cell types identified in parathyroid glands include chief cells, oxyphil cells, water clear cells, and transitional cells. Chief cells usually predominate

with two subgroups, dark and light (or clear, glycogen-containing) cells. The latter are defined by pale eosinophilic vacuolated staining. The dark chief cells are responsible for the synthesis and secretion of PTH.

Parathyroid Adenoma

The first molecular genetic abnormality identified in patients with parathyroid adenoma results from two breaks and an inversion in chromosome 11 that move the 5′ regulatory region of the PTH gene away from the coding sequence to a distinct gene known as proline-rich attachment domain (PRADI). The protein encoded by PRADI is a cyclin, which stimulates cell proliferation without malignant change. The unmutated chromosome, with its 5′ regulatory and coding regions adjacent and unchanged, is presumably the source of excess PTH secretion. This defect occurs in about 5% of parathyroid adenomas. However, up to 25% of parathyroid adenomas show losses of large segments of one allele of chromosome 11, which, in association with deletions or with mutations of the other allele, could lead to adenoma formation. Adenomas are principally monoclonal. In contrast, parathyroid hyperplasia, especially as seen in multiple endocrine neoplasia type 1 (MEN 1), is typically polyclonal, presumably because of an inherited mutation in a tumor suppressor locus on chromosome 11.

Parathyroid Hyperplasia

Multiglandular pHPT or parathyroid hyperplasia is defined as the presence of two or more enlarged glands weighing greater than 50 mg. Multiglandular hyperparathyroidism patients account for approximately 15% to 20% of patients with sporadic primary HPT. Chief-cell hyperplasia occurs more commonly than clear-cell hyperplasia. Grossly, chief-cell hyperplastic glands appear yellow to tan to red–brown, often with small cysts, and one or two glands are significantly larger than the remainder. Clear-cell hyperplastic parathyroid glands are more markedly enlarged than in chief-cell hyperplasia. Histologically, chief-cell hyperplasia is without stromal fat and may be either diffuse or nodular. Lobular parathyroid glands with variable glandular pattern, cord arrangement, and sheets suggest chief-cell hyperplasia. In clear-cell hyperplasia, the cytoplasm is characteristically pale and vacuolated with variable enlarged cells. Multiple parathyroid tumors are more common in patients over 60 years old and in patients with familial HPT. Parathyroid adenomas generally have a follicular arrangement varying mitosis, cell, and nuclear size. A normal or atrophic rim of parathyroid tissue with fat cells external to the hypercellular tissue suggests adenomatous disease, but does occur in multiglandular disease also. In spite of these differences, the histological differentiation of parathyroid adenomas from hyperplasia is very difficult. As such, it is not possible to differentiate between single and multigland parathyroid disease using intraoperative frozen section examination of one gland. Rather all parathyroid tissue is visualized and the intraoperative decision is made on size, color, and consistency of the parathyroid tissue. Unfortunately, attempts to differentiate adenoma from hyperplasia by frozen section of a single gland, continues to be a common error during parathyroidectomy. Recently, this decision has been less difficult due to increased use of intraoperative PTH measurements.

Parathyroid Cancer

The incidence of parathyroid cancer is now estimated to be about 0.1% of the whole population (Hundahl) (13). Patients

Table 4 Distribution of Parathyroid Abnormalities

Type	Frequency (%)
Adenoma	80–85
Double adenoma	1–2
Hyperplasia	10–15
Carcinoma	<1
Parathyroid cyst	1–3
Parathyromatosis	<0.1
Ectopic hyperparathyroidism	Few reported cases

with parathyroid cancer often present with florid signs and symptoms of HPT and marked hypercalcemia. The average serum calcium levels and PTH levels in patients with parathyroid cancer are usually higher compared to benign parathyroid adenoma. Neck masses are palpable in 32% to 69% of patients with parathyroid carcinomas. Intraoperative differentiation between benign and malignant parathyroid tissue is fairly clear because the latter group have a tendency for locally aggressive growth. However, differentiation of parathyroid cancer from atypical parathyroid adenoma by gross inspection is not possible. At operation, parathyroid cancers are often large and hard, and have a whitish capsule that is adherent to adjacent tissues. For the diagnosis of parathyroid carcinoma, it is imperative to have one of the three following criteria: (i) capsular invasion, (ii) metastases to local lymph nodes or distant organs (lung, liver or bone), or (iii) local recurrence following complete resection (not caused by tumor spillage at resection). Histologically, a trabecular growth pattern, numerous mitotic figures, capsular invasion, and marked neovascularization sometimes help distinguish parathyroid carcinoma from adenoma. Parathyroid cancer is treated by an en bloc resection of all the structures surrounding the neoplastic gland. Even for recurrences, surgical resection is generally the most effective treatment for controlling hypercalcemia. Hypocalcemia is the best marker for successful resection of a parathyroid cancer. Recurrences often occur many years after resection of the primary lesion. Thus, lifelong surveillance is necessary. Scant reports exist of partial responses to radiation therapy (5412 cGy) or chemotherapy (14).

Parathyromatosis

Parathyromatosis is a rare entity that usually occurs in patients with secondary HPT or patients with MEN 1 after parathyroidectomy. It is characterized by the finding of multiple nodules of hyperfunctioning parathyroid tissue scattered throughout the neck and mediastinum. The characteristic location of parathyromatosis is in the superior mediastinal fat, tracheoesophageal groove, or at parathyroid autotransplantation sites. The cause of parathyromatosis is unknown, but seeding at surgery, hyperplastic remnant parathyroid tissue, or parathyroid carcinoma are some of the possible causes. Seeding at surgery seems an unlikely cause of this condition because resection of local disease is rarely curative.

Clinical and Biochemical Diagnosis of pHPT

The current clinical presentation of pHPT in the United States bears little resemblance to the "classical primary hyperparathyroidism," described by Albright in the 1930s, which was characterized by nephrolithiasis, osteitis fibrosa cystica, and frequent neuromuscular complications in the majority of patients (15). The biochemical changes associated with pHPT often result in alterations in bone density with a predisposition to urolithiasis, skeletal fractures, neuromuscular weakness, abdominal pain, and vague mood or personality changes. Historically the constellation of these symptoms has been referred to as "stones, bones, groans, abdominal moans, and psychic overtones." Primary HPT is now most commonly diagnosed by the unexpected detection of hypercalcemia by a multichannel autoanalyzer examination performed in patients with no symptoms clearly referable to hypercalcemia or increased PTH levels (16). However, population-based studies suggest that closer evaluation of "asymptomatic" patients with pHPT reveals that

these patients often have neuropsychiatric complaints, including lassitude, fatigue, irritability, and lack of sexual and emotional interests. These patients also have more frequent subclinical abnormalities such as lower total body, spine, and hip bone density and higher serum alkaline phosphatase, cholesterol very low density lipoprotein (VLDL), triglycerides, glucose, urate, and hemoglobin values, compared to age-matched controls. In addition, clinically detected HPT is associated with premature cardiovascular death (17–19). Others have also noted an increased association between pHPT and cardiovascular morbidity, including myocardial and valvular calcifications and hypertension. Further, numerous studies demonstrate regression of cardiac abnormalities such as left ventricular hypertrophy one year after successful parathyroid surgery (20–25).

pHPT is characterized by hypercalcemia in the presence of inappropriately elevated PTH levels. Two-site or intact antibody-based assays have improved the sensitivity for documenting an inappropriately elevated intact PTH level in the serum. These assays demonstrate no cross-reactivity with PTH-related peptide as occurs with earlier C-terminal or mid-regional PTH assays. Intact PTH assays have facilitated the distinction between HPT and other causes of hypercalcemia. In the latter, PTH levels are uniformly suppressed; however, PTH is frankly elevated in approximately 90%, but not all, of patients with pHPT. Even pHPT patients with "normal" PTH levels demonstrate a PTH level that is in the high-normal range, i.e., too high for the concurrent serum calcium. Patients with pHPT and coexisting vitamin D deficiency may also present with normal serum calcium levels, although their PTH levels are high. Vitamin D deficiency, which is not uncommon in adults in the United States, can be demonstrated by serum assays for calcifediol and/or calcitriol. In such patients, correction of the vitamin D deficiency causes an increase in the serum calcium level into the hypercalcemic range. Rarely, a patient with malignancy has an elevated PTH level due to ectopic secretion of native PTH by the tumor. More commonly, hypercalcemia in a patient with a malignancy is associated with the secretion of PTH-related protein, a molecule that does not cross-react with PTH.

Other laboratory findings in patients with pHPT include low or low-normal serum phosphorus (90%), hypercalciuria, hyperchloremia or high-normal chloride (80%), elevated alkaline phosphatase (10%), elevated chloride–phosphorus ratio (≥ 33), and elevated serum uric acid. The average total urinary calcium excretion is at the upper end of normal and only about 40% of all hyperparathyroid patients have hypercalciuria. Serum 25-(OH)D levels tend to be in the lower spectrum of the normal range. Although mean values of 1,25-dihydroxyvitamin D_3 are in the high-normal range, approximately one-third of patients have frankly elevated levels of this hormone. Measurements of the blood urea nitrogen level and serum creatinine level and a urinalysis can document normal renal function and rule out renal failure or calculi. The vitamin D (25-OH) level may be measured if excessive vitamin D intake is suspected. The serum level of 1,25-$(OH)_2D$ is usually in the high-normal range or mildly increased in patients with pHPT.

Bone resorption and bone formation are increased by parathyroid hormone. Biochemical markers of bone turnover provide clues to the extent of skeletal involvement in pHPT. Bone formation is reflected by osteoblast products, including bone-specific alkaline phosphatase activity, osteocalcin, and Type I procollagen peptide, all of which are increased in pHPT. Although the urinary hydroxyproline level is usually elevated in patients with osteitis fibrosa cystica, mild asymptomatic pHPT is typically associated with normal hydroxyproline levels. The blood urea nitrogen and serum creatinine levels must be measured because renal insufficiency alters the interpretation of the serum and urinary calcium measurements. Serum protein electrophoresis is important to exclude multiple myeloma, but patients with multiple myeloma should have a normal intact PTH level.

Benign FHH is the metabolic condition that can most closely mimic HPT biochemically, with increased serum calcium and intact PTH levels. However, patients with FHH usually demonstrate low urinary calcium ($<100\,\text{mg}/24\,\text{hr}$), whereas patients with HPT have normal or elevated urinary calcium levels ($>100\,\text{mg}/24\,\text{hr}$). For this reason, it is important to include a 24-hour urine test for calcium and serum and urinary creatinine measurements in the diagnostic evaluation. However, urinary calcium measurement is not necessary if the patient has previously had blood tests documenting normocalcemia before the onset of primary HPT. In conclusion, pHPT can be accurately and cost-effectively diagnosed by documenting an elevated serum calcium level and an elevated serum level of intact PTH in a patient who is not hypocalciuric.

Serum levels of bone-specific alkaline phosphatase and osteocalcin are also good clinical indicators of increased bone turnover in patients with pHPT, because they are elevated before parathyroidectomy and decrease after parathyroidectomy. If significantly elevated, these markers may be useful in determining the need for parathyroidectomy in patients with mild or asymptomatic hyperparathyroidism (18).

Treatment of pHPT

There is little debate about the need for parathyroidectomy in patients with classic symptomatic pHPT characterized by radiologic manifestations of pHPT (significantly decreased bone density or osteitis fibrosa cystica), nephrolithiasis or nephrocalcinosis, classical neuromuscular disease characterized by generalized fatigue and muscular weakness and easy fatigability (especially quadriceps muscle weakness and fatigability), fracture, and acute pHPT (i.e., hypercalcemic crisis). Other indications for parathyroidectomy are coexisting vitamin D deficiency or inability to ensure long-term follow-up. However, much controversy exists about the appropriate management of patients with asymptomatic or minimally symptomatic pHPT. The National Institutes of Health (NIH) Consensus Conference clearly recommended surgery for patients with significant adverse effects of pHPT, complicating coexistent illnesses, age less than 50, and those in whom consistent long-term follow-up could not be assured. The Consensus Conference agreed that conscientious surveillance may be justified in patients with minimal hypercalcemia and no adverse effects, but it recognized that for many patients, the time and expense involved in rigorous follow-up could outweigh the risks of surgery. More recently the NIH convened another consensus conference. Their recommendations are published in manuscript form (26). A comparison of both recommendations is listed in Table 5.

Surgery for pHPT

Felix Mandl performed the first successful parathyroidectomy on a street-car driver with osteitis fibrosa cystica in 1925. After removal of a $21 \times 15 \times 12\,\text{mm}$ parathyroid gland, the patient's urine cleared within a week and recalcification of his bones was noted on follow-up radiography. In 1926, the first parathyroidectomy in the United States was

Table 5 Recommendations for Surgical Intervention

Measurement	Guidelines (1990)	Guidelines (2002)
Serum Ca (above upper limit of normal)	1–1.6 mg/dL	1.0 mg/dL
24 hr urinary calcium	> 400 mg	> 400 mg
Creatinine clearance	Reduced by 30%	Reduced by 30%
Bone mineral density	z-score < -2.0 (forearm)	t-score < -2.5 any site
Age < 50 years		

performed on a sea captain (Charles Martell); unfortunately he required six operations, including total thyroidectomy, over a seven-year period before an elusive parathyroid adenoma was identified beneath his sternum and removed. His hypercalcemia resolved but he died soon of renal failure after the successful operation. Since then, parathyroidectomy has been demonstrated to successfully cure over 95% of patients with pHPT (27–31).

Technique. Until recently, most surgeons advocated routine bilateral neck exploration and identification of all parathyroid glands. During bilateral neck exploration, abnormal glands are defined by size, weight, color, and consistency.

Recent advances in Sestamibi imaging and rapid intact PTH assay have fueled the development of minimally invasive approaches for parathyroid operative procedures. Minimally invasive approaches have potential for improved cosmetic appearance, elimination of overnight hospital admission, less pain, and shorter convalescence. However, they rely heavily on the availability and accuracy of preoperative localization tests such as high-resolution ultrasonography, Sestamibi scanning, computed tomography (CT), and/or magnetic resonance imaging (MRI) (32). Abnormal glands are then localized at operation. Palpation, intraoperative ultrasonography, and radioactive probe–directed localization (see below) may be useful adjuncts to localize the enlarged glands in the operating room. Controversy abounds regarding the costs of preoperative testing in patients and the potential for missing other hyperplastic parathyroid glands in patients with multiglandular disease when limited exploration is employed, because the incidence of multiglandular disease ranges from 7% to 30%. The sensitivity of Sestamibi scan has been as high as 95% using the single photon emission computed tomography (SPECT) technique and a 3-D display (volume-rendered reprojection for visualization). However, it is associated with a high false-positive rate especially in patients with thyroid nodules. This false-positive rate may be the reason for operative failures in patients who undergo parathyroidectomy based solely on Sestamibi scans.

Irvin and colleagues popularized the use of rapid intraoperative chemiluminescent PTH monitoring to confirm excision of all hyperfunctioning parathyroid tissue. In 61 patients who underwent 63 explorations for pHPT, there was a 54% decrease in the serum PTH level 10 minutes after excision of a parathyroid adenoma in patients who were rendered normocalcemic postoperatively. Their 10-minute assay had a sensitivity of 96%, a specificity of 100%, and a positive predictive value of 97% (33,34). Our group and others have since validated the benefits of rapid intact PTH as a reliable method of ensuring excision of all hyperfunctioning parathyroid tissue (35). Many surgeons now use the threshold of greater than 50% decline in PTH levels 10 minutes after excision, and a decline into the normal range, to confirm adequate parathyroidectomy. If the criteria are not met, it should be assumed that there is additional disease and full neck exploration is indicated.

Many surgeons exploit the property of parathyroid adenomas to retain Sestamibi as a guide to direct resection using radioactive assessment with a hand-held gamma probe (Neoprobe Corp., Columbus, Ohio, U.S.A.). This technique involves excising the suspected parathyroid adenoma previously identified on preoperative Sestamibi scan. After excision, radioactive counts of the excised parathyroid over 20% of background radioactivity in the neck confirm that the excised tissue is the Sestamibi-identified gland. Reports of successful application of this technique indicate an accuracy of up to 95% (36). This technique clearly depends on high sensitivity Sestamibi scans, which can be achieved using SPECT techniques or oblique views. Further, proponents of this method indicate that such patients need to undergo surgery soon after Sestamibi injection. Using these techniques, radio-guided parathyroidectomy has been successful in more than 90% of patients with a positive Sestamibi scan. This technique, however, requires seamless communication between the nuclear radiologists and surgical teams.

Others have used a directed approach based on both preoperative Sestamibi scan and high-resolution ultrasonography, with or without intraoperative PTH measurement. When both the Sestamibi and ultrasound scans are concordant, success rates of 95% to 98% are observed. We have successfully used the directed approach with Sestamibi, ultrasonography, and intraoperative PTH measurement. Our preferred algorithm for evaluating surgical candidates for directed parathyroidectomy is shown in Figure 6. Using this technique, we have been able to perform successful directed parathyroidectomy in 70% of our patients with pHPT with a mean hospital stay of 12 hours (37). In summary, directed parathyroidectomy using any of these approaches can be performed with cure rates equivalent to those seen after conventional bilateral neck exploration. Further, directed parathyroidectomy involves less operating time, morbidity, and cost. Choice of technique should depend on local expertise (radiologic, surgical, laboratory, and pathology), patient choice, and institutional resources.

For patients with multiglandular disease, directed approaches are usually unsuccessful due to inability to localize a single gland preoperatively or decrease the PTH level after excision of a single gland. Such patients require bilateral neck exploration, however controversy exists regarding the extent of parathyroidectomy. Both subtotal parathyroidectomy and total parathyroidectomy with autotransplantation help achieve excellent results in patients with primary HPT due to multiglandular disease. The latter approach is based on the belief by many surgeons that all parathyroids are potentially hyperfunctioning when there is multiglandular disease, even when they are not all enlarged (38).

Ectopic Parathyroid Glands. Although as many as 20% of parathyroid glands in pHPT are located in the mediastinum, most mediastinal parathyroid glands are intrathymic (inferior glands) and can be removed transcervically. Preoperative imaging including sestamibi scintigraphy in combination with an anatomic study such as CT or MRI is necessary to determine the optimal approach. The Cooper™ thymectomy retractor has been useful in facilitating transcervical resection of deep mediastinal ectopic parathyroid glands.

Other options for the management of mediastinal parathyroid glands include the use of anterior mediastinotomy (Chamberlain procedure), mini thoracotomy, video-assisted thoracic surgery, and angiographic ablation (39). Using these techniques, only about 2% of deep mediastinal parathyroid glands cannot be extracted through a cervical incision and have required median sternotomy for removal. Figure 7 shows a mediastinal ectopic parathyroid gland. The importance of accurate, preoperative localization studies prior to undertaking these operative approaches cannot be overemphasized. Multiple preoperative studies are frequently used, and the diagnosis is more certain with two or more concordant studies (40).

Results of Parathyroidectomy. Successful parathyroidectomy results in normalization of serum calcium concentrations and reverses the other adverse effects of the disease. For example, serum levels of PTH, bone-specific alkaline phosphatase, and osteocalcin when elevated before parathyroidectomy, decrease significantly after parathyroidectomy (41). This is manifested by a significant increase in bone mineral density of the spine, femoral neck, hip, and trochanter.

Surgical Treatment of Renal Hyperparathyroidism

Secondary (renal) HPT induced by chronic renal failure is one of the most serious complications for long-term hemodialysis patients. Parathyroidectomy is indicated in patients with secondary renal HPT refractory to medical treatment. However, skeletal deformity, vessel calcification, and remarkable reduction of bone content are irreversible in these patients, so it is important to perform parathyroidectomy prior to the onset of these changes. HPT complicating renal failure is characterized by several pathogenic factors including hypocalcemia, phosphate retention, deficiency of active vitamin D, decreased number of calcitriol receptors in parathyroid cells, and skeletal resistance to PTH action. The purpose of medical treatment is to reduce hyperphosphatemia, elevate the serum calcium level, reduce serum PTH levels, and improve skeletal turnover. However, it is very difficult to maintain a normal serum phosphate level by phosphate restriction, and the use of phosphate binders. Currently, vitamin D (calcitriol) administration is the most promising form of prophylaxis and treatment for secondary HPT. Vitamin D is usually prescribed as an "intermittent high-dose treatment" (42).

Indications and Technique of Parathyroidectomy in Patients with Renal Hyperparathyroidism

Parathyroidectomy may be considered for normocalcemic patients with radiographic evidence of bone disease (osteitis fibrosa cystica), high serum PTH level, imaging studies showing parathyroid glands weighing over 500 mg; and bone metabolic markers or bone scintigraphy showing high rates of bone turnover. Patients with a functioning kidney graft are rarely considered for parathyroidectomy except in circumstances such as the presence of persistent or progressive hypercalcemia, progressive osteodystrophy, nephrolithiasis, or deterioration of graft function. Total parathyroidectomy with a forearm autograft is preferred for renal HPT requiring surgical treatment, because it is convenient and safer to remove the residual parathyroid tissue from the forearm if the HPT recurs compared to a reoperative procedure in the neck. Moreover, the function of the autografted parathyroid tissue can be easily determined by measuring PTH samples from both arms. The removal of all parathyroid

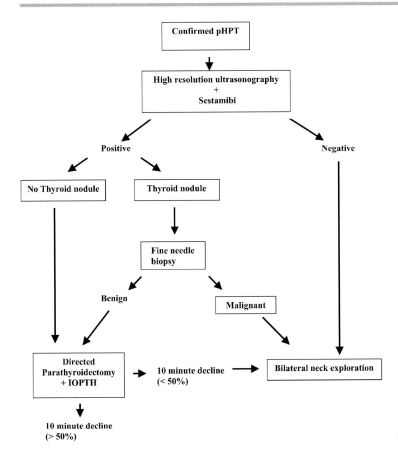

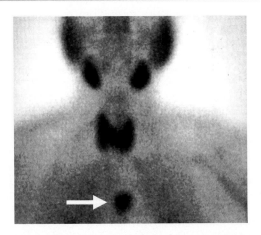

Figure 6   Algorithm for evaluating surgical candidates for directed parathyroidectomy.

tissue, including supernumerary glands, at the initial operation, and choice of adequate parathyroid tissue for the autograft, are important to prevent persistent and recurrent HPT. Supernumerary glands and rudiments of parathyroid tissue are present in 13% to 15% of all individuals. For this reason, concurrent routine thymectomy is recommended during parathyroidectomy for renal hyperparathyroidism. After confirmation of parathyroid tissue by frozen-section examination of each gland, suitable parathyroid tissue is selected for autografting. The parathyroid autotransplants are preferably excised from the smallest gland in each case, avoiding macroscopically visible nodules. The glandular tissue is sliced into $1 \times 1 \times 3$ mm pieces, and approximately 20 to 30 pieces weighing a total of about 90 mg should be used for autotransplantation by implantation into separate pockets in the brachioradialis muscle of the arm, without hemodialysis access.

Calcium replacement therapy is crucial during the first three weeks after operation because PTH secretion from the autografted parathyroid tissue is insufficient and the bone formation is accelerated after parathyroidectomy. Calcium replacement therapy is usually begun after the serum calcium level falls below 3.5 mEq/L, confirming adequate excision of all parathyroid tissue. Initially, intravenous calcium gluconate injection is given, after which oral 1-α-calcitriol and calcium carbonate are given to maintain a normal serum calcium level. After the serum alkaline phosphatase level becomes normal, an adequate amount of vitamin D and calcium salts should be given to prevent recurrent HPT and to avoid adynamic bone disease.

Medical Approaches to pHPT

Because parathyroidectomy is associated with high cure rates and low complication rates, parathyroidectomy is the treatment of choice for most patients with pHPT. A small fraction of patients with pHPT are not candidates for parathyroidectomy. These include elderly, poor

Figure 7   Demonstration of a mediastinal ectopic parathyroid gland.

operative risk patients, and patients who refuse surgery. Acceptable nonoperative alternatives for primary HPT include bisphosphonates, estrogen replacement, and calcimimetics. Oral phosphate treatment has also been examined for this subgroup of patients. However the potential danger of "parathyroid poisoning," caused by deposition of calcium phosphate salts in the kidney and other organs has caused oral or intravenous phosphate therapy to fall out of favor.

Bisphosphonate Therapy of pHPT
Bisphosphonates are analogs of inorganic pyrophosphate in which the central oxygen atom is replaced by a carbon atom, yielding the core structure P-C-P. These agents reduce serum calcium levels by direct inhibition of bone resorption by osteoclasts and caspase-mediated apoptosis of osteoclasts. Oral administration of the potent second-generation bisphosphonate clodronate (dichloromethylene bisphosphonate) reduces serum calcium level to almost normal. The hypocalcemic effect of clodronate waned over time, and the level of PTH rises. The increasing circulating PTH levels consistently observed with bisphosphonate administration points to a fundamental difficulty with such therapy.

Estrogens and Progestins
High doses of estrogen can correct hypercalcemia and hypercalciuria (43). However there are no randomized, controlled trials comparing hormonal therapy with parathyroid surgery. In addition, the effect of hormonal therapy on other symptoms of HPT such as renal stones and neurologic function has not been addressed. Hormonal replacement therapy is further limited to postmenopausal women who have no contraindications to estrogen treatment. Although a randomized trial is needed to resolve the differences between the effects of hormonal replacement therapy and parathyroidectomy on bone, current evidence suggests that medical treatment with estrogens and progestins provides a reasonable alternative to parathyroidectomy for postmenopausal women with primary HPT (especially in those with no other indication for parathyroidectomy and in those who are poor surgical candidates). It is not clear whether postmenopausal estrogen therapy for pHPT offers any advantage over bisphosphonate treatment with regard to bone mass; however, the disadvantage of bisphosphonates is that they may increase the serum PTH level (44). Studies of postmenopausal HPT confirm the benefit of postmenopausal hormone replacement treatment on bone mass and the size of the parathyroid glands (45–47).

Calcimimetics
The newest and potentially most useful class of drugs for the treatment of HPT is calcimimetic agents. Unlike the other therapeutic agents that work primarily by inhibiting bone resorption in response to PTH, the calcimimetics target the calcium-sensing mechanism in the parathyroid glands. The molecular basis of calcium sensing by the parathyroid glands was elucidated with the identification of a calcium receptor on the surface of the parathyroid cell. On binding calcium, the receptor signals the interior of the parathyroid cell to inhibit the secretion of PTH. The predominant intracellular second messenger that carries this signal is intracellular calcium. Thus, an increase in extracellular calcium induces an increase in intracellular calcium, which, in turn, inhibits the secretion of PTH from secretory granules within the parathyroid cell. The calcium receptor is also present in the renal tubule, where it regulates renal calcium excretion, and in

calcitonin-secreting C-cells of the thyroid, where it mediates the stimulation of calcitonin release by hypercalcemia.

Calcimimetic drugs alter the sensitivity of the parathyroid calcium receptor to extracellular calcium. These phenylalkylamine compounds decrease the responsiveness of cells to low extracellular calcium. The net effect of these actions is to increase the sensitivity of parathyroid cells to the suppressive effects of high extracellular calcium, markedly decreasing the rate of PTH secretion at ambient calcium levels of about 1 mmol present in both normal and hyperparathyroid states. The administration of a single 160 mg dose of the calcimimetic, NPS R-568 to postmenopausal women caused a maximal 51% decrease in the serum PTH level. However, there was only a small decrease in the serum level of ionized calcium detected with the administration of NPS R-568. Acute administration of NPS R-568 to dialysis patients achieved a dose-dependent repression of PTH secretion and an increase in calcitonin levels (48). In a placebo-controlled study of 21 dialysis patients treated for 15 days, NPS R-568 significantly decreased the serum PTH level and the serum levels of total and ionized calcium. The serum ionized calcium level fell to less than 1 mmol/L in approximately half of the patients receiving the drug; five patients withdrew from the study because they developed hypocalcemia caused by the drug. In addition, in a patient with parathyroid carcinoma who presented with parathyroid crisis, monotherapy with NPS R-568 controlled the hypercalcemia for two years with no adverse side effects (49). Although NPS R-568 can acutely reduce serum PTH levels, it has a short half-life because it is rapidly metabolized by the liver, thus reducing its clinical usefulness. Second-generation calcimimetics with longer half-lives and a more predictable therapeutic effect are currently in clinical trials in patients with primary and secondary HPT (50). In fact, small studies have documented the efficient lowering of serum PTH in patients with primary hyperparathyroidism, suggesting that this approach may soon gain widespread acceptance (51).

MULTIPLE ENDOCRINE NEOPLASIA SYNDROMES

Multiple endocrine neoplasias are inherited endocrine diseases that manifest in several endocrine glands including the pituitary, parathyroid, thyroid, pancreas, and adrenal glands. Based on a kindred with medullary thyroid carcinoma, pheochromocytomas, and parathyroid hyperplasia, Steiner and his colleagues introduced the term *"multiple endocrine neoplasia"* in 1968 (52). MEN 1 is used to describe the multiple endocrine adenomatosis syndrome described by Wermer, which includes pituitary adenomas, parathyroid hyperplasia, and pancreatic islet tumors. MEN 2 is used to describe the kindred that manifest with medullary thyroid cancer, pheochromocytoma, and either parathyroid hyperplasia (MEN 2A) or ganglioneuromas (MEN 2B). In addition to these syndromes, Foley and his colleagues described an inherited hypercalcemic condition that was distinct from the MEN syndromes, which they termed "familial benign hypercalcemia." In the MEN syndromes, generalized HPT is a common feature. It occurs much more frequently in patients with MEN type 1 as compared to patients with MEN type 2A. Unlike the MEN syndromes, patients with FHH have only hypercalcemia with no associated endocrinopathies. The HPT in patients with either of the MEN syndromes is managed by parathyroidectomy, whereas patients with FHH are managed nonoperatively.

The specific genetic defects associated with MEN type 2 syndromes and FHH have been identified (53).

SUMMARY

Calcium and phosphorus balance are critically important for normal neuromuscular excitation, contraction, and relaxation. When a perturbation in calcium occurs, a corresponding derangement in phosphorus also results. Because an alteration in calcium is the driving force behind consequent phosphorus alterations, a clear understanding of calcium homeostasis is mandatory. Key sites of calcium regulation include absorption from the gut, resorption from bone, and excretion by the kidneys. Thus, hypocalcemia can result from any dysfunction of these processes, such as excess intake and absorption from the intestine, decreased renal excretion, or increased tone resorption. Conversely, hypocalcemia is caused by decreased calcium intake, increased calcium binding in the gut, increased excretion, or decreased bone resorption. The parathyroid glands are the master regulators of these actions. They accomplish these goals by sensing ionized calcium in the blood as well as effecting normal calcium homeostasis through parathormone secretion, which controls bone resorption and calcium excretion by the kidneys.

Primary hyperparathyroidism is the major disorder affecting the parathyroid glands as well as the major disorder responsible for hypercalcemia. Although hypercalcemia can be acutely managed by a variety of medical strategies, when caused by hyperfunction of the parathyroid glands, surgical management is the most effective means of control. This can range from removal of a single gland if an adenoma is involved to resection of 3-1/2 glands if diffuse hyperplasia is the cause of the hyperfunction.

Primary hypoparathyroidism is extremely rare and usually of no consequence to the surgeon. The major reason for hypoparathyroidism in the surgical setting is that the glands have been removed or severely compromised in terms of blood supply during total thyroidectomy. If the former situation occurred, permanent calcium replacement therapy will be required. If the latter circumstance exists, some parathyroid function may ultimately return, but even in this setting, adjunctive calcium replacement treatment is often needed.

REFERENCES

1. Stewart AF. Translational implications of the parathyroid calcium receptor. N Engl J Med 2004; 351:324–326.
2. Thakker RV. Diseases associated with the extracellular calcium-sensing receptor. Cell Calcium 2004; 35:275–282.
3. Brown EM. Physiology and pathophysiology of the extracellular calcium-sensing receptor. Am J Med 1999; 106:238–253.
4. Urena Torres PA, Chanard J. Cinacalcet for secondary hyperparathyroidism in hemodialysis recipients. N Engl J Med 2004; 351:188–189; author reply 188–189.
5. Mallette LE, Coscia AM. Rapid radioimmunoassay for parathyroid hormone: its use in hypercalcemic crisis. South Med J 1984; 77:323–326.
6. Mallette LE. Immunoreactivity of human parathyroid hormone (28–48): attempt to develop an assay for intact human parathyroid hormone. Metab Bone Dis Relat Res 1983; 4:329–332.
7. Palmer FJ, Nelson JC, Bacchus H. The chloride-phosphate ratio in hypercalcemia. Ann Intern Med 1974; 80:200–204.
8. Lendel I, Horwith M. An update from the latest workshop on asymptomatic primary hyperparathyroidism. Otolaryngol Clin North Am 2004; 37:737–749.
9. Ahmad R, Hammond JM. Primary, secondary, and tertiary hyperparathyroidism. Otolaryngol Clin North Am 2004; 37:701–713.
10. Adami S, Marcocci C, Gatti D. Epidemiology of primary hyperparathyroidism in Europe. J Bone Miner Res 2002; 17(suppl 2):N18–N23.
11. Melton LJ III. The epidemiology of primary hyperparathyroidism in North America. J Bone Miner Res 2002; 17(suppl 2):N12–N17.
12. Bilezikian JP, Potts JT Jr. Asymptomatic primary hyperparathyroidism: new issues and new questions—bridging the past with the future. J Bone Miner Res 2002; 17(suppl 2):N57–N67.
13. Hundahl SA, Fleming ID, Fremgen AM, Menck HR. Two hundred eighty-six cases of parathyroid carcinoma treated in the U.S. between 1985–1995: a National Cancer Data Base Report. The American College of Surgeons Commission on Cancer and the American Cancer Society. Cancer 1999; 86:538–544.
14. Favia G, Lumachi F, Polistina F, D'Amico DF. Parathyroid carcinoma: sixteen new cases and suggestions for correct management. World J Surg 1998; 22:1225–1230.
15. Silverberg SJ, Bilezikian JP, Bone HG, Talpos GB, Horwitz MJ, Stewart AF. Therapeutic controversies in primary hyperparathyroidism. J Clin Endocrinol Metab 1999; 84:2275–2285.
16. Lundgren E RJ, Thrufjell E, Akerstrom G, Ljunghall S. Population-based screening for primary hyperparathyroidism with serum calcium and parathyroid hormone values in menopausal women. Surgery 1997; 121:287–294.
17. Hedback GM, Oden AS. Cardiovascular disease, hypertension and renal function in primary hyperparathyroidism. J Intern Med 2002; 251:476–483.
18. Palmer M, Adami HO, Bergstrom R, Jakobsson S, Akerstrom G, Ljunghall S. Survival and renal function in untreated hypercalcaemia. Population-based cohort study with 14 years of follow-up. Lancet 1987; 1:59–62.
19. Nilsson IL, Aberg J, Rastad J, Lind L. Left ventricular systolic and diastolic function and exercise testing in primary hyperparathyroidism-effects of parathyroidectomy. Surgery 2000; 128:895–902.
20. Stefenelli T, Abela C, Frank H, Koller-Strametz J, Niederle B. Time course of regression of left ventricular hypertrophy after successful parathyroidectomy. Surgery 1997; 121:157–161.
21. Stefenelli T, Abela C, Frank H, et al. Cardiac abnormalities in patients with primary hyperparathyroidism: implications for follow-up. J Clin Endocrinol Metab 1997; 82:106–112.
22. Langle F, Abela C, Koller-Strametz J, et al. Primary hyperparathyroidism and the heart: cardiac abnormalities correlated to clinical and biochemical data. World J Surg 1994; 18:619–624.
23. Stefenelli T, Mayr H, Bergler-Klein J, Globits S, Woloszczuk W, Niederle B. Primary hyperparathyroidism: incidence of cardiac abnormalities and partial reversibility after successful parathyroidectomy. Am J Med 1993; 95:197–202.
24. Stefenelli T, Globits S, Bergler-Klein J, Woloszczuk W, Langle F, Niederle B. Cardiac changes in patients with hypercalcemia. Wien Klin Wochenschr 1993; 105:339–341.
25. Stefenelli T, Pacher R, Woloszczuk W, Glogar D, Kaindl F. Parathyroid hormone and calcium behavior in advanced congestive heart failure. Z Kardiol 1992; 81:121–125.
26. Bilezikian JP, Potts JT Jr, Fuleihan Gel H, et al. Summary statement from a workshop on asymptomatic primary hyperparathyroidism: a perspective for the 21st century. J Bone Miner Res 2002; 17(suppl 2):N2–N11.
27. Conroy S, Moulias S, Wassif WS. Primary hyperparathyroidism in the older person. Age Ageing 2003; 32:571–578.
28. Inabnet WB, Fulla Y, Richard B, Bonnichon P, Icard P, Chapuis Y. Unilateral neck exploration under local anesthesia: the approach of choice for asymptomatic primary hyperparathyroidism. Surgery 1999; 126:1004–1009; discussion 1009–1010.
29. Irvin GL III, Molinari AS, Figueroa C, Carneiro DM. Improved success rate in reoperative parathyroidectomy with intraoperative PTH assay. Ann Surg 1999; 229:874–878; discussion 878–879.
30. Peix JL, el Khazen M, Mancini F, Binet A, Berger N, Lapras V. Surgery for primary hyperparathyroidism in 1998. Apropos

of 66 patients and 3 methods of approach. Ann Chir 1252000346–352.

31. Udelsman R, Donovan PI, Sokoll LJ. One hundred consecutive minimally invasive parathyroid explorations. Ann Surg 2000; 232:331–339.

32. Moka D, Voth E, Dietlein M, Larena-Avellaneda A, Schicha H. Technetium 99m-MIBI-SPECT: a highly sensitive diagnostic tool for localization of parathyroid adenomas. Surgery 2000; 128:29–35.

33. Boggs JE, Irvin GL III, Molinari AS, Deriso GT. Intraoperative parathyroid hormone monitoring as an adjunct to parathyroidectomy. Surgery 1996; 120:954–958.

34. Irvin, Molinari AS, Carneiro DM, Rivabem F, Ruel MM, Boggs JE. Parathyroidectomy: new criteria for evaluating outcome. Am Surg 1999; 65:1186–1188; discussion 1188–1189.

35. Gordon LL, Snyder WH III, Wians F Jr, Nwariaku F, Kim LT. The validity of quick intraoperative parathyroid hormone assay: an evaluation in seventy-two patients based on gross morphologic criteria. Surgery 1999; 126:1030–1035.

36. Murphy C, Norman J. The 20% rule: a simple, instantaneous radioactivity measurement defines cure and allows elimination of frozen sections and hormone assays during parathyroidectomy. Surgery 1999; 126:1023–1028; discussion 1028–1029.

37. Burkey SH, Snyder WH III, Nwariaku F, Watumull L, Mathews D. Directed parathyroidectomy: feasibility and performance in 100 consecutive patients with primary hyperparathyroidism. Arch Surg 2003; 138:604–608; discussion 608–609.

38. Proye C, Carnaille B, Quievreux JL, Combemale F, Oudar C, Lecomte-Houcke M. Late outcome of 304 consecutive patients with multiple gland enlargement in primary hyperparathyroidism treated by conservative surgery. World J Surg 1998; 22:526–529; discussion 529–530.

39. Heller HJ, Miller GL, Erdman WA, Snyder WH III, Breslau NA. Angiographic ablation of mediastinal parathyroid adenomas: local experience and review of the literature. Am J Med 1994; 97:529–534.

40. Medrano C, Hazelrigg SR, Landreneau RJ, Boley TM, Shawgo T, Grasch A. Thoracoscopic resection of ectopic parathyroid glands. Ann Thorac Surg 2000; 69:221–223.

41. Tominaga Y, Numano M, Tanaka Y, Uchida K, Takagi H. Surgical treatment of renal hyperparathyroidism. Semin Surg Oncol 1997; 13:87–96.

42. Thorsen K, Kristoffersson AO, Lorentzon RP. Changes in bone mass and serum markers of bone metabolism after parathyroidectomy. Surgery 1997; 122:882–887.

43. Marcus R, Madvig P, Crim M, Pont A, Kosek J. Conjugated estrogens in the treatment of postmenopausal women with hyperparathyroidism. Ann Intern Med 1984; 100:633–640.

44. Strewler GJ. Medical approaches to primary hyperparathyroidism. Endocrinol Metab Clin N Am 2000; 29:523–539, vi.

45. Diamond T, Ng AT, Levy S, Magarey C, Smart R. Estrogen replacement may be an alternative to parathyroid surgery for the treatment of osteoporosis in elderly postmenopausal women presenting with primary hyperparathyroidism: a preliminary report. Osteoporos Int 1996; 6:329–333.

46. Guo CY, Thomas WE, al-Dehaimi AW, Assiri AM, Eastell R. Longitudinal changes in bone mineral density and bone turnover in postmenopausal women with primary hyperparathyroidism. J Clin Endocrinol Metab 1996; 81:3487–3491.

47. McDermott MT, Perloff JJ, Kidd GS. Effects of mild asymptomatic primary hyperparathyroidism on bone mass in women with and without estrogen replacement therapy. J Bone Miner Res 1994; 9:509–514.

48. Antonsen JE, Sherrard DJ, Andress DL. A calcimimetic agent acutely suppresses parathyroid hormone levels in patients with chronic renal failure [Rapid communication]. Kidney Int 1998; 53:223–227.

49. Goodman WG, Frazao JM, Goodkin DA, Turner SA, Liu W, Coburn JW. A calcimimetic agent lowers plasma parathyroid hormone levels in patients with secondary hyperparathyroidism. Kidney Int 2000; 58(1):386–387.

50. Weigel RJ. Nonoperative management of hyperparathyroidism: present and future. Curr Opin Oncol 2001; 13:33–38.

51. Shoback DM, Bilezikian JP, Turner SA, McCary LC, Guo MD, Peacock M. The calcimimetic cinacalcet normalizes serum calcium in subjects with primary hyperparathyroidism. J Clin Endocrinol Metab 2003; 88:5644–5649.

52. Steiner AL, Goodman AD, Powers SR. Study of a kindred with pheochromocytoma, medullary thyroid carcinoma, hyperparathyroidism and Cushing's disease: multiple endocrine neoplasia, type 2. Medicine (Baltimore) 1968; 47:371–409.

53. Herfarth KK, Wells SA Jr. Parathyroid glands and the multiple endocrine neoplasia syndromes and familial hypocalciuric hypercalcemia. Semin Surg Oncol 1997; 13:114–124.

50

Pituitary Dysfunction

Henry Ty and Kathryn Holloway

INTRODUCTION

The pituitary gland secretes hormones that affect the functions of the endocrine organs. These are essential in maintaining the internal homeostasis of the body as it adapts to the environment. They establish communications between distant cells to facilitate the gathering of nutrients, water, and minerals, their metabolism and their use for growth, repair, and reproduction. The function of the pituitary gland ultimately determines the ability to cope with the environment and the chances for a successful propagation of progenies.

Pituitary dysfunction results when there is a relative excess or deficiency in the amount or activity of one or more of its hormones. It can be caused by tumors, vascular lesions, inflammation, infection, trauma, systemic disease, surgery, radiation, medication, congenital abnormalities, or genetic defects. These may involve primarily the hypothalamus, the pituitary gland, or the target endocrine organs. Different causes can produce the same symptoms. The clinical presentation is dependent on how fast the lesion progresses. A tuberculum sella meningioma may cause the insidious development of pituitary deficiency and have few symptoms until it reaches a large size, while pituitary apoplexy may present with sudden loss of consciousness and result in death if untreated. Although hormonal excess is usually caused by a pituitary adenoma, it can be secondary to hypothalamic lesions such as a hamartoma that increases the secretion of pituitary gonadotropins, ectopic sources of hormones such as an adrenocorticotropic hormone (ACTH)-secreting lung tumor, or oversecretion by the target organs. On the other hand, hormonal deficiency, while common in pituitary macroadenomas due to their mass effect on the adjacent normal gland, may be caused by failure of the hypothalamus, target organs, or hormonal receptors.

The diagnosis of pituitary dysfunction necessitates recognition of the part of the hypothalamic-pituitary-target organ axis that is involved. Treatment involves the removal of the cause of the dysfunction, replacement of deficient hormones, and control of hormonal oversecretion. This chapter reviews pituitary physiology and focuses on surgical lesions in the sellar area that causes pituitary dysfunction.

ANATOMY OF THE PITUITARY GLAND

The pituitary gland (hypophysis) is an ovoid organ weighing about 0.6 g. It is approximately 6 mm high, 13 mm wide, and 9 mm long (1). Its width is usually equal to or greater than its length. It is larger in females, especially during pregnancy. It is composed of the anterior and posterior lobes. The larger anterior lobe (adenohypophysis) constitutes about 80% of the hypophysis and is divided into pars distalis, pars intermedia, and pars tuberalis, which partially wraps around the pituitary stalk. The pars intermedia are vestigial in adults. The smaller multinodular posterior lobe (pars nervosa) is attached to the stalk (infundibular stem), which is continuous with the median eminence of the hypothalamus. The pars nervosa, infundibular stem, and median eminence form the neurohypophysis.

The pituitary gland is located within the sella turcica, a bony fossa at the central part of the sphenoid bone, which is lined by dura mater. Anterior to it is the tuberculum sella. Posteriorly, the dorsum sella curves down to form the clivus. The cavernous sinuses are adjacent to the pituitary gland bilaterally (Fig. 1). Within each sinus are cranial nerves III, IV, V_1, V_2, VI, and the internal carotid artery (ICA). The optic chiasm is above the gland and normally is anterior to the infundibulum. The basilar artery and pons are posterior to it. The inferior surface of the gland conforms

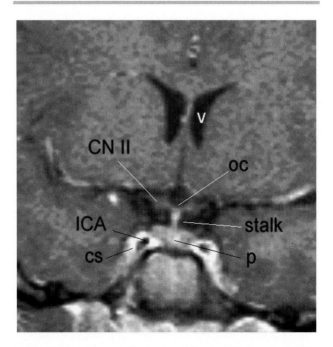

Figure 1 Coronal magnetic resonance imaging showing the pituitary gland (p) with its stalk adjacent to the optic chiasm (oc) and optic nerves (CN II). Lateral to the gland on each side is the cavernous sinus (cs) with the internal carotid artery within it. The frontal horn of the lateral ventricles (v) can be seen.

to the shape of the sellar floor but its lateral and superior margins vary in shape because they are bounded by soft tissue rather than bone. Below the sellar floor is the sphenoid sinus, which separates the gland from the nasal cavity (Fig. 2). Its size, shape, and degree of pneumatization are variable and are important considerations prior to a transsphenoidal surgery.

The diaphragma sella is a thin, rectangular dural structure that forms the roof of the sella turcica. It lies below the plane of the anterior clinoid processes. It has a round to ellipsoid central opening through which the pituitary stalk passes. This opening measures at least 5 mm and is larger than the diameter of the stalk. The arachnoid membrane lies above the diaphragma sella but protrudes through this opening in about half of the patients (2). When the cerebrospinal fluid (CSF) fills the top half of the sella and pushes the gland to the sellar floor, this is called an empty sella, which is not pathologic. A lesion located above the diaphragma sella, e.g., an aneurysm, may protrude downward and appear to be within the sella.

The superior hypophyseal arteries arise from the supraclinoid ICA to supply the median eminence, proximal infundibulum, and the optic chiasm. Their capillaries drain into the hypophyseal portal veins that join another capillary bed in the pars distalis. The inferior hypophyseal arteries arise from the intracavernous ICA to supply the pars nervosa. The hypophyseal veins drain into the adjacent dural sinuses, and eventually to the cavernous and petrosal sinuses. The median eminence has fenestrated capillaries that allow transport of polypeptide hormones. There is no blood brain barrier in the neurohypophysis.

Lesions in the adjacent structures, e.g., hypothalamic tumor, may result in pituitary dysfunction. Similarly, lesions in the sellar area, e.g., pituitary adenoma, may become large enough to compress the surrounding structures such as the optic chiasm and alter their functions.

PHYSIOLOGY OF THE PITUITARY GLAND

The pituitary gland releases hormones that alter the metabolism of their target organs. The hypothalamus in turn controls the pituitary gland by its neural projections to the neurohypophysis and by a vascular network through the adenohypophysis. It secretes releasing hormones and inhibiting factors that regulate the synthesis and release of pituitary hormones. The hormones produced by the pituitary and target organs modulate further secretion from the pituitary and the hypothalamus. This complex integration of neurohormonal functions by both nervous and endocrine systems regulates the metabolic activities that affect homeostasis, growth, development, and reproduction.

The adenohypophysis produces hormones that are stored prior to their release. The parvocellular neurons in the arcuate and paraventricular nuclei of the hypothalamus produce factors that control the release of hormones from the adenohypophysis. These factors are transported from the cell bodies of the paired nuclei, along the tuberohypophyseal (tuberoinfundibular) tract, to the neuronal terminals at the median eminence. They are released into the capillaries of the median eminence and proximal infundibulum in response to action potentials. From here, they travel via the portal vessels to reach the pars distalis. The hypophyseal portal system serves as a vascular connection between the hypothalamus and the adenohypophysis. There is no direct neuronal connection between the two.

The magnocellular neurons of the supraoptic and paraventricular nuclei of the hypothalamus produce vasopressin and oxytocin (OT). The hormones are produced in the cell bodies and are bound to carrier polypeptides called neurophysins. They are transported within membrane-bound vesicles by axoplasmic flow along the supraopticohypophyseal and the paraventriculohypophyseal tracts that arise from the paired nuclei and terminate at the pars nervosa. In response to an action potential, both hormone and neurophysin are released into the capillaries in the neurohypophysis (3).

The hormones secreted by the target organs provide feedback to the hypothalamus and the pituitary gland. Failure of the target organs results in increased secretion of both the releasing hormones and the pituitary hormones. In addition to hypothalamic and feedback inputs, factors secreted within the pituitary gland influence its function. The list of intrapituitary factors has been steadily expanding over the past decade (4). Ongoing studies on the synthesis and secretion of these factors, the regulation of their receptors, and their response mechanisms will add to our understanding of the complex processes that occur within the pituitary gland.

HORMONES OF THE ADENOHYPOPHYSIS

The adenohypophysis produces growth hormone (GH), prolactin (PRL), ACTH, thyroid-stimulating hormone (TSH), follicle-stimulating hormone (FSH), and luteinizing hormone (LH) (Table 1). GH, PRL, and ACTH are polypeptides. TSH, FSH, and LH are glycoproteins that have α and β subunits. They have identical α subunits consisting of 92 amino acids. Their β subunits are different and confer the

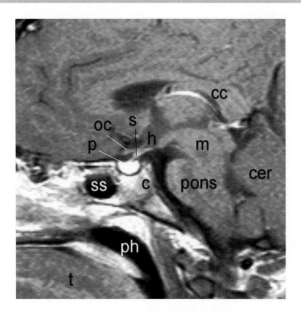

Figure 2 Sagittal MRI showing the pituitary gland (p) connected to the hypothalamus (h) by its stalk (s). Anterior to the stalk is the optic chiasm (oc). Posterior to the sphenoid sinus (ss) is the clivus (c). The corpus callosum (cc), midbrain (m), pons, cerebellum (cer), pharynx (ph), and tongue (t) are identified. *Abbreviation*: MRI, magnetic resonance imaging.

Table 1 Hormones of the Adenohypophysis

Hormones	Target organs	Hypothalamic factors		Feedback inhibition by	Effects
		Stimulated by	Inhibited by		
GH	Liver, bone, epiphyseal growth plate, muscle, adipose tissue, lymphocytes, gonads	GHRH	Somatostatin	IGF-1, GH	Growth, production of IGF-1, decreased glucose metabolism, increased lipolysis and redistribution of fat, increased nitrogen retention
PRL	Breasts, liver, gonads, prostate	TRH, OT, VIP	Dopamine		Mammary gland development, milk secretion, inhibits FSH/LH secretion
ACTH	Adrenal cortex	CRH, ADH	CRIF	Cortisol, ACTH	Cortisol synthesis and secretion, adrenal gland growth and maturation
TSH	Thyroid gland	TRH	Dopamine, somatostatin	Thyroid hormones	Thyroid hormone synthesis and secretion, thyroid gland growth and maturation
FSH	Gonads	LHRH		Estrogen, progesterone, androgens, folliculostatin, inhibin	Females: development of ovarian follicle, secretion of estrogen and inhibin; males: development of testicular tubules, spermatogenesis, secretion of inhibin
LH	Gonads	LHRH		Estrogen, progesterone, androgens, inhibin	Females: luteinization, secretion of progesterone; males: development of Leydig cells, secretion of testosterone

Abbreviations: ACTH, adrenocorticotropic hormone; ADH, antidiuretic hormone; CRIF, corticotropin release inhibiting factor; CRH, corticotropin-releasing hormone; FSH, follicle-stimulating hormone; GH, growth hormone; GHRH, GH releasing hormone; IGF, insulin-like growth factors; LH, luteinizing hormone; LHRH, lutenizing hormone-releasing hormone; OT, oxytocin; PRL, prolactin; TRH, thyrotropin-releasing hormone; TSH, thyroid stimulating hormone; VIP, vasoactive intestinal peptide.

specificity for a particular receptor site. The β subunit becomes biologically active when coupled with the α subunit (5).

GH is a polypeptide with 191 amino acids and occurs in several forms. Its secretion by the somatotrophs is stimulated by GH releasing hormone (GHRH) and inhibited by somatostatin (somatotropin release-inhibiting factor). It has no specific target organ but affects the liver, muscles, adipose tissues, lymphocytes, gonads, and the epiphyseal growth plate. It has early insulin-like effects such as hypoglycemia, increased protein synthesis, glycogenolysis, and lipogenesis. Its predominant effects are diabetogenic or anti-insulin and include decreased glucose transport and metabolism and increased lipolysis and free fatty acid levels (6). It induces insulin resistance in the liver, with or without hyperglycemia, ketonemia, or hyperinsulinemia (7–9). It also redistributes fat, increases nitrogen retention, and promotes body growth. Each GH molecule binds to two cytokine receptors on the membrane of the target organs (dimerization) to activate the Janus kinase (JAK) intracellular tyrosine kinases and the signal transducers and activators of transcription (STAT) proteins (10,11). After phosphorylation, STAT proteins move into the nucleus, bind with DNA, and activate transcription. GH forms complexes with plasma GH-binding proteins, resulting in a longer half-life and a larger volume of distribution (12). Some actions of GH are believed to be mediated by the somatomedins or insulin-like growth factors (IGF), specifically Sm-C or IGF-1 (13). These are peptides that resemble proinsulin and are present in many tissues but mainly in the liver (14). They have insulin-like activity in extraskeletal tissues, promote sulfation in cartilage, and stimulate DNA synthesis and cell multiplication. Their plasma concentration is GH-dependent. They are believed to be mitogens that stimulate clonal growth of the cells that were induced to differentiate by GH (15). With aging, secretion of both GH and IGF is decreased, resulting in loss of muscle mass and increased adipose tissue (16,17).

PRL is the largest of the polypeptide hormones with 198 amino acids. Like GH, it occurs in several forms (18). Its secretion by the lactotrophs is under constant suppression by dopamine but may be enhanced by various PRL-releasing factors including thyrotropin-releasing hormone (TRH) and vasoactive intestinal peptide. It stimulates glandular development and milk secretion of the mammary gland in females. In males, it may be essential for normal spermatogenesis. The main target organ is the breast, although PRL receptors are also present in the liver, ovary, testis, and prostate. These receptors are part of the cytokine receptor superfamily and can be stimulated by GH. During pregnancy, estrogen, progesterone, PRL, and placental mammotropic hormones stimulate breast development together with insulin, cortisol, and thyroid hormones. Lactation is inhibited by high levels of estrogen and progesterone.

Corticotropin (ACTH) is a polypeptide with 39 amino acids. It is formed by proteolytic cleavage of proopiomelanocortin (POMC) into β-lipotropin and pro-ACTH, which is further processed into ACTH, N-proopiomelanocortin, and joining peptide. ACTH is cleaved into α-melanocyte-stimulating hormone and corticotropin-like intermediate lobe peptide. The secretion of ACTH by the corticotrophs is stimulated by corticotropin-releasing hormone (CRH) and vasopressin, and inhibited by glucocorticoids and the recently characterized corticotropin-release inhibiting factor (19). Its target is the zona fasciculata and zona reticularis of the adrenal cortex, where it stimulates the secretion of cortisol. Within minutes, it increases the adrenal blood flow and stimulates the conversion of cholesterol to pregnenolone (5). It is essential not only for adrenal growth and maturation, but also for life. It binds to membrane receptors on the adrenocortical cells with the help of extracellular calcium. This activates adenylate cyclase and increases intracellular cyclic adenosine monophosphate (cAMP) levels, protein kinase A activity, and phosphorylation of proteins that synthesize and release the steroid hormones. Because these are lipophilic, they are secreted shortly after being produced. At very high levels present in Nelson's syndrome or Addison's disease, ACTH can act on melanocytes to increase skin pigmentation.

The thyrotropin (TSH) β subunit consists of 112 amino acids. TSH secretion by the thyrotrophs is stimulated by the thyrotropin-releasing hormone (TRH). A TSH-inhibiting hormone has not been demonstrated. TSH stimulates the production and secretion of thyroid hormones and is essential for the function of the thyroid gland, increasing its size and vascularity. It binds to membrane receptors on the thyroid cell, activating adenylate cyclase and increasing the cAMP levels, protein kinase A activity, and phosphorylation of proteins that regulate thyroid functions (20). The follicular epithelium develops and there is increased iodide transport, thyroglobulin synthesis, and production of T_3 and T_4.

The follitropin (FSH) β subunit consists of 115 amino acids. FSH secretion by the gonadotrophs is regulated by the gonadotropin-releasing hormone, also known as lutenizing hormone-releasing hormone (LHRH). Its secretion is inhibited by estrogen, folliculostatin, and inhibin (21). In females, it stimulates the growth of ovarian follicles and the secretion of estrogen and inhibin. In males, it stimulates Sertoli cells and inhibin secretion, promotes testicular tubule development and spermatogenesis, and controls the number of LH receptors on the Leydig cells. The FSH receptors are in the granulosa cells and the Leydig cells.

The lutropin (LH) β subunit also consists of 115 amino acids. LH secretion by the gonadotrophs is also regulated by LHRH. Its secretion is stimulated by estrogen and progesterone. It initiates the resumption of meiosis and release of the first polar body and is required for ovulation. It causes luteinization of the granulosa cells in the mature ovarian follicle by increasing cAMP levels. There is subsequent production and secretion of progesterone. LH is also known as the interstitial cell-stimulating hormone and is important in the development of the Leydig cells. It stimulates the production and secretion of testosterone (5).

HORMONES OF THE NEUROHYPOPHYSIS

The neurohypophysis secretes arginine vasopressin (AVP) and OT (Table 2). They contain nine amino acids and have both antidiuretic and uterus-contracting properties. AVP has mainly antidiuretic activity but has minimal oxytocic activity. OT has some antidiuretic activity. Both hormones are synthesized as prohormones with their neurophysins in the supraoptic and paraventricular neurons. Their release in the pars nervosa is stimulated by acetylcholine and influenced by cathecholamines and endorphins.

AVP is also known as antidiuretic hormone (ADH). It maintains the blood osmolality within 2% of 282 mOsm/kg by its actions on renal water absorption and thirst (22). Above the osmotic threshold, ADH is secreted. It increases the reabsorption of water at the collecting ducts by binding to V_2 receptors on the peritubular surface. This activates adenylate cyclase, which catalyzes the formation of cAMP, resulting in activation of protein kinases and phosphorylation of aquaporin 2, a water-channel protein that controls

the pore size of the luminal membrane of the collecting duct cells. ADH also stimulates the reabsorption of urea in the inner medullary collecting ducts by a similar mechanism involving the urea transporter 1 protein, which mediates the facilitated diffusion and accumulation of urea (3). Maximal antidiuresis is seen when serum osmolality reaches about 295 mmol/L, at which point thirst becomes more important in lowering osmolality (23). ADH may raise blood pressure through vasoconstriction by binding to the V_1 receptors of the vascular smooth muscle cells. It also stimulates pituitary ACTH secretion.

OT stimulates contraction of uterine and mammary smooth muscles and is important in parturition and milk ejection. It also potentiates the release of ACTH, PRL, FSH, and LH from the adenohypophysis. It binds to G protein–coupled receptors, which are present in the uterine myometrium, mammary gland, pituitary, spinal cord, kidney, thymus, gonads, heart, and vascular endothelial cells (24). This results in activation of protein kinase C and intracellular calcium mobilization. In the myometrial cells, activation of myosin light chain kinase initiates contraction. The onset of labor is triggered by a decrease in progesterone. The uterine contraction that follows stimulates OT secretion, which peaks during delivery. OT is used to induce labor and control uterine hemorrhages.

REGULATION OF HORMONE SECRETION

Many hormones produced by the hypothalamus and adenohypophysis are secreted in pulses with periods of inactivity. GH, PRL, ACTH, and TSH have circadian rhythms (25). The hormones secreted by the hypothalamus control the pituitary cellular proliferation and its hormonal synthesis and release. One hypothalamic hormone may affect more than one pituitary hormone. Both releasing and inhibiting factors interact to modulate their effects. Their secretion is regulated by the interaction of neurotransmitters, neuropeptides, and other hormones.

Somatotropin

GH is secreted in multiple bursts occurring at anytime of the day but usually within the first hour of sleep, reaching its peak levels at night. A delay in the onset of deep sleep delays the onset of the major GH peak. GHRH stimulates GH synthesis and the release of preformed GH by binding to G protein–coupled receptors on the somatotrophs, activating adenylate cyclase and increasing cAMP and intracellular calcium levels. Somatostatin inhibits GH pulsed release by binding to receptors and decreasing intracellular calcium levels (26). Somatostatin has a more dominant effect than GHRH. GH exerts a short-loop negative feedback on the hypothalamus. IGF-1 from the peripheral tissues provides negative feedbacks by enhancing somatostatin release

Table 2 Hormones of the Neurohypophysis

Hormones	Target organs	Stimulated by	Inhibited by	Effects
ADH	Kidneys, vascular smooth muscles	Serum hyperosmolality, rapid intravascular volume depletion, NE , angiotensin II, opiates, nausea, stress, pain	Serum hypoosmolality, fluid overload, ANP, alcohol, phenytoin	Antidiuresis, vasoconstriction, stimulates ACTH secretion
OT	Uterus, breasts	Vaginal distention, suckling of nipples, NE, nausea	Opiates, stress	Uterine contraction, milk ejection

Abbreviations: ACTH, adrenocorticotropic hormone; ADH, antidiuretic hormone; ANP, atrial natriuretic peptides; NE, norepinephrine; OT, oxytocin.

from the hypothalamus and by inhibiting GH gene transcription in the pituitary.

GH secretion is stimulated by fasting, exercise, stress, low insulin levels, and in certain conditions like anorexia, non-insulin dependent diabetes mellitus (IDDM), and liver cirrhosis. It is also stimulated by central α_2-adrenergic agonists(clonidine), acetylcholine agonists, dopamine agonists (levodopa), β_2-adrenergic antagonists (propranolol), opioids, glucagon, arginine, leucine, estrogen, and GH secretagogues like MK-677 (27,28). GH secretion is decreased with obesity, emotional deprivation, aging, hyperglycemia, hyperinsulinemia, and hypothyroidism.

Prolactin

PRL is secreted in a pulsatile manner with its lowest levels at noon that gradually increase in the afternoon. The levels increase further after the onset of sleep and peak at around midnight (29). It is under tonic inhibition by dopamine produced in the hypothalamus. Dopamine inhibits PRL synthesis and release by binding to membrane receptors and inhibiting adenylate cyclase, which results in decreased cAMP, intracellular calcium, and PRL gene transcription in the lactotrophs.

PRL secretion is stimulated by stress, estrogen, TRH, OT, lesions to the hypothalamus or the pituitary stalk, and chronic use of opioids, dopamine antagonists (chlorpromazine, haloperidol, metoclopramide), antidepressants (amitriptyline, fluoxetine), antihypertensives (α-methyldopa, reserpine), H_2-blockers (cimetidine, ranitidine), and calcium channel blockers (verapamil) (30). Medications rarely increase PRL levels to more than 30 to 50 ng/mL (31). PRL levels are higher in premenopausal women than in men and rise during menarche and pregnancy. In postpartum women, suckling also increases PRL levels. Mild PRL elevation caused by increased TRH secretion seen in primary hypothyroidism may take months to normalize even with thyroid hormone replacements. GH-secreting adenoma, chronic renal failure, and hepatic cirrhosis may elevate PRL levels.

Corticotropin

ACTH is secreted in bursts that become more frequent after three to five hours of sleep and peak just prior to and about an hour after awakening. The levels decrease during the day to reach the lowest in the evening. This rhythm is not affected by temporary sleep deprivation as long as the normal sleep pattern is preserved. However, changing time zones alters the rhythm and may take several days to normalize (32). CRH stimulates ACTH secretion by binding to receptors, increasing cAMP levels, protein kinase A activity, and ACTH synthesis and release. This process is potentiated by ADH (33).

Glucocorticoids exert negative feedbacks on the pituitary, hypothalamus, and hippocampus by binding to receptors and forming complexes that affect the genome (34). They inhibit ACTH, CRH, and ADH secretion and synthesis of their mRNAs. A fast feedback within minutes and an intermediate feedback over a few hours target the hypothalamus to reduce CRH secretion and its action on ACTH release. A slow feedback over days reduces gene transcription and peptide synthesis of POMC, a precursor of ACTH (35). Glucocorticoids act on both the mineralocorticoid and the glucocorticoid receptors in the hippocampus. They may injure hippocampal neurons during prolonged stress. The amount of cortisol needed for negative feedback is directly correlated to the level of CRH. ACTH also inhibits its own secretion.

Trauma, burn injury, surgery, fever, hypoglycemia, and stress increase ACTH and cortisol secretion. Fever releases cytokines interleukin (IL) -1, IL-2 and IL-6, which enhance CRH release.

Thyroid-Stimulating Hormone

TSH levels are high during the night and decrease in the morning to low levels in the evening (36). TRH is a tripeptide that stimulates TSH secretion by binding to membrane receptors, with subsequent hydrolysis of phosphatidylinositol, activation of protein kinases, and increase in intracellular free calcium and TSH α and β mRNAs (25). Thyroid hormones inhibit TSH secretion by binding to intranuclear receptors and by inhibiting TRH synthesis in the hypothalamus.

Cold exposure increases TSH secretion. Stress, starvation, infection, and inflammation inhibit TSH secretion. Dopamine and somatostatin also inhibit TSH secretion (37).

Gonadotropins

Both FSH and LH are secreted in a pulsatile manner following an LHRH pulse delivered by the hypothalamus about once every 90 minutes. When the LHRH pulses become more frequent, LH secretion is increased. At slower LHRH pulses, FSH secretion is increased (38,39). During childhood, there is maximal inhibition of LHRH secretion. This intrinsic suppression of LHRH gradually decreases as puberty is reached, resulting in an increased FSH and LH secretion seen in puberty. LHRH causes a sequential release of FSH and LH during the normal menstrual cycle. LHRH action is mediated by receptor binding and G-protein activation on the gonadotrophs (40).

Estrogens, progestogens, and androgens bind to nuclear receptors to modulate FSH and LH secretion. Gonadotropin secretion in both sexes is suppressed by estrogens and androgens. This negative feedback requires an intact hypothalamus and is gender specific and dose dependent. Estrogen and progesterone also exert a positive feedback in women, resulting in a surge of gonadotropins at midcycle, which induces ovulation. This response is not seen in men. In lactating women, elevated PRL can decrease LHRH, LH, and estrogen secretion, resulting in amenorrhea (30). In menopausal women, there is an increase in the production of LH and FSH.

Vasopressin

The release of ADH is mainly controlled by osmoreceptors that are believed to be located in the supraoptic nuclei. Rising osmolality increases ADH secretion, resulting in renal water absorption and lowering of the osmolality. As the osmolality normalizes, further release of ADH is reduced. Baroreceptors located in the carotid sinus, aortic arch, and the heart, mainly in the left atrium, also control ADH secretion by relaying impulses to the supraoptic and periventricular nuclei (41). When blood volume is rapidly depleted by about 10%, ADH is released even when the osmolality is still below threshold.

ADH secretion is stimulated by norepinephrine, angiotensin II, opiates, and prostaglandin E_2. Inflammatory cytokines IL-1, IL-2, and IL-6 induce ADH release. It is also enhanced by hypoxia, hypercapnea, nicotine, cholinergic, and β-adrenergic agents, metoclopramide, barbiturates, carbamazepine, histamine, and halothane (42). Nausea, stress, and pain can trigger ADH release. Adrenal insufficiency lowers the set point for osmotic control, resulting in syndrome of inappropriate antidiuretic hormone (SIADH) secretion, which is reversed by glucocorticoid treatment (25).

Atrial natriuretic peptides (ANP) released from stretched myocytes in the left atrium during fluid overload inhibits ADH release and thirst, and promotes renal sodium excretion and diuresis. ANP also blocks the effects of angiotensin II, including thirst (43). ADH release is suppressed by alcohol, phenytoin, and α-adrenergic agents. Mood, anxiety, and emotional stress influence ADH secretion (42).

Oxytocin

OT release is stimulated by mechanical vaginal distention or suckling of the nipples. During pregnancy, uterine OT receptors are upregulated and a strong uterine sensitivity to OT is seen just before parturition. After parturition, uterine OT binding sites decrease while those in the mammary gland reach their maximum and remain elevated throughout lactation (24). In nursing females, OT results in the milk let-down reflex, which can be conditioned in response to a crying infant. OT secretion is also stimulated by nausea and norepinephrine. It is inhibited by emotional stress and opiates.

HYPOPITUITARISM

The deficiency of one or more pituitary hormones presents with increased mortality. The most common cause in adults is pituitary adenoma (Table 3). Many patients with pituitary macroadenomas (greater than 1 cm in diameter) have hypopituitarism, usually from compression of the pituitary stalk and portal vessels. Other sellar or parasellar lesions cause hypopituitarism by cellular infiltration or mechanical compression of the hypophysis or hypothalamus and by disruption of the hypothalamic-pituitary axis. Head injuries, particularly with fracture of the sella, are known to result in hypopituitarism. Surgical resections of sellar or parasellar tumors may result in transient or permanent hormonal deficiency. Radiation therapy is associated with a high incidence of hypopituitarism. Genetic defects may result in isolated deficiencies of GH, LHRH, TSH, or ACTH (44).

The symptoms vary from mild to severe insufficiency. The most severe involves failure of all pituitary hormones, resulting in panhypopituitarism. There is a wide spectrum of clinical findings. Patients may present with fatigue, weakness, cold intolerance, pale and dry skin, low blood pressure, orthostatic hypotension, regression of secondary sexual characteristics, amenorrhea, or impotence. In children, cessation of growth and delayed puberty are common and mental retardation may ensue. Fever, shock, coma, and death may follow relatively minor stresses due to lack of the ACTH–cortisol response.

These symptoms are similar to those seen in primary target organ failure, which has decreased or absent hormonal

secretion. The main difference is the elevated levels of pituitary hormones seen in primary organ failure. In contrast, hypothalamic or pituitary dysfunction generally presents with low levels of pituitary hormones. Pituitary failure usually presents with a deficiency of GH initially, followed by that of the gonadotropins, and then of ACTH and TSH. An excess of PRL, rather than its deficiency, is more common. Pituitary stalk compression from a mass lesion results in decreased delivery of dopamine and loss of its tonic inhibition of PRL secretion. Moreover, the most common secretory adenoma is a prolactinoma.

The diagnosis of hypopituitarism is made with clinical suspicion. Further imaging and endocrine work-ups help in identifying the specific causes of pituitary failure. Visual examination is essential in detecting peripheral visual loss due to chiasmal compression. Compression of adjacent structures should be evaluated by magnetic resonance imaging (MRI). Although computed tomography (CT) scan is helpful in showing calcifications and the bony anatomy, it is a poor second choice to an MRI (compare Figs. 1 and 3). Endocrine evaluation requires both baseline and stimulated hormone levels. Retesting is indicated in those with likelihood of progression of hypopituitarism, e.g., following radiation, surgery, or those with hypothalamic or pituitary lesions that are being monitored.

Treatment is aimed at removal of the cause and normalization of the hormonal environment. Hypothalamic lesions, even in the best of hands, may only be subtotally resected and usually require hormonal replacement. Endocrine replacement should be as close to normal levels as possible because overtreatment can be deleterious. Surgical removal of a lesion in the sellar and parasellar areas requires a careful consideration of the extent of involvement of the adjacent structures, the patient's risk stratification prior to surgery, and the availability of other treatment options.

Table 3   Causes of Hypopituitarism

Pituitary macroadenoma
Other sellar and parasellar lesions
Trauma
Surgery
Radiation
Pituitary apoplexy
Sheehan's syndrome
Genetic
Idiopathic

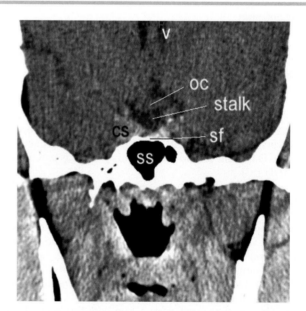

Figure 3   Coronal computed tomography showing the sellar floor (sf) and the pituitary stalk adjacent to the optic chiasm (oc). The sphenoid sinus (ss) is directly inferior to the sella. The cavernous sinus (cs) and lateral ventricles (v) are also seen.

Somatotropin Deficiency

GH deficiency in childhood is usually idiopathic while in adults, it is often due to adenoma, pituitary surgery, or radiotherapy. In children, there is dwarfism, truncal deposition of fat, prominence of the forehead, depressed midfacial development, and delay in dentition or onset of puberty. In adults, there is increased total body fat, lower than normal bone density with increased fracture rate, decreased lean body mass, muscle strength, exercise capacity, and libido, and reduced sense of physical and psychological well-being (45). Patients may complain of being less energetic, with emotional liability and a sense of social isolation.

GH replacement therapy has been used successfully in childhood for several decades. Its use in adults, however, has only recently begun to be evaluated. GH replacement in adults has been shown to reduce fat mass, increase lean body mass, improve physical performance, oxygen uptake, and bone mineral density (46). The recommended starting dose is 0.15 to 0.3 mg SC daily, increasing every four to six weeks based on clinical and biochemical responses (47). At least six months of steady maintenance dose is necessary to determine the benefits of the treatment. Regular measurement of weight, blood pressure, Hb A1c, IGF-1, lipid profile, and fat distribution is taken. Side effects include peripheral edema, arthralgia, and myalgia.

Gonadotropin Deficiency

Gonadotropin deficiency results from a pituitary lesion or deficiency of hypothalamic LHRH stimulation of the gonadotrophs. Hyperprolactinemia may also cause hypogonadal features. The symptoms are similar to those of primary gonadal failure and depend on whether the onset is before or after puberty. Boys present with small genitalia and eunuchoid habitus. Girls have primary amenorrhea and absent breast development. Adolescents present with delayed or arrested puberty. In men, there is reduction of testicular size, loss of facial and body hair, thinning of the skin, decreased bone density and muscle mass, poor libido, impotence, and infertility. Spermatogenesis may be preserved but the seminal volume is reduced. Symptoms develop more slowly and they are diagnosed later than in women. In women, there is amenorrhea, oligomenorrhea, dyspareunia, breast atrophy, and infertility. There is no loss of pubic and axillary hair unless there is concurrent ACTH deficiency.

Gonadotropin replacement is indicated in patients who want to maintain fertility. Otherwise, replacement with progesterone and estrogen for women and testosterone for men is sufficient to maintain the normal body composition, bone density, and sexual function.

Corticotropin Deficiency

This is the most life threatening. Patients may present with hypovolemic shock, fever, and acute abdomen. They may die from trivial illnesses due to vascular collapse and coma. Symptoms include weakness, fatigue, anorexia, weight loss, nausea, diarrhea, headache, orthostatic hypotension, dizziness, and skin pallor. In women, there is loss of pubic and axillary hair. In severe deficiency, there may be hyponatremia, increased insulin sensitivity, and decreased glycogen reserves, resulting in hypoglycemia.

The symptoms of glucocorticoid deficiency are similar to those of Addison's disease. The difference is that only cortisol and adrenal androgens are decreased in ACTH deficiency. The mineralocorticoid secretion, which is regulated by renin and angiotensin, is normal in ACTH deficiency so that adrenal crisis is less common than in Addison's disease. However, in chronic untreated cases, mineralocorticoid deficiency may develop. In contrast to ACTH deficiency, Addison's disease presents with hyperpigmentation of the skin and mucous membranes because of the elevated ACTH levels. Hyponatremia also occurs with Addison's disease and is less common in ACTH deficiency except in the elderly.

Acute cortisol deficiency is a medical emergency that must be considered when patients present with these symptoms, especially with a history of acute headache, pituitary surgery, radiotherapy, or significant head injury. It is important to remember that this may also follow an abrupt cessation of glucocorticoids or ACTH intake, even when they have been given for only a few weeks. To prevent this, steroids are usually tapered over several weeks before being discontinued.

Diagnosis is confirmed by low levels of cortisol and ACTH. Blood samples obtained at 8 A.M., just after the peak of cortisol secretion, are measured for levels of cortisol and ACTH. Cortisol levels below 100 nmol/L with normal or low ACTH levels are consistent with ACTH deficiency. In Addison's disease, the ACTH level is high. In suspected acute adrenal insufficiency, blood samples are sent for evaluation but hormonal replacement is started immediately without waiting for the results.

If an adrenal crisis is suspected, fluid resuscitation with normal saline is done to correct hypotension and electrolyte imbalance. Hydrocortisone 100 mg IV is given immediately and then every six hours (48). When the patient is stable, other tests are performed to determine the cause of adrenal sufficiency. Treatment for ACTH deficiency is similar to that for Addison's disease. Replacement with oral hydrocortisone at 10 mg on awakening and 5 mg at noon, and at 6 P.M. is recommended by some authors (44). The dose may be increased to 10 mg three times daily based on serum cortisol levels. Synthetic glucocorticoids like prednisone and dexamethasone are preferred by some because of their longer duration of action (49). Oral prednisone 5 mg or dexamethasone 0.5 mg is given once daily at bedtime. Clinical symptoms are monitored to avoid over-replacement, which can cause bone loss and Cushing's syndrome. The dose is increased during illness, injury, or surgery. During febrile illness, minor stress, surgery, or injury, the dose is increased two to threefold for about three days. For major surgery or severe illnesses, hydrocortisone 100 mg IV is given every eight hours, with the first dose given before induction of anesthesia. The dose is tapered daily by half to maintenance level, depending on the patient's course.

TSH Deficiency

TSH deficiency (secondary hypothyroidism) occurs relatively late in the course of hypopituitarism and is characterized by malaise, fatigue, weakness, inability to lose weight, weight gain, lack of energy, cold intolerance, dry skin, or constipation. It can also cause moderate hyperprolactinemia. The degree of hypothyroidism depends on the duration of TSH deficiency. The symptoms are similar to those of primary hypothyroidism, but generally are milder because some thyroid hormone is still being produced.

In TSH deficiency, the serum T_4 level is low but most patients will have normal TSH levels (50). In primary hypothyroidism, T_4 level is even lower while TSH level is increased. A TRH test with absent or impaired TSH response is suggestive of TSH deficiency; a normal or delayed response may indicate TRH deficiency.

TSH deficiency is treated with levothyroxine (L-T₄), a prohormone that is converted to T₃. ACTH deficiency must be excluded or treated prior to L-T₄ replacement to prevent any worsening of the symptoms of cortisol deficiency. Oral L-T₄ once a day is started at $100\,\mu g$ in young patients and 25 to $50\,\mu g$ in the elderly or in those with chronic hypothyroidism or ischemic heart disease (51). The dose is adjusted based on the clinical response and free T₄ levels. Chronic over-replacement is associated with osteoporosis and atrial fibrillation. Surgery in hypothyroid patients is associated with increased risks of minor complications as well as heart failure, gastrointestinal, and neuropsychiatric symptoms (52). L-T₄ is given preoperatively to hypothyroid patients.

PRL Deficiency

PRL deficiency results in failure of lactation and reproductive difficulty (30). It is rare except in Sheehan's syndrome wherein pituitary tissues are destroyed. Sheehan's syndrome is secondary to shock, hemorrhage, or sepsis associated with childbirth, which results in spasm of the hypophyseal arteries and necrosis of the adenohypophysis. Pituitary thrombosis and scar formation result in secondary atrophy of the thyroid, adrenal cortex, and ovaries (53). The symptoms of Sheehan syndrome are secondary to the resultant hormonal deficiencies. Prognosis is good with prompt hormonal replacement. No replacement for PRL is required.

Vasopressin Deficiency

ADH deficiency results in neurogenic or central diabetes insipidus (DI). It usually indicates a hypothalamic or stalk disorder and not a pituitary disease. Most of the cases are acquired and result from vascular insufficiency of the pituitary gland, cranial or pituitary surgery, meningitis, encephalitis, suprasellar lesions, or head injury. About 30% are idiopathic, with some patients exhibiting antibodies to ADH-secreting neurons (54). It may also be familial, with autosomal dominant inheritance affecting the processing of the precursor ADH molecule.

Neurogenic DI must be differentiated from nephrogenic DI, which is due to a partial or total unresponsiveness of the renal tubules to ADH. Nephrogenic DI may be genetic, idiopathic, or secondary to chronic renal disease, hypercalcemia, hypokalemia, and use of lithium or mannitol. Hypothalamic diseases such as sarcoidosis may cause excessive inappropriate drinking (primary polydipsia). This condition of polyuria with normal ADH secretion and renal responsiveness is known as dipsogenic DI (23).

DI is associated with hypernatremia and polyuria, with daily urine output usually greater than 3 L. Patients may have polydipsia, nocturia, nighttime thirsts, and hypotension. Those incapable of adequate oral fluid replacement may present with dehydration, hypovolemia, hyperosmolality, fever, hyperpnea, stupor, coma, and death. Evaluation of possible ADH deficiency should be done only after suspected anterior pituitary hormone deficiency is corrected because ACTH deficiency can mask ADH deficiency (44).

Diagnosis is suspected when there is hypernatremia and dilute urine. In milder cases, patients may drink enough to prevent hypernatremia. They can be diagnosed with a water deprivation test. With central DI, plasma osmolality rises with dehydration and urine osmolality remains low. A decrease in urine output after 1-deamino-8-D-arginine vasopressin (DDAVP) administration is diagnostic of central DI. This is in contrast to nephrogenic DI and polydipsic polyuria, which do not respond to DDAVP. In nephrogenic DI, there is a primary defect in the responsiveness to ADH. In polydipsic polyuria, the responsiveness to ADH is decreased by the washout of interstitial solutes including urea.

Patients with DI need careful monitoring of fluid intake and urine output. The treatment of choice for severe central DI is DDAVP, a synthetic analog of ADH, which has increased antidiuretic activity and half-life and minimal pressor activity (55). It is available in oral, intranasal, and parenteral forms. The oral form is not reliably absorbed and the intranasal and parenteral forms are preferred. The dosage varies between the different forms and among patients as well. Milder DI may be managed with oral fluid replacement alone.

SELLAR AND PARASELLAR LESIONS

Various tumors and non-neoplastic lesions arise in the sellar and parasellar areas and present with mass effects on the adjacent structures in addition to hypopituitarism. Most of these are benign but may grow aggressively to involve contiguous structures. Stretching of the diaphragma sella or dural impingement by a macroadenoma produces headache (56). Pressure on the optic chiasm results in a progression from scotomas to bitemporal hemianopia to blindness. Involvement of the cavernous sinus may result in ptosis, diplopia, ophthalmoplegia, facial hypesthesia, or pain. Lesions in the hypothalamus are far less common and may affect the regulation of temperature, appetite, thirst and water metabolism, the sleep–wake cycle, circadian rhythms, the control of autonomic nervous system, emotional expression, behavior, and memory (57). Patients frequently present with DI, obesity, hypogonadism, dysthermia, and sleep disturbances. Children may present with precocious puberty. Frontal lobe involvement may result in anosmia, personality disorders, or seizures. Tumors large enough to involve the third ventricle and occlude the foramina of Monro or the aqueduct of Sylvius may cause hydrocephalus. Hydrocephalus and increased intracranial pressure may cause nausea, vomiting, and eventually coma (Table 4).

MRI is the imaging study of choice. It can delineate the tumor as well as the adjacent structures along three axes (Figs. 4 and 5). For patients who cannot have an MRI, a coronal CT provides images with less soft tissue distinction but with more details on bony structures and calcification. Pituitary microadenomas usually appear hypointense to the normal gland on T1W images and have delayed contrast enhancement. They also appear hypoattenuated within the gland on enhanced and nonenhanced CT (58). Imaging studies are essential in establishing an anatomic diagnosis, in surgical planning, and follow-up evaluations.

A baseline endocrine test consists of PRL, IGF-1, LH, FSH, α subunit, 24-hour urinary free cortisol, am cortisol, ACTH, free T₄, TSH, testosterone (male), and estradiol (female) (59). When clinically indicated, provocative tests such as insulin tolerance test and metyrapone test may be needed to evaluate the pituitary reserve and hypopituitarism. Dynamic tests may also be needed to identify hypersecretion in acromegaly and Cushing's disease. These tests identify hormonal excess or deficiency and establish an endocrine diagnosis.

Any consideration for surgical resection of these lesions must be based on the natural history of the lesion, signs of compression of adjacent structures, need for tissue diagnosis, alternative treatments available, patient safety,

Table 4 Sellar and Parasellar Lesions

Tumors
Pituitary adenoma
    Secretory—PRL, GH, ACTH, TSH, mixed, LH, FSH, α subunit
    Nonsecretory
Craniopharyngioma
Meningioma
Metastasis
Glial tumors
    Glioma
        Optic nerve glioma
        Hypothalamic glioma
        Pilocytic astrocytoma
        High grade glioma
    Granular cell tumor/choristoma
    Trigeminal schwannoma
Germ cell tumors
    Germinoma
    Teratoma
    Embryonal carcinomas
    Endodermal sinus tumor
    Choriocarcinoma
Neuronal tumors
    Gangliocytoma
    Hypothalamic Hamartoma
    Olfactory neuroblastoma
Lipoma
Primary lymphoma
Primary melanoma
Mesenchymal tumors
    Chordoma
    Giant-cell tumor of bone
    Fibroma/fibrosarcoma
    Osteogenic sarcoma
    Hemangiopericytoma
Vascular tumors
    Cavernous angioma
    Hemangioblastoma
    Glomus tumor
Paraganglioma
Plasmacytoma/multiple myeloma
Cysts
Rathke's cleft cyst
Arachnoid cyst
Epidermoid cyst
Dermoid cyst
Echinococcal cyst
Aneurysms
Inflammation
Infiltrative
    Lymphocytic hypophysitis
    Idiopathic granulomatous hypophysitis
    Xanthomatous hypophysitis
    Sarcoidosis
    Langerhan's cell histiocytosis
    Giant-cell granuloma
Infectious
    Pituitary abscess
    Tuberculoma
Pituitary hyperplasia
Empty sella

Abbreviations: ACTH, adrenocorticotropic hormone; FSH, follicle-stimulating hormone; GH, growth hormone; LH, luteinizing hormone; PRL, prolactin; TSH, thyroid stimulating hormone.

and prognosis. The lesions may be removed totally or partially, depending on the possible benefits and weighing against risks of complications and bad outcome. The goals are to safely recover and preserve as much function of the adjacent structures to these lesions as possible, and improve or normalize the endocrine function. Endocrine deficiency is relatively easy to treat with the appropriate replacement. Most tumors in this area are treated with surgery. The exceptions are prolactinomas, asymptomatic tumors in the elderly, and nonsecretory microadenomas. Radiation is used as an adjunctive therapy for subtotal tumor resection, aggressive tumors, recurrence, and in patients with poor surgical risks or failure of medical management (60). The risk of hypopituitarism following radiotherapy must be considered. It occurs in a delayed fashion over 10 years and requires vigilant monitoring for detection and treatment. Long-term risks of conventional radiotherapy include depression, decreased memory, and glioma formation. Stereotactic radiosurgery has recently been used instead of conventional radiotherapy. It offers lesser complications but long-term results are still forthcoming.

Pituitary Adenoma

Pituitary adenoma is the most common neoplasm of the sellar region (61). It is a benign tumor arising within the adenohypophysis. It accounts for about 10% of all intracranial tumors in adults and is found in 6% to 22% of adults during autopsy. More than 50% occur between the third and fifth decades. The incidence is higher in women (62). About 10% of adults with pituitary adenoma are asymptomatic (63). Pituitary adenomas are classified as microadenomas (less than 1 cm in diameter) and macroadenomas. Among the microadenomas, only secretory tumors are of significance. Medication is the primary treatment for prolactinomas. All other adenomas are treated with surgery. Pituitary adenomas present with hormonal dysfunction, mass effects, or both. The dysfunction may be hypopituitarism or hyperpituitarism. A nonsecretory adenoma lacks the early symptoms of hormonal oversecretion and tends to be large when it presents, usually with visual symptoms and hypopituitarism. It is more common in older patients while a secretory adenoma is more common in younger patients.

Some prolactinomas, GH-secreting adenomas, and nonsecretory adenomas are associated with multiple endocrine neoplasia type 1 (MEN-1). Nearly half of MEN-1 patients develop pituitary adenomas. On the other hand, only 1% to 15% of pituitary adenomas have MEN-1 (64). Prolactinoma is the most common adenoma occurring in MEN-1. MEN-1 is an autosomal dominant disorder associated with tumors of the pituitary, parathyroid, and pancreas. A mutated MEN-1 tumor suppressor gene is passed on to the affected individual. Tumor growth is caused by mutation of the remaining normal MEN-1 allele. This loss of heterozygosity of the allele is seen in parathyroid adenomas and islet cell tumors including insulinomas and gastrinomas. These endocrine tumors usually present in young adulthood with high levels of PTH, gastrin, or PRL. These are treatable with medication or surgery. In patients with a pituitary adenoma, calcium levels should be checked to exclude primary hyperparathyroidism.

Prolactinoma

Prolactinoma is the most common type of pituitary adenoma. It usually presents as microadenomas in women and macroadenomas in men. Microadenomas usually occur at the lateral portion of the gland. Overall, microprolactinomas are more common than macroprolactinomas (65). Microprolactinomas present with symptoms of PRL hypersecretion rather than visual symptoms or mass effects.

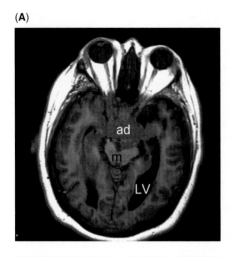

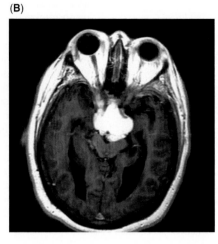

Figure 4 **(A)** Axial T1W MRI shows a large adenoma (ad) compressing the midbrain (m). The lateral ventricles are enlarged because of obstruction at the aqueduct of Sylvius within the midbrain. **(B)** Delayed enhancement of the adenoma with gadolinium.

Women usually seek medical attention earlier because of galactorrhea, amenorrhea, and infertility. They may also present with hirsutism, acne, mood changes, dyspareunia, decreased libido, and osteopenia. Men usually present with impotence, loss of libido, and visual complaints. They may also present with galactorrhea, anxiety, depression, and irritability similar to the mood changes seen in menopausal women (66). The hypogonadism and infertility associated with hyperprolactinemia result from its central inhibitory effects on the pulsatile LHRH secretion and in women, its blockage of the positive feedback of estrogen, which induces the LH surge (67). Adolescents may present with delayed puberty. Some prolactinomas in men and postmenopausal women are asymptomatic when they are first discovered incidentally during imaging studies. Some prolactinomas are mixed adenomas that cosecrete GH, ACTH, TSH, and rarely FSH and/or LH. They may be derived from two different cell lines or from a single cell line, which secretes both hormones. Patients present initially with symptoms of hyperprolactinemia and later on with the clinical picture of the cosecreted hormones.

Diagnosis is based on PRL levels greater than 200 ng/mL and radiologic images of a sellar tumor. The degree of hyperprolactinemia correlates with the size of the prolactinoma. Pregnancy, primary hypothyroidism, renal or hepatic failure, and use of drugs that can cause hyperprolactinemia must be excluded during the initial evaluation. Modest elevation of PRL levels (less than 200 ng/mL) may be secondary to a microprolactinoma or compression of the pituitary stalk by other tumors.

Because most microprolactinomas do not enlarge and some may regress, they may be observed with annual evaluation of PRL levels and MRI studies. Treatment is started when the hypogonadal effects of hyperprolactinemia are present or when the tumor enlarges. Macroprolactinomas, because of their potential for further growth and mass effects, are treated upon diagnosis. The primary therapy for prolactinomas is with bromocriptine, a dopamine agonist. It binds to the D_2 receptors of both normal and prolactinoma cells and normalizes the PRL level in most patients. It also induces regression of the tumor size. Large adenomas disappear with effective medical treatment but will immediately recur when

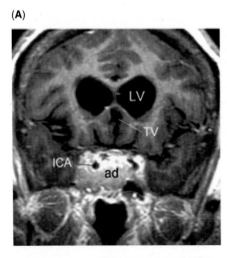

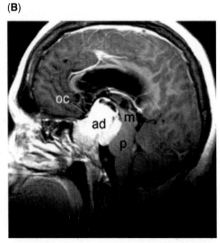

Figure 5 **(A)** Coronal MRI showing the adenoma (ad) with involvement of the cavernous sinus. The internal carotid artery is surrounded by tumor. Note the enlargement of the lateral ventricles and the third ventricle because of hydrocephalus. **(B)** Sagittal MRI showing the same tumor (ad) compressing the optic chiasm (oc), midbrain (m), and pons (p).

the treatment is discontinued. Therefore it is necessary to continue medication for the lifetime of the patient. The hypogonadal symptoms are reversed within months. Long-term treatment has been associated with perivascular fibrosis in some tumors, which may affect subsequent surgery.

Bromocriptine is generally well tolerated. Common side effects include nausea, headache, vomiting, postural hypotension, and nasal congestion (68). These often occur with dose increases and may be relieved by temporarily reducing the dose. In some macroprolactinomas with sellar floor erosion, shrinkage of the tumor may result in CSF rhinorrhea. The effective daily dose is 5 to 7.5 mg taken with meals and is gradually increased from a low starting dose. Cabergoline is an oral dopamine agonist that has less frequent side effects. Its dose is 0.25 to 1.0 mg twice a week. Pergolide, a dopamine agonist used in the treatment of Parkinson's disease, has been used successfully in those who did not respond to bromocriptine.

Surgery is preferred for apoplectic or cystic prolactinomas, which do not respond well to dopamine agonists (69). It is also indicated in patients who do not respond to dopamine agonists, cannot tolerate their side effects, or prefer surgery to lifelong medication. In women with macroprolactinoma, who are planning pregnancy, surgical resection may prevent the consequences of tumor growth that occurs during pregnancy, including apoplexy. Surgery in pregnant women may pose a greater risk for the fetus than continuing bromocriptine during pregnancy. Generally, curative resection with return of PRL levels to normal is likely in microprolactinomas and unlikely in macroprolactinomas. Thus macroprolactinomas will generally require continuous bromocriptine treatment even after resection.

Radiation has been shown to normalize PRL levels and decrease tumor size years after treatment (60). However, it is generally reserved for those who failed combined medical and surgical treatment.

Acromegaly

Acromegaly is a rare, slowly evolving disease that results from excessive GH secretion. The most common cause is a GH-secreting pituitary adenoma, which sometimes cosecretes PRL or other hormones. It may rarely be due to the overproduction of GHRH by a hypothalamic hamartoma, gangliocytoma, or carcinoid tumors in the lungs, pancreas, or GI tract (70). GH hypersecretion results in acromegaly if it occurs after the closure of the epiphysis of the long bones. The soft tissues in the hands and feet are thick. Carpal tunnel syndrome is common. The skin and hair are thickened and sweating may be increased. There is excessive growth of the supraorbital rim, nose, and jaw, resulting in elongation of the face, tooth gaps, macrognathia, and malocclusion. Few patients seek help because the gradual change in appearance may go unnoticed for years. Joint pain and osteoarthritis are common. Although cortical bone is thick, the trabecular bone may be osteopenic. Myopathy with weakness of the proximal muscles may be seen. Often there is enlargement of the tongue, thyroid, heart, liver, spleen, and thymus. MI is a common cause of death. The longer the GH excess remains untreated, the more severe the cardiomyopathy becomes. Left ventricular hypertrophy results in decreased diastolic volumes and diastolic hypertension. These may be irreversible when interstitial fibrosis is present. Patients present with hypertension, atherosclerosis, and congestive heart failure. Diabetes mellitus, sleep apnea, and daytime sleepiness are also common. There is

an increased risk for colonic polyps and GI cancer (71). Regular colonoscopy is recommended.

Diagnosis is confirmed with radiologic images of a sellar tumor and biochemical tests showing elevation of serum IGF-1 and GH. GH levels fluctuate depending on the activities and time of day during sampling. Serum IGF-1 levels, on the other hand, are more constant and reflect the GH secretion of the preceding day (72). Thus, IGF-1 is the preferred screening test. Because IGF-1 levels are normally higher in females, during puberty and pregnancy, and lower in the elderly, the levels are interpreted based on values adjusted for age and sex. An elevated age- and sex-matched IGF-1 level is consistent with acromegaly. GH hypersecretion may be further demonstrated by the oral glucose tolerance test (OGTT). Normally, GH is suppressed after an oral glucose load. Acromegaly is diagnosed when GH levels do not fall below 1 ng/mL two hours after intake of 75 g of glucose (73). Hypercalciuria and hyperphosphatemia are also commonly seen.

Aggressive treatment is important. The main goal is to normalize GH and IGF-1 levels. Transsphenoidal resection is the preferred treatment because with tumor removal, cure may be permanent. It provides good remission and avoids lifelong therapy with medications. Remission is defined by normal IGF-1 levels and GH suppression to less than 1 ng/mL in OGTT. Macroadenomas, which usually present at the time of diagnosis, have lower remission. This is more so when the tumor involves the cavernous sinus, which precludes complete resection. Possible complications include hypopituitarism, DI, CSF leak, and meningitis. When there is failure of remission after surgery, octreotide is usually started. If this is still unsuccessful, dopamine agonists, radiation, repeat surgery, or GH receptor antagonists may be considered (72).

Octreotide is a long-acting somatostatin analogue that inhibits the secretion of GH, glucagon, and insulin. It lowers GH and IGF-1 levels and may shrink the tumor. It relieves the headache, joint pain, sweating, carpal tunnel syndrome, and sleep apnea in acromegalic patients. Its effectiveness is limited but it can be used as primary treatment in patients who refuse surgery or with poor surgical risks. It is also used in an attempt to shrink the tumor prior to surgery. Side effects include GI discomfort, diarrhea, cholelithiasis, and chronic gastritis.

Bromocriptine is used at high doses (20–30 mg/day) to lower GH levels in some acromegalic patients. The mechanism of action is unclear because dopamine normally stimulates GH secretion. Unlike in prolactinomas, bromocriptine is much less effective in GH-secreting adenomas.

Radiation is used as an adjunct and is reserved for recurrence or failure of remission with surgery and medical therapy. It may take years for GH levels to normalize.

Cushing's Disease

Cushing's disease is hypercortisolism secondary to an ACTH-secreting pituitary adenoma. It is more common in women. It comprises the majority of Cushing's syndrome in adults. Cushing's syndrome is characterized by glucocorticoid excess from various causes. It may be due to hypothalamic, pituitary, or adrenocortical tumors, or ectopic tumors secreting ACTH or CRH. Patients present with truncal obesity, loss of muscle bulk, moon facies, buffalo hump, fragile skin, which bruises easily, purple striae, and hirsutism. Hypertension, diabetes mellitus, hypercalciuria, osteopenia, and hypogonadism are common. Frequent infections and hypercoagulability are also seen. Patients may present with anxiety, depression, emotional lability, or psychosis. Cataracts and glaucoma are known complications.

ACTH-secreting pituitary adenomas are usually microadenomas. Diagnosis is made by confirming hypersecretion of cortisol and pituitary ACTH. Hypercortisolism is established by elevated 24-hour urinary free cortisol and failure of dexamethasone to suppress cortisol secretion. Dexamethasone 1 mg given orally at 11 PM normally suppresses the 8 AM serum cortisol level to less than 5 μg/L. In hypercortisolism, the cortisol level is usually greater than 10 μg/L (74). Measurement of late-night salivary cortisol has also been used as a screening test for hypercortisolism (75). Certain conditions of hypercortisolism thought to be due to increased CRH secretion must be excluded. These pseudo-Cushing states include severe stress, illness, depression, renal failure, alcoholism, ethanol withdrawal, and morbid obesity. The CRH test is helpful because these states show poor responsiveness to CRH given following the two-day low-dose dexamethasone suppression test. In contrast, with Cushing's syndrome, serum cortisol becomes elevated 15 minutes after CRH is injected (76).

ACTH excess is readily diagnosed by immunoradiometric assays. Elevated ACTH levels in the presence of hypercortisolism are usually consistent with Cushing's disease when a pituitary adenoma is seen on MRI. In cases wherein no tumor is visualized, a pituitary source of ACTH must be differentiated from other sources including adrenocortical tumors and ectopic ACTH secreted by carcinoma of the lungs, thymus, pancreas, and bronchial carcinoids. Cavernous sinus and inferior petrosal sinus samplings showing higher ACTH levels than in peripheral samples are suggestive of Cushing's disease.

Transsphenoidal resection is the treatment of choice. Exploration may be required for those with negative imaging. The adenomas are usually in the anteromedial areas deep within the gland. Immediate correction of hypercortisolism is seen. Patients are maintained on steroids postoperatively which are tapered gradually over weeks. Microadenomas have better remission and less frequent recurrence compared to macroadenomas.

Radiotherapy is used as primary treatment in patients with poor surgical risks, incompletely resected macroadenomas, or recurrent tumors. Because it may take years before the cortisol levels are normalized, medications are generally used to reduce the cortisol levels after radiation.

Medical therapy is used as an adjunct to radiotherapy. Ketoconazole is an antifungal agent that blocks various enzymes in cortisol production and inhibits pituitary ACTH secretion. It is effective in lowering the cortisol levels. Side effects include gynecomastia and hepatotoxicity. Metyrapone is an inhibitor of 11β-hydroxylase and is used in combination with ketoconazole or aminoglutethimide for more severe cases. Aminoglutethimide blocks the conversion of cholesterol to pregnenolone, decreasing cortisol production. Mitotone is a drug that destroys the adrenal cortex and inhibits steroid production. Other drugs have been used to control ACTH secretion with limited success. These include valproic acid, octreotide, cyproheptadine, and bromocriptine.

In cases wherein surgery, radiotherapy, and medical treatment have failed to control hypercortisolism, bilateral adrenalectomy is an option. Patients will require lifelong steroid replacement. They are also monitored for Nelson's syndrome, which is characterized by a rapidly enlarging pituitary adenoma, elevated ACTH levels, and hyperpigmentation. The treatment of choice for Nelson's syndrome is transsphenoidal resection with or without postop radiation.

Thyrotropinoma

TSH-secreting adenomas are rare, comprising 0.5% to 1% of pituitary adenomas (77). The most common cause of an elevated TSH with an enlarged pituitary gland is primary hypothyroidism with reactive pituitary hyperplasia. Most TSH-secreting adenomas secrete TSH alone, but some may secrete the α subunit. Others cosecrete GH, PRL, or gonadotropins. Most are macroadenomas, which are locally invasive. Patients usually present with goiter and hyperthyroidism, which may have been previously treated with thyroid ablation. Thyroidectomy or radioiodine ablation removes the negative feedback and results in further growth of the TSH-secreting adenoma. Some patients have hyperprolactinemia with acromegaly. Macroadenomas may present with mass effects and hypopituitarism. Diagnosis is suggested by elevated levels of free T_4 and TSH, and CT or MRI showing a sellar tumor.

Treatment is with transsphenoidal resection. The adenoma is usually fibrous and located in the anteromedial portion of the gland. Larger tumors with involvement of adjacent structures are generally less favorable. Thioamines, potassium iodide, or β-blockers are used for short-term control of hyperthyroidism prior to surgery (78). Octreotide and propranolol may also be used prior to surgery. After surgery, T_4 replacement may be needed temporarily or permanently. Other hormonal replacement may be required. Radiotherapy is indicated in patients who refuse surgery, are poor surgical risks, or have failed surgery. Octreotide has been used successfully in shrinking the tumor and normalizing TSH and thyroid hormone levels. This requires continuous therapy.

Gonadotroph Adenoma

Gonadotroph adenomas are common. They comprise about half of all macroadenomas and a large proportion of clinically nonfunctioning adenomas (79). Their hypersecretion is minimal compared to other secreting adenomas. It usually involves FSH and a combination of α and β subunits of FSH and LH. The relative amounts of each incomplete hormone are not consistent among gonadotroph adenomas (80). Patients usually present with headache and visual symptoms. Macroadenomas may result in hypopituitarism and mild hyperprolactinemia. They may be found incidentally on radiologic work-ups. Diagnosis is made with images showing sellar tumor and elevated levels of gonadotropins and their subunits, which are often increased further with the administration of TRH (81).

Treatment is transsphenoidal resection. Most cases have improvement of visual symptoms. Postop hormonal levels are measured and replacement is given as required. Radiotherapy is indicated in patients who decline surgery, have poor surgical risks, or incomplete resection. Medical therapy has not been successful in decreasing tumor size.

Nonsecretory Adenoma

Pituitary adenomas may secrete clinically insignificant amounts of hormone, inactive hormones, or none at all (82). Nonsecretory adenoma is the most common type of macroadenoma. It usually presents with mass effects, hypopituitarism, and mild hyperprolactinemia from stalk effect. Diagnosis is suggested by images of a sellar tumor and absence of hormonal hypersecretion. In patients with a history of primary cancer, pituitary metastasis is possible.

Treatment is aimed at restoring vision and pituitary function by decompressing the adjacent structures. This is usually done with transsphenoidal resection but may require a combined transcranial approach as well. Recurrent tumors are treated with repeat surgery. Radiotherapy is reserved for patients with poor surgical risks or recurrent tumors that are inaccessible by surgery. No medical therapy is effective in decreasing the tumor size. For patients with nonsecretory microadenomas that are discovered incidentally, no treatment is indicated unless there is tumor growth or pituitary dysfunction.

Pituitary Apoplexy

Pituitary apoplexy is a sudden hemorrhagic or ischemic infarction of the pituitary gland or tumor that may result in transient or permanent hypopituitarism. It may be clinically silent or acutely life threatening. It is associated most often with rapidly growing adenomas and less frequently with head injury, bromocriptine therapy, hypertension, and systemic anticoagulation (83). Ischemic infarction of the normal gland may be seen following obstetric hemorrhage (Sheehan's syndrome). Predisposing factors include DM, bleeding disorders, and radiation (5). Patients may present with headache, nausea, vomiting, visual loss, ophthalmoplegia, diplopia, ptosis, mydriasis, fever, stiff neck, stroke, seizure, altered mental status, or coma.

CT or MRI is usually diagnostic. Blood density or intensity in the sellar area with occasional fluid level is seen (Fig. 6). Baseline hormone levels must be obtained. Treatment is directed at replacement of deficient hormones, especially the steroids. Emergent transsphenoidal surgery must be planned if there are visual deficits or altered sensorium. Pituitary function may recover. With modern imaging techniques, hormonal replacement, and surgical decompression, most symptomatic pituitary apoplexy should have a good outcome.

Other Sellar and Parasellar Lesions

Craniopharyngioma is the most common parasellar tumor in children, comprising 5% to 13% of pediatric intracranial tumors (84). Up to one-third occurs in adults, making up 1.2% to 4% of adult intracranial tumors (85). It is a benign, slowly growing encapsulated tumor with cystic and solid components and frequent calcification. It is more commonly suprasellar than intrasellar. Treatment with surgery and radiation is individualized to maximize long-term tumor control while minimizing morbidity.

Meningiomas of the olfactory groove, tuberculum sella, and medial sphenoid wing comprise about 14% of parasellar tumors (86). These are benign, slowly growing well-circumscribed tumors that are usually solid and enhance with contrast. They are more common in women. They usually present with visual symptoms. The majority of these can be resected totally.

Metastatic tumors may be sellar or suprasellar. About 70% involve the neurohypophysis (63). They arise commonly from the lungs and breasts but may also come from the nasopharynx, kidney, and GI tract. They are usually solid and enhance with contrast. Surgery may be indicated for tissue diagnosis and decompression of adjacent structures. The treatment is combined with radiotherapy and chemotherapy for palliation.

A giant aneurysm (greater than 2.5 cm in diameter) of the anterior communicating artery may present as a suprasellar mass with occasional calcification seen on head CT. Aneurysms of the ICA and anterior and posterior communicating arteries in the parasellar and suprasellar areas can present clinically like a pituitary tumor. Compression of adjacent structures may result in visual deficits and hypopituitarism. Rupture into the cavernous sinus may result in an arteriovenous fistula. Angiography is diagnostic. Treatment is with surgical clipping, endovascular coiling, or both.

Lymphocytic hypophysitis is a lymphocytic infiltration of the pituitary gland typically seen in pregnant women or during the postpartum period. The gland is often enlarged due to the lymphocytic infiltrates and may resemble a tumor. The etiology is unknown but may be autoimmune. Many of the patients have immunopathies such as thyroiditis, autoimmune gastritis, and lupus erythematosus (45). Patients present with hypopituitarism and a pituitary mass. Clinical suspicion in a patient with headache, visual disturbance, weakness, and fatigue may prevent possible death from unrecognized adrenal insufficiency. Treatment with steroids has been effective in reducing inflammation. A therapeutic trial with a dopamine agonist may be started to treat hyperprolactinemia but this does not affect the enlargement, which may regress spontaneously. Surgery may be indicated in patients with progressive symptoms of compression or failure of medical treatment.

(A)

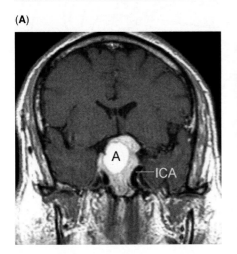

(B)

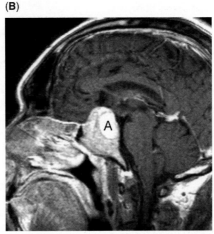

Figure 6 **(A)** Coronal MRI showing acute hemorrhage (A) within the large adenoma. The internal carotid artery on each side of the tumor can be seen. **(B)** Sagittal MRI showing the adenoma eroding through the sellar floor into the sphenoid sinus. The hemorrhage (A) is confined within the tumor.

Sarcoidosis is a granulomatous disease that affects multiple organs. About 5% of patients with sarcoidosis have clinical signs of neurosarcoidosis and less than 1% of patients have symptoms of hypothalamic or pituitary dysfunction (87). Neurosarcoidosis primarily involves the leptomeninges at the base of the brain and posterior fossa, but may also affect the infundibulum and the optic nerves. Surgical biopsy provides a definitive tissue diagnosis. Treatment is with steroids. Cyclophosphamide may be considered for resistant cases (88).

In chronic primary hypothyroidism, pituitary hyperplasia resulting from an increased TRH secretion may mimic the appearance of a tumor. The pituitary gland may become large enough to cause optic nerve compression. Because TRH stimulates PRL, these patients may present with hyperprolactinemia and hypogonadism. An elevated TSH level with low T_3 and T_4 levels in these patients confirm the diagnosis. Treatment with L-T_4 will shrink the pituitary gland to its normal size.

Empty sella syndrome is a condition wherein the subarachnoid space extends into the sella turcica. It is primary if a defect in the diaphragma sella results in herniation of the arachnoid membrane and compression of the pituitary gland against the sellar floor. This generally does alter the parenchymal structure of the compressed pituitary gland. It may be an incidental finding in patients with morbid obesity or pseudotumor cerebri. It is secondary if previous surgery, radiation, or remote tumor infarction (apoplexy) has decreased the volume of the pituitary and caused the sella to be filled with CSF. In these cases, hypopituitarism may be present. No treatment is usually necessary unless there is pituitary dysfunction.

Surgical Approaches to Sellar and Parasellar Lesions

Lesions in the sellar area may be approached transsphenoidally or transcranially. With either approach, intraoperative use of microscope or endoscope is essential to visualization. Fluoroscopy and stereotactic imaging guidance are helpful in localization (Fig. 7).

The transsphenoidal approach is preferable for most pituitary adenomas and cystic lesions (Fig. 8). Even large adenomas with significant suprasellar extension can be completely resected as long as there is no significant constriction at the diaphragma sella, which results in a dumb-bell-shaped tumor. Meningiomas and aneurysms should not be approached with this route. The incision is made either sublabially or endonasally, followed by a submucosal dissection along the cartilaginous septum and the floor of the nasal cavity (Fig. 9). The sellar lesion is reached by removing the wall of the sphenoid sinus and the floor of the sella. The improvement in optics and video technology has allowed the use of endoscopes not only as adjuncts to the microscope but more recently also as the main optical instruments in endoscopic endonasal transsphenoidal surgery. The transsphenoidal approach has the advantages of providing a direct access to the sella, visualization of the pituitary gland and its adjacent lesion, and allowing decompression of the optic chiasm without directly manipulating it.

The transcranial approach is used for meningiomas, aneurysms, and lesions above the diaphragma sella. It may be used as the second stage operation following a transsphenoidal resection. It involves a scalp incision, craniotomy, dural opening, and brain retraction to visualize the sellar and parasellar areas. The angle of the approach may be subfrontal, pterional, subtemporal, or a combination of these.

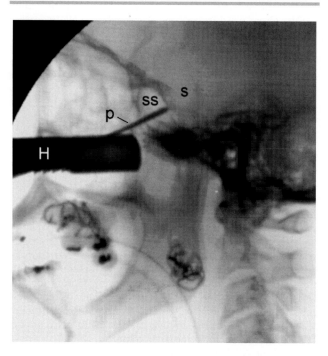

Figure 7 Intraoperative fluoroscopy showing a probe (p) passing through the anterior wall of the sphenoid sinus (ss) and pointing at the floor of an enlarged sella turcica (s). The Hardy speculum (H) rests on the floor of the nasal cavity and provides a corridor through which the sellar tumor can be removed. The endotracheal tube and oropharyngeal packing can be seen.

SYNDROME OF INAPPROPRIATE SECRETION OF ADH

SIADH is a condition of continued secretion of ADH even when the plasma osmolality falls below the threshold. It

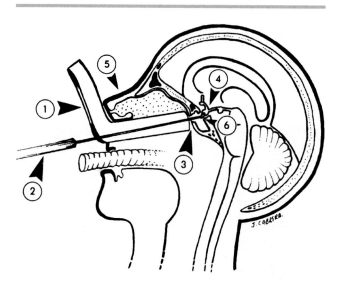

Figure 8 Schematic representation of the transnasal, trans-septal, trans-sphenoidal approach to the pituitary gland. 1, Bivalve speculum in place; 2, ring curette in the sella; 3, open sphenoidal sinus; 4, pituitary gland; 5, resected nasal cartilage; and 6, open sellar floor.

(A)   **(B)**   **(C)**

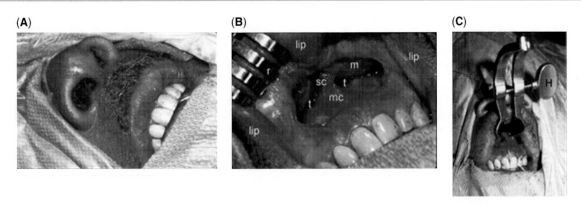

Figure 9 (**A**) Draping for a transsphenoidal procedure. Patient's nose and upper lip remain exposed. (**B**) After a sublabial incision, the mucosa (m) is separated from the maxillary bone to create inferior submucosal tunnels (t). The septal cartilage (sc) will be detached from the maxillary crest (mc) and pushed to the left to enlarge the right anterior tunnel that is being developed. The joining of the tunnels will create a space through which the speculum can be placed. A retractor (r) is holding the upper lip. (**C**) The Hardy speculum (H) in place.

presents with hyponatremia with low plasma osmolality and elevated urine osmolality that is usually higher than plasma osmolality (23). The patient must be euvolemic with normal renal, adrenal, and thyroid functions. Patients remain asymptomatic unless serum sodium decreases rapidly or fall below 115 mmol/L (89). Symptoms include headache, fatigue, nausea, vomiting, anorexia, cramps, ileus, confusion, irritability, seizures, ataxia, and coma. Personality changes, inattentiveness, and forgetfulness may progress to paranoia and delusions.

SIADH may be seen in head trauma, intracranial bleeding, brain tumors, meningitis, encephalitis, porphyria, bronchial carcinoma, and other ectopic tumors producing ADH. Hypothyroidism and hypocortisolism may result in a similar euvolemic hypotonic hyponatremia. Nicotine, morphine, barbiturates, vincristine, and some tricyclic antidepressants stimulate ADH secretion. Phenytoin, chlorpropamide, clofibrate, thiazides, and mono-amine oxidase (MAO) inhibitors may cause SIADH.

Treatment consists of the removal of possible causes of SIADH and restriction of daily water intake to 500 mL. Demeclocycline 600 to 1200 mg/day is used to block the antidiuretic action of ADH. Oral furosemide with salt supplementation may also be used (90). Severe hyponatremia is corrected very slowly to at least 125 mmol/L with hypertonic saline. Rapid correction of hyponatremia must be avoided to prevent central pontine myelinolysis, which usually occurs within a few days after rapid correction and presents with seizures, brain edema, and coma.

SUMMARY

The hypothalamic-pituitary-target organ axis provides an intercellular communication that is essential in maintaining internal homeostasis and metabolism. Its dysfunction affects normal growth, development, and reproduction. Various lesions in the sellar and parasellar areas cause excessive or deficient secretion of pituitary hormones and compression of adjacent tissues. The most common sellar tumor is a pituitary adenoma. Diagnosis is facilitated by modern imaging technology and bioassay techniques. Treatment is aimed at removal of the etiology of hormonal dysfunction or mass

effects, preservation and improvement of pituitary, visual, and neurologic functions, and normalization of the hormonal milieu by controlling hypersecretion or replacing deficient hormones. Current medical therapy provides crucial hormonal replacement and is able to control hypersecretion in prolactinomas and, to a minor extent, in acromegaly. Surgery is still the preferred treatment for acromegaly, Cushing's disease, and most tumors including gonadotropin-secreting adenomas and nonsecretory adenomas. Surgery is usually indicated for tumor debulking, decompression of surrounding structures, or tissue diagnosis. Radiotherapy is used as an adjunctive therapy. With prompt diagnosis and treatment, pituitary dysfunction should not cause undue morbidity or early mortality. Multispecialty care provided by the endocrinologist, neuroradiologist, neuroophthalmologist, neurosurgeon, neuropathologist, and radiation oncologist can increase the chance of leading a normal life.

REFERENCES

1. Abboud CF, Ebersold MJ. Prolactinomas. In: Thapar K, Kovacs K, Scheithauer BW, Lloyd RV, eds. Diagnosis and Management of Pituitary Tumors. New Jersey: Humana Press, 2001:279–294.
2. Asa SL, Kovacs K, Melmed S. The hypothalamic-pituitary axis. In: Melmed S, ed. The Pituitary. Cambridge: Blackwell, 1995: 3–44.
3. Baumann G, Amburn KD, Buchanan TA. The effect of circulating growth hormone-binding protein on metabolic clearance, distribution, and degradation of human growth hormone. J Clin Endocrinol Metab 1987; 64:657–660.
4. Baylis PH. Vasopressin, diabetes insipidus and syndrome of inappropriate antidiuresis. In: DeGroot LJ, Jameson JL, eds. Endocrinology. 4th ed. Philadelphia: W.B. Saunders, 2001: 363–376.
5. Beck-Peccoz P, Amr S, Menezes Ferreira MM, et al. Decreased receptor binding of biologically inactive thyrotropin in central hypothyroidism. Effect of treatment with thyrotropin-releasing hormone. N Engl J Med 1985; 312:1085–1090.
6. Beck-Peccoz P, Persani L. TSH-producing adenomas. In: DeGroot LJ, Jameson JL, eds. Endocrinology. 4th ed. Philadelphia: W.B. Saunders, 2001:321–328.
7. Brabant G, Prank K, Ranft U, et al. Physiological regulation of circadian and pulsatile thyrotropin secretion in normal man and woman. J Clin Endocrinol Metab 1990; 70:4403–4409.

8. Braunstein GD. Hypothalamic syndromes. In: DeGroot LJ, Jameson JL, eds. Endocrinology. 4th ed. Philadelphia: W.B. Saunders, 2001:269–281.

9. Buchfelder M, Fahlbusch R. Thyrotroph adenomas. In: Thapar K, Kovacs K, Scheithauer BW, Lloyd RV, eds. Diagnosis and Management of Pituitary Tumors. New Jersey: Humana Press, 2001:333–342.

10. Cardoso ER, Peterson EW. Pituitary apoplexy: a review. Neurosurgery 1984; 14:363–373.

11. Carroll PV, Christ ER, Bengtsson BA, et al. Growth hormone deficiency in adulthood and the effects of growth hormone replacement: a review. J Clin Endocrinol Metab 1998; 83: 382–395.

12. Carter-Su C, Schwartz J, Smit LS. Molecular mechanism of growth hormone action. Annu Rev Physiol 1996; 58:187–207.

13. Chandler WF. Pituitary tumors. In: Bernstein M, Berger MS, eds. Neuro-oncology the Essentials. New York: Thieme, 2000:399–408.

14. Chapman IM, Bach MA, Van Cauter E, et al. Stimulation of the growth hormone (GH)-insulin-like growth factor I axis by daily oral administration of a GH secretagogue (MK-677) in healthy elderly subjects. J Clin Endocrinol Metab 1996; 81:4249–4257.

15. Cobb WE, Spare S, Reichlin S. Neurogenic diabetes insipidus: management with DDAVP (1-desamino-8-D arginine vasopressin). Ann Intern Med 1978; 88:183–188.

16. Copinschi G, Vanonderbergen A, Lhermitebaleriaux M, et al. Effects of a 7-day treatment with a novel, orally active, growth hormone (GH) secretagogue, MK-677, on 24-hour GH profiles, insulin-like growth factor I, and adrenocortical function in normal young men. J Clin Endocrinol Metab 1996; 81:2776–2782.

17. Corbetta S, Pizzocaro A, Peracchi M, et al. Multiple endocrine neoplasia type I in patients with recognized pituitary tumours of different types. Clin Endocrinol 1997; 47:507–512.

18. Daneshdoost L, Gennarelli TA, Bashey HM, et al. Identification of gonadotroph adenomas in men with clinically nonfunctioning adenomas by the LHβ subunit response to TRH. J Clin Endocrinol Metab 1993; 77:1352–1355.

19. DeBold CR, Sheldon WR, DeCherney GS, et al. Arginine vasopressin potentiates adrenocorticotropin release induced by ovine corticotropin-releasing factor. J Clin Invest 1984; 73:533–538.

20. Decaux G, Waterlot Y, Gennette F, et al. Inappropriate secretion of antidiuretic hormone treated with furosemide. Br Med J 1982; 285:89–90.

21. Desir D, Van Cauter E, Fang VS, et al. Effects of "jet lag" on hormonal patterns. I: procedures, variations in total plasma proteins, and disruption of adrenocorticotropin-cortisol periodicity. J Clin Endocrinol Metab 1981; 52:628–641.

22. Emery D, Kucharczyk W. Imaging of pituitary tumors. In: Thapar K, Kovacs K, Scheithauer BW, Lloyd RV, eds. Diagnosis and Management of Pituitary Tumors. New Jersey: Humana Press, 2001:201–217.

23. Essat S, Melmed S. Clinical review 18: are patients with acromegaly at increased risk for neoplasia? J Clin Endocrinol Metab 1991; 72:245–249.

24. Evans RM. The steroid and thyroid hormone receptor superfamily. Science 1988; 240:889–895.

25. Evans WS, Cronin MJ, Thorner MO. Hypogonadism in hyperprolactinemia. Proposed mechanisms. In: Ganong WF, Martini L, eds. Frontiers in Neuroendocrinology. New York: Raven, 1982:77–122.

26. Faglia G. Prolactinomas and hyperprolactinemic syndrome. In: DeGroot LJ, Jameson JL, eds. Endocrinology. 4th ed. Philadelphia: W.B. Saunders, 2001:329–342.

27. Fried LF, Palevsky PM. Hyponatremia and hypernatremia. Med Clin N Am 1997; 81:585–609.

28. Gerich JE, Lorenzi M, Bier DM, et al. Effects of physiologic levels of glucagon and growth hormone on human carbohydrate and lipid metabolism. Studies involving administration of exogenous hormone during suppression of endogenous hormone secretion with somatostatin. J Clin Invest 1976; 57:875–884.

29. Green H, Morikawa M, Nixon T. A dual effector theory of growth hormone action. Differentiation 1985; 29:195–198.

30. Growth Hormone Research Society. Consensus guidelines for the diagnosis and treatment of adults with growth hormone deficiency: summary statement of the Growth Hormone Research Society Workshop on Adult Growth Hormone Deficiency. J Clin Endocrinol Metab 1998; 83:379–381.

31. Ho KKY. Growth hormone deficiency in adults. In: DeGroot LJ, Jameson JL, eds. Endocrinology. 4th ed. Philadelphia: W.B. Saunders, 2001:520–527.

32. Holl RW, Thorner MO, Leong DA. Intracellular calcium concentration and growth hormone secretion in individual somatotropes: effects of growth hormone-releasing factor and somatostatin. Endocrinology 1988; 122:2927–2932.

33. Horseman ND. Prolactin. In: DeGroot LJ, Jameson JL, eds. Endocrinology. 4th ed. Philadelphia: W.B. Saunders, 2001:209–220.

34. Kacsoh B. Endocrine Physiology. New York: McGraw-Hill, 2000.

35. Kopchick JJ. Growth hormone. In: DeGroot LJ, Jameson JL, eds. Endocrinology. 4th ed. Philadelphia: W.B. Saunders, 2001: 389–404.

36. Kunwar S, Wilson CB. Sellar and parasellar tumors in children. In: DeGroot LJ, Jameson JL, eds. Endocrinology. 4th ed. Philadelphia: W.B. Saunders, 2001:354–360.

37. Ladenson PW, Levin AA, Ridgway EC, Daniels GH. Complications of surgery in hypothyroid patients. Am J Med 1984; 77:261–266.

38. Lipscombe L, Asa S, Ezzat S. Management of lesions of the pituitary stalk and hypothalamus. Endocrinologist 2003; 13(1):38–51.

39. Lissett CA, Shalet SM. Hypopituitarism. In: DeGroot LJ, Jameson JL, eds. Endocrinology. 4th ed. Philadelphia: W.B. Saunders, 2001:289–299.

40. Lo JC, Tyrrell JB, Wilson CB. Corticotroph adenomas. In: Thapar K, Kovacs K, Scheithauer BW, Lloyd RV, eds. Diagnosis and Management of Pituitary Tumors. New Jersey: Humana Press, 2001:317–332.

41. Loriaux DL, McDonald WJ. Adrenal insufficiency. In: DeGroot LJ, Jameson JL, eds. Endocrinology. 4th ed. Philadelphia: W.B. Saunders, 2001:1683–1690.

42. Magalini SI, Magalini SC. Dictionary of Medical Syndromes. 4th. Philadelphia: Lippincott-Raven, 1997.

43. Marshall JC, Kelch RP. Gonadotropin-releasing hormone: role of pulsatile secretion in the regulation of reproduction. N Engl J Med 1986; 315:1459–1468.

44. Mathews LS, Gaddy-Kurten D. Hormone signaling via cytokine receptors and receptor serine kinases. In: DeGroot LJ, Jameson JL, eds. Endocrinology. 4th ed. Philadelphia: W.B. Saunders, 2001:49–57.

45. McKeever PE, Blaivas M, Gebarski SS. Sellar tumors other than adenomas. In: Thapar K, Kovacs K, Scheithauer BW, Lloyd RV, eds. Diagnosis and Management of Pituitary Tumors. New Jersey: Humana Press, 2001:387–447.

46. Melmed S, Jackson I, Kleinberg D, et al. Current treatment guidelines for acromegaly. J Clin Endocrinol Metab 1998; 83:2646–2652.

47. Melmed S. Acromegaly. In: DeGroot LJ, Jameson JL, eds. Endocrinology. 4th ed. Philadelphia: W.B. Saunders, 2001: 300–312.

48. Melmed S. Evaluation of pituitary masses. In: DeGroot LJ, Jameson JL, eds. Endocrinology. 4th ed. Philadelphia: W.B. Saunders, 2001:282–288.

49. Metcalfe P, Jonston DG, Nosadini R, et al. Metabolic effects of acute and prolonged growth hormone excess in normal and insulin-deficient man. Diabetologia 1981; 20:123–128.

50. Molitch ME. Medical therapy of pituitary tumors. In: Thapar K, Kovacs K, Scheithauer BW, Lloyd RV, eds. Diagnosis and Management of Pituitary Tumors. New Jersey: Humana Press, 2001:247–267.

51. Moore KD, Couldwell WT. Craniopharyngioma. In: Bernstein M, Berger MS, eds. Neuro-oncology the Essentials. New York: Thieme, 2000:409–418.

52. Moose BD, Shaw EG. Radiation therapy of pituitary tumors. In: Thapar K, Kovacs K, Scheithauer BW, Lloyd RV, eds. Diagnosis

and Management of Pituitary Tumors. Humana PressNew Jersey2001; 9:269–277.

53. Morley JE. Neuroendocrine control of thyrotropin secretion. Endocr Rev 1981; 2:396–436.

54. Moses AM, Norman DD. Diabetes insipidus and syndrome of inappropriate antidiuretic hormone secretion (SIADH). Adv Intern Med 1982; 27:73–110.

55. Orth DN, Kovacs WJ. The adrenal cortex. In: Wilson JD, ed. Williams Textbook of Endocrinology. 9th ed. Philadelphia: W.B. Saunders, 1998:517–664.

56. Pohl CR, Richardson DW, Hutchinson JS, et al. Hypophysiotropic signal frequency and the functioning of the pituitary-ovarian system in the rhesus monkey. Endocrinology 1983; 112:2076–2080.

57. Quabbe H, Plockinger U. Somatotroph adenomas. In: Thapar K, Kovacs K, Scheithauer BW, Lloyd RV, eds. Diagnosis and Management of Pituitary Tumors. New Jersey: Humana Press, 2001:295–315.

58. Raff H, Raff JL, Findling JW. Late-night salivary cortisol as a screening test for Cushing's syndrome. J Clin Endocrinol Metab 1998; 83:1163–1167.

59. Reavley S, Fisher AD, Owen D, et al. Psychological distress in patients with hyperprolactinaemia. Clin Endocrinol 1997; 47:343–348.

60. Redei E, Rittenhouse PA, Revskoy S, McGivern RF, Aird F. A novel endogenous corticotropin release inhibiting factor. Ann NY Acad Sci 1998; 840:456–469.

61. Reeves W. Brian, Daniel G. Bichet, Thomas EA. Posterior pituitary and water metabolism. In: Wilson JD, ed. Williams Textbook of Endocrinology. 9th ed. Philadelphia: W.B. Saunders, 1998:341–387.

62. Reichlin S. Neuroendocrinology. In: Wilson JD, ed. Williams Textbook of Endocrinology. 9th ed. Philadelphia: W.B. Saunders, 1998:165–248.

63. Rhoton AL Jr. The sellar region. Neurosurgery 2002; 4(suppl): S1–355–374.

64. Rinderknecht E, Humbrel RE. The amino acid sequence of human insulin-like growth factor I and its structural homology with proinsulin. J Biol Chem 1978; 253:2769–2776.

65. Rudman D, Feller AG, Nagraj HS, et al. Effects of human growth hormone in men over 60 years old. N Engl J Med 1990; 322:1–6.

66. Rudman D, Kutner MH, Rogers CM, et al. Impaired growth hormone secretion in the adult population: relation to age and adiposity. J Clin Invest 1981; 67:1361–1369.

67. Saeger W. Tumor-like lesions of the pituitary and sellar region. Endocrinologist 2002; 12(4):300–314.

68. Sanno N, Teramoto A, Osamura Y, et al. Pathology of pituitary tumors. In: Weiss MH, Couldwell WT, eds. Neurosurgery Clinics of North America. Philadelphia: W.B. Saunders, 2003:14(1):25–39.

69. Sassin JF, Frantz AG, Kapen S, et al. The nocturnal rise of human prolactin is dependent on sleep. J Clin Endocrinol Metab 1973; 37:436–440.

70. Schwartz J. Intercellular communication in the anterior pituitary. Endocr Rev 2000; 21(5):488–513.

71. Sherwin RS, Schulman GA, Hendler R, et al. Effect of growth hormone on oral glucose tolerance and circulating metabolic fuels in man. Diabetologia 1983; 24:155–161.

72. Shupnik MA, Ridgway EC, Chin WW. Molecular biology of thyrotropin. Endocr Rev 1989; 10:459–475.

73. Snyder PJ. Gonadotroph adenomas. In: DeGroot LJ, Jameson JL, eds. Endocrinology. 4th ed. Philadelphia: W.B. Saunders, 2001: 313–320.

74. Snyder PJ. Gonadotroph cell adenomas of the pituitary. Endocr Rev 1985; 6:552–563.

75. Stojilkovic SS, Reinhart J, Catt KJ. Gonadotropin-releasing hormone receptors: structure and signal transduction pathways. Endocr Rev 1994; 15:462–498.

76. Suh HK, Frantz AG. Size heterogeneity of human prolactin in plasma and pituitary extracts. J Clin Endocrinol Metab 1974; 39:928–935.

77. Sved AF. Central neural pathways in barorecptor control of vasopressin secretion. In: Schrier RW, ed. Vasopressin. New York: Raven, 1985:443–453.

78. Thapar K, Laws ER Jr. Pituitary surgery. In: Thapar K, Kovacs K, Scheithauer BW, Lloyd RV, eds. Diagnosis and Management of Pituitary Tumors. New Jersey: Humana Press, 2001:225–246.

79. Thorner M, Vance ML, Laws ER Jr, Horvath E, Kovacs K. The anterior pituitary. In: Wilson JD, ed. Williams Textbook of Endocrinology. 9th ed. Philadelphia: W.B. Saunders, 1998:249–340.

80. Van Cauter E, Copinschi G, Turek FW. Endocrine and other biologic rhythms. In: DeGroot LJ, Jameson JL, eds. Endocrinology. 4th ed. Philadelphia: W.B. Saunders, 2001:235–256.

81. Van Wyk JJ, Underwood LE, Hintz RL, et al. The somatomedins: a family of insulin like hormones under growth hormone control. Recent Prog Horm Res 1974; 30:259–318.

82. Vance ML. Diagnosis, management, and prognosis of pituitary tumors. In: Thapar K, Kovacs K, Scheithauer BW, Lloyd RV, eds. Diagnosis and Management of Pituitary Tumors. New Jersey: Humana Press, 2001:165–172.

83. White A, Ray DW. Adrenocorticotropic hormone. In: DeGroot LJ, Jameson JL, eds. Endocrinology. 4th ed. Philadelphia: W.B. Saunders, 2001:221–233.

84. Wiersinga WM. Hypothyroidism and myxedema coma. In: DeGroot LJ, Jameson JL, eds. Endocrinology. 4th ed. Philadelphia: W.B. Saunders, 2001:1491–1506.

85. Yamada S. Epidemiology of pituitary tumors. In: Thapar K, Kovacs K, Scheithauer BW, Lloyd RV, eds. Diagnosis and Management of Pituitary Tumors. New Jersey: Humana Press, 2001:57–69.

86. Yanovski JA, Cutler GB, Chrousos GP, Nieman LK. Corticotropin-releasing hormone stimulation following low-dose dexamethasone administration. JAMA 1993; 269:2232–2238.

87. Yeung VT, Lai CK, Cockram CS, et al. Atrial natriuretic peptide in the central nervous system. Neuroendocrinology 1991; 53:18–24.

88. Ying SY. Inhibins, activins, and follistatins: gonadal proteins modulating the secretion of follicle-stimulating hormone. Endocr Rev 1988; 9:267–293.

89. Young WF Jr. Clinically nonfunctioning pituitary adenomas. In: Thapar K, Kovacs K, Scheithauer BW, Lloyd RV, eds. Diagnosis and Management of Pituitary Tumors. New Jersey: Humana Press, 2001:343–351.

90. Zingg HH. Oxytocin. In: DeGroot LJ, Jameson JL, eds. Endocrinology. 4th ed. Philadelphia: W.B. Saunders, 2001:201–208.

51

Adrenal Glands

Maria A. Kouvaraki, Douglas B. Evans, Ana O. Hoff, and Jeffrey E. Lee

INTRODUCTION

Physicians must always be aware of potential adrenal pathology when evaluating and treating a surgical patient. In this way, they are more likely to detect occult adrenal insufficiency, pheochromocytomas, functioning adrenal adenomas, and aldosteronomas at an early stage. However, this requires physicians to have a fundamental understanding of both the normal and abnormal endocrine functions of the adrenal gland and a working knowledge of the surgical approaches appropriate for the treatment of the range of adrenal tumors. They must also know the natural history of diseases that can affect the adrenal gland. In particular, they must have an understanding of the natural history and epidemiology of incidental masses of the adrenal gland, functioning and nonfunctioning adenomas, pheochromocytomas, and adrenal cortical carcinomas. This will help the surgeon to evaluate thoroughly and critically a patient with an incidental adrenal mass and then, once the diagnosis is established, to recommend the most appropriate treatment. The discussion in this chapter focuses on aspects of adrenal physiology and pathophysiology important in the surgical evaluation of the patient with a known or suspected adrenal mass, adrenal hormone excess, or adrenal hormone deficiency.

EMBRYOLOGY, ANATOMY, AND HISTOLOGY

The adrenal gland is composed of a cortex and medulla that have different embryologic origins. The adrenal cortex arises from the coelomic mesoderm between the fourth and sixth weeks of gestation. The adrenal medulla is derived from cells of the neural crest that migrate to the adrenal cortex. The neural crest also forms the sympathetic nervous system and ganglia. Chromaffin tissue may also develop in extra-adrenal sites, most commonly in the para-adrenal and para-aortic regions. The single most common site where extra-adrenal chromaffin tissue develops is the organ of Zuckerkandl, located adjacent to the aorta near the origin of the inferior mesenteric artery. Although the adrenal cortex is composed initially of an inner zone and a large outer fetal zone, this fetal zone involutes late in gestation and in the early postnatal period, leaving only a thin cortical layer in the mature adrenal gland.

The adrenal glands are paired structures that have a pyramid shape and are located in the retroperitoneum along the superior medial aspect of each kidney. The normal adult adrenal gland weighs approximately 4 to 5 g and has a rubbery consistency. The bright yellow color of the adrenal gland helps to distinguish it from the surrounding retroperitoneal fat. On cut sections, the adrenal gland has two distinct layers: a thin (1–2 mm), bright yellow cortex that envelops an even thinner layer of dark reddish gray tissue, the adrenal medulla. The medulla is soft and constitutes only approximately 10% to 20% of the total weight of the adrenal gland.

The adrenal glands are highly vascularized; they receive arterial blood from branches of the inferior phrenic arteries, the renal artery, and directly from the aorta. The nutrient arteries coalesce and anastomose to form a capsular arterial plexus that sends capillaries coursing through the cortical cells. These capillaries combine to form a venous portal system that drains into the adrenal medulla. There, the vessels come together to join the central adrenal vein. This venous portal system supplies the adrenal medullary tissue with a high concentration of adrenal steroids. Additionally, the adrenal medulla is supplied by arteriae medullae that penetrate directly into the substance of the adrenal medulla. Although some small veins drain from the surface of the adrenal cortex, most arterial blood flows from the capsular plexus, through the cortex, into the medulla, and out of the central vein. The right adrenal vein is short and wide; it exits the gland and immediately enters the posterolateral aspect of the inferior vena cava. The left adrenal vein exits anteriorly and usually drains into the left renal vein, although it occasionally enters the inferior vena cava directly. As a result, it is easier to catheterize the adrenal vein on the left than on the right.

There is a lymphatic plexus within the subcapsular portion of the adrenal cortex and the adrenal medulla that drains into the adjacent para-aortic and renal lymph nodes. Although the adrenal cortex does not appear to be innervated, the adrenal medulla is richly supplied by preganglionic sympathetic nerves that extend from the splanchnic nerve, celiac ganglia, and other plexuses. There is no parasympathetic innervation of the adrenal medulla.

Histologically, the adult adrenal cortex is composed of three zones: an outer zona glomerulosa, a middle zona fasciculata, and an inner zona reticularis. Each zone has distinct histologic features under a light and electron microscope. Aldosterone is produced exclusively in the zona glomerulosa, and cortisol and androgens are produced in the zona fasciculata and zona reticularis. Adrenal medullary cells have a polyhedral shape and are arranged in cords around adrenal portal veins. They contain catecholamines and precipitated chromium salts that stain brown with hematoxylin and eosin. Electron microscopy shows vesicles in the core of these cells that contain epinephrine and norepinephrine. The hormones secreted by the adrenal cortex and the vascular supply to the gland affect adrenal medullary secretion. Adrenal medullary cells are generally clumped around blood vessels coming from the cortex, which provides these cells with a high local concentration of cortisol. Cortisol induces the enzyme phenylethanolamine

N-methyltransferase (PNMT), which converts norepinephrine to epinephrine. The vessels that provide a direct arterial blood supply to the adrenal medulla are surrounded primarily by cells that secrete predominantly norepinephrine.

PHYSIOLOGY

Physiologically, the adrenal gland must be regarded as two separate organs. This is because the cortex and the medulla are regulated by independent control systems and their functions do not overlap.

Adrenal Cortex

The adrenal cortex secretes three major products: glucocorticosteroids (cortisol and corticosterone), mineralocorticoids (aldosterone and deoxycorticosterone), and sex steroids (mainly androgens). The metabolic pathways are shown in Figure 1.

Cortisol

Cortisol is secreted from the zona fasciculata in relatively large amounts (10–20 mg/day). The control of cortisol secretion begins in the central nervous system (CNS). Specifically, neurons from almost every part of the brain converge on the hypothalamus and modulate the release of a 41–amino-acid peptide, corticotropin-releasing factor (CRF), from the hypothalamus. After its release, CRF travels via a direct portal venous system to the anterior pituitary, where it stimulates the synthesis and release of adrenocorticotropic hormone (ACTH), a 39–amino-acid peptide. ACTH secretion shows a diurnal rhythm, with the highest levels occurring early in the morning and the lowest levels occurring late in the afternoon. In turn, under basal conditions, the CNS, via CRF, ACTH, and the adrenocortical cascade, causes a fluctuation in the mean plasma cortisol concentrations, which follows the fluctuation in the ACTH levels. Therefore, a peak plasma cortisol concentration normally occurs in the early morning and a nadir concentration in the late afternoon.

Regulation of Cortisol Secretion

Under basal conditions, plasma cortisol concentrations are maintained within fairly narrow limits by an interplay between the concentrations of circulating cortisol, CRF, and ACTH. In particular, as the cortisol concentration exceeds its physiologic limit, as a result of either endogenous stimulation or exogenous administration, ACTH secretion is suppressed. This suppression of ACTH secretion by cortisol is exerted through three mechanisms: (i) cortisol acts directly on the pituitary to inhibit the synthesis of ACTH, (ii) cortisol suppresses the release of ACTH by CRF, and (iii) cortisol inhibits the synthesis of CRF. This negative feedback effect of cortisol on ACTH release maintains the circulating plasma cortisol level in the normal range.

The stimulation of cortisol secretion by ACTH occurs via a steroidogenic pathway. ACTH's primary action in this pathway is to convert cholesterol to δ-5-pregnenolone.

In general, ACTH and cortisol secretion are increased under conditions of acute stress, fever, pain, or hemorrhage, and this overrides the negative feedback effect of acute endogenous or exogenous hypercortisolemia. Indeed, ACTH secretion increases in proportion to the magnitude of the stress, and the adrenal secretion of cortisol is related linearly to the concentration of ACTH up to a range of 400 to 500 pg/mL. The maximum plasma concentration of cortisol elicited by stress is in the range of 50 to 70 g/dL. Concentrations above 70 to 80 g/dL are distinctly unusual, however, even in the context of longstanding adrenal hyperplasia caused by ectopic ACTH production.

Longstanding cortisol (or synthetic steroid) excess has a lasting suppressive effect on ACTH secretion. In particular, it prevents the ACTH response to stress and other

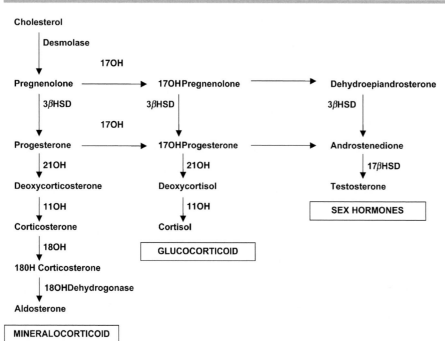

Figure 1 Steroidogenesis in the adrenal cortex.

stimuli. The length of time that excess cortisol or cortisol-like steroids must be administered before the ACTH release is suppressed has not been precisely determined in humans; however, approximately two to three weeks of chronic daily steroid therapy is sufficient to suppress the normal pituitary-adrenal axis. In the case of exogenously administered steroids, the suppressive effect is clearly dose dependent. Once the cortisol excess is abolished, however, either by removing the endogenous source or by stopping the administration of steroids, the return of pituitary-adrenal function follows a fairly predictable pattern; ACTH secretion returns within three to four months, followed a few months later by the restoration of adrenocortical responsiveness and consequent cortisol secretion.

Systemic Effects of Cortisol

Almost every tissue in the body is affected by glucocorticoids. Glucocorticoid-related changes in carbohydrate metabolism have the net effect of producing hyperglycemia. The two primary events responsible for hyperglycemia are decreased peripheral utilization of glucose and increased gluconeogenesis. A separate action of glucocorticoids in the context of carbohydrate metabolism is to increase hepatic glycogen synthesis, which is thought to be insulin dependent. Decreased glucose utilization is due to an inhibition of glucose transport and metabolism (especially in fat cells, resulting from a direct cellular effect of the glucocorticoids) and a resistance to the action of insulin. Glucocorticoids increase gluconeogenesis through several mechanisms, including peripheral and hepatic mechanisms. In particular, glucocorticoids act on muscle to release branched-chain and other glucogenic amino acids, which are then converted to glucose in the liver. Both the lipolytic effect of epinephrine, causing the release of glycerol from fat cells, and the glycogenolytic effect of epinephrine, causing release of lactate from muscle, appear to depend partly on the presence of glucocorticoids. Thus, glucocorticoids provide increased glucogenic amino acids, glycerol, and lactate from the periphery for glucose production in the liver through the process of gluconeogenesis. The permissive effect of glucocorticoids accounts for the dependence of epinephrine and glucagon on these steroids for their gluconeogenic action. Lastly, glucocorticoids have a direct effect on gluconeogenesis, apparently through their induction of several gluconeogenic hepatic enzymes.

The effects of glucocorticoids on immune function are complex and numerous. On the basis of both their in vivo and in vitro effects, as well as those seen in response to both low-dose and high-dose steroid administration, it is evident that almost every aspect of the immune response can be modified by steroid administration. For example, the numbers and distribution of granulocytes and lymphocytes, as well as the function of these cells, are affected either directly or indirectly by glucocorticoids. Excess glucocorticoids also decrease the tensile strength of wounds, suppress contraction of the scar, and delay epithelialization. These effects have been demonstrated in several species, including humans. In vivo studies have also shown that collagen synthesis is decreased as a result of decreased protein synthesis produced by glucocorticoids. Excess or exogenously administered glucocorticoids may also exert effects on bone mineralization (by increasing bone resorption), in the cardiovascular system, in the digestive tract, and on renal function.

Aldosterone

Aldosterone is a steroid secreted in small amounts (100–150 µg/day) from the zona glomerulosa. It is the end product of a steroidogenic pathway that includes corticosterone and deoxycorticosterone. As with glucocorticoids, the specificity of aldosterone's action is determined by its chemical configuration, by the conformational structure and location of steroid receptors, and by postreceptor intracellular events.

The actions of aldosterone are less generalized than those of glucocorticoids because of the more limited tissue distribution of mineralocorticoid, or type I, receptors. Specifically, mineralocorticoid receptors are present in the kidney, colon, heart, brain, and blood vessels. Although corticosterone, deoxycorticosterone, and cortisol may act as mineralocorticoids, mineralocorticoid receptors are selective for aldosterone. Responsible for this selectivity is the enzyme 11β-hydroxysteroid dehydrogenase type 2, which inactivates cortisol to cortisone, thereby allowing aldosterone to bind to the mineralocorticoid receptor (1–3).

Mainly through its effects on the kidneys, aldosterone plays a major role in the regulation of electrolyte excretion and extracellular fluid balance. The mineralocorticoid receptors in the kidneys are located in the distal renal tubule and cortical collecting ducts. The principal effect of aldosterone on the kidney is to increase sodium resorption and potassium secretion in the proximal portion of the collecting tubule of the distal nephron. More specifically, aldosterone increases the number of apical sodium channels, potassium conductance through specific channels, and the synthesis of the ATPase pump. Aldosterone also promotes the secretion of hydrogen ions into the renal tubule, a process that may not necessarily be directly associated with sodium resorption. Aldosterone receptors also control electrolyte balance in the salivary glands and the colonic mucosa.

Chronic aldosterone excess results in depletion of total body potassium levels through increased kaliuresis. Metabolic alkalosis results from a chronic proton deficit. Moreover, excessive aldosterone secretion leads to increased sodium and water retention by the kidneys and to expansion of the extracellular fluid compartment, resulting in suppression of plasma renin activity (PRA). This eventually leads to a higher intravascular volume, which increases cardiac output and blood pressure.

Regulation of Aldosterone Secretion

Physiologically, the principal mechanism controlling aldosterone secretion is the renin–angiotensin system. Renin is released from the juxtaglomerular apparatus of the kidney in response to a decrease in intravascular volume, such as occurs in the setting of hemorrhage, a negative sodium balance, or dehydration. Both a decrease in pressure in the afferent arteriole entering the glomerulus and a decrease in the intratubular sodium concentration at the level of the macula densa will stimulate renin secretion. Renin released into the bloodstream then hydrolyzes a circulating protein substrate derived from the liver to produce angiotensin I. This peptide is then further cleaved in the lung by a converting enzyme to form angiotensin II. Angiotensin II is a potent vasoconstrictor and functions as a trophic hormone in the adrenal zona glomerulosa responsible for the stimulation of aldosterone secretion. A decrease in the intravascular volume therefore results in increased aldosterone secretion. Conversely, in the setting of a replete blood volume, positive sodium balance, or overhydration, secretion is suppressed, which leads to a decrease in aldosterone secretion.

Aldosterone secretion is also directly controlled by the concentration of serum potassium. Specifically, an increase in serum potassium stimulates aldosterone secretion, and a decrease in serum potassium results in a lowering of aldosterone secretion. In the anephric patient without a renin–angiotensin system, the serum potassium level appears to be the primary mechanism controlling aldosterone secretion.

ACTH can also control aldosterone secretion, but to a lesser degree, because the action of ACTH is short lived (less than 24 hours). Such stimulation is normally accompanied by an increase in cortisol secretion. In contrast, angiotensin II and a high serum potassium concentration do not stimulate cortisol production. ACTH alone is not sufficient, however, to restore the full secretory capacity of the zona glomerulosa.

Androgens

The three major androgenic steroids produced by the adrenal cortex are dehydroepiandrosterone (DHEA), DHEA sulfate (DHEAS), and androstenedione, and these androgens have anabolic effects. Quantitatively, DHEA is the most prominent androgenic steroid produced by the adrenal cortex; the synthesis of testosterone by the adrenal cortex is minimal. The androgenic steroids produced by the adrenal cortex are not themselves effective androgens; however, they become so when converted to the potent androgens testosterone and 5α-dihydrotestosterone in peripheral tissues. In women, the peripheral conversion of adrenal androgens is an important source of circulating androgens (one-half of circulating testosterone); in men, most circulating androgen is produced by the testes. The adrenal cortex also produces small amounts of the estrogens, estrone, and estradiol, though most circulating estrogens in women are derived from the ovaries.

Pathologically, the adrenal cortex has the potential to produce virilization, either through the secretion of excess androgens by tumors or as a consequence of enzyme defects that shunt steroidogenesis to favor androgen formation. Excess androgen secretion in adults or children is most commonly due to adrenal tumors; it can also be due to congenital adrenocortical enzymatic defects, which are found primarily in newborns and associated with sexual ambiguity. Androgen secretion by adrenal tumors is usually associated with excess cortisol secretion. Female patients with Cushing's syndrome have masculinizing features, including the coarsening of facial hair and maldistribution of pubic hair into the male pattern. Although aspects of virilization may appear in patients with benign adrenocortical tumors, excessive adrenal androgen production, as evidenced by increased 17-ketosteroid concentrations in the urine, is characteristic of an adrenocortical carcinoma.

Adrenal Medulla

Epinephrine and norepinephrine are the principal secretory products of the adrenal medulla. Dopamine is also secreted by the adrenal medulla, but its physiologic importance is unclear (undetermined functional significance). Enkephalins have recently been identified in the adrenal medulla, and their significance is also unclear. Under basal conditions, approximately 80% of the catecholamine produced by the adrenal medulla is epinephrine derived from the amino acid tyrosine. In this pathway, tyrosine is first converted to dihydroxyphenylalanine (dopa) by tyrosine

hydroxylase, the rate-limiting enzyme in the synthetic pathway. The tyrosine hydroxylase content is increased in response to sympathetic nerve stimulation. Next in the pathway, dopa is converted to dopamine by dopa decarboxylase, and the dopamine, now in catecholamine storage vesicles, is converted to norepinephrine by dopamine β-hydroxylase. PNMT then converts norepinephrine to epinephrine. Interestingly, PNMT depends on high concentrations of cortisol for its activity. Vascular connections leading from the adrenal cortex through the adrenal medulla have been demonstrated; presumably, these carry high concentrations of cortisol to the enzyme.

The effects of adrenomedullary stimulation and sympathetic nerve stimulation are generally similar. In some tissues, however, epinephrine and norepinephrine may produce different effects because of the existence of two types of receptors, α-adrenergic and β-adrenergic receptors. These receptors have differing sensitivities for various catecholamines and therefore produce different responses. α-Receptors are most sensitive to epinephrine and norepinephrine, whereas β-receptors are most sensitive to isoproterenol. The α-receptors are further subdivided into the α_1 group, which causes vasoconstriction, intestinal relaxation, uterine contraction, and pupillary dilation, and the α_2 group, which causes platelet aggregation, vasoconstriction, and presynaptic norepinephrine release. The β-receptors are further subdivided into the β_1 group, which are equally sensitive to epinephrine and norepinephrine and cause cardiac stimulation, intestinal relaxation, and lipolysis, and the β_2 group, which are more sensitive to epinephrine than norepinephrine and cause vasodilation, uterine relaxation, bronchodilation, and presynaptic norepinephrine release.

Catecholamine release has several metabolic effects. In particular, carbohydrate metabolism is affected by alterations in glycogenolysis in the liver and in striated muscle. In this process, β-receptor stimulation activates glycogen phosphorylase and inhibits glycogen synthetase. Concomitantly, gluconeogenesis is increased in the liver by catecholamine (especially epinephrine) secretion. Glycogenolysis produces metabolic precursors for gluconeogenesis such as lactate and pyruvate. In all, glucose levels generally rise as catecholamine secretion increases. In addition, catecholamines result in the stimulation of glucagon secretion and reduction in insulin secretion (by pancreatic islet cells), further contributing to the hyperglycemia observed in states in which catecholamine concentrations are increased.

Hyposecretory states of the adrenal medulla generally produce no recognizable clinical symptoms. The most common causes include destruction of the gland by autoimmune disorders, malignant metastatic disease, or tuberculosis. The surgical removal of the gland can also, obviously, lead to a lack of secretion. In contrast, the hypersecretion of catecholamines from chromaffin cell tumors produces the well-known clinical syndrome discussed below in the section on pheochromocytoma.

NEOPLASMS OF THE ADRENAL GLAND
Neoplasms of the Adrenal Cortex—Benign Neoplasms
Aldosteronoma

Natural History and Presentation

Primary hyperaldosteronism is a clinical syndrome that was first described by Conn in 1954 and results from the hypersecretion of aldosterone (4). Primary hyperaldosteronism occurs in 0.5% to 2.0% of unselected hypertensive patients, but its prevalence may be as high as 5% to 12% in hypertensive populations treated at specialty centers (5–11). Primary hyperaldosteronism is characterized by hypokalemia, suppressed PRA, and the increased urinary excretion of aldosterone (12–14).

The signs of mineralocorticoid excess are generally nonspecific but include fatigue, hypokalemia, and metabolic alkalosis. However, up to 40% of patients with confirmed primary hyperaldosteronism are normokalemic (11,15–17). Hypertension is also almost always present but is frequently mild. Primary hyperaldosteronism is usually diagnosed in hypertensive patients in the third to sixth decades of life. Severe hypokalemia may cause muscle weakness, cramping, palpitations, or polyuria and nocturia. Mild hypernatremia can result from a decreased release of vasopressin caused by plasma volume expansion, and mild hyperglycemia can result from decreased insulin secretion caused by chronic potassium depletion.

Hyperaldosteronism is caused by an aldosterone-producing adrenal adenoma (APA) in approximately 60% of patients and by bilateral adrenal hyperplasia [idiopathic hyperplasia (IHA)] in 40% of patients (18–20). Other rare causes (<2%) of primary hyperaldosteronism include unilateral primary adrenal hyperplasia (PAH), adrenocortical carcinoma, aldosterone-secreting ovarian tumors, and familial hyperaldosteronism (Table 1) (21,22).

There are two types of familial hyperaldosteronism. Familial hyperaldosteronism type I (FH-type I), or glucocorticoid-remediable hyperaldosteronism (GRA), is inherited as an autosomal dominant hybrid gene mapped on 8q22, which is a chimeric gene duplication that results in a gene containing the 3' promoter region from the 11β-hydroxylase gene (ACTH responsive) fused to the 5' coding sequence of the gene that encodes aldosterone synthase. In these patients, the zona fasciculata of the adrenal cortex is able to secrete not only cortisol but also aldosterone under the regulation of ACTH. GRA is characterized by the early onset of severe hypertension that is usually refractory to conventional antihypertensives. However, because aldosterone production is regulated by ACTH, its secretion can be decreased by exogenous steroids. The diagnosis of GRA is based on family history, the finding that dexamethasone

suppresses aldosterone production, and the finding of elevated levels of the hybrid steroids 18-oxocortisol and 18-hydroxycortisol. Genetic testing, however, is the best means of diagnosing the disorder and can be arranged by contacting the International GRA registry (http://www.bwh.partners.org/gra). Familial hyperaldosteronism type II (FH-type II) is an autosomal dominant pattern of APA, IHA, or both. This disorder is not suppressed with exogenous glucocorticoid, and the FH-type I gene is not involved. Recent studies have, however, identified a genetic linkage between FH-type II and chromosomal region 7p22.

Increased mineralocorticoid activity may also be caused by Cushing's syndrome. Cortisol has mineralocorticoid activity (cortisone does not), but normally circulates at a much lower concentration than aldosterone. The urinary free cortisol level, as well as the results of an overnight dexamethasone suppression test, can exclude the diagnosis of Cushing's syndrome. In addition, the long-term use of licorice or chewing tobacco may cause mineralocorticoid hypertension and elevated urinary cortisol levels by inhibiting the enzyme 11-β-hydroxysteroid dehydrogenase, which converts hormonally active cortisol to inactive cortisone.

APAs are unilateral, commonly small (0.5–2.0 cm), and are three times more common in women than in men. They produce 18-hydroxycortisol and 18-oxocortisol, which are 17α-hydroxylated analogues of 18-hydroxycorticosterone and aldosterone. These steroids cannot be synthesized in the normal zona glomerulosa or zona fasciculata. Differentiating unilateral adenoma from bilateral idiopathic hyperaldosteronism is critical, because surgical removal of the adrenal gland is helpful only in the former.

Diagnostic Evaluation

Mineralocorticoid excess should be suspected in any patient with hypertension, unexplained hypokalemia, and metabolic alkalosis, and such patients should be fully evaluated. Although hypokalemia is present in up to 50% of patients with primary hyperaldosteronism, and in almost all patients with GRA, screening for hyperaldosteronism should also be performed in normokalemic patients with severe, resistant hypertension. Prior to biochemical testing, all nonessential medications should be stopped for at least two weeks. However, only few antihypertensive agents (thiazide diuretics, spironolactone, and angiotensin II receptor blockers) actually interfere with the diagnosis of primary hyperaldosteronism and therefore need to be discontinued two weeks prior to the screening tests (15,23–25). Spironolactone, however, should be withdrawn at least four to six weeks before the tests (15,26,27).

The first step in the diagnostic evaluation of primary hyperaldosteronism is to determine a random plasma aldosterone-to-renin ratio. In this test, the PRA should be measured simultaneously with the plasma aldosterone level. The PRA is typically very low in patients with primary hyperaldosteronism and a plasma aldosterone-to-PRA ratio (ARR) exceeding 30 (ng/dL:ng/mL/hr), along with a plasma aldosterone concentration (PAC) exceeding 20 ng/dL, is very sensitive and specific in establishing the diagnosis of primary hyperaldosteronism (11,24,25,28–30). However, if the ARR is higher than 30 ng/dL, then additional studies that can demonstrate the inappropriate secretion of aldosterone can be used to confirm the presence of primary hyperaldosteronism. Either of the following aldosterone suppression tests may be used for this purpose: the intravenous saline suppression test, in which 2 L of normal saline is infused over four hours and then the PAC is measured, and

Table 1 Causes of Primary Aldosteronism

Disorder	Incidence	Genetic basis
APA	60%	Mostly sporadic, rarely familial (AD)
Bilateral IHA	30%	Mostly sporadic, rarely familial (AD)
Unilateral PAH	5%	
ACC	<2%	
Aldosterone-secreting ovarian tumors	<2%	
FH	<2%	
Glucocorticoid-remediable aldosteronism (FH-type I)		Chimeric gene duplication (*CYP11B/CYP18*) (AD)
FH-type II (APA or IHA)		AD

Abbreviations: AD, autosomal dominant; APA, aldosterone-producing adrenal adenoma; IHA, idiopathic hyperplasia; PAH, primary adrenal hyperplasia; ACC, aldosterone-producing adrenocortical carcinoma; FH, familial hyperaldosteronism.

the three-day oral salt loading (100 mmol NaCl/day) test, in which a 24-hour urine collection is obtained on the third day of the test to measure the levels of aldosterone, sodium and potassium, and serum is obtained to measure sodium and potassium. Confirmation of hyperaldosteronism is obtained when PAC is greater than 10 ng/dL (saline-loading test) or urinary aldosterone is greater than 14 µg/24 hr (oral salt-loading test). In the latter test, it is important to demonstrate adequate salt loading; therefore the urinary sodium level should be greater than 200 mEq/24 hr. Potassium supplementation should be given to patients during the salt-loading test because severe hypokalemia can be life threatening and can inhibit aldosterone production in some patients. The captopril test, another confirmatory test, has not been widely used. Table 2 shows all the essential diagnostic tests for the screening and confirmation of primary hyperaldosteronism. An additional test that can be performed early in the evaluation of patients with possible hyperaldosteronism is a 24-hour urine collection for potassium. Patients with primary hyperaldosteronism have inappropriate urinary potassium wasting (>30 mEq/day) as the cause for hypokalemia. This test is most useful when extrarenal losses of potassium are suspected, such as in patients with surreptitious vomiting or laxative abuse.

Once the diagnosis of hyperaldosteronism is established, it is critical to differentiate unilateral APA or unilateral PAH from bilateral hyperplasia of the zona glomerulosa (IHA). Patients with a unilateral APA usually have more severe hypertension, higher plasma aldosterone levels, and therefore more profound hypokalemia; however, these findings cannot accurately differentiate patients with unilateral adenoma from those with idiopathic hyperaldosteronism.

Identifying the cause of primary hyperaldosteronism may require one or more tests. Computed tomography (CT)

and magnetic resonance imaging (MRI) can confirm the presence of a unilateral adrenal nodule, and iodocholesterol (NP-59 or [131]I-6β-iodomethyl-19-norcholesterol) imaging (Fig. 2) and selective adrenal venous sampling for aldosterone measurements can confirm physiologically that the nodule on CT or MRI studies is in fact responsible for the excess aldosterone production. CT may detect a solitary unilateral macroadenoma (>1 cm) and normal contralateral adrenal gland. Additional evaluation is needed, however, in patients with normal-appearing adrenals, minimal unilateral adrenal thickening, unilateral microadenomas (≤1 cm), or bilateral adenomas (44–47). This is because small adrenal microadenomas may be missed on CT scans or misdiagnosed as bilateral idiopathic hyperplasia. There is also a high frequency of nonfunctioning adrenal cortical adenomas in the normal population (2–8%), so the finding of a small adrenal mass on CT or MRI studies does not necessarily establish a diagnosis of a unilateral APA. In these cases, because selective venous sampling is invasive and cannulation of the right adrenal vein is often difficult and occasionally results in adrenal vein thrombosis with adrenal infarction (47,48), we frequently combine adrenal imaging (CT or MRI) with iodocholesterol imaging to confirm the presence of a unilateral functioning adrenal mass. Our current approach to the evaluation of patients suspected of having primary hyperaldosteronism is shown in Figure 3.

Treatment

The treatment of primary hyperaldosteronism depends on the cause. Surgery is of little value in patients with idiopathic hyperaldosteronism, and these patients should therefore be treated medically (48). IHA is best managed medically using the aldosterone antagonist spironolactone.

Table 2   Biochemical Diagnosis of Functioning Adrenal Tumors

Diagnostic study	Diagnostic values	Interpretation	Sensitivity (%)	Specificity (%)
Primary hyperaldosteronism				
Plasma K	Normal or decreased	Exclude hypokalemia[a]	NA	NA
PAC[b] and ARR (31)	PAC >20 ng/dL and ARR >30 ng/dL:ng/ml/hr	Screening test, suggests hyperaldosteronism	90	91
4-hr IV saline-loading test (32,33)	PAC >10 ng/dL	Confirmatory test	96	93
3-day oral salt-loading (34)	Ur Na >200 mEq then Ur ALD >14 µg/24 hr	Confirmatory test	96	93
Cushing's syndrome (selected tests)				
Overnight 1 mg DMS test (35–37)	PC >5 µg/dL	Screening test, suggests hypercortisolism	100	88
Low dose DMS test (38)	PC >5 µg/dL at 9 AM, post-DMS for 48 hr	Alternative screening test, suggests hypercortisolism	98	99
24-hr urine free cortisol (39)	>3 times normal level	Alternative screening test, suggests hypercortisolism	100	98
Salivary cortisol at 11 P.M. (40)	>3.6 nmol/L	Screening test, suggests hypercortisolism	92	100
CRH–DMS test (41,42)	PC >1.4 µg/dL, 15 min post last CRH infusion	Confirmatory test, excludes pseudocushing	100	100
Pheochromocytoma				
Plasma free metanephrines[c] (41,42)	Increased	Screening test, suggests PHEO or PG	99	89
Urine total metanephrines and catecholamines[c] (43)	Increased	Alternative screening test, suggests PHEO or PG	90	98

[a]Mineralocorticoid-induced hypokalemia may inhibit aldosterone production in some patients.
[b]PAC in combination with ARR to exclude hyporeninemic hypertension.
[c]Combined measurements of plasma free metanephrines and urine total metanephrines; urine catecholamines increase the sensitivity to 100% and specificity to 98%.
Abbreviations: ALD, aldosterone; ARR, plasma aldosterone-to-plasma renin activity ratio; CRH, corticotropin-releasing hormone; DMS, dexamethasone suppression; IV, intravenous; K, potassium; PAC, plasma aldosterone concentration; PC, plasma cortisol; PG, paraganglioma; PHEO, pheochromocytoma; Ur, urinary.

(A)

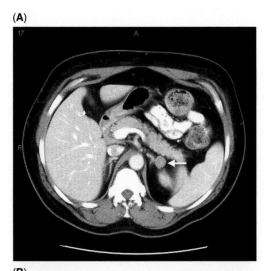

(B)

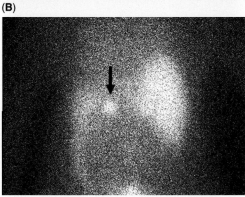

Figure 2 (A) Contrast-enhanced computed tomography of a left-sided aldosteronoma (*arrow*) arising from the lateral limb of the left adrenal gland and measuring 1.7×1.5 cm (H.U. = 7). (B) Results of NP-59 (iodocholesterol) imaging of the same patient. Persistent NP-59 uptake that increased over the observation period in the area of the left adrenal gland is consistent with a functioning adrenocortical adenoma, in this case the patient's aldosteronoma (delayed posterior images obtained at 96 hours).

Most patients can achieve adequate control of their blood pressure with this medication alone or in conjunction with other antihypertensives. However, because it is not a specific blocker of the aldosterone receptor, potential side effects include impotence, decreased libido, and gynecomastia in men and menstrual irregularities in women. Eplerenone is a new selective aldosterone receptor antagonist approved by the U.S. Food and Drug Administration in 2002 for the treatment of hypertension (49). The results of clinical trials comparing this drug with spironolactone in patients with primary hyperaldosteronism have not been published, but the anticipated starting dose in these patients is 50 mg twice daily up to a maximum dose of 200 mg twice daily. If eplerenone proves as effective as spironolactone in controlling blood pressure in patients with IHA, it will have the advantage of not causing the adverse symptoms associated with testosterone receptor blockade.

When an APA is confirmed, the appropriate therapy remains surgical resection. In the three to four weeks before operation, patients should be placed on spironolactone and given potassium supplementation to help normalize fluid and electrolyte balance. Surgery corrects the hypokalemia and lowers the blood pressure in all patients with an APA and unilateral adrenal hyperplasia (PAH); the hypertension resolves in approximately 70% of surgically treated patients (50–54).

Surgical resection can be performed either through an open or a laparoscopic approach. Because nearly all patients with aldosteronomas have relatively small tumors with no malignant potential, they are often excellent candidates for a laparoscopic adrenalectomy (55,56). Laparoscopic adrenalectomy has become the standard surgical approach for patients with APAs because of the lower morbidity, fewer postoperative complications, and equal results in cure rates compared to open adrenalectomy (54). The early results from the surgical resection of an APA are good, and the long-term cure rate is approximately 70% (51,53,54).

Approximately 2% or less of adrenocortical carcinomas (ACC) cause isolated hyperaldosteronism. In the very rare situation of a patient with hyperaldosteronism and a large adrenal mass, an open anterior approach should be taken to facilitate complete surgical resection.

Cortisol-Producing Adenoma

Natural History and Presentation

Cushing's syndrome is the term used to refer to the state of hypercortisolism that can result from a number of different pathologic processes (Table 3). The most common cause of Cushing's syndrome is exogenous steroid administration. Excluding these patients, approximately 70% of the remaining cases of hypercortisolism are secondary to the hypersecretion of ACTH from the pituitary gland, a condition known as Cushing's disease. Most of the time, a small pituitary adenoma is the cause. The ectopic secretion of ACTH, referred to as ectopic ACTH syndrome, is the cause of approximately 15% of cases of Cushing's syndrome and usually results from bronchial carcinoids or small-cell lung carcinomas. Other tumors associated with ectopic ACTH production include pancreatic endocrine neoplasms, medullary thyroid carcinoma, malignant thymoma, and pheochromocytoma. The ectopic secretion of CRF is exceedingly rare but has been reported in a few cases. The hypersecretion of cortisol from the adrenal glands accounts for approximately 10% to 20% of cases of Cushing's syndrome. The underlying cause of Cushing's syndrome is an adrenal adenoma in 50% to 60% of cases, an adrenocortical carcinoma in 20% to 25%, and IHA in 20% to 30%.

The signs and symptoms of hypercortisolism are listed in Table 4; the actions of glucocorticoids are discussed in the previous section on cortisol physiology. The most common symptom of hypercortisolism is weight gain; in adults, cortisol-induced obesity is usually in the classic (truncal) pattern.

Diagnostic Evaluation and Treatment

The evaluation of patients with possible Cushing's syndrome starts with establishing the diagnosis and then determining the etiology.

To establish the diagnosis, a state of hypercortisolism must be documented. The adult adrenal glands secrete on an average 10 to 30 mg of cortisol each day, and the secretion follows a diurnal variation: cortisol levels tend to be high early in the morning and low in the evening. A relatively sensitive initial method for detecting hypercortisolism is the overnight 1-mg dexamethasone suppression test (Table 2). In this test, 1 mg of dexamethasone is taken orally

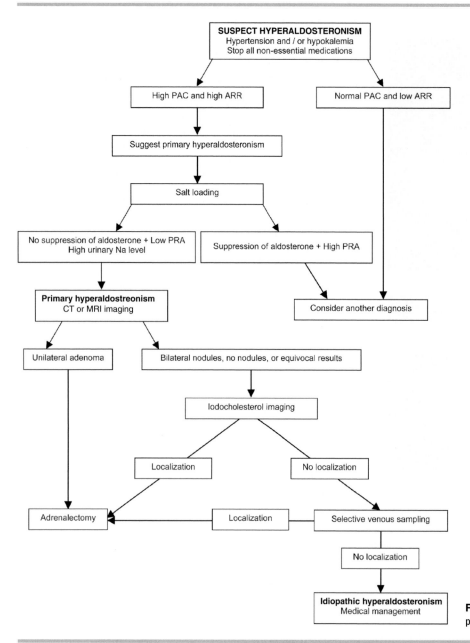

SUSPECT HYPERALDOSTERONISM
Hypertension and / or hypokalemia
Stop all non-essential medications

High PAC and high ARR

Normal PAC and low ARR

Suggest primary hyperaldosteronism

Salt loading

No suppression of aldosterone + Low PRA
High urinary Na level

Suppression of aldosterone + High PRA

Consider another diagnosis

Primary hyperaldostreonism
CT or MRI imaging

Unilateral adenoma

Bilateral nodules, no nodules, or equivocal results

Iodocholesterol imaging

Localization

No localization

Adrenalectomy

Localization

Selective venous sampling

No localization

Idiopathic hyperaldosteronism
Medical management

Figure 3 Algorithm for the evaluation of the patient with suspected primary hyperaldosteronism.

at 11:00 P.M.; normal individuals have a plasma cortisol level of less than 5 µg/dL at 8:00 A.M. the following morning. Failure to suppress the 8:00 A.M. cortisol to <5 µg/dL is consistent with hypercortisolism. However, although this

Table 3 Causes of Cushing's Syndrome

Exogenous steroids
Cushing's disease (due to pituitary adenoma)
Adrenal tumors
   Adrenal cortical adenoma
   Adrenal cortical carcinoma
Primary adrenal cortical hyperplasia
Ectopic ACTH syndrome
Ectopic CRF syndrome

Abbreviations: ACTH, adrenocorticotropic hormone; CRF, corticotropin-releasing factor.

test has a false-negative rate of only 2%, the false-positive rate is 30%. Therefore, although a normal overnight dexamethasone suppression test essentially excludes clinically significant hypercortisolism, an abnormal test result requires further investigation. The two-day low-dose dexamethasone suppression test (dexamethasone, 0.5 mg orally every six hours for 48 hours) can also be used to detect hypercortisolism. In this test, the measurement of plasma cortisol (9 A.M. prior to starting the dexamethasone and 48 hours later) instead of urinary free cortisol provides a higher sensitivity. This test is reported to have a sensitivity and specificity approaching 99% (57). A 24-hour urine collection for the measurement of urinary free (unmetabolized) cortisol is somewhat less sensitive than the overnight and low-dose dexamethasone suppression tests, but it is a useful complementary test because of its specificity. A urinary free cortisol level that is more than three times greater than

Table 4 Clinical Manifestations of Adrenal Cortical Hormone Excess

Cortisol	Androgen	Estrogen	Aldosterone
Truncal obesity	Male pattern baldness	Gynecomastia	Hypertension
Buffalo hump		Breast tenderness	Hypokalemia
Moon faces	Hirsutism	Testicular atrophy	Weakness
Abdominal striae	Voice change	Decreased libido	Polyuria
Hypertension	Breast atrophy		Polydypsia
Glucose intolerance	Libido change		Metabolic alkalosis
Thin skin	Oligomenorrhea		Glucose intolerance
Osteoporosis	Increased muscle mass		
Psychiatric changes			

the upper range of normal is consistent with Cushing's syndrome. Urinary collection for the measurement of 17-hydroxysteroids and a salivary cortisol measurement can also be used (40). Another useful way to detect Cushing's syndrome is to measure the nocturnal plasma cortisol level. Patients with Cushing's syndrome do not show a circadian rhythm in cortisol secretion; therefore, a midnight plasma cortisol concentration greater than 7 µg/dL is suggestive of hypercortisolism.

Cushing's syndrome with mild hypercortisolemia is often indistinguishable from that seen in pseudo-Cushing's states such as depression and alcoholism. The diagnostic accuracy of dexamethasone suppression and corticotropin-releasing hormone (CRH) stimulation tests, when used individually in order to distinguish these conditions, is not greater than 85% (41). In such cases, in order to confirm the presence of Cushing's syndrome, and exclude pseudo-Cushing syndrome, the most useful test is the combined CRH–dexamethasone test (42). Eight oral doses of dexamethasone, 0.5 mg each, are given every six hours. The last dose should be given two hours before IV injection of CRH 1 µg/kg. Response to CRH is seen in all patients with Cushing's syndrome but in none with pseudo-Cushing's state. Thus, plasma cortisol levels more than 1.4 µg/dL, 15 minutes after CRH injection, confirms the existence of Cushing's syndrome and excludes pseudo-Cushing's states.

Upon the confirmation of hypercortisolism, patients should undergo an evaluation to detect its etiology. In a patient with an adrenal mass and hypercortisolism, the only additional biochemical test required is the measurement of ACTH. Plasma ACTH obtained at 8 or 9 A.M. in patients with a cortisol-secreting adrenal tumor plasma ACTH is invariably undetectable (discussed below). Additional tests are necessary when Cushing's disease or ectopic ACTH syndrome is suspected. These tests include the high-dose dexamethasone suppression test, the metyrapone test, and the CRH test (58).

ACTH secretion also follows a diurnal variation, preceding that of cortisol by one to two hours. Levels of ACTH are suppressed (<5 pg/mL) in patients with functioning adrenal adenomas, functioning ACC, or autonomously functioning adrenal hyperplasia. In such cases, the autonomous secretion of cortisol by the pathologic process within the adrenal gland inhibits pituitary ACTH release. ACTH-dependent Cushing's syndrome include Cushing's disease (i.e., a pituitary adenoma–secreting ACTH) and ectopic ACTH secretion (i.e., a nonpituitary tumor–secreting ACTH, such as a metastatic tumor). Patients with Cushing's disease usually have plasma ACTH levels that are elevated or within the upper limits of normal. When there is an ectopic

source of ACTH secretion, the plasma ACTH level is usually markedly elevated. In patients diagnosed with ACTH-dependent Cushing's syndrome, the next step is to distinguish between a pituitary and nonpituitary ACTH–producing tumor by imaging the pituitary gland using MRI. If this shows no obvious pituitary lesion, bilateral simultaneous inferior petrosal sinus sampling is the "gold standard" method to distinguish central (pituitary tumor) from peripheral (nonpituitary tumor) ACTH production (59). In this method, both inferior petrosal sinuses are catheterized, and blood samples are obtained at 0, 2, 5, and 10 minutes following the administration of 1 µg/kg ovine CRH from each inferior petrosal sinus and a peripheral vein, which allows the calculation of an inferior petrosal sinus-to-peripheral ACTH ratio (IPS:P). An IPS:P that exceeds 3 is considered consistent with Cushing's disease.

Patients with evidence of ACTH-independent hypercortisolism should undergo abdominal imaging to evaluate the adrenal glands. Choices for abdominal imaging include CT, MRI, and iodocholesterol scanning. CT has a high sensitivity and is the initial imaging study of choice. However, MRI has a higher specificity than CT, because chemical shift and T2-weighted image analysis can help differentiate adrenal cortical adenomas from primary or metastatic carcinomas and from pheochromocytomas (60–65). A drawback of MRI is that it has a lower resolution and therefore a lower sensitivity than CT. Finally, ^{131}I-6β-iodomethyl-19 norcholesterol (NP-59 or iodocholesterol) can demonstrate uptake in an adrenal adenoma along with suppression of the contralateral gland. If CT and MRI findings are equivocal, iodocholesterol scanning may be helpful in differentiating unilateral adrenal cortical adenoma (unilateral uptake with contralateral suppression) from bilateral micronodular hyperplasia (bilateral uptake) (66).

The appropriate management of hypercortisolism depends on the underlying etiology. Patients with Cushing's disease should undergo transphenoidal resection of their pituitary adenoma, if it is deemed resectable. Bilateral adrenalectomy is rarely indicated and should be reserved for patients who fail to respond to transphenoidal hypophysectomy and external beam radiation therapy (EBRT), and experience end organ injury from the consequences of overt hypercortisolism. If bilateral adrenalectomy is performed, patients require not only perioperative steroid coverage (Tables 5 and 6) but also lifelong replacement of both glucocorticoids and mineralocorticoids. Patients with autonomously functioning bilateral adrenal hyperplasia usually require bilateral adrenalectomy. Patients with ectopic ACTH syndrome should have the underlying malignant lesion identified and resected if possible. Bilateral adrenalectomy

Table 5 Comparison of Steroid Preparations

Steroid	Half-life (hr)	Glucocorticoid activity (relative to cortisol)	Mineralocorticoid activity (relative to cortisol)
Cortisol	8–12	1	1
Cortisone	8–12	0.8	0.8
Prednisone	12–36	4	0.25
Prednisolone	12–36	4	0.25
Methylprednisolone	12–36	5	0
Triamcinolone	12–36	5	0
Betamethasone	36–72	25	0
Dexamethasone	36–72	30–40	0

Table 6   Recommendations for Perioperative Glucocorticoid Coverage

Steroid treatment	HPA axis response	Surgical stress	Perioperative steroid coverage
Currently on steroids			
<10 mg/day[a]	Normal	Any	Not required
>10 mg/day[a]	Suppressed	Minor	25 mg of hydrocortisone at induction
		Moderate	Usual preoperative steroids + 25 mg of hydrocortisone at induction[b] 100 mg/day for 24 hr
		Major	Usual preoperative steroids + 25 mg of hydrocortisone at induction + 100 mg/day for 48–72 hr
High dose[a] (immunosuppression)	Suppressed	Any	Usual immunosuppressive doses during perioperative period
Stopped <3 mo	Suppressed	Any	Treat as if on steroids
Stopped >3 mo	Normal	Any	Not required

[a]Prednisolone dose.
[b]Patients take their usual daily dose with a sip of water preoperatively.
Abbreviation: HPA, hypothalamic-pituitary-adrenal axis.
Source: From Ref. 171.

should be reserved for the small group of patients whose primary tumor is unresectable and whose symptoms of cortisol excess cannot be controlled medically. Bilateral adrenalectomy can be performed laparoscopically, via a posterior approach, or via laparotomy.

Patients with a unilateral cortisol-producing neoplasm of the adrenal gland should undergo adrenalectomy. However, there is no easy way preoperatively to differentiate a benign cortical adenoma from an adrenal cortical carcinoma. As will be discussed in detail in the section entitled "Incidentalomas," neoplasm size and its characteristics on CT or MRI studies can indicate whether its likely benign or malignant. In general, homogeneously enhancing tumors less than 4 cm in size with smooth borders are considered benign. Such tumors (presumed to be functioning cortical adenomas) can be removed laparoscopically (67,68). We currently favor open transabdominal laparotomy for any cortical tumor (functioning or nonfunctioning) that may be an adrenal cortical carcinoma.

Adrenogenital Syndrome–Producing Tumors

Tumors (adenomas or carcinomas) of the zona reticularis produce excessive amounts of androgen or estrogen, leading to the adrenogenital syndrome. The most striking clinical examples of virilizing adrenal tumors are those producing primarily androgens. These tumors may initially go undetected in the adult male, but the female patient shows a deepening of the voice, coarsening of the skin, the thickening and darkening of facial hairs, the assumption of male hair distribution, clitoral hypertrophy, menstrual cessation, and breast atrophy. These tumors may appear in childhood (50% of the cases) and result in precocious puberty in both males and females. At postpubertal ages, the adrenogenital syndrome is far more frequent in females than males.

Rarely, adrenal cortical adenomas or carcinomas produce estrogens. Additionally, peripheral conversion of androstenedione to estrogens can result in feminization in patients with adrenal cortical tumors or adrenocortical enzymatic defects; extra-adrenal tumors or extra-adrenal enzymatic defects can also cause feminization. In such unusual cases, it is usually difficult to detect estrogen excess in the female patient, but menstrual irregularities may lead to a definitive diagnosis based on measurements of plasma or urinary estrogens. The male patient with estrogen excess has a loss of libido and onset of impotency, enlargement of breast tissue (gynecomastia), testicular atrophy, and occasionally softening of facial hair and an alteration in male-pattern hair distribution.

Neoplasms of the Adrenal Cortex—Malignant Neoplasms

Adrenal Corticocarcinoma

Molecular Pathogenesis

Molecular genetic studies have revealed that a variety of genes and chromosomal loci that are abnormal in hereditary syndromes associated with adrenocortical tumors could also be altered in sporadic ACC (69). For example, the *MEN 1* gene, which is responsible for the multiple endocrine neoplasia type 1 (MEN 1) syndrome, is on chromosomal locus 11q13 and encodes the tumor suppressor menin. Comparative genomic hybridization and loss of heterozygosity (LOH) studies have also shown a loss of genetic material in chromosome 11q in sporadic ACCs and their metastatic lesions that was not associated with an *MEN 1* mutation (70–72). LOH at 2p16, the locus for the Carney complex familial cancer syndrome, was also strongly associated with malignant ACCs (70). In addition, mutations in the tumor suppressor gene *p53* on 17p13 or overexpression of the protein product have been detected in approximately 50% of ACCs (73). In children with sporadic ACC, the high frequency of germline *p53* mutations may identify probands of the Li–Fraumeni syndrome, which has obvious genetic-counseling implications. Moreover, IGF1 and IGF2 receptors and their ligands, which are involved in the growth and differentiation of the adrenal cortex, are produced at high levels in functional ACCs, and correlate with the malignant phenotype, suggesting a possible role in ACC tumorigenesis (74). Other genetic abnormalities found in cases of sporadic ACC include a loss of genetic material at 11p15 (Beckwith–Wiedemann syndrome), 9p (p16), 3p [von Hippel Lindau (VHL) syndrome], and 13q (*retinoblastoma* gene), as well as mutations of the *ras* gene. Mutations of genes encoding gip2 and the ACTH receptor have also been found in sporadic ACCs (75,76). Studies examining the proliferative signaling pathways are therefore being performed in an attempt to elucidate the mechanisms of tumor growth; these pathways include those involving Akt/PKB and the mitogen-activated protein kinases.

Epidemiology and Natural History

ACC is a rare disease; there are approximately 150 to 200 new cases reported each year in the United States, and it accounts for only 0.2% of the annual cancer incidence in the United States (69,77). There is a bimodal age distribution, with the incidence peaking in young children and then again in patients between 40 and 50 years of age. Most ACCs are diagnosed at an advanced stage; this is because of the nonspecific nature of the early signs and symptoms. This delay in diagnosis, together with the aggressive histologic behavior of the disease, accounts for the poor prognosis in patients with an ACC (78–81).

Presentation and Diagnosis

Patients with ACC usually present with vague abdominal symptoms secondary to an enlarging retroperitoneal mass or with the clinical manifestations of an overproduction of one or more adrenal cortical hormones. Approximately 60% of these tumors are functional, as shown by biochemical parameters. In particular, 50% secrete cortisol, producing Cushing's syndrome. Another 10% to 20% produce steroid hormones, which can cause hypertension and varying degrees of virilization in females and feminization in males.

The presence of a functioning adrenal mass can be suspected on the basis of history (e.g., hirsutism, acne, weight gain, proximal muscle weakness, or headache), physical examination findings (e.g., cushingoid features, hypertension, or hyperandrogenism), and abnormal routine serum chemistry findings such as hypokalemia and hyperglycemia. The biochemical evaluation of these patients should include (Table 2) screening for a pheochromocytoma (as shown by the plasma metanephrine level), Cushing's syndrome (as shown by the 1-mg overnight dexamethasone suppression test), hyperandrogenism (as shown by DHEAS, androstenedione, and testosterone levels) if there are signs or symptoms, and hyperaldosteronism (as shown by the ARR and serum aldosterone concentration) if hypokalemia and/or hypertension are present (43,82). The results serve to guide perioperative replacement therapy, to exclude the diagnosis of pheochromocytoma, and to identify potential tumor markers useful during postoperative follow-up.

High-resolution abdominal CT and MRI are the best modalities for imaging the adrenal glands. CT can usually identify lesions as small as 7 mm in diameter. MRI may be especially helpful, not only in identifying tumor extension into the inferior vena cava but also in differentiating between various lesions based on the adrenal-to-liver ratio on T2-weighted images. Adenomas usually have ratios of 0.7 to 1.4; malignant lesions, whether primary or metastatic to the adrenal gland, have ratios of 1.4 to 3.0; and pheochromocytomas usually have ratios greater than 3.0. Chest radiography is helpful in ruling out pulmonary metastasis.

Staging

The most widely used staging system for ACC is the Sullivan et al. (83) modification of the McFarlane (84) system. In contrast to most modern staging systems, the Sullivan staging system groups patients with adjacent organ invasion or fixed positive lymph nodes and patients with distant metastatic disease into stage IV. Icard et al. (85) and Lee et al. (79) have suggested a modification to this system, in which patients with locally advanced tumors are classified as having stage III disease, with the stage IV designation reserved for patients with metastatic disease (Table 7). These modifications to the Sullivan staging system more accurately reflect the natural history of the disease and are in agreement with the cancer-staging systems (TNM) used for other solid tumors; the stages also correlate with the correct treatment (surgical or medical) required.

Surgical Treatment

Complete surgical resection is currently the only potentially curative therapy for localized ACC. Approximately 50% of the tumors are localized to the adrenal gland at the time of initial exploration (69). Several recent studies have demonstrated, however, that contiguous organ invasion is common and that therefore adjacent organs frequently need to be resected as part of the primary treatment for a localized ACC (Fig. 4). However, results of at least two series have also demonstrated that although the kidney is frequently removed as part of an en bloc operation, in only a minority of specimens does histologic examination of the resected specimens demonstrate evidence of invasion of the kidney. Further, kidney-sparing complete resection is not associated with decreased survival (79,85,87).

An open transabdominal approach is recommended to provide maximal exposure for complete resection, minimize the risk of tumor spillage, and allow vascular control of the inferior vena cava, aorta, and renal vessels when necessary. A review of the surgical complications in patients with primary ACC confirms that tumor extirpation requires complex operative procedures that are often associated with significant morbidity; despite this, a mortality of only 5% or less has been noted in most contemporary series from large referral centers.

A number of investigators have evaluated predictors of survival following the resection of an ACC. By far the strongest predictor of outcome is the ability to perform a complete resection. The five-year actuarial survival rate is approximately 40% for patients who undergo a complete resection (Table 8). In the experience of the authors, however, neither the need for extended resection nor the presence of tumor thrombus in the inferior vena cava or renal vein predict a poor prognosis, as long as all diseases are completely resected. In contrast, patients who undergo incomplete resection of their ACC, including a less than total resection of the primary tumor or resection of the primary tumor in the face of unresectable distant metastatic

---

Table 7 Staging Systems for Adrenocortical Carcinoma

Stage	Macfarlane (1958) (84)	Sullivan et al. (1978) (83)	Icard et al. (1992) (86)	Lee et al. (1995) (79)
I	T_1 (≤ 5 cm), N_0, M_0	T_1 (≤ 5 cm), N_0, M_0	T_1 (≤ 5 cm), N_0, M_0	T_1 (≤ 5 cm), N_0, M_0
II	T_2 (>5 cm), N_0, M_0	T_2 (>5 cm), N_0, M_0	T_2 (>5 cm), N_0, M_0	T_2 (>5 cm), N_0, M_0
III	T_3 (local invasion without involvement of adjacent organs) or mobile positive lymph nodes, M_0	T_3 (local invasion), N_0, M_0 or T_{1-2}, N_1 (positive lymph nodes), M_0	T_3 (local invasion) and/or N_1 (positive regional lymph nodes), M_0	T_3/T_4 (local invasion as demonstrated by histologic evidence of adjacent organ invasion, direct tumor extension to IVC, and/or tumor thrombus within IVC or renal vein) and/or N_1 (positive regional lymph nodes), M_0
IV	T_4 (invasion of adjacent organs) or fixed positive lymph nodes or M_1 (distant metastases)	T_4 (local invasion), N_0, M_0; or T_3, N_1, M_0; or T_{1-4}, N_{0-1}, M_1 (distant metastases)	T_{1-4}, N_{0-1}, M_1 (distant metastases)	T_{1-4}, N_{0-1}, M_1 (distant metastases)

Abbreviation: IVC, inferior vena cava.

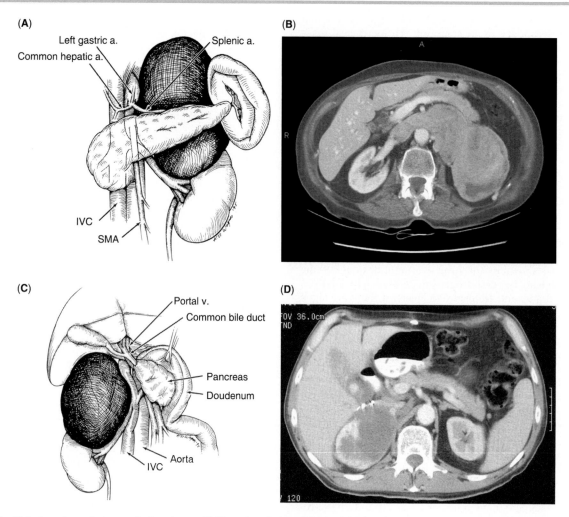

Figure 4 Clinical spectrum of adrenocortical carcinoma. (**A**) Illustration of a large left adrenal carcinoma showing the intimate relationship between the tumor and the origin of the celiac axis and the SMA. *Source*: From Ref. 69. (**B**) Contrast-enhanced CT of a large left adrenal carcinoma extending into the inferior vena cava. *Source*: From Ref. 69. (**C**) Illustration of a large right adrenal carcinoma showing the frequent finding of tumor invasion of the liver (posterior segment of the right hepatic lobe) and the IVC. (**D**) Contrast-enhanced CT of a large right adrenal carcinoma extending into the liver and inferior vena cava. *Abbreviations*: CT, computed tomography; SMA, superior mesenteric artery; IVC, inferior vena cava.

disease, have a uniformly poor prognosis with a median survival of less than one year (Table 9).

Common sites of recurrence include the lungs, lymph nodes, liver, peritoneum, and bones. The complete resection of recurrent disease, including pulmonary metastases, is associated with prolonged survival in some patients and can control symptoms related to excess hormone production. After a potentially curative resection, patients whose tumors were hormonally active should be monitored with interval urinary steroid profiles as well as abdominal and chest imaging studies.

Adjuvant Treatment
No adjuvant treatment for patients with ACC following a complete resection has been demonstrated to prolong survival (96–98). Most investigations of adjuvant treatment for ACC have involved the use of mitotane (*ortho*, *para*-DDD), a derivative of dichlorodiphenyltrichloroethane (DDT) with direct adrenolytic activity (69,97,98). Mitotane not only inhibits steroid production, it also leads to the atrophy of

adrenocortical cells (97,98). The role of mitotane as adjuvant therapy for ACC remains controversial, largely due to the absence of randomized trials (96–98). Given the low incidence of ACC, it is unlikely that future randomized trials will be performed. Nonetheless, anecdotal reports and small series have not documented a clear benefit of mitotane in patients who receive it adjuvantly. A further drawback to the use of mitotane is that it is associated with a number of side effects, most notably gastrointestinal and neuromuscular symptoms. Mitotane also has a narrow therapeutic index, the serum levels must be closely monitored, and exogenous steroid hormone replacement must be instituted to prevent the symptoms of adrenal insufficiency. For these various reasons, it is perhaps most reasonable to consider mitotane as adjuvant therapy for those patients without evidence of disease after a first recurrence, such as after the resection of isolated pulmonary or hepatic metastases. Recently, the results of phase II trials of combination chemotherapy with mitotane have been reported; these combinations have included etoposide, doxorubicin, and

Table 8 Survival of Patients Who Underwent a Potentially Curative Resection for Adrenal Cortical Carcinoma

Reference	Institution or country	Year	No. of patients	Margin analysis	Median follow-up (mo)	Overall survival (mo)	5-Yr actuarial survival (%)
Icard[a] (87)	France	2001	182	No			50
Favia (88)	Italy	2001	23	No			
Harrison (89)	MSKCC	1999	46	No	20	28[b]	56
Khorram–Manesh[a] (90)	Sweden	1998	18	No	85		58
Crucitti (91)	Italy	1996	91	No		28[c]	48
Lee (79)	MDA	1995	16	Yes	43	46[b]	46
Haak (92)	Netherlands	1994	47	No			49
Zografos (93)	Roswell Park	1994	15	No		13[b]	38
Icard[a] (85)	France	1992	127	No			42
Icard (86)	France	1992	31	No		44[c]	45
Pommier[a] (94)	MSKCC	1992	53	No	28	28[c]	47
Gröndal[a] (78,95)	Sweden	1990	22	No			
Henley (95)	Mayo Clinic	1983	31	No			32

[a]Includes patients who underwent resection of synchronous metastatic disease.
[b]Median.
[c]Mean.
Abbreviations: MDA, M.D. Anderson Cancer Center; MSKCC, Memorial Sloan-Kettering Cancer Center.

cisplatin (99) and etoposide, doxorubicin, and vincristine (99). The former trial reported an overall response rate [according to the World Health Organization (WHO) criteria] of 49% (99), and the latter trial showed a response rate of 22% (100). Other investigational studies have used combinations of systemic agents, including cisplatin with gemcitabine (101) and CYC202 (R-roscovitine) (102). Percutaneous image-guided radiofrequency ablation and percutaneous ethanol injection have also been tested for the treatment of liver metastasis (103,104). Finally, EBRT is often used for the palliation for bone metastases.

In summary, resection should only be performed if preoperative imaging studies indicate that a complete margin-negative resection is possible. Rarely is resection indicated for a primary tumor when there is also synchronous metastatic disease. Nonetheless, anecdotal reports indicate that complete resection of limited metastatic disease in good-risk individuals is occasionally clinically beneficial (105,106). However, resection of the primary tumor in the face of unresectable distant metastatic disease is not indicated. Systemic treatment options for patients with unresectable local recurrence or distant metastases include treatment with mitotane, suramin, ketoconazole, and systemic chemotherapy regimens containing cisplatin. Mitotane appears to be most effective when given for the symptomatic control

of hormonally active tumors, because a decrease in serum hormone levels is much more common than a radiographic response. Dose and serum levels of mitotane must be monitored and adjusted to maintain efficacy while minimizing toxicity.

Neoplasms of the Adrenal Medulla
Pheochromocytoma

Pheochromocytoma as a distinct lesion has been recognized for over a century, going back to 1886, when Frankel described his finding of bilateral adrenal tumors at autopsy in an 18-year-old woman who had suffered sudden death. In 1912, Pick described and named the tumor. In 1922, L' Abbé found a pheochromocytoma at autopsy in a 28-year-old woman who had presented with paroxysmal hypertension. In 1926, Rue described the first successful resection of a pheochromocytoma; in 1927, Mayo described the first successful resection in the United States. In 1951, the biochemical basis of the disease was identified by Van Hueller, who demonstrated the increased urinary catecholamine levels.

Etiology and Physiology

Pheochromocytomas, or intra-adrenal paragangliomas, originate from chromaffin cells of the adrenal medulla, whereas paragangliomas arise from extra-adrenal sympathetic chromaffin tissue. Paragangliomas can also arise from parasympathetic ganglia in the head and neck, and these tumors include chemodectomas (carotid body tumors), tumors of the glomus jugulare (affecting the ninth and tenth cranial nerves), ganglioneuromas, and neuroblastomas and ganglioneuroblastomas.

Chromosomal abnormalities common in pheochromocytomas include LOH at chromosomes 1p, 3p, 17p, and 22q. N-*ras* and *c-myc* mRNA can also be overexpressed. The *RET* proto-oncogene and the tumor suppressor gene *VHL* play an important role in the development of pheochromocytomas in MEN 2 kindreds and in patients with VHL, respectively. MEN 2A and 2B, as well as familial (non-MEN) medullary thyroid cancer, are associated with mutations in the *RET* proto-oncogene (107), which maps to chromosome 10q11.2. *RET* mRNA may also be overexpressed in sporadic pheochromocytomas (108). *RET* mutations may have a

Table 9 Patient Survival Following Incomplete Resection[a] of Adrenocortical Carcinoma

Series	Institution or country	Year	No. of patients	Median survival (mo)
Crucitti (91)	Italy	1996	33	16
Lee (79)	MDA	1995	7	8.5
Zografos (93)	Roswell Park	1994	28	2
Icard (85)	France	1992	28	<12
Icard (86)	Cochin	1992	10	<4
Gröndal (78,95)	Sweden	1990	12	10
Henley (95)	Mayo Clinic	1983	14	<6

[a]Patients with incomplete resections included those who underwent incomplete resection of the primary tumor and those who underwent complete resection of the primary tumor in the presence of unresectable distant metastatic disease.
Abbreviation: MDA, M.D. Anderson Cancer Center.

variety of clinical consequences. In Hirschsprung's disease, *RET* mutations include deletions and stop codons that result in the loss of parasympathetic innervation in the distal colon.

In familial medullary thyroid cancer, MEN 2A, and MEN 2B, point mutations in *RET* result in amino acid substitutions, there is no loss of chromosome 10 alleles, and the point mutations probably result in altered regulation of the *RET* tyrosine kinase growth-factor receptor (109). However, the role of *RET* mutations in sporadic pheochromocytomas remains controversial (108,110,111). Mutations in the succinate dehydrogenase family of genes (*SDHD*, *SDHB*, and *SDHC*) are responsible for pheochromocytomas and paragangliomas that are part of the hereditary paraganglioma syndrome (112,113).

A unique characteristic of pheochromocytomas is that they release catecholamines independent of neural stimulation. Because pheochromocytomas possess glucagon receptors, glucagon may mediate this catecholamine release. It is important to keep in mind that events that precipitate a hypertensive crisis in patients with pheochromocytoma can include the administration of glucagon, opiates, intra-arterial contrast material, and sympathomimetics, as well as adrenal biopsy.

Understanding the pathophysiology of pheochromocytoma requires an understanding of catecholamine metabolism. In this pathway, tyrosine is converted to epinephrine from norepinephrine in the adrenal medulla; dopamine represents an intermediary step. Generally, pheochromocytomas produce much more norepinephrine than epinephrine. Exceptions include very small tumors and those tumors in patients with familial endocrinopathies (e.g., MEN 2). Extra-adrenal pheochromocytomas (paragangliomas) are classically pure norepinephrine-producing tumors. The final conversion of norepinephrine to epinephrine is inefficient in most pheochromocytomas, resulting in the production of large amounts of the catecholamine metabolites—3,4-dihydroxymandelic acid, metanephrine, and normetanephrine. All three of these catecholamine metabolites can be converted to vanillylmandelic acid (VMA), and all of these metabolites can be detected in urine.

Natural History

Pheochromocytomas exist in less than 0.1% of hypertensive patients and are usually benign. Pheochromocytomas are one of the most satisfying general surgical diseases to treat, because the five-year survival rate in patients with the benign tumors is approximately 97%, they recur in less than 10% of patients, and the hypertension is cured in 75% of patients. However, malignant pheochromocytomas are associated with a high incidence of recurrence and metastasis, and the five-year survival rate in patients with these tumors is less than 60%.

Pheochromocytoma is known as the 10% tumor. Approximately 10% of pheochromocytomas are bilateral, with some patients presenting with multiple tumors. In addition, 10% of pheochromocytomas occur in extra-adrenal locations, where they are referred to as *paragangliomas*. Extra-adrenal tumors that occur within the abdomen are usually in the organ of Zuckerkandl at the bifurcation of the aorta and occasionally within the bladder wall. Thoracic locations of pheochromocytomas include the posterior mediastinum and the pericardium. Extra-adrenal pheochromocytomas may also occur anywhere along the sympathetic chain because of the presence of chromaffin tissue. Histologic evidence of malignancy is demonstrated in approximately 10%

of patients with pheochromocytomas, though malignancy is more common with extra-adrenal lesions than in those with tumors arising in the adrenal glands. Documenting malignancy can be difficult, however, because invasion of adjacent organs or distant metastatic disease must be present. Adding to this difficulty is the fact that both benign and malignant lesions may penetrate the tumor capsule, invade veins draining the gland, or show cellular pleomorphism, mitoses, and atypical nuclei.

Familial pheochromocytomas have been estimated to account for approximately 10% of cases, though recent data suggest that up to 25% of unselected cases of apparently sporadic pheochromocytomas are in fact hereditary (112,113). Familial tumors are more likely to be benign and bilateral, and less likely to be extra-adrenal and malignant. The familial syndromes associated with pheochromocytomas include MEN types 2a and 2b (risk for pheochromocytoma, 50%) and VHL syndrome (risk for pheochromocytoma, 10%), in which bilateral or multiple tumors are common. There is also a slight risk for pheochromocytoma in patients with neurofibromatosis type 1 (<1%) and MEN 1 syndrome (<1%). Pheochromocytoma can also occur in patients with the hereditary paraganglioma syndrome (mutations in *SDHD*, *SDHB*, and *SDHC* genes), in whom the risk may be as high as 80% (112,113). The hereditary paraganglioma syndrome predisposes to the development of both extra-adrenal and adrenal paragangliomas. For this reason, patients with these syndromes require follow-up and periodic screening for pheochromocytoma, especially before any planned surgical procedure. At The University of Texas M.D. Anderson Cancer Center, our current screening protocol for patients with suspected familial pheochromocytoma or paraganglioma includes genetic testing for the appropriate genes, depending on the patient's personal and family history (113). Once the diagnosis of one of the above-mentioned syndromes has been established by genetic testing, periodic screening of the plasma free metanephrines is done to increase the chances of detecting a familial pheochromocytoma early (114).

Presentation

The classic presentation of a patient with pheochromocytoma includes the five P's: *p*ressure (hypertension), *p*ain (headache), *p*erspiration, *p*alpitations, and *p*allor/diaphoresis. Sustained or paroxysmal hypertension is associated with headache and tachycardia (115,116). Paroxysmal elevation in blood pressure can vary markedly in frequency and duration and can be spontaneous or initiated by a variety of events, including heavy physical exertion and eating foods high in tyramine (e.g., chocolate, cheese, and red wine). Paroxysmal hypertension can occasionally be precipitated by trauma or surgery. The hypertension is characteristically labile and refractory to medical management; the most effective antihypertensive agents in this setting are α-adrenergic receptor blockers, calcium channel blockers, labetalol, and nitroprusside. An unrecognized pheochromocytoma may lead to death as the result of a hypertensive crisis, arrhythmia, or myocardial infarction.

More than half of patients with pheochromocytomas have impaired glucose tolerance, and thus may have symptoms of diabetes mellitus, including polydipsia and polyuria. These symptoms result from the excess catecholamine secreted by the tumor and resolve with tumor resection. Patients with pheochromocytoma are rarely asymptomatic; exceptions include patients with hereditary pheochromocytomas and extra-adrenal paragangliomas.

Diagnostic Evaluation

Pheochromocytoma is diagnosed by documenting the excess secretion of catecholamines. Plasma free metanephrines is the most accurate test to exclude or confirm the diagnosis (43,82). Twenty-four–hour urine collections for the testing of free catecholamines (dopamine, epinephrine, and norepinephrine) and their metabolites (normetanephrine, metanephrine, and VMA) also can be obtained. However, these tests are less sensitive. Moreover, the combination of different tests does not improve the diagnostic yield beyond that of the single test of plasma free metanephrines. Plasma catecholamine determination is only occasionally helpful; clonidine suppression tests may be useful in borderline cases. Provocative tests are potentially hazardous and now obsolete. In addition, although the adrenal glands and the organ of Zuckerkandl produce the enzyme PNMT that converts norepinephrine to epinephrine, pheochromocytomas that arise elsewhere do not contain this enzyme and thus do not produce much, if any, epinephrine. As a result, extra-adrenal pheochromocytomas secrete predominantly dopamine and norepinephrine.

Patients with a biochemically based diagnosis of pheochromocytoma should undergo preoperative localization. This can be done with CT, MRI, or ^{131}I-metaiodobenzylguanidine (MIBG) scanning. MIBG scanning may assist in lateralizing a tumor when no mass is seen on abdominal images, but this virtually never happens with the current CT technology (117). The current practice at M.D. Anderson is to obtain high-quality multidetector (multislice) CT scans, which can detect up to 95% of adrenal masses larger than 6 to 8 mm. MRI may be useful in selected cases because the T2-weighted images can clearly identify chromaffin tissue; the T2-weighted adrenal mass-to-liver ratio of pheochromocytomas or paragangliomas is usually more than 3. This ratio is much higher than that for adrenocortical adenomas, ACCs, or metastases to the adrenal gland. Thus, MRI may provide useful functional (biochemical) information. MIBG imaging may also be helpful in localizing extra-adrenal, metastatic, and/or bilateral pheochromocytomas (117). The particular advantage of this technique is that the radiolabeled amine is selectively picked up by chromaffin tissue and can identify most pheochromocytomas, regardless of their location. MIBG scanning may be used to assess atypical cases, and more commonly to determine the presence or absence of multifocal or recurrent disease. It is rare for MIBG scanning not to be able to localize a pheochromocytoma preoperatively.

Preoperative Preparation

Careful preoperative preparation is required to prevent a cardiovascular crisis during surgery caused by excess catecholamine secretion in a patient with a pheochromocytoma. The cornerstone of this preparation is α-adrenergic receptor blockade and the complete restoration of fluid and electrolyte balance. Phenoxybenzamine is the α-adrenergic–blocking agent of choice, and treatment is usually begun at a dose of 10 mg once or twice a day. The dosage is gradually increased over a two- to three-week period until adequate α-blockade is reached. The total dose should not exceed 1 mg/kg/day. The occurrence of orthostatic hypotension generally indicates the presence of adequate α-blockade. β-Blockade may be instituted after adequate α-blockade and may help prevent tachycardia and other arrhythmias. β-Blockade should not be instituted unless α-blockade has been established; otherwise, the β-blocker will inhibit epinephrine-induced vasodilation, leading to greater hypertension and left heart strain. In addition to the pharmacologic preparation, patients with pheochromocytoma may require the correction of volume depletion and any concurrent electrolyte imbalances. Nifedipine and metyrosine may also be used preoperatively.

Surgical Treatment

When preoperative imaging suggests a benign-appearing pheochromocytoma with a radiographically normal contralateral gland, we currently use a unilateral laparoscopic approach to adrenalectomy. A laparoscopic approach is also appropriate for patients with MEN 2 or VHL, whose disease is limited to one adrenal gland. This is also because of the very rare incidence of malignant pheochromocytoma in these patients. Cortex-sparing adrenalectomy, either open or laparoscopic, has been performed successfully in patients with MEN 2 or VHL who have bilateral pheochromocytomas, thereby avoiding the need for long-term steroid hormone replacement and the risk of Addisonian crisis in most patients (118). Cortical-sparing and laparoscopic adrenalectomy are discussed in more detail later in this chapter.

Nipride is used for the intraoperative management of blood pressure in pheochromocytoma patients because of its rapid response time and short half-life. The surgeon should manipulate the tumor as little as possible and ligate the tumor's venous outflow via the adrenal vein as early in the procedure as possible. Postoperatively, patients should be monitored carefully for at least 24 hours because of the risk for arrhythmias. They should also be watched for hypotension secondary to the compensatory vasodilation that can occur once the source of excess catecholamine stimulation has been removed in the setting of α-blockade. Occasionally, hypertension remains a problem postoperatively, especially in those patients who had sustained hypertension preoperatively. All patients should undergo yearly evaluation postoperatively, which includes measurement of the plasma free metanephrine level or a timed urine collection for total catecholamine determination to exclude recurrence.

Malignant Pheochromocytoma

The most common sites of metastases from malignant pheochromocytoma are bone, liver, and lungs; less commonly, metastases arise in regional lymph nodes. Although the absolute criteria for malignancy are adjacent organ invasion and distant metastatic disease, some general pathologic characteristics can help to identify those tumors that are likely to behave in a malignant fashion. Malignant tumors tend to be larger than their benign counterparts and mitoses tend to be much more frequent in malignant pheochromocytomas. Malignant pheochromocytomas have also been reported to be aneuploid and may exhibit more necrosis than benign tumors. However, it should be emphasized that microscopic vascular or capsular invasion and nuclear pleomorphism are not reliable indicators of malignancy. Patients with known or suspected malignant pheochromocytoma should undergo staging using standard imaging studies and MIBG scanning.

Therapy should be individualized on the basis of the extent of disease. Palliative therapy may include treatment with metyrosine, as well as α- and β-blockade. Resection of malignant pheochromocytoma, including resection of metastases, may be considered in good-risk individuals if the metastases are limited in extent.

The best currently available palliation for patients with unresectable or metastatic pheochromocytoma is α-blockade with phenoxybenzamine; α-methyltyrosine can also be used. The most commonly used chemotherapy regimens for pheochromocytoma are high-dose streptozocin and a combination of cyclophosphamide, vincristine, and dacarbazine (119). The overall response rate to these regimens is approximately 50%. Radiation therapy may effectively palliate symptomatic bony metastases. More recently, there has been some interest in treating metastatic lesions with therapeutic doses of radioactive ^{131}I-MIBG (120). Unfortunately, however, a high percentage of metastatic pheochromocytomas do not take up ^{131}I-MIBG; therefore, the response rate in patients treated with this approach, as manifested by a reduction in urinary catecholamine levels, is only about 50%. Objective responses, as determined by imaging studies, are seen even less frequently. The five-year survival rate in patients with malignant pheochromocytoma is approximately 43%, as compared with a 97% five-year survival rate in patients with benign lesions.

Adrenal Incidentaloma

Natural History and Presentation

Incidental adrenal masses are common; they are found in up to 4% of individuals undergoing abdominal imaging studies and at up to 9% of autopsies (121–126). In evaluating a patient who presents with an incidental adrenal mass, it is therefore important to remember that benign, nonfunctioning adrenocortical adenomas are common, ACCs are extremely rare, and isolated metastases to the adrenal glands from malignant solid tumors occurs occasionally (127–137). Therefore, the three critical questions that must be answered in the evaluation of each patient who presents

with an incidental adrenal mass are: (i) Is the mass primary or metastatic? (ii) Is it functioning or nonfunctioning? and (iii) Is it benign or malignant?

Evaluation

A hormonally active cortical adenoma or pheochromocytoma should be ruled out in all patients with an incidental adrenal mass. To do this, the evaluation should include a history-taking that elicits information about symptoms secondary to a functioning tumor or an underlying malignancy (weight loss, abdominal pain, and rectal bleeding); physical examination (blood pressure; breast, lymph node, pelvic, and rectal examination; and stool analysis for occult blood); and laboratory evaluation (serum potassium concentration, chest radiograph, and mammogram in adult women). A biochemical evaluation should be performed that includes an overnight 1-mg dexamethasone suppression test to exclude Cushing's syndrome. Patients found to have suppressed cortisol levels do not have Cushing's syndrome and do not require further evaluation for this condition. Patients without suppressed cortisol levels, however, should undergo a 24-hour urine collection for the measurement of urinary free cortisol and 17-OHCS and 17-keto-steroid levels. Plasma free metanephrine levels should be measured to exclude pheochromocytoma (Fig. 5). In equivocal cases, further imaging studies may be helpful, such as high-resolution CT of the adrenal glands or MRI to include T1-weighted chemical-shift analysis. We advocate fine needle aspiration biopsy of the adrenal neoplasm only if the patient has a history of a prior malignancy or if there are symptoms, physical examination findings, or biochemical or radiographic

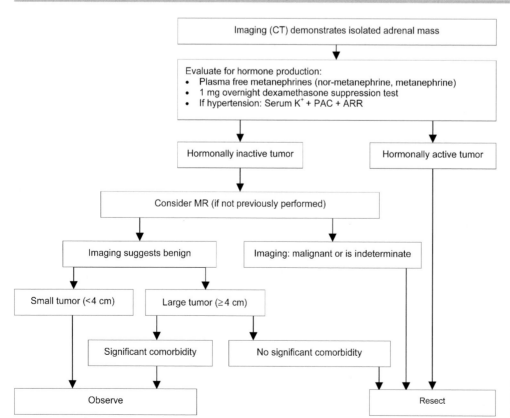

Figure 5 Algorithm for the evaluation of the patient with an incidental adrenal mass.

evidence indicating an underlying malignancy, making an adrenal metastasis the most likely diagnosis (138).

The majority of small incidental adrenal masses are nonfunctioning cortical adenomas. However, we consider it reasonable to screen all patients with incidental adrenal masses for hypercortisolism, as will be discussed below. Screening for androgen or estrogen excess is unnecessary in the absence of specific signs or symptoms suggestive of overproduction of these hormones. Likewise, because the presence of normal serum potassium concentrations and a normal blood pressure virtually exclude a diagnosis of aldosteronoma, we do not recommend screening for aldosterone excess in the absence of these findings.

A controversial area in the evaluation of patients with adrenal masses includes the clinical entity termed "subclinical Cushing's syndrome" (139–143). Between 5% and 25% of patients with incidental adrenal masses have evidence of subclinical Cushing's syndrome, which is defined as the absence of specific clinical manifestations and by an abnormal 24-hour urinary cortisol level, abnormal dexamethasone suppression, a suppressed ACTH level, loss of diurnal variation in cortisol production, or lateralizing findings on NP-59 nuclear medicine scintigraphy. If adrenal insufficiency develops in a patient after the removal of an apparently nonfunctioning incidental adrenal mass, this is also evidence that subclinical Cushing's syndrome was present preoperatively. Although a 24-hour urinary free cortisol test may miss an occasional patient with cortisol overproduction, overnight cortisol suppression with 1 mg of dexamethasone can detect the overwhelming majority of patients with cortisol overproduction due to a minimally functional adrenocortical adenoma. Therefore, the overnight 1-mg dexamethasone suppression test is probably the least expensive, the most convenient, and the most sensitive screening test for hypercortisolism in the patient with an incidental adrenal mass.

A summary of our diagnostic approach in the patient with an incidental adrenal mass is shown in Figure 5. On the day the patient is first evaluated, blood samples are obtained for the measurement of plasma metanephrine, electrolyte, ACTH, and cortisol levels. A 1-mg dose of dexamethasone is then given to the patient, to be taken at 10:00 o'clock that evening. On the following morning at 8:00 o'clock, the patient's blood is drawn for determination of the plasma cortisol level. If the patient's plasma cortisol level is not suppressed below 5.0 μg/dL, the patient undergoes a timed 24-hour urine collection for the measurement of cortisol and 17-hydroxy- and 17-keto-steroid levels. Only in the presence of a low serum potassium level or hypertension do we proceed with further evaluation for possible hyperaldosteronism. We believe this is an efficient yet appropriately thorough schema for the evaluation of patients with incidental adrenal masses. These recommendations are similar to those of the NIH State-of-the-Science Statement on Management of the Clinically Apparent Adrenal Mass ("Incidentaloma") (http://consensus.nih.gov/ta/021/adrenal_mass_consensus.pdf).

The risk of malignancy is related to the size and radiographic characteristics of the incidentaloma. Size, however, is the single best clinical indicator of malignancy in patients with an incidental adrenal mass. ACC accounts for 2%, 6%, and 25% of incidentalomas smaller than 4, 4.1 to 6, and greater than 6 cm in size, respectively. In addition, greater than 90% of ACCs are greater than 6 cm in size, whereas adrenocortical adenomas are rarely greater than 6 cm in size. Although accurate and detailed information regarding the

size distribution of adrenocortical adenomas is not available, the frequency and average size of nonfunctioning adrenal adenomas generally increase with age. This information must be taken into account when evaluating a patient who presents with an incidental adrenal mass.

Treatment
Any hormonally active adrenal neoplasm, regardless of size, should be resected. Furthermore, resection is indicated if the adrenal mass shows radiographic characteristics suggestive of malignancy (heterogeneous density or irregular borders) or if the tumor enlarges during follow-up (144). In general, lesions larger 6 cm should be resected, because 25% of them may be malignant. Observation and follow-up are generally recommended for nonfunctioning tumors smaller than 3 cm in diameter, but the management of tumors between 3 and 6 cm is more controversial (145). This is because, at our own institution and elsewhere, ACCs have been identified in patients whose tumors were smaller than 5 cm. Most of these small tumors, however, had CT or MRI characteristics suspicious for carcinoma. On the basis of individual experience and a review of the literature, recommendations have been made to resect nonfunctioning adrenal masses ranging from 5 cm down to 3 cm. The recent success with laparoscopic adrenalectomy has led some investigators to suggest the surgical removal of even small incidentalomas. We recommend adrenalectomy for all adrenal tumors associated with suspicious radiographic findings regardless of size. In contrast, patients with nonfunctioning tumors between 3 and 6 cm in diameter showing a benign CT appearance may be observed; most appropriately, though, the nature of management should be determined on an individual-basis consideration of patient age and general health. The following may be helpful in evaluating such patients with intermediate-sized, nonfunctioning adrenal masses: (i) CT or MRI, (ii) a more thorough endocrine evaluation, and (iii) consideration of age and comorbidity. Figure 5 provides an overview of our approach to patients with adrenal incidentalomas. These recommendations are similar to those of the NIH State-of-the-Science Statement on Management of the Clinically Apparent Adrenal Mass ("Incidentaloma") (http://consensus.nih.gov/ta/021/adrenal_mass_consensus.pdf).

Adrenal Metastases
Natural History and Presentation
Metastases to the adrenal glands are relatively common. On the basis of autopsy study findings, 42% of lung cancers, 16% of gastric cancers, 58% of breast cancers, 50% of malignant melanomas, and a high percentage of renal and prostate cancers have metastasized to the adrenals at the time of death. However, only rarely is adrenal insufficiency encountered in such patients. In general, more than 90% of the adrenal gland must be replaced with tumor before clinically detectable adrenocortical hypofunction is appreciated. When adrenal insufficiency does occur, it is usually when both adrenal glands are grossly enlarged, as detected by CT.

Evaluation
Evaluation of the patient with an adrenal mass and a history of malignancy starts with an evaluation of hormone production, because some of these patients will have an occult, functioning adrenal tumor unrelated to their prior

malignancy (e.g., a pheochromocytoma) (Fig. 6). In addition, patients with known or suspected adrenal metastases in whom surgical resection is contemplated should undergo ACTH stimulation testing prior to adrenalectomy to document adequate adrenocortical reserve (146–148).

After pheochromocytoma has been excluded, fine-needle aspiration biopsy of a suspicious adrenal mass (i.e., a mass that shows a heterogeneous appearance with a high attenuation value on CT scans) may be helpful in selected patients to confirm a diagnosis of metastasis, particularly in those who are not surgical candidates or who have not yet had their primary cancer resected (145,149). In the absence of signs or symptoms of a malignant solid tumor, unilateral adrenal metastases are uncommon. Indeed, in our recent experience with over 1600 patients, the incidence of metastasis from an occult primary cancer was only 0.2% (four patients). In all four patients, malignancy was suspected on the basis of tumor size, bilateral involvement, and/or symptoms. For these reasons, we do not routinely biopsy patients with small nonfunctioning adrenal tumors in a search for occult metastatic disease (150).

Treatment
Surgery for isolated metastases to the adrenal gland may be considered in highly selected patients. These include good-risk individuals who do not have extra-adrenal disease and who have a history of favorable tumor biology (151–156). A favorable tumor biology is suggested by a long progression-free interval, response to systemic therapy, and a history of isolated metachronous metastases. A long disease-free interval from the time of the primary cancer therapy to the adrenal metastasis suggests the potential for a survival duration adequate to justify adrenalectomy. The site of the primary tumor also appears to affect survival, in that longer median survival times are observed following the resection of metastases from primary kidney, colon, and lung cancers, as well as melanoma, and poorer survival is seen in patients with esophageal, liver, and unknown primary tumors and in patients with high-grade sarcomas.

CONTROVERSIES IN THE SURGICAL MANAGEMENT OF ADRENAL DISEASE
Cortical-Sparing Adrenalectomy
Cortical-sparing adrenalectomy represents a method of limiting the morbidity of adrenal insufficiency associated with total adrenalectomy in selected patients with bilateral pheochromocytoma. Bilateral pheochromocytoma is associated with a variety of inherited disorders, but most commonly with MEN 2A and 2B. MEN 2A and 2B are characterized by the presence of hyperparathyroidism and medullary thyroid cancer, and, in patients with MEN 2B, by a characteristic phenotype (157). Other inherited disorders associated with pheochromocytoma include neurofibromatosis, VHL (retinal angiomatosis and cerebellar hemangioblastoma), and hereditary paraganglioma syndrome (*SDH* gene mutations).

Although, virtually all patients with MEN types 2A and 2B have bilateral adrenal medullary hyperplasia, malignancy is uncommon, occurring in 3.9% of 387 patients from 12 collected series (69). In patients with VHL, malignancy is also uncommon. In particular, although pheochromocytomas occur in 10% to 19% of patients with VHL, and bilateral pheochromocytomas develop in 40% to 60% of these individuals, malignancy occurs in less than 4% (69). Because of this low incidence of malignancy, we currently recommend cortex-sparing adrenalectomy for patients with bilateral pheochromocytoma who have MEN 2 or VHL syndrome (118), to eliminate the requirement for long-term steroid hormone replacement and the resulting risk of Addisonian crisis. A review of our experience with this approach has demonstrated that bilateral adrenalectomy using the cortex-sparing technique is safe and does indeed avoid the need for long-term steroid hormone supplementation postoperatively in the majority of patients. There is, however, an approximately 20% incidence of pheochromocytoma recurrence 10 years or more after a cortex-sparing adrenalectomy, and thus, long-term follow-up is necessary. The adrenocortical reserve should be evaluated in all patients postoperatively (158,159); those patients found to have abnormal adrenocortical reserve should receive supplemental steroid hormone replacement

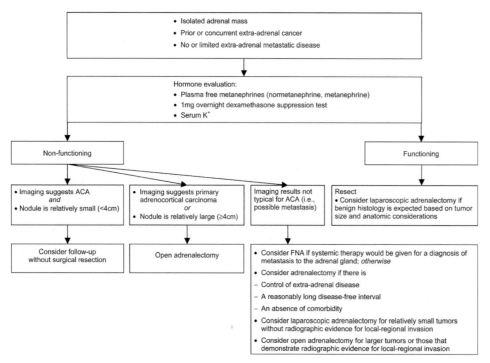

Figure 6 Algorithm for the evaluation and surgical treatment of the patient with extra-adrenal cancer presenting with an adrenal mass. *Abbreviation:* VMA, vanillylmandelic acid.

when undergoing major surgical procedures or when they develop an acute illness (Fig. 7).

The treatment of unilateral pheochromocytoma in patients with MEN 2 has been controversial. Bilateral total adrenalectomy has been advocated by some. However, despite steroid replacement, bilateral total adrenalectomy results in Addisonian crisis in up to 20% of patients. Therefore, in patients with familial pheochromocytoma, we remove only the affected side. Because this management approach is associated with a risk for recurrent metachronous pheochromocytoma, patients undergo annual screening of the contralateral normal adrenal gland. On an encouraging note, malignant pheochromocytoma has not been seen in such patients undergoing annual evaluations at our institution.

Finally, patients with the hereditary paraganglioma syndrome are not candidates for the cortex-sparing procedure because of the increased frequency of malignancy in these tumors.

Laparoscopic Adrenalectomy

Since the first description of laparoscopic adrenalectomy in 1992 (68), use of this approach has expanded such that now it is considered the standard technique for the removal of benign adrenal tumors. Most surgeons use an anterolateral transperitoneal approach; a posterior or lateral flank retroperitoneal approach has also been reported (160,161). A retroperitoneal laparoscopic adrenalectomy is currently indicated in patients with previous abdominal operations who have benign adrenal tumors smaller than 4 cm in diameter (162–164). Carefully selected patients with relatively small adrenal masses who undergo laparoscopic adrenalectomy may experience a more rapid recovery, less discomfort, a faster return to preoperative activity level, and better cosmetic results, as compared with patients who undergo open adrenalectomy.

Patients who should be considered for laparoscopic adrenalectomy include those with aldosterone-producing

adenomas; small (<4 cm) functioning (glucocorticoid- or androgen/estrogen-producing tumors) cortical neoplasms; unilateral, benign-appearing sporadic pheochromocytomas; and pheochromocytomas in the setting of MEN 2 or VHL syndrome. Bilateral laparoscopic adrenalectomy is also feasible for patients with IHA and for patients with hereditary bilateral pheochromocytomas. We urge caution in the use of laparoscopic adrenalectomy for patients with malignant or potentially malignant adrenal tumors. This includes occasional patients with sporadic pheochromocytoma in whom radiographic imaging findings raise a suspicion of malignancy, patients with the hereditary paraganglioma syndrome, and patients with cortical neoplasms (functioning or nonfunctioning) that exceed 4 cm in diameter or with radiographic evidence of malignancy. To reiterate, the reason for operating on patients with nonfunctioning adrenal tumors (incidentalomas) is that they are potentially malignant cortical neoplasms. Therefore, we specifically do not recommend laparoscopic adrenalectomy for patients in whom an ACC is part of the preoperative differential diagnosis.

ADRENAL INSUFFICIENCY

Adrenal insufficiency was first described by Thomas Addison in 1855 (165). In this report, he described 11 patients in whom destruction of the adrenal glands was associated with a fatal outcome; six had tuberculosis, three had metastatic malignancies, one had adrenal hemorrhage, and one had adrenal atrophy. Adrenal insufficiency is rare, with only 39 to 60 cases of chronic primary adrenal insufficiency (Addison's disease) per million population. It is convenient to segregate adrenal insufficiency into that resulting from primary mechanisms (destruction of the adrenal cortex) and that resulting from secondary mechanisms (insufficient stimulation of the adrenal cortex by ACTH) (166).

The most common cause of primary adrenal insufficiency today is autoimmune adrenalitis (80–90%), which can present either as an isolated autoimmune adrenalitis or as a part of the autoimmune polyendocrine syndrome (167). Other etiologies include granulomatous diseases (histoplasmosis and tuberculosis); metastatic cancer (lung cancer and breast cancer) (146–148); hemorrhage [anticoagulant therapy, Waterhouse–Friderichsen syndrome (meningococcemia), *Pseudomonas aeruginosa* infection]; and inherited disorders (X-linked adrenomyeloneuropathy). Finally, acquired immunodeficiency syndrome–associated opportunistic infections are an increasingly frequent cause of adrenal destruction. Unfortunately, primary adrenal insufficiency does not usually become clinically apparent until at least 90% of adrenal cortical tissue is destroyed.

Causes of secondary adrenal insufficiency include withdrawal of long-term exogenous glucocorticoids (the most frequent cause of adrenal insufficiency) and pituitary destruction [e.g., in patients after trans-sphenoidal surgery for pituitary adenoma and in patients with Sheehan's syndrome (postpartum pituitary necrosis)]. Although neither the dose nor the duration of glucocorticoid administration accurately predicts the degree of suppression of the hypothalamic-pituitary-adrenal axis (HPA), theoretically, any patient who has received the equivalent of 20 to 30 mg of prednisone per day for five consecutive days is at risk for adrenal insufficiency. However, although such short glucocorticoid use suppresses the HPA axis, the suppression lasts for only a few days. Patients who have received more than 30 mg of prednisone per day (or

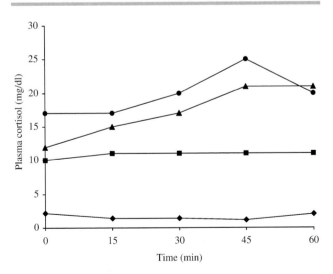

Figure 7 Cosyntropin stimulation test results in selected patients after total and subtotal adrenalectomy for bilateral pheochromocytoma. Patient 1 (♦) underwent total adrenalectomy. Patient 2 (■) underwent subtotal adrenalectomy but required postoperative steroid hormone replacement. Patients 3 (▲) and 4 (●) underwent subtotal adrenalectomy and did not require postoperative steroid hormone replacement. *Source*: From Ref. 118.

7.5 mg of prednisolone or 0.75 mg of dexamethasone per day) for more than three weeks within three months prior to a major stress or a surgical procedure are at risk for adrenal insufficiency and, in the latter case, should receive perioperative glucocorticoid coverage (168–170). Historically, recommendations for perioperative glucocorticoid replacement were based on anecdotal experience and were most likely excessive; a consensus review has now summarized the recommendations for perioperative glucocorticoid coverage (Table 6) (171–173).

Adrenal insufficiency usually has a gradual, insidious onset. However, major physiologic stress, including surgical stress, may precipitate an adrenal crisis. Therefore, a history consistent with chronic primary or secondary adrenal insufficiency should be sought in any patient with suspected acute adrenal insufficiency. Characteristic, though nonspecific, symptoms include fatigue, weakness, listlessness, orthostasis, and weight loss. Gastrointestinal symptoms may include abdominal cramps, anorexia, nausea, and vomiting. Physical examination may reveal evidence of secondary adrenal insufficiency due to prior exogenous steroid hormone administration (Cushingoid features). Alternatively, patients with primary adrenal insufficiency may have hyperpigmentation or vitiligo due to the influence of ACTH and other pro-opiomelanocortin peptides. Hypotension may occur in either primary or secondary adrenal insufficiency. However, the hypotension is characteristically more severe in primary adrenal insufficiency and is due to aldosterone deficiency. In secondary adrenal insufficiency, the hypotension is due to the decreased expression of catecholamine receptors. Abnormal laboratory results include hypoglycemia, hyponatremia, hyperkalemia, azotemia, hypercalcemia, anemia, leukopenia, lymphocytosis, and eosinophilia.

It is essential to consider a diagnosis of acute adrenal insufficiency in critically ill patients with unexplained catecholamine-resistant hypotension, because glucocorticoid replacement can be lifesaving in these patients (169,174). Patients with acute adrenal insufficiency may present in shock, with dehydration and hypotension out of proportion to the severity of the underlying illness or stress. Patients may complain of abdominal pain and manifest abdominal tenderness with fever. Lethargy, confusion, or coma may develop. Signs and symptoms may mimic a surgical abdomen or septic shock.

The treatment of patients in a suspected adrenal crisis should begin immediately. This includes isotonic intravenous fluid replacement and a stress dose of glucocorticoid, which is also administered intravenously. Dexamethasone (4 mg) is preferred over hydrocortisone (100 mg), because it has a long duration of action and does not interfere with the subsequent measurement of serum steroids during ACTH stimulation testing. While waiting for a clinical response to the dexamethasone, one should perform a high-dose ACTH stimulation test. In this test, a baseline serum cortisol level is determined. Cosyntropin (250 μg), a synthetic ACTH subunit, is then given intravenously, and the serum cortisol level is determined 30 and 60 minutes later. A baseline serum cortisol level that exceeds 20 μg/dL (or an increase of > 7 μg/dL over baseline) indicates a normal adrenal reserve; lesser values in the face of a physiologic stress indicate HPA hypofunction (166). Patients in whom adrenal insufficiency is established require initial stress doses of glucocorticoid replacement intravenously (e.g., hydrocortisone, 300 mg/day in divided doses), followed by tapering of the dose to physiologic replacement doses given orally (e.g., hydrocortisone, 10–12 mg/m^2/day in divided doses). Additionally, patients with primary adrenal insufficiency should receive fludrocortisone (50–200 μg/day) to prevent hyponatremia due to mineralocorticoid deficiency.

REFERENCES

1. Funder JW, Pearce PT, Smith R, Smith AI. Mineralocorticoid action: target tissue specificity is enzyme, not receptor, mediated. Science 1988; 242:583–585.
2. Edwards CR, Stewart PM, Burt D, et al. Localisation of 11 beta-hydroxysteroid dehydrogenase—tissue specific protector of the mineralocorticoid receptor. Lancet 1988; 2:986–989.
3. Arriza JL, Weinberger C, Cerelli G, et al. Cloning of human mineralocorticoid receptor complementary DNA: structural and functional kinship with the glucocorticoid receptor. Science 1987; 237:268–275.
4. Conn J. Primary aldosteronism, a new clinical entity. J Lab Clin Med 1955; 45:3–17.
5. Young WF Jr. Minireview: primary aldosteronism-changing concepts in diagnosis and treatment. Endocrinology 2003; 144:2208–2213.
6. Loh KC, Koay ES, Khaw MC, Emmanuel SC, Young WF Jr. Prevalence of primary aldosteronism among Asian hypertensive patients in Singapore. J Clin Endocrinol Metab 2000; 85:2854–2859.
7. Lim PO, Dow E, Brennan G, Jung RT, MacDonald TM. High prevalence of primary aldosteronism in the Tayside hypertension clinic population. J Hum Hypertens 2000; 14:311–315.
8. Fardella CE, Mosso L, Gomez-Sanchez C, et al. Primary hyperaldosteronism in essential hypertensives: prevalence, biochemical profile, and molecular biology. J Clin Endocrinol Metab 2000; 85:1863–1867.
9. Gordon RD, Ziesak MD, Tunny TJ, Stowasser M, Klemm SA. Evidence that primary aldosteronism may not be uncommon: 12% incidence among antihypertensive drug trial volunteers. Clin Exp Pharmacol Physiol 1993; 20:296–298.
10. Stowasser M. How common is adrenal-based mineralocorticoid hypertension? Curr Opin Endocrinol Diab 2000; 7:143–150.
11. Gordon RD, Stowasser M, Tunny TJ, Klemm SA, Rutherford JC. High incidence of primary aldosteronism in 199 patients referred with hypertension. Clin Exp Pharmacol Physiol 1994; 21:315–318.
12. Merrell RC. Aldosterone-producing tumors (Conn's syndrome). Semin Surg Oncol 1990; 6:66–70.
13. Weigel RJ, Wells SA, Gunnells JC, Leight GS. Surgical treatment of primary hyperaldosteronism. Ann Surg 1994; 219:347–352.
14. White PC. Disorders of aldosterone biosynthesis and action. N Engl J Med 1994; 331:250–258.
15. Mulatero P, Rabbia F, Milan A, et al. Drug effects on aldosterone/plasma renin activity ratio in primary aldosteronism. Hypertension 2002; 40:897–902.
16. Ganguly A. Primary aldosteronism. N Engl J Med 1998; 339:1828–1834.
17. Lund JO, Nielsen MD, Giese J. Prevalence of primary aldosteronism. Acta Med Scand Suppl 1981; 646:54–57.
18. Melby JC. Primary aldosteronism. Kidney Int 1984; 26:769–778.
19. Conn JW, Cohen EL, Herwig KR. The dexamethasone-modified adrenal scintiscan in hyporeninemic aldosteronism (tumor versus hyperplasia). A comparison with adrenal venography and adrenal venous aldosterone. J Lab Clin Med 1976; 88:841–856.
20. Conn JW. Part I Painting background. Part II. Primary aldosteronism, a new clinical syndrome, 1954.. J Lab Clin Med 1990; 116:253–267.
21. Grim CE, Ganguly A, Yum MN, Donohue JP, Weinberger MH. Hyperaldosteronism due to unsuspected adrenal carcinoma: discovery during investigation of hypertension in a young woman. J Urol 1981; 126:783–786.

22. Scott HW Jr, Sussman CR, Page DL, Thompson NW, Gross MD, Lloyd R. Primary hyperaldosteronism caused by adrenocortical carcinoma. World J Surg 1986; 10:646–653.

23. Stowasser M, Gordon RD, Rutherford JC, Nikwan NZ, Daunt N, Slater GJ. Diagnosis and management of primary aldosteronism. J Renin Angiotensin Aldosterone Syst 2001; 2:156–169.

24. McKenna TJ, Sequeira SJ, Heffernan A, Chambers J, Cunningham S. Diagnosis under random conditions of all disorders of the renin-angiotensin-aldosterone axis, including primary hyperaldosteronism. J Clin Endocrinol Metab 1991; 73:952–957.

25. Hiramatsu K, Yamada T, Yukimura Y, et al. A screening test to identify aldosterone-producing adenoma by measuring plasma renin activity. Results in hypertensive patients. Arch Intern Med 1981; 141:1589–1593.

26. Gallay BJ, Ahmad S, Xu L, Toivola B, Davidson RC. Screening for primary aldosteronism without discontinuing hypertensive medications: plasma aldosterone-renin ratio. Am J Kidney Dis 2001; 37:699–705.

27. Sawka AM, Young WF, Thompson GB, et al. Primary aldosteronism: factors associated with normalization of blood pressure after surgery. Ann Intern Med 2001; 135:258–261.

28. Hamlet SM, Tunny TJ, Woodland E, Gordon RD. Is aldosterone/renin ratio useful to screen a hypertensive population for primary aldosteronism? Clin Exp Pharmacol Physiol 1985; 12:249–252.

29. Weinberger MH, Fineberg NS. The diagnosis of primary aldosteronism and separation of two major subtypes. Arch Intern Med 1993; 153:2125–2129.

30. Montori VM, Young WF Jr. Use of plasma aldosterone concentration-to-plasma renin activity ratio as a screening test for primary aldosteronism. A systematic review of the literature. Endocrinol Metab Clin North Am 2002; 31:619–632, xi.

31. Blumenfeld JD, Sealey JE, Schlussel Y, et al. Diagnosis and treatment of primary hyperaldosteronism. Ann Intern Med 1994; 121:877–885.

32. Holland OB, Brown H, Kuhnert L, Fairchild C, Risk M, Gomez-Sanchez CE. Further evaluation of saline infusion for the diagnosis of primary aldosteronism. Hypertension 1984; 6:717–723.

33. Kem DC, Weinberger MH, Mayes DM, Nugent CA. Saline suppression of plasma aldosterone in hypertension. Arch Intern Med 1971; 128:380–386.

34. Bravo EL, Tarazi RC, Dustan HP, et al. The changing clinical spectrum of primary aldosteronism. Am J Med 1983; 74: 641–651.

35. Findling JW, Raff H. Diagnosis and differential diagnosis of Cushing's syndrome. Endocrinol Metab Clin N Am 2001; 30:729–747.

36. Cronin C, Igoe D, Duffy MJ, Cunningham SK, McKenna TJ. The overnight dexamethasone test is a worthwhile screening procedure. Clin Endocrinol (Oxf) 1990; 33:27–33.

37. Montwill J, Igoe D, McKenna TJ. The overnight dexamethasone test is the procedure of choice in screening for Cushing's syndrome. Steroids 1994; 59:296–298.

38. Kennedy L, Atkinson AB, Johnston H, Sheridan B, Hadden DR. Serum cortisol concentrations during low dose dexamethasone suppression test to screen for Cushing's syndrome. Br Med J (Clin Res Ed) 1984; 289:1188–1191.

39. Mengden T, Hubmann P, Muller J, Greminger P, Vetter W. Urinary free cortisol versus 17-hydroxycorticosteroids: a comparative study of their diagnostic value in Cushing's syndrome. Clin Investig 1992; 70:545–548.

40. Raff H, Raff JL, Findling JW. Late-night salivary cortisol as a screening test for Cushing's syndrome. J Clin Endocrinol Metab 1998; 83:2681–2686.

41. Yanovski JA, Cutler GB Jr, Chrousos GP, Nieman LK. Corticotropin-releasing hormone stimulation following low-dose dexamethasone administration. A new test to distinguish Cushing's syndrome from pseudo-Cushing's states. JAMA 1993; 269:2232–2238.

42. Yanovski JA, Cutler GB Jr, Chrousos GP, Nieman LK. The dexamethasone-suppressed corticotropin-releasing hormone stimulation test differentiates mild Cushing's disease from normal physiology. J Clin Endocrinol Metab 1998; 83: 348–352.

43. Sawka AM, Jaeschke R, Singh RJ, Young WF Jr. A comparison of biochemical tests for pheochromocytoma: measurement of fractionated plasma metanephrines compared with the combination of 24-hour urinary metanephrines and catecholamines. J Clin Endocrinol Metab 2003; 88:553–558.

44. Young WF Jr, Stanson AW, Grant CS, Thompson GB, van Heerden JA. Primary aldosteronism: adrenal venous sampling. Surgery 1996; 120:913–919; discussion 919–920.

45. Doppman JL, Gill JR Jr. Hyperaldosteronism: sampling the adrenal veins. Radiology 1996; 198:309–312.

46. Magill SB, Raff H, Shaker JL, et al. Comparison of adrenal vein sampling and computed tomography in the differentiation of primary aldosteronism. J Clin Endocrinol Metab 2001; 86:1066–1071.

47. Rossi GP, Sacchetto A, Chiesura-Corona M, et al. Identification of the etiology of primary aldosteronism with adrenal vein sampling in patients with equivocal computed tomography and magnetic resonance findings: results in 104 consecutive cases. J Clin Endocrinol Metab 2001; 86:1083–1090.

48. Young WF Jr, Klee GG. Primary aldosteronism. Diagnostic evaluation. Endocrinol Metab Clin N Am 1988; 17:367–395.

49. Young WF. Primary aldosteronism–treatment options. Growth Horm IGF Res 2003; 13(suppl):S102–S108.

50. Proye CA, Mulliez EA, Carnaille BM, et al. Essential hypertension: first reason for persistent hypertension after unilateral adrenalectomy for primary aldosteronism? Surgery 1998; 124:1128–1133.

51. Celen O, O'Brien MJ, Melby JC, Beazley RM. Factors influencing outcome of surgery for primary aldosteronism. Arch Surg 1996; 131:646–650.

52. Irony I, Kater CE, Biglieri EG, Shackleton CH. Correctable subsets of primary aldosteronism. Primary adrenal hyperplasia and renin responsive adenoma. Am J Hypertens 1990; 3:576–582.

53. Sawka AM, Young WF Jr, Schaff HV. Cardiac phaeochromocytoma presenting with severe hypertension and chest pain. Clin Endocrinol (Oxf) 2001; 54:689–692.

54. Shen WT, Lim RC, Siperstein AE, et al. Laparoscopic vs open adrenalectomy for the treatment of primary hyperaldosteronism. Arch Surg 1999; 134:628–631; discussion 631–632.

55. Marescaux J, Mutter D, Wheeler MH. Laparoscopic right and left adrenalectomies. Surgical procedures. Surg Endosc 1996; 10:912–915.

56. Fletcher DR, Beiles CB, Hardy KJ. Laparoscopic adrenalectomy. Aust N Z J Surg 1994; 64:427–430.

57. Newell-Price J, Trainer P, Besser M, Grossman A. The diagnosis and differential diagnosis of Cushing's syndrome and pseudo-Cushing's states. Endocr Rev 1998; 19:647–672.

58. Findling JW, Doppman JL. Biochemical and radiologic diagnosis of Cushing's syndrome. Endocrinol Metab Clin N Am 1994; 23:511–537.

59. Oldfield EH, Doppman JL, Nieman LK, et al. Petrosal sinus sampling with and without corticotropin-releasing hormone for the differential diagnosis of Cushing's syndrome. N Engl J Med 1991; 325:897–905.

60. Ichikawa T, Ohtomo K, Uchiyama G, Fujimoto H, Nasu K. Contrast-enhanced dynamic MRI of adrenal masses: classification of characteristic enhancement patterns. Clin Radiol 1995; 50:295–300.

61. Mayo-Smith WW, Lee MJ, McNicholas MM, Hahn PF, Boland GW, Saini S. Characterization of adrenal masses (<5 cm) by use of chemical shift MR imaging: observer performance versus quantitative measures. AJR Am J Roentgenol 1995; 165:91–95.

62. Krestin GP, Steinbrich W, Friedmann G. Adrenal masses: evaluation with fast gradient-echo MR imaging and Gd-DTPA-enhanced dynamic studies. Radiology 1989; 171:675–680.

63. Doppman JL, Reinig JW, Dwyer AJ, et al. Differentiation of adrenal masses by magnetic resonance imaging. Surgery 1987; 102:1018–1026.

64. Outwater EK, Siegelman ES, Radecki PD, Piccoli CW, Mitchell DG. Distinction between benign and malignant adrenal masses: value of T1-weighted chemical-shift MR imaging. AJR Am J Roentgenol 1995; 165:579–583.

65. Reinig JW, Doppman JL, Dwyer AJ, Frank J. MRI of indeterminate adrenal masses. AJR Am J Roentgenol 1986; 147:493–496.

66. Yu KC, Alexander HR, Ziessman HA, et al. Role of preoperative iodocholesterol scintiscanning in patients undergoing adrenalectomy for Cushing's syndrome. Surgery 1995; 118:981–986; discussion 986–987.

67. Guazzoni G, Montorsi F, Bocciardi A, et al. Transperitoneal laparoscopic versus open adrenalectomy for benign hyperfunctioning adrenal tumors: a comparative study. J Urol 1995; 153:1597–1600.

68. Gagner M, Lacroix A, Bolte E. Laparoscopic adrenalectomy in Cushing's syndrome and pheochromocytoma. N Engl J Med 1992; 327:1033.

69. Dackiw AP, Lee JE, Gagel RF, Evans DB. Adrenal cortical carcinoma. World J Surg 2001; 25:914–926.

70. Kjellman M, Kallioniemi OP, Karhu R, et al. Genetic aberrations in adrenocortical tumors detected using comparative genomic hybridization correlate with tumor size and malignancy. Cancer Res 1996; 56:4219–4223.

71. Gortz B, Roth J, Speel EJ, et al. MEN1 gene mutation analysis of sporadic adrenocortical lesions. Int J Cancer 1999; 80:373–379.

72. Heppner C, Reincke M, Agarwal SK, et al. MEN1 gene analysis in sporadic adrenocortical neoplasms. J Clin Endocrinol Metab 1999; 84:216–219.

73. McNicol AM, Nolan CE, Struthers AJ, Farquharson MA, Hermans J, Haak HR. Expression of p53 in adrenocortical tumours: clinicopathological correlations. J Pathol 1997; 181:146–152.

74. Gicquel C, Raffin-Sanson ML, Gaston V, et al. Structural and functional abnormalities at 11p15 are associated with the malignant phenotype in sporadic adrenocortical tumors: study on a series of 82 tumors. J Clin Endocrinol Metab 1997; 82:2559–2565.

75. Reincke M, Mora P, Beuschlein F, Arlt W, Chrousos GP, Allolio B. Deletion of the adrenocorticotropin receptor gene in human adrenocortical tumors: implications for tumorigenesis. J Clin Endocrinol Metab 1997; 82:3054–3058.

76. Lyons J, Landis CA, Harsh G, et al. Two G protein oncogenes in human endocrine tumors. Science 1990; 249:655–659.

77. Jemal A, Murray T, Samuels A, Ghafoor A, Ward E, Thun MJ. Cancer statistics, 2003. CA Cancer J Clin 2003; 53:5–26.

78. Grondal S, Cedermark B, Eriksson B, et al. Adrenocortical carcinoma. A retrospective study of a rare tumor with a poor prognosis. Eur J Surg Oncol 1990; 16:500–506.

79. Lee JE, Berger DH, el-Naggar AK, et al. Surgical management, DNA content, and patient survival in adrenal cortical carcinoma. Surgery 1995; 118:1090–1098.

80. Soreide JA, Brabrand K, Thoresen SO. Adrenal cortical carcinoma in Norway, 1970–1984. World J Surg 1992; 16:663–667; discussion 668.

81. Yano T, Linehan M, Anglard P, et al. Genetic changes in human adrenocortical carcinomas. J Natl Cancer Inst 1989; 81:518–523.

82. Lenders JW, Pacak K, Walther MM, et al. Biochemical diagnosis of pheochromocytoma: which test is best? JAMA 2002; 287:1427–1434.

83. Sullivan M, Boileau M, Hodges CV. Adrenal cortical carcinoma. J Urol 1978; 120:660–665.

84. Macfarlane D. Cancer of the adrenal cortex: the natural history, prognosis and treatment in a study of fifty-five cases. Ann R Coll Surg Engl 1958; 23:155.

85. Icard P, Chapuis Y, Andreassian B, Bernard A, Proye C. Adrenocortical carcinoma in surgically treated patients: a retrospective study on 156 cases by the French Association of Endocrine Surgery. Surgery 1992; 112:972–979; discussion 979–980.

86. Icard P, Louvel A, Chapuis Y. Survival rates and prognostic factors in adrenocortical carcinoma. World J Surg 1992; 16:753–758.

87. Icard P, Goudet P, Charpenay C, et al. Adrenocortical carcinomas: surgical trends and results of a 253-patient series from the French Association of Endocrine Surgeons study group. World J Surg 2001; 25:891–897.

88. Favia G, Lumachi F, D'Amico DF. Adrenocortical carcinoma: is prognosis different in nonfunctioning tumors? Results of surgical treatment in 31 patients. World J Surg 2001; 25:735–738.

89. Harrison LE, Gaudin PB, Brennan MF. Pathologic features of prognostic significance for adrenocortical carcinoma after curative resection. Arch Surg 1999; 134:181–185.

90. Khorram-Manesh A, Ahlman H, Jansson S, et al. Adrenocortical carcinoma: surgery and mitotane for treatment and steroid profiles for follow-up. World J Surg 1998; 22:605–611; discussion 611–612.

91. Crucitti F, Bellantone R, Ferrante A, Boscherini M, Crucitti P. The Italian Registry for Adrenal Cortical Carcinoma: analysis of a multiinstitutional series of 129 patients. The ACC Italian Registry Study Group. Surgery 1996; 119:161–170.

92. Haak hr, Hermans J, van de Velde CJ, et al. Optimal treatment of adrenocortical carcinoma with mitotane: results in a consecutive series of 96 patients. Br J Cancer 1994; 69:947–951.

93. Zografos GC, Driscoll DL, Karakousis CP, Huben RP. Adrenal adenocarcinoma: a review of 53 cases. J Surg Oncol 1994; 55:160–164.

94. Pommier RF, Brennan MF. An eleven-year experience with adrenocortical carcinoma. Surgery 1992; 112:963–970; discussion 970–971.

95. Henley DJ, van Heerden JA, Grant CS, Carney JA, Carpenter PC. Adrenal cortical carcinoma—a continuing challenge. Surgery 1983; 94:926–931.

96. Markoe AM, Serber W, Micaily B, Brady LW. Radiation therapy for adjunctive treatment of adrenal cortical carcinoma. Am J Clin Oncol 1991; 14:170–174.

97. Wooten MD, King DK. Adrenal cortical carcinoma. Epidemiology and treatment with mitotane and a review of the literature. Cancer 1993; 72:3145–3155.

98. Vassilopoulou-Sellin R, Guinee VF, Klein MJ, et al. Impact of adjuvant mitotane on the clinical course of patients with adrenocortical cancer. Cancer 1993; 71:3119–3123.

99. Dogliotti L, Sperone P, Berruti A, et al. Multicenter phase II study of mitotane associated with etoposide, doxorubicin and cisplatin in the treatment of advanced adrenocortical carcinoma. Vol. ASCO's Annual Meeting, Chicago, Illinois, 2003.

100. Abraham J, Bakke S, Rutt A, et al. A phase II trial of combination chemotherapy and surgical resection for the treatment of metastatic adrenocortical carcinoma: continuous infusion doxorubicin, vincristine, and etoposide with daily mitotane as a P-glycoprotein antagonist. Cancer 2002; 94:2333–2343.

101. Nagourney RA, Isaacs J, Bosserman L, Sommers BL, Evans SS. Adrenocortical carcinoma therapy with cisplatin & gemcitabine: laboratory and clinical correlates. Vol. ASCO's Annual Meeting, Chicago, Illinois, 2003.

102. Pierga J-Y, Faivre S, Vera K, et al. A phase I and pharmacokinetic (PK) trial of CYC202, a novel oral cyclin-dependent kinase (CDK) inhibitor, in patients (pts) with advanced solid tumors. Vol. ASCO's Annual Meeting, Chicago, Illinois, 2003.

103. Wood BJ, Abraham J, Hvizda JL, Alexander HR, Fojo T. Radiofrequency ablation of adrenal tumors and adrenocortical carcinoma metastases. Cancer 2003; 97:554–560.

104. Hara F, Kishikawa T, Tomishige H, Nishikawa O, Nishida Y, Kongo M. A child with adrenocortical carcinoma who underwent percutaneous ethanol injection therapy for liver metastasis. J Pediatr Surg 2003; 38:1237–1240.

105. Jensen JC, Pass HI, Sindelar WF, Norton JA. Recurrent or metastatic disease in select patients with adrenocortical carcinoma. Aggressive resection vs chemotherapy. Arch Surg 1991; 126: 457–461.

106. Kwauk S, Burt M. Pulmonary metastases from adrenal cortical carcinoma: results of resection. J Surg Oncol 1993; 53: 243–246.

107. Eng C, Clayton D, Schuffenecker I, et al. The relationship between specific RET proto-oncogene mutations and disease phenotype in multiple endocrine neoplasia type International RET mutation consortium analysis. JAMA 1996; 276:1575–1579.

108. Matias-Guiu X, Colomer A, Mato E, et al. Expression of the ret proto-oncogene in phaeochromocytoma. An in situ hybridization and northern blot study. J Pathol 1995; 176:63–68.

109. van Heyningen V. Genetics. One gene-four syndromes. Nature 1994; 367:319–320.

110. Beldjord C, Desclaux-Arramond F, Raffin-Sanson M, et al. The RET protooncogene in sporadic pheochromocytomas: frequent MEN 2-like mutations and new molecular defects. J Clin Endocrinol Metab 1995; 80:2063–2068.

111. Chew SL, Lavender P, Jain A, et al. Absence of mutations in the MEN2A region of the ret proto-oncogene in non-MEN 2A phaeochromocytomas. Clin Endocrinol (Oxf) 1995; 42:17–21.

112. Shapiro SE, Cote GC, Lee JE, Gagel RF, Evans DB. The role of genetics in the surgical management of familial endocrinopathy syndromes. J Am Coll Surgeons. In press.

113. Dluhy RG. Pheochromocytoma—death of an axiom. N Engl J Med 2002; 346:1486–1488.

114. Pacak K, Linehan WM, Eisenhofer G, Walther MM, Goldstein DS. Recent advances in genetics, diagnosis, localization, and treatment of pheochromocytoma. Ann Intern Med 2001; 134:315–329.

115. Bravo EL, Gifford RW Jr. Current concepts. Pheochromocytoma: diagnosis, localization and management. N Engl J Med 1984; 311:1298–1303.

116. Werbel SS, Ober KP. Pheochromocytoma. Update on diagnosis, localization, and management. Med Clin N Am 1995; 79: 131–153.

117. Shapiro B, Copp JE, Sisson JC, Eyre PL, Wallis J, Beierwaltes WH. Iodine-131 metaiodobenzylguanidine for the locating of suspected pheochromocytoma: experience in 400 cases. J Nucl Med 1985; 26:576–585.

118. Lee JE, Curley SA, Gagel RF, Evans DB, Hickey RC. Cortical-sparing adrenalectomy for patients with bilateral pheochromocytoma. Surgery 1996; 120:1064–1070; discussion 1070–1071.

119. Patel SR, Winchester DJ, Benjamin RS. A 15-year experience with chemotherapy of patients with paraganglioma. Cancer 1995; 76:1476–1480.

120. Rose B, Matthay KK, Price D, et al. High-dose 131I-metaiodobenzylguanidine therapy for 12 patients with malignant pheochromocytoma. Cancer 2003; 98:239–248.

121. Abecassis M, McLoughlin MJ, Langer B, Kudlow JE. Serendipitous adrenal masses: prevalence, significance, and management. Am J Surg 1985; 149:783–788.

122. Belldegrun A, Hussain S, Seltzer SE, Loughlin KR, Gittes RF, Richie JP. Incidentally discovered mass of the adrenal gland. Surg Gynecol Obstet 1986; 163:203–208.

123. Bitter DA, Ross DS. Incidentally discovered adrenal masses. Am J Surg 1989; 158:159–161.

124. Copeland PM. The incidentally discovered adrenal mass. Ann Intern Med 1983; 98:940–945.

125. Kobayashi S, Iwase H, Matsuo K, Fukuoka H, Ito Y, Masaoka A. Primary adrenocortical tumors in autopsy records—a survey of "Cumulative Reports in Japan" from 1973 to 1984. Jpn J Surg 1991; 21:494–498.

126. Yamakita N, Saitoh M, Mercado-Asis LB, et al. Asymptomatic adrenal tumor; 386 cases in Japan including our 7 cases. Endocrinol Jpn 1990; 37:671–684.

127. Penn I, Moulton J, Bracken B. Diagnosis and management of adrenal masses: 1987 Du Pont lecture. Can J Surg 1988; 31:105–109.

128. Siekavizza JL, Bernardino ME, Samaan NA. Suprarenal mass and its differential diagnosis. Urology 1981; 18:625–632.

129. Siren JE, Haapiainen RK, Huikuri KT, Sivula AH. Incidentalomas of the adrenal gland: 36 operated patients and review of literature. World J Surg 1993; 17:634–639.

130. Wood DE, Delbridge L, Reeve TS. Surgery for adrenal tumours: is operation for the small incidental tumour appropriate? Aust N Z J Surg 1987; 57:739–742.

131. Thompson NW, Cheung PS. Diagnosis and treatment of functioning and nonfunctioning adrenocortical neoplasms including incidentalomas. Surg Clin N Am 1987; 67:423–436.

132. Staren ED, Prinz RA. Selection of patients with adrenal incidentalomas for operation. Surg Clin N Am 1995; 75:499–509.

133. Katz RL, Shirkhoda A. Diagnostic approach to incidental adrenal nodules in the cancer patient. Results of a clinical, radiologic, and fine-needle aspiration study. Cancer 1985; 55:1995–2000.

134. Bertagna C, Orth DN. Clinical and laboratory findings and results of therapy in 58 patients with adrenocortical tumors admitted to a single medical center (1951 to 1978). Am J Med 1981; 71:855–875.

135. Geelhoed GW, Druy EM. Management of the adrenal "incidentaloma." Surgery 1982; 92:866–874.

136. Herrera MF, Grant CS, van Heerden JA, Sheedy PF, Ilstrup DM. Incidentally discovered adrenal tumors: an institutional perspective. Surgery 1991; 110:1014–1021.

137. Jockenhovel F, Kuck W, Hauffa B, et al. Conservative and surgical management of incidentally discovered adrenal tumors (incidentalomas). J Endocrinol Invest 1992; 15:331–337.

138. Lee JE, Evans DB, Sherman SI, Gagel RF. Evaluation of the incidental adrenal mass. Am J Med 1997; 103:249–250.

139. Laudat MH, Billaud L, Thomopoulos P, Vera O, Yllia A, Luton JP. Evening urinary free corticoids: a screening test in Cushing's syndrome and incidentally discovered adrenal tumours. Acta Endocrinol (Copenh) 1988; 119:459–464.

140. Rosen HN, Swartz SL. Subtle glucocorticoid excess in patients with adrenal incidentaloma. Am J Med 1992; 92:213–216.

141. Huiras CM, Pehling GB, Caplan RH. Adrenal insufficiency after operative removal of apparently nonfunctioning adrenal adenomas. JAMA 1989; 261:894–898.

142. Beyer HS, Doe RP. Cortisol secretion by an incidentally discovered nonfunctional adrenal adenoma. J Clin Endocrinol Metab 1986; 62:1317–1321.

143. Bogner U, Eggens U, Hensen J, Oelkers W. Incidentally discovered ACTH-dependent adrenal adenoma presenting as 'pre-Cushing's syndrome'. Acta Endocrinol (Copenh) 1986; 111:89–92.

144. Barnett CC Jr, Varma DG, El-Naggar AK, et al. Limitations of size as a criterion in the evaluation of adrenal tumors. Surgery 2000; 128:973–982; discussion 982–983.

145. Grumbach mm, Biller BM, Braunstein GD, et al. Management of the clinically inapparent adrenal mass (incidentaloma). Ann Intern Med 2003; 138:424–429.

146. Seidenwurm DJ, Elmer EB, Kaplan LM, Williams EK, Morris DG, Hoffman AR. Metastases to the adrenal glands and the development of Addison's disease. Cancer 1984; 54:552–557.

147. Kung AW, Pun KK, Lam K, Wang C, Leung CY. Addisonian crisis as presenting feature in malignancies. Cancer 1990; 65:177–179.

148. Mor F, Lahav M, Kipper E, Wysenbeek AJ. Addison's disease due to metastases to the adrenal glands. Postgrad Med J 1985; 61:637–639.

149. Saboorian MH, Katz RL, Charnsangavej C. Fine needle aspiration cytology of primary and metastatic lesions of the adrenal gland. A series of 188 biopsies with radiologic correlation. Acta Cytol 1995; 39:843–851.

150. Lee JE, Evans DB, Hickey RC, et al. Unknown primary cancer presenting as an adrenal mass: frequency and implications for diagnostic evaluation of adrenal incidentalomas. Surgery 1998; 124:1115–1122.

151. Lenert JT, Barnett CC Jr, Kudelka AP, et al. Evaluation and surgical resection of adrenal masses in patients with a history of extra-adrenal malignancy. Surgery 2001; 130:1060–1067.

152. Paul CA, Virgo KS, Wade TP, Audisio RA, Johnson FE. Adrenalectomy for isolated adrenal metastases from non-adrenal cancer. Int J Oncol 2000; 17:181–187.

153. Soffen EM, Solin LJ, Rubenstein JH, Hanks GE. Palliative radiotherapy for symptomatic adrenal metastases. Cancer 1990; 65:1318–1320.

154. Reyes L, Parvez Z, Nemoto T, Regal AM, Takita H. Adrenalectomy for adrenal metastasis from lung carcinoma. J Surg Oncol 1990; 44:32–34.

155. Branum GD, Epstein RE, Leight GS, Seigler HF. The role of resection in the management of melanoma metastatic to the adrenal gland. Surgery 1991; 109:127–131.

156. Ettinghausen SE, Burt ME. Prospective evaluation of unilateral adrenal masses in patients with operable non-small-cell lung cancer. J Clin Oncol 1991; 9:1462–1466.

157. Evans DB, Lee JE, Merrell RC, Hickey RC. Adrenal medullary disease in multiple endocrine neoplasia type Appropriate management. Endocrinol Metab Clin N Am 1994; 23:167–176.

158. Mohler JL, Michael KA, Freedman AM, McRoberts JW, Griffen WO Jr. The evaluation of postoperative function of the adrenal gland. Surg Gynecol Obstet 1985; 161:551–556.

159. Chalmers RA, Mashiter K, Joplin GF. Residual adrenocortical function after bilateral "total" adrenalectomy for Cushing's disease. Lancet 1981; 2:1196–1199.

160. Mercan S, Seven R, Ozarmagan S, Tezelman S. Endoscopic retroperitoneal adrenalectomy. Surgery 1995; 118:1071–1075; discussion 1075–1076.

161. Siperstein AE, Berber E, Engle KL, Duh QY, Clark OH. Laparoscopic posterior adrenalectomy: technical considerations. Arch Surg 2000; 135:967–971.

162. Smith CD, Weber CJ, Amerson JR. Laparoscopic adrenalectomy: new gold standard. World J Surg 1999; 23:389–396.

163. Baba S, Miyajima A, Uchida A, Asanuma H, Miyakawa A, Murai M. A posterior lumbar approach for retroperitoneoscopic adrenalectomy: assessment of surgical efficacy. Urology 1997; 50:19–24.

164. Baba S, Ito K, Yanaihara H, Nagata H, Murai M, Iwamura M. Retroperitoneoscopic adrenalectomy by a lumbodorsal approach: clinical experience with solo surgery. World J Urol 1999; 17:54–58.

165. Addison T. On the constitutional and local effects of disease of the supra-renal capsules. London: Highley, 1855.

166. Oelkers W. Adrenal insufficiency. N Engl J Med 1996; 335:1206–1212.

167. Arlt W, Allolio B. Adrenal insufficiency. Lancet 2003; 361: 1881–1893.

168. Krasner AS. Glucocorticoid-induced adrenal insufficiency. JAMA 1999; 282:671–676.

169. Cooper MS, Stewart PM. Corticosteroid insufficiency in acutely ill patients. N Engl J Med 2003; 348:727–734.

170. Axelrod L. Perioperative management of patients treated with glucocorticoids. Endocrinol Metab Clin North Am 2003; 32:367–383.

171. Nicholson G, Burrin JM, Hall GM. Peri-operative steroid supplementation. Anaesthesia 1998; 53:1091–1104.

172. Salem M, Tainsh RE Jr, Bromberg J, Loriaux DL, Chernow B. Perioperative glucocorticoid coverage. A reassessment 42 years after emergence of a problem. Ann Surg 1994; 219: 416–425.

173. Glowniak JV, Loriaux DL. A double-blind study of perioperative steroid requirements in secondary adrenal insufficiency. Surgery 1997; 121:123–129.

174. Lamberts SW, Bruining HA, de Jong FH. Corticosteroid therapy in severe illness. N Engl J Med 1997; 337:1285–1292.

52

The Thyroid Gland

Ronald C. Merrell and Lucian Panait

INTRODUCTION

Despite its small size, the thyroid gland plays a key role in modulating and coordinating a wide variety of metabolic processes within the human body. Although many of the diseases involving this organ can be managed nonoperatively, the surgeon is frequently consulted when swallowing or breathing is adversely affected by an enlarged gland, or when a solitary module is thought to be potentially malignant. Thus, a thorough knowledge of the pathophysiology of this gland is mandatory if correct decision-making is to occur when surgical interventions are being considered. This chapter attempts to provide that understanding.

THYROID ANATOMY
Gross Anatomy

The thyroid gland extends from the level of the middle thyroid cartilage of the larynx superiorly, to the second tracheal ring inferiorly. In normal adults, the thyroid gland weighs 15 to 20 g. It is formed by a left and right lobe connected by an isthmus, which crosses the trachea (Fig. 1). In approximately 80% of individuals, a pyramidal lobe representing a remnant of the thyroglossal duct ascends in the midline. The lateral lobes are bordered by the carotid sheath and the sternocleidomastoid muscles laterally, the strap muscles (sternothyroid and sternohyoid) anteriorly, and the trachea medially. On the posterior aspect of the lobes lie the recurrent laryngeal nerves and the parathyroid glands.

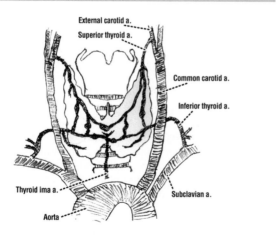

Figure 1 Anatomy of the thyroid gland.

The thyroid gland is surrounded by a loose connective tissue fascia, which results from the division of the deep cervical fascia into an anterior and a posterior sheath. The ligament of Berry tightly attaches the thyroid to the anterior trachea, which causes the thyroid to move with the larynx and trachea while swallowing. The true capsule is made of a thin fibrous layer that sends septae into the gland.

Blood is supplied to the thyroid gland by the superior and inferior thyroid arteries. The superior thyroid artery is the first branch of the external carotid artery. The inferior thyroid artery arises from the thyrocervical trunk off the subclavian artery and approaches the gland inferiorly from a posterolateral direction, behind the carotid sheath. A fifth artery, the thyroidea ima, originates directly from the aortic arch, ascends in the midline, and enters the gland inferiorly. Venous drainage of the thyroid is via subcapsular venous plexuses, which converge to form the superior, middle, and inferior thyroid veins. The superior and middle veins drain into the internal jugular veins, while the inferior ones drain into the brachiocephalic trunks. Of special importance for the surgeon is the middle thyroid vein, unaccompanied by an artery, which is the only structure in the region crossing the carotid sheath anteriorly. It can be safely divided over the carotid artery to reflect the thyroid gland before identification of the recurrent laryngeal nerve.

Lymphatic drainage of the thyroid gland is racemose, but destined for pretracheal, paratracheal, and jugular lymph nodes (1).

The relationship of the thyroid gland to the recurrent laryngeal nerves is extremely important for surgeons. If these nerves are involved in a neoplastic process or injured during surgery, alterations of the voice can occur.

The recurrent laryngeal nerves have a different course on the right and left side. After originating from the vagus nerve, the right recurrent laryngeal nerve loops around the subclavian artery and ascends in the tracheoesophageal groove on the posterior aspect of the thyroid. The left recurrent laryngeal nerve loops around the ligamentum arteriosum at the aortic arch after leaving the vagus, and then ascends along the left tracheoesophageal groove. The recurrent laryngeal nerves cross the inferior thyroid artery in the middle-third of the thyroid gland and may course behind the artery (most of the cases), between its branches, or in front of the artery. The inferior parathyroid glands are located anterior to the nerves, at the junction of the recurrent laryngeal nerves and inferior thyroid artery. The recurrent laryngeal nerves may have several trunks (2). The recurrent laryngeal nerve pierces the cricothyroid membrane to innervate all muscles of the larynx except the cricothyroid. It also supplies sensation to the trachea and subglottic region of the larynx. In rare cases, the nerves may not be recurrent and enter the larynx directly. Injury of the recurrent laryngeal nerve on one side leads to ipsilateral vocal cord paralysis, with the cord lacking tension and resting immobile near its midline position.

The superior laryngeal nerve originates from the inferior (nodose) ganglion of the vagus, just caudal to the jugular foramen of the skull. At the level of hyoid bone, it splits into an external and an internal branch. The internal branch travels parallel and medial to the superior laryngeal artery, passes beneath the thyrohyoid muscle to pierce the thyrohyoid membrane, and supplies sensation to the pyriform fossa and laryngeal mucosa above the vocal cords. In rare cases, this branch can have an inferior and medial position relative to the superior laryngeal artery (3). The external branch of the superior laryngeal nerve descends lying on the inferior pharyngeal constrictor muscle. It travels with the superior thyroid artery and, before this artery branches to approach the superior pole of the thyroid gland, the external branch of the recurrent laryngeal nerve pierces the cricothyroid muscle. If this branch is injured, the cricothyroid is paralyzed and the vocal cords cannot be tensed. As a consequence, the timbre and volume of the voice are diminished and the voice tires easily.

Histology

The thyroid gland is divided by fibrous septae into pseudolobules, which are subdivided into 20 to 40 follicles each. The follicles, spherical in shape, are lined by cuboidal epithelium and have a central core of proteinaceous colloid. In the stroma surrounding thyroid follicles, there are C-cells or parafollicular cells. These cells are more numerous in the upper portions of the thyroid lobes and can be either individual or aggregated in the interfollicular stroma (Fig. 2).

Embryology

Development of the thyroid gland begins in the second branchial arch at the base of the tongue, in the region of the foramen cecum. From here, it descends in the anterior region of the neck, between the fusing halves of the hyoid bone and the larynx. The descent occurs along the

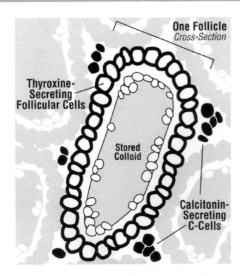

Figure 2 Microanatomy of the thyroid gland.

thyroglossal duct, a structure that will eventually atrophy in normal individuals. During its descent, the thyroid is invaded by cells from the ultimobranchial body from the fourth branchial pouch to populate the gland with the C-cells, or parafollicular cells, that produce calcitonin.

Anomalies of Development

Developmental anomalies may be classified as failure of development, failure of descent, or failure of atrophy of the thyroglossal duct.

The failures of development include thyroid agenesis (athyreosis) or hemiagenesis. Although the pathogenesis of these conditions is not known, it is believed that, at least in some cases, genetic factors might be involved (4).

Failure of descent of thyroid gland results in thyroid tissue being located anywhere along its tract of descent. Although the most common location is the base of the tongue, ectopic thyroid tissue can be sublingual, thyroglossal, or intralaryngotracheal. The presentation depends on the location, and in rare cases these patients can develop ectopic thyroid carcinoma (5,6). The thyroid gland can also descend more caudally, to an intrathoracic location.

When the thyroglossal duct fails to atrophy, the remnants form thyroglossal duct cysts, the most common congenital cervical abnormality. They can be found anywhere in the midline, from the submental region to the suprasternal notch, but are most commonly located in the vicinity of the hyoid bone. These cysts also contain thyroid tissue, which can undergo malignant transformation in 1% of cases (7).

PHYSIOLOGY

The two active thyroid hormones are represented by triiodothyronine (T_3) and tetraiodothyronine (Thyroxine, T_4). Through their secretion, the thyroid gland controls the metabolic rate of most tissues in the body. Regulation of thyroid function is by plasma iodide concentration and hypothalamo-pituitary-thyroid axis.

Iodine Metabolism

The synthesis of thyroid hormones depends on the availability and entry of iodine, one of their major constituents, into the thyroid gland. The sources of iodine in the body are exogenous, from alimentation, and endogenous, from the conservation of degraded thyroid hormones. Organic dietary iodine is converted in the stomach and jejunum to iodide, which is easily absorbed through the intestinal mucosa. Iodide is mainly removed from plasma by the thyroid gland (one-third of iodide concentration) and the kidneys (the remaining two-thirds). Kidney clearance depends on glomerular filtration rate and is not influenced by the plasma hormones or iodide levels.

Synthesis and Secretion of Thyroid Hormones

Synthesis of thyroid hormones is a multistep process, controlled by the secretion of thyroid-stimulating hormone (TSH) from the pituitary gland. This process involves (i) active uptake of iodide into the thyroid cell; (ii) oxidation of iodide to iodine; (iii) efflux of iodine into the follicle and bonding to tyrosine residues in thyroglobulin to form monoiodothyrosines (MIT) and diiodothyrosines (DIT); and (iv) different combinations of MIT and DIT to form active thyroid hormones (T_3 and T_4).

Inorganic iodide is actively transported from plasma into the thyroid follicular cell by a sodium-iodide symporter present in the basolateral plasma membrane. Once inside the cytoplasm, iodide diffuses toward the apical membrane, where it is oxidized under the influence of thyroperoxidase and hydrogen peroxide. It subsequently passes from the thyroid cell into the colloid through a chloride–iodide–transporting protein (8). Here, at the apical membrane, iodine becomes attached to tyrosine residues in the primary sequence of thyroglobulin, a protein produced by the follicular cell and found abundantly in colloid (Fig. 3). Tyrosine iodination gives rise to two molecules, MIT and DIT. Two iodinated tyrosine residues are removed from thyroglobulin and make a dipeptide by a coupling enzyme. MIT and DIT combine to form triiodothyronine (T_3). The combination of two molecules of DIT forms tetraiodothyronine (T_4). Formation of T_3 and T_4 is mediated, at their turn, by thyroperoxidase and hydrogen peroxide. The deiodinated tyrosine has the active carboxyl group. Reverse T_3 is an inactive hormone and has no metabolic functions. It is formed by DIT and MIT, where the monoiodinated tyrosine has the active carboxyl group (Fig. 4).

T_3 and T_4 are stored in the colloid follicle bound to thyroglobulin, but no longer in the primary sequence. For active hormones to be released into the blood, they must cross the thyroid cell. Colloid is taken up by pinocytosis at the apical membrane and, inside the follicular cell, colloid droplets fuse with the lysosomal vesicles to form phagolysosomes, in which proteases hydrolyze thyroglobulin. Subsequently, free T_3 and T_4 are released into the blood. Thyroglubulin hydrolyzation also gives rise to MIT and DIT, which are deiodinated in the follicular cell and the iodine is recycled. T_4 is the dominant product.

Thyroid Hormone Transport and Metabolism

In the blood, thyroid hormone is almost entirely bound to plasma proteins, which act as transporters. Binding proteins include thyroid hormone binding globulin (TBG), thyroid hormone binding prealbumin (TBPA), and albumin. A small quantity of thyroid hormone (0.02%) is unbound and represents the active physiological fraction. Increased TBG levels associated with certain conditions (Table 1) lead to an initial lowering of free hormone concentration.

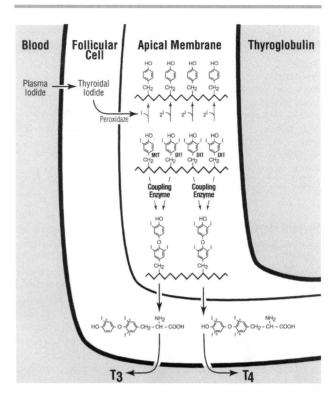

Figure 3 Synthesis of thyroid hormones.

Compensatory mechanisms restore the free hormone levels by raising the total hormone concentration and therefore restoring the euthyroid state.

Although the thyroid secretes more T_4 than T_3 (the T_4:T_3 ratio in the blood is 10:1 to 20:1), T_3 is more active than T_4 and it is less tightly bound to plasma proteins; therefore it enters the extracellular fluid space more quickly. T_4 converts peripherally to T_3, making the thyroid hormone more readily available to the tissues. The peripheral conversion of T_4 also gives rise to the inactive form rT_3 (Fig. 5).

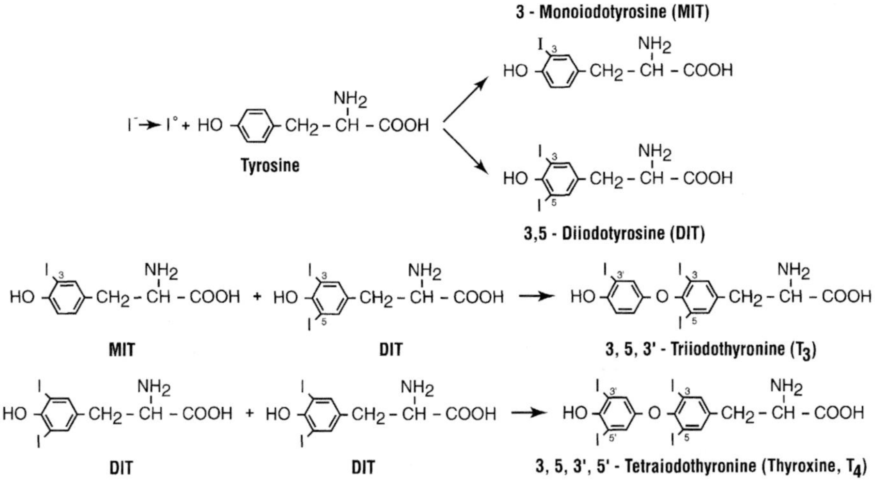

Figure 4 Chemical reactions leading to formation of thyroid hormones.

Table 1 Circumstances Associated with Increased Concentrations of Thyroglobulin

Increased TBG
Pregnancy
Newborn state
Use of oral contraceptives and other sources of estrogen
Use of tamoxifen
Infectious and chronic active hepatitis
Biliary cirrhosis
Acute intermittent porphyria
Perphenazine
Genetic determination

Abbreviation: TBG, thyroid hormone–binding globulin.

Table 2 Conditions Associated with Decreased Peripheral Conversion of T_4 to T_3

Decreased peripheral conversion of T_4 to T_3
Physiologic
Fetal and early neonatal life
Old age
Pathologic
Fasting
Malnutrition
Systemic illness
Physical trauma
Postoperative state
Drugs (propylthiouracil, dexamethasone, propranolol, amiodarone)
Radiographic contrast agents (ipodate, iopanoate)

Thyroid Hormone Action

Thyroid hormones are transported into the cell by an adenosine triphosphate–dependent transport mechanism. Inside the cells, T_3 is the active hormone and it binds to one or more cytoplasmic receptor complexes, which in turn bind to specific regulatory sites on the chromosomes to influence phenotypic expression. There are two classes of thyroid hormone receptors—α and β—each with two isoforms. They are encoded by genes located on chromosomes 17 and 3, respectively. Expression of T_3 receptors is tissue specific, with the liver expressing mostly β receptors, the brain mostly α receptors, and the cardiac muscle both of them.

Thyroid hormone affects most organs and systems in the body, being essential for calorigenesis, by increasing the basal metabolic rate and oxygen consumption rate in all tissues except brain, spleen, and testis. Thyroid hormone modulates intermediary metabolism, by stimulating protein synthesis, glycogenolysis, gluconeogenesis, lipolysis, and synthesis and degradation of cholesterol. It increases the heart rate and myocardial contractility and also increases the total body sensitivity to catecholamines and the number of catecholamine receptors in cardiac muscle. Thyroid hormone also increases bone turnover and stimulates erythropoiesis and steroid hormone release. In childhood, thyroid hormone is essential for normal myelination and development of the nervous system. Thyroid hormone is also essential for normal growth and development.

Thyroid Hormone Elimination

Once inside the peripheral cells, T_3 and T_4 undergo a series of reactions that will ultimately lead to their inactivation and excretion. The most important is deiodination, in which iodine atoms are sequentially removed from the thyronine nucleus. Removal of only one iodine atom from

T_4 yields T_3, and this reaction accounts for almost 80% of T_3 present in the body. It is catalyzed by the type 1 izoenzyme in the liver and kidney and by the type 2 izoenzyme in the pituitary, central nervous system, placenta, and brown fat. In certain conditions, the peripheral conversion of T_4 to T_3 is impaired and may lead to hypothyroidism if a compensatory increase in T_4 production does not follow (Table 2).

After complete deiodination, the free iodine can be recycled in the thyroid or excreted in the kidneys. T_4 and T_3 are also conjugated with glucuronate or sulfate in the liver and then excreted in the bile, thus reaching the small intestine. They can be either excreted or reabsorbed, constituting one enterohepatic circulation.

Regulation of Thyroid Function

Thyroid function is regulated by suprathyroid and intrathyroid mechanisms. The hypothalamic-pituitary-thyroid axis represents the suprathyroid one. TSH is a glycoprotein of 28,000 Da produced by the basophilic cells of the anterior pituitary, and it directly influences thyroid function through multiple mechanisms: (i) thyroid hypertrophy, hyperplasia, and vessel formation; (ii) increased iodine uptake into the follicular cell; (iii) enhanced synthesis of nucleic acids and proteins, including thyroglobulin; and (iv) stimulated synthesis and secretion of thyroid hormones.

TSH secretion from the pituitary gland is regulated by three mechanisms. Secretion is stimulated by thyrotropin-releasing hormone (TRH), a tripeptide from the hypothalamus, and inhibited by somatostatin or raised levels of thyroid hormone in the blood. TRH reaches the pituitary via the hypophyseal portal system and exerts its actions

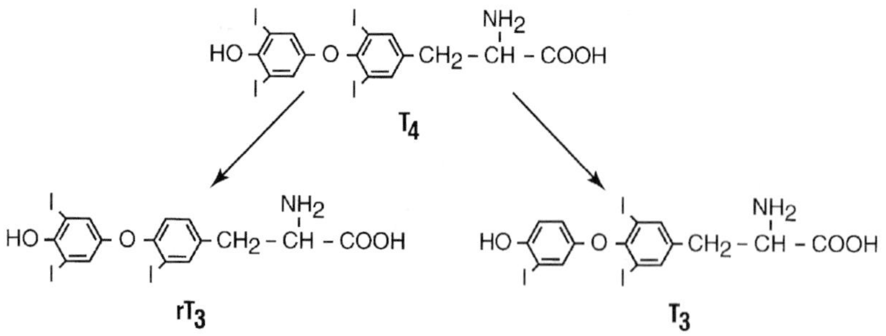

Figure 5 Conversion of thyroxine to triiodothyronine and reverse-triiodothyronine.

through hydrolysis of inositol triphosphate, leading to Ca^{2+} and diacylglycerol activation of protein kinase C. Circulating thyroid hormone also inhibits TRH secretion from the hypothalamus through a feedback loop.

Intrathyroid regulation of thyroid function is also important. Organic iodine concentration in the thyroid gland influences the response to TSH stimulation: low levels of iodine enhance TSH effects on the thyroid, while increased levels inhibit its actions.

Other factors involved in the regulation of the hypothalamo-hypophyseal-thyroid axis in physiologic conditions or in stress include glucocorticoids, tumor necrosis factor-α (TNF-α), interleukins 1 and 6, and interferon-γ (9).

ASSESSMENT OF PATIENTS WITH THYROID DISEASE

The most common complaints that make a patient with thyroid disease present to the physician are related to alteration of thyroid function (either hypo- or hyperfunction) or presence of a mass. Mass and the altered function can be present at the same time.

Signs and Symptoms

Hyperthyroidism, or thyrotoxicosis, is represented by excess circulating levels of thyroid hormone. The common complaints include weight loss with increased appetite, altered mood, irritability, insomnia, heat intolerance, palpitations, amenorrhea or loss of libido, and increased bowel frequency.

Hypothyroidism is characterized by decreased levels of thyroid hormones. Usually, the disease develops progressively and patients seek medical attention late. The symptoms include weight gain, cold intolerance, fatigue, dry skin, menorrhagia, and constipation.

If goiter is present, compression symptoms may be due to the mass effect. These include dysphagia, dyspnea, and choking. Superior vena cava syndrome, although uncommon, can be seen in patients with a large intrathoracic goiter.

Pain is usually not a common presentation in patients with thyroid disease. If present, its characteristics should be noted. Localized pain may suggest either hemorrhage into a colloid nodule or malignancy, especially medullary thyroid carcinoma. Thyroiditis may sometimes present with pain radiating to the ear.

Thyroid disease may present as only a thyroid nodule. Rapid growth of a nodule and changes in the character of the voice are suspicious for malignancy. Voice alteration may occur secondary to vocal cord paralysis due to recurrent laryngeal nerve involvement in a malignant process. However, a benign nodule may grow rapidly after an intralesional hemorrhage, and a benign goiter may stretch the recurrent laryngeal nerve to cause hoarseness.

Patient History

Prior exposure to low doses of ionizing radiation (<1 gray) is associated with an increased frequency of benign thyroid nodules, as well as with increased incidence of thyroid and salivary cancer. This type of exposure was historically applied in infants for thymic enlargement, enlarged adenoids, acne, or tinea capitis. Low irradiation doses are more carcinogenic than the much larger doses used in radiation therapy, which are more likely to cause hypothyroidism.

A family history of benign or malignant diseases of the thyroid is relatively common. This is especially true for medullary carcinoma of the thyroid in multiple endocrine neoplasia (MEN) type II. However, a family history of goiter, thyroiditis, or, rarely, papillary cancer may be encountered. Living in an iodine-deficient area, taking goitrogenic medication, or having relatives with thyroid malformations represent other important factors that may be present in patients with thyroid disease.

Physical Examination

The thyroid gland may not be palpable under normal circumstances. However, it usually can be appreciated by bimanual palpation. The examiner stands behind the seated patient, whose neck is slightly extended. With the examiner's fingers fixed on either side of the trachea, the patient is asked to swallow. The thyroid gland ascends due to its attachments to the trachea. Palpation helps assess thyroid size, thyroid nodules, tenderness, and the consistency of the gland (Fig. 6).

Cervical lymph nodes should also be assessed, both along the carotid sheath and in the posterior triangle of the neck. The presence of enlarged lymph nodes adjacent to a thyroid nodule is highly suggestive of cancer. Sometimes a median lymph node (Delphian node) can be palpated between the isthmus and the cricoid cartilage. It is called Delphian because its presence may predict, like the Delphic oracle, the presence of thyroid cancer when the primary lesion is not palpable.

Laboratory Tests

A large variety of laboratory tests can assess the function of the thyroid gland. However, most of them are only of historical interest and have little importance in the management of thyroid disease.

Ultrasensitive measurement of TSH levels has made this the first-line test for diagnosing hyper- and hypothyroidism (both subclinical and overt), eclipsing all other methods (10). The test, based on nonisotopic immunometric assay, has a sensitivity of 0.02 mIU/L or less. Low TSH implies hyperthyroidism with suppression of the hypothalamo-pituitary-thyroid axis. High TSH implies hypothyroidism

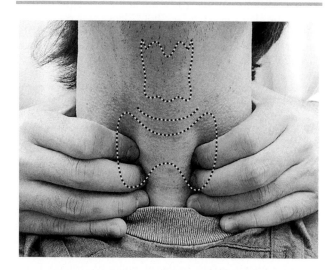

Figure 6 Bimanual examination of the thyroid gland.

Table 3   Thyroid Tests

	Increased	Decreased
Ultrasensitive TSH	Hypothyroidism	Hyperthyroidism
Antiperoxidase	Thyroiditis	N/A
Antithyroglobulin	Graves' disease	
Thyroglobulin	Thyroid malignancy	Thyroidectomy
Thyrocalcitonin	Medullary carcinoma	Thyroidectomy

Abbreviations: TSH, thyroid-stimulating hormone; N/A, not available.

with an appropriate hypothalamo-pituitary response. Ultrasensitive TSH is also the standard way to assess the adequacy of therapeutic thyroid replacement or therapeutic thyroid suppression.

Ultrasensitive TSH may miss the rare patient with either secondary (central) hypothyroidism, or hyperthyroidism due to a TSH-secreting pituitary adenoma or thyroid hormone resistance. Moreover, this test can also be misleading when hypothyroidism was induced in the initial treatment of hyperthyroidism, due to delayed recovery of previously suppressed TSH. When there is any doubt, both TSH and free thyroxine levels (FT_4) should be measured (11).

Thyroid autoantibody tests determine autoimmune thyroiditis. High titers of antithyroid peroxidase antibodies or antithyroglobulin antibodies are encountered in patients with Hashimoto's thyroiditis or Graves' disease.

Serum thyroglobulin is a tumor marker for differentiated thyroid carcinomas. Because thyroglobulin is secreted only by the follicular cell of the thyroid, increased levels in patients after total thyroidectomy suggests the presence of loco-regional recurrence or distant metastases.

Serum calcitonin from C-cells is elevated in medullary carcinoma. If this disease is part of MEN type II, mutations of the RET proto-oncogene may also be detected (Table 3).

Imaging Tests

Radionuclide scanning can demonstrate hypo- or hyperfunctional areas within the thyroid gland, including the function of a palpable thyroid nodule, ectopic thyroid tissue, retrosternal goiter, hemiagenesis of the thyroid, and functioning metastases of thyroid carcinoma. The test employs ^{123}I or sodium [^{99m}Tc] pertechnetate and defines areas within the gland as "cold" or "hot," depending on the concentration of the isotope in that specific area relative to the surrounding tissue. Radionuclide scanning for neoplasm is currently rarely used in clinical practice.

Ultrasonography is useful in assessing the size of the thyroid nodules. It can reliably differentiate between cystic and solid masses, but not between benign and malignant nodules. It is also used to verify the presence of nonpalpable thyroid nodules discovered incidentally by other imaging procedures and to detect cervical lymph nodes in follow-up examination. Ultrasonography may guide the fine needle aspiration biopsy (FNAB). Sequential ultrasonography can assess the progression of a goiter or the regression of the thyroid pathology with resolving inflammation or after medical treatment.

Chest X rays may be helpful in diagnosing a substernal goiter. Computed tomography (CT) and magnetic resonance imaging (MRI) of the neck are not useful in the evaluation of thyroid patients, except in the planning of operations for mediastinal goiter or advanced malignancy. They may give important information when recurrence is suspected but there is no palpable disease in the neck. CT or MRI is strongly indicated by elevation of serum levels of tumor markers such as thyroglobulin or thyrocalcitonin (12).

Fine Needle Aspiration Biopsy

FNAB is a simple and low-risk method used in the assessment of patients with thyroid nodules. Since its introduction into practice in the 1970s, it has become the initial diagnostic test of choice for thyroid nodules. The nodule is pierced with a fine caliber needle and its contents are aspirated into a syringe. The aspirated cells are prepared for cytologic examination. Although the aspiration can be performed by a primary care physician, surgeon, pathologist, or endocrinologist, the accuracy of the test depends on the skills and experience of the cytopathologist.

Two techniques are used for performing FNAB and they yield similar results. In the suction technique, a 22- to 25-gauge needle is attached to a 10- or 20-mL syringe that may, or may not be attached to a "pistol-grip" device. Local anesthesia may be used but an injection of lidocaine to numb the skin for another needle puncture seems unnecessary. The patient may either lie supine, with the neck in hyperextension, or sit. The physician immobilizes the nodule with his nondominant hand, while the needle is advanced rapidly into the nodule. Upon penetration, the needle is moved back and forth multiple times while vigorous negative pressure is applied to the syringe, to dislodge cells and draw them into the needle. The pressure in the syringe must rise to atmospheric pressure before removing the needle to avoid splatter of the material into the syringe chamber. The syringe is then detached from the needle, filled with air, and reattached to extrude the contents of the needle onto the cytology slides. It is recommended that both alcohol-fixed and air-dried smears be prepared with the material extracted from the nodule. The needle and syringe barrel may be rinsed with fixatives to prepare a cellblock after centrifugation of the liquid.

The nonsuction technique is similar, but the thyroid nodule is punctured with a detached needle, which is moved multiple times back and forth within the mass. The needle is then withdrawn and attached to a syringe filled with air, and the content is blown onto the slides for smear preparation.

Either Papanicolaou or hematoxylin and eosin stains may be employed. FNAB is not, however, a substitute for conventional histopathology. Instead, it should be regarded as a component of the diagnostic study of thyroid nodules in combination with clinical, imagistic, and other laboratory data.

Rare complications of the FNAB include bleeding and hematoma formation. Pressure at the aspiration site usually is sufficient. Most importantly, FNAB has not been associated with needle tract implantation of tumor cells.

SICK EUTHYROID SYNDROME

Sick euthyroid syndrome represents a derangement of the thyroid hormone economy in patients with shock, severe illness, trauma, or psychological stress. The abnormality may involve alterations in the peripheral transport and metabolism of thyroid hormones, inappropriate secretion of TSH, or modifications in the function of the thyroid gland. In the most common variant, the sick euthyroid syndrome is characterized by decreased circulating concentrations of T_3 and increased concentrations of rT_3, as a result of impaired conversion of T_4 to T_3 in peripheral tissues. TSH levels in serum are normal, although diminished TSH response to TRH stimulation may be encountered. The abnormalities are of no physiologic importance because the patients are infact euthyroid.

HYPERTHYROIDISM (THYROTOXICOSIS)

Thyrotoxicosis is a disorder of metabolism due to excess thyroid hormone. The cause may be excessive intake of exogenous thyroid hormone or increased secretion of thyroid hormones with loss of the normal feedback inhibition. Graves' disease and toxic multinodular goiter are by far the most common causes of the longer list in Table 4.

Graves' Disease

Graves' disease was first described by Robert Graves of Dublin in 1835. It is the most common form of thyrotoxicosis and is most commonly seen in young women in the third or fourth decade of life. The ratio of women to men is 13:1 and a family history is obtained in 33% of patients. The evidence of this common endocrine disorder is estimated at 1 in 100 people.

Graves' disease is an autoimmune disease where the offending antibody drives the thyroid gland to an excess of secretion. Hyperthyroidism with diffuse goiter is associated with a specific ophthalmopathy. Other extrathyroidal manifestations may include pretibial myxedema, dermopathy, acropathy, and vitiligo.

The thyroid gland is uniformly enlarged, with a smooth consistency and an increased vascularity. Histologically, hyperplasia of the follicular epithelium is present, with columnar appearance and a reduced quantity of colloid. Lymphocytic infiltration with germinal center formation and some regional reactive lymph adenopathy may also be encountered.

Pathogenesis

The pathogenesis of the disease involves antibodies against the TSH receptor on the follicular cell. These antibodies have a stimulatory effect on thyrocytes, leading to increased hormone secretion, hypertrophy, and hyperplasia of the thyroid follicles. Although stimulating TSH receptor antibodies (TSHR-Ab) are unique to patients with Graves' disease, serum of these patients contains a mixture of both blocking and stimulating antibodies (13). These levels of thyroid hormone in patients with Graves' disease are not directly correlated with the TSHR-Ab levels.

Lymphocytic infiltration is common in Graves' disease and these cells are the major source of antibodies (14). Some other locations responsible for antibody production include bone marrow and cervical lymph nodes. Initiation of antibody production in Graves' disease is not clearly understood. Probably a lack of suppressor T-cells leads to multiplication of T-helper cells and subsequent stimulation of TSHR-Ab production from B-cell clones. The intrathyroidal inflammatory cells also produce cytokines, such as interleukin-1, TNF-α, and interferon-γ, which lead to adhesion and activation of local inflammatory cells. Thyrocytes themselves may synthesize other cytokines, which sustain the intrathyroidal autoimmune process (15). However, thyroid follicular cells are not damaged by the lymphocyte infiltration, as in Hashimoto's thyroiditis. The follicular cells are not destroyed because the antibody does not fix complement. This cell preservation might also be explained by the regulation of the apoptotic factor Fas, its ligand, FasL, and the antiapoptotic molecule Bcl-2. The balance of these factors in the infiltrating lymphocytes may lead to their own apoptosis, thus impairing their ability to mediate tissue damage. Contrarily, in the follicular cells, the reduced levels of Fas and increased levels of Bcl-2 probably favor thyrocyte survival and hypertrophy associated with TSHR-Ab (16).

The ophthalmopathy in Graves' disease is probably due to recognition by T-cells of an antigen that cross-reacts with a TSH receptor-like protein, expressed in the periorbital preadipocyte fibroblasts. Lymphocyte infiltration in the extraocular muscles and orbital connective tissue leads to production of cytokines that activate fibroblasts, which secrete hydrophilic glycosaminoglycans, resulting in an increased osmotic pressure, swelling of the extraocular muscles, fluid accumulation, and eventually fibrosis (15).

Predisposition to Graves' disease is determined by genetic, environmental, and endogenous factors in different proportions. The genetic factor is suggested by the presence of disease in homozygous twins and the increased frequency of specific human leukocyte antigens (HLAs) in different populations with Graves' disease: HLA-B8 and HLA DR3 in Caucasian populations, HLA-Bw 35 and HLA-A2 in the Japanese, and HLA-Bw 46 in Chinese populations (17). Psychological stress may trigger Graves' disease. Of the environmental factors, the increased ingestion of iodine seems to play the most important role in initiation of this condition.

Clinical Manifestations

The clinical features of Graves' disease can be divided into signs and symptoms of thyrotoxicosis and those specific to Graves' disease. Common manifestations of hyperthyroidism include hyperactivity, hyper-reflexia, weight loss with increased appetite, irritability, altered mood, insomnia, heat intolerance, increased sweating, warm, moist skin, palpitations, sinus tachycardia, atrial fibrillation, muscle weakness and wasting, oligomenorrhea or amenorrhea, and loss of libido. Diarrhea or increased bowel frequency is the most common abdominal complaint.

Specific manifestations of Graves' disease include goiter, ophthalmopathy, and dermopathy. The goiter is a diffuse enlargement of the thyroid, including the pyramidal lobe, with smooth consistency. Ophthalmopathy includes exophthalmos with proptosis, supraorbital and infraorbital

Table 4 Diseases Associated with Thyrotoxicosis

Causes of hyperthyroidism
Associated with increased thyroid hormone secretion (hyperthyroidism)
Graves' disease
Toxic multinodular goiter
Iodine-induced (Jod–Basedow) thyrotoxicosis
Hyperfunctioning thyroid adenoma
Functioning metastatic thyroid cancer
TSH-secreting pituitary tumors
Struma ovari
Not associated with increased thyroid hormone secretion
Subacute thyroiditis
Trophoblastic tumor (secretes human chorionic gonadotropin with thyroid-stimulating properties)
Thyrotoxicosis factitia (thyroid hormone ingestion)
"Hamburger toxicosis" (ingestion of food prepared from animal thyroid)

Abbreviation: TSH, thyroid-stimulating hormone.

swelling, and chemosis. Skin changes include nonpitting edema of the pretibial region with occasional raised, hyperpigmented, violaceous papules. These physical findings, especially in a young woman, plus a low TSH confirm the diagnosis. TSHR-Ab may be helpful.

Treatment

The goals of treatment in patients with Graves' disease are to restore euthyroidism and to obtain a good control of the symptoms. No therapeutic modality is perfect. Graves' disease is managed by treating the target organ, the thyroid, rather than by addressing the autoimmune process. Treatments include antithyroid drugs, radioiodine, and surgery. The choice of treatment may depend on the age of the patient, the severity of the disease, the size of the goiter and the associated pathology, and regional preferences exist in various parts of the world.

For instance, management of Graves' disease employs the prolonged use of antithyroid drugs in Europe, Asia, New Zealand, Australia, and the former USSR, while radioiodine after antithyroid drugs is preferred in North America (18–22). For failure of medical therapy, surgical ablation is favored in most of the world, while thyroid ablation with radioactive iodine (RAI) is the standard in North America. Initial medical management includes thionamines (antithyroid drugs) in either case.

The antithyroid drugs (propylthiouracil and methimazole) are transported into the follicular cells, where they block thyroid hormone synthesis. Propylthiouracil also blocks the peripheral conversion of T_4 to T_3. Initial dose is 100 to 300 mg propylthiouracil three times a day, or 10 to 30 methimazole three times a day. The dose is dropped when a response is seen, usually in several weeks. Some physicians prefer to add to this regimen 0.05 to 0.1 mg of thyroxine a day, to prevent hypothyroidism (the "block-replace" regimen). Based on the TSH levels, the dose is decreased as euthyroidism is achieved. Propylthiouracil can be used safely during pregnancy, when radioiodine therapy is contraindicated and surgical treatment is not fully embraced by all physicians. The adverse effects of antithyroid drugs include agranulocytosis, hepatitis, vasculitis, thrombocytopenia, rash, arthralgia, and fever. The length of treatment varies between 12 to 24 months in the majority of cases. However, the likelihood of recurrence after treatment is 60% to 70% (15). Therefore definitive therapy is usually required by thyroid ablation method, like radioiodine or surgery.

Surgery is rarely the preferred ablation in the United States, although most authors recommend it for children, very large glands that do not respond well to RAI, those who fail RAI, women in fertility programs likely to conceive in the next year, and those patients who adamantly refuse radiation (23). Ophthalmopathy is not necessarily controlled by operation and mechanistically should not be. Subtotal thyroidectomy is the preferred operation and patients should be euthyroid prior to the operation or at least have a beta-adrenergic blockade. Most patients are euthyroid due to antithyroid drugs. Beta blockade is established prior to operation to prevent thyroid storm.

Thyroid storm is marked by exacerbated symptoms of hyperthyroidism, with tachycardia, hyperpyrexia, congestive heart failure, vomiting, diarrhea, and neurological impairment. If untreated, it can progress to coma. Thyroid storm precipitated in hyperthyroid patients by trauma, infection, or iodine ingestion. All manifestations are apparently mediated by the beta-adrenergic nervous system. If the condition develops, the treatment should take place in an intensive care unit and it employs the use of replacement fluids, antithyroid drugs, beta-blockers, sodium iodate solution or Lugol's solution, hydrocortisone, and a cooling blanket. If the patient is agitated, sedation is recommended.

With preoperative beta blockade, thyroid storm is a preventable complication of surgery for Graves' disease. To prevent thyroid storm, if patients are not completely euthyroid by antithyroid medication prior to operation, very large doses of propranolol are needed to achieve blockade, which is documented by a normal heart rate. Prior to surgery, beta blockade is far more important for a safe operation than a drug-induced euthyroid state. The euthyroid patient may still have a storm, but the patient with beta blockade is secure in this regard. Potassium iodide is a traditional treatment to suppress the thyroid before operation. This tactic also reduces blood flow and may provide some surgical advantage. In fact, a bruit can commonly be heard over the toxic thyroid, which attenuates or disappears on iodine suppression. However, many patients who take oral iodine have gastric distress that may confound the taking of the beta-blocker. Beta blockade is paramount.

Surgical treatment entails subsequent hypothyroidism in about half of patients. Some surgeons prefer total thyroidectomy to avoid recurrence. The operation can be complicated by bleeding, cord paresis, and hypocalcemia. The latter may be due to parathyroid damage or secondary hypoparathyroidism from excess bone metabolism under the influence of thyrotoxicosis.

The more common treatment in the United States calls for RAI and requires no beta blockade. A dosee of 5 to 15 mCi ^{131}I is enough to ablate the gland. The advantage of this medical therapy to permanently correct hyperthyroidism is its ease of dosing and lack of complications. Some authors prefer to use it as a first-line treatment in hyperthyroid patients (24), although the more common approach involves the use of antithyroid drugs first, followed by radioiodine ablation. The most important side effect of radioiodine treatment is hypothyroidism, which occurs in more than 50% at 10 years (25). Less common side effects include worsening of ophthalmopathy and radiation thyroiditis. RAI is contraindicated in pregnancy and children.

Toxic Multinodular Goiter (Plummer's Disease)

Toxic multinodular goiter may complicate long-standing simple goiter. One or more nodules inside the thyroid become hyperfunctional and secrete excess thyroid hormone independent of TSH control. Mutations of the TSH receptors are present in almost all these nodules (26). The condition is more commonly found in the elderly and in iodine-deficient areas. The iodine-deficient goiter will in all likelihood become hyperthyroid if iodine is suddenly reintroduced to the diet.

The clinical presentation is characterized by milder hyperthyroidism symptoms than in Graves' disease and the lack of ophthalmopathy. The thyroid gland is enlarged and nodules can be palpated. Compression symptoms like dysphagia or dyspnea may be present. Laboratory tests show decreased TSH and increased levels of thyroid hormone.

The treatment of choice is thyroidectomy. Antithyroid drugs and beta-blockers are used to control the symptoms prior to operation. Radioiodine therapy is less effective than in Graves' disease. The surgical treatment employs subtotal or total thyroidectomy.

Hot Nodule

Occasionally, thyrotoxicosis is due to a solitary hyperfunctioning nodule. Patients with thyrotoxicosis and a single nodule should have a scan to assess for activity of that nodule. If the single nodule is the cause of thyrotoxicosis, antithyroid drugs and beta-blockers should precede a thyroid lobectomy, which is curative.

HYPOTHYROIDISM

Hypothyroidism is characterized by decreased circulating levels of thyroid hormones. A severe form is represented by myxedema, in which mucopolysaccharides are deposited in the dermis and other tissues. The leading cause of hypothyroidism worldwide is iodine deficiency, although in the United States the most common causes are autoimmune thyroiditis and iatrogenic mechanisms. A more complete classification of the causes of hypothyroidism is listed in Table 5.

Between 60 and 89 years of age 7% of women and 3% of men are hypothyroid (27). Therefore, screening by ultrasensitive TSH is a reasonable measure at this age for subclinical hypothyroidism (28).

Untreated hypothyroidism can progress to myxedema coma, which may be fatal. This condition is associated with hypothermia, stuporous state, respiratory depression, and increased PCO_2.

Decreased levels of thyroid hormones characterize hypothyroidism. The most useful laboratory test is the measure of ultrasensitive TSH, which is increased in primary hypothyroidism and decreased in secondary hypothyroidism.

Table 5   Causes of Hypothyroidism

Primary
  Autoimmune
    Hashimoto's thyroiditis
    Primary idiopathic myxedema
  Iatrogenic
    Thyroidectomy
    ^{131}I therapy
    Antithyroid drugs (aminosalicylic acid, iodides, phenylbutazone,
      iodoantipyrine, lithium)
    Congenital (cretinism)
    Developmental defects
    Heritable biosynthetic defects
    Maternally transmitted (iodides, antithyroid agents, circulating
      antibodies)
  Inflammatory
    Subacute thyroiditis
    Riedel's thyroiditis
  Metabolic
    Iodine deficiency
Secondary
  Pituitary hypothyroidism
    Panhypopituitarism
    Isolated TSH deficiency
  Hypothalamic hypothyroidism
    Congenital defects
    Infection (encephalitis)
    Neoplasm
    Infiltrative (sarcoidosis)
  Peripheral resistance to thyroid hormones

Abbreviation: TSH, thyroid-stimulating hormone.

If autoimmune thyroid disease is present, circulating autoantibodies like antithyroglobulin, antimitochondrial antibodies, or antithyroid-peroxidase may be detected.

Patients with hypothyroidism are treated with thyroid hormone replacement. There is large product variability among the oral thyroid drugs. Levothyroxine (T_4) replacement is between 50 and 200 μg/day, depending on the age of patients and severity of disease. The treatment is monitored by ultrasensitive TSH levels and the clinical response of the patient. Bone resorbtion may be associated with excess thyroid hormone replacement and may limit compliance to therapy (29,30). The end point for thyroid replacement is a drop in TSH and not an arbitrary value for T_4. With this guideline over treatment, metabolic bone disease may be avoided.

THYROIDITIS

Inflammatory disease of the thyroid may be due to a variety of conditions. Riedel's thyroiditis and acute suppurative thyroiditis are rare diseases. Riedel's thyroiditis is characterized by fibrosis of the thyroid and surrounding structures and is sometimes associated with fibrosis of the mediastinum and retroperitoneum, lacrimal ducts, and bile ducts. Patients are euthyroid and have compression symptoms in most of the cases. Treatment may involve the use of steroids, tamoxifen, thyroxine, or surgery.

Acute suppurative thyroiditis is usually preceded by an upper respiratory infection and manifests with tenderness and swelling of the thyroid, localized pain, and general signs of infection. The treatment is represented by intravenous antibiotics and incisional drainage of any abscess, if present. Subacute thyroiditis and Hashimoto's thyroiditis are more common entities, and their characteristics are described below.

Autoimmune Lymphocytic Thyroiditis (Hashimoto's Thyroiditis)

Hashimoto's thyroiditis is a chronic inflammatory disease of the thyroid, and the most common cause of hypothyroidism. It is most frequently encountered in middle age women and is the most common cause of sporadic goiter in children. The disease appears to develop as a result of a complex interaction between predisposing genes and environmental factors (31). Autoimmune factors were proven to play an important role in the pathogenesis of Hashimoto's thyroiditis. The condition may coexist with other autoimmune disease, like pernicious anemia, Sjögren's syndrome, systemic lupus erythematosus, rheumatoid arthritis, adrenal insufficiency, diabetes mellitus, and Graves' disease.

Studies assessing the regulation of apoptosis in endocrine autoimmunity suggest that activation of Fas death receptors and decreased expression of the antiapoptotic molecule Bcl-2 in Hashimoto's thyroiditis can promote thyrocyte apoptosis and gradual reduction in thyrocyte number, leading to hypothyroidism (16).

The clinical manifestations are dominated by the presence of a firm, painless, nontender goiter, which involves symmetrically the entire gland and sometimes also the pyramidal lobe. Compression symptoms, although not common, may be associated. The patients are initially euthyroid, but they become hypothyroid as the disease progresses. This happens due to replacement of thyroid follicles by lymphocytes or fibrous tissue. Thyroid failure is represented by increased levels of TSH and decreased levels of T_4.

Antithyroglobulin and antithyroid peroxidase antibodies are present in most of the cases. In some patients, hyperthyroidism can alternate with hypothyroidism, perhaps due to the intermittent presence of thyroid-stimulating antibodies or disruptions of follicles with random hormone release.

FNAB can confirm the diagnosis and it is recommended when a nodule suggests malignancy. Typical histopathologic findings in Hashimoto's thyroiditis include lymphoid follicles with germinal centers, follicular and Hürthle cells (degenerated epithelial cells), low-to-moderate colloid, and lymphocytes and plasma cells infiltrating the epithelium (32). As lymphocytic infiltration extends, the thyroid tissue degenerates and is progressively replaced by fibrous tissue.

Treatment usually employs the use of thyroxine, which should be administered in the presence of goiter, even if patients are euthyroid. T_4 treatment for six months may reduce the thyroid enlargement by 30% (33).

Patients with thyroiditis are atrocious surgical candidates. Surgical treatment is indicated in the presence of compression symptoms or thyroid pain, unresponsiveness to hormonal replacement therapy, or when cancer is associated (34). No surgeon should express enthusiasm for operation in thyroiditis. The angry gland is adherent, is bloody, and resists removal. Any surgical indication (goiter, hyperthyroidism, or nodules) should be regarded with skepticism if thyroiditis is at issue. Any patient with a tender goiter has thyroiditis until proven otherwise.

Subacute Thyroiditis (De Quervain's, Granulomatous, Giant Cell Thyroiditis)

Subacute thyroiditis is an acute, inflammatory disorder of the thyroid, which is believed to be viral in origin. It usually manifests after an upper respiratory infection. The clinical picture is represented by asthenia, malaise, fever, and unilateral or bilateral thyroid pain. Sometimes the pain is referred to the mandible, ear, or occiput. In some patients, symptoms of thyrotoxicosis may be present due to the disruption of the thyroid follicles by the inflammatory process. Palpation of the gland may reveal uni- or bilateral tenderness and nodularity.

The laboratory findings are represented by elevated erythrocyte sedimentation rate and neutrophilia. In the initial stages of the disease, serum levels of T_3 and T_4 are high, due to leakage of hormones from the gland, and consequently TSH levels are low. Later, as glandular hormones are depleted, patients may pass through a hypothyroid phase, with decreased levels of T_4 and increased TSH. Usually, the clinical picture and lab tests are enough for establishing the diagnosis. However, if FNAB is performed, the histologic examination shows the presence of noncaseous granulomas comprising colloid, inflammatory cells, and multinucleated giant cells. In the nongranulomatous lesions, the cellular inflammatory infiltration leads to disruption of the basement membrane and rupture of the follicles (35).

Treatment employs nonsteroidal anti-inflammatory drugs (NSAIDs), which alleviate the symptoms and allow the disease to run its natural course in an asymptomatic fashion. Beta-blockers may be needed in the initial stages for thyrotoxic patients. In more severe cases, corticosteroids rapidly relieve symptoms in 24 to 48 hours. In rare situations, thyroxine treatment may be used to prevent repeated exacerbations (36). Thyroidectomy, although not part of the routine treatment, should be considered in patients not responsive to the medical treatment or in those with severe dysphagia (37).

Table 6   Types of Thyroid Nodules

Cyst
    Simple cyst
    Mixed cystic-solid nodule
Colloid nodule
Adenoma
    Nonfunctioning or hypofunctioning
    Functioning (hot)
Thyroiditis
Dominant nodule in multinodular goiter
Carcinoma
    Primary
    Metastatic
    Primary lymphoma

De Quervain's thyroiditis usually has a one- to six-week course, after which the symptoms disappear completely. In some cases, the disease lasts longer, with alternating recurrence and remission episodes. Rarely, recurrence may occur years after the initial episode (38). Permanent hypothyroidism may develop in a small number of patients, despite NSAID or corticosteroid therapy (39).

THYROID NODULE

Palpable thyroid nodules are found in 4% to 7% of the general population, but ultrasound shows nodules in 19% to 67% of the population (40,41). A solitary thyroid nodule is a discrete mass within a normal size thyroid or a diffusely enlarged goiter. Dominant thyroid nodules are defined as large nodules in a multinodular thyroid. The prevalence of thyroid nodules appears to increase with age, and women are more affected than men. Different thyroid conditions may present as a thyroid nodule (Table 6).

The vast majority of thyroid nodules are benign and do not require removal. However, the nodules occurring in children and in the elderly have an increased chance of being malignant and the nodules in males are more suspect than those in females. The challenge for the physician is to assess the risk factors for thyroid cancer and to determine the number of patients who will benefit from surgical intervention. Malignancy accounts for 20% of the palpable solitary thyroid nodules in euthyroid patients.

The risk for a solitary or dominant thyroid nodule to be malignant is increased in patients previously exposed to low-dose ionizing radiation of the head and neck or if another family member has thyroid cancer. Moreover, the characteristics of the nodule or the associated symptoms can be highly suggestive of malignancy. Factors associated with an increased risk for thyroid cancer are listed in Table 7.

Table 7   Factors Associated with Increased Risk for Thyroid Cancer

Older male
Exposure to low-dose ionizing radiation
Family member with thyroid cancer or MEN type II or type III
Rapid growth of nodule
Adherence of the nodule to trachea or strap muscles
Compression symptoms (dyspnea, dysphagia)
Horner's syndrome
Hoarseness
Cervical lymphadenopathy adjacent to a thyroid nodule

Abbreviation: MEN, multiple endocrine neoplasia.

Table 8 Diagnostic Groups for Fine Needle Aspiration Biopsy of the Thyroid

Benign thyroid nodule
    Scant cells
    Colloid
Indeterminate thyroid nodule
    Numerous follicular cells, scant colloid
    Consistent with follicular neoplasm
    Hürthle cells
Malignant thyroid nodule
    Papillary
    Follicular
    Medullary
    Anaplastic
    Lymphoma
    Metastatic

Evaluation of Thyroid Nodules

FNAB is the method of choice for evaluating patients with thyroid nodules. The procedure is fast, inexpensive, accurate, minimally invasive, and causes little discomfort to the patient. Since its introduction into clinical practice, FNAB reduced the number of patients who require surgery and increased the percentage of malignant lesions in the excised nodules. The procedure still has limitations, and false-negative results are encountered in some patients. This is why patients with an initial benign FNAB should be followed up, and the procedure repeated if the nodule persists.

Table 8 illustrates the terminology used by most laboratories for reporting the results of the FNAB.

Primary malignant nodules are treated surgically. These lesions, which are highly cellular, may represent an adenoma or a malignancy with well-differentiated follicular cells. These patients should be scanned, and if the nodule is cold, it should be treated surgically. If the nodule is clearly benign as in colloid nodule or inflammatory lesions are present, the patient is followed with serial examinations, and FNAB is repeated if suspicion increases. Even benign nodules are appropriately treated by excision if they become symptomatic. Hürthle cells seen alone reflect a worrisome neoplasm. However, Hürthle cells in the company of inflammatory cells are consistent with thyroiditis.

Management of a solitary thyroid nodule follows the algorithm in Figure 7.

THYROID CANCER

Thyroid cancers have variable histology, patterns of metastasis, and response to therapy. They account for approximately

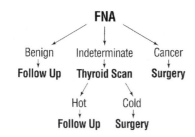

Figure 7 Algorithm for management of patients with a solitary thyroid nodule. *Abbreviation*: FNA, fine needle aspiration.

Table 9 The Number of New Cases and Deaths Per Year for Several Organ Malignancies

Site	New cases per year	Deaths per year
Ovary	23,300	13,900
Pancreas	30,300	29,700
Brain	17,000	13,100
Esophagus	13,100	12,600
Thyroid	20,700	1300

1.5% of all new malignancies. Thyroid cancer is in the middle rank of malignancies in the United States along with ovarian, pancreatic, brain, or esophageal cancers. However, unlike those other diseases, thyroid cancer is a very rare cause of death as shown in Table 9 (42).

Of all thyroid malignancies, 94% are differentiated thyroid carcinomas, that is follicular or papillary carcinomas; 5% are medullary thyroid carcinomas, and 1% are anaplastic (43,44). The chief complaint is usually a palpable solitary nodule, which if properly diagnosed and managed, has a wonderful probability of survival for well-differentiated thyroid cancer. The 10-year survival for thyroid carcinomas is approximately 93% to 98% for the papillary type, 85% to 92% for the follicular carcinomas, 75% to 80% for the medullary, and 13% to 14% for the anaplastic ones (Table 10). These recent reports represent a substantial improvement over statistics from 20 years ago (44,45).

The molecular basis and the genetics of thyroid carcinomas are unclear. The familial inheritance is most obvious in medullary thyroid carcinomas, in which a mutation in the tyrosine kinase proto-oncogene RET, located on chromosome 10, is transmitted in an autosomal dominant way and is present in 98% of the affected family members. However, familial aggregation may be also present in 5% of patients with differentiated thyroid carcinoma, or this condition may be inherited as a component of familial adenomatous polyposis, Gardner's syndrome, or Cowden's disease (43).

Low-dose irradiation of the head or neck for varied conditions favors the development of thyroid carcinomas. The phenomenon was observed after the nuclear accident at Cherbonyl, which led to an increase in the incidence of papillary carcinomas of the thyroid (46,47). RET activation with production of the RET/papillary thyroid carcinoma (PTC) oncogenes is only present in a limited number of patients with papillary carcinomas, and it may also be present in benign thyroid disease (48). Besides the RET/PTC rearrangements, some other mechanisms may be implicated in the etiology of papillary carcinomas. A more complete list of these factors is outlined in Table 11. The RET mutation in MEN may be demonstrated in every cell of the body (germ line), while the mutations in the papillary cancer are limited to the tumor (somatic).

One distinction of follicular adenoma from carcinoma is point mutation in the ras oncogenes and deletion of genes from chromosomes 11 and 3, but none of these findings can have a predictive or diagnostic role.

Table 10 The Incidence and 10-Year Survival Rates for Different Thyroid Carcinomas

	Incidence (%)	10-year survival rate (%)
Papillary carcinoma	80	93–98
Follicular carcinoma	15	85–92
Medullary carcinoma	4–5	75–80
Anaplastic carcinoma	1–2	13–14

Table 11 Factors Associated with the Development of Thyroid Carcinomas

Papillary carcinoma
   RET rearrangements (chromosome 1)-RET/PTC 1, RET/PTC 3
   TRK-A (chromosome 1) overexpression
   Mitogen-activated protein kinase overexpression
   c-myc overexpression
   c-fos overexpression
   c-ras overexpression
   c-erb B2/neu overexpression
   DNA hypermetilation
   Cell cycle dysregulation
Follicular carcinoma
   Ras mutations
   Deletions of genes from chromosome 11q
   Deletion of chromosome 3p
   Pax8-peroxisome proliferator activated receptor recombination
Medullary carcinoma
   RET mutations
Anaplastic carcinoma
   p53 mutations

Abbreviations: RET, rearranged during transfection; PTC, papillary thyroid carcinoma; TRK, tropomyocin receptor kinase.

As stated before, medullary thyroid carcinomas have a high familial aggregation, and RET mutations are a common finding in all family members with the disease. The mutations are also present in some of the patients with clinically sporadic disease.

Mutations of the p53 tumor suppressor gene lead to proliferation of malignant cells and are present in many cancers. Between 60% and 90% of patients with undifferentiated and anaplastic carcinomas also have this mutation (49).

Although different staging systems exist for differentiated thyroid carcinoma, the tumor node metastasis (TNM) classification (Table 12) is the most recommended for use and represents the most useful way to predict death from thyroid cancer. However, other staging systems are in common use (Tables 13 and 14).

Papillary Carcinoma

Papillary carcinoma is the most common form of thyroid cancer. FNAB is usually diagnostic. Papillary carcinomas have pathologic features that make them unique compared with the other forms of thyroid cancer. These include the presence of cuboidal cells with pale and abundant

Table 12 The Tumor Node Metastasis Classification for Thyroid Carcinomas

Primary tumor (T)	
TX	Primary tumor cannot be assessed
T0	No evidence of primary tumor
T1	1 cm or less, limited to thyroid
T2	1.1–4 cm
T3	More than 4 cm, limited to thyroid
T4	Any size, extends beyond thyroid capsule
Nodal involvement (N)	
NX	Nodes cannot be assessed
N0	No regional nodes involved
N1	Regional nodes involved
Distant metastases (M)	
MX	Metastases cannot be assessed
M0	No metastases present
M1	Distant metastases present

Table 13 Stage Grouping for Differentiated Thyroid Carcinomas

Stage	Age <45 years	Age >45 years
I	M0	T1
II	M1	T2-3
III	–	T4 or N1
IV	–	M1

cytoplasm and intranuclear inclusions, called "Orphan Annie" cells. The name comes from a cartoon strip character of the same name who was depicted with large but featureless blank eyes. The stroma may contain calcium deposits known as psammoma bodies. Although the histology of papillary carcinomas resembles the normal histology of the gland to a lesser degree when compared to follicular carcinoma, the prognosis is better in papillary than in the follicular carcinoma.

Unlike most cancers, the papillary carcinomas have a better prognosis if present in younger patients, and are generally more fatal in older patients. In 20% to 30% of cases, the lesion may be multicentric, but this does not affect the prognosis of the disease. Papillary cancer metastasizes by lymphatic spread. However, in advanced forms, papillary tumors may invade neighboring structures or metastasize hematogenously. The presence of metastases in the lymph nodes has little influence on the prognosis, as well. The anomalous features of papillary cancer relative to other malignancies are listed in Table 15.

In 1987, clinicians at the Mayo Clinic found four independent variables for well-differentiated thyroid cancer by multivariable analysis, which affects prognosis. Patient age and tumor grade, extent, and size were the four variables and a score could be assigned (50,51). Indeed younger patients fare better and lymph node metastases are not a significant barrier. At one time, those patients at higher risk were thought to be candidates for more radical surgical treatment. However, no additional benefit at 10-year or 25-year survival can be shown with bilateral resections compared to unilateral operations, even for large tumors.

Treatment of Differentiated Thyroid Carcinoma
Surgical Treatment
Surgery is the treatment of choice for differentiated thyroid carcinoma. The extent of resection varies.

Total thyroidectomy is supported by the following facts: 5% to 10% of recurrences of papillary carcinoma after lobectomy occur in the contralateral lobe (50); postoperative radioiodine treatment is more effective if there is no normal tissue competing in affinity for the iodine; and the thyroglobulin monitoring has a higher specificity as a marker of recurrence if total thyroidectomy was performed. Moreover, the incidence of locoregional recurrence is proved to be lower in total versus unilateral thyroidectomy (52), while,

Table 14 Stage Grouping for Medullary Thyroid Carcinomas

Stage	Characteristic
I	T1
II	T2-4
III	N1
IV	M1

Table 15 Prognostic Features of Papillary Thyroid Carcinoma That Differentiate It from Most Malignancies

Anomalous behavior of papillary carcinoma
Better prognosis in young patients
Better prognosis than follicular cancer, although worse histology
Multicentricity does not affect prognosis
Presence of lymph node metastases does not affect prognosis

Table 16 Tumor Recurrence 10 Years After Initial Surgery for Different Postoperative Approaches in Patients with Differentiated Thyroid Carcinoma

Type of postoperative treatment	Total recurrences (%)
None	40
T_4 alone	22
T_4 + RAI remnant ablation	8

Abbreviation: RAI, radioactive iodine.

in high-risk patients, mortality is moderately decreased after bilateral operations in some reports (53).

A very prudent variant of total thyroidectomy is near-total thyroidectomy. In this maneuver, an inconsequential 50 mg of thyroid tissue at the tubercle of Zuckerkandl is left intact to avoid a tedious dissection of the recurrent laryngeal nerve near its entry into the cricothyroid membrane.

Unilateral thyroidectomy is a highly effective treatment of differentiated thyroid carcinoma. The reasons to support it are the absence of any substantial survival benefits with more extensive procedures, and unaffected prognosis of papillary carcinomas by the multicentricity of the disease. In low-risk patients, the cause-specific mortality and the incidence of distant metastases are not significantly higher if thyroid lobectomy is performed, compared to total thyroidectomy (52). However, leaving one lobe of the thyroid in place has the disadvantage of making the postoperative monitoring with thyroglobulin impossible.

All patients receive T_4 to deprive any remaining tumor cells of the trophic effects of TSH. Therefore, leaving the contralateral lobe does not provide any thyroid function.

The complications of total versus unilateral thyroidectomy are not different (54), especially if a parathyroid autograft is routinely done to prevent hypoparathyroidism (55). Although positive lymph nodes do not have a major influence on the survival rate in papillary carcinoma, removal of palpable nodes is recommended.

Radioiodine Ablation of Residual Thyroid Tissue
Postoperative iodine ablation is advised in patients with differentiated thyroid carcinoma who had an initial tumor larger than 1.5 cm. This treatment was proved to reduce the recurrence of disease in patients of all ages, and to reduce the risk of death from thyroid carcinoma in patients older than 40 years at the time of diagnosis (56). The effects of therapy are less profound if the initial tumor was less than 1.5 cm, unless there is history of radiation exposure, extrathyroid invasion, or metastasis (57).

Postoperative ^{131}I adjuvant therapy in well-differentiated thyroid carcinoma decreases recurrences by elimination of microscopic residual or metastatic disease (44,58,59). Some authors report increased disease-free intervals (60) and prolonged survival with radioiodine therapy (57). Radioiodine is concentrated into the follicular cells, including malignant cells of follicular origin. Once inside the cell, the isotope releases high-energy electrons, which undergo both β and γ decay, resulting in high radiation ablation locally. Gamma rays can also be detected in scanning procedures, for diagnostic purposes. The effective radiation doses are 100 mCi for functioning tissue in the thyroid bed, 150 to 175 mCi for cervical node metastases, 175 to 200 mCi for lung metastases, and 200 mCi for skeletal metastases (61). The tissue dose is 250 Gy when 150 mCi are given. In 80% of cases, all residual malignancies or nodal metastases will be ablated by a radiation dose of 30,000 rad delivered to the residual thyroid tissue or 10,000 ± 2000 rad/lymph node (62).

Because TSH stimulates iodine trapping into the follicular cells, TSH should be driven to higher levels prior to ^{131}I administration (40 pg/mL). Therefore, thyroid hormone replacement therapy should be delayed until after this procedure, and it takes three to four weeks for patients to become profoundly hypothyroid with high TSH. However, T_3 (cytomel) can be given until about a week prior to study and the TSH will still rise. Foods with high concentration of iodine should be avoided, because non-RAI trapping into the thyroid tissue would impede the capture of ^{131}I isotope.

After TSH is stimulated (3–4 weeks), a total body thyroid scan is performed. If there is an uptake of iodine at any site, 150 mCi of RAI are given. Residual thyroid activity in the neck does not imply metastatic disease. Some 25% of patients after anatomically complete thyroidectomy will have some residual activity in ectopic thyroid tissue. Thus, the near total thyroidectomy leaving 50 mg of thyroid tissue does not have any significant impact or raise any grave concerns when there is a small amount of activity on the total body scan.

Thyroid hormone administration is the most important adjunctive measure for differentiated thyroid tumors to reduce local recurrence. This is true if the patient has residual functioning lobe or needs replacement if total thyroidectomy has been done. TSH from the pituitary stimulates the growth of differentiated thyroid carcinoma. Thyroxine (T_4) at a dose of 150 mcg/day is preferred to T_3 for several reasons. T_4 has a longer half-life than T_3 (1 week, compared to 1 day), allowing a sustained suppression of TSH. Another advantage is that cardiac arrhythmias occur less with T_4 than with T_3 (54). However, TSH suppression may still have adverse effects, which include acceleration of osteoporosis, provocation of atrial fibrillation, and cardiac hypertrophy and dysfunction (43).

The effects of different treatments on the number of total recurrences 10 years following total thyroidectomy for differentiated thyroid carcinoma are summarized in Table 16 (57).

Other Therapeutic Options
External beam radiotherapy showed little beneficial value in the management of patients with differentiated thyroid carcinoma, because these tumors are not especially radiosensitive. It may be effective if gross extrathyroidal invasion is present, after incomplete resection, or if the tumor does not take up RAI.

Chemotherapy is used in patients who do not respond to surgery and radioiodine treatment. Doxorubicin, either alone or in combination with other drugs, may improve the survival rate in this category of patients.

Follow-Up of Patients with Differentiated Thyroid Cancer
The long-term follow-up regimen is well established. Thyroglobulin is tested yearly and total body ^{131}I scanning should be performed every three to five years to identify

recurrences. TSH is measured yearly to assess T_4 replacement and suppression. Physical examination yearly helps assess local, nodal, or thyroid bed recurrences.

Follicular Carcinoma

Follicular carcinoma is the other type of differentiated carcinoma of the thyroid. It occurs in older age groups than the papillary type, and it is more frequent in iodine-deficient areas. The FNAB cannot always differentiate between follicular adenoma and carcinoma. The lesion is typically unifocal and surrounded by a capsule. Microscopically, the follicles are present but they contain little colloid. Follicular tumors metastasize hematogenously to bone and lung. Lymphatic spread is uncommon. Follicular carcinoma is also less likely than papillary to take up radioiodine.

Occasionally, FNAB will show follicular cells, but histology of the specimen shows mixed papillary and follicular carcinoma. These mixed tumors do not show a malignant behavior intermediate between papillary and follicular carcinomas. All tumors with any element of papillary cancer behave in the more favorable pattern of papillary lesions.

Hürthle Cell Carcinoma

Hürthle cell carcinoma is considered a variant of follicular cell neoplasm. It is often an aggressive tumor with a worse prognosis than differentiated thyroid carcinoma. Hürthle cell carcinomas originate in the oxyphilic cells of the thyroid, whose function is unknown, and are characterized microscopically by the presence of oxyphilic cells with an increased number of mitochondria.

Contrary to follicular cell carcinomas, Hürthle cell carcinomas are more likely to be multifocal and bilateral, they metastasize more often in the regional lymph nodes, and are even less likely to take up radioiodine. Total thyroidectomy with ipsilateral central neck lymphadenectomy and modified radical neck dissection is the procedure of choice when there is evidence of central or lateral node involvement (63). Postoperative radioiodine ablation of any thyroid remnant is advised, although fewer than 10% of these neoplasms take up ^{131}I. All patients with Hürthle cell carcinoma should be administered thyroid hormones, because most of these tumors have TSH receptors. Like differentiated thyroid carcinomas, Hürthle cell carcinomas produce thyroglobulin. Therefore, postoperative follow-up by measuring serum thyroglobulin levels is effective in detecting tumor recurrences.

Anaplastic Carcinoma

Anaplastic carcinoma is the worst of all follicular cell malignancies and the most aggressive of all thyroid tumors. It is encountered mainly in the elderly, with a peak incidence in the seventh and eighth decades of life. It is slightly more common in women than in men. The tumor occurs more frequently in iodine deficient areas and is associated with a history of goiter or differentiated thyroid carcinoma. Explosive growth may occur, leading to death within a few months after diagnosis.

Microscopically, anaplastic carcinomas are characterized by the presence of different cell populations. Large multinucleated cells or spindle-shaped cells may be encountered. Furthermore, foci of papillary or follicular malignant cells may also be present.

Anaplastic carcinomas metastasize very frequently, by local, lymphatic, and hematogenous ways. Local invasion is aggressive, leading to dyspnea, dysphagia, and dysphonia. Cervical lymph nodes are usually palpable at presentation.

Distant metastases may be present in lungs, pleura, bone, and brain (43).

There is no effective treatment for patients with anaplastic carcinoma. Several approaches have been tried, including combination of surgery, radiotherapy, and chemotherapy, but the results are not satisfactory. The role of the surgery is palliative and its purpose is to maintain the integrity of the aerodigestive tract for as long as possible.

Medullary Thyroid Carcinoma

Medullary thyroid carcinoma arises from the parafollicular (or C) cells of the thyroid. These are neuroectodermal cells derived from the ultimobranchial bodies of the fourth branchial pouch, and more densely populate the superior parts of the thyroid lobes. The condition may occur either as a sporadic form, which accounts for 80% of the cases, or as familial forms. The inherited forms may, in turn, be part of MEN type II and type III syndromes or may occur in a non-MEN setting. MEN type II is characterized by the presence of medullary thyroid carcinoma associated with pheochromocytoma and parathyroid hyperplasia. Hirschsprung's disease and lichen cutaneous amyloidosis may be associated in rare cases. Patients with MEN type III have medullary thyroid carcinoma, pheochromocytoma, ganglioneuromatosis, and marfanoid habitus.

Multicentricity is encountered in 20% to 30% of sporadic cases and in almost all familial ones. Microscopically, medullary thyroid carcinomas have great heterogenicity, with sheets of polygonal or spindle-shaped cells in an amyloid and collagen stroma. Certain staining features make the diagnosis of medullary thyroid carcinoma sure, and these include the presence of amyloid, calcitonin secretory granules, and carcinoembryonic antigen (CEA). The mode of spread may be lymphatic or hematogenous. In 50% of patients, enlarged cervical lymph nodes are noted at initial presentation. The tendency of tumor and the involved lymph nodes to calcify may help in making the diagnosis, when calcification is noted on radiographs of the neck.

Medullary thyroid carcinoma is slightly more common in women than in men. The sporadic form has a peak incidence in the fifth or sixth decades of life, although the disease may appear at younger ages in patients with MEN syndromes. The chief complaint at presentation is a neck mass, which may be associated with cervical lymphadenopathy or compression symptoms. Medullary thyroid tumors may secrete a variety of peptides, including calcitonin, calcitonin gene–related peptide, adrenocorticotrophic hormone, CEA, and serotonin. These lead to unusual symptoms, like diarrhea, Cushing's syndrome, or facial flushing.

The diagnosis is usually made by FNAB. Although serum calcitonin is increased in patients with medullary thyroid carcinomas, routine use of this test is not recommended in the assessment of all patients with thyroid nodules, because the test is not cost-effective. Because it is difficult to distinguish between familial and nonfamilial forms of the disease, RET mutations should be assessed in all newly diagnosed patients. Differentiation between the gene line mutations of the sporadic versus familial forms helps the surgeon decide whether preoperative screening for pheochromocytoma is necessary. If RET testing cannot be performed, serum calcium and 24-hour urinary excretion of metanephrines and catecholamines should be measured before the operation, to exclude the MEN syndrome.

The treatment of patients with medullary thyroid carcinoma consists of total thyroidectomy with bilateral central neck compartment dissection, because these lymph nodes are involved early in the disease. If central lymph nodes are positive at the time of operation, additional prophylactic ipsilateral radical neck dissection is recommended. If the primary tumor is bilateral, then bilateral radical neck dissection is advised (64). Postoperative external beam irradiation may be useful in patients at high risk for regional recurrences. Because these tumors originate from the C-cells, RAI therapy and TSH suppression have no influence on the outcome. Somatostatin may help alleviate associated symptoms (diarrhea, flushing, weight loss, etc.). Postoperative thyroid hormone replacement is of course necessary after thyroidectomy.

The postoperative follow-up is done by measuring the blood levels of calcitonin and CEA. Increased values after the operation alert the surgeon to look for residual disease in the neck and distant metastases. The imaging studies to localize residual or recurrent disease may include ultrasonography, CT, and MRI. Tumor markers may implicate residual disease long before any tumor can be detected by palpation or imaging. In these circumstances, prescriptive ablative surgery offers no advantage over prudent waiting and selective application of surgery or chemotherapy.

SUMMARY

The thyroid gland is of significance to the surgeon in two important respects. First, its dysfunction can adversely affect the perioperative management of a patient requiring surgery, making it mandatory that any physiologic aberration is corrected preoperatively. Second, surgery often plays an important role in managing patients with enlarged glands and hyperthyroid states as well as individuals with thyroid lesions that could be potentially malignant. A thorough understanding of these pathologic states and their current management have greatly benefitted individuals who will need thyroid surgery. Except in unusual circumstances, a good-to-excellent outcome can be expected with minimal morbidity and almost no mortality.

REFERENCES

1. Wiseman SM, Hicks WL Jr, Chu QD, Rigual NR. Sentinel lymph node biopsy in staging of differentiated thyroid cancer: a critical review. Surg Oncol 2002; 11(3):137–142.
2. Hisham AN, Lukman MR. Recurrent laryngeal nerve in thyroid surgery: a critical appraisal. ANZ J Surg 2002; 72(12):887–889.
3. Furlan JC, Brandao LG, Ferraz AR, Rodrigues AJ Jr. Surgical anatomy of the extralaryngeal aspect of the superior laryngeal nerve. Arch Otolaryngol Head Neck Surg 2003; 129(1):79–82.
4. Leger J, Marinovic D, Garel C, Bonaiti-Pellie C, Polak M, Czernichow P. Thyroid developmental anomalies in first degree relatives of children with congenital hypothyroidism. J Clin Endocrinol Metab 2002; 87(2):575.
5. Jimenez OV, Ruiz RR, Davila MA, et al. Intra-laryngeal ectopic thyroid tissue. Report of one case and review of the literature. Acta Otorrinolaringol Esp 2002; 53(1):54–59.
6. Massine RE, Durning SJ, Koroscil TM. Lingual thyroid carcinoma: a case report and review of the literature. Thyroid 2001:1191–1196.
7. Organ GM, Organ CH Jr. Thyroid gland and surgery of the thyroglossal duct: exercise in applied embryology. World J Surg 2000; 24(8):886–890.
8. Nilsson M. Iodide handling by the thyroid epithelial cell. Exp Clin Endocrinol Diab 2001; 109(1):13–17.
9. Reichlin S. Neuroendocrine-immune interactions. N Engl J Med 1993; 329(17):1246.
10. Demers LM, Spencer CA. Laboratory medicine practice guidelines: laboratory support for the diagnosis and monitoring of thyroid disease. Clin Endocrinol 2003; 58(2):138–140.
11. Beckett GJ, Toft AD. First-line thyroid function tests—TSH alone is not enough. Clin Endocrinol 2003; 58(1):20–21.
12. Lawrence W Jr, Kaplan BJ. Diagnosis and management of patients with thyroid nodules. J Surg Oncol 2002; 80(3):157–170.
13. Davies T, Marians R, Latif R. The TSH receptor reveals itself. J Clin Invest 2002; 110(2):161–164.
14. Simchen C, Lehmann I, Sittig D, Steinert M, Aust G. Expression and regulation of regulated on activation, normal T cells expressed and secreted in thyroid tissue of patients with Graves' disease and thyroid autonomy and in thyroid-derived cell populations. J Clin Endocrinol Metab 2000; 85(12):4758.
15. Weetman AP. Graves' disease. N Engl J Med 2000; 343(17):1236.
16. Salmaso C, Bagnasco M, Pesce G, et al. Regulation of apoptosis in endocrine autoimmunity: insights from Hashimoto's thyroiditis and Graves' disease. Ann NY Acad Sci 2002; 966:496–501.
17. Huang M, Wu J, Lee TD, Yang EKL, Shaw K, Yeh C. The association of HLA-A, -B, and -DRB1 genotypes with Graves' disease in Taiwanese people. Tissue Antigens 2003; 61(2):154–158.
18. Ford HC, Delahunt JW, Feek CM. The management of Graves' disease in New Zealand: results of a national survey. N Z Med J 1991; 104(914):251–252.
19. Wartofsky L, Glinoer D, Solomon B, Lagasse R. Differences and similarities in the treatment of diffuse goiter in Europe and the United States. Exp Clin Endocrinol 1991; 97(2–3):243–251.
20. Tominaga T, Yokoyama N, Nagataki S, et al. International differences in approaches to ^{131}I therapy for Graves' disease: case selection and restrictions recommended to patients in Japan, Korea, and China. Thyroid 1997; 7(2):217–220.
21. Gerasimov G, Judenitch O, Zdanova E, et al. The management of hyperthyroidism due to Graves' disease in the former USSR in 1991: results of a survey. J Endocrinol Invest 1992; 15(7):513–517.
22. Walsh JP. Management of Graves' disease in Australia. Aust N Z J Med 2000; 30(5):559–566.
23. Alsanea O, Clark OH. Treatment of Graves' disease: the advantages of surgery. Endocrinol Metab Clin North Am 2000; 29(2):321–337.
24. Solomon B, Glinoer D, Lagasse R, Wartofsky L. Current trends in the management of Graves' disease. J Clin Endocrinol Metab 1990; 70(6):1518–1524.
25. Ginsberg J. Diagnosis and management of Graves' disease. CMAJ 2003; 168(5):575.
26. Luft FC. Toxic thyroid adenoma and toxic multinodular goiter. J Mol Med 2001; 78(12):657–660.
27. Sawin CT, Chopra D, Azizi F, Mannix JE, Bacharach P. The aging thyroid. Increased prevalence of elevated serum thyrotropin levels in the elderly. JAMA 1979; 242(3):247–250.
28. Woolf SH. Laboratory screening tests. In: Woolf SH, Jonas S, Lawrence RS, eds. Health Promotion and Disease Prevention in Clinical Practice. Williams & Wilkins, 1996:85–142.
29. Coindre JM, David JP, Riviere L, et al. Bone loss in hypothyroidism with hormone replacement. A histomorphometric study. Arch Intern Med 1986; 146(1):48–53.
30. Krolner B, Jorgensen JV, Nielsen SP. Spinal bone mineral content in myxoedema and thyrotoxicosis. Effects of thyroid hormone(s) and antithyroid treatment. Clin Endocrinol (Oxf) 1983; 18(5):439–446.
31. Tomer Y, Barbesino G, Greenberg DA, Concepcion E, Davies TF. Mapping the major susceptibility loci for familial Graves' and Hashimoto's diseases: evidence for genetic heterogeneity and gene interactions. J Clin Endocrinol Metab 1999; 84(12): 4656–4664.
32. Kumar N, Ray C, Jain S. Aspiration cytology of Hashimoto's thyroiditis in an endemic area. Cytopathology 2002; 13(1): 31–39.
33. Dayan CM, Daniels GH. Chronic autoimmune thyroiditis. N Engl J Med 1996; 335(2):99–107.
34. Gourgiotis L, Al Zubaidi N, Skarulis MC, et al. Successful outcome after surgical management in two cases of the "painful variant" of Hashimoto's thyroiditis. Endocr Pract 2002; 8(4):259–265.

35. Kojima M, Nakamura S, Oyama T, Sugihara S, Sakata N, Masawa N. Cellular composition of subacute thyroiditis an immunohistochemical study of six cases. Pathol Res Pract 2002; 198(12):833–837.

36. Volpe R. The management of subacute (DeQuervain's) thyroiditis. Thyroid 1993; 3(3):253–255.

37. Duininck TM, van Heerden JA, Fatourechi V, et al. de Quervain's thyroiditis: surgical experience. Endocr Pract 2002; 8(4):255–258.

38. Iitaka M, Momotani N, Ishii J, Ito K. Incidence of subacute thyroiditis recurrences after a prolonged latency: 24-year survey. J Clin Endocrinol Metab 1996; 81(2):466–469.

39. Fatourechi V, Aniszewski JP, Fatourechi GZ, Atkinson EJ, Jacobsen SJ. Clinical features and outcome of subacute thyroiditis in an incidence cohort: olmsted county, Minnesota, study. J Clin Endocrinol Metab 2003; 88(5):2100–2105.

40. Welker MJ, Orlov D. Thyroid nodules. Am Fam Physician 2003; 67(3):559–566.

41. Brander AEE, Viikinkoski VP, Nickels JI, Kivisaari LM. Importance of thyroid abnormalities detected at US screening: a 5-year follow-up. Radiology 2000; 215(3):801.

42. Jemal A, Thomas A, Murray T, Thun M. Cancer Statistics 2002. CA Cancer J Clin 2002; 52(1):23–47.

43. Sherman SI. Thyroid carcinoma. Lancet 2003; 361(9356): 501–511.

44. Hundahl SA, Fleming ID, Fremgen AM, Menck HR. A National Cancer Data Base report on 53,856 cases of thyroid carcinoma treated in the U.S., 1985–1995. Cancer 1998; 83(12):2638–2648.

45. Gilliland FD, Hunt WC, Morris DM, Key CR. Prognostic factors for thyroid carcinoma. A population-based study of 15,698 cases from the Surveillance, Epidemiology and End Results (SEER) program 1973–1991. Cancer 1997; 79(3):564–573.

46. Bandurska-Stankiewicz E, Stankiewicz A, Shaffie D, Wadolowska L. Thyroid cancer morbidity in the Olsztyn region in 1993–1999. Wiad Lek 2001; 54(suppl 1):136–142.

47. Pacini F, Vorontsova T, Molinaro E, et al. Thyroid consequences of the Chernobyl nuclear accident. Acta Paediatr Suppl 1999; 88(433):23–27.

48. Elisei R, Romei C, Vorontsova T, et al. RET/PTC rearrangements in thyroid nodules: studies in irradiated and not irradiated, malignant and benign thyroid lesions in children and adults. J Clin Endocrinol Metab 2001; 86(7):3211–3216.

49. Haugen BR, Woodmansee WW, McDermott MT. Towards improving the utility of fine-needle aspiration biopsy for the diagnosis of thyroid tumours. Clin Endocrinol (Oxf) 2002; 56(3):281–290.

50. Hay ID, Grant CS, Taylor WF, McConahey WM. Ipsilateral lobectomy versus bilateral lobar resection in papillary thyroid carcinoma: a retrospective analysis of surgical outcome using a novel prognostic scoring system. Surgery 1987; 102(6): 1088–1095.

51. Hay ID, Bergstralh EJ, Goellner JR, Ebersold JR, Grant CS. Predicting outcome in papillary thyroid carcinoma: development of a reliable prognostic scoring system in a cohort of 1779 patients surgically treated at one institution during 1940 through 1989. Surgery 1993; 114(6):1050–1057.

52. Hay ID, Grant CS, Bergstralh EJ, Thompson GB, van Heerden JA, Goellner JR. Unilateral total lobectomy: is it sufficient surgical treatment for patients with AMES low-risk papillary thyroid carcinoma? Surgery 1998; 124(6):958–964.

53. Hay ID, McConahey WM, Goellner JR. Managing patients with papillary thyroid carcinoma: insights gained from the Mayo Clinic's experience of treating 2,512 consecutive patients during 1940 through 2000. Trans Am Clin Climatol Assoc 2002; 113:241–260.

54. Clark OH. TSH suppression in the management of thyroid nodules and thyroid cancer. World J Surg 1981; 5(1):39–47.

55. Kikumori T, Imai T, Tanaka Y, Oiwa M, Mase T, Funahashi H. Parathyroid autotransplantation with total thyroidectomy for thyroid carcinoma: long-term follow-up of grafted parathyroid function. Surgery 1999; 125(5):504–508.

56. Mazzaferri EL. Thyroid remnant ^{131}I ablation for papillary and follicular thyroid carcinoma. Thyroid 1997; 7(2):265–271.

57. Mazzaferri EL, Kloos RT. Current approaches to primary therapy for papillary and follicular thyroid cancer. J Clin Endocrinol Metab 2001; 86(4):1447–1463.

58. Varma VM, Beierwaltes WH, Nofal MM, Nishiyama RH, Copp JE. Treatment of thyroid cancer. Death rates after surgery and after surgery followed by sodium iodide I-131. JAMA 1970; 214(8):1437–1442.

59. Samaan NA, Maheshwari YK, Nader S, et al. Impact of therapy for differentiated carcinoma of the thyroid: an analysis of 706 cases. J Clin Endocrinol Metab 1983; 56(6):1131–1138.

60. Samaan NA, Schultz PN, Hickey RC, et al. The results of various modalities of treatment of well differentiated thyroid carcinomas: a retrospective review of 1599 patients. J Clin Endocrinol Metab 1992; 75(3):714–720.

61. Parthasarathy KL, Crawford ES. Treatment of thyroid carcinoma: emphasis on high-dose ^{131}I outpatient therapy. J Nucl Med Technol 2002; 30(4):165–171.

62. Maxon HR, Thomas SR, Samaratunga RC. Dosimetric considerations in the radioiodine treatment of macrometastases and micrometastases from differentiated thyroid cancer. Thyroid 1997; 7(2):183–187.

63. Yutan E, Clark OH. Hürtle cell carcinoma. Curr Treat Options Oncol 2001; 2(4):331–335.

64. Kebebew E, Clark OH. Medullary thyroid cancer. Curr Treat Options Oncol 2000; 1(4):359–367.

53

Endocrine Pancreas

Ronald C. Merrell, Giacomo P. Basadonna, and Cristiana Rastellini

INTRODUCTION

To coordinate the function of metazoan life forms for mutual, organismal benefit, the cells of the organism must communicate. In simple multicellular organisms, electrical coupling, cell-contact events, and the local diffusion of metabolic and messenger molecules are sufficient. Neighboring cells are informed by mass action, allosteric enzyme interactions, or specific binding to receptors. In a larger organism with a circulatory system, coordinating messages in the form of small molecules may flow through the organism to arrive at tissues possessing specific receptors, with complex postreceptor events. Also, neural fibers arborize across great distances to release communicating molecules to specialized receptors when triggered by propagated depolarization of the neuronal membrane (1).

The pancreas demonstrates essentially all the known mechanisms for cellular communication in a metazoan organism. In addition to cell-to-cell interaction among islet cells across gap junctions (Fig. 1), the simplest coordinated function, and complex adrenergic and cholinergic innervation, the pancreas engages in exocrine, paracrine, and endocrine interactions with the remainder of the body (Fig. 2). *Exocrine function* is described as the release of synthesized products into a nonvascular duct for delivery at another anatomic locus. *Paracrine function* is the release of a synthesized product into the extracellular space for delivery by diffusion to a target tissue no more than several microns away. *Endocrine function* is the release of a synthesized product that enters the circulation for transport to a distant target tissue. The intricacy and redundancy of communication pathways for this islet cell mass underscore its crucial role in maintaining glucose homeostasis through the balance of glucose clearance, mediated by insulin, and glucose generation, mediated by glucagon.

In 1869, Paul Langerhans demonstrated the unique features of the islets that now bear his name. These structures, originally viewed as islands in the alien sea of the exocrine pancreas, are now more clearly seen as integral rather than accidental features of the pancreas, with extensive interaction with the exocrine portion of the gland. Von Mering and Minkowski (2) provided evidence for an endocrine function of the pancreas in 1889, when they found that total pancreatectomy led not only to the expected exocrine insufficiency but also to diabetes mellitus. Attribution of endocrine function to the islets followed, seeming to culminate with isolation of insulin and its clinical application for type I diabetes mellitus by Banting and Best in 1922 (3). However, the full richness of islet interaction and regulation was only suggested by the recognition of insulin, and new data continue to enhance the importance of the islets in homeostasis. This chapter describes the endocrine community of the islets of Langerhans, their origins and relationships

(both internal and external), and their role in homeostasis and disease states.

ANATOMY AND EMBRYOLOGY OF THE ISLETS

The islets of Langerhans individually constitute an endocrine community engaged in active collaboration to secure glucose homeostasis. At least four distinct endocrine cells have been identified: (i) *A cells*, which secrete glucagon, a catabolic hormone that raises plasma glucose level; (ii) *B cells*, which produce insulin, an anabolic hormone that lowers plasma glucose level; (iii) *D cells*, which produce somatostatin, a regulatory hormone for A and B cells;

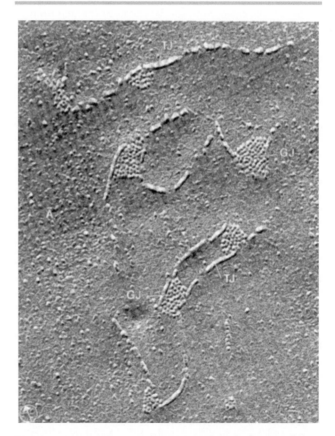

Figure 1 Gap junctions and tight junctions between islet cells suggest the rich transcellular communication between component cells of islets of Langerhans. This freeze-fracture electron micrograph shows extensive cellular contacts between islet cells. *Courtesy:* Lelio Orci, Geneva.

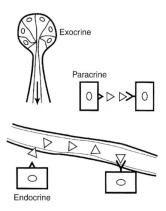

Figure 2 Exocrine delivery of secreted cellular products occurs along ducts that ultimately discharge into the gastrointestinal tract or outside the body. Paracrine secretions reach a target cell solely by diffusion across a short distance (the schematic cell on the left is discharging a substance received by the cell on the right). Endocrine secretions enter the circulation and arrive at a target tissue some distance from the point of origin. (The schematic cell on the left is discharging substance into blood; blood transports the substance to the target cell on the right.)

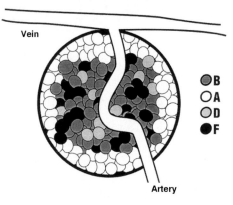

Figure 3 B cells are centrally located in the islet in close approximation to incoming blood supply, whereas A cells are arrayed as a mantle at the periphery of the islet. D and F cells are interspersed. B cell secretions move through the islet toward the periphery before reentering the circulation. This flow determines the opportunity for paracrine interaction among the component cells. The modest suppression by insulin of A cells may be paracrine, whereas the more substantial stimulation of B cells by glucagon must be endocrine. D and F cells could interact with one another, with A cells, or with B cells.

and (iv) *F cells*, which secrete pancreatic polypeptide (PP), a 36–amino acid linear polypeptide. Each cell contains and secretes only one endocrine product. The lettering system for these cells stems from special chemical staining properties of the secretory granules. The letter *C* in the series was reserved for a cell in guinea pig islets, which contained no granules. This cell may have been a degranulated B cell or a precursor cell, but it no longer has any valid stature among its lettered neighbors. Also, the *E cell*, described only in the opossum, must await further study before inclusion in this endocrine community. The cells were lettered in order of discovery, and the missing C and E cells in the islet serve to remind us of the enormous confusion that preceded our current, meager understanding (4). That understanding is based on staining islets with specific antibodies to the various secretory products and then using a variety of tactics to visualize that bound antibody on the secretory granules of the appropriate cell. This staining by immunocytochemistry forms the basis of our current understanding of islet anatomy.

The pancreas arises from foregut endoderm through a dorsal bud, first evident in the 3 mm embryo, and then by a ventral anlage, which is a branch of the liver bud. By clockwise rotation, the ventral structure ultimately fuses with the dorsal structure. The endocrine cells derive from precursors along the pancreatic ductal elements. With immunocytochemistry, A, B, and D cells can be recognized in organized islets by eight weeks of gestation. By 10 to 11 weeks, islets can be identified. The islets organize away from ducts as discrete structures and then grow by cell division throughout fetal life and for the first few years after birth. Islets are not of uniform size in humans, but they average approximately 300 μm (5). The A cells mature first, but at birth the distribution of the cells is the same as in adults: 60% to 70% B cells, 20% to 25% A cells, 10% to 15% D cells, and 5% to 10% F cells (Fig. 3). The distribution of the islets is not completely uniform throughout the pancreas with respect to constituent cells. For example, A and B cells are more numerous in tail islets, and F cells are much more numerous in the pancreatic head. Islets have a direct arterial

blood supply and are so well vascularized that the mass of islets' capillaries is often described as glomerulus-like. Islets' serial sections reveal four patterns of islet endocrine cells and capillaries: (i) a single row of cells between two capillaries, (ii) a double row of cells between two capillaries, (iii) a ring of cells around a cross-sectioned capillary, and (iv) a clump of cells between two capillaries. At least two of these patterns are present in any islet section (6). Ultrastructural studies show that in a normal B cell, insulin granules fill the cytoplasm, and no obvious polarity is evident. After degranulation, however, a clear polarity of insulin granules has been demonstrated, with insulin granules clumped at the opposite side of the arbitrarily defined basal face, where the nucleus is closer to one capillary face. All the B cells around a particular cross-sectioned capillary show the same polarity, with the apical side facing the central capillary (6). These findings could signify a topographic separation of an apical secretory surface and a basal sensing surface for the B cell and possibly the other endocrine cells.

The origin of islet cells has been the subject of spirited debate for nearly 10 years. The islet cells have metabolic and morphotic features shared by all neuroendocrine cells, including amine precursor uptake and decarboxylase (APUD) and neurone-specific enolase. A common embryologic source for all these cells in the neuroectoderm of the neural crest has been proposed (7). However, careful studies in developmental biology refute this origin for pancreatic islet cells and place them firmly in the same lineage as the exocrine cells. For example, elimination of the neural fold before the three-somite stage does not preclude B cell development in rat embryo explants (8). A great majority of the endocrine system derives from the gastrointestinal epithelium, including the pituitary (Rathke's pouch), the thyroid (second branchial arch and ultimo branchial body), and the parathyroid glands (branchial pouches III and IV). Nonetheless, the APUD concept has been of enormous value in predicting the properties of endocrine tissue in a site, on the basis of knowledge of other endocrine systems. Also, the behavior of pathologic endocrine tissue can be

Table 1 Insuloacinar Axis

Hormone	Exocrine effect
Insulin	▲ Uptake of amino acids
	▲ Amylase synthesis
	▲ Cell division
	Permits HCO_3^- release
Glucagon	▼ Enzyme synthesis
	▼ Enzyme release
	▲ HCO_3^- release
Somatostatin	▼ Pancreatic secretion
Pancreatic polypeptide	▼ Release of enzymes

anticipated in less well-known tumors on the basis of knowledge of better-characterized tumors. All cells in an organism have the same genome, and the differentiation of transcription during development can be convergent, so after many different branch points in development, two cells serving similar (e.g., endocrine) functions may be more alike than are cells much closer in developmental lineage.

It is significant that the islets are in the pancreas and develop with the pancreas, because this relationship suggests that islets function along with the remainder of the pancreas. Indeed, there is an insuloacinar axis, which constitutes a portal system that delivers islet hormones in high concentrations to much of the acinar pancreas (Table 1). Insulin increases amylase synthesis, permits bicarbonate secretion, and is permissive for the action of cholecystokinin (CCK). The pancreas in patients with insulin-dependent diabetes is much smaller than normal as a result of atrophy, which may be caused by a relative lack of insulin locally or by the inhibitory effects of excess glucagon, which suppresses enzyme synthesis and release, although it stimulates bicarbonate secretion. The inhibitory effects of glucagon are so pronounced experimentally that this hormone was proposed for the treatment of acute pancreatitis; however, clinical results have not been impressive. Somatostatin and PP are also inhibitory to the exocrine pancreas, and they presumably are active in the insuloacinar axis (9).

PHYSIOLOGY OF THE ISLETS
Insulin and the B Cell

The best studied of the islet cells is the B cell. The nucleus of this cell transcribes messenger RNA (mRNA) for preproinsulin, which is synthesized in the rough endoplasmic reticulum. The amino-terminal signal sequence is cleaved in the lumen of the endoplasmic reticulum, and the 9 kDa product, proinsulin, passes through the Golgi apparatus, where secretory vesicles are assembled. The insulin gene, one of the first human genes to be cloned (10), is 1500 bp long and contains three exons and two introns. The introns can be of variable length: intron 1 varies from 119 bp in chickens to 179 bp in humans, whereas intron 2 can vary from 264 bp in dogs to more than 3500 bp in chickens (786 in humans). The insulin gene exists as a single copy in most species, except in rats and mice, where two copies exist. Interestingly, rat insulin gene I does not have the second intron and exhibits 70% homology with the other copy. In the rat, both genes are present in the same chromosome and appear to be transcribed in equal portions. In mice, the genes are in different chromosomes, but this seems to have no effect on the relatively identical rates of transcription. The location of the insulin gene in humans is on band p15 of the short arm of chromosome 11 (11).

Glucose stimulates insulin biosynthesis as well as secretion. Glucose does indeed regulate insulin biosynthesis

at both translational and transcriptional levels, but there is a time shift in these effects. Thus, transcriptional effects are long term, whereas the translational effects occur in the short term. Some evidence to support this conclusion is that the glucose-stimulated increase in the amount of preproinsulin mRNA is not observed until two hours after glucose administration, and it is then maintained for about 24 hours. On the other hand, after one hour, there is an increase in insulin biosynthesis without a change in the mRNA levels. Glucose also stimulates preproinsulin mRNA levels as well as secretion in human islets (12). The effects of glucose on preproinsulin mRNA levels occur in two phases: an initial short-term phase involving posttranscriptional control, and a long-term regulation under transcriptional control. The insulin vesicles are stored in the cytoplasm in the webbing of the cytoskeleton and, under secretory stimuli, move to the plasma membrane, where the vesicle and plasma membranes fuse to release equimolar concentrations of insulin and C-peptide into the extracellular space. In the storage vesicles, the single chain of proinsulin is doubly cleaved to give the A and B chains of insulin (molecular weight 6 kDa), bonded together by two disulfide bridges and the connecting chain, C-peptide. A third disulfide bond determines the shape of the A chain. In the vesicles, insulin is a hexamer coordinated by two Zn^{2+} ions. During release and dilution, the hexamer dissociates to the active monomeric form (13).

Stored insulin is abundant, and the number of B cells in the normal pancreas far exceeds the number required for insulin release. Even when insulin release is maximally stimulated, the release of more than 5% of the total insulin available is rare. As much as 95% of the normal pancreas can be resected without inducing insulin insufficiency or carbohydrate intolerance. The intracellular signals for the release of insulin are prompted by a movement of Ca^{2+} into the B cell and by the accumulation of the cyclic adenosine monophosphate (cAMP). Glucose enhances Ca^{2+} uptake from extracellular medium, as well as other secretagogues such as glyceraldehyde and sulfonylurea. Glucose may also cause a transient decrease in Ca^{2+} efflux and the closure of K^+ channels, which could cause the opening of Ca^{2+} channels (14). At high glucose concentrations, insulin secretion agonists such as glucagon induce secretion by increasing cAMP concentration through protein phosphorylation. It is convenient to view Ca^{2+} and cAMP as the final events necessary for access to the insulin pool. Access to the Ca^{2+} and cAMP pools, in turn, can be achieved through a variety of routes, either receptor mediated or connected to the metabolism of the B cell (Fig. 4) (15). Pluralistic access to the insulin pool is important to explain even partially the wide range of secretagogues and inhibitors for the release of this crucial hormone. Glucose is one of the most important extracellular signals for insulin release (Table 2). On the other hand, after a normal mixed meal, plasma glucose levels reach only low peak values (6–7 mmol/L). These concentrations of extracellular glucose are usually able to elicit a very weak insulin response. Nevertheless, after ingestion of a mixed meal, a significant insulin response is obtained through different patterns, releasing acetylcholine at parasympathetic synapses of vagal efferents on B cells, and secreting CCK through the neurons that innervate the B cells. CCK, glucagon-like peptide 1, and gastric-inhibitory peptide (GIP) all act on the B cell through the bloodstream. GIP and glucagon-like peptide 1 stimulate adenylate cyclase. Acetylcholine and CCK act on phosphoinositide-specific phospholipase C, causing an increase in both phosphoinositide hydrolysis and the Ca^{2+} concentration.

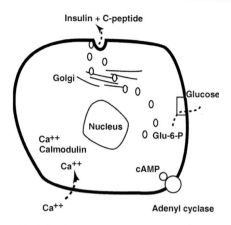

Figure 4 The release of insulin from B cells is controlled at least by intracellular cAMP and Ca^{2+}. Although glucose is the predominant secretagogue for insulin, many other metabolic or receptor-mediated events also modulate insulin secretion. Proinsulin is packaged from the endoplasmic reticulum after synthesis and moves through the Golgi body. Proinsulin is cleaved in the secretory or storage vesicles to yield C-peptide and insulin, which are released in equimolar quantities by exocytosis. *Abbreviation*: cAMP, cyclic adenosine monophosphate.

The B cells are generally concentrated at the center of an islet, in close apposition to the arteriole that penetrates the islet to deliver blood initially to its interior (Fig. 3). These cells are coupled electrically to surrounding cells and have rich gap–junction contacts, transmitting sizable molecules among B cells and other adjacent endocrine cells (16). Table 2 outlines the major secretagogues and inhibitors of insulin release. The insulin leaving the islets, like all islet hormones, reaches the liver through the portal vein. Approximately 50% of insulin is removed on the first pass through the liver, which may be considered the major site of action for insulin.

Table 2 Insulin Release

Secretagogs	Suppressors
Metabolic	Metabolic
Glucose	D-Manno-heptulose
Other hexoses (potentiate)	2-Deoxy-D-glucose
Hexosamines (potentiate)	Diazoxide
Glycolytic products (potentiate)	
Amino acids	Receptor-mediated
Fatty acids	Somatostain
Ca^{2+}(ionic)	α-Adrenergic agonists
Calcium ionophores	
Islet-activating protein	*Suppression of Electrical Activity*
	Cytoskeleton blockade
Receptor-mediated	Diphanylhydantoin
Glucagon	Colchicine
GIP	
β-Endorphin	
β-Adrenergic agonists	
Acetylcholine	
Sulfonylurea	
Gastrin	
Secretin	
CCK	
Coristol	

Abbreviations: GIP, gastric-inhibitory peptide; CCK, cholecystokinin.

The least understood of the mechanisms for insulin release are the metabolic pathways. Clearly, flow of oxygen through the mitochondrial respiratory chain is critical, and lipoxygenase has been implicated (17). It is possible that glucose has a membrane receptor that prompts release in addition to metabolic regulation. Although many hexoses and intermediates are secretagogues or facilitate glucose-mediated insulin release, galactose and 3-O-methylglucose participate in glycolysis but do not promote insulin secretion. Also, some agents that block glycolysis do not block glucose-stimulated insulin release. Therefore, a glucose receptor has been suggested (18). However, the nature of a receptor that responds in a concentration range of 5×10^{-3} to 15×10^{-3} mol/L for glucose is obscure at best. The dissociation constant for hormone receptors favors regulatory interaction at 10^{-8} to 10^{-9} mol/L. The high molecular concentration of glucose that affects insulin regulation is more consistent with allosteric interaction with an enzyme than with cell-surface or cytosolic receptor kinetics. It is clear that glucose metabolites promote insulin exocytosis, which maybe via inhibition of specific protein phosphatases (18a). In general, three routes of stimulation may be distinguished: *metabolic*, typified by glucose and amino acids; *receptor mediated*, typified by acetylcholine; and *ionic*, as in Ca^{2+} ionophores. Vagal stimulatory effects on insulin secretion are dramatic and may induce hypoglycemia with only the sight and smell of food. However, B cells can generally function in glucose homeostasis with or without this extraordinary amount of input. The checks and balances of insulin release are so numerous that failure of the B cell mass with glucose intolerance represents the collapse of a long series of protective endocrine and metabolic mechanisms.

The basal release of insulin averages 4 mU/min (19). This level is biologically quite active. Therefore, insulin is important in basal metabolism and does not simply reduce excursions in the glucose concentration. When an appropriate stimulus is given, insulin is released in two phases.

There is an initial or first-phase peak, which reaches about five times the basal insulin within three to five minutes. This phase deteriorates and a second, sustained phase of insulin release continues for 60 to 70 minutes. This second phase is quantitatively much more substantial (20). The biphasic contour (Fig. 5) suggests that insulin is stored in

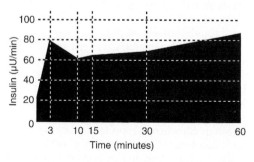

Figure 5 Biphasic release of insulin after glucose stimulation is seen either from isolated islets of Langerhans, as in this figure, or from the in situ pancreas when pulsed with glucose. The initial sharp peak of insulin release at three minutes is followed by sustained insulin release, which peaks at 30 to 60 minutes. The significance of the biphasic nature of insulin secretion is probably great but is poorly understood. Multiple insulin pools have been proposed to explain the discontinuity of insulin release.

at least two compartments under somewhat different controls. Insulin release returns to the basal level after either restoration of ambient glucose to normal levels or exhaustion of the B cell. Physiologic inhibitors do indeed modulate insulin release, but they are not important in a feedback loop. Insulin itself may not be directly involved in feedback, because infused insulin in vivo (21) can reduce insulin output, but no such effect can be demonstrated with isolated islets in vitro (22). All the modulators of insulin release are of modest importance compared with the primacy of glucose as the major regulator of B cell function.

Insulin lowers plasma glucose level principally by facilitating the diffusion of glucose into tissues that have insulin receptors. After interaction with its receptors, a number of protein phosphorylations occur, and the entry of glucose as glucose-6-phosphate is greatly accelerated (23). The hormone promotes glycogen synthesis by reducing cAMP effects on glycogenolysis. Insulin also promotes amino acid uptake and protein synthesis and inhibits protein degradation. Fat synthesis is promoted by means of pyruvate dehydrogenase, and lipolysis is inhibited (24). Insulin promotes the entry of K^+ and Mg^{2+} into cells, even in the absence of glucose (Table 2). The hormone generally supports cell growth and division by metabolic enhancement. Insulin is similar in primary structure to nerve growth factor, other growth factors, and relaxin. The wide array of insulin effects apparently does not have a common postreceptor second messenger. Rather, insulin has multiple intracellular actions after initial binding and internalization of the insulin–receptor complex. Insulin is also associated with a reduction in intracellular cAMP.

Insulin is so critical to the existence of life forms with a circulatory system, and therefore with endocrine relationships, that its primary sequence is conserved with exquisite precision through speciation. Among mammals, there is significant variation only at amino acid residue numbers 8, 9, and 10 of the A chain (25). Human and porcine insulins differ by only one amino acid. Insulin from fishes has significant biologic activity in humans (Fig. 6).

Although most tissues need insulin to modulate the metabolism of glucose, this hormone is not needed by the central nervous system. In fact, insulin does not readily pass the blood–brain barrier. Muscle tissue that has been physically conditioned by exercise has a great reduction in the need for insulin to transport glucose. Quantitatively, the most important site for insulin activity in metabolism is the liver, and the most important site for rapid reduction of plasma glucose is the fat cell mass.

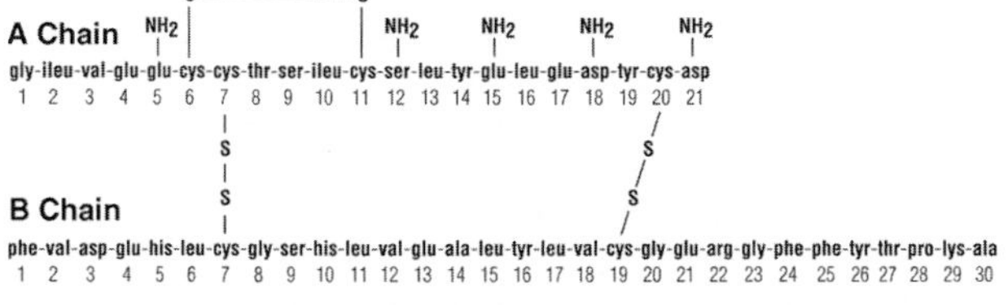

Figure 6 The structure of insulin in all species is quite similar to human insulin, which is shown here. Sequence variation among various species is most prominent at residues 8, 9, and 10 of the A chain. Both A and B chains are derived from the same proinsulin molecule by proteolytic removal of the C-peptide. The three sulfhydryl bridges coordinate the tertiary structure of the molecule.

Glucagon and the A Cell

The complementary hormone to insulin is glucagon, which is secreted by A cells and acts to raise plasma glucose level. Glucagon is a single peptide of 3.485 kDa, which has sequence homology with secretin, vasoactive intestinal peptide (VIP), GIP, growth hormone–releasing factor, and placental lactogen (26). A prohormone is synthesized, which yields glucagon in the secretory granules after proteolytic cleavage. In health, glucagon is clearly as important as insulin, but because it is not of primary importance in any common disease states, its discovery in 1923 received little notice (27). This crucial hormone has until recently been viewed as a probe to the primacy of insulin. However, glucagon in stress is so preponderant in driving catabolic metabolism that new knowledge concerning its actions and properties is received with great anticipation by those wishing to better understand stress physiology.

The principal stimulus for glucagon release is hypoglycemia. The mechanisms of release are probably similar to those of insulin but have been much less studied. Amino acids stimulate the release of both glucagon and insulin. The only gastrointestinal peptide known to stimulate glucagon secretion is CCK. Glucagon release is also prompted by epinephrine by means of α-adrenergic effects. Cortisol, growth hormone, and β-endorphin all promote glucagon release. Glucagon release is suppressed by hyperglycemia, somatostatin, secretin, and insulin. It also exercises feedback inhibition on its own secretion (28). After a glucose challenge, the suppression of baseline glucagon release closely parallels insulin stimulation. The magnitude of the suppression is much greater after oral glucose intake than after intravenous delivery. The mirror image of insulin response is clear.

1. Secretagogues
    a. Hypoglycemia
    b. Amino acids
    c. CCK
    d. α-Adrenergic agonists
    e. Cortisol
    f. Growth hormone
    g. β-Endorphin
2. Suppressors
    a. Hyperglycemia
    b. Insulin
    c. Secretin
    d. Somatostatin

Basal glucagon level is of great importance in countervailing the effects of insulin. At steady state glucose level, basal insulin release describes an oscillation easily measured in portal venous blood. The period of the oscillation is about 10 minutes. Basal glucagon release follows a similar sine-wave variation, 180° out of phase with that of insulin. The oscillatory delivery of insulin and glucagon to the liver cannot be explained on the basis of variable glucose delivery to the islets. Rather, an internal rhythm must be presumed in the islets themselves, one that does not require the circulatory system (29). Despite the extensive communication among the cells within an islet, there is no evidence for linkage among individual islets. However, rhythmic basal insulin release can be seen in cultured islets in vitro. The mechanism for this biologic clock is not known.

Approximately 25% of the portal venous glucagon remains in the liver after one pass. The liver is the most important target tissue for this hormone; in the liver, specific receptors recognize portal venous glucagon and promote a

Table 3   Glucagon Effects

Enhances	Inhibits
Glycogenolysis	Glycogen synthesis
Lipolysis	Lipogenesis
Gluconeogenesis	
cAMP	

Abbreviation: cAMP; cyclic adenosine monophosphate.

rise in intracellular cAMP level. Glycogenolysis follows by enzyme activation by means of protein kinases. On a molar basis, glucagon is 20 to 30 times more potent than epinephrine in stimulating glycogenolysis. Gluconeogenesis is enhanced, whereas lipolysis in both the liver and the periphery is stimulated by this hormone. Glucagon is not as pervasive in its cell membrane effects as insulin. There are, for example, no important ion movements associated with glucagon, and it does not stimulate cell division. In addition to its metabolic effects, however, glucagon is a powerful suppressor of pancreatic exocrine activity and a powerful smooth muscle antagonist in the gastrointestinal tract (Table 3). This property is used mostly in endoscopy and radiology, to temporarily paralyze the gut.

Somatostatin and PP

Somatostatin is released by islet D cells that lie in juxtaposition to, and often between, A and B cells. It was first recognized in the brain as a suppressor of growth hormone release. Somatostatin modulates insulin and glucagon release by inhibiting both. Its regulatory action in the islets may be more paracrine than endocrine. One pathway to the inhibition of insulin release may be by means of somatostatin. The release of somatostatin is prompted by glucose, arginine, leucine, and glucagon (30).

PP is a hormone with a single peptide chain weighing 4.240 kDa and is secreted by the F cells of the islets. PP bears sequence homology to glucagon and secretin. Its potency to promote hepatic glycogenolysis rivals that of glucagon. It also causes gallbladder relaxation, decreases intestinal motility, and suppresses gastric acid secretion. This intriguing peptide, described first in 1968 (31), does not have a clear place in metabolic regulation and gastrointestinal physiology. Assignment of importance or consignment to obscurity must await further investigation.

ISLETS IN HEALTH AND DISEASE

As reviewed in the previous section, the islets of Langerhans regulate metabolism with the object of maintaining plasma glucose level. The principal site for insulin and glucagon to accomplish this mission is the liver. At rest between meals, insulin and glucagon have a balanced, almost harmonic effect. After meals, the hormonal balance shifts according to the chemical nature of the meal to distribute the calorigenic nutrients for efficient use and storage. In prolonged fasting, glucagon is more important to support glucose synthesis from protein by gluconeogenesis and by hydrolysis of glycogen. Glucagon also permits use of the lipid stores. The glucose requirement in fasting is modest, and its provision generates little detriment to body protein. In times of severe stress or injury, glucagon is again important to provide the extra glucose synthesis needed for caloric consumption from protein by gluconeogenesis and by hydrolysis of glycogen. Therefore, the islet cell mass

responds to disease states and metabolic derangements by ensuring a hormonal balance through insulin or glucagon release, which promotes the generation of endogenous fuel substrates.

The disease states of the endocrine pancreas are small in number, although they are significant in terms of medical consequence. There are states of deficiency and neoplasia. The only spontaneous deficiency involves the B cells. No natural deficiency diseases are recognized for glucagon, somatostatin, or PP. However, each cell of the islet may become neoplastic as a benign or malignant tumor, secreting isotopic (entopic) hormone, ectopic hormone, or no hormone.

Diabetes Mellitus

The B cells may be nearly eliminated, as occurs in type I insulinopenic diabetes mellitus, or may be functionally inadequate, as occurs in type II diabetes mellitus. In the latter condition, plasma insulin level may be normal or high, but insulin insensitivity in target tissues hampers glucose clearance, and hyperglycemia develops.

Type I or insulinopenic diabetes mellitus results from the loss of B cells in childhood or early adult life. There is a strong familial tendency in the autosomal recessive mode with variable penetrance. Approximately 25% of patients with diabetes have one or more first-order relatives with the disease. Children whose fathers have diabetes have a 6.1% likelihood of acquiring the disease; offspring of mothers with diabetes have a diabetic incidence of only 1.3%. This disparity is not explained (32). A close association with the antigens HLA-DR3 and HLA-DR4 has been noted. In families at risk for diabetes, the clinical disease is heralded for as long as a year by circulating autoantibodies to islet cells (33), which are frequent in 65% to 85% of patients with diabetes.

Although the detection of anti-islet antibodies is useful for disease prediction, the consensus among investigators is that beta-cell destruction is mediated by T-cells, and not by autoantibodies. Islet-specific T-cell clones have been isolated from the spleen, lymph node, and islets of Langerhans of nonobese diabetic (NOD) mice, and such islet-specific T-cells are capable of inducing diabetes after adoptive transfer into young NOD mice. Evidence of disease "transfer" in human patients is also available with the recurrence of islet beta-cell destruction in pancreas transplanted from a nondiabetic identical twin into a twin with long-term diabetes. The development of frank diabetes is also prefaced by a progressive decline in the first phase of insulin release. In a bold experiment, children with recently diagnosed diabetes were immunosuppressed with cyclosporine. After one year, a startling one-half of those children were in remission and required no insulin (34). These newer data conflict with the previous picture of diabetes developing as an acute illness, with perhaps a viral cause.

There are, in fact, viruses that selectively destroy B cells in animals, and there are numerous B cell–specific toxins. Patients with familial diabetes may not accurately represent the larger number (50–75%) of spontaneous diabetes cases. The final common pathway to the disease is loss of B cells, and a variety of approaches to this path can be imagined. However, among the diabetes-prone families, the recognition of prediabetes as an autoimmune event offers the prospect of immune suppression to delay or eliminate the emergence of overt diabetes. In some patients newly diagnosed with type 1A diabetes, initial insulin therapy may be accompanied by a brief metabolic remission, termed the "honeymoon phase." During this time, low doses of insulin are sufficient to achieve glycemic control. This brief metabolic remission usually lasts for less than one year, and it probably reflects decreased insulin resistance after treatment of severe hyperglycemia. With the discovery of two spontaneous animal models of type 1A diabetes, the NOD mouse and the biobreeding (BB) rat, studies of animal T-cells have contributed to our understanding of the immunopathogenesis of this disease. The development of diabetes in the transplanted pancreas was remarkable in that diabetes recurred within a matter of weeks after organ transplantation. This finding suggests that the immune process that leads to type 1A diabetes remains intact for years after the development of diabetes. In contrast, the development of diabetes usually occurs over years. In human patients, not only is there progressive loss of insulin secretion after intravenous glucose before the diagnosis of diabetes, but also, after the diagnosis of diabetes, C-peptide secretion is progressively lost.

Although insulin deficiency results in diabetes mellitus, several mutant insulins have been characterized. Both [Leu^{B25}] and [Ser^{B24}] insulin have been found in patients with diabetes; the latter results in a milder form of the disease (35). Another important process in the development of type 1 diabetes is the balance between B cell mass destruction through different temporal courses in different patients. In vitro and in vivo data prove that B cells are able to repair themselves after damage. Islets from nonobese diabetic mice, isolated in the prediabetic period, can restore a normal insulin-release pattern in tissue culture. Glucose, nicotinamide, and branched-chain amino acids can enhance B cell ability to repair damage after toxic assault. Better understanding of this process and possible intervention in this delicate mechanism of B cell repair could change the development of type 1 diabetes (36).

Insulinopenic type I diabetes, also called *juvenile-onset diabetes*, accounts for about 10% of the 200,000 new cases of diabetes diagnosed in the United States each year. Before the use of insulin, this acute illness was usually fatal, and the gene pool for diabetic propensity remained small. In the last 60 years, however, the gene pool has enlarged considerably as patients treated for diabetes have more consistently achieved reproductive maturity. What had been a devastating acute illness has now become an important chronic illness. When all patients with diabetes are grouped together, they represent 1% to 5% of the U.S. population. Diabetes is the leading cause of blindness in young Americans, and it is the most frequently reported diagnosis for patients beginning long-term dialysis for renal failure. The clinical ramifications of this disease are so extensive that it is appropriate to consider the condition as a syndrome rather than a single disease.

The most obvious effect of diabetes is hyperglycemia, which reflects the reduced capacity of glucose to enter cells that rely on insulin–receptor occupation for facilitated glucose diffusion. Renal tubular capacity to reabsorb glucose is exceeded at 180 to 200 mg/dL (10 mmol/L), and glycosuria follows. Glucose is osmotically important and causes osmotic diuresis. Hemoconcentration and dehydration follow because of the diuresis. Hyperosmolar effects are significant when the plasma glucose level exceeds 540 mg/dL, where the 30 mmol/L glucose contributes 30 mOsm/L to the plasma osmolarity. Hyperosmolarity leads to coma, and the volume loss caused by osmotic diuresis leads to vascular collapse. Without treatment, hyperglycemia is fatal (Fig. 7).

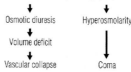

Effects of Hyperglycemia

Figure 7 Effects of hyperglycemia.

The metabolic response to reduced glucose movement into cells is prompt, damaging, and potentially fatal (Fig. 8). Intracellular metabolic compartments perceive the mass-action message of insufficient glucose. Therefore, protein catabolism is accelerated to support gluconeogenesis. Nitrogen loss is massive and is accompanied by substantial loss of potassium. The extra glucose leads to further increases in plasma glucose level. It is important to realize that the potentially fatal glucose level in the plasma of patients with uncontrolled diabetes does not represent ingested carbohydrate that arrives in the circulation directly from the jejunum. Rather, the source of the enormous glucose compartment in the plasma is endogenous, either glycogen or gluconeogenesis. The decrease in intracellular energy substrate also prompts lipolysis. The liberated glycerol participates in gluconeogenesis. Free fatty acids go to the liver, where β-oxidation in the mitochondria is associated with the release of acetoacetate and beta-hydroxybutyrate (ketogenic events). The generation of ketones involves acidic reactions sufficient to produce metabolic acidosis. There are no renal mechanisms to reabsorb these short carbon chains; therefore, ketonuria develops. Also, the ketones are volatile and may escape in expired air, lending a fruity odor to the breath. The released ketones are available for metabolism and energy generation. β-Oxidation is the only event in the diabetic adaptation, which helps to increase the generation of high-energy phosphate bonds. The respiratory response to the metabolic acidosis is hyperventilation in the form of air hunger called *Kussmaul–Kien respiration*. The clinical picture of diabetic ketoacidosis is now complete, with hyperglycemia, dehydration, ketoacidosis, ketonuria, polyuria, and Kussmaul–Kien respiration. If this metabolic nightmare is not corrected by insulin, coma, vascular collapse, and death follow.

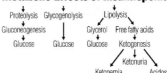

Metabolic Effects of Insulinopenia

Figure 8 When insulin levels are low, insulin mediation of glucose uptake in responsive tissues is greatly reduced, leading to a deficiency of intracellular glucose. The response to diminished intracellular carbohydrate is to increase the export of glucose from the liver by gluconeogenesis or glycogenolysis. In response to meager intracellular energy, substrate lipolysis is encouraged, with export of ketone bodies, acetoacetate, and β-hydroxybutyrate from the liver. Pathologically elevated plasma glucose level, abundant plasma ketones with ketonuria, and the metabolic acidosis that attends ketogenesis is defined as hyperglycemic ketoacidosis.

Type II noninsulin-dependent diabetes mellitus is also called *adult-onset diabetes mellitus* or *nonketogenic diabetes*. This disease is quite distinct from type I diabetes and shares only the common feature of derangement of carbohydrate metabolism tending toward hyperglycemia. The consequences of the hyperglycemia in terms of vascular complications are quite similar in the two diseases. Whereas type I diabetes is marked by profound insulinopenia, type II diabetes is a condition in which the circulating insulin levels may be normal, or even greater than normal. The impact of circulating insulin in regulating total body carbohydrate metabolism is greatly diminished, however, and hyperglycemia develops.

The presence of amyloid deposits, one of the common pathologic features of the islets of patients with type II diabetes, was originally described in 1901 (37). The major component of this amyloid tissue is a protein termed *islet amyloid polypeptide*, which represents a new B cell secretory product whose activities are unknown. The production of the islet amyloid polypeptide is not necessarily the cause of the type II diabetes, but it may be the consequence of a derailed behavior of B cells. Studies seeking a deeper knowledge of this protein are underway (38).

The sensitivity of peripheral tissue receptors for insulin seems greatly diminished in patients with type II diabetes, and there has been considerable confusion regarding whether this disease arises because of any real pathology of the B cells of the islets of Langerhans or whether it indeed represents a receptor problem at the periphery. Although defects in the insulin receptor may cause insulin resistance, the primary cause of insulin resistance in patients with type II diabetes is believed to be in one of the fast-receptor sites, such as the glucose transport system, which is characterized by decreased activity and decreased number of transporters in cases of insulin resistance. Recent studies have shown that an abnormal regulation and expression of a specific glucose transporter isoform, GLUT4, which mediates insulin-stimulated glucose transport in adipose and muscle cells, is responsible for insulin resistance in adipose tissue and possibly muscle tissue as well (39,40). Because insulin secretion and reception are so tightly linked, it is difficult to divorce the two events to obtain a better, if arbitrary, distinction between type I and type II diabetes. Type II diabetes, though, does occur in older patients, with a striking propensity for obese patients. The hyperglycemia and hyperinsulinemia can be resolved in many obese patients simply by lowering the fat stores through a reducing diet. There is a familial tendency in adult-onset diabetes, but it more closely parallels the familial incidence of obesity. Control of hyperglycemia may require supplemental insulin in patients with type II diabetes mellitus, but the use of insulin still should not cause confusion between this illness and the type I variant. In type II diabetes, the insulin is not required to sustain life but merely to better regulate plasma glucose level. Therefore, the term *noninsulin-dependent diabetes mellitus* is still applicable to type II diabetes.

The principal feature of type II diabetes that causes clinical trouble is hyperglycemia. This can be associated with a striking and life-threatening syndrome of hyperosmolar coma when the blood sugar level exceeds 800 mg/dL. The increase in blood glucose level is osmotically quite important and can literally draw water out of the brain cells, resulting in a comatose state. However, ketosis is not associated with this drastic derangement in carbohydrate metabolism in which glucose clearance is so inadequate as to potentially lead to hyperosmolar death.

This lack of ketosis is not completely understood. The dehydration that is associated with the polyuria of hyperosmolar coma has been implicated. It is more likely that the hyperglycemic crisis in type II diabetes is unique because insulin is indeed present in substantial quantities, unlike the situation in the hyperglycemic crisis of type I diabetes. The impact of insulin in diminishing lipolysis is preserved in larger measure in type II diabetes. The adipocytes are 20 to 30 times more sensitive to the antilipolytic effects of insulin than to the facilitated entry of glucose under the influence of insulin. It is therefore likely that, although a hyperglycemic crisis has followed because of poor insulin effect in type II diabetes, lipolysis and thus ketogenesis cannot occur. The treatment of nonketotic, hyperosmolar coma in type II diabetes is directed toward fluid resuscitation and providing sufficient insulin to clear the extracellular compartment of the extraordinary concentrations of free glucose.

Complications of Diabetes

Diabetes is a truly devastating disease in terms of curtailment of longevity and quality of life, as a consequence of its complications, and not as a consequence of its more dramatic metabolic manifestations such as ketoacidosis or nonketotic hyperosmolar coma. It is the leading cause of blindness in young Americans and may soon become the most common diagnosis in patients subject to long-term dialysis programs for end-stage renal disease. Although diabetes affects less than 10% of the population of the United States, it is the eighth leading cause of death. About half of patients with diabetes die of coronary disease, whereas most patients with juvenile-onset diabetes die of ramifications of renal failure. The complications are not inherently different in type I and type II diabetes and may be considered to be neural, vascular, or infectious. These three categories are interrelated but probably independent in their genesis. Nonetheless, they are all related to abnormal glucose metabolism.

Neuropathy is manifested by autonomic motor and sensory problems. The autonomic problems include gastroparesis, impotence, orthostatic hypotension, and diarrhea. Sensory deficits include position sense and pinprick sensation. Radiculopathy is seen, and the pain can be disabling. The sensory deficit problems contribute to lower extremity injury, which does not heal because of poor blood supply. Such extremities tend to become infected because of poor response to bacteria, with consequent limb loss.

The cause of the neuropathy is not well understood and tends to parallel the vascular complications in the course of the natural history of diabetes. However, recent work implicates abnormal metabolism of sugar alcohols through the enzyme aldose reductase. This activity of this enzyme is the rate-limiting step in the pathway to sugar alcohols, and that pathway is confined to Schwann cells, spinal roots, and the lens epithelium. The enzyme is probably not abnormal in patients with diabetes, but mass-action events in hyperglycemia and intracellular glucoprevia activate this otherwise exotic pathway. The nature of the toxicity of sugar alcohols in these tissues has not been elucidated, but inhibition of aldose reductase has been clinically useful in improving autonomic function and in relieving the pain that can be a manifestation of sensory neuropathy (41).

The vascular lesions of diabetes are numerous and perhaps distinct in development. There is an acceleration of atherosclerosis in patients with diabetes along lines that are indistinguishable from the peripheral vascular lesions seen in patients without carbohydrate intolerance. These lesions are associated with the hyperlipemia that accompanies diabetic metabolism. However, disease of small vessels develops along lines that are distinctive to diabetes (42). Capillary basement membranes thicken through the course of diabetes. Although this thickening may be something of an exaggeration of normal aging, its implications for the patient with diabetes are important. If the capillary basal lamina is considered to be the framework for wound healing and the gate that must be passed in the diapedesis of inflammatory cells, the stiff, thickened layer may be seen as a significant part of other diabetic problems. The glycopeptides of basal lamina have not been exclusively studied in diabetes, but the opportunity for abnormal glycosylation is certainly great in hyperglycemia and has been observed in patients with this disease. The covalent addition of glucose molecules to protein normally requires a glycosyl transferase. However, enzymatic glycosylation, like all enzymatically catalyzed reactions, favors through catalysis a reaction that would normally occur without the enzyme, although at a much slower rate. In the presence of persistently high ambient glucose concentrations, glucose molecules apparently can be added to the amino acid backbone of many peptides to create new and potentially pathologic glycopeptides. The glycosylated hemoglobin, hemoglobin A-1-c (HbA1c), is easily measured, and the concentration of this substance in the blood of a patient with diabetes has a direct correlation with the degree of ambient hyperglycemia in recent weeks (43). Therefore, a high HbA1c level means that control of hyperglycemia has been poor not just on the day of blood sampling but in preceding weeks as well. Although HbA1c has not by itself been associated with any malfunction of hemoglobin, the potential importance of glycosylation of other peptides in the evolution of diabetic pathology has been suggested. This glycosylated product can be measured readily and reflects the degree of hyperglycemia and thus the degree of diabetic control in recent weeks. The ultimate significance of glycosylation in diabetic pathology remains to be determined.

Angiopathy in the retina takes the form of microaneurysms of capillaries. These lesions can rupture, with escape of blood and opacification of the eye. Great progress has been made in controlling these lesions by photocoagulating aneurysms with lasers to thrombose them before they burst. Cataract formation is also prevalent in patients with diabetes as a consequence of either derangement of carbohydrate metabolism or accelerated aging.

The renal vasculopathy seen in diabetics was first described by Kimmelstiel and Wilson in 1936. Accumulation of basement membrane material in the mesangium of the glomerulus may be either nodular or diffuse. This glomerulosclerosis leads to proteinuria and eventually to azotemia. All patients with insulin-dependent diabetes who have survived 20 years or longer manifest the microscopic lesion, and half of the patients have significant renal impairment. The kidney may also be affected by hypertension, atherosclerosis, and infection in patients with diabetes. End-stage renal disease in patients with diabetes is treated with dialysis and renal transplantation.

Diagnosis and Treatment of Diabetes

The diagnosis of diabetes is precise and easily accomplished. Patients with polyuria, polydipsia, and weight loss, and especially those with visual disturbances or frequent pyogenic infections, should be evaluated for hyperglycemia. A fasting blood sugar level ≥140 mg/dL on more than one occasion defines carbohydrate intolerance and mandates its evaluation by oral glucose-tolerance testing. After an overnight fast by a patient who has previously had unrestricted calories and unrestricted exercise, 75 g glucose is given by mouth, and the blood glucose level is measured periodically for the next two hours. A value of 200 mg/dL or greater at two hours and at one previous time point defines diabetes mellitus. The test is invalidated by stress from infection, surgery, or trauma; prolonged fasting, prolonged physical inactivity, and glucocorticoid or thiazide administration. Therefore, testing of hospitalized patients as a group is inappropriate. Furthermore, the benefit of diagnosing mild diabetes mellitus in truly symptom-free patients is meager in that no treatment is indicated. Oral glucose-tolerance testing is therefore not a routine screening test (44).

The goal of diabetes management is to keep blood glucose levels as close to the normal range as safely possible. A major study, the Diabetes Control and Complications Trial (DCCT), sponsored by the National Institute of Diabetes and Digestive and Kidney Diseases, showed that keeping blood glucose levels as close to normal as safely possible reduces the risk of developing major complications of type 1 diabetes.

The 10-year study, completed in 1993, included 1441 people with type 1 diabetes. The study compared the effect of two treatment approaches—intensive management and standard management—on the development and progression of eye, kidney, and nerve complications of diabetes. Intensive treatment aimed at keeping HbA1c as close to normal (6%) as possible. HbA1c reflects average blood sugar over a two- to three-month period. Researchers found that study participants who maintained lower levels of blood glucose through intensive management had significantly lower rates of these complications. More recently, a follow-up study of DCCT participants showed that the ability of intensive control to lower the complications of diabetes persists up to four years after the trial ended.

The treatment of type II adult-onset diabetes mellitus in many, if not most, cases involves caloric restriction and weight loss to restore carbohydrate tolerance. If insulin is required, the goals and considerations for treatment become the same as for type I diabetes. The use of oral hypoglycemic agents (e.g., tolbutamide) has been less important recently, because the benefit to patients in the long term has been difficult to document and there has been more than a suggestion that vascular complications are made worse (45). Perhaps oral agents were misused by patients as an apparently simple alternative to the rigors of dieting. Therefore, patients receiving oral agents may have represented a rather noncompliant population. At any rate, when dietary measures fail to control type II diabetes, the use of insulin to manage hyperglycemia is becoming more commonplace.

The goals of diabetic management are to keep blood glucose levels normal, to recognize and treat complications promptly, and to enhance the lifestyle of patients having this disease. A significant advance has been realized in recent years by improved monitoring of plasma glucose levels. Traditionally, patients with diabetes estimated blood glucose control by monitoring the presence of glucose in the urine with test strips impregnated with glucose oxidase or tubules that tested for glucose as a reducing substance. When the plasma glucose level exceeded the maximum for renal tubular reabsorption (180 mg/dL or 10 mmol/L), glucose spill in the urine occurred. The greater the plasma glucose level, the greater was the renal loss. Therefore, the more intense the glucose reaction in urine, the greater was the need for insulin administration. Despite the usefulness of glycosuria monitoring to determine insulin needs in most patients with diabetes, it must be emphasized that its correlation with the status of glucose intolerance is generally unreliable in renal disease, pregnancy, and unstable or brittle diabetes.

Although measurement of urinary glucose is preferred in monitoring patients who do not require insulin, blood glucose measurement at home is becoming the recommended parameter for insulin administration. Capillary blood obtained by finger stick is made to react with glucose oxidase on paper strips and is read by a color chart or in a reflectance meter. Plasma glucose level is usually about 15% higher than these whole-blood measurements. Home blood glucose monitoring offers precise monitoring for extremely close glucose control.

Another tactic to quantitate the precision of glucose control is the measurement of HbA1c. As previously indicated, this glycosylated hemoglobulin is generated by nonenzymatic means, has a relatively long half-life, and is directly proportional to the average ambient glucose level. Chromatographic analysis of HbA1c reflects the accumulation of the glycoprotein in recent weeks above the customary 4% of total hemoglobin. The accumulation of HbA1c is an excellent parameter of glucose control through time.

The use of home glucose monitoring and precise review of management by measuring HbA1c are only appropriate in highly trained patients with diabetes. The training of patients with diabetes to become actively involved in the management of their disease has been greatly promoted and advanced by the American Diabetes Association. From a very early age, the patient is an active participant in therapy, recognition of complications, general health maintenance, and formulating life goals. There are instructional peer group camps for children, instructional programs for all ages, mutual support groups, and active encouragement for patients to understand and question the scientific progress being made in the area of diabetes.

Dietary measures to limit disposable glucose have recently been greatly liberalized to permit the patient with diabetes more freedom. The effect has been to generally improve adherence by better-trained patients to a more acceptable dietary regimen. Carbohydrates constitute 45% to 60% of daily calories, fat provides 30% to 35%, and protein yields 12% to 20%. Total calories are carefully prescribed on the basis of physical activity.

Appropriate insulin therapy necessitates a familiarity with the various forms available. Insulin is purified from beef or pork pancreas and exists in several modifications. When given subcutaneously, regular, crystalline insulin has its onset of action at 30 to 60 minutes, peaks at three to six hours, and has a duration of action of 6 to 10 hours. Neutral protamine Hagedorn (NPH) insulin is complexed for slower absorption and has its onset of action at 1.5 to 3 hours, peaks at 6 to 12 hours, and has a duration of action of 18 to 24 hours. Other forms are available for special purposes, but regular and NPH insulin form the basis for most diabetic management. Some patients acquire allergies to the protein sequence of animal insulin. Porcine insulin differs by only one amino acid from human insulin, but standard preparations are contaminated with proinsulin, which is antigenically quite distinct in the C-peptide region. Porcine insulin can be more

highly purified for allergic patients. Recombinant DNA technology now offers human insulin for therapy in patients with significant allergy to animal insulins.

Maintenance insulin is administered to keep the plasma glucose level below 150 mg/dL and above 80 mg/dL. Insulin is usually administered subcutaneously as a single morning dose, with a supplemental evening dose, as needed. The dosage in type I diabetes varies from 15 to 90 NPH U/day. For the patient without a pancreas, who lacks the countervailing effects of glucagon, 15 to 20 U/day is generally sufficient. The management of ketoacidosis is a special case for insulin administration. The acidosis diminishes tissue sensitivity to insulin. Therefore, extremely large amounts of insulin are required. The objectives in treating ketoacidosis are rehydration, restoration of normal plasma pH, reduction in plasma glucose level, and replacement of glycolytic pathways with ketogenic pathways by moving glucose into cells. Rehydration is commenced with normal saline solution at 1 L/hr until the heart rate, blood pressure, and urinary output suggest an improvement in the volume status. In adults, 2 to 3 L is commonly needed. Hypotonic saline solution (0.45%) is given at a rate of 1 L every two to four hours to resuscitate and reduce the hyperosmolarity that follows the osmotic diuresis and high glucose levels. When plasma glucose level falls to 300 mg/dL, glucose should be added to the intravenous infusion. If the arterial pH is less than 7.1, buffering with intravenous bicarbonate is indicated. As the plasma glucose moves into cells under the influence of insulin, potassium is shifted also. Therefore, vigorous potassium replacement is necessary.

The regimen for insulin administration in ketoacidosis is disputed among clinicians. Basically, the glucose level must be lowered in a patient with rapidly changing insulin sensitivity, but without inducing an overshoot and potentially fatal hypoglycemia. A safe approach calls for 20 U of regular insulin administered intravenously, followed by an insulin drip (100 U in 500 mL of 0.45% saline solution) at 50 to 75 mL/hr. The blood glucose level must be measured every 30 to 60 minutes until the insulin infusion rate stabilizes. The fatal components of ketoacidosis are dehydration and acidosis. There is no need to cause the glucose level to plummet in a short time. In fact, rapid reduction can lead to fluid shifts, resulting in cerebral edema or fatal hypoglycemia.

Insulin administration in the patient with diabetes who is undergoing surgery varies, depending on the complexity of the operation and the time it takes to perform. If the procedure is minor and the operation is performed early in the morning, the insulin dose is delayed until the procedure is completed. For major procedures involving a general anesthetic, a highly workable regimen calls for half the usual morning dose to be given subcutaneously as NPH, continuous 5% dextrose intravenous infusion, and monitoring of the plasma glucose every six hours. Insulin is given to keep the glucose level between 150 and 250 mg/dL. After surgery, insulin dosages according to urinary glucose are not as precise as the dosages administered according to the plasma glucose level. Continuous insulin infusion along with 5% dextrose infusion is appropriate in monitored environments and may replace intermittent insulin administration just before and after the operation. Surgical patients undergoing prolonged operations or undue stress may require 25% or 50% more insulin than usual.

To attain a constancy of plasma glucose level, which is impossible with bolus injection, continuous subcutaneous insulin infusion was recently developed. A programmable pump delivers short-acting regular insulin by means of a subcutaneous cannula. The baseline delivery rate can be increased to cover for the increased carbohydrate absorption after meals. Continuous subcutaneous insulin infusion and home glucose monitoring offer the greatest precision in control of ambient glucose. The precision can be documented by tracking HbA1c levels. However, the impact of this precision on preventing or slowing the development of diabetic complications has not been particularly gratifying (46).

An unstated belief has long prevailed in the management of diabetes that the complications associated with this disease are the consequence of inferior compliance by the patient and therefore of inadequate control of blood glucose level. By implication, perfect control of glucose levels with supplemental insulin should eliminate complications. Although there is some basis for this belief, it cannot be absolutely true. Vascular and retinal complications progress even in patients treated with infusion pumps. To explain the syndrome of diabetes mellitus, there is no reason to propose that the loss of B cells leads to a deficiency of any hormone other than insulin. However, the exquisite balance between insulin and glucagon metabolism that occurs in the patient without diabetes has not been achieved by exogenous insulin delivery. Plasma glucose level is merely a crude approximation of the profound coordination that exists between insulin and glucagon release and its effects on the body's metabolic compartments and the movement of substrate through those compartments.

Until the interaction of A and B cells is more completely understood and mechanically reproducible, transplantation of islets of Langerhans may offer an option for normal glucose homeostasis in patients with diabetes. In rodent models of diabetes caused by streptozocin, syngeneic islets purified from the pancreas of a healthy animal can be transplanted into the liver through the portal vein. Treated animals are permanently replenished and normoglycemic (47,48). Apparently, loss of innervation, acinar relationships, and the introduction of heterotopic relationships do not affect the capacity of the transplanted islets to serve the endocrine needs of affected animals. However, the animals with transplants have a distinct advantage with respect to diabetic rats treated with exogenous insulin. Rats with streptozocin-induced diabetes maintained on a regimen of insulin eventually show retinal and renal changes that resemble those seen in humans. Transplantation of islets of Langerhans can arrest and even reverse these changes (49,50). Therefore, the prospect looms for controlling the diabetic syndrome in its entirety, rather than controlling only the gross excursions of plasma glucose level. The rodent experience with transplantation has been extended to autografts in dogs, but not yet successfully to humans.

Pancreatic islet transplantation is a relatively innovative approach for the treatment of diabetes. This offers the promise of cure in type 1 diabetes mellitus by a simple injection of cellular graft into the liver, with consequent freedom from administration of exogenous insulin, glucose monitoring, and dietary restriction. Furthermore, this approach may prevent, stabilize, or even reverse secondary diabetic complications if applied sufficiently early in the course of the disease (51,52). There has been increased research activity in the field of pancreatic islet transplantation during the last decade (1990–2000). Major experimental findings have been promptly applied to the clinical setting, reporting sporadic successes and relevant information. During the last decade, a drastic increase in clinical islet transplantation cases was observed, with 35 centers worldwide performing 267 allotransplants.

Prevention of surgically induced diabetes in patients undergoing total or partial pancreatectomy, performing an autoinfusion of islets (first reported in 1972 by Najarian and colleagues) demonstrated the feasibility of the procedure in replacing the endocrine function of the pancreas and controlling the glucose homeostasis. Whereas the autotransplants performed achieved an elevated rate of success (53), the treatment of autoimmune diabetes with pancreatic islet transplantation has been unsatisfactory and inconsistent up to 1999 (54,55). Major limitations and the possible interconnection of multiple factors seem to yield this poor result. Reduced mass of islets engrafting, high metabolic demand, immunological graft loss, and diabetogenicity of the immunosuppressive drugs are the crucial aforementioned variables involved and have been responsible for the final outcome.

On comparing the data from auto- and allotransplantation cases, it is clear that the immunological component plays the major role in the failure of establishment and maintenance of insulin independence (53,55). Based on a retrospective analysis, we can extrapolate that in an alloenvironment, a certain critical mass of more than 10,000 fresh islets/kg must be infused into the recipient to potentially achieve normoglycemia. Presumably, the transplanted mass per se is not responsible for graft failure but rather the environmental factors that involve any single injected islet, from the inflammatory response to the systemic insulin resistance of long-term diabetic patient and the specifically toxic effect of the immunosuppression, determine the requirement of a larger amount of cells. The toxic effects of cyclosporine, tacrolimus, and steroids, the regimen followed up to 1999 to protect grafts from rejecting, have been extensively demonstrated in experimental and clinical settings (56–60). Moreover, a dose-related toxicity has been observed in experimental and clinical solid organ and cell transplantation (61–64). The simultaneous transplantation of pancreatic islets and either kidney or liver performed in humans (majority of the total number of allo-islet transplants performed between 1990 and 2000) has always implied a consistently elevated level of immunosuppression to insure the solid organ engraftment and protection. While strategies of minimally toxic nonspecific immunosuppression have been proposed, new specific modulations of the immune system without a diabetogenic effect have been conducted in animal models leading to innovative approaches now available for clinical investigation.

Because of the aforementioned limitations, up to 1999, the promise of islet transplant as a cure for diabetes has been difficult to sustain in worldwide trials, and of the 267 allografts performed over the most recent decade, only 12.4% achieved insulin independence for longer than one week, and only 8.2% beyond one year (65). Improvements in the separation of viable insulin-producing and -secreting cells have permitted renewed attempts at islet cell replacement (66,67). The exponential increase in availability of new and more potent immunosuppressive agents within the past five years offered potential for development of specifically tailored strategies to meet the unique needs of islet transplantation, providing greater immunological protection without diabetogenic side effects (68,69). Several factors seem to limit insulin independence after islet transplantation (55): (i) an inadequate B cell reserve due to a limited islet engraftment mass and immediate cellular loss through apoptotic and other nonimmune inflammatory pathways (70–72), (ii) immunological graft loss through both alloimmune and autoimmune pathways as a result of ineffective immunosuppression (73), and exacerbated by the lack of available tools for early diagnosis of rejection (68,69,74), and (iii) a high islet metabolic demand from preexisting insulin resistance and further compounded by the use of highly diabetogenic immunosuppressive drugs including synergistic toxicity from calcineurin inhibitors and steroids in combination (59,68,69,75).

Recent data from the Edmonton Group have shown 100% success in achievement of sustained insulin independence in 12 consecutive, brittle type 1 diabetic patients receiving solitary islet grafts in conjunction with a novel steroid-free immunosuppressive regimen (76,77). This study has clearly demonstrated that by optimizing all aspects of islet preparation, transplantation, immunosuppression, and posttransplant care, solitary islet transplantation offers minimal risk and now provides good metabolic control with normalization of HbA1c and sustained freedom from exogenous insulin. The immunosuppressive strategy utilized induction with the humanized anti-IL2 receptor monoclonal antibody daclizumab, and a combination of sirolimus and low-dose tacrolimus.

This is the first trial where consecutive diabetic patients are cured from diabetes using a pancreatic islet infusion. Furthermore, these results are providing, following sporadic cases reported by various investigators (54), the consistent result of the autotransplant cases that transplanted pancreatic islets could effectively replace the missing endocrine function.

Islet recipients represent the most attractive patient source for subsequent trials, because the consequences of graft failure will result in the patient's return to insulin injections, rather than the loss of a life-sustaining solid organ graft.

Immunomodulatory procedures could be investigated in islet recipient patients because (i) the procedural risk of islet transplantation is minimal, (ii) graft failure is not life threatening, (iii) conventional immunosuppressive drugs are diabetogenic, and, most importantly, (iv) tolerogenic protocols have shown promise in preclinical NOD and nonhuman primate islet transplant models. Moreover, unique options exist for tolerance induction in islet transplantation, because isolated islets can be pretreated in culture, transplanted to immunoprivileged sites, and potentially transplanted after a delay to permit recipient pretreatment and conditioning with donor antigen.

Unparalleled progress made over the past few years in the conceptual understanding of the mechanisms operative in the induction of allotolerance and restoration of self-tolerance has led to the development of unique and selective immunomodulatory strategies. Prime examples of progress made include: (i) the demonstration of long-term islet allograft survival in nonhuman primates receiving anti-CD40L antibody monotherapy (78), (ii) the induction of robust tolerance to murine islet allografts by alloantigen pretreatment under the cover of short-term anti-CD40L therapy (79), and (iii) the restoration of self-tolerance to B cell autoantigens in overtly diabetic NOD mice by FcR nonbinding anti-CD3 antibodies (80,81). Moreover, blockade of the CD40L/CD40 costimulatory pathway has been shown to prevent inflammatory responses such as cell extravasation, production of inflammatory and chemotactic cytokines, and activation of macrophage effector function (82).

Pancreatic transplantation remains the best method available today to successfully substitute the endocrine pancreas and reverse the diabetic condition to a normal glucose metabolism. Pancreatic transplantation was originally reported in 1967 at the University of Minnesota. Since then,

and especially during the past 10 years, more than 15,000 cases have been reported worldwide. Pancreatic transplantation today carries a five-year patient survival greater than 80%, and a graft survival greater than 70%. Recipients of a pancreas graft for diabetes are insulin free, and recent research shows a positive impact of the new pancreas on the secondary complications of type I diabetes, in particular neuropathy and microangiopathy (83,84). Pancreatic transplantation is currently offered to patients with uremic diabetes in need of a renal transplant or who received a kidney graft in the past. In some selected nonuremic patients with diabetes, affected especially by extremely brittle glucose control, frequent hypoglycemia, and severe neuropathy manifesting as hypoglycemia unawareness, pancreatic transplantation remains the only logical therapeutic alternative. New options in the fight to cure diabetes, such as gene therapy, continue to be aggressively pursued and could become available to prevent the disease entirely in the future.

ENDOCRINE TUMORS OF THE PANCREAS

The rich endocrine resources found within the pancreas can generate a wide variety of syndromes and clinical conundrums when one or more of the cell lines becomes neoplastic (Table 4). The resulting tumors may secrete hormones not normally released from the endocrine pancreas, in which case the secretions are ectopic. Although endocrine tumors of the pancreas are rare, they have taught us a great deal about the nature of endocrinology in health and disease. For example, hypergastrinemia, first described by Zollinger and Ellison in 1955 (85), has, despite its rarity, greatly advanced our understanding of acid-peptic ulceration of the stomach. Proinsulin was first discovered in secretions of an insulinoma and introduced the concept of large-molecular-weight gene products that are subsequently tailored before secretion (4).

Our understanding of the nature of endocrine tumors has been greatly advanced by the APUD concept of Pearse and Polak (86). The capacity to diagnose these tumors has been profoundly enhanced by the availability of radio-immunoassays for the measurement of the endocrine products. Localization of endocrine tumors has been tremendously aided by selective venous catheterization coupled with radioimmunoassay to identify the source of the abnormal concentrations of the hormones found in circulating blood. Localization and logistics for removal of endocrine tumors have been aided considerably by precise arteriography, ultrasonography, and computed tomographic imaging of the pancreas (87). Unfortunately, a significant number of pancreatic endocrine tumors are malignant, with a propensity toward early metastasis. Medical oncology sees islet cell tumors in ways not incompatible with surgeons challenged to ablate or palliate. The reviews in Surgical Clinics of North America (June 2001) provide much details about these challenging tumors (88,89).

Types of Pancreatic Endocrine Tumors
Insulinoma
Insulinomas, the most common of the pancreatic endocrine tumors, arise from the B cells of the islets. Approximately 80% are solitary and benign; the incidence of malignancy is about 10%. The remainder are either multiple benign adenomas or islet cell hyperplasia causing hyperinsulinism.

Table 4 Pancreatic Endocrine Neoplasia

Syndrome/cell of origin	Pathology	Metabolic change	Hormone	Symptoms
B	Adenoma Carcinoma (10%) Hyperplasia	Hypoglycemia Glycogenesis Gluconeogenesis Lipolysis Ketogenesis	Insulin Proinsulin	Those of hypoglycemia
A	Carcinoma (70%) Hyperplasia	Hyperglycemia Glycogenolysis Lipolysis Ketogenesis Gastrointestinal motor changes	Glucagon Enteroglucagon	Dermatitis Ileus Constipation
D	Carcinoma Adenoma	Mixed, mild glucose Biliary Pancreatic exocrine	Somatostatin Insulin Glucagon	Cholelithiasis Steatorrhea Dyspepsia
F	Adenoma	?	PP	None
? Zollinger–Ellison	Carcinoma (80%) Adenoma Hyperplasia	H^+ secretion	Gastrin	Acid-peptic ulceration Diarrhea
? Verner–Morrison	Carcinoma (50%) Adenoma	Intestinal secretion Gastric secretion Hypokalemia	VIP	Diarrhea Hypochlorhydria

Abbreviations: PP, pancreatic polypeptide; VIP, vasoactive intestinal peptide.

In infants, hyperinsulinism is usually a result of adenomatous hyperplasia of B cells (nesidioblastosis). Insulinomas are small; about 40% are 1 cm or less in diameter. Tumors are distributed in almost equal numbers throughout the head, body, and tail of the pancreas. Only 1% or fewer of all insulinomas are ectopic, and these are found close to the pancreas in most instances. Multiple endocrine neoplasia type I syndrome occurs in 10% of patients with insulinomas (see Chapter 51).

The major signs and symptoms of insulinoma are a result of the effects of hypoglycemia (from the hyperinsulinemia) on the central nervous system. These include apathy, sluggishness, irritability, excitement, changes in behavior, and occasionally convulsions and coma. Hypoglycemia also induces a release of epinephrine, which causes sweating, nervousness, tremor, palpitation, hunger, and pallor. The classic diagnostic criteria (Whipple's triad) are still valid. Whipple's triad includes central nervous system symptoms brought on by fasting, a fasting blood glucose level less than 50 mg/dL, and complete reversal of all symptoms by intravenous infusion of glucose.

Insulin levels are high relative to the blood glucose concentration. The insulin-to-glucose ratio is normally less than 0.4, but in patients with insulinoma the ratio is often close to 1 or even greater. The measurement of elevated plasma proinsulin levels is also helpful in the diagnosis of insulinoma. Furthermore, malignant tumors can be differentiated from benign islet cell lesions by documenting the greater percentage of proinsulin in the total insulin immunoactivity typically seen in patients with malignant lesions.

The traditional diagnostic test for insulinoma is the demonstration of fasting hypoglycemia (less than 50 mg/dL). Fasting is continued for 72 hours, or until hypoglycemic symptoms appear. Hypoglycemia occurs in two-thirds of patients by 24 hours and in 95% by 48 hours. During fasting, insulin levels remain elevated in patients with insulinoma because of the autonomous nature of the insulin secretion. Provocation tests for insulin release (e.g., tolbutamide, glucagon, leucine, and arginine) have been used to make the diagnosis of insulinoma but are thought to be of little value, because serum insulin levels can be measured directly. The infusion of secretagogues in healthy patients should not result in pathologically low blood glucose levels. However, secretagogues may provoke an insulinoma to release profoundly pathologic amounts of insulin, with consequent hypoglycemia.

Selective angiography with subtraction and magnification techniques is the best method of preoperative localization of an insulinoma. The success rate of localizing these tumors approaches 90%. Selective pancreatic vein catheterization and venous sampling for insulin assay have also been used, with considerable success, to diagnose and localize the site of insulinomas. Ultrasonography and computed tomography have been used to localize these lesions, but in comparison with the other diagnostic modalities available, they are of limited usefulness. Localization of the small, usually single, benign insulinoma continues to be an issue. When computed tomography fails to find the lesion, percutaneous transhepatic portal catheterization may give very sensitive clues to the site of the tumor. The most useful information comes from intraoperative ultrasound (90). Endoscopic ultrasound has limited ability to localize and characterize insulinomas (91). Localization of metastatic neuroendocrine tumors, suspected by assayable endocrine activity, can be facilitated by single photon emission computed tomography nuclear imaging with ^{111}In-pentetreotide, a somatostatin analog (92).

Because they are predominantly benign, insulinomas are the only pancreatic endocrine tumors that can frequently be cured by surgery. Depending on location, enucleation or distal pancreatectomy is the treatment of choice. It is rarely necessary to perform a pancreaticoduodenectomy as the initial procedure for a small tumor of the head of the pancreas. Laparoscopic resection of benign insulinoma has been described and almost certainly has merit, although the technical aspects are formidable (93–97). Other endocrine tumors are also amenable to laparoscopic resection, especially if they are small and benign (95,97). Even more aggressive pancreatic resection seems feasible (98). The adjunctive therapeutic agent of choice in patients with metastases is streptozocin, with a response rate approaching 50%. In patients in whom persistent hypoglycemia poses a problem after presumably successful removal of insulinoma, and in patients with metastases, diazoxide is frequently effective in suppressing insulin release.

Gastrinoma and Malignant Islet Tumors (Zollinger–Ellison Syndrome)

The first of the endocrine tumor syndromes identified in pancreatic islets was reported by Zollinger and Ellison in 1955 (85). The tumors responsible for this syndrome (gastrinomas) not only occur in pancreatic islets but also may be found as isolated lesions within the proximal duodenum or in its vicinity. The cell that gives rise to gastrinoma has not been identified. Gastrin is not a normal product of the islets of Langerhans. The gastrinoma syndrome results from excessive quantities of gastrin released from these tumors and is usually manifested clinically by virulent acid-peptic ulceration of the upper gastrointestinal tract. Such ulceration may be found in the first portion of the duodenum, where other forms of acid-peptic disease commonly occur; not infrequently, however, ulcers may occur in aberrant regions, such as the distal duodenum and jejunum (98). These ulcers are usually single, but they may be multicentric occasionally. Generally, the ulcer precedes identification of the tumor by three to five years; occasionally, the ulcer itself is totally asymptomatic and is discovered accidentally. In approximately 20% of patients, diarrhea with steatorrhea is the only clinical symptom of the syndrome; this presumably occurs because of excessive acid production of the stomach, which inactivates pancreatic enzymes and thereby inhibits fat digestion and absorption by the duodenum and jejunum.

Approximately one-third of patients with hypergastrinemia caused by gastrinoma have relatives with endocrinopathies. This condition is commonly suspected because of refractory or recurrent acid-peptic disease. Upper gastrointestinal X-ray films frequently show a suspicious multiplicity of ulcers throughout the duodenum and even the proximal jejunum. Hypertrophic mucosal folds are evident in the stomach as a result of the hypergastrinemia. Before the availability of radioimmunoassays that enable measurement of serum gastrin levels, the clinical diagnosis of gastrinoma was made on the basis of gastric analysis. The high volume of gastric secretion in patients with gastrinoma displayed an acid output that approached the physiologic maximum elicited by histamine derivatives. Currently, the diagnosis is made on the basis of the demonstration of hypergastrinemia under fasting conditions. A serum gastrin level in excess of 200 pg/mL is suggestive of this syndrome. When gastrin levels exceed 100,000 pg/mL, extensive tumoral involvement, including hepatic metastasis, is highly probable. For equivocal fasting gastrin levels, provocative testing with secretin has been useful. A rise of at least 100 pg/mL from a fasting baseline following the administration of an intravenous bolus of 2 U/kg secretin is diagnostic of the disease. Gastrin levels may also be elevated in some patients with hyperplasia of the G cells in the antrum. In this circumstance, however, serum gastrin does not change during secretin provocation (99).

Islet tumors of the pancreatic head, which are large and/or malignant, may require pancreaticoduodenectomy for oncologic thoroughness, and long-term survival may follow. However, small benign tumors do not qualify for this radical and complication prone operation. Enucleation can be curative (100). When islet tumors do not secrete enough hormone to produce an endocrine syndrome, they may grow silently to considerable size even if malignant. Extensive surgical resection is appropriate and may lead to long-term survival (101). When malignant islet tumors metastasize to the liver, patients may have a rather long course of treatment made more difficult because of endocrine issues than oncologic issues. However, a hepatic resection of even concurrent hepatic metastases may significantly prolong life, with prompt and durable oblation of the endocrine syndrome (102). Even hepatic debulking seems to offer benefit in terms of the endocrine syndromes and life extension (103). Hepatic metastases of endocrine tumors are also amenable to radiofrequency ablation when resection is not feasible (104). The most pressing issue in the management of gastrinomas is the acid secretion. When medical management is sought, pantoprazole or other proton pump inhibitors are highly effective as a maintenance therapy (105).

The ulcerogenic gastrinoma may be localized in approximately one-third of cases by means of angiography (106). Computed tomography often demonstrates pancreatic tumors if they are larger than 2 cm. Successful localization of pancreatic tumors by computed tomography approaches 32% for primary pancreatic tumors (107). Noninvasive preoperative ultrasonography in the intact patient has not been as successful as desired; however, intraoperative ultrasonography has been successful in identifying lesions otherwise not obvious. Percutaneous transhepatic portal and pancreatic venous sampling for gastrin can also localize the source of systemic hypergastrinemia (108).

Hypergastrinemia caused by gastrinoma is ideally treated by complete resection of the gastrinoma. Unfortunately, this is possible in only approximately 20% of cases, because the gastrinomas may be multiple or metastatic at diagnosis. Until recently, total gastrectomy was uniformly accepted as the treatment of choice to control the acid-peptic disease in patients for whom complete tumor excision was not possible. The concept of end-organ ablation by surgical removal has been challenged with the development of H_2-receptor antagonist therapy and completely repudiated by the introduction of proton pump inhibitors (109). Parietal cell vagotomy can improve the effectiveness of cimetidine therapy (110), but tumor plus end-organ ablation appears to be the only secure procedure to restore serum gastrin levels to normal. Of interest, an effect of the stomach on enhancing tumor growth has been proposed (111); if the stomach is removed, tumor growth is slowed.

Because 80% of gastrinomas are malignant, metastatic disease is not uncommon. Palliation with streptozocin has produced a positive response in about half of the patients with metastatic gastrinoma and other malignant islet tumors so treated. When chemotherapy is invoked for metastatic islet cell tumors, streptozotocin with 5-fluorouracil has been the first-choice drug regimen (112). Somatostain also offers a suppressive effect only on endocrine secretion from islet tumors and also the growth of metastases (113).

Glucagonoma

In glucagonoma, a neoplastic condition of the A cells of the islets of Langerhans, the entopic hormone glucagon is released. These tumors are malignant, approximately, two-thirds of the time, with early metastases to regional lymph nodes or the liver. Distant metastases are uncommon. The tumors are more frequently found in the tail of the pancreas, where there is the largest representation of A cells.

Glucagonoma causes a striking clinical syndrome manifested biochemically by hyperglycemia as a result of hyperglucagonemia. Patients with the syndrome sustain marked weight loss and demonstrate glossitis, frequent venous thrombosis, depression, and diarrhea. The most striking feature of this syndrome is called *necrolytic migratory erythema* (114). This skin lesion consists of erythematous macules and pustules together with flaccid bullae. The necrolytic pattern is present on portions of the skin that are easily traumatized. Histologically, there is superficial epidermal necrolysis and severe inflammation of the dermis with cellular infiltration. There is no explanation for this dermatologic phenomenon, which resolves after resection of the glucagonoma. The patients also demonstrate a normochromic, normocytic anemia. The hyperglycemia is not usually particularly severe. The metabolic consequences of hyperglucagonemia include rapid movement of the plasma amino acids into glucoenogenic pathways in the hepatic cytosol. The consumption of amino acids for gluconeogenesis depletes the circulating pool of amino acids and results in hypoaminoacidemia. This pool is not rapidly replenished by a complementary catabolism of muscle protein. The degree of hyperglucagonemia would be expected to cause a much sharper rise in blood glucose level, but this is partially compensated for by a slight hyperinsulinism that arises because of the hyperglycemia, and also because glucagon is a secretagogue for insulin. Although glucagon does not directly promote loss of muscle protein into the amino acid pool, the brisk gluconeogenesis deprives skeletal muscle of circulating amino acids that might be applied to muscle anabolism. Therefore, muscle wasting and weakness are quite prominent. In many ways, patients with glucagonoma resemble chronically stressed patients who have received inadequate nutritional support.

When the disease is suspected, diagnosis is established by radioimmunoassay for glucagon (115). In cases of a marginal elevation of glucagon level, pathologic overresponse to arginine can be demonstrated. Intravenous tolbutamide similarly causes a spectacular rise in the glucagon level in patients with glucagonoma. Once glucagonoma has been diagnosed, anatomic localization by computed axial tomography has been useful, because the tumors are frequently rather large in their position in the body and tail of the pancreas. Percutaneous transhepatic venous sampling has not been particularly helpful as a diagnostic aid because of the delicate nature of the glucagon assay and the large number of samples needed for adequate localization. Ultrasonography demonstrates these tumors only when they are large and bulky.

Radical surgical resection of the tumor is clearly the most satisfactory treatment for glucagonoma. Unfortunately, surgical resection is frequently palliative because of the presence of hepatic metastases. For unresectable or metastatic glucagonoma, streptozocin can be useful in reducing the size of the tumors, slowing the growth of metastases, and reducing the circulating levels of glucagon (116). The clinical symptoms, such as skin lesions and anemia, are ameliorated by streptozocin; however, the carbohydrate intolerance does not undergo remission, probably because of toxicity of the streptozocin on the B cells of the healthy islets of Langerhans.

Vipoma

Verner–Morrison syndrome was described in 1958 as the third islet-associated syndrome, after insulinoma and the Zollinger–Ellison syndrome (117). These islet cell tumors, called *vipomas*, secrete VIP. It is not clear as to which cell in the normal islet gives rise to this tumor. The secreted product is clearly ectopic, and the 28–amino acid peptide causes watery diarrhea, hypokalemia, and hypochlorhydria or achlorhydria. Only about 100 cases have been described, and in approximately 80% of these, a single tumor of the endocrine pancreas was held responsible for the syndrome. In the remaining 20%, hyperplasia of an uncertain member of the islet cell community was implicated. Ductal proliferation and an increase in the number of cells in the islets have been described in patients with this syndrome. Approximately half of the tumors are benign.

The VIP released by these tumors causes diarrhea, with volume losses in the range of 2 to 10 L/day. Associated potassium wasting, leading to hypokalemia, is observed. Not infrequently, the hypokalemia gives rise to flaccid paralysis and a nephropathy that can lead to renal failure. Hypomagnesemia and mild hypercalcemia have also been described in patients with this syndrome. The clinical effects of excessive VIP secretion are anticipated rather easily because of its known biologic action. VIP has specific receptors on the small-bowel mucosa, and binding of the peptide causes a sharp rise in cAMP, causing the effect of VIP to be similar to that of cholera toxin. The fluid losses are quite similar to those expected in cholera, and Verner–Morrison syndrome has therefore been called *pancreatic cholera*. VIP has substantial sequence homology with other gastrointestinal hormones such as secretin, glucagon, and GIP. Tumors secreting this peptide therefore may (i) enhance the secretion of alkaline fluid by the pancreas, which suggests secretin overactivity; (ii) induce hyperglycemia, which suggests a glucagon effect; and (iii) strikingly suppress gastric acid secretion, like an infusion of GIP. The release of VIP from these tumors can occur in paroxysms, to give pictures of flushing caused by the vasodilatory reaction of VIP, which may lead to some confusion with the carcinoid syndrome.

Diagnosis of the Verner–Morrison syndrome is not easily accomplished, because radioimmunoassay for VIP is not universally available. Further, an extremely similar syndrome is caused by tumors that release prostaglandin E_2. Generally, when the clinical picture of the Verner–Morrison syndrome is encountered, the pancreas is studied by computed tomography, angiography, or ultrasonography for evidence of a pancreatic mass lesion. If a tumor is identified, the preferred treatment is by surgical resection. In the presence of hepatic metastases, high-dose steroids and streptozocin have offered reasonable palliation (7).

PPoma

A few tumors of the endocrine pancreas have been described that apparently secrete only PP. The importance of this is uncertain, because there is no specific metabolic or clinical manifestation of these tumors, called *PPomas*. PP is released in abnormally large amounts by patients who harbor other kinds of non–B islet cell tumors. Therefore, PP has been suggested as a marker for other pancreatic endocrine tumors, especially in families with a propensity toward development of these lesions. Approximately half of all patients with other pancreatic endocrine tumors have an elevation in the PP level. Furthermore, approximately 50% of patients with carcinoid tumors, regardless of site, demonstrate an elevation in the PP level. When they are present, PP-secreting tumors are detected clinically because of the effect of the mass in the pancreas or because of metastases. Therefore, the syndrome of PP-secreting tumors is not necessarily an endocrine syndrome, but one more related to neoplasia. In patients with islet cell tumors, PP is frequently secreted in high concentration in addition to the primary or symptom-producing hormone. Also, the PP level is quite often elevated in the plasma of patients with asymptomatic tumors. Therefore, PP measurement can be used as a tumor marker to screen patients with multiple endocrine neoplasia type 1 syndrome, for the preclinical appearance of an islet cell tumor.

Somatostatinoma

The first case report of a somatostatin-secreting tumor was published in 1977. Approximately 20 cases have now been described (118). These tumors are usually malignant and accompanied by hepatic metastases. Somatostatinomas may be located in the pancreas or duodenum.

Metabolically, somatostatin inhibits numerous endocrine and exocrine secretory functions. Dyspepsia, mild diabetes, and cholelithiasis with steatorrhea constitute the expected pathophysiologic constellation for this endocrine condition. These effects are easily attributable to the inhibitory effects of somatostatin on a wide array of smooth muscle and endocrine secretory events. Somatostatin is inhibitory for essentially all gastrointestinal hormones, including insulin, PP, glucagon, gastrin, secretin, motilin, and GIP. The mild diabetes is directly attributable to inhibition of insulin secretion, whereas diarrhea and steatorrhea are attributable to deficient secretion of pancreatic enzymes. The dyspepsia may be more a motor disturbance in smooth muscle function, because hypochlorhydria is observed when gastric acid studies are performed in patients with somatostatinoma. The reduced muscular tone of the gallbladder presumably leads to gallbladder stasis and the formation of stones. Patients with somatostatinoma also uniformly lose weight, which may be attributable to neoplastic effects or malabsorption. Somatostatinoma may be identified by elevated levels of somatostatin in the blood. Excessive secretion of somatostatin by these tumors can be induced in response to intravenous tolbutamide. These tumors are identified on computed tomography and angiography; if they have not metastasized, the ideal treatment is complete excision.

Other Islet Cell Tumors

Pancreatic islet cell tumors yielding a syndrome related to hypercalcemia have been described. These tumors have undetectable parathyroid hormone levels, so a parathyroid hormone-like substance has been implicated as the causative agent (119). Many of the features of hyperparathyroidism are present, including bone resorption, nephrocalcinosis, nephrolithiasis, peptic ulcer, and psychoneurologic symptoms. Unless the tumor is extirpated, conventional treatment of hypercalcemia is futile, and the patient eventually dies. Adrenocorticotropinomas of the pancreas have been described, and most have produced a clinical Cushing's syndrome (120). Plasma cortisol and urinary 17-hydroxycorticosteroid levels have not been suppressible by the dexamethasone suppression test. Several cases of tumors of the pancreas secreting growth hormone–releasing factor and causing acromegalic symptoms have been described. Acromegaly may regress after tumor extirpation without hypophysectomy (121).

In addition, a variety of non–B islet cell tumors apparently have no secretory products that can be identified. They generate no endocrine syndrome to lead to their diagnosis, even though they constitute approximately 20% of all islet cell tumors and are most commonly discovered by computed tomography or angiography as incidental structures or as the explanation for a larger intra-abdominal mass. These tumors can affect the biliary tree by obstruction, which leads to their discovery in approximately half of affected patients. A tumor marker for these lesions is plasma neurone-specific enolase, a neural isomer of the glycolytic enzyme enolase. The glycolytic pathway in neural tissue could be adversely affected by the lowered pH in neural cells, which is the consequence of intense metabolic activity. The enolase found in other tissues is an allosteric subunit enzyme that dissociates in the cytosolic pH found in neural cells. Neurone-specific enolase is stable in its allosteric confirmation at the pH range associated with neural tissue. This enzyme is common to all APUD and neural cells. In fact, the enzyme is released into the plasma of patients with APUD tumors and can be used as a marker for all APUD tumors (19).

In as many as 80% of patients with nonfunctioning islet cell tumors, histologic examination reveals evidence of malignancy; however, these tumors grow slowly, and even patients with hepatic metastases may have prolonged survival. Surgical removal is generally the preferred treatment; medical therapy with streptozocin yields a good response in patients with metastases.

The endocrine tumors of the pancreas present a challenge to the endocrinologist and surgeon, with the prospect for occasional cure and frequent long-term palliation. Recently, substantial endocrine palliation has been achieved with almost all of the endocrine syndromes by administering long-acting somatostatin to suppress hormone release. Somatostatin is not a chemotherapeutic agent, and no tumor remission has been seen. However, control of the endocrine syndrome in Zollinger–Ellison syndrome, insulinoma, Verner–Morrison syndrome, and glucagonoma represents a spectacular improvement in the treatment of these unfortunate patients.

A knowledge of the islet cell tumors of the pancreas is important to anyone treating pancreatic neoplasia. In fact, all masses in the pancreas are not evidence of hopeless adenocarcinoma of the pancreas. Indeed, pancreatic masses, even those that occlude the common bile duct, deserve careful attention. The identification of a resectable islet cell tumor may indeed be the happy conclusion of a diagnostic workup in which the islet cell tumor was not the leading possibility at the outset of the investigation.

SUMMARY

The endocrine pancreas controls the movement of glucose through the extracellular fluid by regulating the generation of glucose and the facilitated diffusion of glucose into most cells. The islets of Langerhans that comprise the endocrine pancreas constitute a community of at least four cell types that interact in the islets for the purpose of regulating conflicting secretions that either raise or lower the plasma glucose level. The A (glucagon), B (insulin), D (somatostatin), and F (PP) cells respond to a vast number of secretagogues and antagonists to support a hormonal output compatible with an appropriate hormonal presentation, especially to the liver, to guarantee the movement of glucose in response to substrate demand. These cells join a larger number of others strewn along the gastrointestinal tract to secrete the hormonally active gut peptides.

This chapter has outlined the anatomy, embryology, and physiology of the islets. The only known spontaneous deficiency disease of the endocrine pancreas, diabetes mellitus, has been discussed in some detail. The pathophysiology of the functioning neoplasms of these endocrine cells has also been discussed. Although the endocrine neoplasms are quite rare, the metabolic and pathologic sequelae of excess states of these critical hormones serve to reinforce our understanding of metabolism and its hormonal regulation.

REFERENCES

1. Merrell RC. Cell-cell recognition in neuroembryology. In: Bradshaw RA, Schneider DM, eds. Proteins of the Nervous System. New York: Raven Press, 1980.
2. Von Mering J, Minkowski O. Diabetes mellitus nach pancreas extirpation. Arch Exp Pathol Pharmacol 1889; 26:371.
3. Banting FG, Best CHL. The internal secretion of the pancreas. J Lab Clin Med 1922; 7:251.
4. Oyer P et al. Studies on human proinsulin. J Biol Chem 1971; 246:1375.
5. Goldman H, Wong I, Patel YC. A study of the structural and biochemical development of human fetal islets of Langerhans. Diabetes 1982; 31:897.
6. Bonner-Weir S. Morphological evidence for pancreatic polarity of 3-cell within the islets of Langerhans. Diabetes 1988; 37:616.
7. Pignal F et al. Streptozotocin treatment in pancreatic cholera (Verner-Morrison) syndrome. Digestion 1982; 24:176.
8. Rutter WJ et al. An analysis of pancreatic development. In: Papoconstautinoi J, Rutter WJ, eds. Molecule Control of Proliferation and Differentiation. New York: Academic Press, 1978.
9. Henderson JR, Daniel PM, Fraser PA. The pancreas as a single organ: the influence of the endocrine upon the exocrine part of the gland. Gut 1981; 22:158.
10. Bell GI et al. Sequence of the human insulin gene. Nature 1980; 284:26.
11. Espinal J. Understanding Insulin Action. West Sussex (UK): Ellis Horwood, 1989.
12. Hammonds P et al. Regulation and specificity of glucose-stimulated insulin gene expression in human islets of Langerhans. FEBS Lett 1987; 223:131.
13. Farnby B, Schmid-Farmby F, Grodsky GM. Relationship between insulin release and ^{65}zinc efflux from rat pancreatic islets maintained in tissue culture. Diabetes 1984; 33:229.
14. Ashcroft FM et al. Glucose induces closure of single potassium channels in isolated rat pancreatic B-cells. Nature 1984; 312:446.
15. Malaisse WJ, Senor A, Malaisse-Lagae F. Insulin release: reconciliation of the receptor and metabolic hypothesis. Mol Cell Biochem 1981; 37:157.
16. Meda P, Perrelet A, Orci L. Increase of gap junctions between pancreatic B-cells during stimulation of insulin secretion. J Cell Biol 1979; 82:441.
17. Metz SA, Fujimoto WY, Robertson RP. Lipoxygenation of arachidonic acid: a pivotal step in stimulus secretion coupling in the pancreatic beta cell. Endocrinology 1982; 111:2141.
18. Matschinsky FM et al. Glucoreceptor mechanisms in islets of Langerhans. Diabetes 1972; 21:555.
18a. Sjoholm A, Lehtihet M, et al. Glucose inhibit protein phosphatases and directly promote insulin exocytosis in pancreatic β-cells. Endocrinology 2002; 143(2):4592–4598.
19. Prinz RA et al. Serum markers for pancreatic islet cell and intestinal carcinoid tumors. Surgery 1983; 94:1019.
20. Reaven E et al. Effect of age and environmental factors on insulin release from the perfused pancreas of the rat. J Clin Invest 1983; 71:345.
21. Klines I et al. Normal insulin sensitivity of the islets of Langerhans in obese subjects with resistance to its glucoregulatory actions. Diabetes 1984; 33:305.
22. Marincola F et al. The independence of insulin release and ambient insulin in vitro. Diabetes 1983; 32:1162.
23. Tepperman J. Metabolic and Endocrine Physiology. 3rd. Chicago: Year Book Publishers, 1973.
24. McGarry JD, Foster DW. Regulation of hepatic fatty acid oxidation and ketone body production. Am Rev Biochem 1980; 49:395.
25. Dayoff MO. Atlas of Protein Sequence and Structure. Silver Spring, MD: National Biomedical Research Foundation, 1969.
26. Pandol SJ et al. Growth hormone-releasing factor stimulates pancreatic enzyme secretion. Science 1984; 225:326.
27. Kimball CP, Murlin JR. Aqueous extracts of pancreas. III. Some precipitation reactions of insulin. J Biol Chem 1923; 58:337.
28. Itoh M et al. Secretion of glucagon. In: Cooperstein SJ, Watkins D, eds. The Islets of Langerhans. New York: Academic Press, 1981.
29. Goodner CJ, Hom FG, Koercker DJ. Hepatic glucose production oscillates in synchronic with the islet secretory cycle in fasting rhesus monkeys. Science 1982; 215:1257.
30. Efendic S, Luft R. Somatostatin and its role in insulin and glucagon secretion. In: Cooperstein SJ, Watkins D, eds. The Islets of Langerhans. New York: Academic Press, 1981.
31. Kimmell JR, Pollack HG, Hazelwood RL. Isolation and characterization of chicken insulin. Endocrinology 1968; 83: 1323.
32. Warren JH et al. Differences in risk of insulin-dependent diabetes in offspring of diabetic mothers and diabetic fathers. N Engl J Med 1984; 311:149.
33. Srikanta S et al. Pre-type I diabetes: identical endocrinological course dependent of HLA DR types or presence of cytoplasmic anti-islet antibodies. Diabetes 1984; 33:10A.
34. Stiller CR et al. Effects of cyclosporine-type I diabetes: clinical course and immune response. Diabetes 1984; 33:13A.
35. Tager HS. Abnormal products of the human insulin glue. Diabetes 1984; 33:693.
36. Eizirick DL et al. Repair of pancreatic β-cells. Diabetes 1993; 42:1383.
37. Opie EL. The relation of diabetes mellitus to lesion of the pancreas: hyaline degeneration of the islands of Langerhans. J Exp Med 1901; 5:527.
38. Bell RH et al. Molecular defects in diabetes mellitus. Diabetes 1991; 40:413.
39. James DE et al. Molecular cloning and characterization of an insulin-regulatable glucose transporter. Nature 1989; 338:83.
40. Birnbaum MJ. Identification of a novel gene encoding an insulin-responsive glucose transporter protein. Cell 1989; 57:305.
41. Jaspan J et al. Treatment of severely painful diabetic neuropathy with an aldose reductose inhibitor: relief of pain and improved somatic and autonomic nerve function. Lancet 1983; 2:758.
42. Siperstein MD, Unger RH, Madison LL. Studies of muscle capillary basement membranes in normal subjects, diabetic and pre-diabetic patients. J Clin Invest 1968; 47:1973.
43. Koenig RJ, Cerami A. Hemoglobin A, C, and diabetes mellitus. Annu Rev Med 1980; 31:29.
44. Clutter WE. Diabetes mellitus and hyperlipidemia. In: Campbell JW, Frisse M, eds. Manual of Medical Therapeutics. Boston: Little, Brown, 1983.
45. Cornfield J. The university group diabetes program: a further statistical analysis of the mortality findings. JAMA 1971; 217(12):1676–1687.
46. Lauritzen T et al. Effect of one year of near-normal blood glucose levels on retinopathy in insulin-dependent diabetics. Lancet 1983; 1:200.
47. Ballinger WF, Lacy PE. Transplantation of intact pancreatic islets in rats. Surgery 1972; 72:175.
48. Cobb L, Merrell R. Intrasplenic islet autografts: insulin response to IV glucose challenge. Curr Surg 1983; 40:36.
49. Bell RH et al. Prevention by whole pancreas transplantation of glomerular basement membrane thickening in alloxan diabetes. Surgery 1980; 88:31.

50. Gray BN, Watkins E. Prevention of vascular complications of diabetes by pancreatic islet transplantation. Arch Surg 1976; 111:254.

51. Tyden G, Bolinder J, Solders G, Brattstrom C, Tibell A, Groth CG. Improved survival in patients with insulin-dependent diabetes mellitus and end-stage diabetic nephropathy 10 years after combined pancreas and kidney transplantation. Transplantation 1999; 67(5):645–648.

52. Fioretto P, Steffes MW, Sutherland DE, Goetz FC, Mauer M. Reversal of lesions of diabetic nephropathy after pancreas transplantation. N Engl J Med 1998; 339(2):69–75.

53. Rastellini C, Shapiro R, Corry R, Fung JJ, Starzl TE, Rao AS. Treatment of isolated pancreatic islets to reverse pancreatectomy-induced and insulin-dependent type I diabetes in humans: a 6-year experience. Transplant Proc 1997; 29(1–2): 746–747.

54. IPTR Annual Report of the International Pancreas Transplant Registry. IPTR Newslett 1998; 10(1):1–12.

55. Hering BJ, Ricordi C. Islet transplantation for patients with type I diabetes. Graft 1999; 2(1):12–27.

56. Gunnarsson R, Klintmalm G, Lundgren G, et al. Deterioration in glucose metabolism in pancreatic transplant recipients after conversion from azathioprine to cyclosporine. Transplant Proc 1984; 16(3):709–712.

57. Friedman EA, Shyh TP, Beyer MM, Manis T, Butt KMH. Posttransplant diabetes in kidney transplant recipients. Am J Nephrol 1985; 5(3):196–202.

58. Boudreaux JP, McHugh L, Canafax DM, et al. The impact of cyclosporine and combination immunosuppression on the incidence of posttransplant diabetes in renal allograft recipients. Transplantation 1987; 44(3):376–381.

59. Jindal RM. Posttransplant diabetes mellitus—a review. Transplantation 1994; 58(12):1289–1298.

60. Jindal RM, Popsecu I, Schwartz ME, et al. Diabetogenicity of FK506 versus cyclosporine in liver transplant recipients. Transplantation 1994; 58(3):370–372.

61. McGeown MG, Douglas JF, Brown WA, et al. Advantages of low dose steroid from the day after renal transplantation. Transplantation 1980; 29:287.

62. Arner P, Gunnarsson R, Blomdahl S, et al. Some characteristics of steroid diabetes: a study in renal transplant recipients receiving high dose corticosteroid therapy. Diabetes Care 1983; 6(1):23–25.

63. Ricordi C, Zeng Y, Alejandro R, et al. In vivo effect of FK506 on human pancreatic islets. Transplantation 1991; 52(3):519.

64. Rilo HLR, Zeng Y, Alejandro R, et al. Effect of FK506 on function of human islets of Langerhans. Transplant Proc 1991; 23:3164.

65. Brendel M, Hering B, Schulz A, Bretzel R. International Islet Transplant Registry Report. Germany: University of Giessen, 1999:1–20.

66. Linetsky E, Bottino R, Lehmann R, Alejandro R, Inverardi L, Ricordi C. Improved human islet isolation using a new enzyme blend, liberase. Diabetes 1997; 46(7):1120–1123.

67. Lakey JR, Warnock GL, Shapiro AM, et al. Intraductal collagenase delivery into the human pancreas using syringe loading or controlled perfusion. Cell Transplant 1999; 46(7):1120–1123.

68. Shapiro AM, Hao E, Lakey JR, Finegood D, Rajotte RV, Kneteman NM. Diabetogenic synergism in canine islet autografts from cyclosporine and steroids in combination. Transplant Proc 1998; 30(2):527.

69. Shapiro AM, Hao E, Lakey JR, Elliot JF, Rajotte RV, Kneteman NM. Development of diagnostic markers for islet allograft rejection. Transplant Proc 1998; 30(2):647.

70. Kaufman DB, Gores PF, Field MJ, et al. Effect of 15-deoxyspergualin on immediate function and long-term survival of transplanted islets in murine recipients of marginal islet mass. Diabetes 1994; 43(6):778–783.

71. Rosenberg L, Wang R, Paraskevas S, Maysinger D. Structural and functional changes resulting from islet isolation lead to islet cell death. Surgery 1999; 126(2):393–398.

72. Bennet W, Sundberg B, Groth CG, et al. Incompatibility between human blood and isolated islets of Langerhans: a

73. finding with implications for clinical intraportal islet transplantation? Diabetes 1999; 48(10):1907–1914.

74. Kenyon NS, Ranuncoli A, Massetti M, Chatzipetrou M, Ricordi C. Islet transplantation: present and future perspectives. Diabetes Metab Rev 1998; 14(4):303–313.

75. Swift SM, Clayton HA, London NJ, James RF. The potential contribution of rejection to survival of transplanted human islets. Cell Transplant 1998; 7(6):599–606.

76. Drachenberg CB, Klassen DK, Weir MR, et al. Islet cell damage associated with tacrolimus and cyclosporine: morphological features in pancreas allograft biopsies and clinical correlation. Transplantation 1999; 68(3):396–402.

77. Shapiro A, Lakey J, Ryan E, et al. Islet transplant in seven patients with type 1 diabetes mellitus patients using a glucocorticoid free immunosuppressive regimen. N Engl J Med 2000; 343:230–238.

78. Ryan E, Lakey J, Rajotte R, et al. Clinical outcomes and insulin secretion after islet transplantation with the Edmonton protocol. Diabetes 2001; 50(4):710–719.

79. Kenyon NS, Chatzipetrou M, Masetti M, et al. Long-term survival and function of intrahepatic islet allografts in rhesus monkeys treated with humanized anti-CDD154. Proc Natl Acad Sci USA 1999; 96(14):8132–8137.

80. Zheng XX, Markees TG, Hancock WW, et al. CTLA4 signals are required to optimally induce allograft tolerance with combined donor-specific transfusion and anti-CD154 monoclonal antibody treatment. J Immunol 1999; 162(8):4983–4990.

81. Chatenoud L, Primo J, Back JF. CD3 antibody-induced dominant self tolerance in overtly diabetic NOD mice. J Immunol 1997; 158(6):2947–2954.

82. Chatenoud L, Thervet E, Primo J, Back JF. Anti-CD3 antibody induces long-term remission of overt autoimmunity in nonobese diabetic mice. Proc Natl Acad Sci USA 1994; 91(1): 123–127.

83. Grewal IS, Flavell RA. The CD40 ligand. At the center of the immune universe? Immunol Res 1997; 16(1):59–70.

84. Sutherland DER. Pancreas and islet transplantation: an update. Transplant Rev 1994; 8:185.

85. Basadonna GP et al. Morbidity, mortality and long-term allograft function in kidney transplantation alone and simultaneous pancreas/kidney transplantation in diabetic patients. Transplant Proc 1993; 25:1321.

86. Zollinger RM, Ellison EH. Primary peptic ulcerations of the jejunum associated with islet cell tumors of the pancreas. Ann Surg 1955; 142:709.

87. Pearse AGE, Polak MJ. Endocrine tumours of neural crest origin: neurolophomas apudomas and the APUD concept. Med Biol 1974; 52:3.

88. Stark DD et al. Computed tomography and nuclear magnetic resonance imaging of pancreatic islet cell tumors. Surgery 1983; 94:1024.

89. Brentjens R, Saltz L. Islet cell tumors of the pancrease: the Medical Oncologist's Perspective. Surg Clin North Am 2001; 81(3):527–542.

90. Azimuddin K, Chamberlain RS. The surgical management of pancreatic neuroendocrine tumors. Surg Clin North Am 2001; 81(3):511–525.

91. Suzuki K, Takahashi S, Airua K, et al. Evaluation of the usefulness of percutaneous transhepatic portal catherization for preoperative diagnosing the localization of insulinomas. Pancreas 2002; 24(1):96–102.

92. Richards ML, Gauger PG, Thompson NW, et al. Pitfalls in the surgical treatment of insulinoma. Surgery 2002; 132:1040–1049.

93. Lebtahi R, Le Cloirec J, Houzard C, et al. Detection of neuroendocrine tumors: ^{99m}Tc-P829 scintigraphy compared with ^{111}In-pentetreotide scintigraphy. J Nucl Med 2002; 43:889–895.

94. Gramatica L Jr, Herrera MF, Mercardo-Luna A, et al. Videolaparoscopic resection of insulinomas: experience in two institutions. World J Surg 2002; 26(10):297–300.

95. Pietrabissa A, Shimi SM, Vaander Velpen G, et al. Localization of insulinoma by laparoscopic infragastric inspection of the pancreas and contact ultrasonography. Surg Oncol 1993; 2(1):83–86.

95. Gagner M, Pomp A, Herrera MF. Early experience with laparoscopic resections of islet cell tumors. Surgery 1996; 120(6):1051–1054.

96. Sussman LA, Christie R, Whittle DE. Laparoscopic excision of distal pancreas including insulinoma. Aust N Z J Surg 1996; 66(6):414–416.

97. Cuschieri A. Laparoscopic pancreatic resections. Semin Laparosc Surg 1996; 3(1):15–20.

98. Lomsky R, Langr F, Vortel V. Demonstration of glucagon in islet cell adenomas of the pancreas by immunofluorescent technic. Am J Clin Pathol 1969; 51:245.

99. Zollinger RM. The ulcerogenic syndrome. In: Friesen SR, ed. Surgical Endocrinology. Philadelphia: JB Lippincott, 1978.

100. Sarmiento JM, Farnell MB, Que FG, et al. Pancreaticoduodenectomy for islet cell tumors of the head of the pancreas: long-term survival analysis. World J Surg 2002; 26(10):1267–1271.

101. Matthews BD, Heniford BT, Reardon PR, et al. Surgical experience with nonfunctioning neuroendocrine tumors of the pancreas. Am Surg 2000; 66(12):1116–1123.

102. Sarmiento JM, Que FG, Grant CS, et al. Concurrent resections of pancreatic islet cell cancers with synchronous hepatic metastases: outcomes of an aggressive approach. Surgery 2002; 132(6):976–983.

103. Sarmiento JM, Heywood G, Rubin J, et al. Surgical treatment of neuroendocrine metastaes to the liver: a plea for resection to increase survival. J Am Coll Surg 2003; 197(1):29–37.

104. Hellman P, Ladjevardi S, Skogsedi B, et al. Radiofrequency tissue ablation using cooled tip for liver metastases of endocrine tumors. World J Surg 2002; 26(8):1052–1056.

105. Metz DC, Soffer E, Forsmark CE, et al. Maintenance oral pantopyrazole therapy is effective for patients with Zollinger-Ellison syndrome and idiopathic hypersecretion. Am J Gastroenterol 2003; 98(2):301–307.

106. Giacobazzi D, Passaro E. Preoperative angiography in the Zollinger-Ellison syndrome. Am J Surg 1973; 126:74.

107. Dunnick NR et al. Computed tomographic detections of non-beta pancreatic islet cell tumors. Radiology 1980; 135:117.

108. Ingemausson S et al. Pancreatic vein catheterization with gastrin assay in normal patients and in patients with Zollinger-Ellison syndrome. Am J Surg 1977; 134:558.

109. Friesen SR et al. Cimetidine in the management of synchronous crises of MEAI. World J Surg 1980; 4:123.

110. Richardson CT et al. Effect of vagotomy in Zollinger-Ellison syndrome. Gastroenterology 1979; 77:681.

111. Friesen SR. Treatment of the Zollinger-Ellison syndrome. Am J Surg 1982; 143:331.

112. Ramanathan RK, Cnaan A, Hahn RG, et al. Phase II trial of dacarbazine (DTIC) in advanced pancreatic iselt cell carcinoma. Study of the Eastern Cooperative Oncology Group-E6282. Ann Oncol 2001; 12:1139–1143.

113. Fjallsko ML, Sundin A, Westlin JE, et al. Treatment of malignant endocrine pancreatic tumors with a combination of α-interferon and somatostatin analogs. Med Oncol 2002; 19(1): 35–42.

114. Pedersen NB, Jonsson L, Holst JJ. Necrolytic migratory erythema and glucagon cell tumour of the pancreas: the glucagonoma syndrome. Acta Derm Venereol (Stockh) 1976; 56:391.

115. Belchetz PE et al. ACTH, glucagon and gastrin production by a pancreatic islet cell carcinoma and its treatment. Clin Endocrinol 1973; 2:307.

116. Danforth DN et al. Elevated plasma proglucagon-like component with glucagon-secreting tumor: effect of streptozotocin. N Engl J Med 1976; 295:242.

117. Verner JV, Morrison AB. Islet cell tumor and a syndrome of refractory watery diarrhea and hypokalemia. Am J Med 1958; 25:374.

118. Pipeleers D et al. Five cases of somatostatinoma clinical heterogeneity and diagnostic usefulness of basal and tolbutamide induced hypersomatostatinemia. J Clin Endocrinol Metab 1983; 56:1236.

119. Rasbach D et al. Pancreatic islet cell carcinoma with hypercalcemia. Am J Med 1985; 78:337.

120. Abe K et al. Production of calcitonin, adrenocorticotropic hormone, and B-melanocyte-stimulating hormone in tumors derived from amine precursor uptake and decarboxylation cells. Cancer Res 1977; 37:4190.

121. Rosch J et al. Functional endocrine tumors of the pancreas: clinical presentation, diagnosis, and treatment. Curr Probl Surg 1990; 26:309.

54

Multiple Endocrine Neoplasia: Types 1 and 2

Frank J. Quayle and Jeffrey F. Moley

INTRODUCTION

Most tumors of the endocrine system are sporadic and arise within a single gland. However, the multiple endocrine neoplasia (MEN) syndromes are characterized by a predisposition to develop neoplasms in multiple endocrine glands. As in other heritable cancer syndromes, the tumors may be multifocal and bilateral, synchronous or metachronous, and tumor histology varies from hyperplasia to invasive, metastasizing carcinoma.

The MEN syndromes have distinct patterns of clinical expression, and each is associated with germline mutations within specific genes. MEN type 1 (MEN 1) is characterized by parathyroid hyperplasia, pancreatic and duodenal neuroendocrine tumors, and pituitary adenomas. It is associated with mutations in the MEN 1 gene. MEN type 2A (MEN 2A) is characterized by medullary thyroid carcinoma (MTC), pheochromocytoma, and parathyroid hyperplasia, while MEN 2B is distinguished by MTC, pheochromocytoma, mucosal neuromas, and a distinctive *marfanoid habitus*. MEN 2A and 2B are associated with mutations in the rearranged during transfection (RET) proto-oncogene.

In each of these disorders, derangements of normal endocrine physiology manifest clinical symptoms and lead to laboratory abnormalities that can be used to diagnose and follow the underlying disease.

MULTIPLE ENDOCRINE NEOPLASIA TYPE 1
History, Molecular Genetics, and Pathogenesis

The presence of parathyroid, islet cell, and pituitary tumors in the same individual was described as a syndrome by Wermer in 1954 (1). Subsequently, MEN 1 was demonstrated to be heritable, highly penetrant, and to have variable clinical manifestations. The pattern of inheritance is autosomal dominant.

A combination of genetic-linkage analysis and tumor-deletion mapping localized the MEN 1 gene to chromosome 11q13 (2). The frequent loss of heterozygosity seen in MEN 1–associated tumors is consistent with the Knudson two-hit model of oncogenesis, suggesting that the mutant protein is a tumor suppressor (3). In this model, both copies of a tumor-suppressor gene must sustain a mutation before neoplastic transformation occurs. The first mutation is inherited in the germline in affected families and leads to susceptibility within involved tissues. The second occurs as a somatic event, after which the regulatory tumor-suppressor function is lost and clonal expansion and cancer development occur. Conceptually, the multifocal occurrence of tumors in affected endocrine glands is explained by multiple second hits within target tissues.

The MEN 1 gene consists of 10 exons encoding a 2.8 kb transcript, and the 610–amino acid protein product is called "menin" (4). This highly conserved protein is expressed during development and in adults across a variety of tissues. Menin is known to localize to the nucleus and has been demonstrated to bind to the transcription factor JunD, suggesting that its tumor-suppressor function is mediated through inhibition of JunD-activated transcription (5).

Mutations implicated in MEN 1 vary widely and include missense, nonsense, frameshift, and splicing defects found across the MEN 1 gene (6,7). No specific genotype–phenotype correlations have been established, although some evidence suggests that mutations associated with MEN 1 tend to cluster in the codons corresponding to domains in the menin protein that interact with JunD (8).

Clinical Features and Management

Patients with MEN 1 generally develop signs and symptoms in the third or fourth decade of life, and onset in the first decade is rare. MEN 1 is highly penetrant, with 52% of patients demonstrating some aspect of the disease by the age of 20, and 99% by the age of 50 (7). Histologic evidence of hyperplasia or neoplasia can be found in multiple endocrine tissues in nearly all patients with MEN 1 (9). Men and women are affected nearly equally, and no racial predilection has been identified.

Despite high penetrance, MEN 1 demonstrates a wide variability of phenotypic expression, including inconsistent tissue involvement, clinical presentation, clinical course, and prognosis. The most common abnormality is hyperparathyroidism (HPT), found in up to 95% of patients. Pancreatic or duodenal endocrinopathies are found in approximately half of patients, and pituitary adenomas are found in approximately a third, depending on the population studied (Table 1) (10). Less common tumors associated with MEN 1 include adrenocortical adenomas, lipomas, and foregut carcinoid tumors. Each of these tumor types may be present in different combinations, present in different order, and have a different prognosis. Nonetheless, as noted, specific patterns of expression are common within families. The high degree of variability precludes strict definitions of MEN 1. The current working definition of MEN 1 is tumors in two of the three primary sites (i.e., parathyroid, pancreaticoduodenal, and pituitary). Familial MEN 1 is defined by an index MEN 1 case with one or more relatives having tumors in one or more primary sites (11).

The clinical manifestations of disease depend upon the specific tissue involved and hormones produced. Classically, the most common presenting problem was peptic ulcer disease, followed by hypoglycemia (12). In the current era, a large proportion of patients continue to present with

Table 1   Characteristics of Multiple Endocrine Neoplasia Type 1 (MEN 1)

Pituitary tumors
    Prolactinomas
    ACTH-secreting tumors
    Growth hormone–secreting tumors
    Nonfunctional tumors
HPT
Pancreatic islet cell tumors
    Most common
        Gastrinoma
        Insulinoma
    Less common
        VIP-oma
        Glucagonoma
        Somatostatinoma
        Ppoma
        Nonfunctional tumors

Abbreviations: ACTH, adrenocorticotrophic hormone; HPT, hyperparathyroidism; VIP, vasoactive intestinal peptide.

evidence of islet cell tumors, although today the most common presenting problem is HPT. The important principle is that clinical symptoms do not always reflect the degree of underlying involved tissues.

Parathyroid Glands

The most common endocrinopathy in MEN 1 is HPT. Unlike most patients with sporadic HPT, who generally have discrete parathyroid adenomas, the distinguishing feature of HPT in MEN 1 patients is four-gland hyperplasia. This distinction has important ramifications for clinical management. The histologic abnormality is diffuse chief cell hyperplasia.

Elevated serum calcium is commonly the first biochemical abnormality detected in MEN 1. As with sporadic HPT, elevated serum parathyroid hormone (PTH) confirms the diagnosis of HPT. Clinical features of HPT in the setting of MEN 1 are similar to those associated with sporadic disease, including renal lithiasis, bone disease, anorexia, generalized muscle weakness, and gastrointestinal (GI) complaints. In general, patients with MEN 1 have an earlier onset of disease and milder hypercalcemia than those with sporadic HPT.

The challenge in the surgical treatment of HPT in the setting of MEN 1 is balancing the risk of hypoparathyroidism with the risk of recurrent hypercalcemia. Two major strategies have emerged to address this problem (13,14). The first is three and one-half gland parathyroidectomy leaving the remaining half-gland in situ in the neck. This is marked with a clip or nonabsorbable suture to aid in identification in the event of recurrent hypercalcemia. The other option is total four-gland parathyroidectomy with intramuscular autotransplantation of parathyroid tissue into the forearm muscle. In both strategies, parathyroidectomy should include a transcervical thymectomy to remove potential supernumary glands and rests within the cranial horns of the thymus. Residual parathyroid tissue should be cryopreserved to enable a subsequent autotransplant in the event of hypoparathyroidism.

The advantages of the four gland/autotransplant approach are twofold. First, in the event of recurrent or persistent HPT, the source is more easily localized if the glands were transplanted into the forearm. PTH levels drawn from right and left antecubital veins will show if the source of excess PTH is the grafts, or if the source is elsewhere, which would include the neck and mediastinum. Second, if the source of recurrent HPT is the grafts, this can be managed by excising a portion of grafted tissue under local anesthesia, thereby avoiding the complications of reoperative neck surgery. Given the diffuse parathyroid involvement, preoperative imaging studies such as sestamibi scanning or ultrasound are not generally helpful. However, these studies are useful for localization in the event of recurrence. Recurrent hypercalcemia occurs in 20% to 33% of patients with MEN 1, a much higher rate than that seen after surgical management of sporadic disease (13,14). This reflects the diffuse glandular involvement seen in MEN 1 patients.

Due to the association of MEN 1 with diffuse parathyroid hyperplasia, patients discovered to have four-gland HPT should undergo screening for other elements of the syndrome. When MEN 1 patients have concurrent HPT and gastrinoma, the former should be addressed first. Hypercalcemia exacerbates hypergastrinemia, and normalization of serum calcium often helps control gastric acid hypersecretion (14).

Pancreas and Duodenum

Neuroendocrine tumors of the pancreas and duodenum are the second most common feature of MEN 1, ultimately found in 50% or more of patients. These tumors can be hormonally active or silent and can be benign or malignant. Gastrin, insulin, glucagon, vasoactive intestinal peptide (VIP), and pancreatic polypeptide (PP) may be secreted. Nonfunctioning tumors or those that secrete PP are the most prevalent (15). Histologically, the most common findings are multifocal microadenomas or diffuse islet cell hyperplasia throughout the pancreas rather than large isolated tumors. Enteropancreatic tumors become clinically significant either due to mass effect or more commonly due to active hormone oversecretion.

Gastrinomas are the most common clinically functional pancreaticoduodenal tumors in patients with MEN 1 (16). The features of gastrinoma, known as the Zollinger–Ellison syndrome (ZES), include hypergastrinemia, massive gastric acid output, and secondary ulcer disease. The clinical characteristics include epigastric pain, peptic ulcer disease, reflux esophagitis, and secretory diarrhea. In this era, severe ulcer diathesis or secondary complications such as esophageal stricture or perforation are less common. Gastrinomas associated with MEN 1 account for approximately 20% of ZES.

The diagnosis of gastrinoma is defined by concurrent demonstration of gastric acid hypersecretion and elevated fasting serum gastrin levels. Levels greater than 15 mEq/L in patients without prior surgery or greater than 5 mEq/L in patients with a history of ulcer surgery constitutes gastric acid hypersecretion, while levels greater than 100 pg/cc constitute an elevated fasting serum gastrin. If results are equivocal, an abnormal secretin test can confirm the diagnosis, defined as an increase of 200 pg/cc in serum gastrin levels after provocative administration of 2 U/kg of secretin.

The goal of medical management of ZES is limiting secondary complications through control of acid hypersecretion. This is achieved either with histamine 2–receptor antagonists or preferably proton-pump inhibitors. In general, proton-pump inhibitors effectively control the clinical manifestations of ZES. With these medical therapies, secondary complications of ZES and the need for gastric resection for acid reduction in patients with ZES have been nearly eliminated.

The surgical management of gastrinoma in MEN 1 remains a controversial issue. The debate revolves around the efficacy of medical management, the frequency of metastatic disease, and the reduced likelihood of surgical cure. In MEN 1, it is recognized that gastrinomas occur frequently within the wall of the duodenum as multiple microadenomas (17,18), and gastrinomas in the setting of MEN 1 are often malignant with evidence of regional lymph node or hepatic metastases in 50% or greater (19). These suggest that more extensive lymphadentectomy or even pancreaticoduodenectomy might improve the success rate of surgery for ZES in MEN 1. Nonetheless, patients with gastrinoma in the setting of MEN 1 are rarely cured by surgery (20,21). The largest series of these patients demonstrated biochemical evidence of recurrence in 96% within three years and 100% within 10 years (20). Still, 5- and 10-year survival in these patients are 100% and 86%, respectively, illustrating the indolent nature of this disease.

Insulinoma is the second most common clinically evident pancreaticoduodenal tumor in MEN 1, occurring in approximately 10% of patients. The clinical symptoms can be incapacitating and are secondary to neuroglycopenia. These include episodic sweating, dizziness, confusion, or syncope, occurring after fasting periods or exercise. A provocative supervised 72-hour fast will elicit symptomatic hypoglycemia with elevated insulin and C-peptide levels and thus establish the diagnosis. Factitious hypoglycemia due to exogenous insulin administration is the other common cause of episodic hypoglycemia and must be ruled out with assessment of C-peptide levels.

In contrast to gastrinomas, functioning insulinomas in MEN 1 are more amenable to surgery. They are more often single, large enough to be identified, and located within the pancreatic parenchyma. They are less often malignant, and they do not have an ideal medical therapy. Medical therapy consists of diazoxide or octreotide for control of hypoglycemia. However, the preferred treatment of insulinoma in MEN 1 is preoperative localization followed by surgical resection.

Conventional imaging studies, including computed tomography (CT), magnetic resonance imaging (MRI), and ultrasound may localize an insulinoma in these patients. Somatostatin receptor scintigraphy has been reported to successfully identify pancreatic neuroendocrine tumors not visualized using traditional modalities (22). Selective arteriography with injection of calcium gluconate stimulates insulin secretion, and differential insulin concentration within the hepatic veins can be used for regional localization (23). Lastly, endoscopic ultrasound (EUS) is a sensitive imaging modality for small pancreatic endocrine tumors, when performed by an experienced ultrasonographer. This technique may image tumors as small as 0.6 cm within the pancreatic parenchyma (24).

With or without successful preoperative localization, surgical exploration is indicated for insulinoma in MEN 1. The surgical approach includes complete mobilization of the pancreas, careful inspection and palpation of the gland, and intraoperative ultrasound if the tumor cannot be identified. Small insulinomas are often amenable to enucleation, while larger or multifocal lesions may require partial pancreatectomy. If an insulinoma is not evident despite an exhaustive intraoperative search, blind subtotal pancreatectomy is not recommended.

Other functional pancreatic neuroendocrine tumors include glucagonoma, VIP-oma, and somatostatinoma. Glucagonoma is associated with weight loss, glucose intolerance, migratory necrolytic erythema, hypoaminoacidemia,

and normochromic, normocytic anemia. VIP-omas cause profuse diarrhea in the setting of low gastric acid (distinguishing them from gastrinomas). Somatostatinomas have a subtler range of symptoms including mild diabetes, gallbladder disease, weight loss, anemia, steatorrhea, and hypochlorhydria. These tumors are often large at presentation and commonly are malignant.

There is little consensus on the role of surgery for enteropancreatic disease in MEN 1. Exploration is clearly indicated for insulinoma. For other tumors, however, recommendations vary widely. Some groups recommend intervening on tumors larger than 3 cm, based on the higher likelihood of metastatic disease in larger tumors (25). Others recommend intervening for tumors of 1 cm, generally the limit of visualization using conventional techniques (26). Based upon the high malignant potential of these tumors, and the advent of more sensitive imaging techniques like EUS, still others are recommending intervention based solely on clear biochemical evidence of enteropancreatic disease (27). As always, the decision to operate must be based upon weighing the risks to the patient and a reasonable likelihood of benefit.

Pituitary

Pituitary tumors occur in 15% to 50% of patients with MEN 1. They cause symptoms either by local mass effect or through secretion of hormones. Approximately two thirds are microadenomas. Larger adenomas can cause visual disturbances through compression of the optic chiasm, or even hypopituitarism by displacement of the normal pituitary. The most common functional tumor is a prolactinoma that may cause amenorrhea and galactorrhea in women and hypogonadism in men (28). Bromocriptine is the medical treatment for prolactinoma. Growth hormone–producing tumors result in acromegaly. Much rarer are adrenocorticotrophic hormone (ACTH)-secreting tumors causing Cushing's disease. Treatment of pituitary tumors associated with MEN 1 is similar to treatment of sporadic pituitary tumors, which can include medical control of functional tumors, surgery, or radiation. When surgery is performed, a trans-sphenoidal approach is usually employed.

Other Tumors in MEN 1

Foregut carcinoids occur occasionally in the setting of MEN 1. They are often clinically silent until a late stage, are rarely biochemically active, and seem to be more aggressive than their sporadic counterparts. The possibility of removing an occult carcinoid or at-risk tissue is an additional reason for transcervical thymectomy at the time of parathyroid exploration. Aside from this, there are no specific recommendations for managing or screening for MEN 1–related carcinoids. In general, recommendations for resection would be limited to controlling symptomatic disease.

Adrenal cortical lesions are common in MEN 1, but their clinical significance is variable. Most are hyperplastic and nonfunctional, but carcinoma has been described. In general, adrenal lesions in MEN 1 exhibit an indolent course, and it is not clear whether their management should be different from sporadic adrenal masses.

Screening

Screening in MEN 1 involves both genetic testing and biochemical screening for markers of disease. A recent international, multidisciplinary consensus statement addresses both of these issues (11).

Genetic testing is performed through sequence analysis of the MEN 1 gene in an index case to discover the specific mutation. Once a mutation is identified, other members of the kindred can be tested for it. Sequence analysis is successful in 80% to 90% of kindreds (7). Other methods of genetic testing can include linkage and haplotype analysis if sequence analysis is uninformative. Testing can be offered to index cases and their relatives. However, it is important to emphasize that genetic testing is an informative tool only, and families should be educated about the implications, risks, and benefits of test results by an experienced genetic counselor.

Periodic screening of tumor expression in MEN 1 is directed toward early identification of the principal tumor types. This includes evaluating clinical symptoms, biochemical markers, and imaging studies. Based on age-related penetrance, screening should begin in early childhood. Biochemical assays should be performed annually, while imaging studies should be performed every several years.

MULTIPLE ENDOCRINE NEOPLASIA TYPE 2

History, Molecular Genetics, and Pathogenesis

Coincident thyroid cancer and pheochromocytoma was first described in 1932 (29), but the association between the two was not recognized until the early 1960s (30), and the heritable syndrome was not characterized until the late sixties (31). Also in the late sixties, a variant was described, which included mucosal neuromas and a distinct facies (32). Today MEN 2A, MEN 2B, and familial medullary thyroid carcinoma (FMTC) form a constellation of related syndromes whose hallmark is MTC.

The development of a radioimmunoassay for calcitonin in 1970 (33) was pivotal for the study of MTC and MEN 2, because MTC is a cancer of calcitonin-secreting C-cells of the thyroid. Basal and stimulated calcitonin levels are useful markers for the diagnosis and surveillance of MTC.

Linkage analysis localized the predisposition gene for the MEN 2 syndromes to the pericentromeric region of chromosome 10 (34,35). Subsequently, mutations in the RET proto-oncogene at that locus were identified in patients with MEN 2A, FMTC (36), and MEN 2B (37). The majority of mutations in MEN 2A are missense involving one of five cysteine residues in the extracellular domain of the RET protein. Almost all cases of MEN 2B demonstrate a methionine to threonine missense mutation in codon 918.

The RET gene consists of at least 20 exons and is expressed as five major mRNA species. In adults, RET is only expressed in a limited number of tissues including the C-cells of the thyroid, the adrenal medulla, and the central nervous system. The RET protein is a cell-membrane receptor tyrosine kinase. It has three domains: a cysteine-rich extracellular receptor domain, a hydrophobic transmembrane domain, and an intracellular tyrosine kinase catalytic domain. Experiments in knockout mice suggest a critical role for RET in the developing enteric nervous system and the kidneys (38). Its ligands are now known to include glial-derived growth factor and neurturin (39,40). Ligand binding causes RET dimerization, which in turn leads to phosphorylation and activation of the tyrosine kinase domain, and ultimately downstream signaling. It appears that RET regulates cellular growth and proliferation in cells derived from the neural crest. It is highly expressed in MTC, pheochromocytoma, and neuroblastoma.

In contrast to MEN 1, there is no evidence of consistent loss of heterozygosity at the RET locus in MEN 2 tumors.

MEN 2 is caused by "gain of function" mutations in RET. Unlike the tumor suppressor MEN 1, RET is a proto-oncogene in which activating mutations are dominant in the development of neoplasia. In vitro experiments demonstrated the transforming effect of these mutations in NIH 3T3 cells through constitutive activation of the RET tyrosine kinase. RET mutations associated with MEN 2A lead to constitutive dimerization, while those associated with MEN 2B change the tyrosine kinase substrate specificity (41).

Familial Hirschsprung's disease (HSCR) has also been associated with mutations in the RET gene. The implicated mutations have been frameshift or nonsense, leading to gene inactivation or abrogation of the functional RET product (42,43). However, a small subset of MEN 2A families have associated HSCR. These kindreds have associated missense mutations in codons 618 or 620 (44). Thus, HSCR can be associated with either loss-of-function or gain-of-function mutations in the RET gene.

Clinical Features and Management

The hallmark of MEN 2A, FMTC, and MEN 2B is MTC. MTC occurs in nearly all affected persons. Pheochromocytoma occurs in approximately half of MEN 2A and MEN 2B patients. HPT occurs in approximately one quarter of MEN 2A patients, and does not occur in patients with MEN 2B and FMTC (Table 2) (45). The rarer MEN 2B syndrome includes MTC, pheochromocytoma, mucosal neuromas, diffuse ganglioneuromas of the GI tract, skeletal abnormalities, megacolon, and a "marfanoid" habitus. These syndromes demonstrate an autosomal-dominant pattern of heritability; however, both variants may occur de novo in an index patient to affect subsequent generations.

MTC is usually the first expression of MEN 2, and management is directed toward early diagnosis, preventive therapy, or control of advanced disease. In MEN 2A, the peak incidence of MTC occurs in the second or third decade of life, and many cases present earlier. MTC in MEN 2B occurs at a younger age (often in infancy) and is more aggressive than MTC in MEN 2A. Due to the aggressive nature of the disease, MEN 2B kindreds are characteristically small, encompassing only two or three generations. The early age of onset necessitates intervention as soon as the genetic testing reveals the presence of an MEN 2B mutation in the RET gene. Thyroidectomy should be performed as soon as the diagnosis is made, during infancy if possible.

Because of the narrower scope of clinical expression and the reliability of current mutation-analysis techniques, MEN 2 and its related syndromes do not have the same difficulty of classification as MEN 1. A recent international consensus statement points out that criteria for FMTC

Table 2 Characteristics of Multiple Endocrine Neoplasia Type 2 (MEN 2)

MEN 2A
  Medullary carcinoma of the thyroid
  Pheochromocytoma
  HPT
MEN 2B
  Medullary carcinoma of the thyroid
  Pheochromocytoma
  Mucosal neuromas
  Marfanoid habitus
  Typical facies
  Ganglioneuromas of oropharynx and intestinal tract

Abbreviation: HPT, hyperparathyroidism.

should be rigorous enough to exclude MEN 2 with late presentation of secondary tumors. These criteria include more than 10 carriers within a kindred, multiple carriers or affected members over the age of 50, and an adequate medical history (11). These rigorous standards should prevent inaccurately designating a true MEN 2 kindred as FMTC and thereby missing a pheochromocytoma.

Screening of at-risk MEN 2 and FMTC family members by measurement of serum calcitonin or, preferably, by genetic testing for the presence of RET mutations, identifies affected individuals who are offered preventative thyroidectomy. In patients who present with advanced MTC, management is directed toward control of symptoms and bulky disease. Occasionally, patients will present with episodic headache, dizziness, or other symptoms to suggest pheochromocytoma, and symptoms of HPT are unusual presenting findings in the MEN 2 syndromes.

Medullary Thyroid Carcinoma

MTC, overall, is a rare malignancy, comprising 5% to 10% of all thyroid malignancies. Nearly 75% of cases are sporadic, while MEN 2A, MEN 2B, and FMTC constitute the remaining 25% in decreasing order of frequency. MTC is usually the earliest clinical abnormality in MEN 2, diagnosed before or concurrently with pheochromocytoma.

Sporadic MTC is nearly always unilateral, while in patients with MEN 2 or FMTC, it is almost always bilateral and multifocal. The characteristic distribution is multicentric foci of tumor in the middle and upper portions of each thyroid lobe. A diffuse proliferation of C-cells known as C-cell hyperplasia is seen in patients with MEN 2 and FMTC, and is thought to be a malignant precursor to MTC. Parafollicular clusters of increased numbers of C-cells represent the early manifestation of hyperplasia or microinvasive carcinoma that ultimately progresses to multifocal MTC. The presence of bilateral MTC or C-cell hyperplasia strongly suggests the presence of familial disease.

MTC appears grossly as a circumscribed, gritty, whitish-tan nodule. Histologically, it appears as sheets or nests of uniform cells separated by variable amounts of stroma (46). An amyloid-like material is frequently present in the stroma of MTC, and consists of accumulated calcitonin prohormone secreted by tumor cells (47). The presence of this material is a distinctive feature of MTC, but is not uniformly present. Immunohistochemical staining for calcitonin within tumor cells is diagnostic of MTC.

MTC cells are capable of diverse biosynthetic activity and have been reported to secrete (in addition to calcitonin) corticotropin, prostaglandins, melanin, and serotonin. Although rare, paraneoplastic syndromes have been reported with MTC, including Cushing's syndrome and the carcinoid syndrome. The most significant biologically active product of MTC is calcitonin. Clinically, this causes diarrhea in up to 30% of patients, attributed to increased jejunal water and electrolyte secretion secondary to high plasma calcitonin levels. More often, calcitonin secretion is clinically silent. However, it is a reliable tumor marker for the presence of MTC, whether in preoperative screening or postoperative evaluation, and serum levels correspond to burden of disease and response to therapy (48).

Clinically evident MTC most often presents as a palpable thyroid nodule or multinodular thyroid gland. Metastatic disease is suggested by palpable cervical lymph nodes. Fine needle aspiration of thyroid or cervical nodal disease in combination with serum calcitonin makes the diagnosis. Symptoms such as hoarseness, respiratory difficulty, or dysphagia suggest invasion of adjacent structures and imply locally advanced disease. The pattern of metastatic spread is first to local–regional lymph nodes and then to distant organs. The most commonly involved sites of distant metastases are liver, lung, and bone. Metastasis of MTC in MEN 2 commonly occurs in a miliary pattern of diffuse fine deposits, in contrast to sporadic MTC where metastases more often are larger and fewer in number.

Once MTC is clinically evident, the frequency of metastatic disease is high. Patients with a palpable neck mass have an alarmingly high rate of cervical lymph node metastases. In our series, patients with unilateral palpable MTC had nodal metastases in 81% of central nodal compartments, 81% of ipsilateral levels II to V compartments, and 44% of contralateral levels II to V nodes. Patients with bilateral MTC had metastases in 78% of central nodal compartments, 71% of levels II to V nodes ipsilateral to the largest intrathyroid tumor, and 49% of levels II to V nodes contralateral to the largest intrathyroid tumor (49).

Historically, measurement of serum calcitonin levels was used to diagnose occult MTC in MEN 2 patients. This was demonstrated by Melvin et al. who showed that patients with clinically occult MTC had either minimally elevated calcitonin levels, or normal basal calcitonin levels that dramatically increased after calcium infusion (50). Later, pentagastrin infusion alone (0.5 µg/kg over 5 sec) (51), and then calcium followed by pentagastrin infusions (2 mg/kg of calcium gluconate over 1 min followed by 0.5 µg/kg of pentagastrin over 5 sec) (52), were demonstrated to be more potent calcitonin secretagogues. Stimulated plasma calcitonin levels above 300 pg/mL are highly suggestive of MTC, and the diagnosis is virtually assured in patients with stimulated plasma calcitonin levels exceeding 1000 pg/cc.

Although sensitive and specific, provocative testing is expensive and labor intensive and is associated with side effects that affect compliance with annual testing. Identification of RET mutations has enabled direct genetic testing, which can be performed at any age and requires only the collection of a single peripheral blood sample. Clinical data suggest that DNA testing is more accurate for the diagnosis of early MTC. Various groups have reported that patients with RET mutations but normal provocative calcitonin assays often have microscopic MTC (53–57). Today, genetic testing has supplanted stimulated calcitonin assay for the screening of potential MEN 2 carriers, and enables the earliest intervention before the occurrence of MTC.

The operative treatment of MTC is total thyroidectomy. Meticulous removal of all thyroid tissue should be done at the initial operation, because MTC in the setting of MEN 2 is nearly always multifocal and bilateral, and all C-cell containing tissue is at risk for subsequent malignancy. Because MTC develops in essentially all patients with MEN 2 and because thyroidectomy is well tolerated, it can be argued that patients become candidates for thyroidectomy as soon as a RET mutation is identified, regardless of age. Although long-term data are still pending, early thyroidectomy has proven an effective management strategy to prevent metastatic MTC and improve outcomes in patients with MEN 2. An older series of patients undergoing early thyroidectomy reported no evidence of disease in 19 of 22 patients at a mean of 11 years of follow-up (54). A more recent European series reported persistent or recurrent disease at four years of follow-up in only 6 of 71 patients with germline mutations undergoing early thyroidectomy (55).

The treatment failures in both of these studies can be attributed to later operations after biochemical evidence of MTC. In 22 patients with RET mutations but no biochemical evidence of MTC, undergoing prophylactic thyroidectomy, C-cell hyperplasia was discovered in 7, intrathyroidal MTC in 14, and lymph node metastases in 1 (56). These results suggest that early prophylactic thyroidectomy can be curative or preventive in almost all MEN 2 patients.

The recent Consensus Conference on MEN offers stratified guidelines for the timing and specific thyroid management of MEN 2 patients based upon specific codon mutations (11). These reflect genotype–phenotype associations for certain mutations. Codon 883, 918 or 922 mutations (those associated with MEN 2B) are designated as level 3 risks and thyroidectomy with central node dissection is recommended within the first six months of life. Patients with codon 611, 618, 620 or 634 mutations are stratified as level 2 and thyroidectomy with or without central node dissection is recommended before the age of five. Patients with codon 609, 768, 790, 791, 804 or 891 mutations are stratified as level 1 and thyroidectomy is recommended for these patients before the age of 5 or 10 years (little consensus was reached for the management of these patients) (11).

Patients with palpable or clinically evident MTC should undergo central neck dissection (right and left levels VI and VII nodes), and ipsi- or bilateral functional neck dissections with removal of levels II to V nodes (49). The goal of this operation is removal of all nodal tissue from the level of the hyoid bone superiorly to the innominate vessels inferiorly. Management of the parathyroid glands is controversial. Some experts, including the authors, recommend four-gland parathyroidectomy with autotransplantation (58), arguing that central node dissection is extremely difficult if the parathyroid glands are left in place with an adequate blood supply. Other experts recommend leaving the parathyroid glands in situ (57). The unreliability of intraoperative assessment to distinguish involved nodes underscores the importance of removing all central nodal tissue. In our series of 73 neck dissections for palpable MTC, intraoperative palpation of lymph nodes had a sensitivity of 64% and a specificity of 71% for identifying metastatic disease. Thus intraoperative assessment would miss involved nodes 36% of the time (49).

After the initial operation, patients are followed with serial serum calcitonin levels. This and calcium–pentagastrin stimulation readily detect residual or recurrent disease. More than 50% of patients with MTC develop persistent or recurrent disease after primary surgical resection, forming a difficult population to manage. Radioactive iodine and radiation therapy have not been demonstrated to be effective treatment options (59–61). Chemotherapeutic combinations have been ascribed only limited success in case reports (62–64). Currently, there is no accepted systemic therapy for recurrent or metastatic MTC.

MTC often has an indolent biological course, and although early metastases to the cervical lymph nodes may occur, it may remain confined to the neck for many months or years. Some groups have demonstrated biochemical cure of patients with persistent disease after their initial operation, through neck reoperation and meticulous lymph node dissection in approximately one third of cases (65,66). Before neck reoperation is attempted, distant metastatic spread should be assessed. Traditionally, this has been done by CT or MRI scanning of the chest, abdomen, and pelvis. However, a trial involving 41 patients who had persistent or recurrent MTC and who underwent laparoscopic or open

liver examination and biopsy discovered metastatic liver deposits in seven patients with normal CT or MRI examinations (67). Our continued experience has supported these findings, and we currently employ diagnostic laparoscopy in patients being considered for neck reoperation for persistent or recurrent MTC. Cases with distant metastatic disease should be considered individually. In general, we recommend resection of bulky or symptomatic disease.

The prognosis of MEN 2A and 2B is essentially that of the thyroid lesion (68). MTC generally has an intermediate grade of malignancy compared with the more aggressive anaplastic thyroid carcinomas or the more benign papillary or follicular carcinomas. However, MTC exhibits variable biological aggressiveness within the different MEN 2 syndromes and varies, sometimes, from kindred to kindred. Most important, the MTC associated with MEN 2B is very aggressive and patients may die at a young age. MTC in the setting of MEN 2A is more frequently indolent and progresses slowly.

Pheochromocytoma

Pheochromocytomas in patients with MEN 2A and 2B appear in the second or third decade of life. In contrast to sporadic pheochromocytoma where bilateral pheochromocytoma is unusual, approximately 60% of pheochromocytomas in the setting of MEN 2 are bilateral. Most tumors present after or concurrent with the diagnosis of MTC, and are infrequently the initial presenting feature. Historically, sudden death from pheochromocytoma was a frequent occurrence in 2 families, perhaps equaling the mortality from MTC. Today, accurate characterization of the syndrome and identification of carriers, along with improved management of pheochromocytoma have decreased morbidity associated with this aspect of the disease. The spectrum of clinical symptoms ranges from silent disease to dramatic symptoms including headache, episodic diaphoresis, palpitations, and anxiety.

Pheochromocytoma in MEN 2 is nearly always limited to the adrenal medulla and is nearly always benign. Histologically, MEN 2–associated pheochromocytomas have an identical appearance as sporadic pheochromocytoma. However, patients with MEN 2 develop hyperplasia of the adrenal medulla, which may be a precursor of pheochromocytoma. A spectrum of diseases, including nodular or asymmetrical hyperplasia, multiple small pheochromocytomas, or a diffuse thickening of all adrenal medullary tissue, may be observed. This pattern of adrenal involvement is comparable to C-cell hyperplasia within the thyroid gland of patients with MEN 2.

The diagnosis of pheochromocytoma in patients with MEN 2 is made biochemically, as for sporadic pheochromocytoma. This is accomplished by measuring urinary excretion of catecholamines and catecholamine metabolites. A 24-hour collection is obtained for measurement of total urinary catecholamines, epinephrine, norepinephrine, metanephrines, and vanillylmandelic acid. Measurement of serum metanephrines is also an acceptable test. High catecholamine or metanephrine levels warrant a CT or MRI to evaluate the adrenal glands. If anatomic imaging is uninformative or equivocal, ^{131}I-metaiodobenzylguanidine scintigraphy may be performed. This study has been shown to have 90% sensitivity and 95% specificity for pheochromocytoma (69). Elevated catecholamine levels in MEN 2 patients may, however, be due to the presence of adrenal medullary hyperplasia, and imaging may not demonstrate a discreet lesion. In these instances, observation with interval imaging is frequently recommended.

As in sporadic cases, all patients with MEN 2 and pheochromocytoma must receive adequate alpha-adrenergic blockade prior to adrenal surgery to prevent intraoperative adrenergic crisis. Alpha-blockade consists of phenoxybenzamine administered to the point of postural hypotension. Beta-adrenergic blockade can be added to treat secondary tachycardia or arrhythmia, but should not be administered alone to avoid unopposed vasoconstriction.

The definitive treatment of pheochromocytoma is surgical excision. For unilateral disease in the setting of MEN 2, we recommend unilateral adrenalectomy. Proponents of bilateral adrenalectomy argue that adrenal medullary hyperplasia in MEN 2 is almost universally bilateral, there is a substantial risk of subsequent development of pheochromocytoma following unilateral adrenalectomy, and the risk of complications of the anadrenal state should be low. We have found that pheochromocytoma develops in approximately half of the patients with MEN 2 following unilateral adrenalectomy after a mean interval of 12 years. Conversely, we have found that approximately one quarter of patients undergoing bilateral adrenalectomy develop at least one addisonian crisis (70). Our group advocates unilateral adrenalectomy for patients with MEN 2 and a unilateral pheochromocytoma based on the 50% rate of recurrence over a prolonged duration of time, the rarity of malignant pheochromocytoma, effective screening regimens, and the substantial morbidity and mortality associated with the addisonian state. These patients continue to be monitored yearly for the development of a contralateral pheochromocytoma.

Intraoperative considerations include avoidance of hyper or hypotension, early ligation of the adrenal vein, and minimal manipulation of the tumor. Laparoscopic adrenalectomy has become the preferred option for experienced laparoscopic surgeons and patients with well-localized unilateral disease. Comparable or even superior results, with regard to operative time, complication rates, hospital stay, and mortality, have been reported for laparoscopic versus open resection (71,72). Cortical-sparing adrenalectomy, both laparoscopic and open, is a new technique that has been described and advocated for bilateral pheochromocytoma (73,72). This approach is frequently not possible in patients with MEN 2 because of the location of the primary tumor, and the presence of a diffusely thickened gland secondary to hyperplasia.

It is imperative that patients with known or suspected MEN 2 have pheochromocytoma excluded before undergoing any operation, including thyroidectomy for MTC. This is particularly important because the pheochromocytoma may be silent clinically but may place the patient at a severe operative risk. If a patient is found to have concurrent pheochromocytoma and MTC, adrenalectomy should be performed after adequate alpha-adrenergic blockade, followed by thyroidectomy in the next several weeks.

Parathyroid Glands

HPT is the most variable component of the MEN 2A syndrome, occurring in 20% to 30% of patients. It is associated with certain RET mutations, particularly with mutations in codon 634 (74). In general, it is milder in patients with MEN 2A than in those with either sporadic disease or MEN 1. Many patients are asymptomatic and recognition of HPT may stem from the finding of hypercalcemia during routine laboratory studies, or finding one or more enlarged

parathyroid glands at the time of thyroidectomy for MTC in a patient who is normocalcemic. The most common sign of HPT in patients with MEN 2A is the presence of asymptomatic or symptomatic renal stones and more advanced signs, such as osteitis fibrosa cystica or nephrocalcinosis, are unusual.

The parathyroid lesions in MEN 2A consist primarily of generalized chief cell hyperplasia. Still, multiple parathyroid gland enlargements may occur, and it is not infrequent to encounter a single "adenoma." As in sporadic cases or patients with MEN 1, an elevated PTH level confirms the diagnosis. Surgical management of HPT in MEN 2A is somewhat controversial. Options include selective parathyroidectomy (excision of grossly enlarged glands only), subtotal (three and one-half) parathyroidectomy, or total parathyroidectomy with heterotopic autotransplantation of parathyroid tissue into the forearm. The principal arguments against total parathyroidectomy with autotransplantation are that it is associated with unacceptable rates of postoperative hypoparathyroidism and that cure rates for patients with MEN 2A and HPT are excellent with lesser procedures (75,76). In experienced hands, however, autotransplantation is highly successful. The importance of removing all thyroid tissue for the management of MTC in MEN 2A and the attendant difficulty of doing so while keeping the parathyroid blood supply intact argue in favor of total parathyroidectomy. Additionally, HPT in MEN 2A tends to be a multiglandular disease with an increased risk of persistent or recurrent HPT after any procedure. As discussed, recurrent HPT in patients with parathyroid tissue left in situ require neck reexploration and its associated risks. For these reasons, we advocate four-gland parathyroidectomy with heterotopic forearm autotransplantation.

Nonendocrine Manifestations of MEN 2A and 2B

MEN 2A and 2B both have distinct nonendocrine features, evidence of the systemic effects of abnormal RET function. As noted, some families with MEN 2A have associated HSCR, a phenotype that is associated with specific RET mutations (44). HSCR, in this setting, presents in a similar manner to sporadic disease and requires early surgical intervention to manage the distal GI obstruction. Several families with MEN 2A have been described, which feature intercapsular lesions of cutaneous lichen amyloidosis (77). This finding is particularly associated with RET codon 634 mutations (78). These lesions are not malignant, but are associated with pruritis in affected areas.

Patients with MEN 2B develop several striking abnormalities of the musculoskeletal and nervous systems. Unlike patients with MEN 1 or 2A, these patients have a characteristic phenotype, including a tall, thin "marfanoid" body habitus. Patients develop diffuse ganglioneuromatosis of the GI tract. Externally, multiple neuromas are visible on the lips, tongue, and oral mucosa (Fig. 1). Histologically, GI tract ganglioneuromas demonstrate hypertrophy and nerve fiber disarray of the myenteric and submucosal plexuses. Almost all of these patients will demonstrate some degree of GI symptoms, which can include excessive flatulence, abdominal distention, abdominal pain, constipation or diarrhea, difficulty swallowing, and vomiting. Imaging commonly reveals chronic megacolon, and a significant proportion of them require abdominal surgery (79). MEN 2B patients also demonstrate other evidence of neurologic abnormalities, including hypertrophied corneal nerves on slit-lamp examination of the eyes.

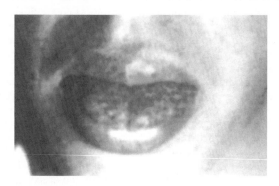

Figure 1   Patient with MEN 2b. Note the small tumors on the tongue and the puffy lips.

Screening

Because MEN 2 is associated with only a limited number of specific activating RET mutations, genetic testing for MEN 2 through DNA sequencing is generally informative. Over 95% of MEN 2 index cases have an identified RET mutation, and the RET locus has not been excluded in any MEN 2 family. Described mutations fall within exons 10, 11, 13, 14, and 15, and so only these exons must be sequenced routinely. Sequencing of the remainder of the gene, haplotype, or genetic-linkage analysis is reserved for families in which initial sequencing is uninformative.

Early intervention in MEN 2 and FMTC dramatically affects outcome, and so mutation analysis is mandated for suspected cases. Any patient with early onset MTC, multifocal MTC, or C-cell hyperplasia should undergo mutation analysis. The same holds true for multifocal pheochromocytoma or adrenal medullary hyperplasia. Some have even advocated more aggressive screening of any patient with MTC or pheochromocytoma. The likelihood of a germline RET mutation in cases of apparently sporadic MTC is 1% to 7% (80), while the likelihood of an underlying hereditary syndrome [MEN 2, von Hippel Lindau (VHL) disease, neurofibromatosis type 1 (NF1), or hereditary pheochromocytoma] in cases of apparently sporadic pheochromocytoma is at least 20% (81). These modest but significant likelihoods form the basis for recommendations that all cases of apparently sporadic MTC undergo RET-mutation analysis, and that all cases of apparently sporadic pheochromocytoma undergo RET, VHL, and NF1 analysis and other screening studies for MEN 2 or VHL.

At risk family members within MEN 2 kindreds must undergo RET-mutation analysis. Before this, family members should speak with a genetic counselor about the implications of genetic testing. Specifically, they should be educated about forms of inheritance, the likelihood of inheriting an autosomal-dominant disorder, risks and benefits associated with genetic testing, and the implications for treatment, including the need for prophylactic thyroidectomy. These sensitive issues are complicated by the fact that many of these patients are children and intervention is necessary at a young age.

For rare patients whose carrier status is in question, or those known carriers who have undergone thyroidectomy, biochemical testing forms the mainstay of screening. These patients should have regular measurement of calcitonin levels to screen for MTC or recurrence. Additionally, serum metanephrine levels screen for pheochromocytoma, and calcium and PTH levels screen for HPT.

SUMMARY

While most tumors of the endocrine system arise sporadically and involve a single gland, a subset of patients present with neoplastic disease involving multiple endocrine tissues. Two clinical syndromes are now well established and develop familiarly in an autosomal-dominant pattern. MEN 1 is characterized by the familial association of tumors involving the pituitary gland, parathyroid glands, and the pancreatic islets. The familial association of MTC and pheochromocytoma has been designated MEN 2. Two variants of MEN 2 are now known to exist. MEN 2A is characterized by the concurrence of MTC, pheochromocytoma, and hyperparathyroidism. The less common but more lethal MEN 2B is characterized by the association of MTC and pheochromocytoma in concurrence with mucosal neuromas, oropharyngeal and intestinal ganglioneuromatosis, and a marfanoid habitus. Because the genetics of these two syndromes have become better classified and various biochemical markers have become available, patients at risk can now be diagnosed earlier allowing less extensive surgical procedures to be employed for management. The lethal outcomes that previously were associated with these syndromes are now exceedingly uncommon, and the focused and expeditious treatment that is now possible has allowed patients with these conditions to enjoy long and productive lives.

REFERENCES

1. Wermer P. Genetic aspects of adenomatosis endocrine glands. Am J Med 1954; 16:363.
2. Larsson C, Skogseid B, Oberg K, et al. Multiple endocrine neoplasia type 1 gene maps to chromosome 11 and is lost in insulinoma. Nature 1988; 332:85.
3. Knudson AG, Hethcote HW, Brown BW. Mutation and childhood cancer: a probabilistic model for the incidence of retinoblastoma. Proc Natl Acad Sci USA 1975; 72:5116.
4. Chandrasekhrappa SC, Guru SC, Manickamp P, et al. Positional cloning of the gene for multiple endocrine neoplasia-type 1. Science 1997; 276:404.
5. Agarwal SK, Guru SC, Heppner C, et al. Menin interacts with the AP1 transcription factor JunD and represses JunD-activated transcription. Cell 1999; 96:143.
6. Agarwal SK, Kester MB, Debelenko LV, et al. Germline mutations of the MEN1 gene in familial multiple endocrine neoplasia type 1 and related states. Hum Mol Genet 1997; 6(7):1169–1175.
7. Bassett JH, Forbes SA, Pannett AA, et al. Characterization of mutations in patients with multiple endocrine neoplasia type 1. Am J Hum Genet 1998; 62(2):232.
8. Wautot V, Vercherat C, Lespinasse J, et al. Germline mutation profile of MEN1 in multiple endocrine neoplasia type 1: search for correlation between phenotype and the functional domains of the MEN1 protein. Hum Mutat 2002; 20(1):35.
9. Majewski JT, Wilson SD. The MEA I syndrome: an all or none phenomenon? Surgery 1979; 86:475.
10. Glascock MJ, Carty SE. Multiple endocrine neoplasia type 1: fresh perspective on clinical features and penetrance. Surg Oncol 2002; 11(3):143.
11. Brandi ML, Gagel RF, Angeli A, et al. Guidelines for diagnosis and therapy of MEN type 1 and type 2. J Clin Endocr Metab 2001; 86:5658.

12. Ballard HS, Frame B, Hartsock RJ. Familial endocrine adenoma-peptic ulcer complex. Medicine 1964; 43:481.

13. Wells SA, Farndon JR, Dale JK, et al. Long term evaluation of patients with primary parathyroid hyperplasia managed by total parathyroidectomy and heterotopic autotransplantation. Ann Surg 1980; 192:451.

14. Norton JA, Cromack DT, Shawker TH, et al. Effect of parathyroidectomy in patients with hyperparathyroidism and multiple endocrine neoplasia type I. Surgery 1987; 102:958.

15. Mutch MG, Frisella MM, DeBenedetti MK, et al. Pancreatic polypeptide is a useful plasma marker for radiographically evident pancreatic islet cell tumors in patients with multiple endocrine neoplasia type I. Surgery 1997; 122:1012.

16. Vieto RJ, Hickey RC, Samaan NA. Type 1 multiple endocrine neoplasias. Curr Probl Cancer 1982; 7:1.

17. Thompson NW, Vinik AI, Eckhuaser FE. Microgastrinomas of the duodenum. Ann Surg 1989; 209:396.

18. Delcore RJ, Cheung LY, Freisen SR. Characteristics of duodenal wall gastrinomas. Am J Surg 1990; 160:621.

19. Norton JA, Doppman JL, Jensen RT. Curative resection in Zollinger-Ellison syndrome: results of a 10 year prospective study. Ann Surg 1992; 215:8.

20. Norton JA, Fraker DL, Alexander HR, et al. Surgery to Cure the Zollinger-Ellison Syndrom. N Engl J Med 1999; 341(9):635.

21. Van Heerden Ja, Smith SL, Miller LJ. Management of the Zollinger-Ellison syndrome in patients with multiple endocrine neoplasia type 1. Surgery 1986; 100:971.

22. Yim JH, Siegel BA, DeBenedetti MK, et al. Prospective study of the utility of somatostatin receptor scintigraphy in the evaluation of patients with multiple endocrine neoplasia type 1. Surgery 1998: 124:1037.

23. Cohen MS, Picus D, Lairmore TC, et al. Prospective study of provocative angiograms to localize functional islet cell tumors of the pancreas. Surgery 1997; 122:1091.

24. Gauger PG, Scheiman JM, Wamsteker EJ, et al. Role of endoscopic ultrasonography in screening and treatment of pancreatic endocrine tumors in asymptomatic patients with multiple endocrine neoplasia type 1. Br J Surg 2003; 90:748.

25. Cadiot G, Vuagnat A, Doukhan I, et al. Prognostic factors in patients with multiple endocrine neoplasia type 1. Gastroenterology 1999; 116:286.

26. Wiedenman B, Jensen RT, Mignon M, et al. Preoperative diagnosis and surgical management of neuroendocrine gastroenteropancreatic tumors: general recommendations by a consensus workshop. World J Surg 1998; 22:309.

27. Doherty GM, Thompson NW. Multiple endocrine neoplasia type 1: duodenopancreatic tumors. J Int Med 2003; 253:590.

28. Carty SE, Helm AK, Amico JA, et al. The variable penetrance and spectrum of manifestations of multiple endocrine neoplasia type 1. Surgery 1998; 124:1106.

29. Eisenberg AA, Wallerstein H. Pheochromocytoma of the suprarenal medulla (paraganglioma): a clinicopathologic study. Arch Pathol 1932; 14:818.

30. Sipple JH. The association of pheochromocytoma with carcinoma of the thyroid gland. Am J Med 1961; 31:163.

31. Williams ED. A review of 17 cases of carcinoma of the thyroid and pheochromocytoma. J Clin Pathol 1965; 18:288.

32. Williams ED, Pollock DJ. Multiple mucosal neuromata with endocrine tumors: a syndrome allied to von Recklinghausen's disease. J Path Bacteriol 1966; 91:71.

33. Tashijian AH, Howland BG, Melvin KEW, et al. Immunoassay of human calcitonin: clinical measurement, relation to serum calcium and studies in patients with medullary carcinoma. N Engl J Med 1970; 283:890.

34. Simpson NE, Kidd KK, Goodfellow PJ, et al. Assignment of multiple endocrine neoplasia type 2a to chromosome 10 by linkage. Nature 1987; 328:528.

35. Norum RA, Lafreniere R, O'Neal LW, et al. Linkage between MEN 2B and chromosome 10 markers linked to MEN 2A. Genomics 1990; 8:313.

36. Mulligan LM, Eng C, Healey CS, et al. Germ-line mutations of the RET proto-oncogene in multiple endocrine neoplasia type 2A. Nature 1993; 363:458.

37. Hofstra RMW, Ladsvater RM, Ceccherini I, et al. A mutation in the RET proto-oncogene associated with multiple endocrine neoplasia type 2B and sporadic medullary thyroid carcinoma. Nature 1994; 367:375.

38. Schuchardt A, D'Agati V, Larsson-Blomber L, et al. Defects in the kidney and enteric nervous system of mice lacking the tyrosine kinase receptor RET. Nature 1994; 367:380.

39. Durbec P, Macos-Gutierrez CV, Kilkenny C, et al. GDNF signaling through the Ret receptor tyrosine kinase. Nature 1996; 381:789.

40. Kotzbauer PT, Lampe PA, et al. Neurturin, a relative of glial-cell-line-derived neurotrophic factor. Nature 1996; 384:467.

41. Santoro M, Carlomagno F, Romano A, et al. Activation of RET as a dominantly transforming gene by germline mutations of MEN2A and MEN2B. Science 1995; 267:381.

42. Romeo G, Ronchetto P, Luo Y, et al. Point mutations affecting the tyrosine kinase domain of the RET proto-oncogene in Hirschsprungs's disease. Nature 1994; 367:377.

43. Edery P, Lyonnet S, Mulligan LM, et al. Mutations of the RET proto-oncogene in Hirschsprung's disease. Nature 1994; 367:378.

44. Borst MJ, VanCamp Jm, et al. Mutational analysis of multiple endocrine neoplasia type 2A associated with Hirschsprung's disease. Surgery 1995; 117:386.

45. Howe JR, Norton JA, Wells SA. Prevalence of pheochromocytoma and hyperparathyroidism in multiple endocrine neoplasia type 2A: results of long-term follow-up. Surgery 1993; 114:1070.

46. Bigner ML, Mendelsohn G, Wells SA, et al. Medullary carcinoma of the thyroid in the multiple endocrine neoplasia IIa syndrome. Am J Surg Pathol 1981; 5:459.

47. Sletten K, Westermark P, Natvig JB. Characterization of amyloid fibril proteins from medullary carcinoma of the thyroid. J Exp Med 1976; 143:993.

48. Tisell LE, Dilley WG, Wells SA. Progression of postoperative residual medullary thyroid carcinoma as monitored by plasma calcitonin levels. Surgery 1996; 119:34.

49. Moley JF, DeBenedetti MK. Patterns of nodal metastases in palpable medullary thyroid carcinoma. Ann Surg 1997; 229:880.

50. Melvin KEW, Miller HH, Tashjian AH. Early diagnosis of medullary carcinoma of the thyroid gland by means of calcitonin assay. N Eng J Med 1971; 285:1115.

51. Hennessy JF, Wells SA, Ontjes DA, Cooper CW. A comparison of pentagastrin injection and calcium infusion as provocative agents for the detection of medullary carcinoma of the thyroid. J Clin Endocrinol Metab 1974; 39:487.

52. Wells SA, Baylin SB, Linehan WM, et al. Provocative agents and the diagnosis of medullary carcinoma of the thyroid gland. Ann Surg 1978; 188:139.

53. Lips CJM, Landsvater RM, Hoppeneer JWM, et al. Clinical screening as compared with DNA analysis in families with multiple endocrine neoplasia type 2a. N Engl J Med 1994; 331:828.

54. Gagel RF, Tashjian AH, Cummings T, et al. The clinical outcome of prospective screening for multiple endocrine neoplasia type 2a: an 18-year experience. N Engl J Med 1988; 318:478.

55. Niccoli-Sire P, Murat A, Baudin E, et al. Early or prophylactic thyroidectomy in MEN 2/FMTC gene carriers: results in 71 thyroidectomized patients. Eur J Endocrinol 1999; 141(5):468.

56. Rodriquez GJ, Balsalobre MD, Pomares F, et al. Prophylactic thyroidectomy in MEN 2A syndrome: experience in a single center. J Am Coll Surg 2002; 195(2):159.

57. Dralle H, Gimm O, et al. Prophylactic thyroidectomy in 75 children with hereditary medullary thyroid carcinoma. World J Surg 1998; 22:744.

58. Herfarth KK-F, Bartsch D, GM, et al. Surgical management of hyperparathyroidism in patients with multiple endocrine neoplasia type 2a. Surgery 1996; 120:966.

59. Samaan NA, Schultz PN, Hickey RC. Medullary thyroid carcinoma: prognosis of familial versus nonfamilial disease and the role of radiotherapy. Horm Metab Res 1989(suppl 21): 20–25.

60. Fife KM, Bower M, Harmer CL. Medullary thyroid cancer: the role of radiotherapy in local control. European J Surg Oncol 1996; 22:588–591.

61. Brierley J, Tsang R, Simpson WJ, et al. Medullary thyroid cancer: analyses of survival and prognostic factors and the role of radiation therapy in local control. Thyroid 1996; 6(4):305–309.

62. Orlandi F, Caraci P, Berruti A, et al. Chemotherapy with dacarbazine and 5-fluorouracil in advanced medullary thyroid cancer. Ann Oncol 1994; 5:763–765.

63. Schlumberger M, Abdelmoumene N, Delisle MJ, et al. Treatment of advanced medullary thyroid cancer with an alternating combination of 5-FU-streptozocin and 5-FU-dacarbazine. Br J Cancer 1995; 71:363–365.

64. Nocera M, Baudin E, Pellegriti G, et al. Treatment of advanced medullary thyroid cancer with an alternating combination of doxorubicin-streptozocin and 5-FU-dacarbazine. Br J Cancer 2000; 83:715–718.

65. Tisell LE, Hansson G, Jansson S, Salander H. Reoperation in the treatment of asymptomatic metastasizing medullary thyroid carcinoma. Surgery 1986; 99:60.

66. Moley JF, Dilley WG, DeBenedetti MK. Improved results of cervical reoperation for medullary thyroid carcinoma. Ann Surg 1997; 225:734.

67. Tung WS, Vesely TM, Moley JF. Laparoscopic detection of hepatic metastases in patients with residual or recurrent medullary thyroid cancer. Surgery 1995; 118:1024.

68. Melvin KEW, Tashjian AH, Miller HH. Studies in familial (medullary) thyroid carcinoma. Recent Prog Horm Res 1972; 28:399.

69. Sisson JC, Frager MS, Valk TW, et al. Scintigraphic localization of pheochromocytoma. N Engl J Med 1981; 305:12.

70. Lairmore TC, Ball DW, Baylin SB, Wells SA. Management of pheochromocytomas in patients with multiple endocrine neoplasia type 2 syndromes. Ann Surg 1993; 217:595.

71. Cheah WK, Clark OH, Horn JK, et al. Laparoscopic adrenalectomy for pheochromocytoma. World J Surg 2002; 26(8):1048.

72. Matsuda T, Murota T, Oguchi N, et al. Laparoscopic adrenalectomy for pheochromocytoma: a literature review. Biomed Pharmacother 2002; 56(suppl 1):126s.

73. Lee JE, Curley SA, Gagel RF, et al. Cortical-sparing adrenalectomy for patients with bilateral pheochromocytoma. Surgery 1996; 120(6):1064.

74. Schuffeneker I, Virally-Monod M, Brohet R, et al. J Clin Endocrinol Metab 1998; 83:487.

75. O'Riordan DS, O'Brien T, Grant CS, et al. Surgical management of primary hyperparathyroidism in multiple endocrine neoplasia types 1 and 2. Surgery 1993; 114:1031.

76. Raue F, Kraimps JL, Dralle H, et al. Primary hyperparathyroidism in multiple endocrine neoplasia type 2A. J Intern Med 1995; 238:369.

77. Gagel RF, Levy ML, et al. Multiple endocrine neoplasia type 2a associated with cutaneous lichen amyloidosis. Ann Intern Med 1989; 111:802.

78. Hofstra RMW, Sijmons RH, et al. RET mutation screening in familial cutaneous lichen amyloidosis and in skin amyloidosis associated with multiple endocrine neoplasia. J Invest Dermatol 1996; 107:215.

79. Cohen MS, Phay JE, Albinson C, et al. Gastrointestinal manifestations of multiple endocrine neoplasia type 2. Ann Surg 2002; 235(5):648.

80. Eng C, Mulligan LM, Smith DP, et al. Low frequency of germline mutations in the RET proto-oncogene in patients with apparently sporadic medullary thyroid carcinoma. Clin Endocrinol 1995; 43:123.

81. Bryant J, Farmer J, Kessler LJ, et al. Pheochromocytoma: the expanding genetic differential diagnosis. J Natl Cancer Inst 2003; 95(16):1196.

55

The Biology of Wound Healing

Dorne R. Yager and Ashley E. Ducale

INTRODUCTION

Wound healing is a fundamental and dynamic response to injury. The process of wound healing involves coordinated interactions between a variety of blood- and parenchymally derived cells, soluble factors, and extracellular matrix. Wounds can be caused by any number of physical insults that disrupt the integrity of a tissue. These include surgical incisions, trauma, thermal injury, and radiation injury. Regardless of the cause, most wounds can be expected to heal in a "timely" fashion. A basic understanding of wound healing is fundamental to surgery. This chapter outlines the basic concepts of the biology of wound healing and provides an introduction to the issues facing and options available for wound care management.

PHASES OF HEALING

The process of normal healing can be viewed as consisting of a cascade of events with four broadly overlapping phases: hemostasis, inflammation, tissue formation, and tissue remodeling. To understand how each phase contributes to healing, a discussion of these various components is in order.

Hemostasis

A direct consequence of injury is local disruption of blood vessels. This triggers three separate responses that work together to stop hemorrhage. Following injury, there is an instantaneous and transient vasoconstriction response by the injured capillaries, thus reducing the flow of blood near the site of injury. A second response involves formation of a platelet plug. Exposure of platelets to fibrillar collagen induces their aggregation at the site of hemorrhage. Serotonin, a vasoconstrictor, adenosine diphosphate, an attractant for platelets, and thromboxane A2, which induces platelet aggregation, degranulation, and vasoconstriction, are all released from stores contained within cytoplasmic granules (1–3).

The third response involves coagulation (4). This consists of two different pathways, intrinsic (originating with the release of factor XII by platelets) and extrinsic (originating with the release of factor III from the damaged tissues). Both clotting pathways eventually converge to activate factor X. Activation of prothrombin activator by factor X leads to the sequential conversion of prothrombin to thrombin, and fibrinogen to fibrin.

Fibrin initially forms a loose mesh, but then factor XIII causes the formation of covalent cross-links, which convert fibrin to a dense aggregation of fibers. Platelets and red blood cells become caught in this mesh of fiber, thus the formation of a blood clot. The resulting fibrin clot enmeshes the platelet aggregate with two consequences: (i) inhibition of further blood loss, and (ii) the formation of a provisional matrix that serves as an initial scaffold for repair. This provisional matrix consists primarily of fibrin, fibronectin, and hyaluronan (5). One final consequence of platelet degranulation is the release of a number of bioactive factors. These include growth factors such as platelet-derived growth factor (PDGF) and transforming growth factor-β (TGF-β) (6). These growth factors attract and direct the functions of the cells involved in the next phase of healing.

Inflammation

Large numbers of neutrophils (polymorphonuclear lymphocytes) begin entering the wound site during the first day following injury. Movement of leukocytes from the circulation into the tissues of the injured site requires three steps. Upon activation by the injury, local endothelial cells express P-selectin and E-selectin, which act to weakly tether circulating leukocytes via their constitutively expressed L-selectin. This loose tethering brings the leukocytes in proximity to chemoattractants and priming factors elaborated by the activated endothelial cells. In response, integrin receptors of the leukocytes are activated and initiate binding to intercellular adhesion molecules and vascular adhesion molecules that are expressed on endothelial cells. Following adhesion, leukocytes then extravasate through the vessel walls and into the damaged tissues (7).

Neutrophils have several functions in the repair process. One function is the debridement of the wound by phagocytosis of invading pathogens and devitalized tissue. Neutrophils possess an extensive armamentarium of degradative enzymes that are prepackaged into several types of granules. These include matrix metalloproteinases (MMPs) such as collagenase and gelatinase, and serine proteases such as elastase and cathepsin G (7). Activated neutrophils are also capable of mounting an enormous respiratory burst (8,9). The resulting reactive oxygen intermediates likely act by inactivating invading microbes and perhaps by activating the proteases contained with the neutrophil granules (10). After phagocytosis of devitalized tissue or microbes, neutrophils undergo apoptosis (11).

Another prominent leukocyte found in wounds is the macrophage. Macrophages are widely distributed in tissues and are primarily derived from circulating monocytes. Macrophages begin appearing at wound sites 48 to 96 hours following injury and participate in the wound's debridement, including phagocytosis of apoptotic neutrophils (12,13).

Macrophages and to some extent neutrophils, elaborate a number of growth factors that promote healing. These include interleukin-1, tumor necrosis factor-α, fibroblast growth factor (FGF), PDGF, and TGF-β (14,15). These factors have diverse effects. They act to modulate the inflammatory process and help direct the events in the subsequent phase of healing. In addition, activated neutrophils and macrophages express inducible nitric oxide synthase (13). Nitric oxide has been implicated in a number of wound-healing events (13).

Fibroplasia (Tissue Formation)

Fibroplasia represents the process by which new tissue comprising cells and matrix fills the wound defect. Stimulated by growth factors from the hemostatic and inflammatory phases, mesenchymal cells differentiate into fibroblasts, begin proliferating, and, using the provisional matrix as a scaffold, begin migrating into the wound site. A major function of fibroblasts is to replace the provisional matrix composed primarily of fibrin and fibronectin with one that is composed primarily of fibrillar collagens and proteoglycans.

Collagens are the principal structural proteins in skin and all other connective tissues. There are at least 19 types of collagen (16). Types I, II, and III make up approximately 90% of the total collagen found in tissues. By virtue of their unique structures, these collagens form fibrils with enormous intrinsic tensile strength. This is mainly due to inter- and intramolecular hydrogen bonding. All collagens consist of three subunits coiled into three-stranded helical structures. A repetitive glycine-proline-x motif is found with high frequency and is necessary for the very tight helical structure of the helical portion of the collagen trimer (17). Glycine, the smallest amino acid, is the only one that can fit into the tight center of the helix. Hydrogen bonding between the –NH of glycine with peptide carbonyls of adjacent polypeptides provide stability for the helical structure.

After their synthesis, collagen monomers are immediately transported into the lumen of the rough endoplasmic reticulum (Fig. 1). There, they are subjected to a series of posttranslational modifications. Hydroxylation of proline and lysine residues occurs in reactions that require oxygen, ferrous iron, α-ketoglutarate, and ascorbate (18). In turn, hydroxylysines become glycosylated (19).

Disulfide bonding between carboxyl termini of the procollagen sequences align the three chains prior to their forming the triple helix. Cleavage of the amino and carboxyl termini of procollagen occurs in the extracellular space as it is secreted. The resulting triple helical molecule, or tropocollagen, begins aggregating into larger structures. Strong,

organized fibrils form by staggered head-to-tail arrangements of the collagen molecules. Lysyl oxidase catalyzes the deamination of lysine that then undergoes intermolecular condensations (20). This cross-linking greatly stabilizes the collagen fibrils. The fibers themselves can form bundles large enough to be viewed by light microscopy (Fig. 2).

The collagens vary in the extent of their helical structures and posttranslational modifications. This allows for a great array of structures and thus, functions. Different collagen types, alone or in combination, are characteristic of different types of tissue. For example, skin and bone comprise mainly type I collagen, while cartilage contains mainly type II collagen (17). Distensible structures such as blood vessels are normally a combination of types III for distensibility and type I for strength. The basal lamina is the thin sheet-like structure upon which most epithelial and endothelial cells attach. Therefore, it is extremely important for the structure and function of organs such as skin, renal tubules, and a whole host of other tissues. Type IV collagen forms an irregular two-dimensional backbone on which the basal lamina is formed.

In addition to collagen, fibroblasts also deposit a large number of other proteins and carbohydrate-based molecules. These include fibronectin and proteoglycans such as deramatan sulfate, chondroitin sulfate, and the nonsulfated glycosaminoglycan, hyaluronan (21).

Angiogenesis

Reestablishment of the blood supply is crucial to provide nutrients and oxygen to the cells involved in repairing the tissue defect and for the continued maintenance of the newly established tissue. Angiogenesis likely initiates immediately after creation of the wound. Exposure of endothelial cells to the extracellular matrix, various cytokines, and possibly hypoxia induces angiogenesis (22–24). Additional cell types also play important roles in angiogenesis. Macrophages release growth factors including acidic and basic FGF (25). Slightly later after wounding, epithelial cells that have been stimulated by hypoxia begin to express vascular endothelial-cell growth factor (26). Together, these growth factors help orchestrate the events involved in angiogenesis.

New capillaries sprout from preexisting small blood vessels (22). Beginning as solid sprouts, capillary buds gradually become hollow to form tubes. These tubes continue being extended until they encounter and merge with another capillary, allowing the circulation of blood. Once the wound is sufficiently vascularized, the process of angiogenesis comes to an end. As the vasculature matures, many of the new blood vessels disintegrate via apoptosis (27).

Epithelialization

Epithelium is a vital component of the skin. It controls fluid loss and protects the host from the external milieu such as invasion of foreign substances such as bacteria and ultraviolet light. Because a wound represents a break in the integrity of the epithelium, these functions are compromised and it becomes important to reestablish this barrier.

The partial thickness wound is an example of a wound that requires almost exclusive healing by epithelialization. These wounds include superficial burns, split-thickness donor sites, and abrasions. As with all other aspects of repair, epithelialization is regulated in part by growth factors. These include epidermal growth factor, transforming growth factor-α, and keratinocyte growth factor (28,29). These growth

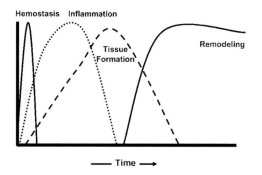

Figure 1 Phases of wound healing: Regardless of the type of injury or the affected tissue, wound healing usually follows a predictable pattern involving overlapping but identifiable phases. The time frame and relative importance of each of the phases are functions of the wound type and environment.

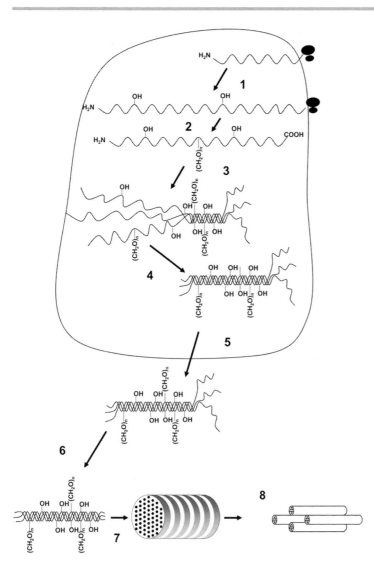

Figure 2 Collagen biosynthesis: Collagen monomers are synthesized on the rough endoplasmic reticulum. As the monomer chain grows, hydroxylation of proline and lysine residues takes place (**1**). In turn, some of the hydroxylysine residues become glycosylated (**2**). The C-terminal domains associate and direct the formation of the triple helix (**3**). The resulting procollagen molecule consists of a large domain with a tight triple helical conformation with the N- and C-terminal domains existing in a nonhelical conformation (**4**). After secretion (**5**), procollagen peptidases remove the terminal domains generating tropocollagen (**6**). Tropocollagen molecules self-assemble into fibrils (**7**), which in turn, further assemble into fibers (**8**).

factors stimulate the activation of the epidermal cells. Soon after wounding, basal epidermal cells at the wound edge or from within hair follicles remaining within the wound itself undergo dissolution of their desmosomes (cell–cell contacts) and their hemidesmosome links to the basement membrane (30). This allows the epidermal cells to begin migrating on the dermal surface. Receptors on the surface of the migrating epidermal cells, called integrins, allow these cells to interact with a variety of extracellular matrix proteins of the provisional matrix, which include fibronectin, vitronectin, and collagen. The expression of several proteases such as collagenase, gelatinase, and plasmin by the migrating epidermal cells is also important (30,31). Other epidermal cells at the wound edge begin to proliferate and migrate into the wound site. The migrating epidermal cells appear to exhibit "contact inhibition" in that they continue to move until a continuous single layer of cells have resurfaced the wound. In simple incisional wounds, this process is completed within 24 hours. At this point, the epidermal cells begin to differentiate into more basal-like cells. These cells then begin proliferating and reestablish the basilar to apical multilayered epithelium. With time, the basal epidermal cells

recreate their attachments to the dermis via hemidesmosomes. This provides resistance to sheer forces.

Remodeling

During this phase, inflammation and fibroplasia come to an end. It is believed that many of the cells involved in the first phases of repair undergo apoptosis, and as a result the scar tissue becomes relatively acellular. Clinically, this is manifested by the scar becoming progressively less pink as the numbers of blood vessels alsodiminish. Net collagen accumulation in the wound reaches a maximum within two to three weeks after wounding. At this time, the tensile strength of the wound is only a small fraction of the bursting strength of uninjured skin. Although there is no further net gain in collagen accumulation, the tensile strength of the wound gradually increases with time (32). This is a reflection of the continuing process of remodeling where the initially synthesized random collagen fibrils are steadily replaced by fibrils that possess greater organization and with more intermolecular cross-links. This process of remodeling requires a carefully maintained equilibrium between degradation of old collagen and synthesis of new collagen (33). In spite of the continual and long-term process of remodeling, the tensile strength of scar tissue only achieves approximately 70% of the strength of normal unwounded skin (32). In addition, scar tissue lacks normal dermal appendages such as hair follicles, sweat glands, and sebaceous glands.

OTHER ASPECTS OF REPAIR

Proteases

Proteases are involved in virtually every process that occurs during repair. For example, thrombin proteolytically converts fibrinogen to fibrin during hemostasis. Thrombin itself is proteolytically converted from prothrombin by factor X. A wide number of proteases participate in wound debridement. These include serine proteases such as neutrophils elastase and cathepsin G and several members of the MMP family. Proteases probably are involved in facilitating the migration of cells from adjacent tissues into the wound site. Proteases also play an essential role in the remodeling of scar tissues.

MMPs are particularly important to the process of repair. As a group, these proteases can enzymatically degrade any protein component found in the extracellular matrix (34). This attribute is particularly important to cells (e.g., fibroblasts, endothelial, and epithelial cells) needing to migrate from the adjacent normal tissues into the wound site. The rate-limiting step in the degradation of collagen is its initial cleavage. There are only three enzymes, all members of the MMP family, capable of initiating the lysis of fibrillar collagen. There is good evidence that all three of these collagenases play a part in the repair of one or more tissues. Because of their overall importance in maintaining tissue homeostasis, the MMPs are subject to regulation at several levels. This includes regulation at the transcriptional level, synthesis as inactive proenzymes that require posttranslational activation, and extracellular inhibition by both MMP-specific and nonspecific inhibitors. Disruption of the regulation of proteases can have important and profound effects on the repair process. Because of the continued activity of proteases, the mature wounds of scorbutic individuals have a significantly increased risk of dehiscence (35). An overexuberant inflammatory response may also play a role in the pathophysiology of chronic wounds (36). A significant number of these wounds contain large amounts of neutrophil-derived proteases that likely inhibit the net deposition of new tissues (37–39).

Contraction

Open wounds, to varying degrees, can contract as they heal. In other words, the surrounding skin has the appearance of being pulled toward the center of the wound. This provides two related advantages: first, there is a reduction in the amount of granulation tissue and ultimately, scar tissue needed to fill the defect; and secondly, the wound is to some extent resurfaced with normal skin and not scar. The mechanisms involved in contraction are poorly understood. There is growing evidence that fibroblasts may assume a myofibroblast-like phenotype (40,41). This is primarily characterized by the expression of large bundles of α smooth muscle actin (40,41). The appearance of myofibroblasts correlates with the process of contraction. Wounds that occur across flexor joints (e.g., the neck) as well as in hollow organs (e.g., esophagus) can also be subject to scar "contracture." In essence, contracture will occur anywhere on the surface of the body where there is not enough loose elastic skin to allow wound closure without contraction (42). Scar contracture can limit the functional range of motion of the involved joint or mechanically block the function of the hollow organ.

WOUND-HEALING PATHOLOGIES

Fibrosis

The disproportionate accumulation of collagen resulting in excessive or abnormal scar is a hallmark of fibrosis. Several fibrotic diseases such as hepatic fibrosis, retroperitoneal fibrosis, chronic fibrotic lung disease, tendon adhesions, and ankylosed joints are associated with significant morbidity and mortality. Some fibrotic conditions occur on the skin surface and often present to the surgeon for treatment. These include hypertrophic scar and keloid. Although both hypertrophic scars and keloid scars are associated with excessive collagen depositions, they are fundamentally different. Excessive scars that remain within the boundaries of the wound are termed "hypertrophic scars" (43). With time, hypertrophic scars typically regress. In contrast, keloids, from the Greek word kelois (or crab), extend beyond the original boundaries of the wound, rarely regress with time, and frequently reoccur following excision (44). The etiologies of hypertrophic scar and keloid are not known. Hypertrophic scarring is a frequent complication in deep partial-thickness and third-degree burns that are allowed to heal without grafting. Dark-skinned individuals are more at risk for forming a keloid and there may be a genetic component. There are no consistently effective treatments for keloid. Intralesional administration of corticosteroids such as triamcinolone often induces some shrinkage of the keloid (43). There have been reports of regression of lesions by treatment with pressure dressings or silicone sheets (43). However, there is no true efficacy for such therapy. Irradiation therapy has fallen into disfavor. Surgical excision followed by steroid injection or steroid injection alone remains the best therapy for treating some keloids.

Chronic Wounds

Chronic wounds can be best described as those wounds that have failed to heal in a timely fashion. Although this definition would seem to also include instances of fibrosis it more often applied to wounds that exhibit "insufficient" healing. The most common chronic wounds are diabetic ulcers, pressure sores, and venous stasis ulcers. As a group, chronic wounds place a significant and growing socioeconomic burden on western societies. These wounds are invariably associated with a number of predisposing conditions that compromise the healing process. However, it has been hypothesized that at least for the majority of chronic wounds (diabetic, stasis, and pressure ulcers), there are three principal common factors—ischemia/reperfusion injury, microbial load, and age (45).

Ischemia/Reperfusion Injury

Ischemia and reperfusion injury have been implicated in the pathophysiology of organ transplantation, hemorrhagic shock, cerebral ischemia, and myocardial infarction (46). Restoration of blood flow to ischemic tissues elicits a cascade of events that include free radical–mediated damage and a cascade of inflammatory events. Although it has not been tested, it seems likely that ischemia/reperfusion injury is involved in the formation of stasis, diabetic and pressure ulcers, and can also contribute to the chronicity of these wounds. A significant number of diabetic, stasis, and pressure ulcers display chronic inflammation (39,47). Inflammation that results from ischemia/reperfusion injury may be further exacerbated by the persistence of devitalized tissue, infection, and intermittent or continuous ischemia. The ensuing exuberant leukocytic response creates an environment rich in degradative enzymes and oxidants that do not have the ability to discriminate between intended targets and normal tissue (7,36). This can interfere with the function of growth factors involved in repair, inhibit the proliferation and migration of cells involved in repair, and impede the deposition of new tissue.

Microbiology

The skin has many important functions, but perhaps, none are as paramount as its providing a physical barrier against microbial invasion. All dermal wounds contain some level of microbial contamination and this is typically polymicrobial (48). In most cases, these microorganisms are not of pathogenic importance. Colonization or contamination represents the state wherein microorganisms are able to overcome local defense strategies and successfully compete but do not provoke clinical symptoms or a detectable immune response. In contrast, a wound infection represents a situation where local and systemic host responses are unable to eradicate the bacteria contaminating the wound. Although there is wide agreement that infection can impede the ability of a wound to heal, the ability to precisely define infection remains problematic. Whether infection occurs is probably dependent on a number of factors including microbial numbers, microbial type(s), wound location, wound size and depth, and the general health and immune status of the individual. Devitalized tissues, foreign bodies, and hematomas can promote the growth of microbes. Tissue that is poorly perfused can become hypoxic and permits the accumulation of acidic products such as lactate. These conditions may promote the growth of microbes.

Microbial virulence is dependent on several factors. The ability to produce toxins can cause further tissue damage. Quantitative and qualitative aspects of the microbial burden may also influence healing. One of the earliest studies attempting to define infection concluded that healing of pressure ulcers was impaired if the bacterial load of fluid exudate exceeded 10^6 CFU/mL (49). More commonly, it has become generally accepted that wounds with microbial loads greater than 10^5 CFU/g of tissue will not heal well (48,50,51). Pathogens such as β-hemolytic streptococci, *Staphylococcus aureus*, *Pseudomonas aeruginosa*, anaerobes, and enteric coliforms produce potentially destructive virulence factors. In spite of this, with the possible exception of the P-hemolytic streptococci, there is little evidence that supports the idea that a single particular type of bacteria is harmful (48,50,52). Instead, it appears that infection and wound-healing problems resulting from it correlate better with diversity (52). This is perhaps a reflection of possible synergy occurring between different types of bacteria.

An ongoing debate has centered on what is the most valuable sampling technique for making a qualitative and quantitative assessment of wound microbiology. It has been proposed that superficial swabs or biopsies provide a reasonably accurate reflection of the microbial flora of a wound (53,54). The rationale for this view is that most if not all microorganisms found in a wound will have originated superficially or from the skin flora. The method is simple and relatively noninvasive. Juxtaposed to this, is the belief that the deep tissue environment of a wound differs sufficiently from the surface to make swab or superficial biopsies of little value (55). Several studies have made a direct comparison of swab and deep tissue biopsy sampling and not found significant differences between the two methods (48,56–58). In spite of this, the use of deep tissue biopsy sampling for determining microbial load remains an accepted approach.

Age

The skin of the elderly is more fragile, and there is a decline in the thickness of the dermis, and rete pegs become smaller and flatter. Healing in the elderly is slower, albeit with less scarring (59). It has been speculated that this may be due in part to a gradual attenuation of the inflammatory/immune response; however, this conflicts with the observation of increased inflammatory cell levels in the aged (60). Levels of MMP-2 and MMP-9 are also increased in acute and chronic wounds of the aged (61). There is also a decreased proliferative potential in fibroblasts and keratinocytes (62).

Other Important Factors

A number of other systemic and local factors or conditions can influence healing. These include nutrition, immunological status, pharmacological impairment, and genetics.

Nutrition

Surgery, trauma, and sepsis induce a protein catabolic state (63). Wound healing is an energy requiring process, and therefore severely malnourished individuals have difficulty in wound healing (64,65). Insufficient carbohydrate and fat intake result in the catabolism of protein as an alternative energy source. Hypoproteinemia, in turn, limits the supply of amino acids that are available for synthesis of new protein at the wound site (66). Inadequate levels of amino acids such as arginine also inhibit the immune response (67). In spite of the recognition of the importance of nutrition to wound healing, there remains no single measure of nutritional adequacy. Serum albumin (minimum of 3.5 g/dL) is an often used indicator of general protein and nitrogen balance.

Several vitamins have important roles in the healing process (64). Ascorbate (vitamin C) is an essential cofactor in the hydroxylation of lysine and proline in collagen synthesis and cross-linking. Scorbutic individuals heal with poor wound strength and have an increased risk of wound dehiscence, because normal baseline collagen synthesis is impaired. Deficiencies in vitamin A, thiamine, zinc, and iron have a negative influence on healing. Vitamins E and C may both act as antioxidants and thus provide some protection from oxidant stress. Alterations in nutrition caused by cancer are also taken into consideration. Cancer typically elevates carbohydrate and protein consumption, and this in turn can impose limits on the nutrients available for repair processes.

Immunologic Status

The immunologic status of an individual can be influenced by genetics, pharmaceutically, and by infection with immunosuppressive agents. The leukocytes of individuals with chronic granulomatous disease are unable to mount an effective respiratory burst and thus do not handle invading microbes as efficiently as normal individuals. Some of the immunosuppressive effects of glucocorticoid steroids probably are responsible for the detrimental effect on healing by this class of agents. Similarly, immunosuppression of transplant recipients may also influence the wound healing of these individuals (68,69). Patients with human immunodeficiency virus (HIV) infection have been found to have impaired wound healing (70). The wounds of patients with HIV infection when measured biomechanically are weaker than those of normal non-HIV controls (69).

Genetic

The wound care provider must be alert to the existence of the possible role of genetics in wound repair. There are several known defects that reduce the numbers of or effectiveness of cells involved in the repair process (e.g., chronic granulomatous disease and leukocyte adhesion deficiency). A number of defects in connective tissue components have been described. These include osteogenesis imperfecta (congenital form of osteopenia resulting from defects in type I collagen); Ehlers-Danlos syndrome (broad group of collagen and collagen processing enzyme defects); epidermolysis bullosa (defects resulting in poor adhesion between the epidermal and dermal layers); and Marfan's syndrome (defects in fibrillin or collagen). Although relatively rare, and variable in manifestation, individuals with connective tissue defects represent a significant challenge to the ability of wounds to heal effectively.

Oxygen

Adequate levels of oxygen at the site of tissue injury are necessary for repair. Tissue hypoxia or anoxia results in cell and tissue death. Without adequate levels of oxygen, neutrophils and monocytes are unable to mount a respiratory burst response (71). Oxygen is also required to support the migration and proliferation of cells involved in tissue formation. Proliferation requires a tissue oxygen tension (pO_2) of 30 mmHg. Collagen synthesis is dependent upon oxygen. It has been shown that wounds with pO_2 less than 20 mm heal poorly, whereas those with pO_2 greater than 40 mm have a better chance of healing in a timely fashion (72,73). The surgeon must be mindful of key factors required to ensure adequate oxygen perfusion of the wound. Pain and hypothermia result in vasoconstriction, which decreases oxygen delivery to the wound bed. Hypovolemia, even in the presence of normal arterial gases can reduce wound oxygen.

Pharmacologic Impairment

There are a variety of agents that while not used directly in the treatment of wounds, may have a significant influence on the repair process. Glucocorticoids possess anti-inflammatory and immunosuppressive functions and have a detrimental influence on leukocyte functions, fibroblast proliferation, and on the synthesis of collagen (74).

Cancer chemotherapy is frequently directed at inhibiting cell proliferation. It seems likely that chemotherapy, especially regimens utilizing multiple agents, could have a negative influence on repair. Surprisingly, there is little evidence suggesting that this is indeed the case. Studies have shown that doxorubicin and 5-fluoruracil can have deleterious effects on wound-healing events (75,76). Chemotherapeutic agents that target tumor angiogenesis may also influence wound healing. This also raises the issue of whether some other commonly used agents that may inhibit angiogenesis as a side effect might also have an impact on wound healing. This could include such agents as Vioxx,

Celebrex, Enbrel, Doxycycline, Captopril, and Furosemide (Lasix) (77–81). Nicotine is a major pharmacologic threat to efficient healing. Nicotine induces vasoconstriction and elevates carboxyhemoglobin levels (82,83). The resulting reduction in oxygen perfusion to the wound has the potential for impairing repair events.

WOUND MANAGEMENT

The management of wounds requires consideration of the wound as well as the patient. As seen from the previous sections, a number of local and systemic factors can interact in a variety of ways to influence wound-healing outcome. In exploring treatment options, wound characteristics such as necrosis, infection, edema, and wound environment, and wound etiology must be assessed.

It is not enough to treat the wound itself. Consideration must be given to the fact that behind each wound is a patient; a patient who may have attendant physical and emotional needs that go beyond the boundaries of the wound itself. To be consistently successful, the healer must treat the patient first and the wound second. Legally, one must record the circumstances of the event, which caused the injury. Will the injury cause a functional impairment at work? Do the patients and their families understand the events of healing that one must expect even after the simplest of lacerations? When can the patient resume normal activities? Time and circumstances of injury are also important. Wounds open for longer than 10 to 12 hours are more prone to infection as the bacterial flora within the wound becomes protected by wound proteinaceous secretions and will not be easily removed by lavage. Did the injury occur in a contaminated environment? This may increase the bacterial burden to the tissues and make debridement and cleaning extremely important. Wound location is also an important consideration. Wounds in the extremities tend to have a slower rate of healing than those of the face.

Cleaning and Debriding

The first steps in the treatment of traumatic wounds are to bring bleeding under control, to cleanse the wound, and to remove foreign material and devitalized tissue. Acceptable agents for irrigation of wounds without gross contamination include physiological saline solutions and Ringer's lactate solution. Irrigants containing antiseptics may be warranted for wounds that are badly contaminated (84). However, they require judicious use, because these agents do not discriminate between microbes and otherwise healthy tissues of the patient.

Debridement involves the elimination of devitalized and contaminated tissues of the wound. Physically removing dead tissue and bacteria from the wound removes an environment that is favorable to microbial growth. There are several methods by which debridement can be accomplished. (i) Mechanical debridement: When changed, moist to dry gauze dressings provide some measure of physically debriding wounds. When performed properly, these dressings are extremely useful in facilitating the debridement of the interstices of deep irregular wounds. It must be taken into consideration that this form of debridement is nonselective, removing both healthy and necrotic tissue, and can be painful. (ii) Autolytic debridement: Use of some barrier-type dressings such as the hydrocolloid alginates promotes the breakdown of necrotic tissue by the body's own white blood cells. However, such treatment may actually increase the bacterial count within the wound and thus increase the incidence of infection and subsequent sepsis. (iii) Sharp debridement: Sharp dissection is by far a more effective and rapid form of debridement (85). However, there are drawbacks that may limit its use. For example, pain and bleeding may be problematical unless the procedure is performed in the operating room. In the very elderly and infirm, when wound closure is not the long-range objective, extensive debridement of a large pressure ulcer is rarely indicated unless a simpler method proves unsatisfactory. (iv) Enzymatic debridement: A notable advantage of this method is that it does not necessitate the same skill level that is required for surgical debridement. This method is widely used in nursing homes and situations where surgical debridement by sharp dissection cannot be performed. Ridding the wound of necrosis using this type of debridement, however, is usually slower than sharp debridement. Overall, the type, consistency, adherence, and amount of necrosis will ultimately influence the debridement method utilized.

Proper aseptic technique in the operating theater can minimize infection from contamination. Prophylactic use of antibiotics during the perioperative period is justified by the premise that the potential benefit outweighs the possible risk of developing and selecting for resistant strains. There is some general agreement as to the use of systemic antibiotics for treating infection involving deeper tissues. Topical antibiotics and antiseptics are frequently used for treating wounds with no or minimal signs of infection. To what extent their use is efficacious is not clear. There is little evidence supporting the usefulness of routine administration of systemic antibiotics to individuals with chronic wounds (86).

Wound Closure

After trauma wounds have been cleaned and debrided, they can be typically closed by direct approximation. Closure by direct approximation (primary closure) facilitates the repair process and usually minimizes scar formation. Wound closure can involve the use of sutures, staples, adhesive tape strips, or tissue adhesives (e.g., cyanoacrylate or fibrin glue). There are two classifications of sutures: absorbable or nonabsorbable. A common example of an absorbable suture is that made from polyglycolic acid polymers. This material maintains its integrity for two to three weeks and induces little inflammatory response. Nylon and silk are typical examples of nonabsorbable sutures. However, many have abandoned silk because it has interstices and may be inflammatory if it remains in the host for a prolonged period of time. Because they are less conducive to wicking, monofilament sutures have the advantage of inducing minimal inflammation. On the other hand, multifilamentous sutures are easier to manipulate. Epithelial tracks followed by scarring can develop in skin sutures left in place longer than 7 to 10 days. However, at this time, the wound has attained only a fraction of strength of unwounded skin. This necessitates a decision whether to compromise cosmesis in lieu of continued support of the direct approximation. Therefore, before the placement of sutures on the surface of the skin, one should try to relieve as much tension on the wound as is possible. Placement of absorbable sutures in the dermis will relieve tension. The skin sutures themselves can be removed after approximately five days without fear of the incision site reopening. Another very popular way of closing skin wounds without the fear of leaving suture marks is to close with a running subcuticular suture of monofilament material such as polypropylene (it is easier to remove than nylon). A running suture can be left in place until one is confident that the incision has gained sufficient tensile strength for removal without wound margin separation.

Delayed Primary Closure

Not all wounds can be immediately closed. In the event of overt or suspected microbial infection, wounds can be left open at the time of injury or surgery. The wounds can then be examined over the course of several days. If there is no evidence of infection, or if it has been brought under control, then the edges can be approximated. Alternatively, wounds can be allowed to heal secondarily. This can require a mixture of granulation tissue formation, re-epithelialization, and contraction. Candidate wounds for secondary closure are encountered in instances of heavy contamination, where there has been significant tissue loss (e.g., pressure ulcers), or in locations where the tissues will not tolerate the strain imposed by approximating the wound edges.

Dressings

A plethora of options are available to the clinician for dressing wounds. Appropriate selection and use of dressings require that the dressing needs of a wound be matched with the dressing type that is optimal for that wound. Simple incisional wounds that have been primarily closed require only simple, clean dressings that provide protective coverage. Since the 1960s, it has become generally accepted that a moist environment is advantageous to the healing of partial-thickness and open wounds (87,88). In the absence of a scab, epithelial cells can proliferate and migrate more efficiently to resurface the wound. Collagen synthesis, angiogenesis, and contraction also appear to benefit from a moist wound environment (89). Appropriate selection of a dressing product is dependent upon the wound type and conditions (90,91).

Partial-thickness wounds such as graft donor sites, abrasions, and first and second degree burns are best treated with semiocclusive dressings. These dressings provide a moist environment that prevents the formation of scab on the wound surface and reduces desiccation. The absence of a scab physically facilitates re-epithelialization and reduces the amount of scar formation. It is also believed that by preventing desiccation, semiocclusive dressings also promote an environment that is more conducive to the migration and proliferation of the cells involved in repair.

A potential problem with semiocclusive dressings is their limited absorption capacity. Excessive fluid accumulation, as might occur during the early phase of repair, can lead to maceration of the wound and surrounding tissues. In these instances, the use of more absorbent dressings such as hydrocolloids is indicated. Hydrocolloids are composed of natural (e.g., gelatin and pectins) or synthetic (polyurethane) hydrophilic materials combined with an adhesive and covered by a semipermeable membrane. Hydrocolloids adhere firmly to the skin surrounding a wound without directly adhering to the wound itself. They are highly absorptive yet maintain a moist wound environment. They also promote some autolytic debridement by virtue of their maintaining a moist environment. Known or suspected infection with anaerobes is a counter indication for the use of occlusive dressings and hydrocolloids. Absorptive fillers are useful in exudative wounds that contain dead space not easily reached by other dressing types. Absorptive fillers can be powders, pads, ropes, or pastes made from alginates, starches, or simple gauzes. Some fillers such as collagen dressings have the advantage of liquefying as they are being absorbed, making them easier to remove. Hydrogels are dressings composed primarily of water. Their primary function is to hydrate relatively dry wounds. These dressings have a cooling effect when applied to superficial burns. They are also recommended for application to wound surfaces that might need to be kept moist (e.g., exposed bone or tendon). Because these dressing do not absorb moisture, they are not particularly useful on exudative wounds.

Cellulose-based gauze dressings are relatively inexpensive and remain the most commonly used type of wound dressing. Gauze is useful in large exudative wounds that require frequent dressing changes. Gauze can also be used to facilitate mechanical debridement. However, gauze has a propensity to dry out and adhere tightly to the wound bed.

Several new dressings intended to provide features that go beyond providing physical protection and moisture control have become available. These include several dressings that possess antimicrobial properties (e.g., iodine or silver releasing dressings). Dressings based on the glyosaminoglycan and hyaluronan have recently entered the market. Hyaluronan is a major component of the provisional matrix and probably is involved in the formation of a highly hydrated environment that promotes cell proliferation and migration. Another dressing product based on a composite of denatured bovine collagen and oxidized regenerated cellulose can seemingly reduce levels of proteolytic activity in wounds. This product probably acts as a competitive inhibitor by introducing a large amount of substrate for the proteases that may be present in a wound.

Skin Grafts, Flaps, and Skin Substitutes

Skin grafting provides an effective means of treating burns and some chronic wounds. When first placed onto a well-vascularized bed, the graft receives nutrients by passive diffusion from the underlying tissue. With time, revascularization of the graft occurs primarily from ingrowth of capillaries from the underlying tissues. Skin grafts are classified as partial or split-thickness (0.01–0.015 in. in thickness) and full-thickness grafts. Partial-thickness grafts consist of a layer of epidermis and some dermis. The donor site heals primarily by re-epithelialization from the edges and from islands of keratinocytes that proliferate and migrate out from the hair follicles and other dermal appendages. In contrast, full-thickness grafts include all of the epidermis and dermis. For grafting to be successful, the recipient site must be well vascularized and microbial contamination minimized. In addition, the graft must make complete and stable contact with the recipient site (seroma or hematoma formation will compromise a graft's survival). In general, partial-thickness grafts have better survival rates than full-thickness grafts and the donor sites also heal more readily. However, wounds treated with full-thickness grafts are subject to less contraction.

Skin grafts are not a viable option in wounds that are heavily contaminated with bacteria or lack a well-vascularized base. In these cases, flaps are used to close the wound. Skin flaps differ from grafts in that the intrinsic blood supply of the donor tissue remains intact or the blood supply is reestablished surgically at the time of transfer. There are essentially two types of flaps. Random-pattern flaps receive their blood supply from a number of vessels located within the subdermal plexus. Random-pattern flaps are limited in size because of the limited nature of their blood supply. In contrast, an axial-pattern skin flap receives its blood supply from a major vessel. In some instances where the axial vessel enters the underlying muscle, the muscle and the overlying skin can be elevated as a single musculocutaneous flap.

The development of skin substitutes offers a possible alternative to autografting and allografting of skin. Substitutes range in complexity from nonliving allogeneic acellular matrices to cultured, allogeneic, bi-layered human skin equivalents derived from neonatal skin. INTEGRA® is a collagen matrix covered with a thin sheet of silicone, which can be placed into a fresh wound bed and allowed to vascularize. The silicone is then removed and the vascularized collagen matrix is covered with a very thin split-thickness skin graft. The use of this material has been successful in skilled hands. However, two procedures are required and "take" is variable. Some reports suggest that there is a reduction in hypertrophic scarring from this method. Other skin substitutes currently marketed include Dermagraft and Apligraf®. The use of skin substitutes in chronic wounds has shown a measure of success. However, their cost is high compared to conventional therapies.

Perfusion/Hyperbaric Oxygen Therapy

Ischemic wounds heal poorly. A hypoxic environment is not conducive to the proliferation, migration, and function of cells involved in the wound-healing process; whereas, it favors the growth of anaerobic microbes. There is now some evidence that hyperbaric oxygen (HBO) therapy involving the intermittent inhalation of 100% oxygen at pressures greater than 1 atm can improve wound-healing outcome (92,93). Increased oxygen tension may promote leukocyte microbicidal functions, angiogenesis, and fibroblast proliferation. At present, HBO therapy should be restricted to wounds involving acute traumatic ischemia, infection by clostridial organisms, necrotizing soft tissue infections, and selected nonhealing problematic wounds.

Vacuum-Assisted Wound Closure

Developed in the past decade, vacuum-assisted closure has experienced a rapid growth in acceptance (94,95). A foam dressing is applied to the wound and the wound sealed with an occlusive dressing. Low-level (125 mmHg) negative pressure is then cyclically applied. This approach is effective in accelerating closure of open acute wounds and in successful application of skin grafts (96). The mechanism(s) by which this device assists healing is not clear. Candidate mechanisms include removal of interstitial pressure, restoration of blood flow and perfusion, removal of cytotoxic factors and proteases, and mechanical induction of wound-healing activity.

Treatment of Chronic Wounds

Chronic wounds are broadly defined as open wounds that have failed to heal in a timely (i.e., three months) fashion. As a group, chronic wounds place a significant and increasing socioeconomic burden on Western societies. These wounds are almost invariably associated with predisposing conditions that compromise the healing process. The pathophysiologies of chronic wounds are complex and diverse. Underlying conditions can be neurological, metabolic, vascular, psychiatric, or perhaps most commonly, a combination of these factors. Successful management of chronic wounds is generally dependent upon recognition of and concomitant treatment of the underlying causes for the chronic wound. A large percentage of chronic wounds are associated with chronic inflammation. This may be the result of persistence of devitalized tissue, infection, and intermittent or continuous ischemia. The ensuing exuberant leukocytic response creates an environment rich in degradative enzymes and oxidants that do not have the ability to discriminate between intended targets and normal tissues. This concept has led to some recent interest in developing strategies that modulate the inflammatory component of chronic wounds. Debridement removes devitalized tissue and reduces the microbial burden, and antibiotics (topical or systemic) are used to control infection. Management of the nutritional and pharmacological state of the individual helps set the stage for healing. As addressed below, specific approaches are used to treat chronic wounds resulting from pressure, venous insufficiency, and diabetes.

Leg Ulcers

Leg ulcers can occur in individuals displaying lower limb arterial or venous insufficiency. Smoking, hyperlipidemia, hypertension, obesity, and age all predispose individuals to local tissue ischemia in the lower limbs with a greatly increased risk of retarded wound healing. Treatment requires addressing the need for adequate perfusion along with cleaning and debriding of the wound site.

More than half of all leg ulcers are directly the result of increased pressure in the venous system. Most venous hypertension is a reflection of the insufficiency of the valves in the deep venous system and the lower perforating veins (97). Valvular incompetence negates the ability of the calf muscle pump to aid in the return of blood to the heart from the lower limbs. The capillaries are subjected to increased tension and become malformed. There is leakage of plasma proteins resulting in a protein-rich edema and the appearance of discontinuous fibrin cuffs. Microthrombi form, occlude the capillaries, and activated leukocytes accumulate. The resulting edema likely contributes to a localized tissue hypoxia. Eventually, this hypoxia in conjunction with the activated leukocytes leads to a breakdown of tissue, resulting in a venous stasis ulcer.

Initial treatment involves cleansing and debridement of proteinaceous exudate. Compression therapy aimed at controlling edema and the venous hypertension itself is essential. The first objective in treating ulcers resulting from arterial insufficiency is to improve perfusion. This requires surgical interventions including grafting, percutaneous transluminal angioplasty, thrombolysis, and placement of stents.

Diabetic Ulcers

There are approximately 15 million diabetics in the United States. The yearly incidence of foot ulcers in diabetics is between 2% and 3% (98). In poorly controlled diabetes, collagen and other proteins are subject to nonenzymatic glycosylation events. This can result in disrupted function of proteins within the tissues. As a consequence, neuropathy resulting in unrecognized pressure and tissue trauma, in conjunction with arterial insufficiency caused by atherosclerotic occlusion of the tibioperoneal arteries, is the likely cause of diabetic foot ulcers.

Angiopathy probably contributes to the poor healing quality often associated with diabetic wounds. There is an impairment in granulocyte chemotaxis and phagocytic function. The absolute numbers of capillaries are lower in diabetics and differ from nondiabetics in morphology.

The risk of infection in diabetic wounds is substantially greater than it is for the wounds of nondiabetics.

Effective treatment of diabetic ulcers involves utilizing a combination of approaches. Control of glucose levels is paramount for successful therapy. In the case of foot ulcers, devices that off-load pressure from susceptible areas may be necessary. Aggressive sharp debridement, restoring circulation, and microbial control are also important. Topically applied recombinant PDGF (Becaplermin gel) has been demonstrated to be an aid in the healing of diabetic ulcers (99).

Pressure Ulcers

Pressure and shear forces over bony prominences have a key role in the formation of pressure ulcers. Individuals immobilized as the result of general anesthesia, sedation, coma, and spinal injury are at significant risk. Prolonged pressure occludes the microcirculation, producing ischemia. Ischemic damage initially occurs in the fat and deep muscles. Skin is relatively resistant to ischemia; thus small skin ulcers often cover large areas of subcutaneous necrosis. There is leakage of plasma proteins and accumulation of activated leukocytes. As a result, there is release of significant levels of active proteases and reactive oxygen metabolites.

The National Pressure Ulcer Advisory Panel has developed a staging system for classifying pressure ulcers. This system is detailed below:

Stage I. Nonblanchable erythema of intact skin, the heralding lesion of skin ulceration.

Stage II. Partial-thickness skin loss involving epidermis and/or dermis. The ulcer is superficial and presents clinically as an abrasion, blister, or shallow crater.

Stage III. Full-thickness skin loss involving damage or necrosis of subcutaneous tissue that may extend down to, but not through, underlying fascia. The ulcer presents clinically as a deep crater with or without undermining of adjacent tissue.

Stage IV. Full-thickness skin loss with extensive destruction, tissue necrosis, or damage to muscle, bone, or supporting structures.

Other Chronic Wound Types

Radiation

Exposure to irradiation damages the DNA of tissues. To minimize damage to normal cells, dosage is fractionated and administered in tangential fields. In spite of this, irradiation can result in rapid death of cells or prevent them from proliferating normally. Due to their exposure to radiation, fibroblasts that migrate into a site damaged by radiation are themselves morphologically abnormal. In addition, these fibroblasts synthesize elevated levels of collagen, which probably have an important role in the characteristic fibrosis of irradiated tissues. Healed irradiated skin has fewer dermal appendages (e.g., hair follicles and sebaceous glands), the walls of blood vessels are thickened, and the vessel lumens have a tendency to become occluded. The epidermis is thin and there are alterations in pigmentation. Therefore, radiated skin is more prone to bacterial invasion and infection. Once irradiated skin has broken down, the best treatment is to bring in new blood supply. This is accomplished by excision of as much radiated tissue as possible and replacement with vascularized tissue either in the form of a pedicle flap or free tissue transfer to restore blood supply to the radiated area. If one must perform elective surgery through radiated skin, it is best to do the same to avoid potential catastrophic results.

Marjolin's Ulcer

This condition often presents as a chronic wound, but is indeed a squamous cell carcinoma that has developed in an old scar from a burn wound or trauma (100,101). These lesions are very aggressive with a high rate of metastasis. After a metastatic work-up, treatment consists of total local excision followed by appropriate reconstructive coverage.

The Future of Wound Healing

Research in wound healing is one of the most exciting areas for investigative young surgeons to consider as part of their careers. Although there has been great progress over the past two decades, the possibilities remain enormous. The use of growth factors, skin substitutes, novel antimicrobials, and biologically active dressings has only begun in the last decade and there is much room for improvement. There are also the potential benefits from gene therapy. One example would be to modulate the inflammatory phase of repair. There is a wealth of evidence that in the absence of infection, wound healing is accelerated, and has a better outcome when inflammation is inhibited or prevented (102–104). As the process of wound healing is more completely understood, it should become possible to design new strategies for the treating of problem wounds and perhaps even improving the healing of otherwise normal wounds.

SUMMARY

Wounds can be caused by a wide variety of insults that disrupt the integrity of a tissue. Factors influencing the healing process include hemostasis, associated inflammation/infection, underlying nutrition and immune status, and the adequacy of blood flow to enable the necessary provision of nutrients and oxygen to the cells involved in repairing the tissue defect. The individual response of a given wound to these various parameters will dictate the efficiency and speed of overall healing and the appearance of the resultant scar. Wounds that can be closed primarily generally result in rapid epithelialization through the effective production of collagen and its cross-linking. Wounds that need to be left open to heal in a more delayed fashion undergo the same process of collagen maturation, but the overall time required for this is usually prolonged when compared to its closed counterpart. Ultimately, though, the resultant scar is amazingly small due to a concomitant wound contraction. The principles of wound management to effect optimal healing are well established so that even the most complex and challenging wound can be expected to heal with a good-to-excellent result. In those wounds that do not respond to standard management strategies, additional approaches for care, such as skin grafts, flaps, and skin substitutes, have often proved helpful.

REFERENCES

1. Esmon CT. Cell mediated events that control blood coagulation and vascular injury. Ann Rev Cell Biol 1993; 9:1.
2. Williams TJ, Peck MJ. Role of prostaglandin-mediated vasodilatation in inflammation. Nature 1977; 270:530.
3. Boucek RJ. Factors affecting wound healing. Otolaryngol Clin North Am 1984; 17:243.
4. Dahlback B. Blood coagulation and its regulation by anticoagulant pathways: genetic pathogenesis of bleeding and thrombotic diseases. J Intern Med 2005; 257:209.
5. Clark RA. Fibrin and wound healing. Ann NY Acad Sci 2001; 936:355.
6. Ross R, Glomset J, et al. A platelet-dependent serum factor that stimulates the proliferation of arterial smooth muscle cells in vitro. Proc Natl Acad Sci USA 1974; 71:1207.
7. Weiss SJ. Tissue destruction by neutrophils. N Engl J Med 1989; 320:365.
8. Babibr BM. Oxygen-dependent microbial killing by phagocytes (second of two parts). N Engl J Med 1978; 298:721.
9. Babior BM. Oxygen-dependent microbial killing by phagocytes (first of two parts). N Engl J Med 1978; 298:659.
10. Reeves EP, Lu H, et al. Killing activity of neutrophils is mediated through activation of proteases by K+ flux. Nature 2002; 416:291.
11. Theilgaard-Monch K, Knudsen S, et al. The transcriptional activation program of human neutrophils in skin lesions supports their important role in wound healing. J Immunol 2004; 172:7684.
12. Leibovich SJ, Ross R. The role of the macrophage in wound repair. A study with hydrocortisone and antimacrophage serum. Am J Pathol 1975; 78:71.
13. Park JE, Barbul A. Understanding the role of immune regulation in wound healing. Am J Surg 2004; 187:11S.
14. Leibovich SJ, Ross R. A macrophage-dependent factor that stimulates the proliferation of fibroblasts in vitro. Am J Pathol 1976; 84:501.
15. Gillitzer R, Goebeler M. Chemokines in cutaneous wound healing. J Leukoc Biol 2001; 69:513.
16. Nimni ME. Collagen: structure, function, and metabolism in normal and fibrotic tissues. Semin Arthritis Rheum 1983; 13:1.
17. Prockop DJ, Kivirikko KI. Collagens: molecular biology, diseases, and potentials for therapy. Ann Rev Biochem 1995; 64:403.
18. Hutton JJ Jr, Trappel AL, et al. Requirements for alpha-ketoglutarate, ferrous ion and ascorbate by collagen proline hydroxylase. Biochem Biophys Res Commun 1966; 24:179.
19. Blumenkrantz N, Rosenbloom J, et al. Sequential steps in the synthesis of hydroxylysine and the glycosylation of hydroxylysine during the biosynthesis of collagen. Biochim Biophys Acta 1969; 192:81.
20. Siegel RC, Pinnell SR, et al. Cross-linking of collagen and elastin. Properties of lysyl oxidase. Biochemistry 1970; 9:4486.
21. Hassell JR, Kimura JH, et al. Proteoglycan core protein families. Ann Rev Biochem 1986; 55:539.
22. Folkman J, Klagsbrun M. Angiogenic factors. Science 1987; 235:442.
23. Tonnesen MG, Feng X, et al. Angiogenesis in wound healing. J Investig Dermatol Symp Proc 2000; 5:40.
24. Richard DE, Berra E, et al. Angiogenesis: how a tumor adapts to hypoxia. Biochem Biophys Res Commun 1999; 266:718.
25. Koch AE, Polverini PJ, et al. Induction of neovascularization by activated human monocytes. J Leukoc Biol 1986; 39:233.
26. Berse B, Brown LF, et al. Vascular permeability factor (vascular endothelial growth factor) gene is expressed differentially in normal tissues, macrophages, and tumors. Mol Biol Cell 1992; 3:211.
27. O'Reilly MS, Holmgren L, et al. Angiostatin: a circulating endothelial cell inhibitor that suppresses angiogenesis and tumor growth. Cold Spring Harb Symp Quant Biol 1994; 59:471.
28. Nanney LB, Sundberg JP, et al. Increased epidermal growth factor receptor in fsn/fsn mice. J Invest Dermatol 1996; 106:1169.
29. Thomas KA. Fibroblast growth factors. FASEB J 1987; 1:434.
30. Singer AJ, Clark RA. Cutaneous wound healing. N Engl J Med 1999; 341:738.
31. Pilcher BK, Dumin JA, et al. The activity of collagenase-1 is required for keratinocyte migration on a type I collagen matrix. J Cell Biol 1997; 137:1445.

32. Forrester JC, Zederfeldt BH, et al. Wolffs law in relation to the healing skin wound. J Trauma 1970; 10:770.

33. Kuzuya M, Iguchi A. Role of matrix metalloproteinases in vascular remodeling. J Atheroscler Thromb 2003; 10:275.

34. Parks WC. Matrix metalloproteinases in repair. Wound Repair Regen 1999; 7:423.

35. Lind J. In: Kincaid A, Donaldson A, eds. Treatise of the scurvy. 1st ed. Edinburgh, Sands, Murray and Cochran, 1753:192–196.

36. Nussler AK, Wittel UA, et al. Leukocytes, the Janus cells in inflammatory disease. Langenbecks Arch Surg 1999; 384:222.

37. Yager DR, Nwomeh BC. The proteolytic environment of chronic wounds. Wound Repair Regen 1999; 7:433.

38. Yager DR, Zhang LY, et al. Wound fluids from human pressure ulcers contain elevated matrix metalloproteinase levels and activity compared to surgical wound fluids. J Invest Dermatol 1996; 107:743.

39. Yager DR, Chen SM, et al. Ability of chronic wound fluids to degrade peptide growth factors is associated with increased levels of elastase activity and diminished levels of proteinase inhibitors. Wound Repair Regen 1997; 5:23.

40. Gabbiani G. The myofibroblast in wound healing and fibro-contractive diseases. J Pathol 2003; 200:500.

41. Hinz B, Gabbiani G, et al. The NH2-terminal peptide of alpha-smooth muscle actin inhibits force generation by the myofibroblast in vitro and in vivo. J Cell Biol 2002; 157:657.

42. Ehrlich HP. Scar contracture: cellular and connective tissue aspects in Peyronie's disease. J Urol 1997; 157:316.

43. Alster TS, Tanzi EL. Hypertrophic scars and keloids: etiology and management. Am J Clin Dermatol 2003; 4:235.

44. Datubo-Brown DD. Keloids: a review of the literature. Br J Plast Surg 1990; 43:70.

45. Mustoe T. Understanding chronic wounds: a unifying hypothesis on their pathogenesis and implications for therapy. Am J Surg 2004; 187:65S.

46. Anaya-Prado R, Toledo-Pereyra LH, et al. Ischemia/reperfusion injury. J Surg Res 2002; 105:248.

47. Nwomeh BC, Yager DR, et al. Physiology of the chronic wound. Clin Plast Surg 1998; 25:341.

48. Bowler PG, Duerden BI, et al. Wound microbiology and associated approaches to wound management. Clin Microbiol Rev 2001; 14:244.

49. Bendy RH Jr, Nuccio PA, et al. Relationship of quantitative wound bacterial counts to healing of decubiti: effect of topical gentamicin. Antimicrob Agents Chemother 1964; 10:147.

50. Robson MC, Stenberg BD, et al. Wound healing alterations caused by infection. Clin Plast Surg 1990; 17:485.

51. Murphy RC, Robson MC, et al. The effect of microbial contamination on musculocutaneous and random flaps. J Surg Res 1986; 41:75.

52. Trengove NJ, Stacey MC, et al. Qualitative bacteriology and leg ulcer healing. J Wound Care 1996; 5:277.

53. Armstrong DG, Liswood PJ, William J, et al. Stickel Bronze Award. Prevalence of mixed infections in the diabetic pedal wound. A retrospective review of 112 infections. J Am Podiatr Med Assoc 1995; 85:533.

54. Levine NS, Lindberg RB, et al. The quantitative swab culture and smear: a quick, simple method for determining the number of viable aerobic bacteria on open wounds. J Trauma 1976; 16:89.

55. Robson MC. Wound infection. A failure of wound healing caused by an imbalance of bacteria. Surg Clin North Am 1997; 77:637.

56. Bill TJ, Ratliff CR, et al. Quantitative swab culture versus tissue biopsy: a comparison in chronic wounds. Ostomy Wound Manage 2001; 47:34.

57. Bornside GH, Bornside BB. Comparison between moist swab and tissue biopsy methods for quantitation of bacteria in experimental incisional wounds. J Trauma 1979; 19:103.

58. Lookingbill DP, Miller SH, et al. Bacteriology of chronic leg ulcers. Arch Dermatol 1978; 114:1765.

59. Marcus JR, Tyrone JW, et al. Cellular mechanisms for diminished scarring with aging. Plast Reconstr Surg 2000; 105:1591.

60. Cohen BJ, Cutler RG, et al. Accelerated wound repair in old deer mice (*Peromyscus manicularus*) and white-footed mice (*Peromyscus leucopus*). J Gerontol 1987; 42:302.

61. Ashcroft GS, Horan MA, et al. Age-related differences in the temporal and spatial regulation of matrix metalloproteinases (MMPs) in normal skin and acute cutaneous wounds of healthy humans. Cell Tissue Res 1997; 290:581.

62. Ashcroft GS, Mills SJ, et al. Ageing and wound healing. Biogerontology 2002; 3:337.

63. Biolo G, Toigo G, et al. Metabolic response to injury and sepsis: changes in protein metabolism. Nutrition 1997; 13:52S.

64. Russell L. The importance of patients' nutritional status in wound healing. Br J Nurs 2001; 10:S42, S44.

65. Williams JZ, Barbul A. Nutrition and wound healing. Surg Clin North Am 2003; 83:571.

66. Thompson WD, Ravdin IS, et al. Effect of hypoproteinemia on wound disruption. Arch Surg 1938; 36:509.

67. Barbul A, Lazarou SA, et al. Arginine enhances wound healing and lymphocyte immune responses in humans. Surgery 1990; 108:331.

68. Davis PA, Corless DJ, et al. Increased risk of wound complications and poor healing following laparotomy in HIV-seropositive and AIDS patients. Dig Surg 1999; 16:60.

69. Davis PA, Wastell C. A comparison of biomechanical properties of excised mature scars from HIV patients and non-HIV controls. Am J Surg 2000; 180:217.

70. Lord RV. Anorectal surgery in patients infected with human immunodeficiency virus: factors associated with delayed wound healing. Ann Surg 1997; 226:92.

71. Sen CK, Khanna S, et al. Oxygen, oxidants, and antioxidants in wound healing: an emerging paradigm. Ann NY Acad Sci 2002; 957:239.

72. LaVan FB, Hunt TK. Oxygen and wound healing. Clin Plast Surg 1990; 17:463.

73. Drucker W, Pearce F, et al. Subcutaneous tissue oxygen pressure: a reliable index of peripheral perfusion in humans after injury. J Trauma 1996; 40:S116.

74. Howes EL, Plotz CM, et al. Retardation of wound healing by cortisone. Surgery 1950; 28:177.

75. Graf W, Ivarsson M, et al. The influence of early postoperative intraperitoneal chemotherapy on human wound healing. J Surg Res 1994; 57:394.

76. Noh R, Karp GL, et al. The effects of doxorubicin and mitoxantrone on wound healing. Cancer Chemother Pharmacol 1991; 29:141.

77. Dicker AP, Williams TL, et al. Targeting angiogenic processes by combination low-dose paclitaxel and radiation therapy. Am J Clin Oncol 2003; 26:e45.

78. Fife RS, Sledge GW Jr, et al. Effects of tetracyclines on angiogenesis in vitro. Cancer Lett 2000; 153:75.

79. Gilbertson-Beadling S, Powers EA, et al. The tetracycline analogs minocycline and doxycycline inhibit angiogenesis in vitro by a non-metalloproteinase-dependent mechanism. Cancer Chemother Pharmacol 1995; 36:418.

80. Qiu JG, Factor S, et al. Wound healing: captopril, an angiogenesis inhibitor, and Staphylococcus aureus peptidoglycan. J Surg Res 2000; 92:177.

81. Weis M, Heeschen C, et al. Statins have biphasic effects on angiogenesis. Circulation 2002; 105:739.

82. Mall T, Grossenbacher M, et al. Influence of moderately elevated levels of carboxyhemoglobin on the course of acute ischemic heart disease. Respiration 1985; 48:237.

83. Sepkovic DW, Haley NJ, et al. Cigarette smoking as a risk for cardiovascular disease. III: Biochemical effects with higher nicotine yield cigarettes. Addict Behav 1983; 8:59.

84. European Pressure Ulcer Advisory Panel. Pressure Ulcer Treatment Guidelines, 2005.

85. Steed DL. Foundations of good ulcer care. Am J Surg 1998; 176:20S.

86. O'Meara SM, Cullum NA, et al. Systematic review of antimicrobial agents used for chronic wounds. Br J Surg 2001; 88:4.

87. Winter GD. Formation of the scab and the rate of epithelisation of superficial wounds in the skin of the young domestic pig. J Wound Care 1995; 4:366.

88. Hinman CD, Maibach HI. Effect of air exposure and occlusion on experimental human skin wounds. Nature 1963; 200:377.

89. Seaman S. Dressing selection in chronic wound management. J Am Podiatr Med Assoc 2002; 92:24.

90. Choucair M, Phillips T. A review of wound healing and dressing materials. Wounds: A Comp Clin Res Pract 1996; 8:165.

91. Kannon GA, Garrett AB. Moist wound healing with occlusive dressings. A clinical review. Dermatol Surg 1995; 21:583.

92. Zamboni WA, Wong HP, et al. Evaluation of hyperbaric oxygen for diabetic wounds: a prospective study. Undersea Hyperb Med 1997; 24:175.

93. Bouachour G, Cronier P, et al. Hyperbaric oxygen therapy in the management of crush injuries: a randomized double-blind placebo-controlled clinical trial. J Trauma 1996; 41:333.

94. Argenta LC, Morykwas MJ. Vacuum-assisted closure: a new method for wound control and treatment: clinical experience. Ann Plast Surg 1997; 38:563.

95. Fleischmann W, Strecker W, et al. Vacuum sealing as treatment of soft tissue damage in open fractures. Unfallchirurg 1993; 96:488.

96. Blackburn JH, Boemi L, et al. Negative-pressure dressings as a bolster for skin grafts. Ann Plast Surg 1998; 40:453.

97. Mekkes JR, Loots MA, et al. Causes, investigation and treatment of leg ulceration. Br J Dermatol 2003; 148:388.

98. Frykberg RG. Epidemiology of the diabetic foot: ulcerations and amputations. Adv Wound Care 1999; 12:139.

99. Steed DL, Goslen JB, et al. Randomized prospective double-blind trial in healing chronic diabetic foot ulcers. CT-102 activated platelet supernatant, topical versus placebo. Diab Care 1992; 15:1598.

100. Fleming MD, Hunt JL, et al. Marjolin's ulcer: a review and revaluation of a difficult problem. J Burn Care Rehabil 1990; 11:460.

101. Stankard CE, Cruse CW, et al. Chronic pressure ulcer carcinomas. Ann Plast Surg 1993; 30:274.

102. Dovi JV, He LK, et al. Accelerated wound closure in neutrophil-depleted mice. J Leukoc Biol 2003; 73:448.

103. Ashcroft GS, Mills SJ, et al. Role of Smad3 in the hormonal modulation of in vivo wound healing responses. Wound Repair Regen 2003; 11:468.

104. Flanders KC, Major CD, et al. Interference with transforming growth factor-beta/Smad3 signaling results in accelerated healing of wounds in previously irradiated skin. Am J Pathol 2003; 163:2247.

56

Breast: Physiologic Considerations in Normal, Benign, and Neoplastic States

Rakhshanda Layeeque and V. Suzanne Klimberg

INTRODUCTION

The breast is a modified sweat gland that is unique to the mammalian species. It is therefore also called the mammary gland. The breast is a functional part of the reproductive system, which is subject to a variety of neuroendocrine stimuli dictating specific morphology and physiology at various stages of life. An understanding of the interplay of the morphology and physiology of the breast and the many endocrine and paracrine controls is essential to study the pathophysiology and management of benign and neoplastic disorders. In the present chapter, we cover the morphological, endocrine, paracrine, and genetic aspects of the various stages of development, function, and involution of human breast tissue. Using this information, special attention is directed to its clinical application in the diagnosis and management of both benign and malignant conditions.

PHYSIOLOGY OF DEVELOPMENT

The development of the human breast begins in the fifth week of gestation and progresses through 10 stages until birth (1). Further development continues throughout childhood, puberty, adulthood, and pregnancy. Menopause marks the beginning of involution of the breast glandular tissue. All these stages are associated with specific alterations in local and systemic neuroendocrine changes.

Embryology to Childhood

During the fifth week of fetal development, the ectodermal primitive milk streak, called the "galactic band" (Stage 1), appears from the axilla to the groin along the milk line on the embryonic trunk (2). Normally the galactic band regresses except in the region of the thorax where it develops to form the "mammary ridge" (Stage 2). At seven to eight weeks, the mammary ridge thickens further marking the Stage 3 called the "milk hill stage." This is followed by the invagination of the ridge into the thoracic mesenchyme (Stage 4—disc stage) and then rapid growth (Stage 5—globular stage). As the invagination progresses through the 10- to 14-week period, the ridge flattens, marking Stage 6 also known as the "cone stage." Between 12 and 16 weeks of gestation, the mesenchymal cells differentiate to form the smooth muscle of the nipple-areolar complex. During the same time, the epithelial cells form buds (Stage 7—budding stage), which then branch into 15 to 20 strips of epithelium at the end of 16 weeks, marking the branching stage (Stage 8). These strips become the secretory alveoli (3). The secondary mammary anlage then develops followed by differentiation of the hair follicle, sebaceous glands, and sweat glands. Only the sweat glands develop fully at this time, along with the growth of special apocrine glands around the nipple, called the Montgomery glands. The developmental stages described thus far are independent of hormonal influences.

In the third trimester between the 20th and 32nd week of pregnancy, the placental sex hormones enter the fetal circulation and induce canalization of the epithelial strips (Stage 9—canalization stage). During 32 to 40 weeks, the parenchyma differentiates, with development of lobuloalveolar structures containing "colostrum" (Stage 10—endvesicle stage). At this time, the mammary gland mass rapidly increases and the nipple-areolar complex forms with pigmentation. In the neonate, the stimulated mammary tissue secretes colostral milk. This secretion declines over three to four weeks postpartum owing to the withdrawal of placental hormones, causing involution of breast tissue (4).

During childhood, the end vesicles become further canalized and develop into ductal structures, which further grow isometrically with the stroma and the rest of the body until puberty in both sexes (5). The lymphatics grow simultaneously with the ductal system and maintain connection with the subareolar plexus (physiology of drainage and clinical relevance is discussed in the section "Blood flow and Lymphatic drainage"). Abnormalities ranging from inappropriate regression of the galactic band to gross maldevelopment of the pectoral region account for various clinical anomalies.

Puberty to Adulthood

Puberty in girls begins on an average between 10 and 12 years of age and is under the influence of hormones controlled by the hypothalamic-pituitary-ovarian axis (Fig. 1). The development of the breast, as evaluated by external appearance, parenchymal mass, and differentiation is subject to individual variation (6). At the onset of puberty, the rudimentary gland begins to show signs of growth, both in the glandular tissue and stroma. Glandular growth entails multiple divisions of primary and secondary ducts to form club-shaped terminal end buds. Cleavage of terminal end buds gives rise to new branches and alveolar buds. Approximately 11 alveolar buds form a lobular unit called type 1 or virginal lobule (lob 1). This is the predominant lobule found at this point. Through adulthood, the process of sprouting of new alveolar buds continues under the influence of ovarian hormones and some of the lob 1 further divides and differentiates to form lobule 2 (lob 2). These are smaller and more numerous, approximating 47 in

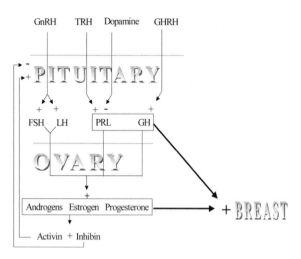

Figure 1 Neuroendocrine control of breast development. *Abbreviations*: GnRH, gonadotropin releasing hormone; TRH, thyrotropin releasing hormone; GHRH, growth hormone releasing hormone; FSH, follicle stimulating hormone; LH, leutinizing hormone; PRL, prolactin; GH, growth hormone.

number, and dominate in late teens, declining after the mid-twenties. Continuous proliferation gives rise to mature ductules or alveoli in lobule 3 (lob 3), containing 80 lobules per unit (7). The distribution of lob 1, 2, and 3 in the breast is dictated by parity, age, and menopause (Fig. 2). Nulliparous women have mostly lob 1, while in parous women lob 3 is most common, decreasing in number after the fourth decade (8). Thereafter lob 3 progressively converts back to lob 1. As the number of pregnancies increase, the number of cycles of lobular differentiation increases and lowers the risk of cancer (discussed in the clinical implications of the section on Menopause).

The Endocrine Control of Development

Numerous hormones and factors secreted by the pituitary, adrenals, thyroid, and ovaries influence the development of the breast (Fig. 1). The ovary, the major determining factor of mammary development, functions under the control of hypothalamic activity (9). During infancy, the secretion of gonadotropin-releasing hormone (GnRH) is centrally inhibited and slowly increases, achieving pulsatile release at puberty (10). The frequency and amplitude of GnRH release controls the synthesis and release of pituitary-luteinizing hormone (LH) and follicle-stimulating hormone (FSH). LH and FSH bind ovarian receptors and trigger the release of androgens during infancy and childhood. During puberty and adulthood the androgen production is mostly replaced by that of estrogen, progesterone, inhibin, and activin (8,9,11). Activin and inhibin are glycoproteins produced by the ovary, which have a feedback control over the pituitary synthesis of FSH and LH, which in turn modulate ovarian steroidal synthesis in conjunction with prolactin (PRL) and growth hormone (GH). This function is also affected by epinephrine from the adrenal medulla (10). GH has positive regulation over ductal development but estrogen and progesterone are essential for normal growth (12,13). Estrogen and progesterone induce proliferation by stimulation of DNA synthesis. Endocrine disturbances of these hormones can therefore be reflected in abnormalities of mammary development.

Changes During Menstrual Cycle

The histology of mammary stroma and epithelium is normally subject to changes dictated by endocrine variations during the menstrual cycle (Fig. 3) (14). The breast passes through five histologic phases during a normal menstrual cycle, viz: early follicular, follicular, luteal, secretory, and menstrual phase. The early follicular phase occurs from day 3 to day 7 in a 28-day cycle. The low level of estrogen at this point is associated with compact alveoli with poorly defined lumina and single cell type embedded in dense stroma. As the level of estrogen rises during the follicular phase (day 8–14), the epithelium exhibits sprouting with increased cellular mitoses and differentiation into three cell types: luminal, basal myoepithelial, and intermediate cells. Ovulation marks the beginning of the luteal phase, when progesterone synthesis reaches maximum and a second estrogen peak occurs. During this phase, the mammary ducts dilate and alveolar epithelial cells differentiate into

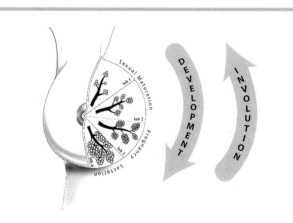

Figure 2 Changes in lobular structure during various phases of mammary development and involution.

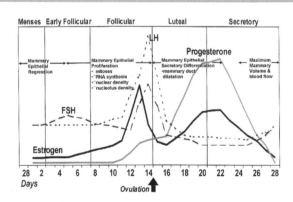

Figure 3 Mammary responses to endocrine changes during menstrual cycle. Mammary epithelial proliferation begins as estrogen level rises and secretory differentiation is caused by rising progesterone level such that maximal breast volume is achieved at the end of secretory phase. A sharp decline in serum concentration of sex steroids causes mammary epithelial regression.

secretory cells. The stromal density decreases markedly to allow for ballooning of alveolar cells as the luminal proteins and glycogen accumulate. Increase in endogenous estrogen also has a histamine-like effect on microcirculation (15), resulting in an increased maximal blood flow three to four days before menstruation. This may in part contribute to premenstrual breast fullness and pain. The maximum number of alveoli and maximum lobule volume occur in the secretory phase (16). There is active protein synthesis and apocrine secretion at this time with peak mitotic activity following the progesterone peak and the second estrogen peak (17,18). The menstrual phase marks the rapid decline in circulating sex steroids, causing diminution of secretory activity by the acinar cells. The regression of epithelium never reaches the premenarche baseline because the new cycle begins and interrupts the process; thus the final regression ensues at menopause (7).

Local Factors and Paracrine Control of Development

In addition to the systemic mammotrophic hormones, normal mammary development entails complex local cell–cell interactions and paracrine influences (19,20). These effects are mediated by a variety of growth factors including epidermal growth factor (EGF), transforming growth factor beta (TGF-β), fibroblast growth factor (FGF), and the wingless type (Wnt) gene families (21–24). TGF-α, a member of the EGF family, may influence ductal growth as well as alveolar differentiation. It has been localized at the actively growing end of the mammary alveolar buds in mice (21). Similarly, FGF-1 and FGF-2 have a role in promoting ductal development during puberty (22). FGF-1 is expressed in the ductal epithelium, while FGF-2 has been localized in the mammary stroma at the onset of ovarian function. These factors contribute to the mesenchymal and epithelial development and may also have a role in neovascularization of the developing gland. Wnt gene family encodes a myriad of glycoproteins, many of which are expressed in the developing mouse mammary gland, suggesting their role in normal development (25,26).

The local growth factors are regulated just like the circulating hormones and act in conjunction with them to control mammary growth and differentiation.

Clinical Implications

Various clinical scenarios can result from abnormalities of intrauterine development, maturation, or pubertal growth.

Congenital Anomalies

The most common abnormality observed in both males and females is an accessory nipple or polythelia (Fig. 4). This results from incomplete regression of the galactic band. Less frequently, accessory breast tissue is also present, called polymastia (Fig. 5), which can function during pregnancy (27). Mutations in the t-box family of transcription factors, normally activated during embryogenesis, can result in hypoplasis (underdevelopment) or amastia (nondevelopment). A wide variety of unilateral or bilateral involvement of these abnormalities may be seen (28), e.g., Poland syndrome, which comprises unilateral hypoplasis of the breast, thorax, and pectoral muscles.

A normal observation, which is often thought to be an abnormality, is when the newborn secretes colostral milk, as a result of maternal hormonal influence (29). Secretion

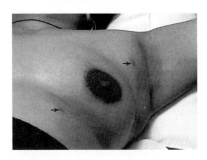

Figure 4 Polythelia. Arrows point to the two accessory nipple-areolar complexes.

declines rapidly within three to four weeks as the endocrine influence is withdrawn and is of no clinical significance.

Anomalous Maturation

The breast development progresses slowly through childhood with a sudden growth spurt in puberty, called thelarche. Premature thelarche is defined as development of the breast before the age of eight without other signs of puberty. Usually bilateral, it occurs within the first few years of life and resolves spontaneously within three to five years, with no adverse sequelae (30). While maternal hormones may initially affect infant breast growth, persistent mammary growth is suggested to result from infantile FSH, LH, and estradiol (31,32). Serum androgen levels (33), free estrogen levels (34), and altered FSH levels (35) have been implicated, as because occurs before the pubertal surge of estrogens.

Breast development under the age of eight, associated with other signs of puberty, is defined as precocious puberty. Abnormality of the hypothalamic-pituitary-ovarian axis, resulting in end-organ hyperfunction, is the main pathophysiology. This may be caused by hypothalamic or pituitary hyperfunction, called central precocious puberty (36), or ectopic excess production of estrogen (37), called peripheral precocious puberty. Investigation and treatment of the underlying pathology is essential to halt the process. This involves a thorough history and physical examination and assessment of serum gonadotropin and sex steroid levels to identify the endocrine defect and its cause so that targeted therapy can be offered.

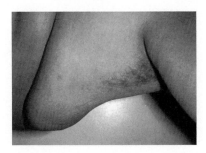

Figure 5 Accessory breast tissue in the anterior axillary fold.

Abnormalities of Pubertal Development

Several normal variants of breast development may occur at puberty, which may be a source of embarrassment but do not carry any significant clinical risk. These include initial unilateral development and asymmetry (Fig. 6) that disappears or becomes less obvious during adulthood (32).

Adolescent, juvenile, or virginal hypertrophy is a postpubertal continuation of epithelial and stromal growth, which results in breasts weighing up to three to eight kilograms. The diagnosis should be limited to severe breast enlargement resulting in physical limitations. The condition is usually bilateral but unilateral presentation is also seen, suggesting the role of local factors. There is an association with ancillary breast tissue in the axilla (38). Drugs like penicillamine have been implicated but hypertrophy does not regress after withdrawal (39). Serum endocrine profile is usually normal; however endocrine manipulation with bromocriptine, tamoxifen, danazol, and medroxyprogesterone has been reported (40,41).

Male gynecomastia presents around 13 to 14 years of age, when pubertal changes have established a male pattern (42). Gynecomastia presents as a small mound of breast tissue directly under the nipple, which represents proliferation of ductal and stromal tissue without evidence of lobuloalveolar differentiation (4). An initial rise in estrogen levels, altered ratios of peripheral and central androgens to estrogens, increased diurnal periods of estrogen excess, and peripheral aromatization of androgens have been implicated (31). Drugs like marijuana and cimetidine may contribute to gynecomastia (43). Altered endocrine profile resulting from gonadal tumors and altered metabolism from liver dysfunction must be ruled out because they require urgent treatment (44,45).

Failure of estrogen production leads to insufficient ductal development. This may result from failure of the ovaries or from lack of stimulation by the hypothalamic-pituitary axis. The most common cause of primary ovarian failure is the Turner syndrome of gonadal dysgenesis and requires early institution of cyclical estrogen therapy to minimize sexual infantilism (46). Intrinsic errors in aromatase activity and steroid biosynthesis may also result in failure of development of female sexual characteristics and virilization (46,47). Hypogonadotropism may result from isolated GnRH insufficiency, space-occupying lesions of the brain, or genetic abnormalities.

Persistent high IGF levels in tall girls have been implicated in their predisposition toward breast cancer, while high adipose-derived estrogen has been hypothesized to cause earlier differentiation of ductal epithelium, thereby protecting obese girls against breast cancer (48).

Blood Flow and Lymphatic Drainage

The blood supply of the breast is derived from internal mammary and lateral thoracic arteries, augmented by perforators from the third, fourth, and fifth intercostal arteries and minor contributions from the vascular network around the scapula. Generally, the blood flow through the breast is similar to the rest of the systemic circulation; however an endocrine-dependent increase in microcirculation is seen with estrogen peaks of menstrual cycle and pregnancy (15).

The lymphatic drainage of the breast follows two main pathways. Most breast tissue drains centripetally into the subareolar plexus and then into the axilla via large lymph trunks to the axilla (49). Embryologically, about 25% of lymphatics arise from the breast lobules, leave the posterior surface of the breast, and pass through the pectoral and intercostal muscles to reach the internal mammary lymph nodes (50). The lymphatic flow through the breast is dictated physiologically by a very fine equilibrium between intra- and extralymphatic pressure (51). This has implications in the metastatic spread of tumor, as well as the clinical utility of sentinel lymph node biopsy techniques.

Clinical Implications

Altered mammary blood flow has significant impact on benign conditions and malignant lesions of the breast. The increase in circulation during the luteal phase of the menstrual cycle has been implicated in causing premenstrual breast tenderness (27).

Angiogenic factors are not only expressed by breast cancer cells, but the plasma levels of these factors have also been correlated with local and metastatic recurrence potential (52). Blood flow through the tumor is directly related to prognosis, suggesting the role of altered vascular physiology in causing metastasis and death (53). Recently, the mammary hypervascularity in the nulliparous woman has been implicated in enhancing her risk toward the development of breast cancer (54).

Lymph node involvement is the single most important prognostic factor in breast cancer. Recently, sentinel lymph node biopsy techniques have been used to exactly stage the lymph nodes in breast cancer. Optimal use of this technique requires precise understanding of the physiology of lymph flow. Slight changes in lymphatic pressures within the breast, caused by the volume or particle size of the material used for sentinel lymph node mapping, can alter equilibrium pressures and compromise identification or cause identification of incorrect nodes (51).

PREGNANCY

Mammary growth and differentiation during pregnancy is directed toward preparation for lactation. During the first three to four weeks of pregnancy, marked ductular sprouting occurs, with some branching and lobular formation (Fig. 2). During the first five to eight weeks of pregnancy, breast enlargement is significant, with dilatation of superficial veins, heaviness, and increasing pigmentation of the nipple-areolar complex. During the second trimester, lobular proliferation and differentiation exceeds ductal sprouting. This results in the formation of the more differentiated lobule 3 (lob 3) and lobule 4 (lob 4) (Fig. 2). Lob 3

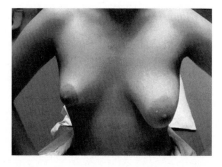

Figure 6   Asymmetry of the breast during pubertal development.

outnumbers the more primitive lob 1 and lob 2 by the end of first trimester, having up to 10 times more alveoli per lobule compared to lob 1 (8). Lob 3 is the dominant structure in all parous women until menopause.

From the second half of pregnancy, the breast enlargement is attributable to progressive dilatation of alveoli differentiating into acini containing colostrum, as well as myoepithelial hypertrophy replacing adipose tissue. Abnormalities of lobuloalveolar differentiation at this stage can cause problems with lactation.

Endocrine Control During Pregnancy

The mammary ductal, lobular, and alveolar growth during pregnancy occurs under the influence of placental sex steroids, human placental lactogen (HPL), PRL, and human chorionic gonadotropin (Fig. 7). These effects can be reproduced in experimental animals when high estrogens and progesterone inhibit the release of PRL-inhibiting factor (PIF), causing a rise in PRL release (55). PRL secretion increases throughout pregnancy and stimulates epithelial growth and secretion (56). Ductular sprouting and branching is mainly under the influence of estrogen while lobular differentiation is under the influence of progesterone (27). HPL, biologically related to PRL, is secreted during the second half of pregnancy and reaches a concentration that is 30 times higher compared to PRL by the end of gestation (57). HPL contributes toward PRL effects of lobuloalveolar differentiation and final maturation of the mammary gland (58).

During pregnancy, PRL primes the breast for lactation; however the initiation of lactogenesis is inhibited by the presence of progesterone. Although estrogen and progesterone are necessary for PRL receptor expression, paradoxically, progesterone reduces the binding and antagonizes the positive effects of PRL at its receptor (59).

Local Factors and Paracrine Control

The EGF family–related neuregulins are expressed in the stroma of the mammary gland during pregnancy (60). Neuregulins have been shown to stimulate alveolar development and secretory activity, suggesting a potential role in mediating PRL activity. In addition, the changing temporal and spatial expression pattern of TGF-α in the breast during pregnancy also suggests that it may function in mediating lobuloalveolar development (61). TGF-α is upregulated in ductal epithelium as well as stromal fibroblasts in pregnancy, signifying its paracrine role in directing hormonal morphogenesis. Mutations in other factors including activins, inhibins, and members of TGF-β family result in an inhibition of alveolar development during pregnancy (62). Recently, a decrease in integrin factor alpha 2 was demonstrated in the luminal epithelium of expanding acini during pregnancy (63).

Clinical Implications

Gravid hypertrophy is the rapid and massive enlargement of the breast during pregnancy. The reason for this hyperresponsiveness to gestational hormones is unknown; however its appearance is a risk factor for recurrence in future pregnancies (41).

Most clinical conditions encountered during pregnancy also exist in nonpregnant patients. Conditions peculiar to pregnancy include lobular hyperplasia and galactoceles (64). An important pathophysiological event during pregnancy is enhanced growth of preexisting lesions, along with generalized mammary development (65). Another lesion peculiar to pregnancy is a breast infarct resulting either spontaneously or from overgrowth of hormone-responsive fibroadenoma (66,67).

Bloodstained nipple discharge during pregnancy is common (Fig. 8). Long-term follow-up of these women revealed neither cancer nor a benign lesion (68). It has been contemplated that rapid ductal proliferation and hypervascularity may be responsible (69). Having said that, bloodstained discharge should be worked up on the same grounds as in nonpregnant women.

PHYSIOLOGY OF LACTATION

While the first half of pregnancy is marked by significant ductal proliferation and lobuloalveolar proliferation giving rise to lob 3, the second half of gestation involves the final maturation of the gland into the secretory organ of lactation mainly comprising lobule 4 (lob 4) structures (Fig. 2). At the beginning of second trimester, the mammary alveoli, but not the ducts, lose the superficial layer of A cells. This monolayer differentiates into the colostrum-cell layer during the third trimester and accumulates eosinophilic cells, plasma cells, and leukocytes around the alveoli.

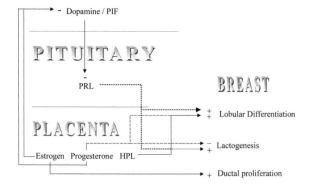

Figure 7 Endocrine control of mammary development and differentiation during pregnancy and lactation. *Abbreviations*: PIF, pituitary inhibitory factor; PRL, prolactin; HPL, human placental lactogen.

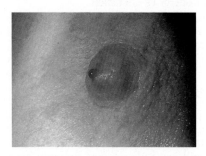

Figure 8 Bloodstained discharge from the nipple during pregnancy. The work-up of this patient did not reveal any pathology.

LACTOGENESIS

The synthesis and secretion of milk products is termed "lactogenesis." Lactogenesis comprises two stages. Stage I is the synthesis of unique milk components. This is accompanied by morphological changes in the alveolar epithelial cell structure, geared toward protein synthesis. Changes include increased DNA and RNA of nuclei, abundant mitochondria and ribosomes, and rough endoplasmic reticulum, along with prominent Golgi apparati. Complex protein, milk fat, and lactose synthetic pathways are activated but with minimal secretion into the alveolar lumen (70,71). Urine lactose concentration, a marker of this synthetic activity, has confirmed that this process begins between 15 and 20 weeks of gestation (72). The alveoli distend with colostrum and along with increased vascularity contribute to the increase in breast volume seen in the later part of gestation. Lob 4 thus formed during pregnancy lasts throughout lactation.

Stage II of lactation is the onset of copious milk secretion during the first four days postpartum (73). This involves a seemingly carefully programmed set of changes in milk composition and volume. Initially, the colostrum provides nutritional elements along with passive immunity. Maternal immunity is transferred to the infant via antibodies, primarily of the immunoglobulin A type, as well as leukocytes including effector and memory T-lymphocytes (74). After a few days of colostrum secretion, transitional milk follows, which has less total protein and less immunoglobulin. The ultimate product is mature milk that comprises fat and protein suspended in a lactose solution secreted in paracrine fashion. Mature milk secretion begins 30 to 40 hours postpartum and averages 1 to 2 mL/g of breast tissue per day (72). The rate of lactation remains constant for the first six months of breast-feeding (75). The stromal lymphatics increase during lactation; interepithelial gaps widen to allow for direct uptake of particles and fluids and improve clearance from the breast (76).

After weaning, the breast involutes and returns to a state resembling that of prepregnancy. The lobules decrease in size with a decrease in the number of alveoli per lobule. The postlactation involution process involves two phases. The first phase is reversible and is associated with accumulation of milk. It is triggered either by the physical distortion of the luminal epithelial cells or by accumulation of apoptosis-inducing factors in the milk (77). The second phase is marked by active tissue remodeling, including destruction of basement membranes and alveolar structure, with irreversible loss of differentiated lactational function of the mammary gland (78).

Endocrine Control of Lactation

PRL is the principal hormone for the synthesis of milk proteins and the maintenance of lactation (5). PRL works via membrane receptors in the mammary epithelial cells. Production of casein, the primary milk protein, ceases in the absence of PRL (58). This hormone is secreted throughout pregnancy and peaks around delivery. However, presence of the PIF and luteal and placental sex steroids, especially progesterone, prohibits PRL from achieving its full lactational effect (Fig. 7). Glucocorticoids work along with PRL to differentiate mammary epithelium and stimulate milk synthesis and secretion. Both glucocorticoids and their receptors are increased in late pregnancy and during lactation. Progesterone binds the glucocorticoid receptor and acts as a glucocorticoid antagonist (71).

After parturition, an immediate withdrawal of placental lactogen and sex steroids occurs. Luteal production of steroid hormones also ceases. At this point, the secretion of PIF decreases from the hypothalamus, causing an increase in the release of PRL from the pituitary. Subsequent physiologic increases in sex steroids, resulting from ovulatory cycles, do not inhibit the effect of PRL. PRL, along with GH, insulin and cortisol, converts the mammary epithelial cells from the presecretory to the secretory state. Other secretogogues identified for PRL include thyrotropin-releasing hormone (TRH) (79), vasoactive intestinal peptide (VIP) (80), and local factors EGF (81) and FGF (82). Oral TRH may improve lactation in partially breast-feeding women (83). Extrapituitary synthesis of PRL occurs in the mammary gland and contributes to the high levels of hormone secreted in the milk. Maturation of the fetal and newborn hypothalamic neuroendocrine system may be modulated by PRL secretion in the amniotic fluid and milk, respectively (84).

Local Factors and Paracrine Control

Cell-to-cell interactions play an important regulatory role in lactational differentiation and milk synthesis. It has been demonstrated that each breast has an independent rate of milk synthesis, suggesting a key role of local and paracrine factors in modulating mammary function. As synthesis of milk products is induced, direct regulatory effects of milk proteins (in addition to PRL) such as lactoferrin and lactoglobulin on local growth factor pathways and epithelial proliferation have been observed (85). Milk proteins are encoded for by the specific consensus sequence in their promoters, called the milk box (86). These genes have specifically programmed expression. Defective expression may lead to altered milk composition (87,88). The transcription factor that activates milk protein synthesis has been termed as "mammary growth factor (Mgf)," which belongs to the signal transducers and activators of transcription family (89). The regulation of the expression of casein gene depends on the balance of activation by Mgf and inhibition by other local proteins (90,91).

Complete mammary differentiation and milk secretion depend not only on proper endocrine stimulation, but also on proper adhesion to the basement membrane through integrins (92) and to each other through occluding cytoskeletal organized tight junctions (93). Moreover, the rate of milk secretion is independent of PRL concentration. Luminal volume may have a rate-limiting effect by altering the interaction between the basement membrane and the lactocyte, causing PRL receptor inhibition (92). A specific compound has now been identified and termed as "feedback inhibitor of lactation (FIL)." FIL has been shown to inhibit lactocyte differentiation, disrupt Golgi vesicle secretions, and inhibit protein synthesis in lactocytes (94).

Involution of the mammary epithelium involves apoptotic cell death. This is a genetically programmed process implemented by genetically directed local factors (95). Disintegration of the tight junctions has been implicated in induction of involution (96). This results from an altered balance between mammary survival factors such as integrins (97) and programmed cell death factors such as proteases (98), which take effect through cell–matrix interaction. The principal enzyme family in the signaling pathway during alveolar epithelial cell death is the aspartate-specific cysteine proteases, called caspases (99). Another important factor in causing programmed cell death is the upregulation of insulin-like growth factor–binding protein

5 (IGFBP-5). This protein vividly binds with the IGF and inactivates it, thereby compromising IGF-mediated cell survival (100,101). The balance between these cell-survival and cell-death factors can be affected by stress and disease states, causing abnormalities of lactation and involution.

BREAST-FEEDING

Upon commencement of breast-feeding, the removal of milk is aided by active ejection. This involves the milk let-down reflex stimulated by the infant suckling (Fig. 9). Sensory nerve endings of T4, T5, and T6 are stimulated by the tactile sensation at the nipple-areolar complex. Impulses pass through the sensory nerves of the dorsal root to the spinal cord. These impulses are then relayed to the hypothalamus via the dorsal, lateral, and ventral spinothalamic tracts. Two separate efferent signals are initiated: the release of PIF is inhibited, which allows the unimpeded secretion of PRL from the anterior pituitary, and simultaneously oxytocin synthesis and release is activated at the paraventricular nucleus in the posterior pituitary. PRL maintains the synthesis of milk. Oxytocin acts on the myoepithelial cells, which contract and eject milk from the alveoli into the lactiferous ducts and sinuses. Milk ejection is uniquely effected by oxytocin, and mammary ductal pressures up to 25 mmHg may be seen with peak blood levels of oxytocin (27). Oxytocin can also be released in response to anticipation of nursing in the presence of a crying infant (58).

An understanding of the mechanisms of lactation helps in the identification and treatment of problems associated with breast-feeding.

Clinical Implications

Physiological changes in the endocrine environment during normal lactation have clinical relevance with contraception and cancer prevention. Breast-feeding suppresses fertility by initial complete inhibition of GnRH and LH release, followed by erratic secretion associated with increased inhibin secretion by the ovary and a prolonged period of anovulatory cycles (102). A decrease in risk of cancer, resulting from breast-feeding is in part attributable to enhanced differentiation of lobular structure (discussed under clinical

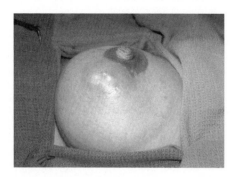

Figure 10   Breast abscess during lactation; notice edema and erythema of the breast with a collection below the nipple.

implications of section on Menopause); molecular events such as increased production of anticarcinogenic molecules during lactation have also been documented (103).

Various clinical scenarios arise as a result of altered endocrine and local physiology during lactation. The onset of lactation can be delayed if the endocrine withdrawal at the end of pregnancy is altered by unscheduled cesarean section or interruption of milk let-down reflex by inadequate suckling stimulus (104). Because progesterone inhibits lactation, high postpartum levels maintained by the retained placenta may inhibit lactogenesis (105). Other causes of compromised lactation include type I diabetes mellitus (106) and maternal stress (107). Rare causes of lactational failure include Sheehan's syndrome, lymphocytic hypophysitis, and isolated or pituitary-related hypoprolactinemia (29).

Galactorrhea is common and is defined as inappropriate secretion of milky fluid in the absence of pregnancy or breast-feeding for more than six months. It is usually bilateral and involves multiple ducts. Amenorrhea is often associated with galactorrhea (108). Endocrine disorders causing hyperprolactinemia or hyperresponsiveness to normal PRL levels also cause galactorrhea (109). Drug-induced hyperprolactinemia can also cause galactorrhea, which usually resolves over time after use of the drug is discontinued (110). Pituitary tumors, hypothalamic lesions (111), adrenal insufficiency (112), Cushing's syndrome (113), acromegaly (114), renal failure (115) and paraneoplastic syndrome (116) may also cause galactorrhea.

Mammary infection is relatively common during lactation. Mastitis is the generalized infection of the breast. Breast abscess may result from a localized collection of purulence, usually occurring in areas of inadequate emptying during nursing (Fig. 10). *Staphylococcus aureus* and streptococci are the most common organisms causing mammary infections, usually entering from the infant's throat through the nipple abrasion (117).

Lactating adenoma is a rare lesion arising during pregnancy and lactation. It presents as a breast mass and excision is often necessary for a definitive diagnosis of this benign lesion and confident exclusion of cancer (118,119).

PHYSIOLOGY OF INVOLUTION

Postlactational involution is accompanied by dramatic apoptosis; however the alveolar structure is largely maintained and the gland reorganizes for another cycle of

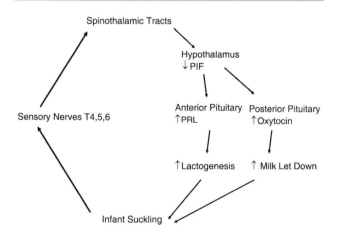

Figure 9   Neuroendocrine reflexes involved in breast-feeding. *Abbreviations*: PIF, pituitary inhibitory factor; PRL, prolactin.

lactation. Definitive involution takes place as the ovarian function declines at menopause.

Menopause

Declining ovarian function through premenopause and menopause leads to regression of epithelial structures and stroma of the mammary gland. Menopause is marked by an increase in lob 1, and a decline in lob 2 and lob 3, such that all women have mostly lob 1 by the end of the fifth decade of life (Fig. 2). Independent of age, nulliparous women have 65% to 80% lob 1, 10% to 35% lob 2, and 0% to 5% lob 3. Lobules in parous women, from postlactational involution to the fourth decade, are 70% to 90% of lob 3. Thereafter, mammary involution starts and after menopause the distribution of lobule structure is the same as in nulliparous women (8). Otherwise, the menopausal regression is the same in both parous and nulliparous women. The climacteric phase from age 45 to 55 has a moderate decrease in glandular epithelium. The postmenopausal phase is characterized by apoptosis of glandular epithelium and replacement of interlobular stroma by fat and intralobular tissue by collagen. Only residual islands of ductal tissue remain scattered throughout the fibrous tissue and fat.

Endocrine Control of Involution

Multihormonal withdrawal is responsible for changes of menopause. The estrogen- and progesterone-induced proliferation and differentiation ceases and programmed cell death ensues.

Local Factors and Paracrine Control

There is little understanding of local influences dictating involution. Tumor suppressor gene p53 has been shown to have a proapoptotic role in secretory mammary epithelium (95). Other local factors involved in cell death have been studied in the setting of postlactational involution, and have been discussed above.

Clinical Implications

One of the most significant clinical entities in the postmenopausal woman is breast cancer. Although cancer may occur in young (1 in 20,000 women at 20 years of age), premenopausal and pregnant women, the incidence rises to one in eight women by the age of 80.

The pattern of lobular differentiation dictates the proliferative index of mammary epithelium, thereby influencing its vulnerability toward cancer. The highest proliferative activity is observed in lob 1 of the breasts of young nulliparous women. Progressive differentiation to lob 2 and lob 3 under hormonal control and full differentiation to lob 4 during lactation results in a significant drop in proliferative activity. Postmenopausal women return to lob 1, and in nulliparous women these lob 1 have a higher proliferative index. Thus, all postmenopausal women are more susceptible to carcinogens, nulliparous women being at greater risk.

CLINICAL APPROACH TO BREAST PATHOLOGY

Clinical evaluation of breast disease is directed toward confident exclusion of cancer at presentation and assignment of the risk of developing one in future. To achieve this, a schematic approach involving a comprehensive relevant history taking, detailed physical examination, and rational work-up of presenting symptoms is necessary.

History Taking

An understanding of physiological and genetic risk factors for breast cancer, discussed previously in this chapter, assist in obtaining a comprehensive history to characterize an individual's risk of breast cancer. Detailed inquiry should include age, parity, and menstrual and nursing histories. The age at menarche and cyclical alterations in breast pain or masses, which occur with menses, are significantly related to benign or malignant disease.

Previous surgical and medical history, particularly of treatments involving alterations in endocrine environment, is very important. These include oophorectomy, hysterectomy, adrenalectomy, and other pelvic surgeries and use of exogenous estrogens, contraceptives, or other steroids. Previous surgeries on the breast and the histopathological diagnosis from any biopsies must be recorded. Malignant or premalignant lesions in the past increase the patient's risk of breast cancer. Social history should focus on ascertaining the amount of caffeine, nicotine, and alcohol intake. These factors are specifically related to mastalgia.

Details of the presenting symptoms such as pain, mass, or nipple discharge should be obtained. The relationship of the presenting symptom to the menstrual cycle is important; hormone-sensitive lesions may be associated with mastodynia with breast fullness and swelling in the immediate premenstrual and postmenstrual periods. Inquiry into growth characteristics of a mass and its association with any possible constitutional symptoms must be made. The spontaneity and nature of nipple discharge and whether or not it is bilateral or multiductal should be ascertained.

In addition to the hereditary factors, the determinants of breast cancer risks may be related to the patient's environment and cultural background that is common to patient's family. This may give rise to aggregations of cancer clusters in families. Thus, a complete family history must be obtained to determine if an individual is at hereditary or familial risk of breast cancer. If a diagnosis of breast cancer is suspected or already known, constitutional symptoms of anorexia, weight loss, skeletal pain, fever, or chest pain must be recorded because they indicate advanced regional and systemic disease.

An insight into a woman's postmenopausal symptoms helps in selecting appropriate therapy for breast cancer and simultaneous management of its side effects.

Physical Examination

Breast examination involves inspection, palpation, and checking for systemic disease. Inspection should be done from the front as well as lateral position to note any asymmetry, changes in skin color, retraction, or ulceration. The examination should be conducted with patient's arms by her side, held behind her head, and on her hips, with contraction of pectoral muscles to enhance the contour and identify any subtle signs.

Inspection

Edema of the skin should be recorded; it may be focal or diffuse and may or may not be associated with erythema. Skin edema results from lymphatic obstruction. Although edema with redness is generally a feature of mastitis or breast abscess, the possibility of inflammatory carcinoma should be borne in mind. Sometimes, the edema produces a skin texture change, with prominent skin pores resembling the skin of an orange, hence the name peau d'orange. Skin dimpling results either from entrapment of Cooper's ligaments or from direct infiltration of dermis by the tumor, and is therefore an ominous sign. Inspection of the entire breast with full abduction of shoulders and while contracting pectoral muscles is necessary to pick up subtle dimpling caused by deeper lesions, especially in large breasts. Some chronic inflammatory conditions may cause skin tethering but carcinoma must be ruled out if this sign exists.

The bilateral symmetry of the nipple-areolar complex should be documented; nipple inversion may result from central tumors infiltrating into the surrounding ducts just before they open to the exterior. Scales and erosion of the nipple may reflect Paget's disease.

The physician must make note of all the surgical scars and their locations. They help in interpreting parenchymal scars on mammograms and planning future incisions if required.

Palpation

The breast is a sensitive organ and the physician must be insightful of this fact lest the palpation be a painful experience and the patient lose confidence in the physician. A systematic gentle palpation of all quadrants and nipple-areolar complex should be carried out with the patient fully relaxed in the supine position with arms extended and shoulders externally rotated. The object of palpation is to detect masses that are separate from the rest of the parenchyma. Once a mass is detected, its shape, consistency, edges, tenderness, and mobility are recorded. Well-circumscribed, painful, mobile, and smooth masses are usually benign; while lesions with indistinct borders, restricted mobility, or fixity to the skin or chest wall should be considered malignant. However, the distinction between benign and malignant lesions is often impossible on the basis of physical examination.

The examination of the breast is incomplete without palpation of the regional lymph nodes in the axilla and the supraclavicular fossa. Examination of the axillae should be done with a patient in sitting position, with the shoulder girdle completely relaxed. Gentle pressure with fingertips demonstrates the enlarged nodes. The size and location of palpable nodes and whether or not they are matted should be recorded. The sensitivity and specificity of clinical examination of the axillary lymph nodes is 70%. The supraclavicular fossa should be palpated with the neck completely relaxed. Pressure effects of large nodes in the neck should be noted.

Systemic Evaluation

A thorough systemic examination is carried out to detect metastatic disease. Cachexia may be obvious from the general health status. Alterations of gait or restricted ambulation may result from metastatic bone disease involving spine and pelvis. Respiratory distress can result from lung involvement from cancer or malignant pleural effusion. Mediastinal lymphadenopathy may manifest as superior vena caval obstruction. These are signs of very advanced disease. However, metastatic disease can exist without obvious manifestations. Spine and ribs should be palpated for tender spots. Lungs should be percussed and auscultated; liver should be palpated and span should be measured; surface and edge should be checked for smoothness if they are palpable. Shifting dullness should be checked to rule out ascites.

Metastatic disease is unlikely to exist in the absence of axillary lymph node involvement.

WORK-UP OF COMMON CLINICAL SYMPTOMS

All patients presenting to the breast clinic should undergo a complete history taking and physical examination emphasizing the specific features outlined above. A thorough history and examination can reasonably narrow the differential diagnoses to a few considerations, and systematic work-up of the pertinent symptoms yields a confident final diagnosis and appropriate treatment. The approach to common clinical scenarios encountered in the office setting is described below.

Mastalgia

Mastalgia is the most common presenting symptom of women attending specialized breast clinics or general practice (120). It is generally believed not to be a symptom of breast cancer; however, about 7% of patients with breast cancer have breast pain as one of their presenting complaints (121). Therefore, a complete physical examination and age-appropriate screening must be carried out for all patients presenting with mastalgia. The responsibility of the physician does not end with a confident exclusion of cancer because mastalgia can be a distressing symptom significantly compromising the patient's quality of life. The severity and association of pain with the menstrual cycle should be ascertained. A daily breast pain chart that employs the visual analogue scale is used at the author's institution for at least two menstrual cycles to characterize the degree of mastalgia into mild to moderate and severe and temporal relation into cyclical and noncyclical. It is important to distinguish between cyclical, noncyclical, and chest wall pain because their response to therapy is different (122). Various nutritional, endocrine, and molecular events have been implicated in the etiology of mastalgia and therefore, no single therapeutic approach has been identified to ameliorate this vexing problem (123). However, a methodical approach toward evaluation and treatment based on the classification of mastalgia suffices for most patients (Fig. 11). History of associated symptoms such as masses or nipple discharge should be documented. Dietary pattern, smoking, and associated pregnancy should be recorded. A detailed physical examination should be performed to exclude masses and focal tenderness of costochondritis

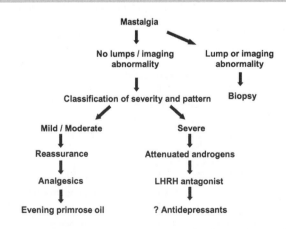

Figure 11 Clinical approach to mastalgia. *Abbreviation*: LHRH, luteinizing hormone–releasing hormone.

and bursistis, which may be mistaken for mastalgia. Most patients respond to counseling and reassurance that they do not have cancer. Dietary modifications emphasizing on decreasing caffeine intake and smoking are helpful. Oral analgesics like nimesulide may be helpful (124). Severe cyclical mastalgia has been associated with abnormal levels of some essential fatty acids (125) and has been shown to respond to gamma-linolenic acid (Evening Primrose Oil) (126). Hormonal manipulation with androgen analogues and luteinizing hormone–releasing hormone antagonists should be reserved for severe and acute cases because of serious side effects. Refractory cases should be evaluated for other pathology. Some patients respond to antidepressant treatment.

LUMP

A breast mass is second only to mastalgia as a presenting symptom to the breast clinic. A lump in the breast is the most anxiety-provoking discovery for the woman. However, not all lumps reported by the patient are confirmed during a surgical evaluation (127). After a thorough history and physical examination, as described above, and age-appropriate imaging evaluation (mammogram over age 40 and ultrasound under age 40), the clinician can reasonably ascertain whether the lump is benign or malignant in nature. However, the false-negative rate of clinical and imaging assessment is too high to settle without a biopsy. Therefore, a core needle biopsy is recommended for all palpable lesions. Further management of the lump is based on the triple assessment, viz. clinical evaluation, imaging criteria (see below) biopsy results (Fig. 12). Lumps smaller than 1 cm in size can safely be subjected to expectant management if the triple test is negative. Larger or suspicious lumps must be excised for confident exclusion of cancer. Once cancer is diagnosed, appropriate oncological staging and treatment should follow.

Nipple Discharge

Nipple discharge accounts for 5% of referrals to the breast clinic (128) and around 7% of all breast surgeries (129). The objective of evaluating nipple discharge in the office setting is to identify surgically significant nipple discharge. To be significant, a discharge should be true, spontaneous, persistent, and nonlactational. It is often uniductal, although significant discharge can involve multiple ducts. When duct excision is carried out for significance derived by these

criteria, about one-fourth of cases have a malignant or premalignant lesion as the etiology (129). The characteristics of the discharge also need to be defined: whether it is milky, multicolored and sticky, purulent, clear (watery), serous (yellow), serosanguinous (pink), or sanguinous (bloody). Hemoccult testing may help to discover occult blood in secreted fluid. Around 10% of patients with bloodstained nipple discharge have a malignant lesion. Another important correlation between malignancy and isolated nipple discharge is the patient's age; in one series of patients undergoing excision for isolated nipple discharge, malignancy was present in 3%, 10%, and 32% in the below 40, 40 to 60, and over 60 age group, respectively (130).

History and physical examination should concentrate on identifying the significant discharge and assessing systemic problems that may cause bilateral multiductal discharge. Bilateral spontaneous milky discharge is galactorrhea, which may result from conditions altering the endocrine profile (pituitary adenoma, chronic hepatic failure paraneoplastic syndromes, etc.) or from certain medications. Breast examination should emphasize identifying the presence of an associated breast mass. Of all cases eventually diagnosed as cancer, only 13% do not have a mass (129). Firm pressure around the areola helps identify the dilated duct by discharge from the nipple upon compression. The location of the discharging duct on the nipple should be carefully recorded. Age-appropriate screening with mammography must be performed and suspicious lesions must be addressed; however, the sensitivity and specificity of mammography are 57% and 62%, respectively (131). Other nonoperative modalities have been investigated to avoid surgery for benign conditions. These include nipple aspirate cytology, ductography, retroareolar sonography, ductoscopy, and magnetic resonance imaging, with variable success rates. The sensitivity of cytology ranges between 11% and 75%, while specificity is between 86% and 96% (131,132). The sensitivity and specificity of ductography range between 0% to 70% and 62% to 90%, respectively (131,132). Ductoscopy identifies 81% of malignancies. The most recent technique used to evaluate nipple discharge is magnetic resonance imaging, which has been shown to correlate with the histopathological diagnosis 73% of the time (133). However, the negative predictive value of none of these investigations is 100%. Therefore, although they may be useful adjuncts in evaluation of nipple discharge, they cannot preclude excisional biopsy for significant discharge. Figure 13 depicts a practical approach for working up patients presenting at the clinic with nipple discharge.

Breast Imaging

Two imaging techniques are commonly used to evaluate potential breast pathology: mammography and ultrasonography. Of the two, mammography is more commonly employed. It can be used as a screening technique in women at risk for breast cancer but in whom no physical abnormalities are palpated, or to help establish a diagnosis in women who present with a palpable mass or other breast abnormality. The standard approach is to use film screen mammography, which is performed in a fashion similar to other X rays, with black and white radiographs being produced, which are viewed on a light box. Xeroradiography takes an electrostatic image of the breast and converts it to a blue on white photocopy image for viewing. The standard film screen imaging uses a slightly less radiation dose than xeroradiography and has proved to be just as effective in diagnosing breast

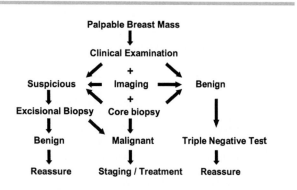

Figure 12   Clinical work-up of a breast mass.

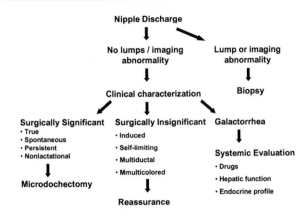

Figure 13 Clinical approach to nipple discharge.

cancer. Because of the high-quality radiologic images that are now available with modern film screen mammography, this technique has largely replaced xeromammography.

Mammography is very sensitive in detecting breast pathology. Although some concern was previously expressed about radiation exposure when used repeatedly as a screening technique, careful evaluation of this concern has proved that it is not an issue in women of screening age. Thus, current recommendations are that all women 50 years of age or older undergo mammography once yearly regardless of whether the physical examination is negative. Women in high-risk groups (e.g., mother had breast cancer) should be screened at least every other year, starting at age 40, and annually when they reach age 50. Mammographic findings suggestive of malignancy include masses, architectural distortions, asymmetric densities, and microcalifications (Fig. 14).

Despite the high sensitivity of mammography in detecting abnormalities, its specificity is considerably less. Only about 25% of lesions that cannot be palpated on physical examination turn out to be cancer. Previously, a suspicious lesion resulted in a woman being subjected to open surgical biopsy utilizing needle location to make a definitive diagnosis. With modern stereotactic techniques, these lesions can now be biopsied percutaneously using specialized computer and X-ray equipment to guide the biopsy needle to a mammagraphically suspicious lesion. Because multiple biopsies of the lesion in question can be obtained using this technology, the presence or absence of malignancy can be ascertained with a high degree of accuracy (greater than 95%), obviating the need for open biopsy.

Ultrasonography uses acoustic waves to image the breast. For cancer screening, it is totally ineffective. However, it can be quite useful for distinguishing between cystic and solid lesions. For example, in a woman with a palpable mass on physical examination or a nonpalpable mass on mammographic evaluation, which appears benign, ultrasound evaluation can help confirm its cystic or solid nature. If it proves to be cystic, biopsy to rule out malignancy is usually not needed.

TREATMENT OF BENIGN BREAST PATHOLOGY

Benign breast diseases incorporate a wide spectrum of conditions presenting with or without acute symptom. Broadly,

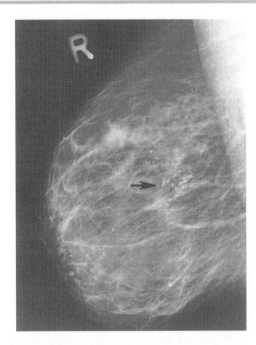

Figure 14 Typical appearance of microcalcifications in breast carcinoma. These calcifications (*arrow*) are irregular in size and shape and occur in small clusters or in linear configurations.

three main categories of benign problems are clinically encountered, viz. inflammatory conditions, aberrations of normal development, and proliferative lesions. The latter category is further stratified into high or low risk according to the risk they incur toward development of cancer in the future. The following is an account of clinical approach toward the management of these conditions.

Inflammatory Conditions

Acute mastitis and breast abscess most commonly affect women between the ages of 15 and 50. The condition can occur in lactational or nonlactational setting. Staphylococci or streptococci are the most common organisms responsible for infection, and gain entry through disruption of the nipple-areolar complex. Diffuse inflammatory response throughout the breast constitutes "mastitis," whereas a localized collection of pus, most commonly in the subareolar region, represents an "abscess."

Mastitis is treated with appropriate antibiotics, e.g., penicillin derivatives, and with supportive therapy like antipyretics and analgesics. Focal heat compresses may benefit the local pain. Abscess requires urgent surgical drainage. Thorough debridement through a circumareolar incision (or multiple incisions) should be done keeping dependent drainage in mind. All loculi of pus must be broken to ensure hygienic drainage. Open drainage system is sometimes necessary to ensure continuous adequate drainage from the entire cavity.

The chronic inflammatory conditions with abscess formation are less common. The differential diagnosis includes chronic infection and malignancy. Tuberculosis is the most common cause of chronic mastitis (134). Tuberculosis may clinically and mammographically resemble malignancy. Biopsy of the breast mass is useful to diagnose the condition, because the yield of acid-fast bacilli culture is very low. A combination of antituberculous drugs is essential to treat mammary tuberculosis. Granulomatous lobular mastitis is associated with noncaseating granulomata confined to the breast lobule that some times responds to treatment with steroids (135).

Aberrations of Normal Development

Nonproliferative lesions of the breast present with various clinical and imaging abnormalities. These include cysts, apocrine changes, fibrocystic changes, mild hyperplasias, and other epithelium-related calcifications (136). On most occasions, the biopsy is done to exclude malignancy, and no further management is required (137). Occasionally, breast cysts can be symptomatic with a lump, pain, and infection requiring aspiration excision and antibiotic treatments. A cyst presenting with rapid refilling after repeated aspirations must be excised to exclude intracystic cancer (138).

Fibrocystic disease refers to a condition in which the breast undergoes a variety of fibrocystic changes characterized by micro or macro cyst formation, fibrous alterations, metaplasia of apocrine glands and ductal or lobular hyperplasia. Clinically, the breasts are often lumpy on palpation and the range symptomatically from intermittent dull achiness to marked pain and tenderness. Severe cystic disease giving rise to tender mastopathy may respond to hormonal manipulation with estrogen modulators or testosterone derivatives (139). However, no hormonal correlation between fibrocystic changes and breast pain has been conclusively identified.

Proliferative Lesions

Proliferative lesions of the breast require careful clinical and pathological evaluation to ascertain their association with atypia. This discrimination is important because women with proliferative lesions without atypia have a slightly higher risk of developing cancer (1.5–2 times), while those with atypia have a substantially higher risk (3.5–5 times) toward malignancy compared with the general population (140). Proliferative lesions without atypia include moderate florid hyperplasia of the usual type: intraductal papilloma, sclerosing adenosis, and fibroadenoma. Most of these lesions are incidental microscopic findings. Fibroadenomas and occasionally sclerosing adenosis may present as palpable lumps. Fibroadenomas, especially, may reach sizes of 1 to 2 cm and on palpation appear smooth and rubbery. Once the pathological evaluation of an imaging or palpable abnormality concordantly establishes the diagnosis of one of these lesions, no further treatment is usually necessary. Large fibroadenomas are occasionally removed for cosmesis.

On the contrary, lesions with atypia (atypical ductal hyperplasia or atypical lobular hyperplasia) need to be completely excised if the diagnosis is based on core needle biopsy because up to 30% of lesions are histologically upgraded to malignant lesions upon complete excision (141). Other proliferative lesions that require complete excision to exclude associated malignancy include radial scars, lobular carcinoma in situ (a neoplastic lesion that is generally considered to be benign), and papillomatosis. Once the diagnosis of cancer is excluded after complete excision, the risk toward subsequent malignancy must be discussed with the patient, including information regarding risk modification (142) and chemoprevention (143).

TREATMENT OF MALIGNANT BREAST PATHOLOGY

Historically, two opposing views concerning the natural history of breast cancer have been put forth (144). Some physicians postulate that it is a systemic disease at inception and surgery has little impact on the risk of death from cancer. Others argue that it is often localized at the time of diagnosis and that timely extirpation of the tumor reduces the risk of death. Randomized controlled trials indicate that screening, adjuvant systemic therapy, and adjuvant radiotherapy can reduce the risk of mortality from breast cancer. The best outcome of treatment for breast cancer can be achieved by careful planning of the workup and therapy at the time when the diagnosis is suspected. The following is an account of the staging system, surgical principles, and the principles of adjuvant therapy that should be employed to plan a rational treatment.

Surgical Principles

A century ago, Halsted published his first report on radical mastectomy for breast cancer (145). At that time, this procedure was truly an appropriate solution to the problem. The typical presentation of breast cancer then was what would qualify as locally advanced disease today. Moreover, the systemic treatment available today was nonexistent. A later report showed that this extensive surgery did improve local recurrence rates, making Halsted mastectomy the standard of treatment at that time. The procedure performed by Halstead was known as a radical mastectomy, which involved total removal of the breast with its underlying pectoralis muscles and the associated axillary lymph nodes. Fisher's work in the 1950s concentrated on lymphatic-venous channel communications in the drainage of the breast (146). This led to the belief that cancer may already be a systemic disease by the time a clinical diagnosis is established. This conclusion led to clinical trials on adjuvant treatment.

As adjuvant systemic treatment developed, the real value of the extent of surgery for local treatment was again questioned. Individual reports of breast-conserving surgery (BCS) appeared in the 1950s and 1960s (147,148). Subsequently, six randomized prospective controlled trials were undertaken (Table 1) (149–154). The largest of the BCS trials was recently updated with a 20-year follow-up (155). The results continue to show the equivalence of BCS followed by radiotherapy with that of mastectomy. This trial required microscopically negative margins; however many ipsilateral recurrences occurred several years after treatment, which may represent residual tumor foci not detected at the time of original surgery. The real importance of these findings is that BCS is feasible in many patients and all attempts should be made to obtain negative margins. Positive margins do not necessarily mean that mastectomy is indicated and patients can have another procedure to revise the surgical margin if possible without grossly compromising the cosmetic outcome.

Some tumors are still more suitable for mastectomy than BCS. There is a cutoff tumor size limit to dictate mastectomy. The breast size and the tumor size should be kept in mind when judging if adequate margins can be obtained while maintaining the cosmetic outcome. Extensive multiple cancers of the breast are best treated with mastectomy. Locally advanced tumors can be subjected to preoperative systemic chemotherapy to achieve BCS (156). Patients who do not respond to preoperative chemotherapy or in whom radiation therapy is contraindicated are suitable candidates

Table 1   Clinical Trials of Mastectomy vs. Breast-Conserving Therapy

| Study | No. of cases | Treatment | Margins | 10 year survival (%) | |
				Mastectomy	BCS
NSABP B-06	1845	MRM vs. BCS + DXRT	Negative	82 (LN+), 66 (LN−)	92, 75
Milan	701	RM vs. BCS	2–3 cm	83	85
NCI	237	TM vs. BCS	–	85	89
EORTC	903	MRM vs. BCS+DXRT	1 cm	73	79
IGR	180	MRM vs. BCS+DXRT	2 cm	91	95
Danish	1153	MRM vs. BCS+DXRT	Negative	82	79

Abbreviations: NSABP, National Surgical Adjuvant Breast and Bowel Project; NCI, National Cancer Institute; EORTC, European Organization for Research and Treatment in Cancer; IGR, Institut Gustave-Roussy; MRM, modified radical mastectomy; BCS, breast-conserving surgery; DXRT, radiotherapy; RM, radical mastectomy; TM, total mastectomy.

for mastectomy. In summary, most early breast cancers should be considered for BCS. If margins are extensively involved, especially after surgical revision, mastectomy may have to become the appropriate option. If margins are only focally positive, a second revision may provide adequate local control. If mastectomy is deemed to be the best management option, it is far less radical than in the days of Halstead. It often involves removing the breast and sparing the pectoralis muscles or at worst removing the pectoralis minor muscle but sparing the pectoralis major. The degree of axillary node dissection is also less radical.

Preoperative Biopsy

Regardless of whether the patient presents with a palpable lump or an imaging abnormality on mammography or ultrasound, such as microcalcifications or a density, it is always desirable to obtain a preoperative pathological diagnosis to plan the surgical approach. This can be achieved on an out-patient setting with a core biopsy guided by ultrasound (preferable if the lesion is sonographically visible) or stereotaxis (if the lesion is only visible on mammogram) (157). If a preoperative diagnosis is not possible for technical or logistic reason, excision of the lesion is indicated as if it was a carcinoma. The excision is guided by clinical examination (for palpable lesions), ultrasound (for sonographically visible lesions) (158), or radiological needle localization (for lesions visible only on mammogram) (159). In any event, incision should be placed directly over the lesion (discussed under the section "incision") and the specimen should be appropriately oriented (discussed under the section "specimen orientation"). Excision should ensure a wide margin of normal tissue around the lesion so that chances of reoperation for margin clearance are minimized in the event that it is a cancer.

Incision

The incision should be placed directly over the tumor mass. Circumareolar incisions to preserve cosmetic outcome should not be used unless the tumor lies directly beneath the areola. Although it is a cosmetically desirable incision, any need to tunnel toward the mass exposes healthy tissue to tumor seeding, increases the risk of incomplete removal of a known carcinoma, and makes revision of margins extremely difficult. The use of curvilinear versus radial incisions is debatable. In the National Surgical Breast and Bowel Project (NSABP) workshop report, radial incisions were advised for the lower-half lesions and curvilinear incisions were suggested for the upper-half tumors. We believe that a radial incision is cosmetically superior and provides an excellent approach toward cancer resection with adequate margins because tumor grows centripetally along the ducts.

Flaps

The subcutaneous tissue contains a network of blood vessels that nourish the skin. If this layer is removed by creating flaps that are too thin, a broad flat scar results, collapsing inwards and creating a saucer-like defect. If the tumor is close to the skin, it is preferable to excise a wider ellipse of skin together with underlying tissue down to the tumor rather than create thin flaps. This approach provides an excellent anterior resection margin as well as a cosmetically superior result.

Specimen Orientation

Correct orientation of the specimen for the pathologist is the key element in breast surgery for cancer. It is important not only for resection of known malignant lesions for proper margin evaluation, but also for diagnostic excisions lest they turn out to be cancer on final pathology. Every institution should have a standard method of orientation well known to surgeons as well as the pathologists; at least three anatomical directions should be marked for complete orientation. At the author's institution, the superior aspect of the specimen is always marked with a short silk stitch while the lateral aspect is marked with a long silk stitch; the posterior margin is inked. Such marking allows precise evaluation of reporting on the margins so that any positive margins can be accurately reresected.

Hormone Receptor Analysis

In addition to a thorough microscopic analysis of breast cancer, measurement of steroid hormone receptors on a portion of the tumor should also be performed. Current immunochemical techniques are highly accurate and can assess both the proportion of tumor cells staining positively for the receptors, and the intensity of this staining. Although estrogen and progesterone receptors are routinely evaluated, estrogen activity seems to correlate best with outcome. The higher the measured value of ER activity, the better patient outcome. The reason for this is incompletely understood, but women in this group usually have malignancies that are more differentiated, exhibiting both nuclear and histologic grades that are more compatible with long-term survival.

A further reason for knowing a patient's ER activity relates to the potential benefit that could accrue from using tamoxifen as adjuvant therapy. Tamoxifen is an "antiestrogen" drug and has been shown to prolong the disease-free interval in postmenopausal ER-positive women with histologically positive nodes, as well as in premenopausal and postmenopausal ER-positive women with negative nodes. Although tamoxifen is associated with an increased risk of developing uterine cancer, this risk overall appears to be quite low. Despite this risk, tamoxifen is clearly less toxic than standard chemotherapy so that it has become the treatment of choice for postmenopausal women with node-positive, ER-positive tumors (see below). Further, in women receiving tamoxifen as adjuvant therapy for breast cancer, a reduction in the incidence of a second-primary breast cancer in the contralateral breast has been noted.

Staging

Staging refers to the grouping of patients according to the extent of their disease, so that appropriate treatment recommendations can be made and adequate estimates of prognosis can be provided. In addition, the staging system provides a framework for reporting treatment outcomes and thereby permits the efficacy of new treatments to be assessed. The most widely used staging system for breast cancer is the TNM (tumor, nodes, and metastasis) classification provided by the American Joint Committee on Cancer (AJCC). Changes in the staging system are periodically required to incorporate new diagnostic and therapeutic advances that affect risks of disease recurrence and patient survival. The new criteria for breast cancer TNM staging have been implemented by AJCC since January 2003 (Table 2) (160).

The exact tumor size is obtained from the pathological measurement of tumor in the excised specimen. Caution must be exercised to include the tissue resected during core needle biopsy; sometimes the entire lesion is excised during preoperative biopsy and no residual tumor is identified in the lumpectomy specimen, in which case the tumor size should be measured from the biopsy specimen.

The most important prognostic factor and staging criteria is the lymph node status (161). Clinical examination of the axilla is notoriously inaccurate for lymph node staging. Approximately 30% of patients with palpable lymph nodes prove to be node negative following axillary dissection, and about 30% of clinically node-negative patients have nodal involvement (162). Axillary lymph node dissection has been the standard method of evaluating the lymph node status in breast cancer patients for many years. However, more than half of the patients treated today for breast cancer have node-negative disease, and the axillary lymph node dissection procedure has significant complications (163).

The current standard approach to assess the lymph node status is changing from complete axillary lymph node dissection to sentinel lymph node biopsy (164). The sentinel lymph node is the first lymph node to receive lymphatic drainage from a tumor. This provides more accurate evaluation of one or several target nodes rather than the entire axillary tissue specimen. The technique of performing sentinel lymph node biopsy has been evolving. Blue dye and/or radiocolloid is injected at a target site (varies with institution and preference) and allowed to drain to the sentinel node, which is then identified visibly (blue dye), by gamma probe (radioisotope), or both and then excised. The consensus statement made by experts in this field reports best results with the use of both radioisotope and the blue dye to identify the sentinel nodes (165). At the author's institution, subareolar injection of both radioisotope and blue dye is performed for sentinel lymph node biopsy (166). Theoretically, sentinel node–negative patients should not require complete axillary dissection. However, the overall long-term

Table 2 AJCC Staging System for Breast Cancer—2003

Primary tumor (T)

TX	Primary tumor cannot be assessed
T0	No evidence of primary tumor
Tis	Carcinoma in situ (ductal or lobular), or Paget's disease without evidence of tumor
T1	Tumor less than 2 cm in greatest dimension
T2	Tumor greater than 2 cm but less than 5 cm in greatest dimension
T3	Tumor greater than 5 cm in greatest dimension
T4a	Tumor of any size with extension into chest wall
T4b	Tumor of any size with extension into skin, or setallite skin nodule or peau d' orange
T4c	T4a and b
T4d	Inflammatory carcinoma

Regional lymph nodes (N)

NX	Regional lymph nodes cannot be assessed
N0	No lymph node metastasis
N1	Metastasis in 1–3 nodes-axillary and/or internal mammary by sentinel node biopsy (not clinically)
N1mi	Micrometastasis (greater than 0.2 mm, less than 2.0 mm)
N2	Metastasis in 4–9 axillary nodes, or clinically + internal mammary nodes without axillary nodes
N3	Metastasis in more than 10 axillary nodes, or inftaclavicular nodes, or clinically + internal mammary nodes with + axillary nodes, or ipsilateral supraclavicular nodes

Distant metastasis (M)

M0	No detectable distant disease
M1	Distant disease detectable clinically or by imaging including contralateral axillary nodes

Stage groupings

Stage 0	TisN0M0
Stage I	T1N0M0
Stage IIa	T0N1M0, T1N1M0, T2N0M0
Stage IIb	T2N1M0, T3N0M0
Satge IIIa	T0N2M0, T1N2M0, T2N2M0, T3N1M0, T3N2M0
Srage IIIb	T4, N0M0, T4N1M0, T4N2M0
Satge IIIc	Any T N3
Stage IV	Any T Any N M1

Abbreviation: AJCC, American Joint Committee on Cancer.

effects on survival, local recurrence, and morbidity of omitting axillary clearance have not been fully elucidated. The NSABP-32 trial, which was initiated in October of 1998 has randomized patients with negative sentinel nodes to no further axillary treatment or follow-up axillary dissection (167). The results of this trial will answer the above-mentioned questions and delineate whether sentinel node biopsy should become the national standard of care.

Adjuvant Systemic Therapy

The conceptual approach toward the treatment of breast cancer has changed from the late 1800s to the present time. The earlier Halstedian concept emphasized that breast cancer slowly grows locally and spreads via lymphatics and subcutaneous facial planes; hence the extensive local en bloc removal of all these tissues should affect cure. Only 12% of patients treated by Halstead survived 10 years and attempts to perform even more radical resections failed to improve the outcome, leading to the belief that it is a systemic disease from the outset. Efforts were then directed toward identifying systemic treatment that could target the nonmanifest systemic disease left behind after local resection of tumor. The type of treatment administered after surgery has always been guided by the experience accumulated from treating patients with metastases. In 1896, Beatson reported on two premenopausal women with metastatic breast cancer, who improved after oophorectomy (168). This approach became a common therapy for women with metastatic breast cancer, and trials involving oophorectomy or radiation-based ovarian ablation were started (169). In the 1950s, chemotherapy was incorporated in the postoperative treatment of breast cancer patients (170). The first randomized clinical trials of adjuvant therapy were performed in the 1970s in North America and Europe. A series of trials showed that adjuvant chemotherapy increased disease-free survival and overall survival rates (171), that polychemotherapy was better than single-agent therapy (172), that adjuvant tamoxifen improved overall survival rates in postmenopausal women (173), and that ovarian ablation prolonged disease-free survival in premenopausal women (174).

At present, the role of adjuvant systemic treatment is well established for early-stage breast cancer, but the benefits in disease-free survival and overall survival are of small magnitude. The Early Breast Cancer Trialists Collaborative Group (EBCTCG) conducted a series of overviews focusing on randomized clinical trials to detect these small benefits. The first EBCTCG meta-analysis was based on pooled raw data from 75,000 women who participated in 133 clinical trials conducted worldwide between 1957 and 1985 (175). This review showed that at 10-year follow-up, adjuvant chemotherapy reduced the risk of recurrence by 22% to 37% and the risk of death by 14% to 27%, depending on age. An update of the EBCTCG overview concluded that anthracycline-based chemotherapy regimens are superior to the regimens that do not contain anthracycline (176). Ovarian ablation resulted in improved survival rates among premenopausal women, with a risk reduction similar to that of adjuvant chemotherapy (177). Five years of tamoxifen therapy reduced the risk of recurrence and death in ER-positive women regardless of age (178). It is however important to understand that all these benefits are reported in terms of relative risks and may actually incur very small benefit in patients with low risk of recurrence and death. The single most important predictor of risk of recurrence and death is the status of lymph nodes; in lymph node–negative patients, the tumor size and grade and receptor expression status are important in dictating recurrence and death. All these factors and other comorbid conditions should be kept in mind to compute a given patients risk of recurrence and death so that the absolute benefit of adjuvant treatment can be presented to the patient. Patients with low risk of recurrence and death from tumor or high risk of death from other illnesses may not be good candidates for adjuvant treatment. Web-based computer softwares (e.g., adjuvantonline.com) have been developed to assist in the computation of a given patient's risk of tumor recurrence and death and the potential benefit from hormonal or chemotherapy.

Aromatase inhibitors (agents that block the conversion of androgens to estrogens) are an effective second-line hormonal therapy for patients with breast cancer. They have been used in the treatment of metastatic disease for a long time and are now rapidly moving into the adjuvant setting. Results of a multi-institutional and multinational study of anastrazole versus tamoxifen, alone and in combination (ATAC Trial), have recently been published (179). The combination arm was stopped because of significant side effects. The hazard ratio for recurrence at four years was 0.86 in favor of anastrazole. Anastrazole was also found to have a superior therapeutic index except for musculoskeletal disorders, which had a relative risk of 1.5 in the anastrazole arm.

The other area of significant advancement is the findings of molecular biology on breast cancer pathogenesis, which have reached therapeutic application on several fronts. The most studied molecule is the human EGF 2 (HER-2), which is an overexpressed gene in 25% to 30% of invasive cancers and associated with a worse prognosis (180). Trastuzumab is a humanized monoclonal antibody that binds to HER-2 with great affinity, resulting in growth arrest of HER-2 overexpressing cancer cells. It has been shown to be effective in the metastatic setting (181), but trials studying its role in the adjuvant setting are underway.

As the advances in adjuvant treatment are being made, the armamentarium of therapeutic options is likely to increase. The physician must present all the risk and benefits to the patients and involve them in the decision-making process regarding adjuvant treatment. The quality of life for patients undergoing adjuvant treatment is not well defined (182), and prospective studies are clearly needed.

Adjuvant Local Therapy

In the last 20 years, BCS for cancer has become more acceptable and is commonly coupled with radiation therapy for local control of disease. After the results of six randomized trials from the United States and Europe (Table 1), radiation therapy to the breast has become an integral part of early breast cancer treatment. These trials reported that the rates of local and regional recurrences, distant metastasis, and overall survival were not significantly different between mastectomy and breast conservation coupled with radiation. Moreover, in an updated meta-analysis of data, Morris et al. found that the pooled odds ratio for overall survival at 10 years favored BCS and radiation therapy over mastectomy (183).

Whether radiation therapy is required for every patient after BCS for invasive cancer is still unresolved. In a phase II single-arm trial, the Joint Center of Radiation Therapy selected patients with favorable prognosis to follow-up after breast conservation without radiation (184). The inclusion criteria included tumor size less than 2 cm, histologically negative nodes, no extensive intraductal component, no lymphovascular invasion, and pathologically 1 cm negative margins. The trial was closed prematurely because of a 16% local recurrence at a median follow-up of 56 months. Several randomized trials compared BCS alone versus adjuvant radiation therapy; the rate of local failure in the radiation therapy group was reduced by an average of 85% (Table 1). Despite these findings, the use of partial mastectomy and tamoxifen without breast irradiation might be appropriate in a select group of patients, particularly those older than 70 years of age with small ER positive tumors excised with wide margins. In a retrospective study of 122 patients treated with partial mastectomy and systemic therapy without breast irradiation therapy, Nemoto et al. showed that overall local failure rate was 19% (185). The rate of recurrence correlated with the size of the tumor and age of the patient; lowest failure rate being in women older than 70, having tumors of size less than 1 cm.

The goal of adjuvant radiation therapy after mastectomy is the sterilization of subclinical disease in the chest wall. Many studies showed that the rate of local failure is reduced when mastectomy is coupled with adjuvant radiation; however deaths related to cardiopulmonary causes in the radiation arm make adjuvant radiation of chest wall unfeasible for all patients with mastectomy. Fowble et al.

analyzed 627 patients enrolled in an Eastern Cooperative Oncology Group adjuvant chemotherapy study, in which radiation therapy was not used, to identify patients who would benefit from adjuvant radiation after mastectomy (186). In patients with four to seven positive lymph nodes, the isolated local failure rate was 10% and 31% for tumors less than and greater than 5 cm in size, respectively. Other unfavorable prognostic indicators for local recurrence included negative ER status, pectoral fascia involvement, and tumor necrosis. Two trials [British Columbia (187) and Danish Breast Cancer (188)] have shown a significant increase in disease-free and overall survival after chest wall radiation following mastectomy in patients with lymph node–positive disease and large tumors. Therefore, the indications for post-mastectomy radiation therapy to the chest wall include the presence of four or more positive lymph nodes, extracapsular extension, and tumor stage of T3 or more.

Techniques of radiation therapy have improved over time and late cardiac deaths are much less common now. Newer advances are being made in the area of partial breast irradiation by concentrating on primary tumor site with an objective to minimize complications and affect local control. These techniques are still in trial phases and should not be used outside of study setting.

SUMMARY

The breast is a functional part of the reproductive system and as such is subject to a variety of specific morphologic and physiologic changes at various stages of life, which are under neuroendocrine control. Understanding these variations is essential if appropriate treatment of its multifarious disorders is to be effectively administered, and the natural history of benign and malignant diseases adequately conceptualized. Although most diseases of the breast are benign and can be effectively managed with relatively simple supportive measures and reassurance, the fear of malignancy is the driving force that brings the majority of patients to a physician. Fortunately, our understanding of breast cancer has evolved considerably from the days of Halstead so that its systemic nature is now universally accepted. Thus, the radical, mutilative procedures that were previously performed, based on the assumption that breast cancer was primarily a local disease, have been replaced with breast-sparing procedures with equally good outcomes. In fact, as our knowledge of the biology of breast cancer has increased, breast conservation surgery in conjunction with adjuvant treatment when needed has enabled most patients with this disease to enjoy long-term survival. As the genetics underlying breast cancer development becomes better clarified, it is envisioned that even more precise treatment will be possible by specific gene manipulation.

REFERENCES

1. Russo J, Hu YF, Silva ID, et al. Cancer risk related to mammary gland structure and development. Microsc Res Tech 2001; 52:204–223.
2. Hamilton NJ, Boyd JD, Mossman HW. Human Embryology. Cambridge, U.K.: Heffer, 1968:428–432.
3. Hughs ESR. Development of mammary gland. Ann R Coll Surg Eng 1950; 6:99–105.
4. Howard BA, Gusterson BA. Human breast development. J Mammary Gland Biol Neoplasia 2000; 5:119–137.
5. Horseman ND. Prolactin and mammary gland development. J Mammary Gland Biol Neoplasia 1999; 4:79–88.
6. Russo J, Russo IH. Development of the human breast. In: Encyclopedia of Reproduction. New York: Academic, 1998; 3:71–97.
7. Russo J, Russo IH. Development of human mammary gland. In: Neville M, Daniel CW, eds. The Mammary Gland. New York: Plenum Press, 1987:67–79.
8. Russo J, Rivera R, Russo IH. Influence of age and parity on the development of the human breast. Breast Cancer Res Treat 1992; 23:211–218.
9. Russo IH, Russo J. Role of hormones in cancer initiation and progression. J Mammary Gland Biol Neoplasia 1998; 3:49–61.
10. Yen SSC. Clinical endocrinology of reproduction. In: Baulieu E-E, Kelly PA, eds. Hormones: From Molecules to Disease. New York: Chapman and Hall, 1990:445–459.
11. Tong S, Wallace EM, Burger HG. Inhibins and activins: clinical advances in reproductive medicine. Clin Endocrinol (Oxf) 2003; 58:115–127.
12. Brisken C, Park S, Vass T, et al. A paracrine role for the epithelial progesterone receptor in mammary gland development. Proc Natl Acad Sci USA 1998; 95:5076–5081.
13. Zeps N, Bentel JM, Papadimitriou JM, et al. Estrogen receptor-negative epithelial cells in mouse mammary gland development and growth. Differentiation 1998; 62:22–26.
14. Vogel PM, Georgiade NG, Fetter Bf, et al. The correlation of histologic changes in the human breast with the menstrual cycle. Am J Pathol 1981; 104:23–34.
15. Zeppa R. Vascular response of the breast to estrogen. J Clin Endocrinol Metab 1969; 29(5):695–700.
16. Hussain Z, Roberts N, Whitehouse GH, et al. Estimation of breast volume and its variation during the menstrual cycle using MRI and stereology. Br J Radiol 1999; 72:236–245.
17. Longacre TA, Bartow SA. A correlative morphologic study of human breast and endometrium in the menstrual cycle. Am J Surg Pathol 1986; 10:382–393.
18. Ferguson DJ, Anderson TJ. Morphological evaluation of cell turnover in relation to the menstrual cycle in the "resting" human breast. Br J Cancer 1981; 44:177–181.
19. Cunha GR, Hom YK. Role of mesenchymal-epithelial interactions in mammary gland development. J Mammary Gland Biol Neoplasia 1996; 1:21–35.
20. Robinson GW, Karpf AB, Kratochwil K. Regulation of mammary gland development by tissue interaction. J Mammary Gland Biol Neoplasia 1999; 4:9–19.
21. Snedeker SM, Brown CF, Di Augustine RP. Expression and functional properties of transforming growth factor alpha and epidermal growth factor during mouse mammary gland ductal morphogenesis. Proc Natl Acad Sci USA 1991; 88(1):276–280.
22. Jackson D, Bresnick J, Dickson C. A role for fibroblast growth factor signaling in the lobulo-alveolar development of the mammary gland. J Mammary Gland Biol Neoplasia 1997; 2(4):385–392.
23. Daniel CW, Robinson S, Silberstein GB. The transforming growth factors beta in development and functional differentiation of the mouse mammary gland. Adv Exp Med Biol 2001; 501:61–70.
24. Smalley MJ, Dale TC. Wnt signaling in mammalian development and cancer. Cancer Metastasis Rev 1999; 18(2):215–230.
25. Tepera SB, McCrea PD, Rosen MJ. A beta-catenin survival signal is required for normal lobular development in the mammary gland. J Cell Sci 2003; 166(pt 6):1337–1349.
26. Buhler TA, Dale TC, Kieback C, et al. Localization and quantification of Wnt-2 gene expression in mouse mammary development. Dev Biol 1993; 155(1):87–96.
27. Osborne M. Breast development and anatomy. In: Harris LM Jr, Morrow M, Osborne CK, eds. Diseases of the Breast. New York: Lippinkott & Wilkins, 2000:1–13.
28. Rohrich RJ, Hartley W, Brown S. Incidence of breast and chest wall asymmetry in breast augmentation: a retrospective

analysis of 100 patients. Plast Reconstr Surg 2003; 111(1): 1513–1523.

29. Rosenbloom A. Breast Physiology: normal and abnormal development and function. In: Bland KCEI, ed. The Breast: Comprehensive Management of Benign and Malignant Diseases. Vol. 1. Philadelphia: W.B. Saunders, 1998:38–50.

30. Mills JL, Stolley PD, Davies J, et al. Premature thelarche. Natural history and etiologic investigation. Am J Dis Child 1981; 135:743–745.

31. Laurence DJ, Monaghan P, Gusterson BA. The development of the normal human breast. Oxf Rev Reprod Biol 1991; 13:149–174.

32. Sloand E. Pediatric and adolescent breast health. Lippincotts Prim Care Pract 1998; 2:170–175.

33. Murakami M, Kawai K, Higuchi K, et al. Correlation between breast development and hormone profiles in puberal girls. Nippon Sanka Fujinka Gakkai Zasshi 1998; 40:561–567.

34. Radfar N, Ansusingha K, Kenny FM. Circulating bound and free estradiol and estrone during normal growth and development and in premature thelarche and isosexual precocity. J Pediatr 1976; 89:719–723.

35. Stanhope R, Abdulwahid NA, Adams J, et al. Studies of gonadotrophin pulsatility and pelvic ultrasound examinations distinguish between isolated premature thelarche and central precocious puberty. Eur J Pediatr 1986; 145:190–194.

36. Styne D. Puberty. In: Greenspan F, Gardner D, eds. Basic and Clincal Endocrinology. New York: McGraw-Hill, 2001:547–574.

37. Bongiovanni AM. An epidemic of premature thelarche in Puerto Rico. J Pediatr 1983; 103:245–246.

38. Frantz A, Wilson JD. Endocrine disorders of the breast. In: Wilson JDFD, Kronenberg HM, Larsen PR, eds. Williams Textbook of Endocrinology. Philadelphia: WB Saunders, 1998: 877–900.

39. Finer N, Emery P, Hicks BH. Mammary gigantism and D-pencillamine. Clin Endocrinol (Oxf) 1984; 21:219–222.

40. Lafreniere R, Temple W, Ketcham A. Gestational macromastia. Am J Surg 1984; 148:413–418.

41. Baker SB, Burkey BA, Thornton P, et al. Juvenile gigantomastia: presentation of four cases and review of literature. Ann Plast Surg 2001; 46:517–526.

42. Lee PA. The relationship of concentrations of serum hormones to pubertal gynecomastia. J Pediatr 1975; 86:212–215.

43. Thompson DF, Carter JR. Drug-induced gynecomastia. Pharmacotherapy 1993; 13:37–45.

44. Kuhn JM, Mahoudeau JA, Billaud L, et al. Evaluation of diagnostic criteria for Leydig cell tumors in adult men revealed by gynecomastia. Clin Endocrinol (Oxf) 1987; 26:407–416.

45. Kirschner MA, Cohen FB, Jespersen D. Estrogen production and its origin in men with gonadotrophin-producing neoplasms. J Clin Endocrinol Metab 1974; 39:112–118.

46. Grumbach M, Conte F. Disorders of sex differentiation. In: Wilson J, Foster D, eds. Williams Textbook of Endocrinology. Philadelphia: WB Saunders, 1992:853–951.

47. Morishima A, Grumbach MM, Simpson ER, et al. Aromatase deficiency in male and female siblings caused by a novel mutation and the physiological role of estrogens. J Clin Endocrinol Metab 1995; 80:3689–3698.

48. Hilakivi-Clarke L, Forsen T, Eriksson JG, et al. Tallness and overweight during childhood have opposing effects on breast cancer risk. Br J Cancer 2001; 85:1680–1684.

49. Sappey MPC. Injection preparation et conservation des vaisseaux lymphatiques. These pour le dectorat en medicine, no 241. Paris: Rignoux Imprimeur de la Faculte de Medicine, 1834.

50. Turner-Warwick RT. The lymphatics of the breast. Br J Surg 1959; 46:574–582.

51. Tanis PJ, Neiweg OE, Olmos RAV, Kroon BBR. Anatomy and physiology of lymphatic drainage of the breast from the perspective of sentinel node biopsy. J Am Coll Surg 2001; 192(3):399–409.

52. Nishimura R, Nagao K, Miayama H, et al. Higher plasma vascular endothelial growth factor levels correlate with menopause, overexpression of p53, and recurrence of breast cancer. Breast Cancer 2003; 10(2):120–128.

53. Osanai T, Wakita T, Gomi N, et al. Correlation among intratumoral blood flow in breast cancer, clinicopathological findings and Nottingham Prognostic index. Jpn J Clin Oncol 2003; 33(1):14–16.

54. Simpson HW, McArdle CS, George WD, et al. Pregnancy postponement and childlessness leads to chronic hypervascularity of the breasts and cancer risk. Br J Cancer 2002; 87(1): 1246–1252.

55. Chepko G, Smith GH. Three-division competent, structurally-distinct cell populations contribute to murine mammary epithelial renewal. Tissue Cell 1997; 29(2):239–253.

56. Chepko G, Smith GH. Mammary epithelial stem cells: our current understanding. J Mammary Gland Biol Neoplasia 1999; 4(1):35–52.

57. Tyson JE, Hwang P, Guyda H, et al. Studies of prolactin secretion in human pregnancy. Am J Obstet Gynecol 1972; 113:14–20.

58. Speroff L, Glass RG, Kase NG. The Breast. Clinical Gynecologic Endocrinology and Infertility. Baltimore: Lippincott Williams & Wilkins, 1999:600–641.

59. Kelly PA, Djiane J, Postal-Vinay MC, et al. The prolactin/growth hormone receptor family. Endocr Rev 1991; 12: 235–251.

60. Yang Y, Spitzer E, Meyer D, et al. Sequential requirement of hepatocyte growth factor and neuregulin in the morphogenesisand differentiation of the mammary gland. J Cell Biol 1995; 131:215–226.

61. Liscia DS, Merlo G, Ciardiello F, et al. Transforming growth factor-alpha messenger RNA localization in the developing adult rat and human mammary gland by in situ hybridization. Dev Biol 1990; 140(1):123–131.

62. Robinson GW, Henninhausen L. Inhibins and activins regulate mammary epithelial cell differentiation through mesenchymal-epithelial interactions. Development 1997; 124:2701–2708.

63. Suzuki R, Atherton AJ, O'Hare MJ, et al. Proliferation and differentiation in the human breast during pregnancy. Differentiation 2000; 66(2–3):106–115.

64. Scott-Conner CEH. Diagnosing and managing breast disease during pregnancy and lactation. Medscape Womens Health 1997; 2(5):1.

65. Slavin JL, Billson R, Ostor AG. Nodular breast lesions during pregnancy and lactation. Histopathology 1993; 22(5):481–485.

66. Jiminez JF, Rickey RO, Cohen C. Spontaneous breast infarction associated with pregnancy presenting as a palpable mass. J Surg Oncol 1986; 32(3):174–178.

67. Harigopal M, Mudrovich SA, Hoda SA, Rosen PP. Secondary tumors in mammary adenolipomas: a report of 2 unusual cases. Arch Pathol Lab Med 2003; 127(3):e151–e154.

68. Scott-Conner CE, Schorr SJ. The diagnosis and management of breast problems during pregnancy and lactation. Am J Surg 1995; 170(4):401–405.

69. Lafreniere R. Bloody nipple discharge during pregnancy: a rationale for conservative treatment. J Surg Oncol 1990; 43: 228–230.

70. McCarty K, Nath M. Breast. In: SS S, ed. Histology for Pathologists. Philadelphia: Lippincott-Raven, 1997:71–82.

71. Kaplan CR, Schenken R. Endocrinology of the breast. In: Mitchell G, Bassett L, eds. The Female Breast and Its Disorders. Baltimore: Williams & Wilkins, 1990:22–44.

72. Cregan MD, Harttman PE. Computerized breast measurement from conception to weaning: clinical implications. J Hum Lact 1999; 15:89–96.

73. Neville MC, Morton J. Physiology and endocrine changes underlying human lactogenesis II. J Nutr 2001; 131 911 0: 3005s–3008s.

74. Kelleher SL, Lonnerdal B. Immunological activities associated with milk. Adv Nutr Res 2001; 10:39–65.

75. Kent JC, Mitoulas L, Cox DB, et al. Breast volume and milk production during extended lactation in women. Exp Physiol 1999; 84:435–447.

76. Ohtani O, Shao XJ, Saitoh M, et al. Lymphatics of the rat mammary gland during virgin, pregnant, lactating and post-weaning periods. Ital J Anat Embryol 1998; 103:335–342.

77. Marti A, Feng Z, Altermatt HJ, et al. Milk accumulation triggers apoptosis of mammary epithelial cells. Eur J Cell Biol 1997; 73:158–165.

78. Lund LR, Romer J, Thomasset N, et al. Two distinct phases of apoptosis in mammary gland involution: proteinase-independent and -dependent pathways. Development 1996; 122:181–193.

79. Yan GZ, Pan WT, Bancroft C. Thyrotropin-releasing hormone action on the prolactin promoter is mediated by the POU protein pit-1. Mol Endocrinol 1991; 5:535–541.

80. Bredow S, Kacsoh B, Obal F Jr, et al. Increase of prolactin mRNA in the rat hypothalamus after intracerebroventricular injection of VIP or PACAP. Brain Res 1994; 660:301–308.

81. Pickett CA, Gutierrez-Hartmann A. Ras mediates Src but not epidermal growth factor-receptor tyrosine kinase signaling pathways in GH4 neuroendocrine cells. Proc Natl Acad Sci USA 1994; 91:8612–8616.

82. Porter TE, Wiles CD, Frawley LS. Stimulation of lactotrope differentiation in vitro by fibroblast growth factor. Endocrinology 1994; 134:164–168.

83. Tyson JE, Perez A, Zanartu J. Human lactational response to oral thyrotropin releasing hormone. J Clin Endocrinol Metabol 1976; 43:760–768.

84. Ben-Jonathan N, Mershon J, Allen D, et al. Extrapituitary prolactin: distribution, regulation, functions, and clinical aspects. Endocrine Rev 1997; 17:639–669.

85. Bezault J, Bhimani R, Wiprovnick J, Furmanski P. Human lactoferrin inhibits growth of solid tumors and development of experimental metastases in mice. Cancer Res 1994; 54(9): 2310–2312.

86. Hennighausen L. Signal networks in the mammary gland: lessons from the animal models. In: Dickson RB, Salomon DS, eds. Hormones and Growth Factors in Development and Neoplasia. New York: Wiley-Liss, 1998:239–277.

87. Greenberg MM, Wolfe J, Rosen JM. Casein gene expression: from transfection to transgenics. In: Dickson RB, Lippman ME, eds. Genes, Oncogenes and Hormones. Boston: Kluver, 1991:379–398.

88. McKnight RA, Burdon T, Pursel VG, Shamay A, Wall RJ, Hennighausen L. The whey acidic protein. In: Dickson RB, Lippman ME, eds. Genes, Oncogenes and Hormones. Boston: Kluver, 1991:399–406.

89. Wakao H, Gouilleux F, Groner B. Mammary gland factor (Mgf) is a novel member of the cytokine regulated transcription factor gene family and confers the prolactin response. EMBO J 1994; 13:2182–2188.

90. Happ B, Groner B. The activated mammary gland specific nuclear factor (Mgf) enhances in vitro transcription of the beta-casein gene promoter. J Steroid Biochem 1993; 47: 21–30.

91. Altiok S, Groner B. β-casein mRNA sequesters a single-stranded-nucleic acid-binding protein which negatively regulates the β-casein gene promotor. Mol Cell Biol 1994; 14(90):6004–6012.

92. Streuli CH, Edwards GM. Control of normal mammary epithelial phenotype by integrins. J Mammary Gland Biol Neoplasia 1998; 3:151–163.

93. Nguyen DD, Neville MC. Tight junction regulation in the mammary gland. J Mammary Gland Biol Neoplasia 1998; 3(3):233–246.

94. Daly SE, Owens RA, Hartmann PE. The short-term synthesis and infant-regulated removal of milk in lactating women. Exp Physiol 1993; 78:209–220.

95. Jerry DJ, Dickinson ES, Roberts AL, Said TK. Regulation of apoptosis during mammary involution by the p53 tumor suppressor gene. J Dairy Sci 2002; 85(5):1103–1110.

96. Shamay A, Shapiro F, Mabjeesh SJ, Silanikove N. Casein-derived phosphopeptides disrupt tight junction integrity, and precipitously dry up milk secretion in goats. Life Sci 2002; 70(23):2707–2719.

97. Prince JM, Klinowska TC, Marshman E, et al. Cell matrix interactions during development and apoptosis of the mouse mammary gland in vivo. Dev Dyn 2002; 223(4):497–516.

98. Strange R, Metcalfe T, Thackray L, Dang M. Apoptosis in normal and neoplastic mammary gland development. Micros Res Tech 2001; 52(2):171–181.

99. Marti A, Graber H, Lazar H, et al. Caspases: decoders of apoptotic signals during mammary involution. Caspase activation during involution. Adv Exp Med Biol 2000; 480: 195–201.

100. Tonner E, Barber MC, Travers MT, et al. Hormonal control of insulin-like growth factor-binding protein-5 production in the involuting mammary gland of the rat. Endocrinology 1997; 138(12):5101–5107.

101. Tonner E, Allen G, Shkreta L, et al. Insulin-like growth factor binding protein-5 (IGFBP-5) potentially regulates programmed cell death and plasminogen activation in the mammary gland. Adv Exp Med Biol 2000; 4880:45–53.

102. McNeilly AS. Lactational control of reproduction. Reprod Fertil Dev 2001; 13(7–8):583–590.

103. Covington C, Mitchell-Gieleghem A, Lawson D, et al. Presence of carotenoid, an anticarcinogenic marker, in nipple aspirates postlactation. Adv Exp Med Biol 2001; 501: 143–152.

104. Chapman DJ, Perez-Escamilla R. Identification of risk factors for delayed onset of lactation. J Am Diet Assoc 1999; 99: 450–454.

105. Anderson AM. Didruption of lactogenesis by retained placental fragments. J Hum Lact 2001; 17(2):142–144.

106. Arthur PG, Kent JC, Hartmann PE. Metabolites of lactose synthesis in milk from diabetic and nondiabetic women during lactogenesis II. J Pediatr Gastroenterol Nutr 1994; 19: 100–108.

107. Dewey KG. Maternal and fetal stress are associated with impaired lactogenesis in humans. J Nutr 2001; 131(11): 3012s–3015s.

108. Forbes A, Hennemen P, Griswold G, et al. A syndrome, distinct from acrorriegamenorrhea, and low follicle-stimulating hormone excretion. J Clin Endocrinol 1951; 12:1087–1094.

109. Archer DF. Current concepts of prolactin physiology in normal, and abnormal conditions. Fertil Steril 1977; 28:125–134.

110. Frantz AG. Prolactin. N Eng J Med 1978; 298:201–207.

111. Blackwell RE. Diagnosis and management of prolactinimas. Fertil Steril 1985; 43:5–16.

112. Kelver M, Nagamani M. Hyperprolactinemia in primary adrenal cortical insufficiency. Fertil Steril 1985; 44:423–425.

113. Mahesh VB, Pria SD, Greenblatt RB. Abnormal lactation with Cushing's syndrome-a case report. J Endocrinol 1969; 29: 978–981.

114. Nabarro JD. Acromegaly. Clin Endocrinol (Oxf) 1987; 26: 481–512.

115. Sievertsen GD, Lim VS, Nakawatase C, et al. Metabolic clearance and secretion rates of human prolactin in normal subjects and in patients with chronic renal failure. J Clin Endocrinol Metab 1980; 50:846–852.

116. Turkington RW. Ectopic production of prolactin. N Eng J Med 1971; 285:1455–1458.

117. Petrek JA. Abnormalities of the breast during pregnancy and lactation. In: Harris LM Jr, Morrow M, Osborne CK, eds. Diseases of the Breast. New York: Lippinkott & Wilkins, 2000: 63–66.

118. Choudhury M, Singal MK. Lactating adenoma-cytomorphologic study with review of literature. Indian J Pathol Microbiol 2001; 44(4):445–448.

119. Baker J. Lactating adenoma: a diagnosis of exclusion. Breast J 2001; 7(5):354–357.

120. Nichols S, Water WE, Wheeler MJ. Management of female breast disease by Southhampton general Practitioner. Br Med J 1980; 281:1450–1453.

121. Preece PE, Baum M, Mansel RE, et al. The importance of mastalgia in operable breast cancer. Br Med J 1982; 248: 1299–1300.

122. Maddox PR, HarrisonBJ, Mansel RE, Hughes LE. Non-cyclical mastalgia: Improved classification and treatment. Br J Surg 1989; 76:901–904.

123. Klimberg VS. Etiology and management of breast pain. In: The Breast: Comprehensive Management of Benign and Malignant Diseases. Vol. 1. Philadelphia: WB Saunders, 1998.

124. Gabrielli G, Binazzi P, Scaricabarozzi L, Massi GB. Nime sulide in the treatment of mastalgia. Drugs 1993; SI:137–139.

125. Gateley CA, Maddox PR, Pritchard GA, et al. Plasma fatty acid profiles in benign breast disorders. Br J Surg 1992; 79:407–409.

126. Mansel RE, Pye JK, Hughs LE. Effects of essential fatty acids on cyclical mastalgia and non-cyclical breast disorder. In: Horrobin DF, ed. Omega-6 Essential Fatty Acids: Pathophysiology and Roles in Clinical Medicine. New York: Willey-Liss, 1990:557–649b.

127. Morrow M, Wong S, Venta L. The evaluation of breast masses in women younger than forty years of age. Surgery 1998; 124:634–641.

128. Dixon JM, Mansel RE. Symptoms assessment and guidelines for referral. ABC of breast diseases. Br Med J 1994; 309:722–726.

129. Leis HP Jr. Management of nipple discharge. World J Surg 1989; 13(6):736–742.

130. Seltzer MH, Perloff LJ, Kelly RL, Fitts WT. Significance of age in patients with nipple discharge. Surg Gynecol Obstet 1970; 131:519–522.

131. Simmons R, Adamovich T, Brennan M, et al. Non-surgical evaluation of pathologic nipple discharge. Ann of Surg Oncol 2003; 10(2):113–116.

132. Baitchev G, Gortchev G, Todorova A, et al. Intraductal aspiration cytology and galactography for nipple discharge. Int Surg 2003; 88(2):83–86.

133. Oral SG, Dougherty CS, Reynolds C, et al. MR imaging in patients with nipple discharge: initial experience. Radiology 2000; 216(1):248–254.

134. Haagenson CD. Anatomy of the mammary gland. In: Haagenson CP, ed. Diseases of the Breast. 3rd ed. Philadelphia: WB Saunders, 1986:1–23.

135. Howell JD, Barker F, Gazet JC. Granulomamtous lobular mastitis; report of a further two cases and a comprehensive literature review. Breast 1994; 3:119–123.

136. Hamed H, Fentiman IS. Benign breast disease. Int J Clin Pract 2001; 55(7):464–464.

137. Dupont WD, Page DL. Risk factors for breast cancer in women with benign breast disease. N Eng J Med 1985; 312:146–151.

138. Drukker BH, de Mendonca WC. Fibrocystic change and fibrocystic disease of the breast. Obstet Gynecol Clin North Am 1987; 14(3):685–702.

139. Norlock FE. Benign breast pain in women: a practical approach to evaluation and treatment. J Am Med Womens Assoc 2002; 57(2):95–80.

140. Schnitt SJ, Connolly JL. Pathology of benign breast disorders. In: Harris LM Jr, Morrow M, Osborne CK, eds. Diseases of the Breast. New York: Lippinkott & Wilkins, 2000; 75–93.

141. Liberman L. Percutaneous image-guided core biopsy. Radiol Clin North Am 2002; 40(3):483–500.

142. Salih AK, Fentiman IS. Breast Cancer prevention. Int J Clin Pract 2002; 56(4):267–271.

143. Kinsinger LS, Harris R, Woolf SH, et al. Chemoprevention of breast cancer: a summary of the evidence for the US Preventive Services Task Force. Ann Intern Med 2002; 137(1):59–69.

144. Jatoi I. Breast cancer: asystemic or local disease? Am J Clin Oncol 1997; 20:536–539.

145. Halsted WS. The results of radical operations for the cure of carcinoma of the breast. Ann Surg 1907; 56:1–19.

146. Fisher B, Fisher ER. Transmigration of lymph nodes by tumor cells. Science 1966; 152:1397–1398.

147. Peters V. Wedge resection and irradiation, effective treatment in early breast cancer. JAMA 1967; 200:134–139.

148. Crile G. Results of conservative treatment of breast cancer at 10 and 15 years. Ann Surg 1975; 182:26–29.

149. Fisher B, Bauer M, Margolese R, et al. Five year results of a randomized clinical trial comparing total mastectomy and segmental mastectomy with or without radiation in treatment of breast cancer. N Eng J Med 1985; 312:665–673.

150. Veronesi U, Sacrozi R, Del Vecchio M, et al. Comparing radical mastectomy with quadrentectomy, axillary dissection and radiotherapy in patients with small cancers of the breast. N Eng J Med 1981; 305:6–11.

151. Jacobson JA, Cowan KH, D' Angelo T, et al. 10 year results of a comparison of conservation with mastectomy in the treatment of stage I and II breast cancer. N Eng J Med 1995; 332:907–911.

152. Van Dongen JA, Bartelink H, Fentimen IS, et al. Randomized clinical trial to assess the value of breast-conserving therapy in stage I and II breast cancer, EORTC 10801 Trial. Monogr Natl Cancer Inst 1992; 11:15–18.

153. Srrazin D, Le M, Arriagada R, et al. Ten year results of a randomized trial comparing a conservative treatment to mastectomy in early breast cancer. Radiother Oncol 1989; 14:177–184.

154. Cady B. Another editorial perspective. Ann Surg Oncol 1998; 5:103–104.

155. Fisher B, Anderson S, Bryant J, et al. Twenty-year follow-up of a randomized trial comparing total mastectomy, lumpectomy and lumpectomy plus irradiation for the treatment of invasive breast cancer. N Eng J Med 2002; 347:1233–1241.

156. Fisher B, Brown A, Mamounas E, et al. Effect of preoperative chemotherapy on local-regional disease in women with operable breast cancer: findings from National Surgical Adjuvant Breast and Bowel Project B-18. J Clin Oncol 1997; 15:2483–2493.

157. Helbich TH, Matzek W, Fuchsjegar MH. Stereotactic and ultrasound-guided breast biopsy. Eur Radiol 2004; 14(3):383–393.

158. Gittleman MA. Single-step ultrasound localization of breast lesion and lumpectomy procedure. Am J Surg 2003; 186(4):386–390.

159. Abrahamson PE, Dunlap LA, Amamoo MA, et al. Factors predicting successful needle-localized breast biopsy. Acad Radiol 2003; 10(6):601–606.

160. Singletary SE, Allred C, Ashley P, et al. Revision of the American Joint Committee on Cancer staging system for breast cancer. J Clin Oncol 2002; 20:3262–3636.

161. Dent DM. Axillary lymphadenectomy for breast cancer. Arch Surg 1996; 131:1125–1127.

162. Sacks NPM, Baum M. Primary management of carcinoma of the breast. Lancet 1993; 342:1402–1408.

163. Jatoi I. Management of the axilla in primary breast cancer. Surg Clin North Am 1999; 79(5):1061–1073.

164. Edge SB, Niland JC, Bookman MA, et al. Emergence of sentinel node biopsy in breast cancer as standard-of-care in academic comprehensive cancer centers. J Natl Cancer Inst 2003; 95(20):1514–1521.

165. Schwartz GF, Guiliano AE, Veronesi U. Proceeding of the consensus conference of the role of sentinel lymph node biopsy in carcinoma or the breast April 19–22, 2001, Philadelphia, PA, USA. Breast J 2002; 8(3):124–138.

166. Smith LF, Cross MJ, Klimberg VS. Subareolar injection is a better technique for sentinel lymph node biopsy. Am J Surg 2000; 180:434–438.

167. Krag D. Current status of sentinel lymph node surgery for breast cancer. J Natl Cancer 1999; 91:302–303.

168. Beatson GT. On the treatment of inoperable cases of carcinoma of the mamma: suggestions for a new method of treatment, with illustrative cases. Lancet 1896; ii:104–107.

169. Taylor GW. Artificial menopause in carcinoma of the breast. N Eng J Med 1934; 211:1138–1142.

170. Nissen-Meyer R, Kjellgren K, Manson B. Preliminary report from the Scandinavian Adjuvant Chemotherapy Study Group. Cancer Chemother Rep 1971; 55:561–566.

171. Bonadonna G, Valagussa P, Moliterni A, et al. Adjuvant cyclophospharnide, methotrexate, and fluorouracil in node-positive breast cancer: the results of 20 years of follow-up. N Eng J Med 1995; 332:901–906.

172. Bonadonna G, Valagussa P, Rossi A, et al. Ten-year experience with CMF-based adjuvant chemotherapy in respectable breast cancer. Breast Cancer Res Treat 1985; 5:95–115.

173. Nolvadex Adjuvant Trial Organization. Controlled trial of tamoxifen as adjuvant agent in management of early breast cancer: interim analysis at four years. Lancet 1983; 1:257–261.

174. Fisher B. Status of adjuvant therapy: results of the National Surgical Adjuvant Breast Project studies on oophorectomy, postoperative radiation therapy and chemotherapy. Other comments concerning clinical trials. Cancer 1971; 28:1654–1658.

175. Early Breast Cancer Trialists Collaborative Group. Systemic treatment of early breast cancer by hormonal, cytotoxic, or immune therapy: 133 randomized trials involving 31000 recurrences and 24000 deaths among 75000 women. Lancet 1985; 339:1–15.

176. Early Breast Cancer Trialists Collaborative Group. Polychemotherapy for early breast cancer: an overview of the randomized trials. Lancet 1998; 352:930–942.

177. Early Breast Cancer Trialists Collaborative Group. Ovarian ablation in early breast cancer: overview of the randomized trials. Lancet 1996; 348:1189–1196.

178. Early Breast Cancer Trialists Collaborative Group. Tamoxifen for early breast cancer: an overview of the randomized trials. Lancet 1998; 351:1451–1467.

179. Cizick J. The ATAC ('Arimidex', tamoxifen, alone or in combination) trial in postmenopausal women with early breast cancer-updated efficacy results based on a median follow-up of 47 months. Breast 2003; 12(suppl 1):S47.

180. Slamon DJ, Clark GM, Wong SG, et al. Human breast cancer: correlation of relapse and survival with amplification of the HER-2/neu oncogene. Science 1987; 235:177–182.

181. Slamon D, Leyland-Jones B, Shak S, et al. Addition of Herceptin (humanized anti HER-2 antibody) to first-line chemotherapy for HER-2 overexpressing metastatic breast cancer markedly increases anticancer activity: a randomized, multinational controlled phase III trial. Proc Am Soc Clin Oncol 1998; 17:377a.

182. Bernhard J, Hurny C, Coates AS, et al. Quality of life assessment in patients receiving adjuvant therapy for breast cancer: The International Breast Cancer Study Group (IBCSG) approach. Ann Oncol 1997; 8:825–835.

183. Morris A, Morris R, Wilson J, et al. Breast-conserving therapy versus mastectomy in early-stage breast cancer: a meta-analysis of 10 year survival. Cancer J Sci Am 1997; 3:6–12.

184. Schnitt S, Hayjman J, Gelman R, et al. A prospective study of conservative surgery alone in the treatment of selected patients with stage I breast cancer. Cancer 1996; 77:1094–1100.

185. Nemoto T, Patel J, Rosner D, et al. Factors affecting recurrence in lumpectomy without irradiation for breast cancer. Cancer 1991; 67:2079–2083.

186. Fowble B, Gray R, Gilchrist K, et al. Identification of a subgroup of patients with breast cancer and histologically positive axillary nodes receiving chemotherapy who may benefit from post-operative radiotherapy. J Clin Oncol 1988; 6:1107–1117.

187. Ragaz J, Jackson S, Le N, et al. Adjuvant radiotherapy and chemotherapy and chemotherapy in node positive premenopausal women with breast cancer. N Eng J Med 1997; 337:956–962.

188. Overgaard M, Hansen P, Overgaard J, et al. Postoperative radiotherapy in high-risk premenopausal women with breast cancer who receive adjuvant chemotherapy. N Eng J Med 1997; 337: 949–955.

57

Hernias of the Abdominal Wall and Its Contents

Philip E. Donahue

INTRODUCTION

"Hernia" (a Latin term for "rupture") is a descriptive term for the protrusion of abdominal cavity contents through an opening or defect in the fascial and muscular layers of the abdominal wall. The abdominal wall is the locus of many opposing physical forces, which ordinarily remain in balance according to established mechanical principles; when this balance is disrupted a hernia appears. While physical breakdown or defect of the abdominal wall is present in all hernias, nutritional, environmental, and congenital cofactors can also be implicated in their appearance. Therefore, the term "rupture" is literally correct for a minority of hernias that appear in the abdominal envelope. Most hernias appear unheralded as anatomic sites predisposed to weakening by virtue of position, function, or structure succumb to natural forces. The most common hernias occur in males as a result of the patent processus vaginalis present in the majority of full-term infants, and persisting in some 25% throughout life, with or without symptoms; approximately 5% of groin hernias appear in women, whose inguinal canal contents are less likely to contain a patent canal (of Nuck) (1–3). Other hernias occur at various stress points within the abdominal wall, including the midline, "rings," foramina, and other natural openings or potential defects. Many hernias will require surgical repair, although there is renewed interest of late in the natural history of unoperated adult hernias that are minimally symptomatic or asymptomatic, because the incidence of hernia strangulation in such patients is quite low. The results of prospective randomized studies comparing nonoperative treatment ("watchful waiting") for minimally or asymptomatic groin hernias with elective surgical repair will provide important evidence for clinicians and for administrators of health care organizations (4,5).

Until recently, hernia repair was always performed in an intuitive way—suture approximation of tissues at the border of the hernia defect. This "old-fashioned" approach, performed in various ways since the Middle Ages, was reasonably successful and performed worldwide until the latter half of the last century, when three major developments were shown to have benefits in terms of patient acceptance and overall success. The concepts embodied by "tension-free" repair combined with advances in prosthetic materials have revolutionized the repair of primary and recurrent hernias worldwide (6,7). The abdominal wall, unfortunately, for patients with huge hernias, still contains unsolved problems and challenges for future generations of hernia surgeons.

The clinical signs and symptoms of hernia presentation in a given patient are remarkably varied, as are the anatomic findings observed in the operating room. Experience teaches the lesson that the appearance of groin structures differs markedly in individuals, especially in the presence of stretching, edema, or distortion of the boundary structures. As a result, surgeons find hernia repair challenging, especially when sliding, strangulated, or recurrent hernias are encountered. Although the overwhelming majority of patients have an uneventful convalescence and prompt return to gainful employment after hernia repair, an unfortunate few will be plagued by a complication of the procedure. If infection, hernia recurrence, or persistent groin pain develops after hernia repair, an entire new world of problems arises for the patient and his or her surgeon. Hernia repair is a major surgical event, undervalued by many in the community, including surgeons, which demands technical awareness and precise skill in performance. The evaluation and care of patients postoperatively often challenges the collective wisdom of the most experienced practitioner. Most of these problems are not life threatening, and most can be solved by attention to the basic facts of hernia science; however, taking hernias for granted is a recipe for disaster. This chapter will highlight the important developments that have occurred during the past several decades in our understanding of hernia formation and how this knowledge is used in the modern practice of herniorrhaphy (6,7).

CONCEPTS AND DEFINITIONS

An abdominal wall hernia exists when tissues protrude through a defect (congenital or acquired) in the musculofascial supports of the abdominal wall, including the endoabdominal fascia, the innermost layer, which lines the entire abdominal cavity. The transversalis fascia on the anterior abdominal wall and groin is the boundary between the peritoneum and the intra-abdominal contents and the abdominal wall, through which the hernia protrudes; if a sac is not present, the hernia consists of preperitoneal fat protruding through a weakened or defective transversalis fascia (8,9). A standard nomenclature is useful in classifying different types of hernias and evaluating the contents of the hernia. A hernia that can be returned to the abdominal cavity is said to be "reducible" in contrast to an "irreducible" or "incarcerated" hernia, which remains present despite physical manipulation. Incarcerated hernias, regardless of their size, may be present for years without causing problems, but their contents are always at some risk for vascular compromise ("strangulation") if edema, hernia contents, or boundary structures interfere with blood supply. When incarcerated hernias are (or become) extremely painful or are accompanied by systemic signs such as vomiting, fever, or prostration, the hernia repair becomes a relative surgical emergency, because ischemic or infarcted tissues may be present.

The term "sliding" hernia describes a hernia in which an organ, usually a hollow viscus, is part of the hernia sac. Sliding hernias pose particular problems for management, because inadvertent perforation of the cecum or sigmoid colon, the most common sliding components, can easily occur during manipulation and dissection of the hernia sac. When an incarcerated hernia cannot be easily reduced, the hernia sac is opened to facilitate the reduction of hernia contents; needless to say, perforation of the intestine markedly increases the risk of infection and restricts the possible use of prosthetic materials to achieve a "tension-free" repair. Sliding hernias often cannot be diagnosed preoperatively, but can be suspected in very large hernias, because any organ attached to the retroperitoneum can be pulled through the internal ring with the hernia contents.

A "Richter" hernia is an incarcerated hernia containing a portion of the circumference of the bowel as opposed to an entire loop or segment of intestine; if the incarcerated portion of bowel becomes strangulated and necrotic, a life-threatening process unfolds without the signal events of a large groin mass or bowel obstruction which generally accompany incarcerated inguinal hernias. Richter hernias occur most commonly with inguinal hernias, followed by femoral and umbilical hernia sites; a "Littre's" hernia contains a Meckel's diverticulum.

A "ventral" hernia is any hernia developing in the ventral abdominal wall, including umbilical, epigastric, and incisional hernias, as well as the Spigelian hernia. "Groin" hernias develop in the inguinofemoral region, including direct and indirect inguinal hernias, as well as femoral hernias.

An "internal" hernia is one containing a loop of intestine protruding through a congenital or acquired orifice within the abdominal cavity, such as defects in the intestinal mesentery, the boundaries of various structures including the foramen of Winslow and the sciatic foramen. Congenital omphalomesenteric connections or postoperative adhesions, as well as postoperative "spaces" such as "retroanastomotic" hernias following antecolic gastrojejunal anastomosis (Peterson hernia) can result in internal hernia formation. Any of these defects may allow a loop or several loops of intestine to become trapped and occasionally strangulated as a result of twisting and peristaltic activity, and may not become symptomatic for years after the initial operation. Parenthetically, the Peterson hernia, thought to have disappeared largely as a result of the decreased incidence of ulcer operations, now has a modern counterpart in the aftermath of Roux-en-y gastric bypass performed laparoscopically (10). A new constellation of unusual hernias has been described, often recognized by postoperative radiographic studies, which provide previously unparalleled insights regarding the presence of internal hernias (11–13).

Internal hernias are generally not diagnosed before surgery, but should be considered in the differential diagnosis of painful abdominal crisis, or small bowel obstruction in the virgin abdomen. Internal hernias comprise about 1% of all hernias, and are recognized in up to 1% of autopsies (11).

PATHOPHYSIOLOGY OF HERNIA DEVELOPMENT

Hernias may develop in any of the structures supporting or surrounding the abdominal cavity. They may be encountered where a previous fetal communication existed between the abdominal cavity and some distant site, when an embryologic canal fails to obliterate, when maldevelopment of a supporting structure occurs, when dilation of a normally situated hiatus results, and when the mesenchymal supporting structures constituting a portion of the body wall become attenuated for some reason. Common sites for abdominal wall hernias include the groin, the umbilicus, the linea alba, various parts of the diaphragm, the lumbar region, along adjacent foramina in the pelvis where blood vessels and nerves exit, and within previously performed surgical incisions. All of these sites are natural foci for stretching, weakening, or rupture as a result of natural, pathologic, or traumatic causes.

Patent Processus Vaginalis and Omphalomesenteric Duct

The role of congenital factors in the development of hernia is reflected by the incidence of hernia in neonates and infants. Umbilical hernias occur where the umbilical ring has failed to obliterate the embryologic opening of the allantoic duct, which is ordinarily prevented by growth of the contiguous fascia of the linea alba. Similarly, indirect inguinal hernias (also called oblique hernias) arise due to the presence of an unobliterated processus vaginalis, the peritoneal connection between the abdominal cavity and the scrotum. A corresponding weakness and potential space exist in the canal of Nuck in the female, which accompanies the fibers of the round ligament through the inguinal canal. The peak incidence of indirect inguinal hernia occurs during infancy, when over 50% of males have a patent vaginal process. Congenital factors also play a role in the development of direct inguinal hernias, which occur between the superior pubic ramus and the arching border of the transversus abdominis muscle, medial to the deep inferior epigastric vessels. Patients with a high-arching lower border of the transversus abdominis aponeurosis (conjoined tendon) are at an increased risk for the development of this type of hernia (2,3). The appearance of hernia, however, depends upon other factors, as shown by autopsy findings of a patent processus vaginalis in 20% of individuals without any clinical evidence of a hernia before death (14–16). Similarly, the incidence of contralateral patency of the processus vaginalis in patients who have undergone repair of an inguinal hernia indicates that patency of this structure does not necessarily lead to inguinal herniation. Further, patency of the canal/diverticulum of Nuck in women occurs without clinical appearance of hernia, as shown by incidental herniography after hysterosalpingography (17,18).

The high incidence of patency of the processus vaginalis is one reason why bilateral exploration of the groin has been recommended in children found to have clinical evidence of unilateral groin hernia. Laparoscopic tools have shown that 30% to 50% of children have a patent processus vaginalis when examined by direct vision, a much higher rate than shown by air insufflation of the peritoneal cavity (19–21). Because meta-analysis has shown only 7.0% of hernia development during five-year follow-up, parents and surgeons have been led to reconsider the routine exploration of the contralateral side, which is sometimes recommended; watchful waiting, an option that has come to the fore in the adult hernia arena, is an option that avoids the low but unavoidable risk of damage to the vas deferens or spermatic artery, with subsequent testicular atrophy (22,23).

Altered Collagen Metabolism

Important causes of hernia development that cannot be easily defined are related to the "wear and tear" of living itself, including such stresses as repetitive local trauma, degenerative changes associated with increased or constant intra-abdominal pressure, and altered collagen synthesis; all of these are possible etiologic factors in patients developing hernias in middle and older age (24,25). Renewed interest in the biochemical and structural aspects of herniology has followed the description of some of the molecular and cellular elements of the protective fascia and collagenous tissues that normally prevent the formation of hernia. Collagen, the major constituent of the various aponeuroses and fascial structures of the body wall, has been studied intensively. Interestingly, collagen, like all other tissues in the body, is in a state of dynamic equilibrium in which there appears to be a constant synthesis of this substance,is matched by a parallel and constant rate of degradation. When Peacock and Madden (26) studied the transversalis fascia medial to the contralateral internal inguinal ring in patients with unilateral hernia, they compared rates of collagen synthesis and collagenolysis in both inguinal regions and found that the rates of both the processes were increased markedly. These findings of an earlier era were thought to support the concept that an abnormality of local collagen metabolism might be a factor in the eventual appearance of a hernia, and have yet to be expanded in a modern setting.

Further support for the view that abnormal collagen underlies hernia formation is provided by studies of hydroxyproline (the major amino acid constituent of collagen) content in the rectus muscle aponeurosis of patients with and without groin hernia. Fibroblasts cultured from the anterior rectus sheath of these patients proliferated poorly, incorporating labeled precursors at a much lower rate than control specimens (24). Additional studies have focused on the procollagen content of the dermal matrix in patients with primary and recurrent hernias of the groin and abdominal wall and have shown a decreased amount of procollagen III mRNA in cultured fibroblasts. This abnormality in the transcriptional regulation of collagen in hernia patients may indeed affect the appearance of frank hernias, as may other abnormalities such as a difference in the relative proportion of collagen and elastic fibers in the transversalis fascia of patients with direct inguinal hernias.

Malnutrition

The specific effects of malnutrition on the evolution of hernias of the groin or other parts of the abdominal wall are as yet undefined. If the collagenous structures that guard the abdominal wall are vital living structures that constantly experience remolding and resynthesis, there is a balance between synthesis and destruction of these supporting structures that could conceivably be altered by one's nutritional status. Other systemic factors such as uremia have definite effects on nutrition, and are interwoven with other mechanical factors in patients who develop hernias (27–29). In the surgical clinic of any large public hospital, many individuals with adult-onset hernias and malnutrition are encountered suggesting a correlation between these conditions; in the absence of experimental data, however, the routine use of supplemental vitamins or other adjunctive nutritional elements is not indicated. Sailors in the 18th century learned that the absence of citrus fruits on long voyages led to systemic signs, including bleeding gums, periosteal pain, and weakness; an additional element of this "scurvy" was the onset of hernias or ruptures of healed scars. Later, a specific effect of vitamin C on collagen maturation was described, allowing a reasonable explanation of the observed effects in these patients. A similar condition occurring naturally is lathyrism, a disease resulting from ingestion

of the flowering sweet pea. The active agent in the pea, beta-amino-proprionitrile, prevents the maturation of collagen and is capable of causing the appearance of groin hernias in young rats and mice (25,26,30–32). Interestingly, groin hernias developed in animals less than a month old, which were given sweet pea seeds in their diet in contrast to older rats, which did not develop hernias when fed with a similar diet. These examples of how nutrition may influence the formation of hernias are of particular importance, illustrating the effect of environmental factors on the natural balance between collagen synthesis and breakdown, which is sometimes accompanied by the appearance of hernia (33).

Defects in collagen maturation and synthesis are present in patients with excessive numbers of hernias or recurrent herniations (vide supra), and may be related in some way to critical vitamin or mineral deficiencies, altered immunity or resistance to infection, or underlying systemic disease. Further, altered levels of circulating enzymes in patients with emphysema add another dimension to the possible role of biologic factors in hernia formation. In a provocative article by Cannon and Read (34), serum elastolytic and antiproteolytic activity in smokers and nonsmokers was measured. Earlier work had confirmed the systemic effects of chronic smoking on elastin and collagen, the essential components of all anatomic support structures, utilizing a positive correlation between skin wrinkles in smokers or those exposed to secondary smoke as the basis for their conclusion. In this study, it was found that smokers had the potentially undesirable combination of increases in proteolytic activity combined with reductions in alpha$_1$-antitrypsin, a major naturally occurring circulating antiprotease, possibly adversely affecting the synthesis: degradation equilibrium of groin collagen toward collagen degradation and hernia formation.

Mechanical Stress

The reaction of the abdominal wall to extreme tension or hydrostatic challenge provides some insight into hernia formation, because there is a linear and sequential relationship between the presence of stress (e.g., cirrhosis with ascites and chronic peritoneal dialysis exert hydrostatic forces pushing toward the exterior, whereas morbid obesity produces additional forces that exert continuous pull on the abdominal wall) (28,29). The fact that hernias appear with regularity provides ample testimony about the stress, although it is impossible to determine which site will become a hernia prospectively. The stress of repetitive exercise in athletes may be a cause of hernia as shown by the results of herniography to define the cause of obscure groin pains in young athletes; the hernia discovered included abnormalities in the obturator canal and incipient hernia defects at the inguinal ring that could not be diagnosed by other means (35). These individuals had severe pain that prevented their usual physical activity; yet they had an unremarkable initial examination (14,17). The utility of herniography in experienced centers provides a noninvasive method for documentation of hernia, which is extremely useful at times, and which could be performed widely. However, the technique is resource intensive (and expensive) and requires highly motivated examiners and patients, but is not applicable to all patients (36).

Ultrasonography (US) is a noninvasive method for the examination of the inguinal canal, which has yielded impressive sensitivity and specificity data regarding the presence or absence of hernia in the hands of some (37,38).

Because of variable accuracy and other confounding issues, US has not supplanted clinical judgment in the selection of patients for inguinal hernia repair. Laparoscopic examination is indeed more sensitive in demonstrating the presence of all varieties of inguinal hernia, but the success of identifying hernias is also tempered by the small but real possibility of injury to the spermatic artery or vas deferens, if an asymptomatic hernia is repaired as a result of an incidental discovery. While the percentage chance of injury is impressively small according to published reports, the potential effects on an individual patient and his family are vast, prompting many surgeons to recommend repair of only those hernias that are symptomatic. The utility of the ultrasound examination is proven mainly in the postoperative period, when problems such as seroma, recurrence, or prosthesis displacement can be identified (39). Recent data suggest that up to 90% of patent processes will close spontaneously, and add support to the notion that a "watchful waiting" approach is appropriate for asymptomatic patients, that is now being proposed in the prospective evaluation of adults (4,5). Other issues such as the cost–benefit analysis of routine ultrasonographic studies remain unresolved, but it is hard if not impossible to demonstrate the value added by an unnecessary test.

In the absence of compelling data, experienced surgeons can be comfortable in relying upon the physical exam as the gold standard in determining which patients require operative treatment of hernia; suspected hernias which cannot be demonstrated can be managed by watchful waiting and reexamination. A persistent complaint of severe groin pain or intermittent bulge is usually a reliable indicator for surgical exploration of potential hernia sites. Happily for the moment, the use of adjunctive tests for the diagnosis of groin and other hernias is not required for the simple fact that they do not provide reliable evidence in many cases.

Iatrogenic Factors

Several iatrogenic factors may result in the subsequent development of a hernia. A conventional open-appendectomy may damage innervation of the muscular constrictors of the internal ring shutter mechanism, allowing later herniation of abdominal contents through a patent processus vaginalis. In one report, laparoscopic views of the internal inguinal ring shortly after acute appendicitis and subsequent appendectomy demonstrated poor-to-absent contraction of the internal ring during coughing or straining. The possibility of a temporary neuropraxia related to surgical trauma could have been responsible, but there is a threefold greater incidence of right inguinal hernia in men who had undergone appendectomy (40).

During surgical exposure of the common femoral artery and the distal external iliac artery for various types of vascular procedures (e.g., aortofemoral bypass), the inguinal ligament and the musculoaponeurotic borders of the inguinal ring must be divided. If closure of the abdominal wall is made with attention to reconstruction of the specific layers of the abdominal wall, including the internal ring, these hernias can be avoided. When the important layers are missing or deficient, the use of mesh reinforcement in the preperitoneal position is definitely indicated at present. Some individuals with severe groin pain after vascular access operations have no discrete hernia sac, but instead possess a lax internal ring that allows preperitoneal fat to bulge (herniate) through it; these individuals are comparable to adults with a symptomatic lipoma of the cord, who

often have pain indistinguishable from frank groin hernia, and who do extremely well with removal of the lipoma and reconstruction of the floor of the inguinal canal (41).

Increased hydrostatic intra-abdominal pressure associated with chronic ambulatory peritoneal dialysis (CAPD) frequently results in hernia development (28,29). An incidence rate of 20% to 50% depends upon the length of follow-up, with most of the hernias occurring in the groin and umbilicus. Hernias may also occur at the exit site of the dialysis catheter, or at other weak points in the abdominal lining. Because the groin is the most frequent site, there is no doubt that congenital factors have set the stage for the appearance of the hernia in this area; because renal failure per se has a deleterious effect on collagen metabolism, a multifactorial causality due to increased abdominal pressure, poor wound healing, and defective or suboptimal collagen synthesis exists (29,35).

Hernia may also appear at trocar sites or at points of egress of various tubes and drainage devices; advances in trocar technology, which avoid cutting the fascia (bladeless or dilating devices), have reduced but not eliminated the possibility of late hernia, and not surprisingly hernias have been reported after closure of port sites.

TYPES OF ABDOMINAL WALL HERNIAS

Groin Hernias

Hernias may develop in any structure supporting the intra-abdominal contents. Most of these involve the anterior abdominal wall, and the vast majority occur in the inguinofemoral region. Of hernias occurring in the groin, the indirect inguinal variety is most frequently encountered (50–60%), with direct inguinal hernias representing 25% to 35% and femoral hernias comprising approximately 5% to 10%. Because of the frequency of groin hernias, an understanding of their anatomy, clinical presentation, and surgical management is important for any student of surgery (9).

Indirect Inguinal Hernia

Indirect hernias are protrusions of weakened transversalis fascia, fat, or abdominal contents through a defect in the internal ring. The internal ring, at one end of the inguinal canal, is the transit point for gonadal tissue in males, or for the round ligament in females, and lies lateral to the deep epigastric artery and vein (Fig. 1A). Indirect hernia occurs 20 times more commonly in males compared to females, representing retention or incomplete obliteration of the embryologic processus vaginalis, which accompanies the testicle in its descent into the scrotum; in females, the indirect hernia is related to a persistent canal of Nuck, which is adherent to the round ligament.

Normally the processus vaginalis obliterates postnatally except for the tunica vaginalis portion that covers the testicle; a patent processus vaginalis is either a "communicating hydrocele" or an indirect inguinal hernia is present. Whether the hernia is evident at birth or in the months thereafter depends upon other factors. A hernial sac that tracks into the scrotum is a *complete* indirect inguinal hernia. The peak incidence of indirect inguinal hernia recurrence is at birth or shortly thereafter, with a second peak occurring in the teen years and in early adulthood (22,23).

Direct Inguinal Hernia

Direct hernias arise medial to the deep epigastric artery and somewhat inferior to the internal inguinal ring due to a frank defect or diffuse weakening of the transversalis fascia, in a

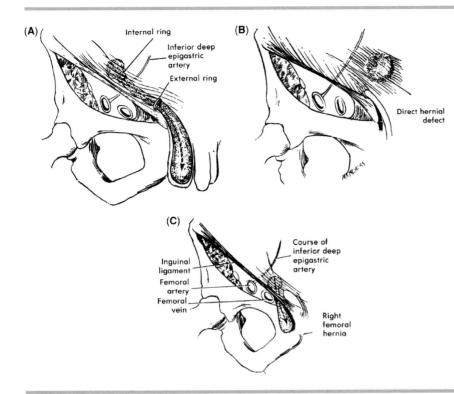

Figure 1 (**A**) Right indirect inguinal hernia. Hernial sac begins at the internal inguinal ring lateral to the inferior deep epigastric artery and exits from the inguinal canal at the external ring to descend into the scrotum. The sac lies anteromedial to the cord structures. (**B**) Right direct inguinal hernia. Hernial sac arises in Hesselbach's triangle medial to the inferior deep epigastric artery and just above the pubic tubercle. It does not descend into the scrotum. (**C**) Right femoral hernia. Hernial sac arises below the inguinal ligament and medial to the femoral vein. *Source*: From Ref. 42.

triangular space known as Hesselbach's triangle (Fig. 1B). Hesselbach's triangle is bounded laterally by the inferior epigastric artery, medially by the lateral border of the rectus sheath, and inferiorly by the inguinal ligament. Direct hernias occur later in life than congenital groin hernias, often after the age of 35. They are usually due to a weakened transversalis fascia as opposed to an opening in the transversalis, which occurs in a minority of cases. In contrast to an indirect inguinal hernia in which the neck of the hernia may be narrow and incarceration always a potential problem, the neck with direct hernias is wide, and incarceration is infrequent. Direct hernias are more common in males.

Sliding Hernia

A sliding hernia is one in which a viscus comprises part of the hernia sac, and is the term applied to slippage of part of an abdominal organ through a hernia orifice, and is common in huge groin hernias. On the right side, the appendix and cecum are commonly seen, while on the left side, the sigmoid colon is a common participant in this type of hernia. In females with inguinal hernia, the fallopian tube and ovary are commonly involved.

Femoral Hernia

A femoral hernia develops as a peritoneal outpouching through an enlarged femoral ring (Fig. 1C). This space is the most medial compartment of the femoral canal, and is bounded below by the inguinal ligament, above by the pubic bone, and medially by the lacunar ligament. The sac of a femoral hernia is always medial to the femoral vein and may progress to the level of the foramen ovale. Because the neck of a femoral hernia is narrow, incarceration and strangulation is always a risk. Femoral hernias occur more often in females for unknown reasons, possibly due to stretching of the pelvic supports during pregnancy.

Clinical Presentation

The usual complaint that brings a patient to the physician's attention when a groin hernia is present is a bulge or a problem with pain, either of which may be persistent or intermittent. The pain is due to compression or irritation of contiguous structures by the hernia. The characteristics of the pain are variable; while usually localized to the groin, it may be sharp, aggravated by a change in position or straining. The pain is often relieved by cessation of the physical activity that precipitated it. When hernia contents are incarcerated, persistent pain may reflect the onset of strangulation in the trapped contents; the presence of systemic signs or symptoms such as elevated temperature, tachycardia, vomiting, and abdominal distention must be recognized as urgent signals by clinicians, if catastrophic consequences due to intestinal necrosis are to be avoided. Symptoms of chronically incarcerated segments of intestine are highly variable, ranging from none to those of bowel obstruction.

Diagnosis of Hernia

Groin hernias are sometimes extremely difficult to diagnose and at other times quite apparent. The standard maneuver to diagnose a groin hernia is based on digital palpation of the floor of the inguinal canal. The patient should initially stand while visual inspection of the groin is conducted. The physician examines the external genitalia to check for any localized swellings along the spermatic cord on either side, or for abnormalities in the testicle or scrotal contents. In a female, there may be palpable swelling noted on the symptomatic side. In any case, ipsilateral swelling in a groin in which pain is apparent requires definite explanation, and the inference that a hernia is present becomes quite tenable. However, inflammation of the vas deferens and seminal vesiculitis must always be considered in the differential diagnosis.

When examining the floor of the inguinal canal in the male, there are three prerequisites for a complete examination: first, invagination of the scrotal skin along the axis of the canal allowing digital palpation of the external inguinal ring. The external ring is a landmark for examination; its size or consistency has nothing to do with the hernia itself. Secondly, digital palpation of the floor of the canal and the overlying spermatic cord are performed to ascertain any apparent weakness. A weakness or mass in the region of the external ring is usually indicative of a direct hernia. Finally, examination of the face of Hesselbach's triangle itself is performed. After the preliminary palpation to determine whether exquisite tenderness is present, the examining finger is withdrawn 5 to 10 mm, and the patient is asked to "push down" or "strain" for 5 to 10 seconds to increase intra-abdominal pressure. Next, the patient is asked to give a gentle cough. A positive response is a palpable "tap" against the fingertip (suggestive of an indirect hernia) or along the medial side of the finger (indicative of a direct hernia), caused as the distended hernia sac transmits the cough-induced increase in pressure. Alternatively, a "gurgle" of peritoneal fluid may be appreciated passing beneath the examining finger.

What Next?

When there is no palpable hernia defect, no history of groin lump or mass, and no ultrasound findings or positive peritoneography indicative of hernia. If no previous operation has been performed, the author advises the patient that there may be a hernia present, but that a groin strain or stretch might also be present; analgesics, tincture of time, and warm soaks (tub baths) are recommended during a six- to eight-week observation period. If the pain is unchanged or worse after that time, surgical exploration of the groin can be justified even when the examiner has no absolute evidence that a hernia exists; this would not be the case if noninvasive testing could detect all hernias. Patients must have realistic expectations however, and understand that the operation might not resolve the pain issue; the overall incidence of chronic groin pain or discomfort is high enough, approximately 1.0%, that some experienced surgeons have recommended routine division of the ilioinguinal nerve during hernia repair (43). As with any condition with a low frequency, individual surgeons have limited experience with this problem; further, because there is no clear cause for the problem, responses to treatment are highly individualized.

The differential diagnosis of postoperative pain includes ilioinguinal nerve entrapment or neuroma, nonspecific pain syndrome, or inflammation of the pubis or cord contents. In the presence of a typical pain syndrome but negative physical examination in the early postoperative period, one or several injections (local anesthesia combined with triamcinolone acetate) may resolve the issue; if pain persists despite exclusion of other causes, surgical re-exploration of the groin is performed early if there is radiation of pain to the leg or medial thigh, attempting to remedy nerve entrapment or encroachment. Because the scarified groin is hostile to reexploration as a rule, the patient must know that some numbness in the groin or proximal leg might result; this type of patient is extremely challenging, and requires all of the interpersonal and scientific skills of the surgeon and pain-management team. Some individuals will have persistent postoperative discomfort despite everyone's best efforts. In a world in which litigious patients sometimes have no tolerance for postoperative discomfort,

the informed surgeon should make certain that the risk of chronic pain is well understood and documented to the patient. If the patient is an adolescent, the discussion regarding risk of testicular atrophy should also be documented. Duplex ultrasound is invaluable at times in demonstrating that spermatic artery function is normal in a postoperative patient, and can relieve much of the mental anguish of patient and surgeon alike.

In contrast to most inguinal hernias that can be diagnosed with a minimum of difficulty, the femoral hernia is often a diagnostic challenge. It may appear as a subtle mass lesion in the inguinal crease, somewhat medial to the femoral artery, and may be quite small (approximately 1.0 cm diameter); in obese individuals, the hernia may be clinically occult. In such situations, the general condition of the patient will have to serve as a guide for the specific management plan undertaken. Patients who experience an unexplained acute onset of local pain in the femoral region, or develop pain or tenderness in a groin mass may have an incarcerated hernia and should have prompt surgical exploration. Inattention to sentinel signs places the patient at extreme risk for strangulation of hernia contents with subsequent complications.

Surgical Management

Until recently, hernias in the groin were considered, with rare exceptions (e.g., terminal malignant disease), as indications for surgical repair to prevent complications such as incarceration and strangulation. This concept has been challenged by modern surgeons and by health system analysts in the context of "watchful waiting" as discussed earlier (4,5). The prospective trials that will be reported in the next few years will shed light on an important (and expensive from a resource-utilization perspective) topic; the importance of these studies to the community at large is immense, and the surgeons who devised these trials deserve our thanks and recognition.

The anatomy of the groin hernia is defined in terms of the various "fasciae, aponeuroses, and ligaments" present; a fascia is a condensation of connective tissue into a definable, homogenous layer that varies from a thin layer to an easily observed stout structure (9). An aponeurosis is a tendinous insertion of a major muscle composed of strong, individual, collagenous fiber bundles. A ligament is any definable tissue "banding" two or more structures, whether bony or visceral, and may refer to structures of either areolar or aponeurotic consistency. The transversus abdominis aponeurosis is the dense connective tissue at the boundary of that specific muscle; the transversalis fascia, in contradistinction, is a separate connective tissue entity that lines the entire abdominal cavity, and is the first anatomic boundary that visceral structures stretch or pass through as they herniate through a defect in the abdominal wall. Transversalis fascia has little anatomic strength, and cannot form an anatomic basis for hernia repairs; instead, all herniated structures are restored to their anatomic position behind the transversalis fascia prior to suture repair of the hernia by approximation of neighboring tendinous aponeuroses and ligaments that can hold sutures properly (9). Formerly, the repair of all common groin hernias was designed to permanently eliminate anatomic defects by means of sutures placed into adjacent solid structures; recently this concept has been supplanted by the recognition that the appearance of a hernia is a declaration that tissues cannot withstand the tension or force exerted at the specific hernia site. At present, therefore, "tension-free" approaches, which eliminate or minimize the tension by a variety of mechanisms have been widely adopted, with resulting improvement in long-term success of hernia repairs (7,44,45).

Groin Hernia Anatomy

The aponeurosis of the external oblique muscle inserts at the pubic tubercle and has a flattened medial portion, which curves beneath the floor of the inguinal canal, and is termed the "inguinal ligament". The inguinal ligament abuts fascia of the transversus abdominis muscle as a contiguous but separate structure. The lacunar ligament is a triangular portion of the inguinal ligament, which extends from the posterior border of the inguinal ligament downwards to the pectineal fascia (1 cm below the pectin); it is separate and superficial to the ileopubic tract. These anatomic details are illustrated in Figure 2.

Before the tension-free concept was widely recognized, the rationale for hernia repair was reconstruction of the separate layers of the abdominal wall, "preserving" (at least from a theoretical perspective) the "shutter" mechanism effected by the muscles of the abdominal wall. Analogously as a camera shutter mechanism, the oblique muscles comprising the internal ring move simultaneously in different planes, constricting the internal ring in so doing. As a result, the superior and inferior crus of the internal inguinal ring compress the internal ring and spermatic cord, narrowing the aperture of Hesselbach's triangle. The end result is continuous protection for the two most vulnerable areas of the groin: posterior wall of the inguinal canal, where direct hernias appear, and the entrance to the canal itself, through which "oblique" herniation occurs.

Anterior Repair—Groin Hernia

Inguinal Hernias. The goal of repair in the modern era is the creation of a tension-free union between the arching transversalis abdominus aponeurosis (and adherent fascia) above and the ileopubic tract below; the best way to achieve tension-free status is interposition of a piece of mesh between the boundaries of the weakened floor of the inguinal canal. Whether this approach (the Lichtenstein repair) is supplemented with a "plug," is a matter of personal preference and choice; either approach has the benefit of a lower recurrence rate (0.5–1.0% vs. 5–8%) compared to conventional repair.

For both direct and indirect inguinal hernias, the repair is carried out through a transverse skin incision positioned above (approximately 2 cm) and parallel to the inguinal ligament, to prevent injury to the iliohypogastric and ilioinguinal nerves (Fig. 3). For hernias lateral to the inferior epigastric vessels (i.e., indirect inguinal hernias), the communication that exists between the peritoneal cavity and the hernial sac is obliterated, with or without excision of the sac. Very large or vascularized sacs can be left in situ with the expectation that they will gradually disappear; aggressive dissection of these sacs is mentioned only to be condemned, because of the risk of damage to the fragile blood supply of the vas deferens (Fig. 4).

In infants and children, high ligation of the sac is usually all that is required; in older children and adults, some reconstruction of the musculoaponeurotic structures is generally performed (Marcy repair) to tighten the internal inguinal ring around the cord structures. Occasionally, an indirect inguinal hernia will be encountered, which has been present for many years and has enlarged to such an extent that a good portion of the supporting structures medial to the internal ring has been destroyed. In this situation, a definitive tension-free repair will be required, following the principles described below, for the repair of a direct inguinal hernia.

The cremaster muscle fibers surrounding the spermatic cord can usually be spared, thus avoiding circumferential dissection of the internal inguinal ring. Through careful dissection, the attenuated floor of the inguinal canal is exposed or excised; the original Bassini repair included excision of the attenuated floor, and provided direct exposure of the edge

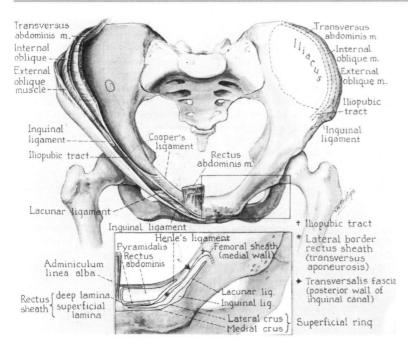

Figure 2 Left pelvis: Origins of the three flat muscles are shown. The oblique and transversus muscles arise from the iliacus fascia and iliopectineal arch (not shown). Inset shows the insertions of the muscle layers of the groin into the pubis. Right pelvis: Internal oblique is not shown, but would arch above the spermatic cord to insert into the rectus sheath. *Source*: From Ref. 46.

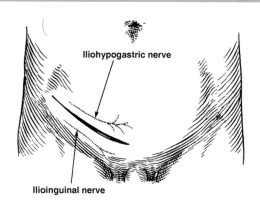

Figure 3 Skin incision is made approximately 2 cm above the inguinal ligament in a gentle curve following Langer's lines. *Source:* From Ref. 47.

of the attenuated fascia. The repair must obliterate or bridge the defect by suture or prosthetic patch as the first goal and prevent recurrence as the second goal. Suture repairs help achieve the first goal well by the transversus/transversalis complex above the ileopubic tract below (Fig. 5) with interrupted nonabsorbable suture material; tension-free repairs, as we now recognize, are far superior in preventing recurrence of hernias. In the past, surgeons utilized various "relaxing incisions" to achieve a relatively tension-free approach; however, when all tension is removed by a bridge or patch of synthetic material as in the Lichtenstein approach (a literally "tension-free" repair), the result is superior to any purely mechanical approach described (Fig. 6). Formerly, surgeons debated the merits of several maneuvers to reduce the stresses created by hernia repair, including the Tanner "slide" procedure, one of the approaches for reducing tension by means of a relaxing incision (43). Incision along the internal oblique portion of the anterior rectus sheath allows the lateral portion of this sheath and its attached transversus arch to "slide" inferolaterally, so as to close a large inguinal hernial

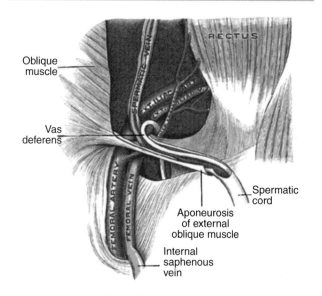

Figure 4 Spermatic artery.

defect; (Figs. 7 and 8) while the utility of relaxing incisions is widely accepted, the wide use of mesh repairs has made relaxing incisions less important (43).

When repairing direct hernias, the surgeon should consider the simultaneous presence of an indirect hernia, which will exist in many of the patients; the spermatic cord should be inspected to demonstrate the junction of the obliterated vaginal process with the peritoneum at the internal ring.

Synthetic Mesh, Plugs, and Patches
At present, it is apparent that routine mesh insertion lowers recurrence rates substantially; in groin hemiorrhaphy, mesh insertion results in an expected recurrence rate of 0.5% to 2.0% versus 7% to 12% when mesh is not employed. The choice of mesh is a matter of judgment, and the flat mesh prosthesis of Lichtenstein, and the various "plugs" and patch devices are commonly employed (7,44). Surgeons, formerly preoccupied with creative uses of endogenous ligaments and tissues to repair hernia defects, now apply the mesh prostheses with confidence that the problem will be solved. The routine use of mesh in adults is the most important advance in hernia repair in the last 50 years. In children or young adults primary repair consisting of sac excision—with or without the Marcy "plastic repair or the internal ring," is still practiced widely (50).

Femoral Hernias. Although femoral hernias are less commonly encountered than inguinal hernias, surgical repair is the treatment of choice. The principles underlying inguinal hernia repair also apply to femoral hernias. Usually the same type of skin incision is used; the sac, once identified, is reduced of its hernial contents, divided, and ligated at its neck; and the entrance into the femoral canal giving rise to this entity is obliterated. This can be accomplished by attaching the transversus/transversalis complex to Cooper's ligament to close off the empty space in the femoral canal.

Posterior Repair
The posterior approach to the transversalis/transversus layers of the abdominal wall (Fig. 9) has been advocated by several surgeons over the past 60 years, but predominantly by Nyhus et al. (52). This technique, when properly applied, is extremely useful in the repair of three major types of hernia: (i) the recurrent inguinal hernia, (ii) the primary femoral hernia, and (iii) incarcerated hernias of all types.

Surgeons unfamiliar with the posterior appearance of groin structures may have difficulty in defining the proper tissue planes, but the widespread interest in laparoscopic hernia repairs has served to educate the surgical community regarding the preperitoneal repair. Many surgeons have abandoned the laparoscopic approach, because the overall risks and benefits are unproven and the cost is high; proponents of the repair are extremely enthusiastic about its benefits, but cannot demonstrate any superiority of the repair when compared head-to-head with open surgical techniques.

When performed as an open procedure, the skin incision is placed transversely, 2.0 cm above and parallel to the inguinal ligament. After the incision to the level of the rectus sheath is deepened, the anterior fascia layer of this sheath is incised, and the rectus muscle retracted toward the midline. The exposed transversalis fascia is then incised to gain access to the preperitoneal space; this space always has a variable amount of fat present, and the appearance of fatty tissue is the signal that the proper plane has been entered. The incision through the abdominal musculature is widened toward the anterior iliac spine, to pass about 2.0 cm above

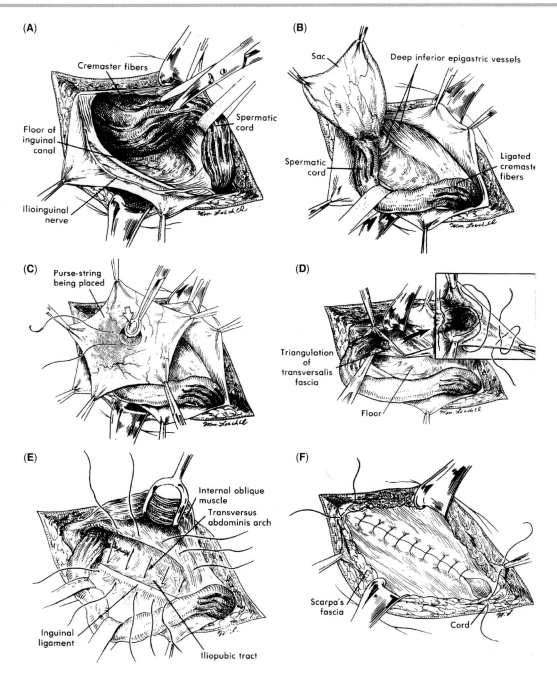

Figure 5 **(A)** Steps in the repair of a right indirect inguinal hernia. The external oblique aponeurosis has been opened. The cord is freed from the inguinal floor. The freed ilioinguinal nerve is seen overlying the retracted lower leaflet of the external oblique aponeurosis. The cremaster muscle is being dissected free of the cord. **(B)** Peritoneal sac must be dissected free of the cord and the abdominal wall at the internal abdominal ring. **(C)** Technical detail of high ligation of the sac is important in an orderly repair. The peritoneum must be freed of omentum, and adherent viscera must be detached. Appendices epiploicae or omentum must not be caught in the closure. **(D)** Components of the transversus abdominis lamina must be accurately identified and closed at the internal ring. Triangulation of the transversalis fascia (shown here) is a useful detail to help achieve accurate closure at the internal ring. **(E)** Transversus abdominis arch is sutured to the iliopubic tract and inguinal ligament. **(F)** External oblique aponeurosis is closed over the spermatic cord. Slight imbrication of this structure gives an excellent closure. Scarpa's fascia is then closed with interrupted sutures of 3–0 plain catgut, and the skin edges approximated with sutures or sterile strips. *Source*: From Ref. 47.

the internal inguinal ring. When this has been accomplished, the posterior inguinal wall is bared of fatty and areolar tissue from the line of incision to the superior pubic ramus. If the deep epigastric vessels obscure proper exposure, they can be ligated and divided as needed.

After the posterior inguinal wall has been exposed, the herniated structures are identified and reduced. If there is an incarcerated hernia, it is prudent (and easy) to inspect all portions of incarcerated bowel for signs of ischemia or infarction. If there is any doubt concerning these possibilities, the surgeon can easily observe the tissues in question until he/she is satisfied about the need for surgical resection. After the walls of the hernial defect have been identified, the repair is fashioned to approximate the margins of

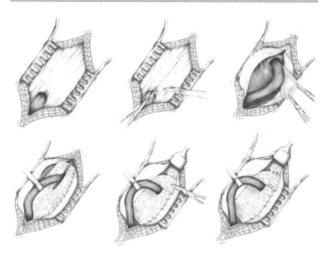

Figure 6 Lichtensein Repair. *Source:* From Ref. 48.

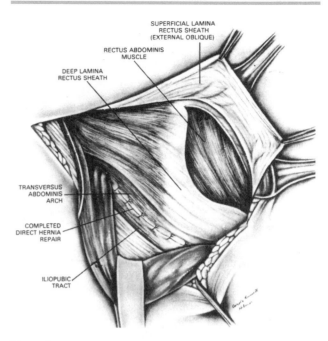

Figure 8 Completed direct hernia repair demonstrates that the relaxing incision allows the transversus abdominis to slide inferiorly. As the relaxing incision opens, the rectus muscle is exposed, but the overlying intact superficial lamina (external oblique aponeurosis) of the rectus sheath supports the muscle externally while the intact fascia posteriorly shields the potential hernial defect. *Source:* From Ref. 49.

the defect with interrupted sutures of permanent material or bridge the hernia defect with a suitably large prosthetic patch. As with the anterior approach to hernia repair, the internal ring and spermatic cord must also be examined to ensure that an additional oblique hernia is not present; the vas deferens is pushed to the lateral margin of the operative field, and overlapped widely by the preperitoneal mesh. This practice of "lateralization" as opposed to the construction of a "keyhole" aperture in the mesh may have less tendency to constrict the vas deferens in the postoperative period.

The posterior approach is strongly recommended for the repair of a recurrent hernia, because it provides an

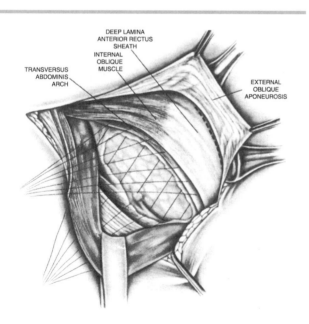

Figure 7 External oblique aponeurosis (superficial lamina rectus sheath) has been dissected medially and superiorly to the line of fusion with rectus sheath. Placement of a relaxing incision in the deep lamina of rectus sheath (transversus abdominis and internal oblique aponeurosis) is shown by dotted line. *Source:* From Ref. 49.

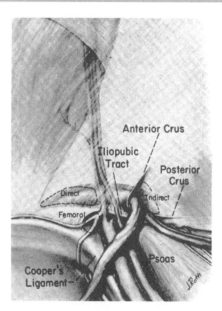

Figure 9 The preperitoneal exposure of the posterior inguinal wall displays the important structures that form the boundaries of groin hernias. Repair of hernial defect(s) is readily accomplished by suture, after preliminary reduction of the hernia. If an indirect hernial sac extends into the scrotum, it is not necessary that the entire distal sac be removed. Note that application of mesh is quite easy, because the posterior wall is completely exposed. *Source:* From Ref. 51.

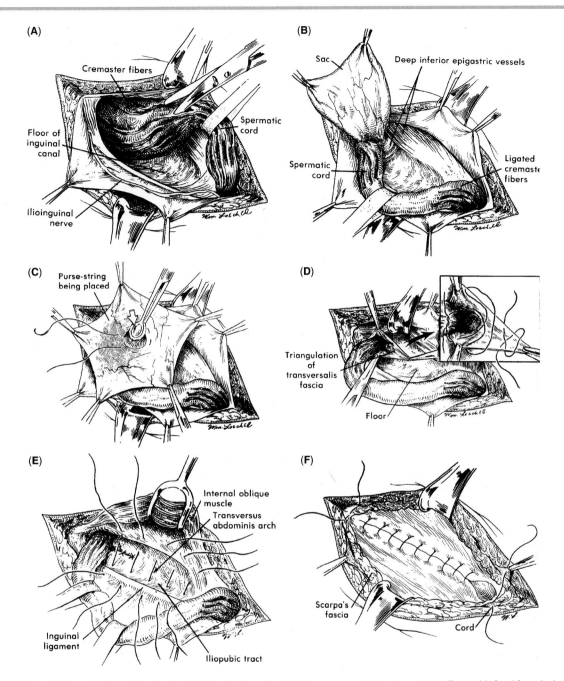

Figure 5 **(A)** Steps in the repair of a right indirect inguinal hernia. The external oblique aponeurosis has been opened. The cord is freed from the inguinal floor. The freed ilioinguinal nerve is seen overlying the retracted lower leaflet of the external oblique aponeurosis. The cremaster muscle is being dissected free of the cord. **(B)** Peritoneal sac must be dissected free of the cord and the abdominal wall at the internal abdominal ring. **(C)** Technical detail of high ligation of the sac is important in an orderly repair. The peritoneum must be freed of omentum, and adherent viscera must be detached. Appendices epiploicae or omentum must not be caught in the closure. **(D)** Components of the transversus abdominis lamina must be accurately identified and closed at the internal ring. Triangulation of the transversalis fascia (shown here) is a useful detail to help achieve accurate closure at the internal ring. **(E)** Transversus abdominis arch is sutured to the iliopubic tract and inguinal ligament. **(F)** External oblique aponeurosis is closed over the spermatic cord. Slight imbrication of this structure gives an excellent closure. Scarpa's fascia is then closed with interrupted sutures of 3–0 plain catgut, and the skin edges approximated with sutures or sterile strips. *Source*: From Ref. 47.

the internal inguinal ring. When this has been accomplished, the posterior inguinal wall is bared of fatty and areolar tissue from the line of incision to the superior pubic ramus. If the deep epigastric vessels obscure proper exposure, they can be ligated and divided as needed.

After the posterior inguinal wall has been exposed, the herniated structures are identified and reduced. If there

is an incarcerated hernia, it is prudent (and easy) to inspect all portions of incarcerated bowel for signs of ischemia or infarction. If there is any doubt concerning these possibilities, the surgeon can easily observe the tissues in question until he/she is satisfied about the need for surgical resection. After the walls of the hernial defect have been identified, the repair is fashioned to approximate the margins of

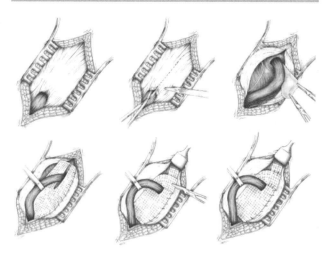

Figure 6 Lichtensein Repair. *Source:* From Ref. 48.

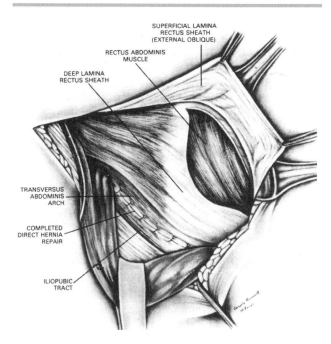

Figure 8 Completed direct hernia repair demonstrates that the relaxing incision allows the transversus abdominis to slide inferiorly. As the relaxing incision opens, the rectus muscle is exposed, but the overlying intact superficial lamina (external oblique aponeurosis) of the rectus sheath supports the muscle externally while the intact fascia posteriorly shields the potential hernial defect. *Source:* From Ref. 49.

the defect with interrupted sutures of permanent material or bridge the hernia defect with a suitably large prosthetic patch. As with the anterior approach to hernia repair, the internal ring and spermatic cord must also be examined to ensure that an additional oblique hernia is not present; the vas deferens is pushed to the lateral margin of the operative field, and overlapped widely by the preperitoneal mesh. This practice of "lateralization" as opposed to the construction of a "keyhole" aperture in the mesh may have less tendency to constrict the vas deferens in the postoperative period.

The posterior approach is strongly recommended for the repair of a recurrent hernia, because it provides an

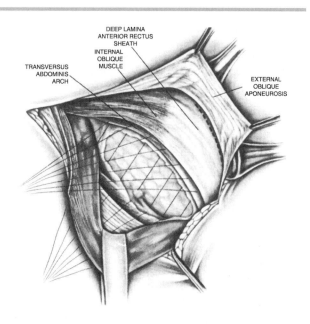

Figure 7 External oblique aponeurosis (superficial lamina rectus sheath) has been dissected medially and superiorly to the line of fusion with rectus sheath. Placement of a relaxing incision in the deep lamina of rectus sheath (transversus abdominis and internal oblique aponeurosis) is shown by dotted line. *Source:* From Ref. 49.

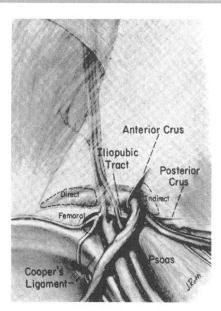

Figure 9 The preperitoneal exposure of the posterior inguinal wall displays the important structures that form the boundaries of groin hernias. Repair of hernial defect(s) is readily accomplished by suture, after preliminary reduction of the hernia. If an indirect hernial sac extends into the scrotum, it is not necessary that the entire distal sac be removed. Note that application of mesh is quite easy, because the posterior wall is completely exposed. *Source:* From Ref. 51.

opportunity to perform the operation in virgin tissue, which is clearly a distinct advantage over any anterior approach. As with all recurrent hernias, a synthetic mesh buttress should be sutured to the posterior wall (Fig. 10), the only caveat regarding mesh in the preperitoneal space is the avoidance of sutures near the femoral nerve or the lateral femoral cutaneous nerve.

Laparoscopic Repair—Abdominal Wall and Groin Hernia

Laparoscopic Approaches to Groin Hernia Repair. Laparoscopic hernia repair, which evolved rapidly following the first demonstration of the feasibility of this approach in the early 1980s, is now being widely performed in many hospitals. The earlier success of posterior approaches to hernia repair, incorporating the concepts of tension-free repair as propounded by Lichtenstein (7), Stoppa, Condon and Nyhus, and Read (44), sets the stage for the rapid development and popularity of this approach. At this time it is clear that early recurrence rates after laparoscopic hernia repair are at least comparable, but possibly worse than those observed following open herniorrhaphy. The recent Type I evidence favoring open repair over laparoscopic hemiorrhaphy is of immense interest in this regard (53).

Several innovative approaches have been attempted in laboratory and clinical settings: plugs, double-patches, intraperitoneal onlay of mesh (IPOM), preperitoneal patch, self-expanding patches, etc. All of these are variations on the theme of the current best approaches regarding hernia repair elucidated above; in 2005, the important components of these repairs are that they are tension-free, and reinforced with synthetic mesh (Figs. 11–13). IPOM appeared satisfactory in both laboratory and clinical settings when first introduced; presently it continues to be reported with enthusiasm in sporadic reports, but possible concerns about mesh in the peritoneal cavity still persist.

The attraction of the totally extraperitoneal (preperitoneal) approach to groin hernia repair is real, but there is still the problem of gaining access without entering the peritoneal cavity and the risk of injury to structures in the vicinity. It is hard to predict whether this approach will become a favored one with surgeons at large, because of technical difficulties.

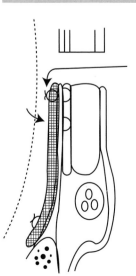

Figure 10 Large arrow illustrates the approach to the preperitoneal space, above the inguinal canal. Small arrow shows the preliminary repair of the hernia defect before insertion of the "regional" prosthetic reinforcement that extends from the primary incision to the pubic ramus and from the midline to lateral of the internal ring.

Laparoscopy, per se, puts the patient at some risk for injury to small intestine, either immediately during the operation, or as a late complication due to the contiguous synthetic mesh materials employed in the hernia repair. If the prolene or marlex mesh is used, there is concern about adhesions or irritation of adjoining organs, similarly as that observed following insertion of these artificial agents in abdominal wall repairs. Additional injuries have been rarely noted in other structures, including hollow organs (vas deferens, urinary bladder, and colon), nerves (ilioinguinal, genitofemoral, lateral femoral cutaneous, and femoral), and vessels (iliac artery and vein and femoral artery and vein). While operative injuries are higher after laparoscopic procedures than following open operations, the advantage of being able to return to work earlier is appreciated by many patients, and many patients (who have had both approaches) favor the use of minimally invasive means. The earlier return to full activity with minimal pain is compelling for some but not all patients; whether the increased cost of performing hernial repair by this means can thus be justified or will continue to be supported by providers is still uncertain (53,54). Which minimally invasive approach to hernial repair will become the most desired cannot be predicted at this time. It is clear that this approach has unique risks, and that some of the problems with laparoscopic procedures are unknown; long term follow-up and analysis of these problems will clarify the issue for a worldwide group of interested surgeons and patients.

Complications

There are many possible problems that may develop following inguinofemoral herniorrhaphy as summarized in Table 1. These should be recognized and discussed with the patient in a direct and supportive way, because the patient's initial reaction will often be one of suspicion and fear that something bad may happen. Several complications related to the hernia repair itself need to be considered.

Swollen Testicle. The swollen testis is a major concern for patients undergoing groin hernia repair, may be due to venous engorgement or lymphatic congestion secondary to the repair itself, compromise to the arterial blood flow as a result of intraoperative trauma, a subfascial hematoma, or a missed hernia (such as an indirect inguinal hernia when a direct hernia was being repaired). In these troubling cases, the management is usually guided by evaluating the overall clinical picture over a period of time. It will usually resolve over a period of 4 to 12 weeks, and the patient will only need the mature guidance of the surgeon during this interval to allay any fears that he may have. In those situations in which the blood supply to the testicle has been compromised, late atrophy of the testis will be noted; this complication is not rare, yet the true incidence is hard to determine because of limited follow-up studies in most reported series of patients undergoing groin herniorrhaphy. Occasionally, an acute infarction of the testicle will develop postoperatively, which will require immediate surgical intervention and eventual orchiectomy; there is never an indication for immediate excision, however, and the availability of duplex ultrasound is of immense value in determining viability (i.e., adequate arterial blood flow) of the affected testis. Ultrasound can also distinguish between "normal" and abnormal masses in the groin after herniorrhaphy (55).

Pain. Occasionally, a patient will develop a persistent pain following groin herniorrhaphy. Most of the pain is of the

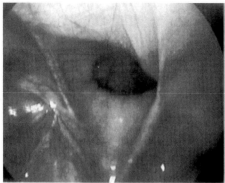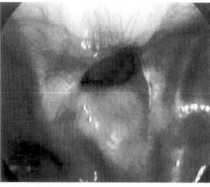

Figure 11 Laparoscopic view illustrates the major advantages of this approach: the vas deferens, testicular vessels, and surrounding structures are seen with clarity and definition, which is not possible by other means.

rapidly subsiding variety, and the pain is usually manageable for three to five days postoperatively. The tension-free repairs are remarkably free of pain in most patients by the second day, although many complain of residual discomfort for several weeks. By the third or fourth week, there is only a residual tenderness to deep palpation, and by three to four months, there are no symptoms referable to the operation. The presence of a "healing" ridge of tissue along the line of incision may be a concern to patients and their families, but reassurance that this is a commonly encountered phenomenon is usually all that is required.

The importance of non-narcotic analgesics, heating pads, and avoidance of unnecessary stress is very important during the first week after operation. Some patients, conditioned to self-denial and personal effort, may believe they can and should ignore and "work through" the pain, but this is unrealistic and unnecessarily taxing to their family and medical supervisors.

Occasional patients have persistent complaints that can be quite troublesome and that can prove difficult to assess and treat successfully. The physical examination is very useful because it gives precise information about the possible sources of pain. For example, if the testicle is swollen or inflamed or if the epididymis is quite tender, a genitourinary infection might be suspected. Alternatively, the floor of the inguinal canal may be painless, whereas the pubic tubercle area is exquisitely tender. Is this an indication of periostitis of the pubic bone? Is this due to a suture that was placed to effect adequate repair? Usually, the surgeon is not sure, but in such cases, no specific intervention

aside from local care, anti-inflammatory medications, and local treatments is needed. After at least three to four months have passed, the acute perioperative reaction has usually subsided and most subjective complaints will have disappeared.

When persistent pain is found along the floor of the inguinal canal (but not at the internal ring), the possibility of a trapped nerve or neuroma must be considered; the problem for the surgeon is that the degree of pain is hard to assess immediately postoperatively. If a patient has excruciating pain immediately after operation, reoperation should be considered; if there is a radiation in the dermatome of the ilioinguinal nerve, the case for reoperation becomes even stronger. If the pain is less intense, but is persisting beyond two to three weeks, and centered along the floor of the inguinal canal, an injection of 2 to 3 mL of 1% xylocaine can be made at the point of tenderness to determine whether the groin discomfort disappears. If so, a "trigger" point has been identified, and the site can be injected with a mixture of cortisone (triamcinolone acetate 40 mg/mL with 1.0% xylocaine) and local anesthesia. Most patients will respond to this type of treatment with a clear decrease in symptoms and not require more than two injections. If unsuccessful, the patient has shown him/herself to be part of a special group of patients with chronic, moderately severe groin pain, for which there is often not a definite cure. Surgical excision of the superficial scar tissue and nerve tissue is indicated at some point, but most patients prefer to have initial treatment through a pain clinic approach.

(A)   **(B)**

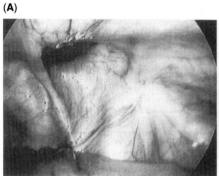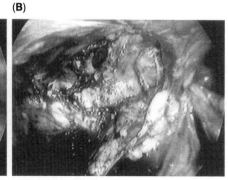

Figure 12 (A) View from the peritoneum reveals a right indirect inguinal hernia. After exposure of the collagenous supports, which will serve as an anchor for the prosthetic mesh, it is easy to plan a safe and effective repair of the defect. The tension-free approach will be used, with fixation only to the pubic ramus and the superior aspect of the transversus arch. **(B)** Landmarks that must be clearly identified include Cooper's ligament, the spermatic vessels and vas deferens, and the iliopubic tract.

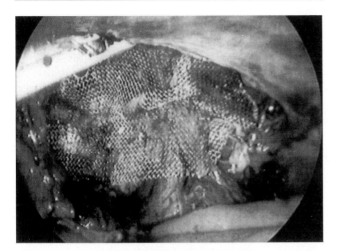

Figure 13 The essential concept governing mesh placement is that the mesh should be large enough to cover all potential hernia sites. The anchoring of the mesh is probably less important than previously thought, because the mesh will be held firmly by inflammatory adhesions postoperatively. When sutures or staples are used, none are placed inferior to the iliopubic tract and the lateral aspect of the internal ring is avoided. Staples placed in the iliopubic tract lateral to the internal ring may jeopardize branches of the femoral nerve.

Nerve Injury After Laparoscopic Repair. Laparoscopic hernia repairs provide unique risks for nerve injury due to the proximity of important nerves to the mesh, sutures, or staples utilized in repair. The femoral nerve, lateral femoral cutaneous nerve, genital branch of genitofemoral nerve, and ilioinguinal nerves have all been reported as injured during these operations. Caution in staple and mesh placement will

Table 1 Local or Regional Complications After Repair of Groin Hernias

Acute
Wound infection/hematoma
Ilioinguinal/iliohypogastric nerve injury
Preperitoneal hemorrhage
Femoral vein/artery laceration or trauma
Thrombosis femoral vein/pulmonary embolus
Transection of vas deferens
Ligation of spermatic artery
Perforation of viscus (sliding hernia)
Nonclosure of internal ring
Loss of domain of erstwhile incarcerated structures
Scrotal ecchymosis/hematoma
Swollen testis
Missed hernia
Urinary retention

Chronic
Recurrent hernia
Hernia in a contiguous area
Late wound/suture sepsis (>5 to 10 years later)
Neuroma
Testicular atrophy
Hydrocele
Pseudoaneurysm of femoral artery
Groin pain
Loss of cremasteric reflex
Periostitis of pubis
Sexual dysfunction

minimize the risk of these complications, but cannot prevent all postoperative problems.

Hernia Recurrence. The most important complication directly relating to the repair itself is that of hernia recurrence. Because of the mobility of our society and the consequent difficulty of following patients over the long term, the actual incidence of recurrence is probably not known. Most series would suggest that this incidence is somewhere between 2% and 10%. In a 22-year analysis of inguinal and femoral hernias repaired by McVay and Chapp (8), a 3.2% recurrence rate in over 1200 cases was noted. Almost 40% of the recurrences occurred after five years following the initial operation, illustrating the constraints of short evaluation periods. The best results ever reported in terms of recurrence rates are those from specialty groups such as the Shouldice Clinic and the Lichtenstein Hernia Institute (7). The Shouldice repair is performed through an anterior incision and includes maneuvers to ensure adequate exposure of the internal inguinal ring followed by an overlapping repair of the floor of the inguinal canal. The principles of this repair are narrowing of the internal ring and a multilayer reinforcement of the transversalis fascial layer. This repair is made without relaxing incisions and maximizes tension in the hernia site. Despite the lack of prosthetic mesh insertion, several authors have reported less than a 1% recurrence rate with this technique, regardless of whether primary or recurrent hernias were being treated.

The tension-free approaches of Lichtenstein and others have achieved similar results, and have been used by surgeons throughout the land as previously discussed.

Umbilical Hernia

Umbilical hernias occur where the umbilical ring has failed to obliterate the opening of the allantoic duct. The majority of these hernias are congenital in origin and are particularly common in Afro-American infants. Most of these hernias close spontaneously by the ages of four to six and almost never become incarcerated or strangulated, and therefore, infant congenital umbilical hernias rarely require surgical closure. Exceptions to this stance include hernias that are symptomatic, those in which the umbilical ring is excessively large so that external trauma poses a threat, and those that have demonstrated no significant closure by six years of age.

Umbilical hernias may also develop in adults. When they occur in this population, a number of predisposing factors appear to give rise to their development, including abdominal distention secondary to massive ascites from underlying disease such as Laennec's cirrhosis; induced ascites as occurs in patients undergoing CAPD, in patients who are pregnant, and in those who are obese; and in certain situations where there may be abnormal or defective collagen synthesis secondary to nutritional deficiencies or advancing age (10). Because many of these hernias have a small neck, the risk of incarceration and strangulation remains a continuing threat. Thus, most of these hernias should be surgically repaired, which can be easily accomplished through an infraumbilical or supraumbilical skin incision in which the sac is removed and the fascial edges surrounding the hernial defect are directly approximated with nonabsorbable sutures.

Hernias of the Linea Alba

In addition to the umbilical hernia, a number of other hernial defects traverse the linea alba. These hernias usually occur between the xiphoid process and the umbilicus, in which case they are termed as "epigastric" hernias; occasionally they may appear below the umbilicus. Hernias of the linea alba are usually small, often multiple, and typically contain preperitoneal fat. Their presentation clinically is often deceptive and may be apparent only as pinpoint convexities overlying the erect patient's linea alba. If the physical examination is negative, but the patient's complaint is persistent pain in this region anatomically, surgical exploration may be required to provide a definite diagnosis. The most cogent explanation for their development is the anatomy of the linea alba, a complex network of the three musculoaponeurotic components of the rectus sheath, which varies considerably in its inherent strength. There are at least three recognizable patterns of decussation of these fibers in the midline, all of which may be aggravated by marked distention of the abdominal wall. In addition, there are discreet areas midway between the xiphoid process and umbilicus that are subjected to repetitive stresses by phrenic aponeurotic bands that insert in the midline fascia; perhaps these latter structures eventually weaken the midline fascia and therefore help explain the location of most hernias in this area. Like umbilical hernias, repair of hernias involving the linea alba consist of excision and closure of the hernial sac and direct approximation of the edges of the defect in the fascia, with nonabsorbable sutures.

Spigelian Hernia

The spigelian hernia develops through a defect in the spigelian fascia (named after the Flemish anatomist Spieghel who described it in the 1600s). The locus of intersection of the semilunar and semicircular lines, the spigelian point, just lateral to where the lower one-third of the rectus fascia (Fig. 14). The development of a hernia in this area is often subtle; as an interparietal hernia, which does not penetrate the external oblique layer, it frequently presents a diagnostic challenge. Persistent pain and tenderness, and occasionally a palpable mass along the rectus muscle may be found. Most of the difficulty in the diagnosis results from the fact that these hernias are usually intramural, so that they may track from their site of origin in almost any direction, being covered by the external oblique muscle. Consequently, they are not obvious as hernial defects traversing the abdominal wall. US has been demonstrated to be of value in the diagnosis of spigelian hernia and for the evaluation of patients with unexplained abdominal wall pain; however, US has been supplanted by computerized axial tomography because it achieves the twofold goal of examination of the abdominal wall and intra-abdominal contents.

Since incarceration and strangulation may occur with spigelian hernias, they should be surgically repaired when diagnosed. Such repair is accomplished through a transverse incision over the site of origin, with division of the external oblique fascia for proper exposure of the hernial defect. Because the defect involves the aponeurosis of the transverse abdominus and internal oblique muscles, conventional repair involves approximation of these two fascial layers and subsequent closure of the divided external oblique fascia. Laparoscopic repair of these defects is also highly successful, and has the added advantage of not weakening the abdominal wall in the process.

Laparoscopic Ventral Hernia Repair

The tension-free approach has achieved moderate success in the repair of large ventral hernias, although the technical challenges of successful repair require the skill of an

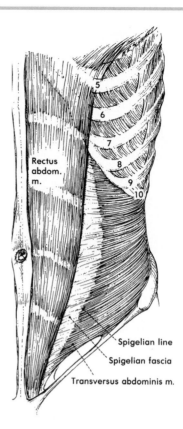

Figure 14 The rectus muscle aponeurosis extends from the fourth, fifth, and sixth ribs. The hernias along the lateral border of the rectus muscle do not penetrate the external oblique layer.

advanced laparoscopic surgeon. In general, the hernias of the abdominal wall can be treated successfully if there is sufficient overlap of mesh onto the abdominal wall, and if sufficient fixating sutures are placed through and through the abdominal wall. The newly available mesh materials, which include a smooth surface (to face the intestines) and a rough edge (to face the fascia and become incorporated), have been popular and have achieved the goals of successful hernia repair and minimal complications. The presence of a seroma is an ongoing concern, but with patience and periodic aspiration, these collections eventually disappear. If infection occurs, the mesh must be removed, but this occurs in less than 2% of cases.

Lumbar Hernia

Hernias arising in the lumbar region through the posterior abdominal wall are called *lumbar* or *dorsal* hernias. One of two sites is generally involved. The superior lumbar triangle, also called Grynfeltt's triangle, is the most common site of origin; the inferior lumbar triangle (also called Petit's triangle) is less frequently involved. The common clinical presentation is usually a mass in the flank that may or may not be associated with pain. On palpation, this mass is generally reducible, and incarceration and strangulation are usually not problems. Most lumbar hernias represent incisional hernias occurring in old nephrectomy incisions, but they may on occasion occur spontaneously. Surgical repair with approximation of the fascial edges of the hernia defect is the treatment of choice.

Pelvic Hernias

A variety of rare hernias may occur through the various foramina in the pelvic floor through which nerves and blood vessels pass into the buttocks or out of the pelvis. Various intra-abdominal structures may make up the hernial contents, small bowel being particularly frequent. The two common types of pelvic hernias include those that pass through the greater sciatic foramen and the obturator foramen. The diagnosis of these types of hernia is often first made at the time of surgery, when a portion of intestine becomes incarcerated, necessitating abdominal exploration. Occasionally an obturator hernia will be diagnosed as a swelling in the upper and medial aspect of the thigh associated with pain radiating to the medial aspect of the knee in the distribution of the obturator nerve (i.e., Howship-Romberg sign). In a patient in whom a sciatic or obturator hernia is suspected, herniography provides confirmation. Both types of hernias are usually repaired through an abdominal approach in which the hernial sac and its contents are reduced (with resection of necrotic bowel if indicated) and primary closure of the fascial defect is performed. Another type of pelvic hernia may occur when there is a defect in the levator sling in the floor of the pelvis. A protrusion through this defect is called a *perineal hernia* and usually appears as a bulge just lateral to the midline perineal raphe. These hernias are usually secondary to a previous surgical procedure such as an abdominoperineal resection or a prostatectomy. Repair involves fascial closure of the perineal defect, usually through a combined abdominal and perineal approach. Perineal hernias are often asymptomatic, but depending on their location they may be associated with pain on sitting or a variety of urinary complaints, predominantly dysuria.

Incisional Hernia

An incisional hernia is one that develops through a surgical incision in the abdominal wall. These hernias most commonly involve incisions of the anterior abdominal wall, although they may be responsible for other types of hernias such as those occurring in the lumbar region (from a previous nephrectomy incision) and in the perineal region (from a previous abdominoperineal resection). The hernia may appear clinically shortly following the placement of the initial incision or develop many years thereafter. When arising in the anterior abdominal wall, incisional hernias are more commonly encountered in vertical than in transverse incisions.

A variety of etiologic factors are involved in the development of incisional hernias that can generally be grouped under the two broad headings of poor postoperative wound healing or postoperative wound infection. Any factor related to poor surgical technique can result in inadequate wound healing. Whether sutures are placed too close to the edges or are tied too tightly so as to necrose the involved tissues, poor wound healing may result. Other contributing factors relating to surgical technique include knots becoming untied, use of the wrong type of suture material for a particular incision, suture damage due to shearing stresses, wound hematomas from poor hemostasis, and the placement of drains through the incision itself, all of which may adversely affect healing. Further, if the incision has not been closed properly and the patient develops a problem with increased intra-abdominal pressure (secondary to such factors as hiccupping, abdominal distention, and postoperative coughing), undue strain may be placed on the suture line that ultimately may give way. Finally, wound infections increase the risk of subsequent incision hernia, particularly if the infection

extends to the level of the fascia. Thus any factor contributing to the development of a wound infection also influences the likelihood of recurrent incision hernia.

The treatment of incisional hernias is similar to that of other hernias. At present, the major question is whether mesh reinforcement should be used in all patients. When a mesh is used, the underlay or sublay technique is the most desirable, with the latter term (sublay) being used to indicate the positioning of the mesh within the rectus sheath, behind the muscle, and in front of the posterior component of the sheath (56–58). If a mesh must be used to bridge intra-abdominal defects, the use of smooth mesh surfaces such as Goretex or Composix is recommended. In all cases, it is now apparent that the mesh requires fixation with sutures that traverse the abdominal wall, and these should be placed at intervals of approximately 5.0 cm whether the repair is performed open or closed (59). Similarly, the mesh should overlap healthy fascia for a suitable distance (3–6 cm) to allow the buttressing effect to be most effective. There is no level 1 evidence available to distinguish the difference between 3.0 and 6.0 cm, and there are other issues such as the presence of boundary structures that are not friendly to suture placement, such as pericardium, costochondral junction, os pubis, etc., which can compromise gratuitous descriptions of "necessary" margins (60–62). In some cases, the goal of avoiding direct contact of mesh with intestines is impossible, but there is reasonable evidence that the mesh materials can be safely implanted without excessive risk of intestinal fistula as a complication (61,62).

Parastomal Hernias

A variant of the incisional hernia is that which occurs through the same fascial opening created for a colostomy or ileostomy. This type of hernia is termed as a "parastomal hernia" and usually occurs when the stomal opening is placed lateral to the rectus muscle. Often this type of hernia can be managed by tightening the fascial defect around the stoma with interrupted sutures. When this is not possible, the colostomy or ileostomy should be taken down and moved to a new site, preferably through the rectus muscle. The remaining fascial defect from the previously placed ostomy is then closed from within the peritoneal cavity. There is a laparoscopic alternative here as well, with the advantage of totally isolating the stoma from the operative field, allowing the use of mesh to buttress the repair without incurring the automatic contamination of the operative site.

Diaphragmatic Hernias

A number of hernias may occur within the diaphragm that separates the thoracic from the abdominal cavity. These hernias may be congenital, in which case they arise through defects or apertures resulting from developmental abnormalities, or they may be acquired through enlargement of preexistent apertures or disruption of points of weakness. A congenital diaphragmatic hernia represents an arrest in the development of some portion of the diaphragm (Fig. 15). Posterolateral defects in the pleuroperitoneal membrane (the foramen of Bochdalek) occur on the left side in 70% to 85% of the cases and allow abdominal viscera to readily migrate into the left thorax; while most present as surgical emergencies of the newborn period, with substantial mortality rate due to accompanying respiratory distress, occasional cases present in adult life. The clinical presentation of this type of hernia and the physiologic principles underlying its management are discussed in detail in

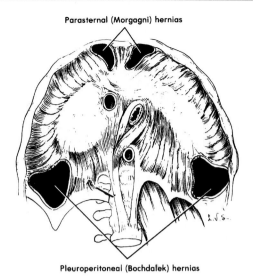

Figure 15 Sites of congenital diaphragmatic herniation. *Source*: From Ref. 63.

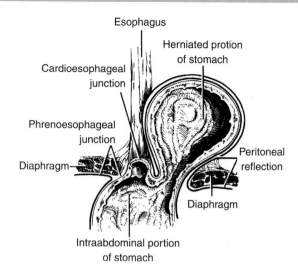

Figure 16 Paraesophageal hernia. *Source*: From Ref. 63.

Chapter 14. Another type of congenital hernia is that which results from failure of fusion anteriorly of the sternal and costal portions of the diaphragm. The resulting midline defect creates a hiatus, known as Morgagni's foramen, through which a hernia may occur. When normal fusion results, only the internal mammary vessels pass through this area and continue into the abdomen as the superior epigastric vessels. When the defect remains, however, various portions of bowel (usually small bowel) or omentum may herniate through this abnormal hiatus. In contrast to the Bochdalek hernia, which clinically presents at birth, most hernias protruding through Morgagni's foramen do not become symptomatic until middle age or later. Often their presence is first shown by a mechanical bowel obstruction with intestinal strangulation and mediastinitis. These hernias should be repaired as soon as they are diagnosed, usually by a transabdominal approach.

Of the acquired types of hernias that may affect the diaphragm, the most common is the sliding hiatus hernia, which may or may not be associated with esophagitis. This type of hernia is discussed in detail in Chapter 14. Less commonly encountered clinically is the parahiatal hernia, also called the paraesophageal hernia (Fig. 16). Because the esophagogastric junction is not disturbed in this condition, esophagitis is not a problem, although heartburn is not unusual as a presenting complaint due to poor esophageal emptying. Usually the presenting symptoms are vague epigastric and lower chest pain that may be aggravated on recumbency. With this type of hernia, all or part of the stomach may herniate into the thorax adjacent and to the left of the gastroesophageal junction. Radiologically, this type of hernia may give the appearance of an upside-down stomach on barium contrast study. Paraesophageal hernias are often associated with the complications of ulceration and bleeding and not uncommonly become incarcerated and at times even strangulated. For many years, the most prudent method of management was thought to be immediate repair of the hernia; however, because many patients survive for years without these complications, the necessity of routine closure in asymptomatic patients has been questioned (64). When symptoms occur, however, the repair should be performed promptly. Often in our clinic, patients who are operated upon discover the importance of their symptoms only when they experience the joy of being normal again in the postoperative period; as a result, I usually find that patients have chronic discomfort or digestive difficulties which can be reasonably expected to disappear by operative treatment; interestingly, the best results are reported by surgeons who routinely employ mesh prostheses in reconstruction of the esophageal hiatus (65). This interesting phenomenon is one that explains our bias toward operating on large hernias once discovered; occasionally, however, if there is a truly asymptomatic patient, we simply describe the possible risks and ask the patient and family to stay in touch periodically.

One additional type of acquired hernia of importance is that produced by rents in the diaphragm, which may result from penetrating or blunt trauma. Because of the protective effects of the liver on the right side, these traumatic hernias almost always occur on the left side and can result in considerable respiratory embarrassment from herniation of abdominal viscera into the left chest, if they are of sufficient size. Surgical repair of the diaphragmatic tear with reduction of the herniated viscera into the abdomen is the treatment of choice.

SUMMARY

Hernias of the abdominal wall are commonly encountered in the practice of surgery and may arise in any structure surrounding or supporting the contents of the abdominal cavity. These hernias are particularly common anteriorly, with the vast majority arising in the groin. Other sites of relatively frequent occurrence include the umbilicus and previous incisions. The clinical presentation of a hernia usually consists of an obvious bulge at the site of the hernial defect, and is often associated with pain. Less commonly, an unexplained intestinal obstruction may be the presenting finding, in which a segment of bowel has become trapped in the hernial defect. Because hernias generally do not resolve spontaneously (an exception being the congenital umbilical hernia), surgical repair has until recently been the treatment of choice once the diagnosis has been established; this concept has been the subject of rethinking, and the role of observation has achieved new currency in modern parlance.

Hernial repairs consist of careful identification of the hernial boundary, reduction of the hernial sac contents, and in many but not all cases, excision of the sac itself. The hernial defect is then repaired by approximating its edges with sutures in one of several ways—with interrupted or continuous, permanent, or absorbable sutures. When the hernial defect is so large that primary closure without tension is impossible, a tension-free repair is performed; the choice of repair is left to the experience and judgment of the surgeon. Anatomic approaches such as "component separation" are sometimes used, but most often, a prosthetic material of some type is utilized. Further, the routine use of a mesh in groin hernias is now well established, and has led to a much-improved outcome for patients with groin hernias. Whether the mesh has a comparable role in umbilical and incisional hernias is not as clear, despite the wide use of mesh in these sites. The key to any successful hernia repair is an understanding of the underlying anatomy and its restoration to normalcy. With this principle in mind, most hernias can be repaired without difficulty and a good-to-excellent result can be expected.

REFERENCES

1. Hughson W. The persistent or preformed sac in relation to oblique inguinal hernia. Surg Gynecol Obstet 1925; 41:610–618.
2. Keith A. On the origin and nature of hernia. Br J Surg 1924; 11:455–460.
3. Anson BJ, Morgan EH, McVay CB. Surgical anatomy of the inguinal region based upon a study of 500 body-halves. Surg Gynecol Obstet 1960; 111:707–724.
4. Fitzgibbons RJ, Jonasson O, Gibbs J, et al. A clinical trial to determine if watchful waiting is an acceptable alternative to routine herniorrhaphy in patients with minimal or no hernia symptoms. J Am Coll Surg 2003; 196:737–742.
5. Read RC. Milestones in the History of Hernia Surgery – Prosthetic repair. Hernia 2004; 8(1):8–14. Epub Hernia 2003: Oct 28.
6. Toki A, Watanabe Y, Sasaki K, Tani M, Ogura K, Wang ZQ. Adopt a wait-and-see attitude for patent processus vaginalis in neonates. J Pediatr Surg 2003; 38:1371–1373.
7. Amid PK. Lichtenstein tension-free hernioplasty: its inception, evolution, and principles. Hernia 2004; 8(1):1–7. Epub 2003, Sep 20.
8. McVay CB, Chapp JD. Inguinal and femoral hernioplasty-the evaluation of a basic concept. Ann Surg 1958; 148:499–510.
9. Condon RE. The anatomy of the inguinal region and its relationship to groin hernia. In: Nyhus LM, Condon RE, eds. Hernia. 4th. Philadelphia: JB Lippincott Co., 1995:16–72.
10. Higa KD, Ho T, Boone KB. Internal hernias after laparoscopic Roux-en-Y gastric bypass: incidence, treatment and prevention. Obes Surg 2003; 13(3):350–354.
11. Armstrong O, Letessier E, Genier P, Laserre P, Le Neel JC. Internal hernia. Report of nine cases. Hernia 1997; 1:143–145.
12. Nikfarjam M, Christophi C. Internal hernia traversing the lesser sac. Ann Coll Surg Hong Kong 2003; 7:99.
13. Nishida S, Pinna AG, Nery JR, et al. Internal hernia of the small bowel around infrarenal arterial conduits following transplantation. Clin Transplant 2002; 16:334–338.
14. Gullmo A, Broome A, Smedberg S. Herniography. Surg Clin N Am 1984; 64:229.
15. van Wessem KJ, Simons MP, Plaisier PW, Lange JF. The etiology of indirect inguinal hernias: congenital and/or acquired? Hernia 2003; 7(2):76–79. Epub 2003 Mar 18.
16. Gullmo A. Herniography: the diagnosis of hernia in the groin and incompetence of the pouch of Douglas and pelvic floor. Acta Radiol Suppl (Stockh) 1980; 361:1–76.
17. Gullmo A. Herniography: the diagnosis of hernia in the groin and incompetence of the pouch of Douglas and pelvic floor. Acta Radiol Suppl 1980; 361:1–76.
18. Gullmo A. Herniography. World J Surg 1989; 13:560–568.
19. DuBois JJ, Jenkins JR, Egan JC. Transinguinal laparoscopic examination of the contralateral groin in pediatric herniorrhaphy. Surg Laparosc Endosc 1997; 7:384–387.
20. Rescorla FJ, West KW, Engum SA, Scherer LR III, Grosfeld JL. The 'other side' of pediatric hernias: the role of laparoscopy. Am Surg 1997; 63:690–693.
21. Wulkan ML, Wiener ES, VanBalen N, Vescio P. Laparoscopy through the open ipsilateral sac to evaluate the presence of contralateral hernia. J Pediatr Surg 1996; 31:1174–1176.
22. Miltenburg DM, Nuchtem JG, Jaksic T, Kozinetiz C, Brandt ML. Laparoscopic evaluation of the pediatric inguinal hernia-a meta-analysis. J Pediatr Surg 1998; 33(6):874–879.
23. Miltenburg DM, Nuchter JG, Jaksic T, Kozinetz CA, Brandt ML. Meta-analysis of the risk of metachronous hernia in infants and children. Am J Surg 1997; 174:741–744.
24. Read RC. Attenuation of rectus sheath in inguinal herniation. Am J Surg 1970; 120:610–614.
25. Peacock EE Jr. Biology of hernia. In: Nyhus LM, Condon RE, eds. Hernia. 2nd ed. Philadelphia: JB Lippincott Co., 1978.
26. Peacock EE Jr, Madden JW. Studies on the biology and treatment of recurrent inguinal hernia. II. Morphological changes. Ann Surg 1974; 179:567–571.
27. Colin JF, Elliot P, Ellis H. The effect of uraemia upon wound healing: an experimental study. Br J Surg 1979; 66:793–797.
28. Karahan OI, Taskapan H, Tokgoz B, Coskiun A, Utas C, Gulec M. Continuous ambulatory peritoneal dialysis. Acta Radiol 2002; 43:170–174.
29. Engeset J, Youngson GG. Ambulatory peritoneal dialysis and hernia complications. Surg Clin N Am 1984; 64:385–392.
30. Zheng H, Si Z, Kasperk R, et al. Recurrent inguinal hernia: disease of the collagen matrix? World J Surg 2002; 26:401–408. Epub 2002 Jan 02.
31. Si Z, Bhardwaj R, Rosch R, et al. Impaired balance of type I and type III procollagen mRNA in cultured fibroblasts of patients with incisional hernia. Surgery 2002; 131:324–331.
32. Rodrigues AJ Jr, Rodrigues CJ, da Cunha AC, Jin Y. Quantitative analysis of collagen and elastic fibers in the transversalis fascia in direct and indirect inguinal hernias. Rev Hosp Clin Fac Med Sao Paulo 2002; 57:265–270. Epub 2003 Feb 17.
33. Hiebert CA. Gastroesophageal reflux and ascorbic acid deficiency. Ann Thorac Surg 1977; 24:108–112.
34. Cannon DJ, Read RC. Metastatic emphysema, a mechanism for acquiring inguinal herniation. Ann Surg 1981; 194:270–278.
35. Kesek P, Ekberg O, Westlin N. Herniographic findings in athletes with unclear groin pain. Acta Radiol 2002; 43:603–608.
36. Heise CP, Sproat IA, Starling JR. Peritoneography (Herniography) for detecting occult inguinal hernia in patients with inguinodynia. Ann Surg 2002; 235:140–144.
37. Dattola P, Alberti A, Dattola A, Giannetto G, Basile G, Basile M. Inguino-crural hernias: preoperative diagnosis and postoperative follow-up by high-resolution ultrasonography. A personal experience. Ann Ital Chir 2002; 73:65–68.
38. Lilly MC, Arregui ME. Ultrasound of the inguinal floor for evaluation of hernias. Surg Endosc 2002; 16:659–662. Epub 2001 Dec 17.
39. Hata S, Takahashi Y, Nakamura T, Suzuki R, Kitada M, Shimano T. Preoperative sonographic evaluation is a useful method of detecting contralateral patent processus vaginalis in pediatric patients with unilateral inguinal hernia. J Pediatr Surg 2004; 39(9):1396–1399.
40. Arnbjornsson E. Development of right inguinal hernia after appendectomy. Am J Surg 1982; 143:367–369.
41. Lilly MC, Arregui ME. Lipomas of the cord and round ligament. Ann Surg 2002; 235:586–590.
42. Soper RT. Abdominal hernia. In: Liechty RD, Soper RT, eds. Synopsis of Surgery. 5th. St. Louis: Mosby, 1985.

43. Dittrick GW, Ridl K, Kuhn JA, McCarty TM. Routine ilioinguinal nerve excision in inguinal hernia repairs. Am J Surg 2004; 188(6):736–740.

44. Rutkow IM. The PerFix plug repair for groin hernias. Surg Clin N Am 2003; 83(5):1079–1098.

45. Read RC. The contributions of Usher and others to the elimination of tension from groin herniorrhaphy Hernia. 2005 (Epub ahead of print).

46. Condon RE. Anatomy of the inguinal region and its relation to groin hernia. In: Nyhus LM, Condon RE, eds. Hernia. 2nd ed. Philadelphia: JB Lippincott, 1978.

47. Ponka JL. Hernias of the Abdominal Wall. Philadelphia: WB Saunders, 1980.

48. Coll JR. Surg Edin 2001; 46:349–353. http: www.edu.rcsed.ac.uk.

49. Condon RE. Anterior iliopubic tract repair. In: Nyhus LM, Cordon RE, eds. Hernia. 2nd ed. Philadelphia: JB Lippincott, 1978.

50. Scott NW, McCormack K, Graham P, Go PM, Ross SJ, Grant AM. Open mesh versus non-mesh for repair of femoral and inguinal hernia. Cochrane Database Syst Rev 2002(4):CD002197.

51. Nyhus LM. The preperitoneal approach and iliopubic tract repair of inguinal hernia. In: Nyhus LM, Condon RE, eds. Hernia. 2d ed. Philadelphia: JB Lippincott, 1978.

52. Nyhus LM, Pollak R, Bombeck CT, Donahue PE. The preperitoneal approach and prosthetic buttress repair for recurrent hernia: the evolution of a technique. Ann Surg 1988; 208:733–37.

53. Neumayer L, Giobbie-Hurder A, Jonasson O, et al. Open mesh versus laparoscopic mesh repair of inguinal hernia. N Engl J Med 2004; 350(18):1819–1827. Epub 2004 Apr 25.

54. Rutkow IM. Demographic and socioeconomic aspects of hernia repair in the United States in 2003. Surg Clin N Am 2003; 83(5):1045–1051.

55. Amid PK. Radiologic images of meshoma: a new phenomenon causing chronic pain after prosthetic repair of abdominal wall hernias. Arch Surg 2004; 139(12):1297–1298.

56. de Vries Reilingh TS, van Geldere D, Langenhorst B, et al. Repair of large midline incisional hernias with polypropylene mesh: comparison of three operative techniques. Hernia 2004; 8(1):56–59. Epub 2003 Oct 28.

57. Bauer JJ, Harris MT, Gorfine SR, Kreel I. Rives-Stoppa procedure for repair of large incisional hernias: experience with 57 patients. Hernia 2002; 6(3):120–123. Epub 2002 Jul 13.

58. Schumpelick V, Klinge U, Junge K, Stumpf M. Incisional abdominal hernia: the open mesh repair. Langenbecks Arch Surg 2004; 389(1):1–5. Epub 2003 Mar 06.

59. Eid GM, Prince JM, Mattar SG, Hamad G, Ikrammudin S, Schauer PR. Medium-term follow-up confirms the safety and durability of laparoscopic ventral hernia repair with PTFE. Surgery 2003; 134(4):599–603; discussion 603–604.

60. Vrijland WW, Jeekel J, Steyerberg EW, Den Hoed PT, Bonjer HJ. Intraperitoneal polypropylene mesh repair of incisional hernia is not associated with enterocutaneous fistuia. Br J Surg 2000; 87(3):348–352 (see comment by Amid P. Br J Surg 2000; 87(10):1436–1437).

61. Ujiki MB, Weinberger J, Varghese TK, Murayama KM, Joehl RJ. One hundred consecutive laparoscopic ventral hernia repairs. Am J Surg 2004; 188(5):593–597.

62. Carbonell AM, Kercher KW, Matthews BD, Sing RF, Cobb WS, Heniford BT. The laparoscopic repair of suprapubic ventral hernias. Surg Endosc 2004 (Epub ahead of print).

63. Grimes OF, Way LW. Esophagus and diaphragm. In: Way LW, ed. Current Surgical Diagnosis and Treatment. 7th ed. Los Altos, CA: Lange Medical Publications, 1985.

64. Stylopoulos N, Gazelle GS, Rattner DW. Paraesophageal hernias: operation or observation? Ann Surg 2002; 236:492–501.

65. Frantzides CT, Madan AK, Carlson MA, Stavropoulos GP. A prospective, randomized trial of laparoscopic polytetrafluoroethylene (PTFE) patch repair vs simple cruropiasty for large hiatal hernia. Arch Surg 2002; 137(6):649–652.

58

Pathophysiology of Thermal Injury

Ronald M. Barton, Evan R. Kokoska, David J. Wainwright, and Donald H. Parks

INTRODUCTION

Thermal injury elicits major pathophysiologic alterations beyond the obvious cutaneous manifestation. Although the burn wound itself can present unique challenges in terms of therapeutic management and is responsible for the high incidence of infection that occurs in thermally injured patients, a number of metabolic aberrations and associated dysfunction of various organs are also commonly encountered, which directly contribute to morbidity and mortality. The magnitude of these latter derangements has led to the proposal that the burn patient is the universal trauma model with the greatest dysregulation of homeostasis of any injury (1,2). Major progress has been achieved in recent years in understanding many of the pathophysiologic mechanisms that occur in burn injury, and has facilitated patient management and improved survival. Such progress has been attributed to the development of specialized burn centers, increased investigative efforts in burn research, and the development of the team concept in patient management (3).

THE BURN WOUND

Biophysics of Thermal Injury

When skin is heated, damage occurs from the transfer of thermal energy. The magnitude of this tissue destruction is a function of both the quantity of heat transferred and the speed at which it dissipates. These factors are determined by the physical properties of the burning agent, the recipient tissue that is burned, and the incipient environment.

Burning Agent

The temperature and duration of exposure to the burning agent are the most important determinants of the degree of injury. For a specific level of injury, there is an inverse relationship between these two parameters (4,5) (Fig. 1). As the temperature is reduced, a progressively longer exposure time is required to inflict the same injury. At a theoretic "threshold temperature," the heat source would have to be applied for an infinite time. Temperatures below this "threshold" do not result in tissue damage, regardless of the duration of application. The exposure interval is related not only to the actual removal of the offending agent but also to the rate at which the heat source loses its energy to the environment. For example, at lower temperatures at which duration is important, a different degree of injury results when a metallic object and liquid are exposed to the same temperature. The liquid loses its heat more slowly.

Recipient Tissue

Certain physical properties of the heated object are also important in determining the extent of damage. These parameters reflect how much energy must be expended to raise the temperature of the object and how efficiently and quickly the heat is transferred. Skin, because of its high water content, has a high specific heat and a low thermal conductivity. Thus slow overheating of the tissues and delayed dispersion of the energy result. This is illustrated by measuring the temperature 1 mm below the skin surface after a 10-second scald burn (Fig. 2). There is an initial rapid, but not immediate, rise in temperature as the heat is applied. Even more dramatic is the length of time required for the temperature to return to baseline values. In this way, heat damage may continue after the offending agent is removed. Heat energy is lost primarily by conduction to the surrounding tissues, with removal of the circulating blood making only a small contribution (7).

Environment

Heat dissipation occurs not only through adjacent tissue but also into the surrounding environment. Heat loss is therefore maximized in a cooler environment. For example, the rapid application of cold water to burned skin has been shown to decrease the severity of the injury by rapidly reducing the elevated tissue temperature (8). There is also evidence that cooling the burn wound minimizes edema (9,10) by decreasing the amount of histamine released (11)

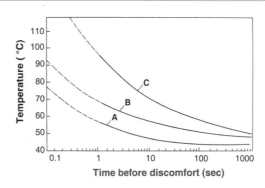

Figure 1 Relationship between temperature and the duration of contact for first-degree (A), second-degree (B), and third-degree (C) injuries. *Source:* From Ref. 4.

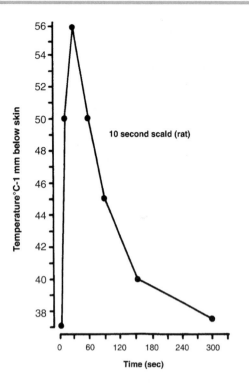

Figure 2   Temperature curve measured by a thermocouple 1 mm below the skin surface during a 10-second scald. The skin's low thermal conductivity results in a slow dispersion of the energy, leading to an additional tissue injury subsequent to the removal of the offending agent. *Source*: From Ref. 6.

through the stabilization of the mast cell membrane (12). Preservation of the dermal microcirculation has likewise been demonstrated by immediate cooling of the thermally injured tissues (9,10), presumably through a reduction in thromboxane production (13).

Histopathology of the Burn Wound

The severity of a burn injury is determined by the anatomic surface area involved and the pathologic depth. *A first-degree burn* is characterized by a painful erythematous and edematous skin. Histologically, vasodilation is present in the dermal microvasculature, and there is an increase in the interstitial fluid volume secondary to increased permeability. If the insult is more severe, necrosis of the epidermis occurs, and blistering of the skin is found clinically. A hyperemic response is again observed in the vessels within the dermis, accompanied by extravasation of fluid. In this instance, the fluid accumulates not only within the connective tissue of the dermis, but also at the dermal–epidermal junction leading to vesicle formation. The composition of the blister fluid has been extensively examined by a number of investigators (14–17). Compounds with a relatively low molecular weight (i.e., electrolytes, urea, glucose, and antibiotics) diffuse freely into the tissues and are found in the same concentrations in the serum, interstitial fluid, and blister fluid. On the other hand, low-molecular-weight proteins that are generally found only in small concentrations in tissue fluid have been shown to attain up to 80% of their plasma concentration within the vesicles. Significant quantities of intracellular enzymes and purine/pyrimidine compounds are also found, reflecting the extent of cellular

damage. Elevated concentrations of several chemical mediators (i.e., prostaglandins) have also been reported in the blister fluid.

In a *partial-thickness injury* or *second-degree burn*, the epidermal appendages are preserved and are responsible for resurfacing the wound. The epithelium in the surviving sweat glands and hair follicles multiplies and begins to migrate across the wound, coverage being complete within 7 to 14 days. This injury is typically painful because of direct nerve-ending damage coupled with the release of irritant chemical mediators into the wound.

An even greater thermal insult leads to additional thermal necrosis. The cellular components are irreversibly damaged, and the connective tissue is sufficiently disrupted that it is unable to fulfill its function of support and protection. If this extends to a depth below the level of the epidermal appendages, a *full-thickness injury* or *third-degree burn* has occurred. Reepithelialization is only possible from the wound edge, a process that would take a considerable length of time for even small defects. A dry, leathery appearance is seen clinically, because the tissues have lost their ability to retain water. This wound is painless because the nerve endings have been destroyed.

Pathophysiology of the Burn Wound
Major Mediators

Prior to discussing the specific derangements involved with burn injuries, a brief review of the major mediators produced, both local and systemic, is warranted (Table 1). As a general principle, under normal conditions these mediators, at low levels, are required to maintain proper blood flow and host immunity. However, either prolonged low levels or sustained elevations following injuries such as burns can be detrimental, both within the local site and at distant organ sites.

Cytokines are low-molecular-weight glycoproteins that act as intercellular messengers in an autocrine, paracrine, or endocrine fashion. They are synthesized de novo in response to potential threats to the organism (antigens, lipopolysaccharides, etc.), must bind receptors, as they are unable to penetrate cell membranes (18), and are not governed by a major negative feedback loop (19). Cytokines are difficult to detect, because they are bioactive at extremely low concentrations, and their levels do not always correlate with the degree of injury (19). Some effects of cytokines are clearly beneficial, but they may become counterproductive during derangements in the body's homeostatic responses. Imbalances may lead to immunosuppression, and excessive activity has correlated with injurious effects (20).

Eicosanoids are produced through the metabolism of arachidonic acid, an unsaturated fatty acid essential in nutrition. Prostaglandins and thromboxanes are generated through the action of cyclooxygenase, whereas 5-lipooxygenase converts arachidonic acid to leukotrienes. A variety of prostaglandin end products have been identified in the burn wound, and many appear to have divergent effects (21). For example, prostaglandin E_2 (PGE_2) and prostacyclin (PGI_2) are vasodilators and inhibit platelet aggregation, whereas thromboxane A_2 (TXA_2) is a potent vasoconstrictor and promotes platelet aggregation. A steady-state relationship exists between these oppositely functioning prostanoids (e.g., PGE_2 and PGI_2 vs. TXA_2) in uninjured tissues. However, a traumatic stimulus may disrupt this balance and favor increased production of a particular group of eicosanoids. Several different isoforms of cyclooxygenase have been recognized: a

Table 1 Local and Systemic Mediators of Burn Injuries

Mediators	Major sources	Major actions	
		Immunologic	*Metabolic*
Cytokines			
IL-1	Monocytes, macrophages	Activate B- and T-cells, natural killer cells, PMNs, and macrophages	Fever, APP production, catabolism, wound healing, and anemia (19,20)
IL-2	T-lymphocytes	Cell-mediated immunity, enhanced cytotoxic T-cell function	Hypermetabolism (19)
IL-6	Macrophages, PMNs, fibroblasts	B-cell proliferation, immunoglobulin production	Hepatic APP production (19)
TNF (cachectin)	Macrophages, endothelial cells	PMN release, margination, and activation	Catabolism, APP production, and fever (19)
Eicosanoids			
PGE_2, PGI_2	Endothelial cells, macrophages, PMNs	Vasodilation, increased vascular permeability, and immunosuppression (PGE_2) (19,20,27–29)	
TXA_2, TXB_2	Platelets, macrophages	Vasoconstriction, platelet aggregation, and local tissue ischemia (30–32)	
LTB_4, LTC_4, LTD_4	Mast cells, macrophages, PMNs	Increased vascular permeability, potent PMN chemoattractant (LTB_4), and small airway constriction (LTC_4, LTD_4) (20,34)	
Nitric oxide	Endothelial cells, macrophages	Low levels: vasodilation High levels: Cytotoxic, vascular decompensation (22,35,36)	
Oxygen free radicals	PMNs	Lipid peroxidation (increased cell membrane permeability and fluidity) (19,20)	
Complement			
C3a, C5a		Anaphylaxis	
C3b		Opsoninization	
C5b		Increased vascular permeability and smooth muscle contraction	
C6 to C9		Cytotoxic (20)	
Acute phase proteins	Hepatocytes	Inactivate proteases, scavenge oxygen free radicals, and modulate wound healing (37)	

Abbreviations: APP, acute phase protein; IL, interleukin; LT, leukotriene; PG, prostaglandin; PMN, polymorphonuclear leukocyte; TX, thromboxane; TNF, tumor necrosis factor.

constitutively expressed (Cox-1) and inducible (Cox-2) form. However, the role of these two differentially expressed enzymes following burn injury remains to be completely characterized.

Burns are also associated with enhanced nitric oxide formation. Similar to cyclooxygenase, nitric oxide is generated from two isoforms of nitric oxide synthase: a constitutive and inducible form. Under basal conditions, low levels of nitric oxide provide a continuous state of active vasodilation and inhibit platelet and polymorphonuclear leukocyte (PMN) adhesion to the endothelium (22). After major injury, however, inducible nitric oxide synthase activity is significantly upregulated by stimuli such as elevated temperature (23) and tumor necrosis fator (TNF) or interleukin-1 (IL-1) released from activated macrophages (22). Excessive nitric oxide is associated with circulatory failure and vascular decompensation.

PMNs and macrophages are primarily responsible for phagocytosis of necrotic tissue. In the phagosome of the neutrophil, superoxide anion radicals and hydrogen peroxide are produced in large quantities to oxidize the ingested debris. These free radical species are normally rendered harmless by the action of superoxide dismutases and catalases that convert them to harmless products including oxygen and water. However, following burn injury, oxygen-derived free radicals are generated secondary to both ischemia/reperfusion via activation of xanthine oxidase (19) and histamine released from stimulated mast cells (24), and it has been postulated that a sufficient quantity of these substances may escape into the interstitial fluid, where the necessary enzymes for their reduction are present in only small amounts (25). These radicals not only increase

capillary permeability directly but also may induce peroxidation of tissues and can also result in enhanced prostaglandin release by their action on the phospholipid bilayer of the cell membrane (26). Complement acts to attract PMNs and degranulate mast cells and further increases oxygen free radical synthesis in addition to the other actions (20) depicted in Table 1.

Progressive Ischemia

An important conceptual model of the burn wound is that proposed by Jackson (38). He described three zones of graded thermal trauma (Fig. 3). Centrally, the "zone of coagulation" is an area of irreversible tissue destruction. Temperatures in this region are extreme and lead to immediate cell death, the depth of necrosis being directly dependent on the quantity of heat transferred. On the periphery, a "zone of hyperemia" exists, where vasodilation and permeability changes are present. Here the tissues are viable and generally heal uneventfully. The "zone of stasis" lies between these two areas. In this zone, the flow through a microvasculature is sluggish or has ceased, leading to progressive ischemia and cell death (39). Jackson (38) conceived that these changes were a direct effect of the heat energy on the tissues, and that eventual tissue necrosis within the zone of stasis was inevitable within 24 to 48 hours. However, other investigators believe that the tissues in this region have not been permanently damaged and thus possess the potential for a full recovery (40). Any deterioration is the result of a combination of physical factors and local inflammatory processes leading to persistent stasis and ischemia with conversion to a "zone of coagulation".

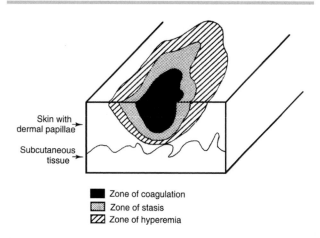

Skin with dermal papillae →

Subcutaneous tissue →

■ Zone of coagulation
▨ Zone of stasis
▨ Zone of hyperemia

Figure 3 Jackson's three zones of graded thermal injury. *Source*: From Ref. 6.

Systemic Factors

The progressive nature of the dermal ischemia occurs secondary to the influence of both systemic and local factors as outlined in Table 2. Depletion of the intravascular volume from fluid leaking into the injured tissues diminishes the filling pressure of the left ventricle and in turn the perfusion pressure within the microcirculation. However, even prior to measurable decreases in plasma volume, there is an alteration in ventricular compliance and a decrease in myocardial contractility (41). This direct myocardial toxicity is thought to be related to the release of a "myocardial depressant factor," although no such factor has been identified chemically (42,43). Other proposed mediators contributing to early myocardial depression resulting in the "ebb" phase following burn injury include TNF (44), interleukins, antidiuretic hormone (ADH), oxygen free radicals (45–47), and nitric oxide (22). Constricting eschar in circumferential burns of the extremities can also lead to reduced perfusion pressures in distally burned tissues (48).

Local Factors

Local factors can be categorized into intraluminal, extraluminal, and those associated with changes in the vessel wall itself. Within the lumen of blood vessels, cellular debris may accumulate, leading to a reduction in the functional

Table 2 Factors Contributing to Progressive Ischemia

Systemic factors
  Diminished circulating volume
  Myocardial depression
  Constricting eschar
Local factors
  Intraluminal
    White blood cell margination
    Platelet microthrombi/microemboli
    Erythrocyte agglutination
  Vessel wall changes
    Endothelial cell shape
    Vasoconstriction
      Direct
      Through chemical mediators
  Extraluminal
    Interstitial edema

diameter for flow. White blood cells respond to the thermal injury with increased margination along the vessel wall. As fluid leaks out of the intravascular space, hemoconcentration occurs, which may encourage erythrocyte aggregation and agglutination, further diminishing local blood flow. Platelet microthrombi and microemboli have also been observed to block the microvasculature within the injured area (49). Release of tissue thromboplastin from the injured tissues and the platelet-aggregating properties of thromboxane are both believed to contribute to the generation of these products of coagulation. Despite these observations, the use of anticoagulants has been unsuccessful in reducing the extent of tissue damage (50). Outside the vessel wall, the interstitial tissue pressure slowly increases, because the lymphatics are unable to contend with the enhanced and continual fluid extravasation. This leads to the compression of the microvasculature within this region and a subsequent reduction in flow.

The vessel wall itself contributes to the reduction of nutrient flow by structural changes in the endothelial cells and vasoconstriction. As a response to direct damage or ischemia, the endothelial cells are less able to regulate their internal electrolyte balance. Water therefore enters the cells, and the cells' normally hexagonal shape assumes a more spherical form (51). In this way the thickness of the vessel wall increases and impinges on the diameter of the lumen. The vasoconstriction is likely the result of a multitude of factors. Increased sympathetic tone and TXA_2 release appear to be the most important causes. Because the changes in the caliber of the lumen secondary to vessel wall alterations are often transient (49), the other pathophysiologic changes detailed above probably play a more important role in reducing blood flow.

For the cells within the zone of stasis to survive, nutrient flow within the microvasculature must be maintained. By preserving these tissues, one may prevent a partial-thickness injury from becoming a full-thickness injury and therefore requiring grafting. Clinically, this is achieved by maintaining the vascular volume and, in turn, the perfusion pressure through adequate resuscitation with intravenous fluids at the time of initial treatment. Similarly, wound care is important to prevent dehydration and infection that can contribute to increasing the depth of injury. There is evidence that, by preserving an intact blister or covering the denuded partial-thickness injury with a skin substitute, dehydration of the exposed dermis is minimized, and maximal tissue preservation is achieved (40,52). More recent attempts at pharmacologic manipulation of the offending chemical mediators have been made to preserve and/or reestablish the flow in this vascular bed. Several studies have demonstrated that TXA_2 is the responsible agent for many of the progressive ischemic changes seen in the dermal microcirculation, and that selectively inhibiting its production can prevent necrosis and attenuate hemodynamic disturbances (27,53,54).

Cellular Alterations

In areas of irreparable damage, cell membranes are disrupted with the escape of intracellular contents. The connective tissue proteins undergo denaturation, and the water content is lost, leaving a solid amorphous substance. This fusion of the dermal and epidermal heat-damaged tissue is referred to as coagulation necrosis. As a reaction to the presence of this damaged and necrotic tissue, a marked inflammatory response characterizes the early phase of the burn wound. In locations where destruction is less extensive, cellular ultrastructure remains intact; however, function is often compromised. Resting membrane potentials are found to be above normal (greater than $-90\,mV$) in this region, and cellular swelling is observed histologically (55). This is likely the result of decreased adenosine triphosphate (ATP) production from tissue ischemia (56,57). The function of the ATP-dependent sodium pump is impaired, permitting a shift of sodium and water into the cell, further compounding the loss of intravascular volume. A specific example of this is the altered function of the endothelial cells, the shape of which has been changed in response to a local thermal insult (51), as discussed earlier in this chapter.

A toxin derived from the cell membranes of burned skin has also been described (58). This burn toxin, called lipid protein complex (LPC), is a complex of lipids and proteins fused together by the effect of thermal injury. LPC has been associated with erythrocyte hemolysis (59,60), immunosuppression (61), and generalized membrane and mitochondrial damage (62). The injurious effects of LPC are thought to be unrelated to lipid peroxidation (63) or bacteria (64), and can be neutralized with antiserum (58). However, the best treatment appears to be the removal of the burn wound.

Fluid Shifts in the Wound

The inflammatory response typical of heat-damaged tissues is characterized by tremendous edema formation. Although various physical and chemically mediated factors are responsible, the fluid efflux depends on the restoration of adequate blood flow to the injured area. Perfusion is maintained by a combination of fluid resuscitation and local vasodilation, the latter following an initial period of transient sympathetic vasoconstriction. The magnitude and the time course of the tissue edema are subject to the timing and volume of fluid resuscitation (65).

The cause of the increased fluid extravasation is multifactorial, with a tremendous amount of synergism between the responsible mechanisms. These can be broadly grouped into two major categories: (i) those that affect the permeability or "leakiness" of the vessel wall and (ii) those whose effect is mediated through alteration of the Starling forces (Table 3).

Physical Factors

The ease by which fluid, solutes, and macromolecules can exit the vessel lumen is influenced directly by architectural changes in the vessel wall and indirectly by a variety of chemical mediators. Vasodilation opens the endothelial gaps, promoting the efflux of fluid. The damaged endothelial cells exhibit an increase in both the number of intracellular vacuoles and the number of open intercellular junctions

(66), the latter secondary to these cells and assuming a more spherical shape (51). These findings are first observed in the venules and later in the capillary bed. Because more channels are open along the vessel wall than exist normally, the outflow of fluid naturally increases.

Humoral Correlates

The release of vasoactive substances is perhaps the most important cause of the increased permeability seen in the early burn wound. The effect of these agents is primarily on endothelial cells of the microvasculature where they cause both an increase in the number and an increase in size of the channels. This allows a number of macromolecules to enter the interstitial compartment, and thus increases the amount of fluid escaping from the vessel lumen. Proteins of up to $150\,\text{Å}$ have been shown to escape into the interstitial compartment, resulting in a decreased intravascular oncotic pressure (67,68). Studies have demonstrated that the integrity of the microvasculature to macromolecular leak is restored by 8 to 12 hours following thermal injury. Hence, at 12 hours postinjury, some clinicians initiate colloid infusions in their resuscitation regimens (69).

A variety of mediators have been implicated in the generation of these permeability changes, but the most important appear to be the prostaglandins, leukotrienes (27–29), and oxygen free radicals (20). Kinins (70) and serotonin (71) released from platelets have been shown to play only a minor role. A stimulus for the mediator response is the connective tissue protein that has been modified by thermal injury. Its effect on activating the complement and clotting mechanisms leads to the generation of the various mediator compounds. Specifically, the C3 and C5 components of complement are responsible for mast cell histamine release and PMN recruitment, whereas the C9 component initiates prostaglandin release from platelets (26). The permeability changes seen within the burn wound take on a biphasic pattern (72) (Fig. 4). The initial increase is primarily caused by the action of histamine (73) and the direct thermal

Table 3 Causes of Edema Formation

Vessel wall changes
  Vasodilation
  Heat-induced damage
  Vasoactive substances
Altered Starling forces
  Increased capillary hydrostatic pressure
    Vasoconstriction
    Partial blockage (platelets, white blood cells, red blood cells)
  Decreased intraluminal colloid osmotic pressure
  Increased interstitial colloid osmotic pressure
  Lymphatic obstruction

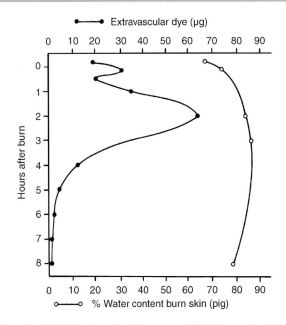

Figure 4 Biphasic pattern of capillary permeability. *Source:* From Ref. 6.

damage to the microvasculature. The specific cause of the second, more prolonged phase is less clear, but is likely the result of prostaglandin and leukotriene release and oxygen free radical generation.

The use of specific histamine H_2 receptor blockers (e.g., cimetidine) in reducing the early phase of edema formation has been successful in animals (74,75); however, their clinical use seems to be ineffective in this regard (76) and is occasionally associated with undesirable side effects (77). These findings are consistent with the fact that histamine is not responsible for the longer, more pronounced phase of increased permeability; therefore its inhibition is unlikely to have an appreciable effect. Topical ibuprofen, as cyclooxygenase inhibitor, has been reported to decrease burn edema (78).

If molecular oxygen is reintroduced to previously underperfused tissue, oxygen-derived free radicals such as hydrogen peroxide and superoxide will be produced, which can result in further tissue damage. However, persistent tissue hypoxia will result in cell death. Therefore the burn patient becomes a victim of the "oxygen paradox" (79). Accordingly, other work directed toward decreasing permeability changes following burns has involved either blocking or scavenging oxygen free radicals. Permeability changes have been attenuated with xanthine oxidase inhibitors (44,80–82), but these trials have not been effective when inhibition is attempted after the burn (83). More promising is the use of vitamin C (a free radical scavenger) during fluid resuscitation, which, when initiated two hours after injury, in an animal model, has been associated with decreased burn wound edema and fluid requirements (84).

Starling Forces

In normal tissues, the balance of the Starling forces results in a slight efflux of fluid from the intravascular to the extravascular compartment (Fig. 5). A steady state is maintained by resorption of this fluid through lymphatic channels. The lymphatic route is also the only avenue by which proteins can be returned to the vascular space to maintain the oncotic pressure gradient between the interstitial and intravascular compartments. In the burn wound these forces are altered so that this extravasation of fluid is greatly enhanced. Within the capillary lumen, hydrostatic forces are increased above normal. The opening of the precapillary sphincters allows the arterial pressure to be transmitted directly to this vascular bed. In addition, intraluminal pressures rise proximal to a partial obstruction to flow caused by platelet microthrombi/microemboli, white blood cell margination, and red blood cell debris. In contrast, capillary intravascular osmotic pressure is decreased by the loss of colloid molecules into the interstitial space (especially albumin), whereas the extravascular osmotic activity rises, which tends to pull fluid out of the vessels (14). Heat-denatured collagen is thought to be responsible for this effect. This denatured protein tends to hold the fluid within the interstitial space, thereby delaying resorption. Initially, the lymphatics increase their flow to compensate for this additional interstitial volume; however, the maximal effect of this flow is achieved within one hour following thermal injury. Not infrequently, blockage or destruction of the lymphatic channels delays resorption of the increased interstitial volume, further compounding this problem. Although tissue pressures rise as the quantity of edema fluid increases (85), this alteration is not sufficient to counteract the forces responsible for flow out of the vessels.

Nonburn Wound Edema

In large burns (i.e., over 40% body surface area), edema is observed in both burned and nonburned tissues. Increased capillary permeability of distant vascular beds may be caused by the systemic effect of chemical mediators released from the damaged tissue (29,68,86). Excessive white blood cell

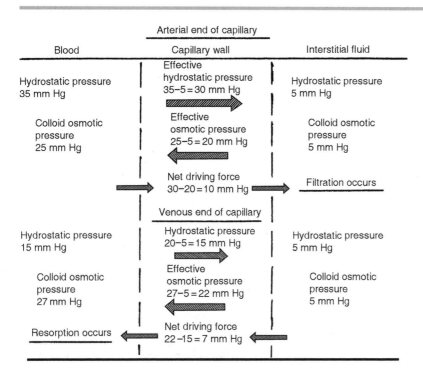

Figure 5 Starling forces.

margination in the nonburned microcirculation has also been considered as a possible cause (87). Demling et al. (24,88) have proposed that intravascular hypoproteinemia may be responsible for this effect. They suggested that the plasma oncotic pressure is lowered not only by protein loss through the burn wound, but also by dilution from the crystalloid solutions used in burn resuscitation. By administering colloid during the resuscitative period, they noted that the edema observed in nonburned tissues was significantly diminished.

Systemic Inflammatory Response Syndrome

Following burn injury, the generalized release of systemic mediators can eventually lead to multiple systems organ failure and death. As mentioned earlier, although some of the effects of cytokines are clearly beneficial, imbalances and excessive activity are universally detrimental, as the body's homeostatic responses become counterproductive. One hypothesis that summarizes the development of the systemic inflammatory response syndrome (SIRS) involves the "two hit" theory. The initial insult (burn injury or gut ischemia) primes the inflammatory factories (cellular elements such as PMNs and macrophages). Subsequent challenge, either by endotoxemia (from gut or wound) or persistent gut ischemia, acts as the "second hit" that initiates a prolonged, exaggerated release of inflammatory mediators resulting in hemodynamic instability and tissue injury (19). A simplified diagram is depicted in Figure 6.

A growing body of evidence currently suggests that infection is not necessary for the development of SIRS. Fewer than half of septic-appearing patients who subsequently die have untreated infections (3,53,90,91), and the overall relationship between endotoxemia and survival is poor (58). It is becoming increasingly clear that devitalized tissue (denatured protein and bacterial products) and gut ischemia are important stimuli for the inflammatory response (3,90).

Changes in intestinal permeability and the promotion of bacterial translocation are evident shortly after a burn injury (90,92). The mucosal injury is mediated in large part by oxygen free radicals derived from increased xanthine oxidase activity (90) as a result of decreased mesenteric blood flow and ischemia/reperfusion and does not appear to be related to bacteria, as germ-free rats demonstrate similar responses (90). Even in the absence of translocating organisms or endotoxin into the portal circulation, gut mucosal damage is injurious through the activation of the gut-associated lymphoid tissue (GALT) (18). The GALT, in addition to the burn wound, serves as a primary site for PMN priming and cytokine release (90). Gut ischemia also results in the release of eicosanoids (93) and complement (94).

Efforts directed toward preventing SIRS by mediator antagonism have been largely disappointing in part because of the enormous costs and the difficulty detecting circulating levels of the various cytokines. Several studies have been stopped, and the results remain unpublished as a result of safety concerns (18). Trials with TNF and IL-1 antagonism have demonstrated no survival benefit (95,96). Currently, there is no "magic bullet" cure for SIRS, and future work involves combination therapy (18). Attempts toward decreasing bacterial translocation, including selective gut decontamination, have demonstrated decreases in infectious complications but no affect on survival (97). Others have reported a decrease in bacterial translocation through preservation of intestinal perfusion with vasodilators (nitroprusside) and TXA$_2$ inhibitors (98,99). However, the best means of preserving mucosal integrity and minimizing GALT activation likely involves early delivery of enteral nutrients (90).

METABOLIC ALTERATIONS

After the "ebb" phase that immediately follows a major burn and involves circulatory depression, local tissue and gut ischemia, and wound edema, patients develop a "flow" phase, which includes an elevated resting consumption of oxygen, coupled with increased nitrogen losses, autocannibalism (100), insulin resistance, hyperglycemia, and futile substrate cycling (101). Management of burn patients during the "flow" phase can be just as challenging as during the acute resuscitation.

Hypermetabolic Response

The insult of a major burn results in a greater elevation of the metabolic rate than is observed in all other forms of trauma (Fig. 7). The hypermetabolic response to thermal injury,

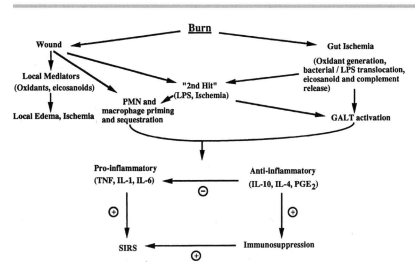

Figure 6 Mediator interactions following burn injury. *Abbreviations*: GALT, gut-associated lymphoid tissue; IL, interleukin; LPS, lipopolysaccharide; PG, prostaglandin; PMN, polymorphonuclear leukocyte; SIRS, systemic inflammatory response syndrome, TNF, tumor necrosis factor. *Source*: From Ref. 89.

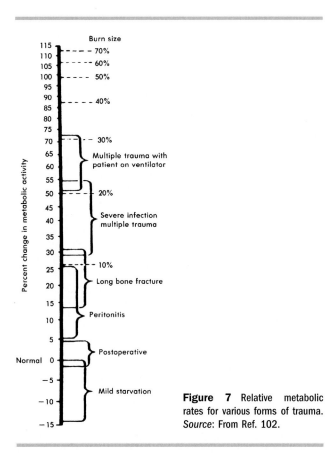

Figure 7 Relative metabolic rates for various forms of trauma. *Source:* From Ref. 102.

which generally begins within 48 hours after injury, appears to be associated with an intrinsic elevation in body core temperature as a result of a direct resetting of the hypothalamic temperature-regulating mechanism. The resetting of the central core temperature to 38.5°C occurs between the 5th and 15th day postinjury. This remains elevated for up to two months (103). The zone of neutrality, or ambient temperature at which energy expenditure is minimal, is increased in burn patients from 27–29°C to 30–32°C (104). Evidence supporting this contention relates to the observations that unburned skin remains vasoconstricted even when ambient temperatures are increased and evaporative losses are minimized (105,106). On the other hand, although the hypermetabolic state does not depend on changes in ambient room temperature, it does appear to be sensitive to such alterations, because heat production and the energy cost of healing a large surface area can be reduced by keeping patients in a warm environment (107,108). Factors mediating postburn hypermetabolism include inflammatory agents (IL-1, IL-6, TNF, eicosanoids, and oxygen free radicals) (109) and counter-regulatory hormones (catecholamines, cortisol, and glucagon) (110,111). The central nervous system appears to be important for this response, as it is decreased in patients with neurologic impairment (112–114). Of additional interest, Hart et al. reported, in pediatric patients who underwent delayed excision, that aggressive feeding was required for the full expression of burn-induced hypermetabolism. However early treatment did improve the net balance of leg skeletal muscle protein (115).

The magnitude of the hypermetabolic response reflects the extent of the thermal injury. It increases over the first week following injury and decreases in response to wound healing and the diminishing size of the burn

wound. During this time, a protein catabolic state is produced that is characterized by increased urinary nitrogen loss, which is associated with protein degradation proportional to the severity of the burn. The hypermetabolic state generates a net caloric deficit. Although much of that deficit can be met through the use of fat deposits, the oxidation of fat requires simultaneous oxidation of carbohydrates. Once glycogen stores are exhausted, protein catabolism becomes the obligatory source of the carbohydrate (116). In the process of gluconeogenesis, muscle protein is expended to liberate alanine and glutamine (116,117). Without exogenous nutritional support, skeletal muscle becomes a prime target organ of the catabolic process (106).

Postinjury Catabolism

The postinjury period is characterized by prolonged protein catabolism (particularly in muscle), negative nitrogen balance, hyperglycemia, lipolysis, hepatic fat deposition, and weight loss, all of which vary according to the extent of thermal injury. Derangements in the counter-regulatory hormones contribute to this "autocannibalism" (Fig. 8). Although it remains in a nonsteady state for weeks, the catabolic state ultimately reaches a plateau and does not change in response to caloric replacement (119,120). For a 50% total body surface area burn, the magnitude of catabolism may be twice that which normally occurs following an injury. Weight loss develops because of a breakdown of lean body mass. The loss of 300 to 600 g of body weight per day can be equated to a daily loss of 75 to 150 g of protein (121). Although treatment with calories and nitrogenous source does not affect breakdown of muscle protein, it can increase in synthesis.

This apparent metabolic paradox can be appreciated by briefly reviewing the cycle through which carbohydrates are produced and used. Gluconeogenesis uses amino acids, principally alanine and glutamine. The source of these two gluconeogenic amino acids is skeletal muscle. Although the source appears to be obligatory, exogenous amino acids can either decrease muscle efflux or contribute to increased muscle synthesis (122). The increase in conversion of alanine to glucose is accompanied by a reduction in the incorporation of exogenous alanine into protein and an increase in the release and synthesis of alanine by muscle (30). At the same time, a reduction in circulating branched-chain amino acids suggests that the administration of exogenous amino acids, especially those of the branched-chain variety, may stimulate de novo synthesis of alanine and glutamine by skeletal muscle (123).

The process of gluconeogenesis from skeletal muscle substrates requires energy. In this process, skeletal muscle uses fatty acid substrates (124). Meanwhile, glucose from the liver's new stores is only partially used in the periphery, being converted to a three-carbon precursor, which in turn must return to the liver for reconversion into new glucose. The process of reconversion, referred to as the Cori cycle, also requires fatty acid substrates (125). Although increased lipolysis and lipid mobilization occur in the burn patient, exogenous administration of fatty acids appears to be of little nutritional value and may be related to variation in the body's ability to clear lipids when in a state of stress (126), Following thermal injury, it has been noted that a diet consisting of 5% to 15% of the nonprotein calories as fat is optimal, and that a diet consisting of more is deleterious (127). In humans, the inhibition of triglyceride lipase by insulin may lead to a futile cycle of triglyceride metabolism (128). Immediately after a burn, for example, there is increased lipoprotein lipase activity and clearance of triglycerides,

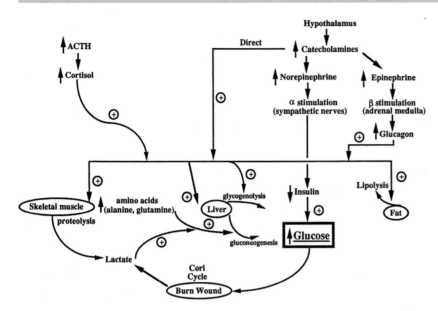

Figure 8 Hormonal interactions following burn injury. *Abbreviations*: ACTH, adrenocorticotropic hormone. *Source*: From Ref. 118.

as insulin levels fall and glucagon and glucose levels rise. In response to plasma triglycerides, lipase activity increases. However, the resulting free fatty acids cannot be used without carbohydrates and eventually must be reesterified to triglycerides. For a more detailed discussion of these considerations, see Chapter 1.

Therapeutic Implications

The dramatically increased metabolic expenditure following thermal injury must be compensated by increased nutritional support to avoid the plethora of potential complications associated with nutritional deficiency. Energy requirements in terms of caloric needs can be calculated according to the formula below proposed by Curreri et al. (124).

$$25 \text{ kcal/kg of body weight } +$$
$$40 \text{ kcal/percent of body surface burned}$$

Carbohydrate is the major source of calories and contributes to nitrogen sparing. The major carbohydrate form is glucose, and it must be administered with nitrogen-containing nutrients to improve nitrogen balance and allow more calories to be used for the restoration of nitrogen balance. Approximately 20% of caloric requirements should be protein or amino acid equivalents; improved survivals have been demonstrated with a 100:1 calorie-to-nitrogen ratio diet (129), and patients may require up to 2 to 2.5 g protein/kg/day. Essential fatty acids must also be provided, and 2% to 4% of daily caloric requirements should consist of linoleic acid (102). In addition to preventing a state of fatty acid deficiency, fat also provides extra calories and may provide a protein-sparing effect (130). Overfeeding, however, may be just as detrimental as underfeeding. Burn catabolism cannot be overcome by massive overfeeding. Infusion rates of 6000 kcal/day did not improve nitrogen balance, but instead led to hepatic steatosis (131) and increased carbon dioxide production (115,132). Disproportionate lipids may lead to hyperlipidemia, hypoxia, impaired immune function, and increase mortality (133).

In patients with large burns, enteral tube feeding is almost always necessary to achieve nutritional goods. Most patients, when left to their own dietary habits, do not consume adequate nutrients orally. Generally a high-calorie, high-protein diet should be administered in addition to the calculated tube requirement. Early enteral feeding has been determined to be safe (134) and has been shown to improve survival by preserving the intestinal mucosal barrier (130) and attenuating elevations of glucagon, cortisol, and catecholamines (128,135). Further, vitamin and mineral requirements must be provided in all nutritional programs. Glutamine and arginine supplementation has been associated with improved immune function, intestinal growth, and wound healing. Oxandrolone, an anabolic analog of testosterone has been found to improve the net balance of protein by improving muscle protein synthesis and lean mass in burned children. This may be related to changes in gene expression (136). Indiscriminate use of total parenteral nutrition in the face of a functioning gut is not justified as it is fraught with immune defense impairment (137) and increased infectious complications (138,139).

Daily weight gain is the most effective single index for assessing the adequacy of nutritional support and must be continually monitored. Nitrogen balance studies generally are inaccurate when large open wounds exist, and indexes of immunologic status and visceral protein pool have not been shown to accurately predict specific nutritional deficiencies (102). Indirect calorimetry (metabolic cart) estimates energy expenditure and therefore nutritional requirements by analyzing inspired and expired gases and calculating the oxygen consumption and carbon dioxide production. However, this technique is expensive, difficult in nonintubated patients, and associated with the error of extrapolating a 20-minute study to 24 hours (130).

ORGAN SYSTEM ALTERATIONS

Cardiovascular Responses

The initial "ebb" phase following burn injury is likely caused by a combination of hypovolemia and myocardial depression

(140) and consists of a fall in cardiac output of 50% of normal or greater. This response occurs within minutes of injury, and there is a loss of myocardial contractility and altered ventricular compliance even prior to measurable decreases in plasma volume or after adequate fluid resuscitation (41,141,142). Suggested mediators of this cardiac dysfunction include a myocardial depressant factor (43), TNF (43), interleukins, ADH, oxygen free radicals (45–47), and nitric oxide (22). Myocardial depressant factor, although still not fully identified chemically, is produced by the pancreas during circulatory shock (143) and has negative effects on the cardiovascular, splanchnic, and reticuloendothelial systems (144).

Most of these responses tend to normalize as plasma volume is restored through resuscitative efforts, although the cardiac output generally returns to normal and may actually exceed normal values before complete restoration of plasma volume is achieved. This resultant hyperdynamic circulatory response (or "flow" pattern) appears to complement the hypermetabolic response previously discussed, and both appear to reflect an effort of the body to heal the injured wound. During this phase, excessive catecholamine secretion may lead to cardiomyopathy, focal necrosis, and myocarditis (145,146). Studies using selective β-adrenergic blockade demonstrated a decrease in myocardial oxygen requirements while preventing the resulting changes in lipid kinetics (147). Further, Herndon et al. have shown in burned children that giving propranolol in sufficient dosage to decrease the heart rate by 20%, decreased the hypermetabolism and reversed the protein catabolism (148). Although postburn hypermetabolism cannot be completely reversed, the use of continuous low-dose insulin infusion, propranolol, and oxandrolone is cost effective and has low toxicity (149).

Renal Responses

The burn patient is initially in a state of antidiuresis. In the presence of a hyperdynamic circulatory response, oliguria occurs as a result of increased and inappropriate ADH secretion. It has also been shown that glomerular vessels become constricted, prolonging transit time through the kidney and decreasing urinary output. Metabolism within the kidney appears to increase, as evidenced by a consistent uptake of glucose, whereas renal plasma flow remains essentially unaltered (150,151).

Despite the glomerular vascular changes, renal complications are relatively uncommon in thermally injured patients because of the improved knowledge of resuscitation since 1980. The initial renal lesion following burn injury appears to be biphasic proteinuria. The initial phase includes a mild, transient albuminuria followed in four to seven days by a proteinuria with a relatively low albumin composition (152). Any relationship between the proteinuria and the subsequent development of renal failure remains unclear. When renal failure does ensue, it proceeds characteristically with polyuria in the face of a rising serum creatinine.

Oliguric renal failure is quite rare. When it occurs, it develops early and appears to be related to inadequate resuscitation. In contrast, the more common polyuric renal failure generally arises in the second or third week following the burn injury and does not seem to be caused by hypovolemia. The findings of low urinary sodium and high urinary potassium indicate intact distal tubular function. These observations indicate that burn-related dysfunction in the glomerulus and proximal tubule presents the distal nephron with a solute load, producing a "downstream"

diuresis (153). The cause of this form of renal failure remains unknown, and it is unique to the burn patient.

Endocrine Responses

A complex endocrine response is elicited by thermal injury that probably is related to peripheral nervous system stimulation of the hypophysial-hypothalamic axis of the brain that then in turn intricately interacts with metabolic, immune, and other body systems (154). Pain, through the release of neuropeptides by sensory C fibers, may be a major stimulatory event for the hormonal response (20). Sustained, elevated levels of adrenocorticotropic hormone (ACTH) from the anterior pituitary gland have been reported throughout the acute phase of thermal injury and only decrease to normal as the burn wound heals (155). If one uses measurements of plasma cortisol as an index of ACTH secretion, however, no consistent patterns have been noted in burn patients (156). The activity of the thyroid gland is decreased following injury, and thyroid-stimulating hormone is decreased relative to the availability of thyroid hormones (157). Thyroxine (T_4) and triiodothyronine (T_3) blood levels are generally low in burn injury, although a less pronounced decrease in T_4 and a transitory increase in reverse T_3 have been identified (156,158). However, there are no data to support thyroid supplementation. The "flow" phase is likely not thyroid dependent as thyroprivic experimental models also demonstrate a catabolic/hypermetabolic burn response (159–161).

Growth hormone secretion is inconsistent in burn patients, but often is elevated following thermal injury. Recent work has been directed toward hormonal modulation in an attempt to improve wound healing. Exogenous growth hormone administration improves the healing time of donor sites in children and accelerates healing after extensive burns, (162,163) but may exacerbate hyperglycemia and insulin resistance (164). Studies by Rose and Herndon have reported that recombinant growth hormone, when administered to burned children in a dose of 2 mg/kg/day, improves skin graft donor site healing and shortens hospital stay by up to 33%. Its anabolic action is related to improving protein synthesis by increasing insulin-like growth factor I (IGF-I) levels (165). Other work with IGF-I supplementation in burn patients showed preservation of lean body mass and gut function without altering glucose metabolism (166). Follicle-stimulating hormone and luteinizing hormone secretion are depressed in burn patients, whereas prolactin secretion may be suppressed in children but elevated in adults (167). The significance of these observations remains unknown.

ADH measurements reveal high levels in both blood and urine of adults and children during the first week after burn injury. ADH release is normally modulated by osmoreceptors of the supraventricular and supraoptic nuclei in the hypothalamus, volume receptors in the right atrium, and the carotid bodies. However, oversecretion is apparently independent of plasma and urine osmolality and volume but related closely to the severity of the thermal injury (168).

Glucocorticoids, mineralocorticoids, and 17-ketosteroids are the major hormonal groups secreted by the adrenal cortex. Cortisol is high in burn patients with loss of the normal circadian rhythm, particularly in the first week following thermal injury. This elevation is believed to be essentially unrelated to ACTH hypersecretion but does relate closely to the size of the burn (60). Aldosterone is secreted in markedly increased amounts and produces sodium retention and increased potassium loss, which persists for many weeks in adults with major burns (168). The 17-ketosteroids are also elevated in burn patients as measured in the urine, but the significance of this finding is unknown.

Epinephrine and norepinephrine synthesis, under hypothalamic control, are dramatically increased in thermal injury, as detected in serum and urine of burn patients, and are major mediators of the hypermetabolic response (169). Immunoreactive insulin is elevated following thermal injury, and this elevation persists until healing of the burn wound. Insulin hypersecretion is usually accompanied by elevated glucose in the blood, implying a relative insulin resistance (170). Plasma glucagon levels are also elevated and appear to play a key role in the hypermetabolic response (171). It is thought that glucagon released from alpha cells of the pancreas is more influential in producing postburn hyperglycemia than the so-called insulin resistance (172). A synergy exists between cortisol, glucagon, and catecholamines that contributes to the increases in glycolysis, gluconeogenesis, proteolysis, and lipolysis observed during the postburn hypermetabolism/catabolism (Fig. 8).

RESISTANCE TO INFECTION

The causes of death have changed with the progression of burn management. In the 1940s to 1950s most patients died of burn shock. With more vigorous fluid resuscitation protocols, wound sepsis became the major killer in the 1960s to the 1970s. However, the development of burn centers, topical and systemic antibiotics, nutritional support, and earlier burn wound excision has considerably decreased the mortality caused by wound sepsis. Currently, pulmonary infection remains the most common cause of death in hospitalized burn patients. Resistance is impaired in these patients through disruption of the skin's mechanical barrier and defects in the body's immune system. Fauci (173) has conveniently classified the body's defense capabilities into the categories of nonspecific immune system and specific immune system. Although many defects in the capacity to resist infection have been defined in thermally injured patients, direct relationships between burning and immunologic alterations are complex and unclear and have eluded successful therapeutic intervention. However, it is clear that postburn patients demonstrate generalized immunosuppression. Allografts in burn victims survive longer than expected (174). Both in vivo and in vitro measurements of immune function are abnormal; these include decreased delayed type of hypersensitivity responses (175), cytolytic responses (176), and mixed lymphocytic responses (177).

Disruption of the Mechanical Barrier

Loss of the morphologic and physiologic integrity of the skin as a result of thermal injury allows access of microorganisms to deeper tissues and the systemic circulation. Not only is devitalized tissue a nutritious medium for the growth of bacteria, but thermally injured skin may also be a source of circulating substances or toxins that can contribute to multifaceted, systemic alterations, including impairment in the synthesis of secretory immunoglobulins, bone marrow depression, and myocardial depression (14,31,168,178). As discussed earlier, decreased meseneric blood flow also contributes to these systemic effects following burn injury through bacterial/endotoxin translocation into the portal circulation and/or priming of the cellular elements within the GALT.

Impairment of the Nonspecific Immune System

Phagocytic cell activity and accumulation are enhanced in response to tissue injury through an inflammatory reaction characterized by increased vascular permeability. This appears to be mediated by vasoactive amines, prostaglandins, C-reactive proteins, and other components of inflammation (179). In addition, the release of chemotactic substances from injured tissues or through the influence of gram-negative organisms enhances the attraction of phagocytes to invading microorganisms. Should bacteria not be contained at the site of invasion, the fixed macrophages, particularly in the regional lymph nodes, may prove effective in killing invading bacteria.

Opsonins are antibodies that enhance the phagocytic process by rendering the microorganisms more susceptible to phagocytosis. Complement and fibronectin are characterized opsonins. Complement is a system of serum proteins that participates in inflammation and phagocytosis and in neutralizing viruses, enhancing leukocyte chemotaxis, and killing bacteria. Fibronectin is a glycoprotein existing in a soluble circulating form in the plasma and a relatively insoluble form in connective tissue. Fibronectin enhances macrophage phagocytosis and may prevent organ failure through inhibition of fibrin aggregation among other functions. Other undefined regional defense mechanisms also participate in protecting the host from hostile microorganisms.

The presence of major thermal injury adversely affects this nonspecific inflammatory system. Both circulating and fixed phagocytic cells, with or without the help of opsonizing factors, are functionally impaired following a major burn. Not only is phagocytic activity decreased in burn injury, but bacteriocidal activity is also decreased, and chemotaxis is impaired through decreased complement activation (180,181).

Impairment of the Specific Immune System

The specific immune system includes both humoral and cellular components and their respective products. The production of specific antibody requires a complex interaction of many cell types. Once an antigen is recognized, it is processed by macrophages and presented to thymic-dependent lymphocytes (T-cells). T-cells proliferate and in turn activate bursal-dependent lymphocytes (B-cells) that ultimately produce a specific antibody to the antigen. Stimulated T-lymphocytes have other important functions such as antigen memory storage, direct cytotoxic effects, and production of mediators of immune reactivity regulating both the specific and nonspecific immune responses. Antibody formation is also influenced by a specific subset of T-cells known as T-helper cells and a second subset known as suppressor T-cells. Suppressor T-cells generally modulate responses, preventing uncontrolled immune reactions by inhibiting T-cell stimulation of antibody production.

In patients with burns of more than 20% of their total body surface area, essentially all immune functions are affected. Overall, there is a decrease in total lymphyoctye populations, an impairment in the functional capacity of T-cells, and an activation of suppressor T-cells (182). This depresses T-cell—generated responses, including production of cytotoxic cells, B-cell activation, and recruitment of uncommitted lymphoid cells. Immunoglobulin (Ig) synthesis is also decreased, particularly IgG production, in contrast to IgM and IgA, which are little altered.

Some investigators suggest that there exists an intracellular T-cell defect (182). Burn injury also interferes with the signalling pathways responsible for T-cell activation and effector response generation (89). This has been associated with the release of hormones (glucocorticoids and catecholamines) (183) and the systemic release of PGE$_2$ by activated macrophages. Although the precise mechanisms are unknown, PGE$_2$ decreases IL-2 production and, hence, T-cell activation (184–186). Trials investigating IL-2 and indomethacin (a cyclooxygenase inhibitor) administration in burned mice have demonstrated an improved survival (187). Others have used polymixin B, which neutralized the effects of lipopolysaccharides and may decrease macrophage activation. Although they observed a reversal of the unfavorable T4/T8 ratio and a decrease in endotoxin concentration, there was no change in survival or outcome (188,189).

PULMONARY CONSEQUENCES OF THERMAL INJURY

Pulmonary alterations as a result of thermal injury occur in response to direct pulmonary injury caused by the inhalation of the products of combustion and indirectly as a response to cutaneous burns alone.

Inhalation of the Products of Combustion

Inhalation injury accounts for the vast majority of deaths in fires, and is responsible for the high mortality in patients who survive and are admitted to hospitals. The following classification has proven useful in categorizing the various disorders related to inhalation injury and is based on mechanisms of disease (190):

1. Carbon monoxide poisoning
2. Smoke toxicity
   a. Direct injury caused by
      i. Hot gases
      ii. Super-heated particulate matter
      iii. Conversion of gases to acid and alkali
   b. Smoke poisoning caused by thermodegradation of
      i. Natural substances
      ii. Synthetic substances

Carbon Monoxide Poisoning

Carbon monoxide is a clear, colorless, odorless gas produced by the incomplete combustion of organic fuels. Carbon monoxide has an affinity for hemoglobin that is approximately 250 times that of oxygen and shifts the oxyhemoglobin dissociation curve to the left. Thus the oxygen that remains bound to hemoglobin is not readily available to cells, resulting in a decreased tissue oxygen tension that is considerably lower than that seen with simple hypoxia alone (Fig. 9). The toxic effect of carbon monoxide may be the result of this hypoxia alone or its binding to heme-containing proteins at the cellular level (191). Carbon monoxide impairs the cytochrome chain through competition with oxygen for cytochrome a$_3$ and has been observed to have a direct toxic effect on mammalian lung tissue (192). Carbon monoxide also binds to cardiac and skeletal muscle, producing carboxymyoglobin that dissociates slower than carboxyhemoglobin. This circumstance may become apparent during initial treatment as a rebound type of response. Pure carbon monoxide poisoning produces no grossly detectable lung pathologic alteration, although, histologically, alveolar type II cellular organelles are physically altered (193).

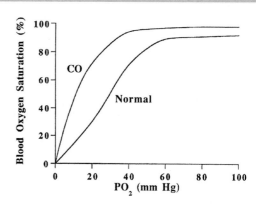

Figure 9 Oxygen–hemoglobin dissociation curve. Note the shift to the left in the presence of carbon monoxide, indicating that oxygen is more tightly bound to the hemoglobin molecule. *Abbreviation*: PO$_2$, partial pressure of oxygen.

The clinical symptoms of carbon monoxide poisoning range from dyspnea and headache at levels in excess of 10% to 20% to coma and death, when inspired air contains levels of 60%. Cherry red skin discoloration is usually not apparent because of facial burning, but a high index of suspicion based on the history of burning in an enclosed space, orofacial burns, and nasal hair singeing suggests the diagnosis. A laboratory carboxyhemoglobin determination confirms the diagnosis, and treatment consists of rapid evacuation from the toxic source and the administration of 100% oxygen, preferably by endotracheal tube, in symptomatic poisoning. The half-life of carboxyhemoglobin in room air is approximately 210 minutes, but during 100% oxygen administration it can be reduced to 40 to 60 minutes. Hyperbaric oxygen has been proposed as a treatment modality in severe poisoning on the basis of a rapid decrease in the half-life of carboxyhemoglobin and clinical evidence of improved neurologic recovery (194). However, the logistics of caring for patients with significant burns within the confines of oxygen chambers is difficult.

Smoke Toxicity

Direct Injury

Direct heat injury as a result of inhalation of hot gases is extremely rare below the vocal cords because of the efficiency of heat dissipatory reflexes (195). However, parenchymal injury to the epithelium in distal air passages may be observed by the inhalation of a superheated system that has 4000 times the heat capacity of air. Super-heated particulate matter and soot that is not filtered out in the proximal airways may also produce local thermal burns in the alveoli (196). Corrosive acids and alkalis resulting from the reaction of sulfur and nitrogen oxides adherent to soot particles with lung surface water also produce direct, local parenchymal injury (190).

Smoke Poisoning

The incomplete combustion of both natural and synthetic products in smoke produces noxious gases that are inhaled and elicit both local and systemic effects. The magnitude of injury is dependent on the type of noxious gas inhaled, its concentration and solubility, and the duration of exposure. Water-soluble chemicals such as ammonia, sulfur dioxide, chlorine, and hydrogen chloride tend to dissolve in the upper respiratory tract, whereas lipid-soluble gases such as the aldehydes, phosgene, and nitric oxide tend to reach more distal lung radicals (197). Cyanide, a product of the combustion of synthetic materials such as polyurethane, produces its effects through systemic absorption and direct cellular poisoning.

The effect of inhaled toxic products includes direct epithelial destruction, mucosal edema, ciliary paralysis, and surfactant deficiency, the latter resulting from injury to type II alveolar epithelial cells (198,199). Cast formation occurs causing obstruction, which leads to atelectasis, air trapping, and an increased risk for barotrauma. Pulmonary alveolar macrophages secrete chemotoxins producing leukocyte sequestration, which in turn release proteolytic enzymes and oxygen free radicals that potentiate pulmonary injury from the microvascular side (193). Concurrently, there is an increase in exudation of protein-rich plasma that encourages bacterial overgrowth. Subsequent pathologic alterations depend on the severity and character of the inhalation and include a fulminant adult respiratory distress syndrome, pulmonary edema, bronchial pneumonia, and sepsis, all of which contribute to the high mortality rate observed in patients with inhalation injury.

The diagnosis of smoke inhalation is based primarily on history, blood gas analysis, carboxyhemoglobin, and cyanide determinations, as well as on special procedures, including bronchoscopy, xenon clearance, and pulmonary function tests. Physical examination and chest X-ray films, although essential, may be misleading, particularly under acute conditions when a paucity of physical signs tend to be the rule in severe inhalation injury.

Careful monitoring of patients suspected of sustaining smoke poisoning is essential. In less severe injuries, treatment consists of the use of humidified air, vigorous pulmonary toilet, and the judicious use of bronchodilators. The early use of aerosolized heparin and acetylcysteine has been useful in preventing mucous plugs and improves pulmonary function (200). Because heparin is ineffective in lysing mucous plugs that have already formed, aerosol administration of tissue plasminogen activator (TPA), which lyses fibrin clots, was studied by Enkhbaatar et al. The study showed, in sheep subjected to cotton smoke, that the administration of 2 mg of TPA improved the pulmonary abnormalities and could be clinically useful (201). Immediate intubation is warranted if signs of laryngeal edema are present (hoarseness or stridor). Rigid bronchoscopy may be required for pulmonary cast removal. Pressure-control ventilation (permissive hypercapnea) may be attempted when pulmonary failure progresses despite conventional volume ventilation.

High-frequency jet ventilation may be beneficial by decreasing barotrauma and improving airway clearance through the maintenance of patent distal airways. High frequency oscillatory ventilation (HFOV) has been utilized in the neonatal intensive care unit for infants with respiratory distress syndrome for many years and has recently been used in adult burn patients with ARDS in an attempt to avoid "ventilator-induced lung injury" (202). Cartotto et al. reported a retrospective study of 25 patients with a 28% incidence of inhalation injury, who had severe oxygenation failure from ARDS following 4.8 days of conventional mechanical ventilation (CMV). After switching from CMV to HFOV, there were significant improvements in the PaO_2/FiO_2 ratio within one hour and in the oxygenation index within 24 hours. HFOV was used for an average of six days and was continued during 26 operations in 14

patients (203). Nitric oxide inhalation has also shown some advantages. Invasive monitoring to include pulmonary wedge pressure and thermodilution cardiac output parameters is often essential, particularly when positive end-expiratory pressure is used. Corticosteroids and prophylactic antibiotics are ineffective (204).

Indirect Pulmonary Injury

Pulmonary edema following pure cutaneous burning without inhalation injury relates to alterations in the pulmonary microvasculature. Hemodynamic alterations related to resuscitation, increased capillary permeability, and alterations in blood flow characteristics as a result of cutaneous thermal injury may contribute to indirect lung damage. Patients with major thermal injury and noninhalation pulmonary dysfunction have been shown to have consistently high concentrations of fragment D resulting from fibrinogen degradation. This phenomenon is associated with systemic complement depletion and platelet aggregation with release of platelet products that may cause increased translocation of water and protein from the pulmonary microcirculation contributing to the development of an ARDS picture (205). In addition, activated complement may stimulate leukocyte aggregation, resulting in trapping of these aggregates in the pulmonary microcirculation. These leukocytes may then produce toxic oxygen metabolites that may also contribute to the development of ARDS. Later, pulmonary alterations generally relate to the onset of sepsis and may also manifest themselves as ARDS or bronchial pneumonia. Trials involving the administration of aerosolized free radical scavengers (dimethyl sulfoxide and N-acetylcysteine) have decreased lung fluid accumulation (206). However, current therapies are primarily directed toward supportive intervention, and mortality from the pulmonary manifestations of burns remains high.

PHYSIOLOGIC CONSIDERATIONS IN MANAGING THE BURN PATIENT
Fluid Resuscitation

The pathophysiologic alterations caused by the fluid losses in acutely burned patients require volume replacement to preserve vital functions and to prevent hypovolemic shock. Fluid losses as a result of increased capillary permeability in injured and noninjured tissues are greatest in the first 24 hours following burning and diminish thereafter. Accompanying intravascular deficits also must be corrected but generally are less responsive to resuscitative efforts until the volume losses from "capillary leaking" are adequately controlled; 20% to 30% of infused crystalloid remains within the vascular system (207).

The optimal approach to fluid resuscitation remains controversial in terms of both the volume of fluid to be administered and its composition. A wide variety of fluid replacement formulas have been proposed (208–212), each with its advocates, differing primarily from one another with respect to salt and colloid content. Virtually all formulas are based on patient weight and the extent of skin surface burned. Only burns reaching a depth of second degree or greater are considered in these calculations. The fluid formulas provide guidelines for the resuscitation of burn patients and are altered according to the response to treatment. The two most widely used formulas are the modified Brooke formula (2 mL/kg/% burn) and the Parkland Formula [(also called the Baxter formula) 4 mL/kg/% burn] (213).

The effectiveness of administered fluid in early burn resuscitation with regard to its colloidal or noncolloidal content remains unresolved. Advocates of colloid-containing fluids recognize their potential use in maintaining plasma oncotic pressure and intravascular volume. Those opposed to such solutions emphasize the increased capillary permeability in the first 24 hours after thermal injury that results in leakage of plasma protein, particularly albumin, into the interstitium. It is argued that adding exogenous protein (i.e., colloid) to the extravascular protein pool raises this interstitial oncotic pressure further, and thereby prevents restoration of an adequate circulating blood volume. Furthermore, controlled trials have demonstrated that colloid use has no effect on clinical outcome (214,215). There is general agreement, however, that the administration of colloid-containing fluids during the second 24 hours following the burn, and thereafter, is associated with intravascular colloid retention and thus decreased fluid requirements.

In contrast to the colloid controversy, sodium ion administration appears to be essential to successful resuscitation. Balanced salt solutions are quite popular and effective, although the use of hypertonic saline solutions has been recommended (211). Hypertonic saline (sodium concentration = 250 mmol/L) reduces volume requirements, may be useful in patients with limited cardiovascular reserve but requires careful monitoring (216), and is associated with increased renal failure and death (217). When employed, hypertonic saline is dependent on careful dosing interval and infusion rates (218).

Burn resuscitation involves walking a physiologic tightrope: under-resuscitation risks low perfusion of the burn wound as well as the hepatic and splanchnic circulation, while over-resuscitation may lead to pulmonary edema, prolongation of mechanical ventilation, the need for escharotomies, and release of abdominal compartment syndrome. Holm et al. (219) used transpulmonary thermo-dilution (TTD) for hemodynamic monitoring to compare goal-directed therapy guided by invasive monitoring with standard care (Parkland/Baxter formula). Fluid infusion during the first 24 hours following burn was significantly different between the two groups. The Parkland patients received a mean of 16,232 mL Ringer's lactate, which was very close to the estimated volume for the first 24 hours (15,988 mL). The TTD patients received a mean of 27,064 mL of Ringer's lactate with an estimated mean Parkland volume in this group being 17,306 mL. The results showed no significant difference in preload or cardiac output parameters. Their findings also included that "the additional crystalloid fluid that was infused in the treatment group was lost from the intravascular space, and had no noticeable effect on the plasma volume." The authors suggest that the manipulation of the capillary permeability is an area that ought to be investigated. Pruitt, in an editorial states that "adequate resuscitation has been succeeded by 'fluid creep,' (220) producing excessive resuscitation in the apparent belief that if some fluid is good, lots of fluid will be even better" (221).

In order to accurately resuscitate the burn patient, there must be a careful estimate of the percent total body surface area that has sustained a second- or third-degree burn. The "rule of nines" (Figs. 10 and 11) divides the adult body surface into single or multiples of 9% (e.g., arm = 9%, anterior trunk = 18%, leg = 18%, and head = 9%). However, it must be modified for children in whom the head is proportionally a greater percentage and the legs are relatively smaller. The Lund and Browder chart is a more accurate

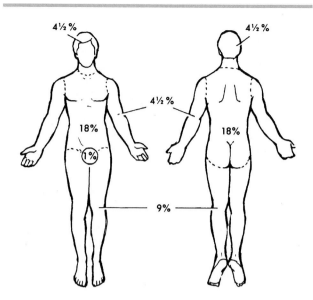

Figure 10 "Rule of nines" for adults. Rapid estimation of extent of burn injury can be accomplished by using the "rule of nines" as an approximation of body surface areas involved. *Source*: From Ref. 212.

way to estimate TBSA burned (222). The "surface area graphic evaluation" diagram is a computer-based method in which the computer mouse is used to trace the area burned on a template. The program will compute the TBSA burned, based upon the individual patient's body weight and height, and the resuscitation volume required according to the Parkland formula. It is available on the Internet at http://www.sagediagram.com and there is a version for personal data assistants. Patients with second- and third-degree burns involving greater than 15% of their body surface area should receive parenteral fluids, and the effectiveness of resuscitation should be monitored precisely.

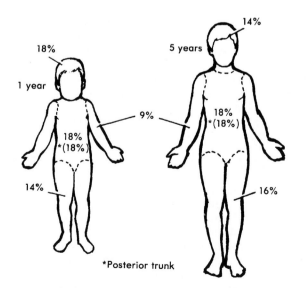

Figure 11 Modified "rule of nines" for ages 1 and 5 years. Adult proportions assumed at age 15. *Source*: From Ref. 212.

An Approach to Resuscitation

The replacement program that we use has proven to be convenient and successful over many years of application and is described here. In this program, fluid losses and daily maintenance requirements are related to the total body surface area and the surface area burned (in m^2) as calculated from a standard height–weight nomogram. This approach has proven to be highly accurate and allows standardization of fluid therapy in managing both adults and children. During the first 24 hours following burning, fluid requirements are calculated as follows:

$2000 \ mL/m^2$ of body surface/24 hr

(maintenance requirements)

$+ \ 5000 \ mL/m^2$ of body surface burned/24 hr

(fluid losses)

One half the calculated volume is infused in the first eight hours following burning, and the remainder in the subsequent 16 hours. Patients should also be given either H_2 blockers or proton pump inhibitors to prevent the development of Curling's ulcers.

For such resuscitation, a single, standard solution for intravenous therapy is used with adaptation to the patient's needs as necessary. This solution consists of:

Lactated Ringer's solution in 5% dextrose and water

$+ \ 12.5$ g of salt-poor albumin per liter

We have found such a solution to be ideal. This isotonic protein-containing fluid ensures the provision of lactate to combat any systemic acidosis and an adequate carbohydrate load to ensure protein sparing. Because of the hyperkalemia associated with tissue injury and increased aldosterone, addition of potassium to this solution during the first 48 hours after burning is inappropriate and may be detrimental.

During the second 24 hours following burning, fluid requirements generally decrease and are calculated on the basis of the following formula:

$1500 \ mL/m^2$ of body surface area/24 hr

(maintenance requirements)

$+ \ 4000 \ mL/m^2$ of body surface area burned/24 hr

(fluid losses)

Such requirements are administered in equal hourly aliquots during this 24-hour period. Oral alimentation is instituted as soon as possible in the form of elemental diets initially, and the intravenous fluid needs are decreased proportionately. In most cases, oral fluid administration completely replaces intravenous therapy at the end of 48 hours following burning, allowing the removal of the intravenous catheter.

Daily fluid requirements after the initial 48 hours of fluid resuscitation generally remain the same as those for the second 24 hours; but as the burn wounds are covered and healing commences, requirements are generally diminished, and fluid therapy is revised accordingly. Initial oral alimentation is usually administered through a nasogastric feeding tube that is retained for several days thereafter to ensure adequate oral nutrition. Until the convalescent phase is well underway, H_2 blockers or proton pump inhibitors should be continued to protect the stomach from the development of a Curling's ulcer. Patients should be started on regular meals as soon as such alimentation can be adequately tolerated.

Monitoring Fluid Resuscitation

The effectiveness of the resuscitation program must be constantly monitored and altered if deviations from the expected course are noted. Among the most useful physical signs to determine the adequacy of resuscitation are the general state of alertness of the patient and the stability of pulse and blood pressure, including peripheral perfusion characteristics. The urine output (by means of an indwelling urinary catheter) is the most readily obtained measure of effectiveness of resuscitation, and a urine volume of 30 to 50 mL/hr in the adult and 20 to 40 mL/m^2 of total body surface area per hour in children are expected. A significantly higher urine output may indicate overhydration or other complications (e.g., polyuric renal failure and excessive glucose loading), because in the acutely burned patient an antidiuretic state caused by multiple factors, including ADH secretion, is present.

Baseline laboratory studies should be obtained at the time of admission and repeated at 12 to 24 hours or more frequently as needed. Among the values to be obtained initially are a complete blood cell count; serum levels of sodium, potassium, chloride, and bicarbonate; a blood urea nitrogen and creatinine, urine protein, and serum protein electrophoresis; and arterial blood gases. An initial hemoconcentration is expected, regardless of the resuscitation program instituted; and therefore an elevated hematocrit and slight elevation of other parameters may be identified. Metabolic acidosis is particularly significant in children and may indicate inadequacy of resuscitation.

A chest X-ray examination, electrocardiogram, and complete urinalysis are usually performed on admission and repeated only as indicated during the subsequent course. Invasive monitoring with Swan-Ganz catheters or central venous lines is not routinely performed except in elderly patients, patients with cardiovascular compromise, or patients with inhalation injury requiring mechanical ventilation. Inotropic agents may be required if cardiac output remains poor, despite adequate volume resuscitation. However, this is generally considered to be a poor prognostic sign.

The timely administration of carefully monitored parenteral fluids to the acutely and extensively burned patient facilitating the body's own compensatory physiologic alterations prevents early complications, minimizes physiologic disturbances, and provides a basis on which future care of the acutely burned patient depends.

Management of the Burn Wound

After fluid resuscitation has been successfully ensured, attention is next directed to the burn wound itself. The wound is cleansed with a suitable antiseptic solution such as povidone-iodine (Betadine) and debrided of foreign matter, necrotic tissue, and any blebs or vesicles that may be present. Because hypothermia may be a problem during this debridement period, overhead radiant energy sources are usually used to minimize the loss of body heat.

Because the burn wound is essentially an extensive area of coagulation necrosis with accompanying ischemia from the underlying thrombosis of the local microcirculation, this avascular dead tissue is an excellent bacterial culture medium that can rapidly become a source of bacterial growth and the development of sepsis from hematologic dissemination of microorganisms. For this reason, topical antimicrobial agents are applied directly to the wound during the early period after the burn. In the historical development of burn management during the past several decades, a variety of agents have been developed for this purpose, each with its particular advantages and disadvantages. Presently four such agents are in use at burn centers across the United States as summarized in Table 4. Each of these agents, in varying degrees, satisfies the characteristics of an ideal topical agent, which include (i) antibacterial activity that is both broad spectrum in nature and nontoxic locally or on absorption, (ii) resistance to the development of strains of bacteria that would not be covered, (iii) adequate permeation and the maintenance of continuing activity in the burn eschar, (iv) absence of pain on application, and (v) absence of adverse effects on the behavior of the wound, including its healing properties.

Silver, in various forms, has been used as an effective antiseptic dating back to 1000 BC (224–227). Silver nitrate solution has been used for decades, but is not without clinical problems and it tends to stain all that it touches. Other compounds of silver such as silver sulphadiazine, silver sulphadiazine chlorhexidine, silver sulphadiazine with cerium nitrate as well as products like Acticoat (Westaim Biomedical, Inc.) and Silverlon (Argentum Medical, L.L.C.) release silver into the wound in a controlled fashion. In an investigational setting, silver is toxic to fibroblasts, but when used clinically its toxic effects are modified in concentrations, which are bactericidal.

Of the agents currently available, 1% silver sulfadiazine is the most popular among burn specialists and is our choice. This drug is essentially nontoxic, is easy to apply and soothing to the patient, and has a broad spectrum of antimicrobial activity and minimal problems with the development of resistant strains. Its only major disadvantage is its limited penetration through the eschar and its relative ineffectiveness when deep eschar colonization with microorganisms has already occurred. When the latter circumstance exists, a gentamicin cream is usually substituted if the cultured organisms are sensitive. Mafenide (11.1%) also diffuses well through devascularized tissues but is unfortunately associated with metabolic acidosis because of carbonic anhydrase inhibition. Silver sulfadiazine is applied in a thin layer (usually 1 mm thick) two or three times daily, using a sterile glove or tongue depressor. Although some specialists leave the treated burn wound open to the air, we generally apply a thin layer of fine mesh gauze impregnated with the cream over the treated burn area and further retain it with a net-like dressing (212). This approach allows patients to move about freely and

guarantees contact of the cream with the burn wound at all times. At the present time, all first-degree and superficial second-degree burns are managed in this fashion, enabling spontaneous reepithelization to occur.

For deep second-degree burns and all third-degree burns, "early" surgical excision is now considered the procedure of choice and is associated with a decreased mortality (228–230). Barret argued for early (within the first 24 hours of injury) excision of the burn wound and coverage with autograft or homograft. The early excision group was compared with patients who were initially treated at another institution and transferred to their hospital and underwent excision and grafting at day 6 post injury. The early excision group had lower bacterial counts and greater skin graft take (231). Although the authors make a valid point that the longer the burn eschar remains in place, the greater the bacterial colonization and lower the graft take, they did not answer the question whether excision during the first 24 hours is superior to excision at 48 to 72 hours in patients initially treated in the same institution. A laboratory study by Chen et al. in rats showed that the early excision group (at 30 minutes after the injury followed with immediate allogenic skin graft) did not show significant changes in the nitric oxide and endothelin-1 levels in plasma (232).

For deep partial-thickness burn wounds, a technique called *tangential excision* is used. This technique involves the excision of the necrotic surface of a burn by removing shavings of eschar until a pattern of pinpoint deep dermal bleeding is reached and then immediately autografting the excised surface. The rationale underlying this approach is that the removal of the zone of coagulation protects the viable elements in the zone of stasis and thereby exposes a surface that readily accepts an autograft.

One of the limiting factors in the amount of body surface area burn that can be excised during a single operative procedure is the amount of blood loss. Historically, 20% of the TBSA could be excised at one time. With the advent of the subeschar infiltration of epinephrine containing solution, the 20% limit may be increased. Multiple studies have demonstrated the safety and efficacy of this technique, some reporting almost a 70% reduction in blood loss per unit area excised without causing cardiac arrhythmias or anesthetic problems (233) Of additional interest, fibrin sealant derived from human plasma has been found to accelerate hemostasis on spilt-thickness donor sites in a multicenter prospective, open label, Phase III, randomized, comparative clinical trial. There were no adverse events reported with the use of fibrin sealant (234).

Table 4 Topical Antimicrobial Agents

Characteristics	Silver nitrate (0.5%)	Mafenide	Silver sulfadiazine	Organic iodine
Type of preparation	Aqueous solution	Cream	Cream	Foam
Method of wound care	Closed	Open or closed	Open or closed	Open or closed
Allergic reactions	None	10%	10%	5%
Pain on application	None	Severe	None	Moderate
Amount absorbed	None	5%	1%	Variable
Associated complications	Significant losses of sodium and potassium into wet dressings, methemoglobinemia	Acidosis, hyperventilation caused by renal carbonic anhydase inhibition	None	None
Fungal overgrowth	–	Often	Often	Often
Bacterial resistance	Bacteriostatic	Rare	Rare	Occasional
Cost	Inexpensive	Moderate	Moderate	Moderate

Source: From Ref. 223.

For full-thickness burns, excision is carried down to the level of the fascia, and an autograft is then placed on the exposed base. These aggressive surgical approaches to burn management have demonstrated several advantages to the more traditional methods of debridement using various proteolytic enzymes, the most popular of which has been sutilains (Travase). Such advantages have included improved function of extremities (particularly hands), a better cosmetic result, a definite decrease in the incidence of hypertrophic scarring after the burn, and a considerable reduction in hospitalization time.

In the event that a patient may have extensive body burns limiting the amount of nonburn areas that can be used for the acquisition of skin grafts, temporary coverage of the surgically debrided burn may be obtained with various biologic dressings, including amnion or porcine xenografts. Another innovative approach has been the use of artificial skin. Several types of synthetic skin have been evaluated investigationally. Of these, the bilaminate membrane appears to be the most useful (235). This substance (called Integra® Dermal Regeneration Template; Ethicon-Endo-Surgery, Inc., Cincinnati, OH, U.S.A.) consists of reconstituted collagen with a silicon synthetic epidermis. Application of Integra® to the debrided burn surface results in vascularization of the collagen layer with the production of an underlying neodermis. When donor sites become available, the silicon synthetic epidermis is stripped from the underlying collagen, and an autograft is placed on the neodermis. In order to study the safety and effectiveness of Integra®, a multi-institutional study was undertaken involving 216 burn injury patients who were treated at 13 burn care facilities in the United States. The mean take rate of Integra® was 76.2%, while the incidence of invasive infection was 3.1% and that of superficial infection 13.2% (236).

Cultured epidermal cells from a 2 cm² skin harvest have also been investigated as another option for skin coverage in the hope that these cells might produce growth factors that would enhance the healing process. The use of cultured epithelial autografts (CEA) for life-threatening burns has been in the clinical armamentarium since 1981 (237). Skin biopsies from the unburned skin are grown in tissue culture into thin sheets. The autografts are ready for placement on the burn wound within two to three weeks. While obviating the need for donor sites, CEAs have potential downsides; they are fragile and must be handled very carefully under aseptic conditions. The initial take is often 80% to 90%, with a decrease in subsequent coverage due to the susceptibility to form bullae from shear forces, even months after application. The successfully engrafted CEA will provide a mechanical barrier, but often is fragile and more susceptible to trauma than ordinary meshed split-thickness skin grafts (238). Further, this therapy is very expensive, with estimates of the cost of sheets of CEA ranging from $1000 to $13,000/% body surface area covered (239,240).

A unique problem that occasionally develops with deep second-degree or third-degree circumferential burns, especially when involving the extremities or trunk, is the resulting tourniquet effect. This occurs because the elastic membrane of the dermis is destroyed with these types of burns and no longer allows the skin to stretch, which is necessary to accommodate the underlying edema formation. In the chest, such circumferential eschar formation may prevent normal respiration. If not corrected, the rapid development of respiratory acidosis may ensue. When this problem exists, incision through the eschar should be carried out and deepened into the subcutaneous fat to effect adequate release of the constricted tissue. This can be accomplished by making vertical anterior axillary line incisions that are curved medially to the level of the suprasternal notch. In addition, transverse incisions at the level the diaphragm effect further release of the constricted tissue. In the extremities, eschar constriction often results in decreased venous outflow from the affected part and in time jeopardizes the arterial inflow. Ischemia then results which may be manifest by decreased capillary refill of the nail beds, severe pain within the involved muscle compartment of the extremity, or the development of motor and/or sensory deficits. Often, elevation of the affected extremity may allay the need for escharotomy, but continuous monitoring of the peripheral pulse, usually with an ultrasound detector, must be assured. If this cannot be guaranteed, lateral longitudinal incisions through the burn eschar should be made to the level of the subcutaneous fat to release the pressure in the constricted muscle compartments. Both extremity escharotomies and those involving the chest can generally be performed without the assistance of anesthesia, because the burn wound is usually insensitive to painful stimuli.

SUMMARY

The disruption of the physiologic equilibrium of the human organism by thermal injury varies with the extent and depth of the burn. The burn wound is characterized by a central irreversible zone of coagulation necrosis surrounded by reversible altered tissues that may be irreversibly compromised by progressive ischemia as a result of systemic factors such as hypoperfusion and local factors such as prostaglandin derivatives. Major fluid shifts caused by permeability alterations occur as a result of physical changes in the microcirculatory ultrastructure and local release of vasoactive substances. Such alterations disrupt normal Starling forces and potentiate fluid losses. Additional fluid extravasation in unburned tissues contributes to the hypovolemic state and may relate to increased capillary permeability and plasma oncotic pressure alterations.

Thermal injury induces a state of marked hypermetabolism mediated by catecholamines and requires an intense nutritional replacement program to overcome the potentially deleterious consequences of malnutrition. The initial fall in cardiac output observed in burns ("ebb" phase) is followed by an intense hyperdynamic circulatory response ("flow" phase). A state of antidiuresis is induced, and the hormonal milieu of the body is dramatically altered in concert with the metabolic and immune alterations.

Resistance to infection is severely compromised in thermally injured patients through alterations in both nonspecific and specific immune systems. Thermally altered tissue allows access of microorganisms and provides a medium for bacterial growth. Phagocytic activity is decreased along with bacteriocidal activity within the phagocytes. T-cell populations are decreased in peripheral blood, and suppressor T-cell activity is increased, whereas T-helper cell activity and other beneficial responses are depressed.

Smoke inhalation is responsible for the majority of deaths in fires. Carbon monoxide poisoning is the most common mechanism of injury; if treated quickly enough with oxygen, a successful outcome can be realized. Smoke toxicity as a result of direct injury to the airways or smoke poisoning caused by inhalation of thermodegradation of natural and synthetic substances is less well understood. Therapy has been primarily directed toward supportive care. Until the pathophysiology of this pulmonary injury is better understood, the prognosis for these patients will remain poor.

Understanding the pathophysiologic events that occur in response to a burn has significantly improved care of the burned patient over the past several decades not only by decreasing morbidity but also by enhancing survival. Particularly germane in this regard has been the recognition of the need for aggressive fluid resuscitation in the first 24 hours following burning and the importance of controlling bacterial colonization of the burn wound with its potentially deleterious effects should infection and sepsis supervene.

REFERENCES

1. Montgomery BJ. Consensus for treatment of the sickest patients you'll ever see. JAMA 1979; 241:345.
2. Pruitt BA Jr. The Scudder oration on trauma. Bull Am Coll Surg 1985; 70:2.
3. Demling RH. Burns. N Engl J Med 1985; 313:1389.
4. Lawrence JC, Bull JP. Thermal conditions which cause skin burns. J Inst Mech Eng 1976; 5:61.
5. Moritz AR, Henriques FC. Studies of thermal injury. II. The relative importance of time and surface temperature in the causation of cutaneous burns. Am J Pathol 1947; 23:695.
6. Moncrief JA. The body's response to heat. In: Artz CP, et al., eds. Burns: A Team Approach. Philadelphia: WB Saunders, 1979.
7. Lepenye G, Novak J, Nemeth L. The biophysics of thermal injury. Acta Chir Plast 1978; 20:77.
8. Wilson CE, et al. Cold water treatment of burns. J Trauma 1963; 3:477.
9. deCamara DL, Raine T, Robson MC. Ultrastructural aspects of cooled thermal injury. J Trauma 1981; 21:911.
10. Raine TJ, et al. Cooling the burn wound to maintain microcirculation. J Trauma 1981; 21:394.
11. Boykin JV, Crute SL. Mechanisms of burn shock protection after severe scald injury by cold-water treatment. J Trauma 1982; 22:859.
12. deCamara DL, Heggers JP, Robson MC. Response of mast cell granules to thermal injury. Surg Forum 1981; 32:560.
13. Heggers JP, et al. Cooling and the prostaglandin effect in the thermal injury. J Burn Care Rehabil 1982; 3:350.
14. Arturson G, Mellander S. Acute changes in capillary filtration and diffusion in experimental burn injury. Acta Physiol Scand 1964; 62:457.
15. Heggers JP, et al. Evaluation of burn blister fluid. Plast Reconstr Surg 1980; 65:798.
16. Nanto V, Viljanto J. Observations on the chemical composition of the blister fluid of burned patients. Acta Chir Scand 1962; 124:19.
17. Shakespeare PG, Levick PL, Vaitheespara RB. Proteins in blister fluid. Burns 1978; 4:254.
18. Foex BA. The cytokine response to critical illness. J Accid Emerg Med 1996; 13:154.
19. Youn Y, LaLonde C, Demling R. The role of mediators in the response to thermal injury. World J Surg 1992; 16:30.
20. Gibran NS, Heimbach DM. Mediators in thermal injury. Semin Nephrol 1993; 13:344.
21. Trang LE. Prostaglandins and inflammation. Semin Arthritis Rheum 1980; 9:153.
22. Szabo C, Thiemermann C. Invited opinion: role of nitric oxide in hemorrhagic, traumatic, and anaphylactic shock and thermal injury. Shock 1994; 2:145.
23. Bernard C, et al. Elevated temperature accelerates the induction of nitric oxide synthesis in rat macrophages. Eur J Pharmacol 1994; 270:115.
24. Demling RH, Kramer GC, Harm B. Role of thermal injury–induced hypoproteinemia on edema formation in burned and, nonburned tissue. Surgery 1984; 95:136.
25. Arturson G. Pathophysiology of the burn wound. Ann Chir Gynecol 1980; 69:178.
26. Sasaki J, Cottam G, Baxter C. Lipid peroxidation following thermal injury. J Burn Care Rehabil 1987; 4:251.
27. Robson MC, et al. Increasing dermal perfusion after burning by decreasing thromboxane production. J Trauma 1980; 20:722.
28. Anggard E, Jonsson CE. Efflux of prostaglandins in lymph from scaled issue. Acta Physiol Scand 1971; 81:440.
29. Harms BA, et al. Prostaglandin release and altered microvascular integrity after burn injury. J Surg Res 1981; 31:274.
30. Aulick LH, Wilmore DW. Leg amino acid turnover in burn patients. Fed Proc 1978; 37:536.
31. Asko-Seljavaara S, Sundell B, Rytomaa T. The effect of early excison on bone-marrow cell growth in burned mice. Burns 1976; 2–3:140.
32. Arturson G. Anti-inflammatory drugs and burn edema formation. In: May R, Dogo G, eds. Care of the Burn Wound. Basel: Karger, 1981.
33. Herndon DN, Abston S, Stein MD. Increased thromboxane B_2 levels in the plasma of burned and septic burned patients. Surg Gynecol Obstet 1984; 159:210.
34. Lewis R, Austen F, Soberman R. Leukotrienes and other products of the 5-lipoxygenase pathway. N Engl J Med 1990; 323:645.
35. Lepoivre M, et al. Alterations of ribonucleotide reductase activity following induction of the nitrite-generating pathway in adenocarcinoma cells. J Biol Chem 1990; 265:141.
36. Nathan CF, Hibbs JB. Role of nitric oxide synthesis in macrophage antimicrobial activity. Curr Opin Immunol 1991; 3:65.
37. Biffil WL, et al. Interleukin-6 in the injured patient: marker of injury or mediator of inflammation. Ann Surg 1996; 224:647.
38. Jackson DM. The diagnosis of the depth of burning. Br J Surg 1953; 40:588.
39. Branemark PI, et al. Microvascular pathophysiology of burned tissue. Ann N Y Acad Sci 1968; 150:474.
40. Zawacki BE. Reversal of capillary stasis and prevention of necrosis in burns. Ann Surg 1974; 180:98.
41. Horton JW, White J, Baxter CR. The role of oxygen-derived free radicals in burn-induced myocardial contractile depression. J Burn Care Rehabil 1988; 9:589.
42. Dobson EL, Warner GF. Factors concerned in the early stages of thermal shock. Circ Res 1957; 5:69.
43. Raffa J, Trunkey DD. Myocardial depression in acute thermal injury. J Trauma 1978; 18:90.
44. Endo S, et al. Plasma tumour necrosis factor-alpha (TNF) levels in patients with burns. Burns 1993; 19:124.
45. Gong KS, Wang CH, Zhu HN. Effect of peripheral injection of arginine vasopressin and its receptor antagonist on burn shock in the rat. Neuropeptides 1990; 17:17.
46. Liu XS, et al. Clinical significance of the change of blood monocytic interleukin-1 production *in vitro* in severely burned patients. Burns 1994; 20:302.
47. Till GO, et al. Oxygen radical dependent lung damage following thermal injury of rat skin. J Trauma 1983; 23:269.
48. Clayton JM, et al. Sequential circulatory changes in the circumferentially burned limb. Ann Surg 1977; 185:391.
49. Boykin JV, Eriksson E, Pittman RN. Microcirculation of a scald burn: an "in vivo" experimental study of the hairless mouse ear. Burns 1981; 7:335.
50. Robson MC, et al. The effect of heparin on dermal ischemia after burning. Burns 1979; 5:620.
51. Nozaki M, et al. Permeability of blood vessels after thermal injury. Burns 1980; 6:213.
52. Miller TA, White WL. Healing of second degree burns. Comparison of effects of early application of homografts and coverage with tape. Plast Reconstr Surg 1972; 49:552.
53. DelBeccaro EJ, et al. The use of specific thromboxane inhibitors to preserve the dermal microcirculation after burning. Surgery 1980; 87:137.

54. Huang YS, Li A, Yang ZC. Roles of thromboxane and its inhibitor anisodamine in burn shock. Burns 1990; 4:249.

55. Baxter CR. Fluid volume and electrolyte changes in the early post-burn period. Clin Plast Surg 1974; 1:693.

56. Carney SA, Hall M, Ricketts CR. The adenosine triphosphate content and lactic acid production of guinea pig skin after mild heat damage. Br J Dermatol 1976; 94:291.

57. Hershey FB, et al. Effect of ATP on glucose metabolism of thermally injured skin in vitro. J Trauma 1971; 11:931.

58. Allgower M, Schoenenberger GA, Sparkes BG. Burning the largest immune organ. Burns 1995; 21:S7.

59. Loebl EC, et al. The mechanism of erythrocyte destruction in the early post burn period. Ann Surg 1973; 178:681.

60. Loebl EC, et al. Erythrocyte survival following thermal injury. J Surg Res 1974; 16:96.

61. Dobke MK, et al. Oxidative activity of polymorphonuclear leukocytes after thermal injury. Eur Surg Res 1982; 14:107.

62. Schoenenberger GA, et al. Experimental evidence for a significant impairment of host defense for gram-negative organisms by a specific cutaneous toxin produced by severe burn injuries. Surg Gynecol Obstet 1975; 141:555.

63. Sparkes BG, et al. Plasma levels of cutaneous burn toxin and lipid peroxides in thermal injury. Burns 1990; 16:118.

64. Schoenenberger GA, et al. Isolation and characterization of a cutaneous lipoprotein with lethal effects produced by thermal energy in mouse skin. Biochem Biophys Res Commun 1971; 42:975.

65. Demling RH, et al. The study of burn wound edema using dichromatic absorptiometry. J Trauma 1978; 18:124.

66. Cotran RS, Majno G. The delayed and prolonged vascular leakage in inflammation. I. Topography of the leaking vessels after thermal injury. Am J Pathol 1964; 45:261.

67. Arturson G. Microvascular permeability to macromolecules in thermal injury. Acta Physiol Scand 1979; 463(suppl):111.

68. Arturson G, Jonsson CE. Transcapillary transport after thermal injury. Scand J Plast Reconstr Surg 1979; 13:29.

69. Carvajal HF. A physiologic approach to fluid therapy in severely burned children. Surg Gynecol Obstet 1980; 150:379.

70. Arturson G. The plasma kinins in thermal injury. Scand J Clin Lab Invest 1969; 24(suppl):153.

71. Baxter CR, et al. Excretion of serotinin metabolites following thermal injury. Surg Forum 1963; 14:61.

72. Hayashi H, et al. Endogenous permeability factors and their inhibitors affecting vascular permeability in cutaneous Arthurs reactions and thermal injury. Br J Exp Pathol 1964; 45:419.

73. Horakova Z, Beaven MA. Time course of histamine release and edema formation in the rat paw after thermal injury. Eur J Pharmacol 1974; 27:305.

74. Brimblecombe RW, et al. Histamine H_2 receptor antagonists and thermal injury in rats. Burns 1976; 3:8.

75. Yoshioka T, et al. Cimetidine inhibits burn edema formation. Am J Surg 1978; 136:681.

76. Burge PD, Gilbert SJ. Effect of a histamine H_2 receptor antagonist on the swelling of the burned hand. Burns 1979; 6:30.

77. Watson WC, Kutty PK, Colcleugh RG. Does cimetidine causi-ileus in the burned patient? Lancet 1977; 2:720.

78. Demling R, LaLonde C. Topical ibuprofen decreases early post burn edema. Surgery 1987; 102:857.

79. Horton JW. Free radicals and lipid peroxidation mediated injury in burn trauma: the role of antioxidant therapy. Toxicology 2003; 189:75.

80. Demling RH, LaLonde C. Early post burn lipid peroxidation: effect of ibuprofen and allopurinol. Surgery 1990; 107:85.

81. Friedl H, et al. Mediator induced activation of xanthine oxidase in endothelial cells. FASEB J 1989; 3:2512.

82. Oldham K, et al. Activation of complement by hydroxyl radical thermal injury. Surgery 1988; 104:272.

83. Saez JC, et al. Superoxide radical involvement in the pathogenesis of burn shock. Circ Shock 1984; 12:229.

84. Tanaka H, et al. Hemodynamic effects of delayed initiation of antioxidant therapy (beginning two hours after burn) in extensive third-degree burns. J Burn Care Rehabil 1995; 16:610.

85. Kingsley NW, Stein JM, Levenson SM. Measuring tissue pressure to assess the severity of burn induced ischemia. Plast Reconst Surg 1979; 63:404.

86. Cottam GL, Mitchell MD, Baxter CR. Measurement of 13,14-dihydro-keto-prostaglandin F and 11-deoxy-13,14-dihydro-keto-11,16-cyclo prostaglandin E_2 in human plasma following therma, injury. J Burn Care Rehabil 1984; 5:324.

87. Ferguson M, Eriksson E, Robson MC. Effect of methyl-prednisolone on oedema formation after a major burn. Burns 1979; 5:293.

88. Demling RH, et al. Effect of nonprotein colloid on postburn: edema formation in soft tissues and lung. Surgery 1984; 95:593.

89. Sayeed MM. Alterations in cell signalling and related effector functions in T lymphocytes in burn/trauma/septic injuries. Shock 1996; 5:157.

90. Deitch EA, Rutan R, Waymack JP. Trauma, shock, and gut translocation. New Horiz 1996; 4:289.

91. Goris RJ, Boekhorst T, Nuytinck J. Multiple organ failure: generalized autodestructive inflammation. Arch Surg 1985; 120:1109.

92. Morris SE, Navaratman N, Herndon DN. A comparison of effects of thermal injury and smoke inhalation on bacterial translocation. J Trauma 1990; 30:639.

93. Myers S, et al. Elevated PGI and PGE in the rat ileum following mild hypotension. J Trauma 1988; 28:1202.

94. Hill J, et al. Soluble complement receptor type 1 ameliorates the local and remote organ injury after intestinal ischemia-reperfusion in the rat. J Immunol 1992; 149:1723.

95. Fisher CJ, et al. Influence of an anti-tumour necrosis factor monoclonal antibody on cytokine levels in patients with sepsis. Crit Care Med 1993; 21:318.

96. Fisher CJ, et al. Recombinant human interleukin 1 receptor antagonist in the treatment of patients with sepsis syndrome. JAMA 1994; 271:1836.

97. Van Saene HKF, Stoutenbeek CC, Stoller JK. Selective decontamination of the digestive tract in the intensive care unit: current status and future prospects. Crit Care Med 1992; 20:691.

98. Herndon DN, Ziegler ST. Bacterial translocation after thermal injury. Crit Care Med 1993; 21:S50.

99. Tokyay R, et al. Effects of thromboxane synthetase inhibition on postburn mesenteric vascular resistance and the rate of bacterial translocation in a chronic porcine model. Surg Gynecol Obstet 1992; 174:125.

100. Arturson G. The pathophysiology of severe thermal injury. J Burn Care Rehabil 1985; 6:129.

101. Wolfe RR, et al. Effect of severe burn injury on substrate cycling by glucose and fatty acids. N Engl J Med 1987; 317:403.

102. Goodwin CW. Metabolism and nutrition. Crit Care Med 1985; 1:97.

103. Rose JK, Herndon DN. Advances in the treatment of burn patients. Burns 1997; 23(suppl 1):S19.

104. Wilmore DW, et al. Effect of ambient temperature on heat production and heat loss in burn patients. J Appl Physiol 1975; 38:593.

105. Caldwell FT. Energy metabolism following thermal burns. Arch Surg 1976; 111:181.

106. Wilmore DW, et al. Alterations in hypothalamic function following thermal injury. J Trauma 1975; 15:697.

107. Pruitt BA Jr. The burn patient. II. Later care and complications of thermal injury. Curr Probl Surg 1979; 16:1.

108. Wilmore DW, Aulick LH. Metabolic changes in burned patients. Surg Clin N Am 1978; 58:1173.

109. Deitch EA. The management of burns: current concepts. N Engl J Med 1990; 323:1249.

110. Bessey PQ, et al. Combined hormonal infusion stimulates the metabolic response to injury. Ann Surg 1984; 200:264.

111. Wilmore DW, et al. Catecholamines: Mediator of the hypermetabolic response to thermal injury. Ann Surg 1974; 180:653.

112. Hume DM, Egdahl RH. The importance of the brain in the endocrine response to injury. Ann Surg 1959; 150:697.

113. Woolf PD, et al. The adrenocortical response to brain injury: correlation with the severity of neurological dysfunction, effects of intoxication and patient outcome. Alcoholism 1990; 14:917.

114. Ziegler MG, Morrisey EC, Marshal LF. Catecholamine and thyroid hormones in traumatic injury. Crit Care Med 1990; 18:253.

115. Hart DW, Wolf SE, et al. Effects of early excision and aggressive enteral feeding on hypermetabolism, catabolism, and sepsis after serve burn. J Trauma 2003; 54(4):755.

116. Long CL. A response to trauma and infection: metabolic changes and immunologic consequences. J Burn Care Rehabil 1985; 6:188.

117. Moati F, et al. Biochemical and pharmacological properties of a cardiotoxic factor isolated from the blood serum of burned patients. J Pathol 1979; 127:147.

118. Muller MJ, Herndon DN. Hormonal interactions in burned patients. Semin Nephrol 1993; 13:391.

119. Bartlett RH, et al. Nutritional therapy based on positive caloric balance in burn patients. Arch Surg 1977; 112:974.

120. Wolfe RR, et al. Response of proteins and urea kinetics in burn patients to different levels of protein intake. Ann Surg 1983; 197:163.

121. Newsom TW, Mason AD Jr, Pruitt BA Jr. Weight loss following thermal injury. Ann Surg 1973; 178:215.

122. Freund H, et al. The role of the branched-chain amino acids in decreasing muscle catabolism in vivo. Surgery 1978; 83:611.

123. Blackburn GL, et al. Branched chain amino acid administration and metabolism during starvation, injury, and infection. Surgery 1979; 86:307.

124. Curreri PW, et al. Dietary requirements of patients with major burns. J Am Diet Assoc 1974; 65:415.

125. Wilmore DW. Carbohydrate metabolism in trauma. J Clin Endocrinol Metab 1976; 5:731.

126. Long JM III, et al. Effect of carbohydrate and fat intake on nitrogen excretion during total intravenous feeding. Ann Surg 1977; 185:417.

127. Mochizuki H, et al. Optimal lipid content for enteral diets following thermal injury. J Parenter Enteral Nutr 1984; 8:638.

128. Mochizuki H, et al. Mechanism of prevention of postburn hypermetabolism and catabolism by early enteral feeding. Ann Surg 1984; 200:297.

129. Alexander JW, McMillan B, Stinnett J. Beneficial effects of aggressive protein feeding in severely burned children. Ann Surg 1980; 192:505.

130. Deitch EA. Nutritional support of the burn patient. Crit Care Clin 1995; 11:735.

131. Lowry SF, Brennan MF. Abnormal liver function during parenteral nutrition: relation to infusion excess. J Surg Res 1979; 16:300.

132. Askanazi J, Rosenbaum SH, Hyman AI, Silverberg PA, Milic-Emili J, Kinney JM. Respiratory changes induced by the large glucose loads of total parenteral nutrition. JAMA 1980; 243:1444.

133. Nghia MV, et al. Effects of postoperative carbohydrate over-feeding. Am Surg 1987; 53:632.

134. McDonald WS, Sharpe CW Jr, Deitch EA. Immediate enteral feeding in burn patients is safe and effective. Ann Surg 1991; 213:177.

135. Mochizuki H, et al. Reduction of postburn hypermetabolism by early enteral feedings. Curr Surg 1985; 42:121.

136. Wolf SE, Thomas SJ, Dasu MR, et al. Improved net protein balance, lean mass, and gene expression changes with oxandrolone treatment in the severely burned. Ann Surg 2003; 237(6):801; discussion 810–811.

137. Mainous MR, Block EF, Deitch EA. Nutritional support of the gut: how and why. New Horiz 1994; 2:193.

138. Detsky AS, et al. Perioperative parenteral nutrition: a meta-analysis. Ann Intern Med 1987; 107:195.

139. McGeer AD, Detsky AS, O'Rourke K. Parenteral nutrition in cancer patients undergoing chemotherapy: a meta-analysis. Nutrition 1990; 6:233.

140. Carleton SC, Tomassoni AJ, Alexander JK. The cardiovascular effects of environmental traumas. Cardiol Clin 1995; 13:257.

141. Baxter CR. Intracellular electrolyte exchange in early postburn period. Am Burn Assoc 1967; 12:40.

142. Horton JW, Baxter CR, White DJ. The effects of aging on the cardiac contractile response to unresuscitated thermal injury. J Burn Care Rehabil 1988; 9:40.

143. Lefer AM. Interaction between myocardial depressant factor and vasoactive mediators with ischemia and shock. Am J Physiol 1987; 252:R193.

144. Squandrito F, et al. Reduction of myocardial leukocyte accumulation and myocardial infarct size following administration of BAY u3405, a thromboxane A_2 receptor antagonist, in myocardial ischaemia-reperfusion injury. Agents Actions 1993; 39:143.

145. Joshi W. Effects of burns on the heart. JAMA 1970; 211:2130.

146. Linares HA. A report of 115 consecutive autopsies in burned children, 1966–1980. Burns 1982; 8:263.

147. Maggi SP, et al. Beta-1 blockade decreases cardiac work without affecting protein breakdown or lipolysis in severely burned patients. Surg Forum 1993; 75:1081.

148. Herndon DN, Hart DW, Wolf SE, et al. Reversal of catabolism by beta-blockade after severe burns. N Engl J Med 2001; 345(17):1223.

149. Pereira C, Murphy K, Jeschke M, Herndon DN. Post burn muscle wasting and the effects of treatments. Int J Biochem Cell Biol 2005; 37(16):1948–1961.

150. Aulick LH, et al. Visceral blood flow following thermal injury. Ann Surg 1981; 193:112.

151. Wilmore DW. Effect of injury and infection on visceral metabolism and circulation. Ann Surg 1980; 192:491.

152. Shakespeare PG, et al. Proteinuria after burn injury. Ann Clin Biochem 1981; 18:353.

153. Planas M, et al. Characterization of acute renal failure in the burned patient. Arch Intern Med 1982; 142:2087.

154. Dolovek R. The endocrine response after burns: Its possible correlations with the immunology of burns. J Burn Care Rehabil 1985; 6:281.

155. Popp MB, et al. Anterior pituitary functioning thermally injured male children and young adults. Surg Gynecol Obstet 1977; 145:517.

156. Vaughn GM, Mason AD Jr, Shirani KZ. Hormonal changes following burns: An overview with consideration of the pineal gland. J Burn Care Rehabil 1985; 6:275.

157. Vaughan GM, Pruitt BA Jr. Thyroid function in critical illness and burn injury. Semin Nephrol 1993; 13:359.

158. Becker RA, Wilmore DW, Goodwin CW. Free T_4, free T_3 and reverse T_3 in critically ill, thermally injured patients. J Trauma 1980; 20:713.

159. Caldwell FT, et al. Metabolic response to thermal trauma of normal and thyroprivic rats at three environmental temperatures. Ann Surg 1959; 150:976.

160. Herndon DN. Mediators of metabolism. J Trauma 1981; 21:701.

161. Sellers EA, You SS, You RW. The influence of adrenal cortex and thyroid on the loss of nitrogen in urine after experimental burns. Endocrinology 1950; 47:148.

162. Gilpin DA, et al. Recombinant human growth hormone accelerates wound healing in children with large cutaneous burns. Ann Surg 1994; 220:19.

163. Herndon DN, et al. Effects of recombinant human growth hormone on donor site healing in severely burned children. Ann Surg 1990; 212:424.

164. Daughaday WH. The anterior pituitary. In: Wilson JD, Foster DW, eds. William's Textbook of Endocrinology. Philadelphia: WB Saunders, 1985.

165. Rose JK, Herndon DN. Advances in the treatment of burn patients. Burns 1997; 23(suppl 1):S19.

166. Cioffi WG, et al. Insulin-like growth factor-1 lowers protein oxidation in patients with thermal injury. Ann Surg 1994; 220:310.

167. Moltei LB, et al. Prolactin, corticotropin, and gonadotropin concentrations following thermal injury in adults. J Trauma 1984; 24:1.

168. Davies JWL. Physiological Responses to Burning Injury. New York: Academic Press, 1982.

169. Wilmore DW. Nutrition and metabolism following thermal injury. Clin Plast Surg 1974; 1:603.

170. Wolfe RR. Glucose metabolism in burn injury: a review. J Burn Care Rehabil 1985; 6:408.

171. Vaughn GA, et al. Nonthyroidal control of metabolism after burn injury: possible role of glucagon. Metabol Clin Exper 1985; 34:637.

172. Bingham HG, et al. Burn diabetes: a review. J Burn Care Rehabil 1982; 33:179.

173. Fauci A. Host Defense Mechanisms Against Infection: Current Concepts/Scope Publication. Kalamazoo, MI: Upjohn, 1978.

174. Branch CD, Wilkins CF, Ross FP. The coagulum contact method of skin grafting in the treatment of burns and wounds. Surgery 1945; 19:460.

175. Pietsch LB, Meakins JL, Gotto D. Delayed hypersensitivity response: the effect of surgery. J Surg Res 1977; 22:228.

176. Markely K, Smallman ET. Effect of burn trauma in mice on the generation of cytotoxic lymphocytes. Proc Soc Exp Biol Med 1979; 160:468.

177. Ninneman JL. Suppression of lymphocyte response following thermal injury. In: Ninneman JL, ed. The Immune Consequences of Thermal Injury. Baltimore: Williams & Wilkins, 1981.

178. Schoenenberger GA. Burn toxins isolated from mouse and human skin: their characterization and immunotherapy effects. Monogr Allergy 1975; 9:72.

179. Daniels JC, et al. Serum protein profiles in thermal burns. II. Protease inhibitors, complement factors, and C-reactive protein. J Trauma 1972; 14:153.

180. Munster AM, Winchurch RA. Infection and immunology. Crit Care Clin 1985; 1:119.

181. Warden GD, Mason AD, Pruitt BA Jr. Evaluation of leukocyte chemotaxis in vitro in thermally injured patients. J Clin Invest 1974; 54:1001.

182. Munster AM. Alteration of the immune system in burns and implications for therapy. Eur J Pediatr Surg 1994; 4:231.

183. Berczi I. Neuroendocrine defense in endotoxin shock (a review). Acta Microbiol Hung 1993; 40:265.

184. Chouaib S, et al. Analysis of prostaglandin E_2 effect on T lymphocyte activation: abrogation of prostaglandin E_2 inhibitory effect by the tumor promotor 12.0 tetradecanoyl phorbol-13 acetate. J Clin Invest 1987; 80:333.

185. Chouaib S, et al. The mechanisms of inhibition of human IL2 production: PGE_2 induction of suppressor T lymphocytes. J Immunol 1984; 132:1851.

186. Goodwin JS, Bankhurst AD, Messner RP. Suppression of human T cell mitogenesis by prostaglandin: existence of a prostaglandin-producing suppressor cell. J Exp Med 1977; 146:1719.

187. Horgan PG, et al. Effect of low dose recombinant interleukin 2 plus indomethachin on mortality after sepsis in a murine burn model. Br J Surg 1990; 77:401.

188. Munster AM, et al. Reversal of postburn immunosuppression with low-dose polymixin B. J Trauma 1986; 26:995.

189. Munster AM, et al. Translocation: true pathology or phenomenology. Ann Surg 1993; 218:321.

190. Trunkey DD. Inhalation injury. Surg Clin N Am 1978; 58:1133.

191. Dolan MC. Carbon monoxide poisoning. CMAT 1985; 133:392.

192. Rhodes ML. The effect of carbon monoxide on mitochondrial enzymes in pulmonary tissue. Am Rev Respir Dis 1971; 103:906.

193. Herndon DN, Thompson PB, Traber DL. Pulmonary injury in burned patients. Crit Care Clin 1985; 1:79.

194. Myers RAM, et al. Value of hyperbaric oxygen in suspected carbon monoxide poisoning. JAMA 1981; 246:2478.

195. Moritz AR, Henriques FC Jr, McLean R. The effects of inhaled heat on lungs: an experimental investigation. Am J Pathol 1945; 21:311.

196. Cox ME, et al. The Dellwood fire. Br Med J 1955; 1:942.

197. Crapo RO. Smoke inhalation injuries. JAMA 1981; 264:1694.

198. Beal DD, Lambeth JR, Conner GH. Follow-up studies on patients treated with steroids following pulmonary thermal and acrid smoke injury. Laryngoscope 1967; 78:396.

199. Pruitt BA Jr, Erickson MD, Morris A. Progressive pulmonary insufficiency and other pulmonary complications of thermal injury. J Trauma 1975; 15:369.

200. Cone JB. What's new in general surgery: burns and metabolism. J Am Coll Surg 2005; 200(4):607.

201. Enkhbaatar P, Murakami K, Cox R. Aerosolized tissue plasminogen inhibitor improves pulmonary function in sheep with burn and smoke inhalation. Shock 2004; 22(1):70.

202. Dreyfuss D, Saumon G. Ventilator induced lung injury: lessons from experimental studies. Am J Respir Crit Med 1998; 157:294.

203. Cartotto S, Ellis M, Gomez A, et al. High frequency oscillatory ventilation in burn patients with the acute respiratory distress syndrome. Burns 2004; s30(5):453R.

204. Monafo WW. Initial management of burns. N Engl J Med 1996; 335:1581.

205. Curreri PW. Supportive therapy in burn care. J Trauma 1981; 21(suppl):724.

206. Nguyen TT, et al. Current treatments of severely burned patients. Ann Surg 1996; 223:14.

207. Sokawa J, et al. The relationship between experimental fluid therapy and wound edema in scald wounds. Ann Surg 1981; 193:237.

208. Baxter CR, Shires GT. Physiologic response to crystalloid resuscitation of severe burns. Ann N Y Acad Sci 1968; 150:874.

209. Cope O, Moore FD. The redistribution of body water in the fluid therapy of the burned patient [footnote]. Ann Surg 1947; 126:1013.

210. Evans EI, et al. Fluid and electrolyte requirements in severe burns. Ann Surg 1952; 135:804.

211. Monafo WW. The treatment of burn shock by the intravenous and oral administrations of hypertonic lacated saline solution. J Trauma 1970; 10:575.

212. Parks DH, Carvajal HF, Larson DL. Management of burns. Surg Clin N Am 1977; 57:875.

213. Cioffi WG. What's new in burns and metabolism. J Am Coll Surgeons 2001; 192(2):241.

214. Goodwin CW, et al. Randomized trial of efficacy of crystalloid and colloid resuscitation on hemodynamic response and lung water following thermal injury. Ann Surg 1983; 197:520.

215. Hall KV, Sorensen B. The treatment of burn shock: results of a 5-year randomized, controlled clinical trial of Dextran 70 vs. Ringers lactate solution. Burns 1978; 5:107.

216. Gunn ML, et al. Prospective, randomized trial of hypertonic sodium lactate versus lactated Ringer's solution for burn wound resuscitation. J Trauma 1989; 29:1261.

217. Huang PP, et al. Hypertonic sodium resuscitation is associated with renal failure and death. Ann Surg 1995; 221:543.

218. Pruitt BA. Does hypertonic burn resuscitation make a difference. Crit Care Med 2000; 28:277.

219. Holm M, Mayr J, Tegeler F. A clinical randomized study on the effects of invasive monitoring on burn shock resuscitation. Burns 2004; 30(8):798.

220. Engrav LH, Colescott PL, Kemalyan N, et al. A biopsy of the use of the Baxter formula to resuscitate burns or do we do it like Charlie did it? J Burn Care Rehabil 2000; 21:91.

221. Pruitt BA. Protection from excessive resuscitation: "Pushing the Pendulum Back" [Editorial]. J Trauma 2000; 49(3):567.

222. Lund CC, Browder WL. Healing of second-degree burns: comparison of effects of early application of homografts and coverage with tape. Plast Reconstr Surg 1972; 49:552.

223. Curreri PW. Burns. In: Polk HC, Stone HH, Gardner B, eds. Basic Surgery. Norwalk, CT: Appleton-Century-Crofts, 1987.

224. Russell AD, Hugo WB. Antimicrobial activity and action of silver. Prog Med Chem 1994; 31:351.

225. Klasen HJ. Historical review of the use of silver in the treatment of burns. Part I. Early uses. Burns 2000; 26:117.

226. Klasen HJ. A historical review of the use of silver in the treatment of burns. Part II. Renewed interest for silver. Burns 2000; 26:131.

227. Poon VK, Burd A. In vitro cytotoxicity of silver: implication for clinical wound care. Burns 2004; 30:140.

228. Burke JF, Bandoc CC, Quinby WC. Primary burn excision and immediate grafting: a method for shortening illness. J Trauma 1974; 14:389.

229. Desai MH, et al. Early burn wound excision significantly reduces blood loss. Ann Surg 1990; 211:753.

230. Herndon DN, et al. A comparison of conservative versus early excison: therapies in severely burned patients. Ann Surg 1989; 209:546.

231. Barret JP, Herndon DN. Effects of burn wound excision on bacterial colonization and invasion. Plast Reconstr Surg 2003; 111(2):744.

232. Chen X, Soejima K, Nozaki, et al. Effect of early wound excision on changes in plasma nitric oxide and endothelin-1 level after burn injury: an experimental study in rats. Burns 2004; 30(8):793.

233. Robertson RD, Bond P, Wallace B, et al. The tumescent technique to significantly reduce blood loss during burn surgery. Burns 2001; 27:835.

234. Nervi C, Gamelli RL, Greenhalgh DG, et al. A multicenter clinical trial to evaluate the topical hemostatic efficacy of fibrin sealant in burn patients. J Burn Care Rehabil 2001; 22(2):99.

235. Burke JF, et al. Successful use of a physiologically acceptable artificial skin in the treatment of extensive burn injury. Ann Surg 1981; 194:413.

236. Heimbach DM, Warden GD, Luterman A, et al. Multicenter postapproval clinical trial of Integra dermal regeneration template for burn treatment. J Burn Care Rehabil 2003; 24(1):42.

237. Atiyeh BS, Gunn SW, Hayek SN. State of the art in burn treatment. World J Surg 2005; 29:131.

238. Boyce S. Principles and practices for treatment of cutaneous wounds with cultured skin substitutes. Am J Surgery 2002; 183(4):445.

239. Rue LW, Cioffi WG, McManus WF et al. Wound closure and outcome in extensively burned patients treated with cultured autologous keratinocytes. J Trauma 1993; 34:662.

240. Munster AM, Weiner SH, Spence RJ. Cultured epidermis for coverage of burn wound: a single center experience. Am Surg 1990; 211:676.

59

Physiologic Problems in the Pediatric Surgical Patient

Daniel J. Ostlie, Shawn D. St. Peter, Sheilendra S. Mehta, and George K. Gittes

INTRODUCTION

The care of the pediatric surgical patient can be a daunting task, both technically and clinically. To paraphrase, as many others have, "children are not little adults." Specifically, congenital anomalies, differences in nutritional requirements, thermoregulation and energy expenditure, and continued maturation of specific organ systems result in a continuum of constant changes in these patients. Additionally, the management of neonatal patients is immensely complex and, in most aspects, altogether different. Successful management requires a complete understanding of the normal physiologic and anatomic differences in relation to the pathophysiology, and leaves little room for error. Driven by these physiologic differences and the breadth of disease processes seen in this population, pediatric surgery has, over the last century, matured into a surgical subspecialty.

The purpose of this chapter is to familiarize the general surgeon with the physiologic, thermoregulatory, biochemical, and nutritional changes that occur at birth and in the newborn period, through later stages of development. Understanding these principles will aid in the initial management of these patients. A brief diagnostic and management overview of several of the most common congenital and acquired neonatal and pediatric surgical diseases will also be discussed.

PHYSIOLOGIC CONSIDERATIONS

Pediatric surgery encompasses the care of neonates, infants, children, and adolescents. The physiologic characteristics of these subpopulations vary, with the most significant differences existing in neonatal and infant patients. To better categorize neonates and infants, an understanding of the gestational age and birth weight is critical. Preterm infants are defined as those having a gestational age of less than 38 weeks, with an age-appropriate birth weight. Term infants have gestational ages between 38 and 42 weeks, and infants with more than 42 weeks gestation are considered post-term. The relationship between birth weight and gestational age describes the different subgroups of neonates and infants. Small for gestational age (SGA) infants weigh less than the 10th percentile expected for their gestational age and, conversely, large for gestational age infants weigh more than the 98th percentile for their gestational age. SGA babies usually result from intrauterine stress, regardless of cause. They have little reserve fat, higher metabolic rates, and reduced hepatic glycogen stores. Understandably, they are subsequently predisposed to hypothermia and hypoglycemia. Low birth weight and very low birth weight (VLBW) infants are premature and weigh less than expected. Stress related to surgical disease and other perinatal events combined with the physiologic immaturity of the VLBW and micropremature ($< 800\,g$) neonatal patients make these neonates particularly susceptible to minor changes that may have dramatic effects, requiring urgent identification and management to prevent catastrophic outcomes.

GLUCOSE, FLUID, AND ELECTROLYTE MANAGEMENT

Fetal serum calcium, magnesium, and glucose levels are tightly controlled via placental filtration and absorption. Management of pediatric surgical patients requires an understanding of the changes in the levels of electrolytes and glucose, and the loss of body water, all of which occur after birth.

Hypoglycemia/Hyperglycemia

The primary source of glucose in the immediate newborn period is hepatic glycogen stores. Typically, a healthy term infant will maintain a normal glucose level ($> 40\,mg/dL$) for two to three hours prior to requiring exogenous glucose. There is little gluconeogenesis to provide additional glucose; therefore, the infant must receive nutrition via enteral or parenteral routes at this time.

SGA, VLBW, and premature infants are particularly susceptible to neonatal hypoglycemia ($< 40\,mg/dL$), and should be monitored carefully during the first 48 hours of life. Infants that require surgical intervention and are unable to utilize enteral feeds should receive 10% dextrose solutions and have ongoing glucose monitoring. Occasionally, an infant will have persistent or more significant hypoglycemia. In these instances, dextrose solutions of up to 50% may be used via central access only. Typically, hypoglycemia does not persist beyond two to three days. However, the addition of surgical or medically related stress can perpetuate the process. In this instance, frequent serum and urine monitoring with appropriate adjustment of the dextrose concentrations is required for optimal management.

In the absence of total parenteral nutrition (TPN), severe prematurity, or sepsis, hyperglycemia is a rare event in the newborn period. However, when present, it can have significant deleterious effects. Electrolyte and fluid management becomes difficult due to water and electrolyte losses secondary to glucosuria, and intraventricular hemorrhage and retinopathy of prematurity are seen more frequently in infants with hyperglycemia (1). Management is based on reducing the dextrose concentration and, rarely, utilizing insulin to reduce the blood sugar.

Calcium

Newborn, and particularly preterm, infants are susceptible to hypocalcemia during the first 24 to 48 hours of life. Late in gestation, the fetus is exposed to high calcium levels due to the rapid transport of calcium across the placenta during the third trimester, for development and growth of the unborn infant. This high serum calcium concentration results in suppression of parathormone and relative hypoparathyroidism, predisposing to postnatal hypocalcemia. Parathormone levels reach normal by around 48 hours after birth, which explains why serum calcium concentrations usually begin to rise to normal at this time.

Predisposition to hypocalcemia, which is defined as an ionized calcium level of less than 1 mg/dL, is seen in several subpopulations. Preterm infants, surgical patients, and infants of complicated pregnancies are at increased risk for developing hypoglycemia. Newborns requiring exchange transfusion or large transfusions of citrated blood are also at increased risk, along with those that receive bicarbonate. Because of similar clinical pictures, it is sometimes difficult to differentiate hypocalcemia from hypoglycemia. Symptomatic hypocalcemia presents with jitteriness, myocardial depression, seizures, and cyanosis. A distinctive hallmark of hypocalcemia, as opposed to hypoglycemia, is increased muscle tone. Treatment is based on calcium supplementation during the period of relative hypoparathyroidism. Ten percent calcium gluconate, dosed at 1 to 2 mL/kg over 10 minutes, is effective in most cases. When asymptomatic hypocalcemia occurs, the infants should be managed with supplemental calcium gluconate added to the maintenance fluids. The usual dose is 5 to 10 mL/kg/day of the 10% solution.

Magnesium

As with calcium, magnesium is actively transported across the placenta, and their metabolism is interrelated because of their similar molecular weight and electronic charge characteristics. Infants at risk for hypomagnesemia mirror those at risk for hypocalcemia. Symptoms of hypocalcemia that do not respond to treatment, particularly seizures, should immediately raise the concern of hypomagnesemia, and prompt a measurement of serum magnesium level. Effective treatment is 25 to 50 mg/kg of magnesium sulfate, repeated every six hours until normal serum magnesium levels are achieved.

Fluid and Electrolytes

The relationship between total body water (TBW), intracellular body water (IBW), extracellular fluid (ECF), and percentage of body weight is classically depicted in Friis–Hansen's graphic representation from gestation to 12 years of age (Fig. 1). At birth, the TBW of the newborn is 78%, and drops to 73–75% by day 5 of life. This decline continues during the ensuing 18 months, at which time the TBW reaches adult levels (~60%). As seen in Figure 1, the decline of ECF levels follow the decline seen in TBW levels, while levels of IBW increase appropriately beginning at about five months gestation and reaching stable ratios at about 12 to 18 months. Infants born premature have higher percentages of TBW and ECF (Fig 1). This places the premature infant in a physiologic state that requires TBW offloading while simultaneously needing to transition fluid from the ECF to the IBW. The premature infant is adept at accomplishing this task, and is usually able to unload excess water by one week of age, even in the presence of significant fluid variations (2).

Renal function is dependent on glomerular filtration rate (GFR) and the concentrating capacity of the nephron. In newborns, the GFR is significantly less than that seen in adolescents or adults, and the ability of the newborn nephron to

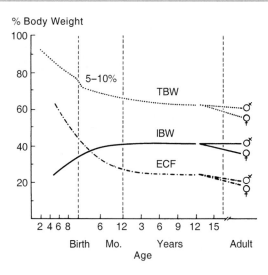

Figure 1 Friis-Hansen's graphic representation of the relationship between total body, extracellular, and intracellular water to percentage of body weight from early gestation to adulthood. *Abbreviations*: TBW, total body water; IBW, intracellular body water; ECF, extracellular body water.

concentrate urine is about 50% of the adult (3). At term, the GFR is 21 mL/min/1.73 m². The GFR triples to approximately 60 mL/min/1.73 m² over the next two weeks and reaches normal adult rates (~80 mL/min/1.73 m²), by two years of age. Due to a diminished response of the newborn tubule to antidiuretic hormone, the typical newborn is only able to maximally concentrate urine to 600 mOsm, about 50% of a normal adults' concentrating capacity. Conversely, their ability to rid themselves of excess free water is superior to adults in that they can excrete urine of 30 to 50 mOsm/kg when needed.

The maintenance of sodium and potassium is accomplished primarily in the distal tubule. While potassium excretion is rarely problematic, sodium excretion is significantly limited in term infants. The limitation is thought to be related to a defect in the distal tubule to limit resorption, because infants readily conserve sodium when needed. Consequently, term infants can easily become hypernatremic, especially when they receive exogenous sodium. For this reason, newborns are generally maintained on a one-fourth normal saline (NS) intravenous (IV) unless other factors necessitate a different concentration. However, preterm infants are considered "salt wasters" due to their inappropriate sodium excretion, regardless of sodium intake. As such, normal daily sodium replacement is dependent on the gestational age and physiologic condition of the infant. Preterm and ill infants may require up to 5 mEq/kg/day, while the healthy term infant will only need 2 mEq/kg/day of sodium. Actual replacement should be based upon laboratory measurements of serum and/or urine sodium as needed.

Accurate assessment and management of fluid status in pediatric surgical patients is dependent on the amount of insensible fluid losses and the fluid requirements based on the physiologic and surgical stressors endured by the infant. Insensible losses comprise transepithelial water loss and respiratory losses, and total on average 12 mL/kg/day. If the infant is receiving humidified air, whether via endotracheal route or hood/cannula, their respiratory losses are essentially zero. However, if the patient is breathing room air, the clinician can approximate respiratory losses to be 4 to 5 mL/kg/day. More importantly, the vast majority of insensible losses occur across the cutaneous epithelium, termed "transepithelial water loss." The volume lost via the transepithelial route is inversely proportional to the gestational age of the infant. Premature infants have been noted to lose as much as 130 mL/kg/day; however, for term infants, the volume lost through the skin is only approximately 7 mL/kg/day. As with ventilation, losses through the transepithelial route can be virtually eliminated by placing the infant under an impervious hood with 100% humidity. In circumstances of severe prematurity, this technique is invaluable for the management of fluid therapy.

With regard to optimal fluid requirements for infants, the volume needed is, again, entirely dependent on the physiologic state of the newborn. For fluid requirement considerations, surgical diseases in infants can be divided into three groups: moderate, severe, and sepsis/peritonitis. Infants with moderate surgical conditions (e.g., atresias, Hirschsprung's disease, imperforate anus, and colostomy) generally require approximately 80 mL/kg/day. Those with severe conditions (volvulus, abdominal wall defect, and exstrophy) require approximately 50% more volume (120 mL/kg/day), and those with severe sepsis or necrotizing enterocolitis (NEC) with perforation will require still more volume (140 mL/kg/day), due to the third space losses associated with the ongoing responses to illness. Optimal fluid management is often difficult to assess in these patients. Frequently, serial body weight is used as a guide to fluid management. One should caution against using body weight as the cornerstone of fluid assessment, however, because third space losses are inevitable and can mimic fluid overload, whereas, in reality, more fluid is required for tissue and organ perfusion. Measurement of urine output in combination with serial body weights is a much better guide for optimal fluid status and organ/tissue perfusion. Generally, a minimum of 2 mL/kg/hr urine output is required to ensure perfusion and solute excretion in most pediatric surgical patients. Urine concentration is also a helpful tool in this patient population. A goal for urine osmolality should be 250 to 290 mOsm/L, with a specific gravity of 1.010 to 1.103.

THERMOREGULATION

Temperature regulation in pediatric surgical patients has implications beyond just the metabolic demands placed on the infant to maintain a level of normothermia. Hypothermia predisposes to coagulation abnormalities, inappropriate response to pharmacologic therapy, and cardiac instability. Newborn infants are predisposed to hypothermia primarily because of their large surface area in relation to body weight. The ability of the newborn to maintain a normal core body temperature is predicated on the utilization of brown fat catabolism, the supply of which is limited. Although infants can produce heat by shivering, it is ineffective and places the newborn under extreme metabolic demands, which cannot be sustained. Therefore, it is of paramount importance that the surgeon caring for these patients be aware of these limitations and prepared to provide thermoregulation when needed. Radiant heat loss (infant warmer than its surroundings) over their large surface area is the most important and significant heat loss mechanism, especially in VLBW and other preterm infants. This heat loss is drastically diminished via the use of automatic servo-controlled incubators

that adjust the ambient temperature to a range based on standard thermal nomograms for weight and gestational age. Radiant warmers are often utilized as the infant matures; however, the surgeon should remain cognizant of heat losses associated with convection (air currents over surface areas) and higher insensible water losses associated with these warmers. Heat regulation during transport to the operating suite and during surgical procedures can be difficult to manage. Surgical procedures are often required for correction of abnormal physiologic or anatomic conditions in these patients. Cold stress can be severe during these circumstances, and normothermia should be maintained via appropriate room temperatures, warming blankets, warmed irrigation fluids, and radiant warmers during the operation, if needed.

PULMONARY AND CARDIAC TRANSITIONAL PHYSIOLOGY

The changes that occur within the circulatory and respiratory organ systems of the fetus during transition to extrauterine life are critical to normal physiologic function as a newborn. The fetal circulation is adapted to deliver oxygenated blood from the placenta to the systemic organs and tissues, avoiding the pulmonary circulation, because during this stage of development, no oxygenation occurs within the pulmonary capillary bed. Oxygenated blood from the placenta passes through the liver into the inferior vena cava, via the ductus venosus, and enters the right atrium where it mixes with deoxygenated blood from the superior vena cava. The pulmonary circulation is avoided via the foramen ovale and ductus arteriousus, which allow blood to be redirected from the right to the left atrium and from the pulmonary artery to the aorta, respectively (Fig. 2). During the fetal phase, this phenomenon is aided by elevated pulmonary artery pressures.

During the transitional phase of newborn physiology, there is a dramatic and rapid decline in pulmonary artery pressure that results from expansion of the neonatal alveoli associated with the initiation of breathing by the infant. This drop in pulmonary artery pressure leads to lower the right-sided heart pressures and subsequent closure of the foramen ovale, eliminating the right-to-left shunt that had existed during the fetal phase, and thus directing blood through the pulmonary vascular bed. The ductus arteriosus spontaneously closes in normal newborns during the first 48 to 72 hours post delivery. The closure of the ductus arteriosus is the result of rapid increases in pO_2, as well as the absence of prostaglandin E_2 and I_2.

With regard to pulmonary physiology, the critical components include adequate alveolar expansion and efficient gas exchange. Alveolar expansion occurs with the initial inspiratory efforts of the newborn, which can be as high as -70 mmHg. However, expansion is ineffective if the alveoli are unable to remain open due to increased surface tension, the result of insufficient surfactant. Surfactant is a phospholipid produced by Type II pneumocytes, beginning at about 26 week's gestation and continuing through delivery. Surfactant allows for lower effective alveolar distending pressures by decreasing surface tension, thereby requiring lower ventilatory pressure to inflate the alveoli and simultaneously decreasing the propensity for alveolar collapse between breaths. Inadequate surfactant results in the need for higher negative inspiratory force, and predisposes to neonatal respiratory support and hyaline membrane disease.

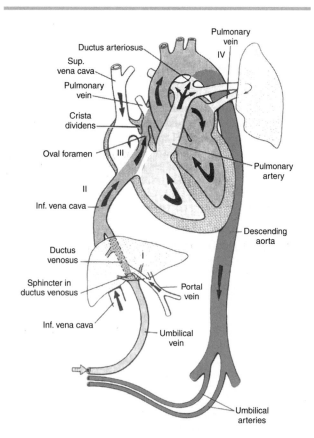

Figure 2 Schematic depiction of fetal blood flow. Blood returns to the fetus from the placenta and is shunted through the liver to the suprahepatic inferior vena cava via the ductus venosus. Blood flow bypasses the pulmonary circulation via its redirection through the right atrium directly to the left atrium through the foramen ovale, and from the pulmonary artery to the descending aorta via the patent ductus arteriosus. Closure of these shunts occurs during fetal transitional physiology.

NUTRITIONAL SUPPORT

The nutritional demands of the newborn are unique, and the addition of surgical stress requires special attention to the patient to ensure that appropriate energy sources are provided for normal growth and development while simultaneously ensuring recovery from the required operation. A full-term newborn should gain 25 to 30 g/day, or double his weight during the first four months of life (4). The growth patterns for a preterm infant are completely different than those for the term infant. Normally, the preterm infant would receive their nutritional needs via the placenta during the third trimester, the phase of rapid growth and significant caloric requirements, leading to adequate nutrient accumulation for postnatal life. Unfortunately, when an infant is born prematurely, they have not had the advantage of complete growth and development, and simultaneously lack the nutrient reserve normally expected of a term infant. Compared to the normal 10% body weight loss seen in term infants, the preterm infant can be expected to lose approximately 15% of their body weight during the first one to two weeks. After the initial weight loss, the preterm infant greater than 27 weeks gestation needs to gain about 35 g/day (5).

The scope of this chapter is not sufficient to allow for a complete description of the nutritional requirements and/or

subtle changes that are necessary for surgical recovery. However, basic guidelines can be provided. Generally, a 1 kg infant has only a four-day reserve, while a full-term infant can survive about one month without nutritional support (6). The daily caloric requirements for pediatric surgical patients are dependent on their level of development and the surgical stress imposed upon them. The hypermetabolic state seen after illness and surgery must be compensated for in relation to the normal nutritional requirements for growth and development. Increased oxygen delivery is needed in these patients, and the cost of this delivery is an increased demand for energy to meet the oxygen demands. Consequently, demands for protein and carbohydrate energy are increased. However, excessive caloric resuscitation can lead to immunosuppression, and it is therefore critical to have a global understanding of the nutritional needs of these infants (7). The full-term infant will require approximately 100 to 120 kcal/kg/day, with 2 to 3.5 g/kg/day of protein, for normal growth. A preterm infant needs more calorie (140–150 kcal/kg/day) and protein synthesis (3–4.5 g/kg/day) for ongoing growth and development.

Providing nutrition via the enteral route is superior to that via the parenteral route. Frequently, especially in surgical patients, enteral feeding is not possible; however, even small amounts of enteral feeds are advantageous. Preservation of intestinal integrity is facilitated by enteral feeds, and that integrity assists in preserving the intestinal epithelial barrier, by helping to maintain absorptive processes and inhibiting the entry of potentially toxic luminal contents (8). Enteral feeds can eliminate the need for central venous access and the subsequent complications associated with insertion and management of central venous catheters. Additionally, septic complications develop more often in infants receiving parenteral nutrition than in those receiving enteral feeds (9,10).

Optimal carbohydrate delivery is based upon maintaining normal serum glucose levels and preventing the complete utilization of glycogen stores. The primary site of glycogen storage in infants is the liver. Following a meal, circulating levels of glucose gradually fall over the ensuing four hours. After this time, the neonate must begin to utilize hepatic stores to prevent hypoglycemia. These stores can be sufficient for up to 12 hours in the full term infant, but may only last a few hours in the premature patient. Therefore, supplemental carbohydrates must be provided to the surgical patient that is unable to initiate enteral feeds shortly after operation. Also, sufficient carbohydrate delivery provides a protein-sparing substrate, as in its absence somatic protein breakdown occurs in an effort to produce more glucose. Generally, prevention of hypoglycemia due to inadequate reserve and synthetic capacity requires 6 to 8 mg/kg/min continuous infusion of a dextrose solution. This concentration can be increased when central access is available; however, one must remember the detrimental effects of hyperglycemia in relation to fluid loss as a result of exceeding the renal tubular glucose resorption capacity leading to an osmotic diuresis, especially in light of potential stress-induced insulin-resistance.

The normal diet of newborns provides adequate quantities of fat to provide calories and essential fatty acids. In the presence of an ileus or other reasons preventing enteral nutrition, the nutritional needs supplied via fats must be provided through TPN. In general, fats should comprise 30% to 50% of all nonnitrogenous calories. Linoleic acid is essential in all newborns and children for the development of cell membranes and the central nervous system as well as the production of prostaglandins and thrombaxanes. Two to four percent of all dietary energy should come from this essential amino acid. The daily fat requirements are usually provided through either 10% or 20% formulations. Twenty percent formulations appear superior in that they contain twice the triglyceride content of 10% lipids with similar phospholipid content, which have been shown to be associated with cholesterol and low-density lipoprotein accumulation (11).

SPECIFIC PEDIATRIC SURGICAL CONDITIONS

Infantile Hypertrophic Pyloric Stenosis

One of the most common surgical diagnoses encountered by the pediatric surgeon is idiopathic pyloric stenosis (IPS). It is the most common cause of gastric outlet obstruction in infants. Although it was first described in 1717, it was not accepted as a true clinical entity until Hirschprung reported two cases in 1888 (12). Prior to the development of an effective operation (Ramstedt in 1912) to relieve the obstruction created by the hypertrophied pylorus, the mortality rate for infants affected by IPS approached 100% (13).

The etiology of IPS remains unknown. Current research focuses on biochemical and neurodevelopmental anomalies. Diminished or absent levels of nitric oxide, which is critical for intestinal relaxation, may be a contributing factor. Levels of nitric oxide synthase have been found to be abnormal in a subset of patients with IPS, however this abnormality is not always present, and no clearly causative abnormality has been identified (14,15). Regardless of mechanism, it is likely that IPS is predominantly an acquired disease, because studies have shown that the pylorus in infants that develop IPS are normal at birth (16,17).

The traditional presentation of IPS is the development of nonbilious vomiting between 2 and 10 weeks of life, with a peak at about four weeks. The vomiting may initially be confused with gastroesophageal reflux (GER) or feeding/formula intolerance, and it is not uncommon for the infant to have changed formulas several times prior to diagnosis. Eventually, the vomiting will become projectile in nature, which prompts the diagnosis of IPS. Historically, the diagnosis has been confirmed via physical exam, with the classic exam finding of a mobile firm mass in the right upper quadrant described as an "olive." More recently, the diagnosis is usually made with ultrasound. Ultrasonic criteria for IPS are a pylorus channel length of greater than 16 mm with a pylorus muscle thickness of 4 mm or pyloric diameter of 14 mm (18). One should be cautioned regarding ultrasonic diagnosis of IPS in that it is entirely user-dependent, and experience is critical in ensuring the correct diagnosis.

Critically important in infants with IPS is their preoperative management. Frequently these patients are significantly malnourished and dehydrated, and fluid resuscitation with electrolyte correction is of utmost importance prior to proceeding with the operation. Electrolyte abnormalities include elevated bicarbonate levels, hypochloremia, and hypokalemia resulting from contraction alkalosis. Benson defined three levels of severity of metabolic derangement based on serum carbon dioxide content (slight: < 25, moderate: 26–35, and severe: > 35 mEq/L) (19). Fluid resuscitation should begin with a 10 to 20 mL/kg bolus of NS which can be repeated, if needed, depending on clinical and physical exam response (skin turgor, mucous membranes, and anterior fontanelle). Maintenance fluid therapy should consist of 0.45 NS at 1.5 times the normal calculated maintenance requirements until normal volume status and electrolyte composition is achieved. Potassium replacement should be withheld until volume status is appropriate, usually defined as urine output of more than 1 mL/kg/hr. Serum electrolytes should be monitored every six hours to guide fluid and electrolyte replacement, with operative correction delayed until electrolyte and dehydration abnormalities have been corrected.

The surgical management of IPS is predicated on the division of the pylorus muscle, which results in relief of the gastric obstruction. This pyloromyotomy can be performed in an open or laparoscopic fashion, and the results of both techniques are excellent. The pyloromyotomy is initiated just proximal to the duodenopyloric junction and carried well onto the antrum. The key to success in the performance of a complete myotomy is "breaking" the concentric musculature that is causing the obstruction. The transition to normal depth of circular muscle is usually apparent on the antral aspect; however, one must approach the duodenal aspect with caution, as the duodenal mucosa may evaginate into the pyloric muscle, predisposing to mucosal perforation during the pyloromyotomy. Acceptable perforation rates are approximately 1% to 4%, and if the complication does occur, the pyloromyotomy should be closed, and a second pyloromyotomy should be performed on the opposite aspect of the pylorus. An alternative approach here is to perform primary closure of the mucosal perforation with omental patch. Both approaches to mucosal perforation repair have reported similar results (20,21). There is significant institutional variation with regard to postoperative management. Our practice is to withhold feedings until the infant has recovered from their anesthetic. Oral feedings are usually begun at about two hours postoperatively. Gradual concentration advancement is used, utilizing the two-hour volume requirements. Pedialyte is initiated at twice the hourly volume requirements every two hours for two consecutive feedings. If the infant tolerates the pedialyte feeds, the concentration is advanced to half strength formula or breast milk at the same volume and feeding schedule. Again, if the feedings are tolerated for two consecutive feeds, the concentration is advanced to full strength and subsequently to ad lib volumes if two consecutive full-strength feeds are tolerated. Most children are discharged by 24 to 36 hours postoperatively.

Abdominal Wall Defects

Prior to Robert Gross' initial description of a staged closure for large abdominal wall defects in 1948 (22), survival of infants born with these congenital anomalies was rare, and literature reports of survivors primarily included small defects in otherwise healthy newborns. Developmental anomalies of the abdominal wall in newborns are classified as either omphalocele or gastroschisis defects, which can be differentiated quickly based on clinical findings (Table 1).

Gastroschisis

Gastroschisis (Greek for "belly cleft") defects usually are found to the right of a normally located umbilical cord. The fascial defect is normally small (2–4 cm), which limits organ herniation to primarily intestine. The small defect also predisposes the herniated intestine to vascular compromise. There is no peritoneal sac to protect the herniated organs, so they are in direct contact with amniotic fluid, which leads to the development of an intense inflammatory process. For this reason, the intestine is edematous with an associated serositis and a thickened, foreshortened mesentery (Fig. 3). The extent of intestinal herniation varies and may

Table 1 Clinical Characteristics of Gastroschisis and Omphalocele

Clinical finding	Gastroschisis	Omphalocele
Location	To the right of umbilicus	Through the umbilicus
Fascial defect size	Small (usually < 5 cm)	Variable (up to 10 cm)
Peritoneal sac	None	Present (can rupture)
Cord attachment	To the left	Onto the sac
Associated anomalies	Rare	Common
Intestinal atresia	Common	Rare
Bowel characteristics	Thick, edematous "peel"	Normal
Bowel ischemia	Occasionally	Rare
Herniated organs	Intestine, liver (rarely)	Intestine, liver (commonly)
Intestinal malrotation	Present	Present

include the small and large intestine as well as the stomach, and rarely the liver. Associated anomalies are uncommon in infants with gastroschisis. However, intestinal atresias are seen in approximately 10% of patients, and infants with gastroschisis are more often premature or SGA (23).

Controversy exists regarding the etiology of gastroschisis. Most investigators agree that the defect is definitely a separate entity, rather than a ruptured omphalocele. The lack of associated anomalies (commonly seen in omphalocele) supports this concept. Generally, it is believed that the defect is the result of a vascular accident or a rupture of the amniotic membrane at the base of a hernia of the umbilical cord (24,25).

Care of the newborn with gastroschisis must begin immediately after birth. These infants should all be cared for at an institution specializing in neonatal and pediatric care, and all require admission to the neonatal intensive care unit (NICU). Fluid and heat losses are substantial due to exposed intestine. Immediately after delivery, the herniated intestine should be placed into an impervious bag to limit these losses. Gastric decompression should be instituted to prevent intestinal dilation secondary to swallowed air. IV access is obtained and fluid replacement/resuscitation is begun. A 20 mL/kg of 5% dextrose in lactated ringers is given over the first hour, followed by 1.5 times maintenance volumes per hour, with fluid boluses as needed. These infants may require two to three times the normal maintenance fluid needs for their age, due to losses associated with the exposed intestine. Fluid management should be based on urine output and acid–base normalization. Occasionally, colloid replacement is utilized to improve retention of intravascular volume, due to the losses from the exposed surface of the intestine. Temperature regulation should be achieved with a radiant, warmer if necessary. Broad-spectrum antibiotics should be used in all gastroschisis patients to decrease the risk of infection after peritoneal exposure to vaginal and environmental organisms.

Operation should be performed as soon as the infant has been stabilized. Repair should focus on protecting the eviscerated intestine via a staged or primary closure. Primary closure is obtained in approximately 75% of patients. The technique for primary closure involves the reduction of the viscera and closure of the fascial defect, which may need to be enlarged slightly. The fascia is approximated in a single layer using permanent interrupted sutures. The subcutaneous tissues are approximated, followed by the skin, which is closed in a subcuticular fashion. The umbilicus should be reconstructed at the appropriate location using a purse string technique, with tacking of the skin to the fascia using the same suture (Fig. 4).

Due to the lack of the intestine being present in the abdomen during development, there is often significant loss of abdominal domain. In these cases, primary closure may be impossible, or may lead to prohibitive intraabdominal pressures placing the abdominal viscera at ischemic risk. Staged closure utilizing a silo is best undertaken in these patients. The intestine is placed in the silo, which may be hand sewn or prefabricated, and the silo is hung from the radiant warmer to place the intestine in a dependent position (Fig. 5). Care should be taken to place the intestine into the silo without rotation of the mesentery, which would lead to vascular compromise. The silo is compressed sequentially over the ensuing three to seven days, with complete closure performed after the abdominal domain has been recovered. Prosthetic closures should be avoided, as they have been shown to have increased risk for sepsis (26).

Prior to the development of central TPN, the survival of gastroschisis patients was dismal due to the prolonged

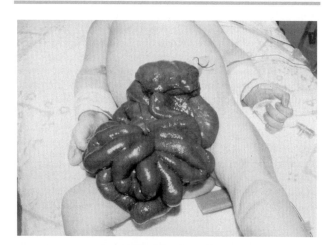

Figure 3 This photograph shows an infant with gastroschisis and the classic intestinal "peel" and edematous bowel with shortened mesentery. Also, the umbilical cord inserts superior and medial to the fascial defect.

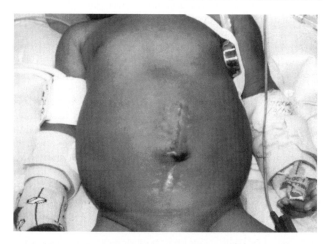

Figure 4 The skin closure after reduction and closure of a gastroschisis is shown. Occasionally, it is necessary to open the skin superiorly and inferiorly to allow for reduction of the herniated organs. The umbilicus is then reconstructed to allow for a more normal location and appearance.

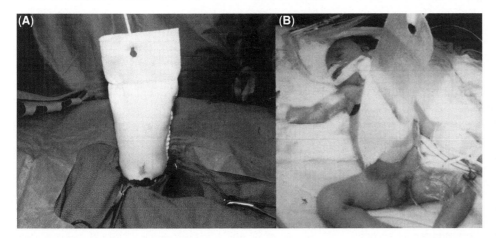

Figure 5 The placement of a silo for gradual reduction of the herniated viscera is shown. (**A**) The silo has been hand sewn and secured to the fascia of the abdominal wall. (**B**) A prefabricated silo is secured to the fascia with the intestine visualized inside. In both cases, the silo is hung to allow for dependent pressure of the viscera. External pressure results in reduction over the ensuing three to seven days, at which time delayed primary closure can be accomplished.

adynamic ileus that developed from the chemical peritonitis and surgical closure. Inability to initiate enteral feeds for as much as 30 days or longer in some patients places these infants in a position of TPN dependence. TPN use is number one determinant for the significant improvement in survival over the last 30 years in infants with gastroschisis. Therefore, infants with gastroschisis should receive central venous access (Hickman catheter or peripherally inserted central catheter line), and initiate TPN after stabilization of their metabolic and surgical stressors. Although intestinal motility returns in all these infants, intestinal transit time is prolonged for up to six months following closure. Additionally, malabsorption is commonly seen and may prompt prolonged TPN use as an adjunct to enteral feeds, to ensure adequate caloric intake until normalization of the motility and absorptive process occurs (27). With advancement in neonatal care, TPN, and closure techniques, the current expected survival for infants born with gastroschisis approaches 95%. Most morbidity and/or mortality are related to sepsis, complications related to prolonged TPN, bowel obstruction, or closure complications (23).

Omphalocele

An omphalocele is a central defect of the umbilical cord. The cord itself arises from the peritoneal sac that surrounds the herniated organs of the omphalocele. The fascial defect can range from small umbilical cord hernias to large "giant" omphaloceles that may be more than 10 cm (Fig. 6). Herniated organs will include the large and small bowel, stomach, and frequently liver. As a result of the large defect and herniation of most of the abdominal viscera, the abdominal cavity is frequently small and underdeveloped in infants with omphalocele, especially giant omphaloceles. The management of these infants is technically and clinically challenging. In approximately 15% of cases, the sac of the omphalocele may rupture (28). If the rupture occurs early during the fetal development, the visceral contents will be exposed to the amniotic fluid and, as in gastroschisis, will be edematous with serositis and shortened mesentery. In this instance, the defect can be differentiated from a gastroschisis by the position of the cord and the remnant of the omphalocele sac.

The embryologic consequences that result in the development of an omphalocele are not understood. Duhamel first described his theory, which is still believed by most researchers, in 1963 (29). He postulated that omphaloceles were the result of failure of body wall morphogenesis, specifically abnormal fusion of the cephalic, lateral, and caudal folds of the developing abdominal wall. Failure of these folds to close results in a central "classic" omphalocele, an epigastric omphalocele, or an omphalocele inferior to the umbilicus, respectively. An epigastric omphalocele is usually part of the pentology of Cantrell syndrome, which includes a cleft sternum, an anterior diaphragmatic defect, and absence of pericardium and intracardiac defects. Hypogastric defects are seen with exstrophy, cloacal, and imperforate anus defects. Regardless of location, the defect is covered with a peritoneal sac, and its development may be initiated by failure of the intestine to return to the abdomen after the period of growth it undergoes in the extracelomic position. Another, less accepted, theory to explain the omphalocele development is that of abnormal migration of body wall myotomes.

The management of infants born with omphalocele is similar to that of newborns with gastroschisis with regard to the abdominal wall defect. However, in more than 50%

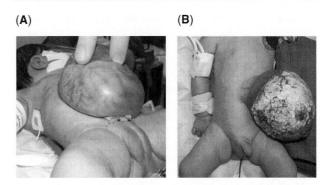

Figure 6 Two infants with omphalocele defects are shown. (**A**) A moderate-sized omphalocele with liver and intestine contained within the sac. Note the umbilical cord originating from the omphalocele sac. (**B**) A giant omphalocele that has been treated with an escharating agent to allow for epithelialization. The omphalocele was later closed in multiple operations, with sequential closure of the large ventral hernia defect.

of cases, there will be an associated anomaly, and these anomalies will require individual attention. The most common associated anomalies are congenital heart defects followed by chromosomal trisomies (13–15,18,21), and Beckwith–Weidemann syndrome (macroglossia, hypoglycemia, and gigantism) (30). Genitourinary, musculoskeletal, neurologic, and gastrointestinal anomalies have also been reported in association with omphalocele.

Similar to infants suffering from gastroschisis, these infants should be cared for in a facility equipped to manage the complex congenital anomalies that are frequently encountered. Although not as severe, water and heat loss are the initial physiologic concerns in these infants. By placing the omphalocele, or lower body if necessary, in a sterile impervious bag, these losses can be minimized. Initial fluid resuscitation is similar to that for gastroschisis. Broad-spectrum antibiotics and gastric decompression should be instituted immediately after birth. Once the resuscitation is accomplished, operation is delayed to allow the evaluation for other anomalies. Renal and spinal ultrasounds are obtained, along with a chest radiograph and an echocardiogram to evaluate for any congenital heart defects. Subspecialty consultation is requested for any abnormal findings, and chromosomal analysis with genetic consultation is obtained in most patients.

Surgical closure of the defect is pursued after the evaluation is complete. When possible, primary closure is performed. The sac should be left intact if possible, to maintain a sterile intraperitoneal environment. The fascia of the abdominal wall is meticulously dissected from the sac, and subsequently closed using interrupted permanent sutures. Manual stretching of the abdominal wall is sometimes necessary to allow for reduction of the herniated viscera. Care should be taken with reduction of the liver, as in these infants the hepatic capsule is exceedingly thin and prone to rupture or tearing, which can lead to life-threatening hemorrhage. If the omphalocele cannot be closed primarily, the management is similar to that of gastroschisis. A silo is placed followed by sequential compression of the omphalocele in the NICU over the ensuing five to seven days to allow for rerecruitment of the abdominal domain. Definitive closure is subsequently performed when possible. Rarely, in cases of giant omphalocele, the fascia cannot be approximated due to the severe underdevelopment of the abdominal cavity, despite sequential compressions. In these instances, several nonoperative strategies have been used. Most commonly, epithelialization of the omphalocele sac is promoted with the use of an escharating agent such as silver nitrate or silver sulfadiazine, or with the placement of split-thickness skin grafts (Fig. 6). The resultant ventral hernia is closed at a later date, and, oftentimes, will require multiple operations over an extended period. Immediately following closure, the infant remains intubated and often paralyzed for 24 to 48 hours. A prolonged ileus should not be expected, as the intestine has not suffered the insult seen in gastroschisis. Enteral feeds can usually be started within seven days, and malabsorption or delayed transit is not common. Survival for infants with omphalocele is not as high as for gastroschisis, primarily due to morbidity and/or mortality related to the associated anomalies.

Necrotizing Enterocolitis

NEC is the most common gastrointestinal emergency in newborns affecting approximately 5% of neonates admitted to the NICU (31,32). It is a predominantly a disease of prematurity with less then 10% of cases occurring in term infants (32,33).

Pathogenesis

NEC is multifactorial in origin. The most frequently implicated clinical variables contributing to the development of NEC include enteral feeds, ischemia, enteric microorganisms, and attenuated host defense systems (i.e., prematurity). Experimental studies in an animal model have shown that a combination of asphyxia, formula feeds, and bacteria results in a very high rate of NEC (34). In this model, asphyxia was clearly the most significant instigating factor with formula feeding less important. Enteral bacterial colonization was not a significant determinant. However, the relative impact of each of these variables has not been clinically defined for NEC in humans.

Since the early descriptions of NEC, enteral feeding had been considered an important etiologic factor in the development of NEC, because 90% of cases occurred after the initiation of feeds (35,36). Initiation of feeds produces a spectrum of physiologic changes within the gastrointestinal tract including the introduction of organisms and increased oxygen demand of the gut (37,38). The type of flora and range of byproducts they produce, as well as the interactions of these variables with the gut mucosa will be affected by the type of substrate used for feeding. Breast milk significantly reduces the risk of NEC (39,40). Maternal milk contains a variety of immunomodulators, including degradative enzymes for some of the most important inflammatory communication molecules behind the propagation of disease in NEC (41,42). When maternal breast milk is not available, the use of human donor milk has also been shown to be associated with a significantly reduced relative risk of NEC (43). However, a superior rate and mode of milk feeding has not been clearly established (44).

The role of ischemia in NEC development appears to be important, but not clearly defined. Necrotic lesions seen in NEC bowel specimens appear to be the result of ischemia; however, episodes of systemic hypoxia are not always present in neonates developing NEC, which implicates mechanisms of local ischemia or vasoconstriction. Mechanisms of local ischemia also remain to be delineated. Angiotensin-mediated pathways have been proposed as a theoretical participant in local vasoconstriction, and it is known that intestinal vasculature is rich in angiotensin receptors (45,46). In experimental models of shock, ischemic colitis secondary to mesenteric vasoconstriction has been shown to be irresponsive to adrenergic blockade but abolished by inhibition of angiotensin converting enzyme (47).

Microorganisms are also felt to contribute to NEC. Bacterial endotoxin has been shown in experimental models to act through and/or with the release of inflammatory mediators to cause intestinal necrosis and a clinical syndrome similar to NEC (48,49). However, it is unlikely that microbes are causative, because there is little consistency in the bacterial strains cultured from the stool and blood of NEC patients. These cultures range widely including gram-positive, gram-negative bacteria, anaerobes, and even viruses with very few reported epidemic strains (50–53). Moreover, cultures from NEC patients are usually representative of the fecal flora within the NICU, and analysis of these trends has revealed no significant correlation between the disease and either age of the infant or intestinal site of disease (53,54). Therefore, bacteria in the gut of NEC infants become opportunistic participants in the disease process taking advantage of the premature gut injured by ischemia in the presence of substrate.

Gut immaturity, enteric substrate, ischemia, and microorganisms contribute to initiation of NEC. After initiation, elaboration of inflammatory mediators results in the activation of responses from polymorphonuclear neutrophils (PMNs). Activated PMNs release proteolytic enzymes, free radicals, and conduct local phagocytosis all causing direct tissue injury. In addition, they further propagate the release of inflammatory mediators, which increase vascular permeability, activate complement and leukocytes, and stimulate leukocyte migration leading to subsequent tissue injury (55–57).

The activation of inflammatory mediators contributes to systemic effects similar to those seen with systemic inflammatory response syndrome. Inflammatory pathways promoting the pathologic findings of NEC continue to evolve, but two communication molecules in particular, tissue necrosis factor-alpha (TNF-α) and platelet-activating factor (PAF) have been shown in multiple animal studies to result in ischemic bowel necrosis similar to NEC (58–60).

The release of TNF-α facilitates local injury and promotes distant organ dysfunction (61,62). PAF further increases TNF-α expression, and activates gene transcription through the nuclear factor-κB (NF-κB). NF-κB, is a ubiquitous transcription factor which accounts for the gene expression of cytokines, chemokines, growth factors, immunoreceptors and cell adhesion molecules (35,36,63–66). Specifically in the intestine, NF-κB activation causes an increase in mucosal permeability, endotoxemia and tissue necrosis (45).

Clinically, the most significant risk factor of a newborn being stricken with NEC is the severity of prematurity (67–74). Its incidence is inversely related to gestational age, and the age-specific attack rate declines sharply after 35 weeks gestational age (69). Similarly, the incidence and severity of NEC are higher in neonates with smaller birth weight, and VLBW infants who develop NEC are more likely to require surgery (72,73,75–79). Congenital heart disease, particularly hypoplastic left heart syndrome and truncus arteriousus, with episodes of poor systemic perfusion of shock has also been shown to be significantly associated with NEC (80). Umbilical artery catheterization had previously been suggested as an etiologic agent of NEC (81); however, accumulating evidence does not support this notion (82). Polycythemia, exchange transfusions, maternal cocaine use, and enteral theophylline have all been implicated as risk factors, but confirmatory data has been conflicting (83–88). However, antenatal theophylline administered to high-risk mothers does appear to subsequently increase the risk of NEC in premature infants (89). It has been shown that newborns with general physiologic compromise, prolonged hypotension, persistent respiratory distress, septicemia, and hypothermia have been shown to significantly increase the incidence of NEC and have a higher risk of developing NEC (74,90–93).

Presentation

Early systemic signs of NEC include mild temperature instability, apnea, bradycardia, and lethargy. Acidosis and thrombocytopenia appear as the disease worsens, followed ultimately by neutropenia, disseminated intravascular coagulation, sepsis syndrome, and cardiovascular collapse (Fig. 7).

Ileus is the initial clinical finding, and usually presents as feeding intolerance, increased residual gastric volume, mild abdominal distension, and bilious emesis.

Gastrointestinal mucosal deterioration leads to the presence of blood in the stool, starting with guiaic-positive stools that can progress to frank bleeding and bright-red blood per rectum. Physical exam findings include abdominal distension proceeding to local peritoneal signs and generalized peritonitis as the NEC worsens. Other advanced physical signs include discoloration of the anterior abdominal wall with cellulitis of the skin and a palpable abdominal mass, most often in the right lower quadrant. Physical findings of NEC are usually necessary to draw attention to the possible diagnosis, because the earliest signs such as mild temperature instability, apnea, bradycardia, and lethargy are nonspecific.

Early in the clinical course, abdominal films may be normal or show mild ileus. Progression of disease leads to the development of pneumatosis intestinalis. Late radiographic signs include portal venous air, ascites, and pneumoperitoneum. In the setting of NEC, pneumatosis and portal venous air are pathopneumonic; however, the absence of these signs offers little comfort that NEC is not present or progressing. The specificity of both pneumatosis and portal venous air for the presence of NEC is extremely high at about 100%, while the sensitivity of these signs remains quite poor, about 44% for pneumatosis and 19% for portal venous air (94).

Treatment

Once the diagnosis of NEC is considered, enteral feedings should be stopped, and parenteral nutrition is initiated. Conservative management includes nasogastric tube placement, broad-spectrum antibiotics, precise fluid management, and aggressive monitoring, with frequent clinical and radiographic assessment. The necessity for invasive intervention is usually evident within 24 hours. If this level of illness is not reached, conservative management as described above should be continued. Although no data exists regarding length of antibiotic usage, usually 10 to 14 days is employed, during which enteral feedings are held.

The decision for intervention is less dogmatic, but pneumoperitoneum is considered an absolute indication for invasive treatments. Portal venous gas and persistent metabolic acidosis are poor prognostic indicators and usually lead to surgical exploration. Additionally, fixed-loops of bowel on plain films, a palpable abdominal mass, abdominal wall erythema, positive peritoneal fluid cultures, or progressive illness are relative indications.

Operative management is first based upon the extent of diseased bowel found at laparotomy. In focal disease with isolated perforation, limited resection with proximal enterostomy is the historical standard, but primary anastomosis has been advocated by some authors as an alternative (95–98). Advocates of primary anastomosis making note of the high morbidity of enterostomy in neonates report that length of hospital stay, time to full feeds, and length of ventilator requirements are all shorter in patients treated with primary anastomosis (97,98). However, routine use of primary anastomosis has produced inferior survival rates compared to proximal enterostomy (98); therefore, the gold standard remains resection of the diseased segment followed by proximal enterostomy.

The presence of diffuse regions of necrosis presents a more posing circumstance. Extensive intestinal involvement with NEC not only increases mortality, but also places survivors at higher risk of the long-term sequelae such as more frequent bowel movements, fecal incontinence, short bowel

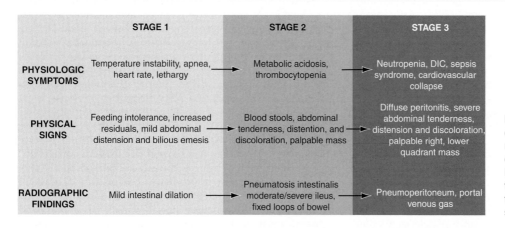

	STAGE 1	STAGE 2	STAGE 3
PHYSIOLOGIC SYMPTOMS	Temperature instability, apnea, heart rate, lethargy	Metabolic acidosis, thrombocytopenia	Neutropenia, DIC, sepsis syndrome, cardiovascular collapse
PHYSICAL SIGNS	Feeding intolerance, increased residuals, mild abdominal distension and bilious emesis	Blood stools, abdominal tenderness, distention, and discoloration, palpable mass	Diffuse peritonitis, severe abdominal tenderness, distension and discoloration, palpable right, lower quadrant mass
RADIOGRAPHIC FINDINGS	Mild intestinal dilation	Pneumatosis intestinalis moderate/severe ileus, fixed loops of bowel	Pneumoperitoneum, portal venous gas

Figure 7 Bell's modified criteria are composed of physical exam findings, clinical symptoms, and radiographic changes. Although these findings exist in a continuum from minimal to severe, the combination of all three predicts the stage and progression of disease.

syndrome, dependence on parenteral nutrition, and progressive liver failure (78,99–101). It has, therefore, become surgical priority to minimize the amount of bowel removed when extensive involvement is encountered at laparotomy.

One method of accomplishing this goal entails resection of only clearly nonviable bowel with proximal stoma formation and a second-look operation within 36 hours (102). Others have proposed no resection at the time of initial exploration when extensive disease is encountered, but simply proximal enterostomy, allowing for demarcation of all nonviable bowel (103,104). Another approach described to avoid the possible loss of length associated with stomal closure has been termed the "clip and drop-back" technique, which involves resection of only obvious nonviable segments, placing surgical clips on the ends of remaining bowel and closing the abdomen, leaving closed blind ends of intestine with no anastomosis or proximal stoma (105).

In the face of severe NEC with a clinically unstable neonate, primary peritoneal drainage has been advocated to facilitate stablization and delay or avert the need for laparotomy (106–109). Peritoneal drainage is accomplished at the bedside with local anesthesia by percutaneous placement of one or two drains into the peritoneal cavity, usually through the right lower quadrant. As most patients will require laparotomy after drainage, some authors view peritoneal drainage as part of resuscitation of the critical NEC patient (110–112). Mortality rates in patients treated with primary peritoneal drainage or initial laparotomy drainage are comparable, and meta-analysis of the studies available to date fail to demonstrate which initial approach is superior (113,114). Primary peritoneal drainage should be considered a useful adjunct in resuscitating critically ill NEC infants, particularly very small premature infants, however, will likely not serve as an alternative to laparotomy, which is usually necessary after clinical stabilization (107,111,115).

Intestinal Atresias

Duodenal Atresia

Duodenal atresia is reported to occur in approximately 1 in 2500 live births. Developmental insults during the 8th to 10th week of gestation can lead to duodenal obstruction in the form of atresia, web, or stenosis. Duodenal atresia is the most common form of duodenal obstruction, followed by stenosis and webs.

The diagnosis of duodenal atresia can be made prenatally. Ultrasonic findings of polyhydramnios (secondary to

high intestinal obstruction) and a dilated stomach and duodenum are highly suggestive of duodenal obstruction. Postnatally, the infant usually develops bilious vomiting, several hours after birth. Due to the proximal location of the obstruction, distention may not be present. Bilious, or persistent nonbilious, vomiting should prompt an abdominal film, which will show the classic double bubble sign, which represents the dilated stomach and duodenum. Most commonly, the abdominal film will show a gasless abdomen beyond the double bubble, suggesting atresia. However, the presence of gas distally should raise the suspicion of a duodenal stenosis or web, and contrast UGI should be obtained to rule out malrotation as a cause of bilious vomiting.

The management of duodenal atresia, stenosis, or web is surgical. Operation should be undertaken once the fluid and electrolyte abnormalities have been corrected, and an echocardiogram has been obtained to evaluate for congenital heart defects. Gastric decompression should be instituted during this time. The operation is begun with a right upper transverse incision. The abdomen is opened and explored. Attention should be paid to the position of the portal vein, as a preduodenal portal vein can be found, and lead to dire consequences if inadvertently entered. The duodenum is mobilized, and the distal collapsed segment adequately exposed for anastomosis to the dilated proximal portion. A diamond-shaped anastomosis is the preferred technique for duodenoduodenostomy, which is the optimal procedure for duodenal atresia, regardless of cause (annular pancreas, duodenal atresia, stenosis, or web). A transverse duodenotomy is made in the dilated proximal segment, followed by a vertical duodenotomy in the distal segment. A single or two-layer anastomosis is performed depending on surgeon's preference.

Postoperatively, gastric decompression is continued until the return of bowel function. Central venous catheterization is obtained, and TPN is begun and continued until adequate enteral feeds are established. Patient survival should exceed 90%, with most morbidity and/or mortality associated with a congenital heart defect.

Jejunoileal Atresias

Jejunoileal atresias are congenital defects resulting in segmental absence of intestinal lumen. They are generally categorized into four types. Type I is a simple mucosal obstruction or web with mural continuity. These are thought to result from embryologic failure of recanalization during the cord stage. Recent data suggests that a defect in smooth muscle actin production within the circular layer of muscularis propria is present in the proximal gut of patients with Type I lesions (116). Type II lesions consist of an atretic cord bridging the two ends of connected bowel. Type IIIa atresias involve complete separation of the bowel ends with a wedge shaped defect in the mesentery, while Type IIIb lesions, referred to as an "apple-peel" or "Christmas tree" deformity, are the same atretric configuration with the distal small bowel spiraled concentrically around an ascending branch of the ileocolic artery. Type IV lesions involve multiple Type III atresias. Types II–IV are felt to be secondary to mesenteric vascular events occurring during fetal development in utero.

Although mostly speculation, a range of causes for transient vascular occlusion during intestinal development has been proposed including intussusception, volvulus, internal herniation, embolus, herniation through abdominal wall defects, or complications of meconium ileus. Unlike the true atresia of the duodenum and esophagus, there is a relatively low rate of associated anomalies ($<10\%$) in infants with intestinal atresia. However, the presence of intestinal atresia does place the infant at a substantially increased risk of having a cystic fibrosis (CF) defect (117). It is therefore reasonable to consider testing all patients with intestinal atresia for the CF mutation. Consistent with the hypothesized causes of a vascular event, patients with gastroschisis have about 10% incidence intestinal atresia (118). The location of atresia is equally distributed between the ligament of Treitz and ileocecal junction, with colon atresia rarely seen.

The disease is sporadic, and no clinical risk factors for the development of intestinal atresia have been defined. However, recent evidence raises the question of an increased incidence of intestinal atresia with the maternal use of pseudoephedrine alone, or in combination with acetaminophen (119).

Overall mortality of infants with intestinal atresias is approximately 10%; however, it is considerably higher for jejunal than for ileal atresia (120–123). The mortality rates continue to decline with time, experience, and improved neonatal care (89). For those patients who gain independence from parenteral nutrition, the long-term prognosis in terms of development and survival is excellent (124,125).

Infants with intestinal atresia present with clinical signs of obstruction including bilious emesis and abdominal distension. Antenatal diagnosis is made in only about one-third of the cases, and most are proximal lesions with polyhydramnios (116,126). At physical examination, the degree of abdominal distension may predict the level of atresia, with worsening distension the more distal the atresia. Likewise, the level can be suggested by the radiographic findings on plain films. The presence of more than two air-filled lumens suggests obstruction beyond the duodenum, with more "bubbles" predicting a more distal lesion. No air is typically seen in the colon or rectum. An upper gastrointestinal series is usually superfluous and adds an unnecessary risk of aspiration.

Surgical treatment must first address establishing intestinal continuity. Anastomosis is usually challenging because of an enormous size discrepancy between the dilated proximal bowel and the atrophic, unused distal segment. The classic method for circumventing the size discrepancy is resection of the grossly dilated segment followed by an end-to-end anastomosis (127,128). However, if extensive resection is required or there is a sparse total length of small bowel present, resection of the dilated

segment may place the child at risk for short bowel syndrome. Alternatively, simple end-to-end anastomosis without resection may cause a functional obstruction within the dilated segment, because the grossly overdistracted sarcomeres within the musclaris propria are unlikely to regain normal peristaltic function (129). As an alternative, deflating proximal enterostomy has been successfully applied to decompress the dilated segment prior to staged anastomosis (130,131). While the staged procedure preserves bowel length, it substantially increases hospital stay, prolongs parenteral nutrition requirement, and increases the rate of postoperative complications (124,131). Therefore, plication with tapering enteroplasty of the dilated segment to mechanically reduce the size of the lumen is the currently suggested technique utilized to preserve length while alleviating the functional obstruction (132,133). Surgical plication of the dilated segment has been shown to result in faster return of peristalsis in the affected region, especially in the immediate postoperative period (134–136).

When multiple atresias are present, maintaining maximal bowel length may be particularly difficult. Several authors have reported utilizing intraluminal stenting of intervening nonatretic segments of bowel without anastomosis. This resulted in spontaneous sutureless anastomoses, allowing the child to tolerate oral feeds (137–139).

Unique approaches to minimal access techniques have been reported for both duodenal and jejunoileal atresias. An umbilical approach utilizing a ring retractor to stretch the umbilical ring and gain exposure to repair isolated jejunoileal atresias has been reported, and may shorten postoperative recovery and improve cosmesis (140). Laparoscopic repair of duodenal atresia is being performed by some authors, and it is likely that this approach will find utility in the treatment of intestinal atresias (141,142).

Currently, a lack of comparative trials to delineate a superior operative approach to the patient with intestinal atresia allows for and/or requires careful consideration of the technical options, given the findings at laparatomy. The principles of primary importance are maximizing bowel length and assuring functional integrity of the remaining bowel while if at all possible, minimizing postoperative recovery time.

Hirschsprung's Disease

Hirschsprung's disease (HD), properly termed "congenital aganglionosis," is manifest by an absence of the enteric ganglia along a variable length of the gastrointestinal tract. Neuron cell bodies derived from the neural crest follow distal progression within the developing gut. In humans, neural-crest–derived cells first appear in the mesenchyme of the developing esophagus at about four weeks gestation. Their migration is in a craniocaudal direction, and they reach the transverse colon by eight weeks and the rectum by 12 weeks gestation (143). The migration of these cells is dependent upon the presence of matrix proteins like fibronectin and hyaluronic acid while other molecules such as laminin and collagen Type IV assure navigation upon the proper matrix. Failure of craniocaudal descent of neural crest-derived ganglia may be minimal, thus limiting disease only to the anal canal, but the severity of disease is defined by the proximal level of aganglionosis.

Bowel motility creates a predictable pattern of propulsion via coordinated contraction stimulating reflex relaxation of adjacent segments. An intact enteric nervous system, with both sympathetic and parasympathetic components is the framework of communication upon which these serpentine muscular functions are possible. The absent ganglia in HD would normally provide the postsynaptic connection for parasympathetic nerve fibers from the spinal cord (S2-4) within the submucosal (Meissner's) and intermyenteric (Auerbach's) plexi. The functional physiologic defect is abnormal reflex relaxation within the region of aganglionosis producing tonic contraction. The contracted segment is a barrier to normal peristaltic propulsions, thus creating a partial or complete obstruction at the level of aganglionosis.

The common presentation in the newborn is failure to pass meconium within the first 24 hours of life. However, this presentation is not uniform as only about 50% of cases are diagnosed in the neonate. HD may manifest simply as constipation or show more significant signs of obstruction with feeding intolerance, abdominal distension, and/or emesis. Plain films are usually nonspecific with multiple gas-filled loops of bowel, but may be more suggestive with substantial proximal rectal or distal colonic dilation. Barium enema is often valuable at identifying the level of demarcation between contracted distal bowel and proximal dilatation. Infrequently, this transition zone may not be present in the first few weeks of life. The combination of rectosigmoid transition zone, retention of barium, and stool mixed with barium appear to offer superior accuracy in the diagnosis of HD than any of these features alone, and comparison films 24 to 48 hours after the enema help to differentiate HD from meconium plug syndrome (144). If the diagnosis is suspected from history and physical and basic radiographic work-up, rectal biopsy is the definitive test. Suction rectal biopsy can be performed safely at the bedside without anesthesia in neonates and infants. The suction biopsy tip is placed 2 to 3 cm above the dentate line, and biopsies in multiple quadrants are obtained to provide a specimen of mucosa and submucosa. Adequate tissue for diagnosis is obtained by suction rectal in about 90% of cases (145). Histologic criteria for diagnosing HD include absence of ganglion cells and hypertrophied myenteric axons in the submucosa with routine hematoxylin and eosin staining. The quantity of acetylcholine esterase can be assessed by specific staining to increase diagnostic accuracy, and is routinely employed in equivocal cases (146). The importance of a pathologist experienced in ruling out HD from a suction rectal specimen has been emphasized by several authors, as has the value of communication between such a pathologist and the pediatric surgeon. Failure to reach a diagnostic conclusion mandates a full-thickness rectal biopsy.

Operative treatment is predicated on the principle of overcoming the functional obstruction without a permanent colostomy. Traditionally, a temporary "leveling" colostomy determining the precise level of aganglionosis is performed upon diagnosis. Six to twelve months later, continuity is reestablished with a low, end-to-end colorectal (Swenson), a retrorectal, side-to-side colorectal anastomosis (Duhamel), or an endorectal pull-through coloanal anastomosis (Soave). Over the past 20 years, there has been a progressive movement toward a single-stage primary endorectal pull-through in the neonate without temporary diversion (147–161). Primary surgical treatment was initially approached by combined abdominal and perineal approach with comparable success when compared to the traditional two-stage approach (147–152). Subsequently, the abdominal component of the operation was performed laparoscopically (153–155), and, most recently, a transanal, one-stage endorectal pull-through has been described (156–160).

Total colonic aganglionosis represents a severe form of HD, wherein distal migration of enteric cells from neural crest origin terminates above the level of the colon. This occurs in less then 10% of HD patients, and is naturally associated with much higher morbidity and mortality (162–166). The disease prognosis correlates inversely with the proximal level of disease, with the most severe disease extending to the esophagus, a lesion not compatible with survival (165–169).

Physicians involved in the care of HD patients should be cognizant of Hirschsprung's-associated enterocolitis (HAEC), which occurs in about 25% of the HD population (166,170). Patients more often develop HAEC prior to definitive surgery, although it may recur or strike de novo after the operation (170,171), and risk is correlated with the distance of aganglionosis (168,172). Patients presenting with HAEC usually present with abdominal distension, explosive diarrhea, vomiting, fever, lethargy, rectal bleeding, and shock in decreasing order (172). Abdominal films may be nonspecific, and although pneumatosis intestinalis and perforation can occur, HAEC usually follows a more indolent course than NEC (170–173). The disease may recur, and while severity does not increase with the number of attacks, the mortality does (170). Mortality in these circumstances is related to the development of sepsis, underscoring the importance of early recognition and treatment.

Meconium Ileus

Meconium ileus is a term for small bowel obstruction caused by viscous enteric content. The great majority of patients presenting with meconium ileus have CF as the primary diagnosis. The genetic defect in CF disables production of a cell membrane ion channel termed the "CF transmembrane conductance regulator," which is a chloride channel. Defective chloride permeability impairs movement of electrolytes across cell membranes, grossly attenuating the water content of secretions, making for abnormally viscous secretions. Negative functional effects are seen in the lungs, pancreas, liver, and gut. Within the gut, the defect results in thick, viscid, high-protein, low-carbohydrate meconium, which may accumulate in the terminal ileum creating an obstruction. Meconium ileus is rare without CF, and may be related to delayed development of the gut motility pacemakers, the interstitial cells of Cajal (174).

Initial presentation of meconium ileus is failure to pass meconium follow by typical signs of obstruction with abdominal distension and bilious vomiting. Plain films demonstrate multiple loops of dilated small bowel. In the clinical scenario of an obstructed newborn with multiple dilated loops of bowel on plain films, meconium ileus needs to be differentiated from an atresia. The offending inspissated meconium may encase small bubbles of air producing the radiographic presence of a ground glass or soap bubble appearance in the right lower quadrant, which can help diagnose meconium ileus. Ultrasound can identify echogenic material within the bowel to separate meconium ileus from an atresia (175). Barium enema reveals an unused microcolon as seen in ileal atresia, and with reflux of contrast into the terminal meconium, concretions will be identified and will confirm the diagnosis of meconium ileus.

Clinically, meconium ileus is broadly categorized as either complicated or uncomplicated. Complicated meconium ileus is compounded by the presence of volvulus, atresia, perforation, and/or giant cystic meconium peritonitis. In these cases, operative exploration is necessary to manage the complications as well as the meconium ileus.

Hypertonic contrast enema is the treatment of choice in simple, uncomplicated cases. Intraluminal hypertonic solution draws water from the mucosa via osmosis to facilitate breaking up of the viscid material, and the progress can be visualized under fluoroscopy. The consequent fluid shifts should be anticipated, and an infusion of crystalloid (20 mL/kg) should be given during the procedure to prevent intravascular volume depletion. Comparative studies of the available hypertonic contrast agents have found Gastrografin to be most effective in relieving the meconium obstruction (176). After instillation of the Gastrografin, the infant will pass portions of the diluted meconium for up to 48 hours. Plain films can be repeated for 12 to 24 hours to assess progress. Successful relief of obstruction can be followed with oral *N*-acetylcysteine in an effort to prevent recurrence. When feedings are initiated, supplemental pancreatic enzymes should be included for CF-positive patients.

If the meconium obstruction is resistant to dilution, or there is a complicated disease, an operation is indicated. The principle of nonoperative management, breaking up the meconium to relieve obstruction, is maintained at operation. The most common surgical approach involves an enterostomy, proximal to the obstruction for the introduction of a catheter, followed by an aggressive flushing of the ileum with a hypertonic solution through the catheter (177–181). In resistant cases, the tube can be left behind as a tube enterostomy to allow for repeat irrigation if needed. If the meconium is refractory to these measures, a resection may be necessary. In this case, maintaining bowel length is the first priority. Enterostomy can be used to allow washing the bowel for a period of time to assure resolution. Operations described for this purpose include double-barreled enterostomy (Mikulicz), distal chimney enterostomy (Bishop–Koop procedure), proximal chimney enterostomy (reverse Bishop–Koop), and side-by-side enterostomy; however, these techniques are not frequently necessary.

Esophageal Atresia and Tracheoesophageal Fistula

Esophageal atresia (EA) with or without tracheoesophageal fistula (TEF) is seen in about 1 in 3000 births, with males and females affected equally. Although initially described in 1697 by Thomas Gibson, the exact embryogenesis is still not fully understood (182). Traditionally, the more accepted theories suggest an abnormal development of the laryngotracheoesophageal groove with persistent communication between the esophagus and the trachea. More recently, with the development of the adriamycin-induced murine model of EA/TEF, along with embryonic microdissection techniques, a new mechanism of embryogenesis has been suggested (183). From these studies, it has been suggested that the fistula tract begins as a trifurcation of the tracheal anlage, which subsequently fistulizes to the stomach, indicating that the fistula tract is actually of respiratory origin with pseudostratified columnar epithelium present in the early embryonic period. As the fetus with EA/TEF matures, this fistula tract undergoes metaplasia to squamous epithelium. This respiratory origin may explain the presence of respiratory epithelium seen in the fistula tract of neonates with EA/TEF and is also consistent with the poor motility of the distal esophagus seen in many of the patients who have undergone surgical correction of the defect (184,185). Further study of the patterning genes of foregut formation have suggested defects in several signaling pathways such as fibroblast growth factor (FGF) and sonic hedgehog (Shh) signaling, which appear to be important in the temporal and spatial pattern of expression of normal esophageal and tracheal formation (186–188).

There are five variants of EA/TEF (Fig. 8). Often included in this classification is esophageal stenosis which is very uncommon. The most common variant is EA with distal TEF (85% of cases). Other types include EA without a TEF (8%), EA with a proximal TEF (2%), EA with both a proximal and a distal TEF (3%), and a TEF without EA (the so-called "H" or "N"-type fistula). There also appears to be an association of EA/TEF with chromosomal abnormalities including trisomy 18 and 21. In addition, EA/TEF may occur as part of the VACTERL (vertebral, anal, cardiac, tracheoesophageal, renal, and limb) association in about 10% of the patients. Accordingly, investigation to identify the presence of other anomalies must be completed prior to definitive surgical therapy, particularly because the mortality rate is usually determined by the presence of some of these other anomalies.

The diagnosis of EA may be suggested on prenatal ultrasound by the presence of polyhydramnios and reduced intraluminal fluid of the fetal gut, with a small or indistinct fetal stomach. However, the predictive value of prenatal ultrasound is low. The use of fetal magnetic resonance imaging in patients with suspicious ultrasonographic findings may help confirm the diagnosis, and has been shown to be relatively safe (189). In contrast, antenatal diagnosis of EA is usually quite straightforward. Infants present with

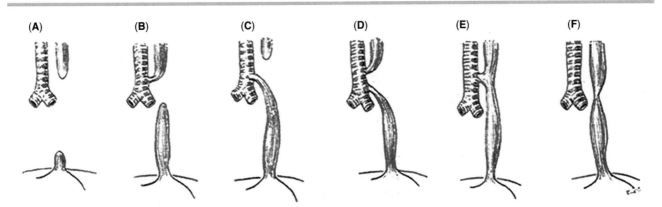

(A)   **(B)**   **(C)**   **(D)**   **(E)**   **(F)**

Figure 8 The six variants of esophageal atresia (EA), tracheoesophageal fistula (TEF) are depicted. (**A**) Pure EA without TEF, (**B**) Proximal TEF with distal EA. (**C**) Proximal EA with distal TEF (the most common variant), (**D**) Proximal and distal TEF, (**E**) H or N type TEF, and (**F**) Esophageal stenosis.

excessive salivation requiring frequent suctioning. Tachypnea and cough may develop as a result of aspiration from overflow of the proximal pouch or from reflux through the TEF. Early feeding will produce almost immediate regurgitation, and cyanosis may develop as a result. When the diagnosis is suspected, a 10 to 12 French orogastric tube may be inserted into the proximal pouch. The inability to pass the catheter into the stomach confirms the diagnosis. The diagnosis may be less obvious with an N-type fistula, where there is no EA. These infants will present with symptoms of aspiration typically following feeding. Often the diagnosis is not made until years later, while in the interim, the patient suffers from a persistent cough associated with recurrent pneumonia. An upright radiograph should be performed as part of the initial work-up. Typically, it will demonstrate the presence of the catheter in the proximal pouch, defining the level of the EA. In addition, air may be seen in the stomach and small intestines indicating the presence of a fistula. Likewise, absence of air in the stomach indicates a pure EA.

The diagnosis of TEF may be less obvious with an N-type fistula where there is no esophageal atresia. These latter infants will present with symptoms of aspiration typically following feeding. Often the diagnosis is not made until years later, while in the interim the patient suffers from a persistent cough associated with recurrent pneumonia.

Once the diagnosis of EA/TEF in an infant is confirmed, the catheter in the proximal pouch should be placed on continuous suction to prevent distention and subsequent aspiration. The baby should also be placed in semi-Fowler's position. The infant should then undergo a full evaluation for the presence of other anomalies. This begins with a thorough physical examination. Careful evaluation of the anus (for patency) and extremities (for limb defects) should be done. The vertebral column and heart contour must be evaluated on plain radiographs. An echocardiogram is important in all patients to identify congenital heart defects and laterality of the aortic arch, which is critically important in surgical planning. Renal ultrasonography is also obtained to evaluate for renal anomalies. On occasion, rigid bronchoscopy may be performed to identify the location or presence of a fistula (especially in an N-type fistula).

While looking for other anomalies, the infant's medical condition should also be evaluated in preparation for surgical management. Fluid and electrolyte normalization should be accomplished, and antibiotics initiated. The presence of severe congenital heart defects, or significant pulmonary disease may delay plans for immediate operative repair. Rather, in these unstable patients, an emergent gastrostomy may be performed, with the definitive repair delayed until the patient's clinical condition improves. For full-term or near full-term infants with mild anomalies and without evidence of significant pulmonary disease, operative therapy may be undertaken shortly after birth.

The operative repair is traditionally performed via an extra-pleural or trans-pleural thoracotomy incision (third or fourth intercostals space) made on the side opposite the aortic arch. In general, the extra-pleural approach is preferred because there is no risk of empyema formation, if an anastomotic leak occurs in the postoperative period. A drain in the extra-pleural space will allow evacuation of any leakage with little clinical consequence in most cases. Upon exploration, the azygous vein is identified within the mediastinum and divided. This allows access to the esophagus and the trachea. The proximal esophageal pouch usually has excellent intramural blood supply originating

from the thyrocervical trunk. For this reason, the proximal pouch can be mobilized extensively without compromise to its integrity. However, the dissection should be carried out rather carefully to identify any proximal pouch fistulas. In contrast to the proximal esophageal segment, the blood supply to the distal esophagus is more segmental with branches originating from the aorta. This limits extensive mobilization of the lower esophageal segment. Tension and excessive mobilization of the distal segment may lead to poor healing resulting in an anastomotic leak, or stricture formation. The fistula is identified and divided close to the trachea taking care not to compromise the tracheal lumen. The trachea is closed with 5–0 or 6–0 interrupted silk suture. A primary end-to-end anastomosis of the esophagus is performed in a full-thickness fashion using interrupted silk sutures. A Silastic stent may be placed across the anastomosis extending from the stomach to the oral cavity, where it is secured as it exits the nares. A small drain is left in the retropleural space prior to closure of the thoracotomy incision. A thorascopic approach to the repair of EA/TEF has been described and appears to be feasible. The main issue appears to be the technical difficulties related to the intracorporeal suturing required to complete the esophageal anastomosis. Although the rate of esophageal narrowing at the anastomosis does appear to be somewhat higher than in the historical controls, the actual long-term outcome of this procedure will become clear as more thorascopic cases are performed (190).

In infants with isolated EA, the distal segment of the esophagus is usually short, leaving a long gap between the proximal and distal segments of the esophagus. This long gap makes primary repair impossible. The infant is usually taken for a gastrostomy and bronchoscopy under the same anesthesia. The bronchoscopy may reveal an occluded proximal or distal fistula, in which case a primary repair may be indicated. The infants that demonstrate true isolated EA are treated with a gastrostomy by which they are able to receive enteral feeds. The proximal pouch is then allowed to elongate with a sump tube in place with the definitive repair delayed for several months as adequate length is gained in the proximal esophageal segment. If the patient still fails to gain length in the esophagus, complete cervical esophageal mobilization via a collar incision followed by circular myotomies in the proximal segment may allow adequate lengthening for primary anastamosis. On rare occasion, if the patient still lacks the length in the esophagus for a primary anastomosis, an interposition colon or gastric tube may be required. Neither colon nor stomach function as well as the native esophagus, and are used in the rare case where all other efforts at esophageal lengthening are unsuccessful.

In patients with the N-type TEF, the repair involves a simple division of the fistula, which is generally performed through a cervical incision. The use of bronchoscopy to place a catheter into the fistula can aid in identifying the fistula tract from the outside during the operative exploration. Careful dissection is important to avoid a recurrent laryngeal nerve injury.

Postoperatively, patients are maintained nil per os (NPO), with a contrast study performed around day 7. If no leak is seen, oral feeds may be started. Once the child demonstrates adequate weight gain while tolerating full feeds, he or she can be discharged with regular follow-up. During long-term follow-up, particular attention should be made to the development of symptoms of dysphagia, GER, anastomotic stenosis, and recurrence of the TEF

(191,192). Abnormal peristalsis in the distal esophagus is almost always present. GER is also quite common, and severe reflux may lead to a Barrett's esophagus or chronic aspiration. In these instances, aggressive medical management must be initiated as soon as the diagnosis is apparent. For cases refractory to medical therapy, a fundoplication may be helpful. Stricture formation is not uncommon and may require periodic dilatation. Long-term follow-up also reveals delayed gastric emptying, which further exacerbates GER symptoms (192). Overall, most children do well with a survival rate reported in the 90% range. The majority of the mortality is related to the severity of congenital heart defects and chromosomal abnormalities. Late deaths usually result from tracheomalacia, aspiration, and reactive airway disease (193).

Congenital Diaphragmatic Hernia

Congenital diaphragmatic hernia (CDH) continues to be one of the more challenging diagnoses of pediatric surgery (Fig. 9). CDH occurs in 1:3000 births, with a slight female predominance (194). The issues of pulmonary complications continue to be a dilemma in the management of patients with CDH, maintaining a mortality rate as high as 60%, and significant morbidity in those who survive (195). There is a 10% incidence of other congenital abnormalities, primarily chromosomal, cardiac, and neurological defects. It is the presence of these abnormalities that are responsible for the high mortality seen immediately after birth in some of these patients. Familial cases have also been reported, although the vast majority of the cases appear to be spontaneous.

Our understanding of how and why this defect develops during embryogenesis remains quite obscure. Traditionally, it was believed that the pulmonary complications of

CDH were a result of failure of the diaphragm to close as the midgut makes its normal return to the abdomen from the yolk sac, during the tenth week of gestation. The herniation of the abdominal viscera into the thorax was then thought to lead to compression of the lung impeding proper lung growth. This theory was supported by lamb animal model studies, where an artificial hernia created in the diaphragm led to similar pathologic findings seen in abnormal lungs of human neonates with CDH (196). Recent rodent model studies provide increasing evidence that the pulmonary hypertension and lung hypoplasia precede the development of the diaphragmatic defect (197–199). Observations from these studies have shown that almost all of the embryos appear to have some degree of pulmonary hypoplasia, with a diaphragmatic hernia occurring in only 40% to 60% of the treated embryos (199). This model also explains the lung hypoplasia seen in both the ipsilateral and contralateral lungs. The fact that there is more severe hypoplasia seen on the ipsilateral side may be explained by the presence of the abdominal contents in the chest, causing further compression of an already hypoplastic lung (196). Other studies have implicated defects in the molecular mechanisms FGF-10 and Shh of normal branching morphogenesis, as being responsible for the lung hypoplasia as an initial event (201,202). It has also been shown that the pulmonary vasculature, including the number of arteriole branches, as well as the arteriolar muscularization in CDH patients is distinctly abnormal.

The left posterolateral diaphragm hernia (Bochdalek hernia) represents the most common site for CDH, and defects in this region represent 85% of all cases. The less common anterolateral defects (Morgagni hernias) present more commonly on the right side and represent about 15% of the hernias. At presentation, patients with CDH typically have varying degrees of hypoxia and acidosis. The lungs are physically small and functionally immature. Gas exchange is poor, resulting in worsening hypoxia after birth. The hypertrophied muscular layers of the pulmonary arterioles increase vascular resistance adding to the pulmonary hypertension. This vicious cycle of the hypoxia and acidosis, both contribute to the persistent pulmonary hypertension of the newborn. As a result, there is persistent fetal circulation with a right to left shift through the foramen ovale and the ductus arteriosus.

The diagnosis of CDH is usually made before birth with the prenatal ultrasonography. The presence of polyhydramnios may prompt this study. A prenatal diagnosis allows for preparation of therapy and provision of perinatal counseling. After birth, respiratory distress is apparent with tachypnea and cyanosis, which may develop immediately after clamping the umbilical cord, or may not be obvious until several hours after birth. Typically, the degree of respiratory distress worsens as the infant continues to breathe. The swallowed air distends the gut, which due to its location in the chest makes lung expansion even more difficult. Prompt endotracheal intubation is required along with orogastric tube decompression of the gut in the chest. Masked ventilation should be avoided as it may distend the stomach further. Physical examination may reveal a scaphoid abdomen with an increased chest diameter. There may be decreased breath sounds bilaterally, with the presence of bowel sounds within the chest. A plain radiograph of the chest usually confirms the diagnosis via the presence of the gastric tube within the affected thorax. Once the diagnosis is made, an echocardiogram should be obtained to evaluate for the presence of congenital heart defects and to determine the degree of right-to-left shunting.

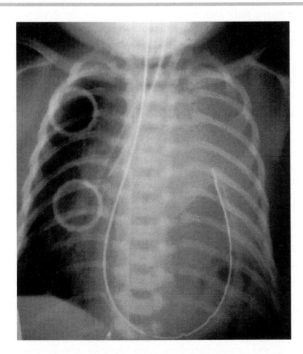

Figure 9 A typical chest radiograph in a newborn with left congenital diaphragmatic hernia. Significant findings include mediastinal shift to the right (note the tracheal deviation identified by the endotracheal tube), bowel gas in the left chest, and the "classic" finding of the nasogastric tube looping upward into the left hemithorax.

The concept that all patients with CDH require immediate surgical repair is no longer the approach to the management of these patients. It appears that improving oxygenation, while avoiding barotrauma prior to surgical intervention has a better overall outcome (203). Aggressive resuscitation with fluids and electrolytes should be used to correct any underlying acidosis, with careful monitoring of the patient's fluid status to provide adequate resuscitation and at the same time to avoid volume overloading. Cardiac dysfunction with hypotension may necessitate the use of ionotropes. The degree to which the pulmonary hypertension improves will determine the timing of surgery. In instances where the patient does not respond to conventional ventilation, high-frequency oscillatory ventilation and nitrous oxide administration may be used (204). Permissive hypercapnia has also been utilized to minimize the degree of barotrauma (205). The use of surfactant therapy has been suggested in the management of CDH, but its use has not been shown to improve overall survival in controlled clinical trials (206). If after all these efforts the patient still fails to respond, extracorporeal membrane oxygenation (ECMO) may be instituted. ECMO allows respiratory support without concerns of barotrauma or oxygen toxicity. Careful selection must be used in choosing patients for ECMO, as it carries significant morbidity and/or mortality. Systemic anticoagulation is necessary and any contraindication to heparin must be taken into consideration. In general, as the patient's condition improves, he or she is weaned from ECMO and operative repair performed; alternatively, the repair can be performed while the patient remains on ECMO.

The surgical repair of CDH is usually performed via a subcostal incision. A reduction of the hernia contents is performed, and if a hernia sac is present, it is excised. The defect in the diaphragm is repaired primarily if possible. If the defect is too large, a prosthetic material or muscle flap may be used. The abdominal incision can then be closed in the usual fashion. In some instances, the abdominal closure may create undue tension on the diaphragm, which may lead to impaired lung ventilation in the postoperative period. In such cases, the abdominal fascia can be closed using a prosthetic patch or the skin approximated with a ventral hernia repair performed at a later date. Alternatively, a "silo" can be used with sequential down sizing and delayed closure of the fascia once the tension is relieved. The postoperative management in these patients involves close ventilatory support and management with serial arterial blood gases. Particular attention is needed in the immediate postoperative period as the surgery may exacerbate pulmonary hypertension and further perpetuate the right-to-left shunting. ECMO may have to be reinstituted for severe cases.

Although the overall mortality of CDH has improved with the institution of the various ventilation techniques described earlier, a single management strategy has yet to be clearly defined. In addition, several experimental techniques are under investigation to better manage this devastating congenital anomaly. Specifically, some fetal interventions have been attempted involving in utero tracheal occlusion surgery. The benefit of this technique has been shown in animal models, but has failed to show a survival advantage in human neonates (207,208).

As the mortality rate continues to decline, the long-term complications of patients who survive CDH repair are becoming more apparent. Foregut dysmotility is increasingly being recognized. GER has been reported in as high as 50% of patients (209). Diaphragmatic hernia recurrence is common, particularly in patients who required a synthetic patch to close the diaphragmatic defect (206). As our management techniques for CDH improves, the significance of the long-term complication will become more apparent. For this reason, extended close follow-up should be maintained in all patients surviving CDH repair.

Malrotation

In the fifth week of gestation, the primitive gut elongates and opens ventrally into the yolk sac, where it remains until the 10th week. During this time, the midgut rotates approximately 270 degrees in a counterclockwise direction, along the superior mesenteric artery (SMA), with the omphalomesenteric duct at the apex (Fig. 10). The prearterial portion of the gut then elongates and forms the duodenum from its proximal portion, while the distal portion of the prearterial segment rotates behind the SMA, and becomes fixed at the ligament of Treitz. The proximal postarterial segment then rotates in a counterclockwise direction anterior to the SMA to end upon in the right lower quadrant. This portion of the gut gives rise to the terminal ileum and cecum, with its distal end extending to the level of the midtransverse colon. By the 12th week of gestation, portions of the gut become fixed to the posterior body wall. This fixation results in an oblique, broad-based small bowel mesentery, extending from the ligament of Treitz to the cecum. When the process of rotation and fixation does not occur properly, the midgut is at risk of forming a volvulus and producing intestinal ischemia (210). The diagnosis of malrotation refers to any abnormality that occurs in this developmental process of rotation and fixation.

Nonrotation refers to the early arrest of rotation of the duodenojejunal loop, so that the segment of bowel remains on the right side of the abdomen. The result is that the small intestine remains on the right side of the abdomen, with the colon on the left, and the cecum near the midline. In contrast, "incomplete rotation" refers to an arrest of the duodenojejunal loop after it has partially rotated around the SMA but has yet to ascend to its normal position. The duodenojejunal junction resides to the right of the midline, and the cecum, which fails to rotate anterior to the SMA, usually remains to its left, in the upper abdomen. In both, nonrotation and incomplete rotation, the patient may present with symptoms that result from duodenal obstruction, which develops from the peritoneal attachments of the cecum, which cross over the duodenum and attach to the posterior abdominal cavity. These bands are the so-called Ladd's bands. In addition, because the SMA vascular pedicle is narrow, a midgut volvulus may occur, with subsequent symptoms of intestinal ischemia (211,212).

Typically, the diagnosis of malrotation is made in the first year of life, with males presenting slightly more often than females. However, patients may remain asymptomatic into adulthood, where the diagnosis is made incidentally during an evaluation for other reasons. Upon further questioning, these patients often reveal ongoing symptoms that may have gone unrecognized. Regardless of the age at presentation, it is generally accepted that all cases of malrotation should undergo correction despite the absence of symptoms (213). Correction of the malrotation will reduce the chance of midgut volvulus with subsequent intestinal ischemia or death.

The duodenal obstruction resulting from the Ladd's bands produces bilious vomiting. The main concern in the neonate with bilious emesis is the possibility of midgut

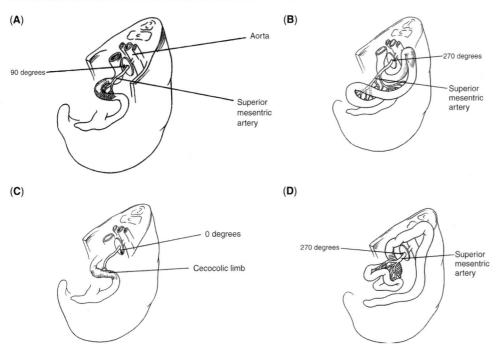

Figure 10 A diagrammatic representation of the embryonic rotational events of the intestine. **(A)** The duodenojejunal limb begins to the right of the superior mesenteric artery (SMA). **(B)** After completion of the 270 degrees counterclockwise rotation, the duodenojejunal limb now lies to the left of the midline and slightly higher than its starting point. **(C)** The cecocolic limb initially begins directly inferior to the SMA and with rotation **(D)** migrates counterclockwise to its normal position in the right lower quadrant. *Abbreviation*: SMA, superior mesenteric artery.

volvulus, and it is this diagnosis that requires an aggressive investigative approach. If the bowel supplied by the SMA is compromised, the patient may require an extensive resection of the infarcted segment, which often leads to an extremely high morbidity and mortality. Therefore, any infant that presents with bilious vomiting should be considered as having a diagnosis of malrotation until proven otherwise. Other symptoms that may be present include abdominal distention with pain, and guaiac-positive stools. In late stages of intestinal ischemia, metabolic acidosis with a coagulopathy and shock may ensue.

The diagnosis of malrotation is usually made with an upper gastrointestinal contrast study. In patients with malrotation without midgut volvulus, the contrast study reveals that the duodenojejunal junction fails to cross the midline and lies lower than normal. When volvulus is present, a partial or complete obstruction of the second/third portion of the duodenum is seen. The duodenum may show a "corkscrew effect," which represents the point of volvulus around the superior mesenteric vessels. In addition, plain films may show gastric and proximal duodenal distention with little or no air in the distal small bowel. A barium enema may demonstrate an abnormally positioned cecum. This finding may not be totally reliable in the infant, because the cecum usually occupies a higher position than in older children.

In the symptomatic patient with a new diagnosis of malrotation, the management should be guided to prepare the infant for emergent operation. The patient should be resuscitated with IV fluids and given IV antibiotics. The stomach should be decompressed, urine output should be closely monitored, and electrolytes should be corrected.

At laparotomy, a Ladd's procedure is performed (214). This procedure includes the division of the Ladd's bands causing obstruction of the duodenum, widening of the base of the mesentery, appendectomy, and placement of the duodenum into the right gutter of the abdomen and the cecum into the left upper quadrant. A laparoscopic approach to the

Ladd's procedure has been described with some reported advantages. Some of these advantages include less postoperative pain, decreased postoperative ileus, and a shorter hospital stay. The laparoscopic approach should be limited to cases where there is no evidence of midgut volvulus, as ischemic bowel is extremely friable and requires gentle manipulation of the involved segments (215). The volvulus is usually a result of a clockwise twisting of the bowel, so the reduction of the bowel should be performed in a counterclockwise direction. Once this is complete and the Ladd's bands are divided, the duodenum should drop inferiorly toward the right lower quadrant, and the cecum falls to the left. The appendix is removed to avoid confusion in the event that appendicitis should develop later in life. In situations where the bowel is infarcted, a resection of the involved intestine should be performed. If there is concern for bowel viability after detorsion, a second look operation can be planned 24 hours later.

If the patient is diagnosed prior to bowel ischemia, the prognosis is excellent with a normal life expectancy. In contrast, infants that require extensive bowel resection have a significantly higher mortality rate, and may suffer from the horrible consequences of a short bowel syndrome.

SUMMARY

This chapter has attempted to show that "children are not little adults" but present unique challenges in perioperative management should a surgical procedure become necessary. These challenges are related to the specific changes that occur in physiology, thermoregulations, biochemistry, and nutrition, which commence at both following the in utero state and continue into the newborn period and throughout later stages of development. Common problems that occur in the pediatric populations have been discussed with these considerations in mind. A thorough understanding of these pathophysiologic perturbations and their clinical presentations not only is critical to enabling early diagnosis but also is likewise crucial, if correct and expeditions treatment is to be employed with an acceptable morbidity and a negligible mortality.

REFERENCES

1. Garg R, Agthe AG, Donohoe PK, Lehman CU. Hyperglycemia and retinopathy of prematurity in very low birth weight infants. J Perinatol 2003; 23:186–194.

2. Lorenz JM, Kleinman LI, Kotagal UR, et al. Water balance in very low birth weight infants: relationship to water and sodium intake and effect on outcome. J Pediatr 1982; 101:423–432.

3. Aperia A, Broberger O, Herin P, et al. Postnatal control of water and electrolyte homeostasis in pre-term and full-term infants. Acta Paediatr Scand 1983; 305:61–65.

4. Marian M. Pediatric nutritional support. Nutr Clin Pract 1993; 8:199–200.

5. Rose J, Gibbons K, Carlson SE, Koo WWK. Nutrient needs of the preterm infant. Nutri Clin Pract 1993; 8:226–232.

6. Heird W, Driscoll J, Schullinger J. Intravenous alimentation in pediatric patients. J Pediatr 1972; 80:351–355.

7. Letton RW, Chwals WJ, Jamie A, et al. Early postoperative alterations in infant energy use increases the risk of overfeeding. J Pediatr Surg 1995; 30:988–993.

8. Pang KY, Bresson JL, Walker WA. Development of the gastrointestinal mucosal barrier. Evidence for structural differences in microvillous membranes from newborn and adult rabbits. Biochim Biophys Acta 1983; 727:201–208.

9. Kudsk KA, Croce M, Favian T, et al. Enteral versus parenteral feeding. Effects on septic morbidity after blunt and penetrating abdominal trauma. Ann Surg 1992; 215:503–511.

10. Moore FA, Moore EE, Kudsk KA, et al. Clinical benefits of an immune-enhancing diet for early postinjury enteral feeding. J Trauma 1994; 37:607–615.

11. Haumont D, Deckelbaum RJ, Richelle M, et al. Plasma lipid and plasma lipoprotein concentration in low birth weight infants given parenteral nutrition with twenty or ten percent lipid emulsion. J Pediatr 1989; 115:787–793.

12. Hirschprung H. Falle von angeborener pylorus stenose. Jb Kinderheilk 1888; 27:61–62.

13. Ramstedt C. Zur operation der angeboren pylorus stenose. Med Klinik 1912; 8:1702–1704.

14. Takahashi T. Pathophysiological significance of neuronal nitric oxide synthease in the gastrointestinal tract. J Gastroenterol 2003; 38:421–430.

15. Subramaniam R, Doig CM, Moore L. Nitric oxide synthase is absent in only a subset of cases of pyloric stenosis. J Pediatr Surg 2001; 36:616–619.

16. Wallgren A. Preclinical stage of infantile hypertrophic pyloric stenosis. Am J Dis Child 1946; 72:371–374.

17. Rollins MD, Shields MD, Quinn RJ, et al. Pyloric stenosis: congenital or acquired? Arch Dis Child 1989; 64:138–139.

18. Keller H, Waldermann D, Greiner P. Comparison of preoperative sonography with intraoperative findings in congenital hypertrophic pyloric stenosis. J Pediatr Surg 1987; 22:950–952.

19. Benson CD, Alpern EB. Preoperative and postoperative care of congenital pyloric stenosis. Arch Surg 1957; 75:877–879.

20. Hulka F, Harrison MW, Campbell TJ, et al. Complications of pyloromyotomy for infantile hypertrophic pyloric stenosis. Am J Surg 1997; 1173:450–452.

21. Royal RE, Linz DN, Gruppo DL, et al. Repair of mucosal perforation during pyloromyotomy: surgeon's choice. J Laparoendosc Surg 1995; 30:1430–1432.

22. Gross RE. A new method for surgical treatment of large omphalocele. Surgery 1948; 24:277–292.

23. Snyder CL. Outcome analysis for gastroschisis. J Pediatr Surg 2000; 35:1253–1256.

24. Hoyme HE, Jones MC, Jones KL. Gastroschisis: abdominal wall disruption secondary to early gestational interruption of the omphalomesenteric artery. Semin Perinatol 1983; 7:294–298.

25. DeVries PA. The pathogenesis of gastroschisis and omphalocele. J Pediatr Surg 1980; 15:245–251.

26. Swartz KR, Harrison MW, Campbell TJ, et al. Selective management of gastroschisis. Ann Surg 1985; 203:214–218.

27. Grosfeld JL, Weber TR. Congenital abdominal wall defects: gastroschisis and omphalocele. Curr Prob Surg 1982; 19:157–213.

28. Knight PJ, Buckner D, Vassey LE. Omphalocele: treatment options. Surgery 1981; 89:332–336.

29. Duhamel B. Embryology of exomphalos and allied malformations. Arch Dis Child 1963; 38:142–147.

30. Drongowski RA, et al. Contribution of demographic and environmental factors to the etiology of gastroschisis: a hypothesis. Fetal Diagn Ther 1991; 6:14–27.

31. Pokorny WJ, Garcia-Prats JA, Barry YN. Necrotizing enterocolitis: incidence, operative care, and outcome. J Pediatr Surg 1986; 21:1149–1154.

32. Kliegman RM, Fanaroff AA. Neonatal necrotizing enterocolitis: a nine-year experience. Am J Dis Child 1981; 135:603–607.

33. Wiswell TE, Robertson CF, Jones T, et al. Necrotizing enterocolitis in full-term infants. A case control study. Am J Dis Child 1988; 142:532–535.

34. Caplan MS, Hedlund E, Adler L, Hsueh W. Role of asphyxia and feeding in a neonatal rat model of necrotizing enterocolitis. Pediatr Pathol 1994; 14:1017–1028.

35. Read MA, Whitley MZ, Gupta S, et al. Tumor necrosis factor alpha-induced E-selectin expression is activated by the nuclear factor-kappa B and c-JUN N-terminal kinase/p38 mitogen-activated protein kinase pathways. J Biol Chem 1997; 272:2753–2761.

36. Shu HB, Agranoff AB, Nabel EG, et al. Differential regulation of vascular cell adhesion molecule 1 gene expression by specific NF-kappa B subunits in endothelial and epithelial cells. Mol Cell Biol 1993; 13:6283–6289.

37. Mannick E, Udall JN Jr. Neonatal gastrointestinal mucosal immunity. Clin Perinatol 1996; 23:287–304.

38. Udall JN Jr. Gastrointestinal host defense and necrotizing enterocolitis. J Pediatr 1990; 117:S33–S43.

39. Lucas A, Cole TJ. Breast milk and neonatal necrotising enterocolitis. Lancet 1990; 336:1519–1523.

40. Kosloske AM. Breast milk decreases the risk of neonatal necrotizing enterocolitis. Adv Nutr Res 2001; 10:123–137.

41. Caplan MS, Amer M, Jilling T. The role of human milk in necrotizing enterocolitis. Adv Exp Med Biol 2002; 503:83–90.

42. Kelleher SL, Lonnerdal B. Immunological activities associated with milk. Adv Nutr Res 2001; 10:39–65.

43. McGuire W, Anthony MY. Donor human milk versus formula for preventing necrotising enterocolitis in preterm infants: systematic review. Arch Dis Child Fetal Neonatal Ed 2003; 88:F11–F14.

44. Robel-Tillig E, Vogtmann C, Bennek J. Prenatal hemodynamic disturbances—pathophysiological background of intestinal motility disturbances in small for gestational age infants. Eur J Pediatr Surg 2002; 12:175–179.

45. Hsueh W, Caplan MS, Qu XW, Tan XD, De Plaen IG, Gonzalez-Crussi F. Neonatal necrotizing enterocolitis: clinical considerations and pathogenetic concepts. Pediatr Dev Pathol 2003; 6:6–23.

46. Sechi LA, Valentin JP, Griffin CA, Schambelan M. Autoradiographic characterization of angiotensin II receptor subtypes in rat intestine. Am J Physiol 1993; 265:G21–G27.

47. Bailey RW, Bulkley GB, Hamilton SR, Morris JB, Haglund UH. Protection of the small intestine from nonocclusive mesenteric ischemic injury due to cardiogenic shock. Am J Surg 1987; 153:108–116.

48. Hsueh W, Gonzalez-Crussi F, Arroyave JL. Platelet-activating factor: an endogenous mediator for bowel necrosis in endotoxemia. FASEB J 1987; 1:403–405.

49. Gonzalez-Crussi F, Hsueh W. Experimental model of ischemic bowel necrosis. The role of platelet-activating factor and endotoxin. Am J Pathol 1983; 112:127–135.

50. Kliegman RM, Fanaroff AA, Izant R, Speck WT. Clostridia as pathogens in neonatal necrotizing enterocolitis. J Pediatr 1979; 95:287–289.

51. Mollitt DL, Tepas JJ III, Talbert JL. The microbiology of neonatal peritonitis. Arch Surg 1988; 123:176–179.

52. Rotbart HA, Nelson WL, Glode MP, et al. Neonatal rotavirus-associated necrotizing enterocolitis: case control study and prospective surveillance during an outbreak. J Pediatr 1988; 112:87–93.

53. Mollitt DL, String DL, Tepas JJ III, Talbert JL. Does patient age or intestinal pathology influence the bacteria found in cases of necrotizing enterocolitis? South Med J 1991; 84:879–882.

54. Peter CS, Feuerhahn M, Bohnhorst B, et al. Necrotising enterocolitis: is there a relationship to specific pathogens? Eur J Pediatr 1999; 158:67–70.

55. Flick MR, Perel A, Staub NC. Leukocytes are required for increased lung microvascular permeability after microembolization in sheep. Circ Res 1981; 48:344–351.

56. Weiss SJ, Curnutte JT, Regiani S. Neutrophil-mediated solubilization of the subendothelial matrix: oxidative and nonoxidative mechanisms of proteolysis used by normal and chronic granulomatous disease phagocytes. J Immunol 1986; 136:636–641.

57. Baird BR, Cheronis JC, Sandhaus RA, Berger EM, White CW, Repine JE. Oxygen metabolites and neutrophil elastase synergistically cause edematous injury in isolated rat lungs. J Appl Physiol 1986; 61:2224–2229.

58. Caplan MS, Sun XM, Hsueh W. Hypoxia causes ischemic bowel necrosis in rats: the role of platelet-activating factor (PAF-acether). Gastroenterology 1990; 99:979–986.

59. Zhang C, Hsueh W, Caplan MS, Kelly A. Platelet activating factor-induced shock and intestinal necrosis in the rat: role of endogenous platelet-activating factor and effect of saline infusion. Crit Care Med 1991; 19:1067–1072.

60. Hsueh W, Caplan MS, Sun X, Tan X, MacKendrick W, Gonzalez-Crussi F. Platelet-activating factor, tumor necrosis factor, hypoxia and necrotizing enterocolitis. Acta Paediatr Suppl 1994; 396:11–17.

61. Colletti LM, Kunkel SL, Walz A, et al. The role of cytokine networks in the local liver injury following hepatic ischemia/reperfusion in the rat. Hepatology 1996; 23:506–514.

62. Remick DG, Colletti LM, Scales WA, McCurry KR, Campbell DA Jr. Cytokines and extrahepatic sequelae of ischemia-reperfusion injury to the liver. Ann N Y Acad Sci 1994; 723:271–283.

63. Collins T, Read MA, Neish AS, Whitley MZ, Thanos D, Maniatis T. Transcriptional regulation of endothelial cell adhesion molecules: NF-kappa B and cytokine-inducible enhancers. FASEB J 1995; 9:899–909.

64. Read MA, Whitley MZ, Williams AJ, Collins T. NF-kappa B and I kappa B alpha: an inducible regulatory system in endothelial activation. J Exp Med 1994; 179:503–512.

65. Shimizu H, Mitomo K, Watanabe T, Okamoto S, Yamamoto K. Involvement of a NF-kappa B-like transcription factor in the activation of the interleukin-6 gene by inflammatory lymphokines. Mol Cell Biol 1990; 10:561–568.

66. Scheinman RI, Cogswell PC, Lofquist AK, Baldwin AS Jr. Role of transcriptional activation of I kappa B alpha in mediation of immunosuppression by glucocorticoids. Science 1995; 270:283–286.

67. Kanto WP Jr, Wilson R, Breart GL, et al. Perinatal events and necrotizing enterocolitis in premature infants. Am J Dis Child 1987; 141:167–169.

68. Wilson R, Kanto WP Jr, McCarthy BJ, et al. Epidemiologic characteristics of necrotizing enterocolitis: a population-based study. Am J Epidemiol 1981; 114:880–887.

69. Wilson R, Kanto WP Jr, McCarthy BJ, Burton A, Lewin P, Feldman RA. Age at onset of necrotizing enterocolitis: an epidemiologic analysis. Pediatr Res 1982; 16:82–85.

70. De Curtis M, Paone C, Vetrano G, Romano G, Paludetto R, Ciccimarra F. A case control study of necrotizing enterocolitis occurring over 8 years in a neonatal intensive care unit. Eur J Pediatr 1987; 146:398–400.

71. Yu VY, Joseph R, Bajuk B, Orgill A, Astbury J. Perinatal risk factors for necrotizing enterocolitis. Arch Dis Child 1984; 59:430–434.

72. Lemons JA, Bauer CR, Oh W, et al. Very low birth weight outcomes of the National Institute of Child health and human development neonatal research network, January 1995 through December 1996. NICHD Neonatal Research Network. Pediatrics 2001; 107:E1.

73. Uauy RD, Fanaroff AA, Korones SB, Phillips EA, Phillips JB, Wright LL. Necrotizing enterocolitis in very low birth weight infants: biodemographic and clinical correlates. National Institute of Child Health and Human Development Neonatal Research Network. J Pediatr 1991; 119:630–638.

74. Ryder RW, Shelton JD, Guinan ME. Necrotizing enterocolitis: a prospective multicenter investigation. Am J Epidemiol 1980; 112:113–123.

75. Stoll BJ, Kanto WP Jr, Glass RI, Nahmias AJ, Brann AW Jr. Epidemiology of necrotizing enterocolitis: a case control study. J Pediatr 1980; 96:447–451.

76. Covert RF, Neu J, Elliott MJ, Rea JL, Gimotty PA. Factors associated with age of onset of necrotizing enterocolitis. Am J Perinatol 1989; 6:455–460.

77. Snyder CL, Gittes GK, Murphy JP, et al. Survival after necrotizing enterocolitis in infants weighing less than 1000g: 25 years' experience at a single institution. J Pediatr Surg 1997; 32:434–437.

78. Rowe MI, Reblock KK, Kurkchubasche AG, Healey PJ. Necrotizing enterocolitis in the extremely low birth weight infant. J Pediatr Surg 1994; 29:987–990.

79. Fasching G, Hollwarth ME, Schmidt B, Mayr J. Surgical strategies in very-low-birthweight neonates with necrotizing enterocolitis. Acta Paediatr Suppl 1994; 396:62–64.

80. McElhinney D, Hedrick H, Bush D, et al. Necrotizing enterocolitis in neonates with congenital heart disease: risk factors and outcomes. Pediatrics 2000; 106:1080–1087.

81. Bunton GL, Durbin GM, McIntosh N, et al. Necrotizing enterocolitis. Controlled study of 3 years' experience in a neonatal intensive care unit. Arch Dis Child 1977; 52:772–777.

82. Davey AM, Wagner CL, Cox C, Kendig JW. Feeding premature infants while low umbilical artery catheters are in place: a prospective, randomized trial. J Pediatr 1994; 124:795–799.

83. Lopez SL, Taeusch HW, Findlay RD, Walther FJ. Time of onset of necrotizing enterocolitis in newborn infants with known prenatal cocaine exposure. Clin Pediatr (Phila) 1995; 34:424–429.

84. Hein HA, Lathrop SS. Partial exchange transfusion in term, polycythemic neonates: absence of association with severe gastrointestinal injury. Pediatrics 1987; 80:75–78.

85. Carmi D, Wolach B, Dolfin T, Merlob P. Polycythemia of the preterm and full-term newborn infant: relationship between hematocrit and gestational age, total blood solutes, reticulocyte count, and blood pH. Biol Neonate 1992; 61:173–178.

86. Werner EJ. Neonatal polycythemia and hyperviscosity. Clin Perinatol 1995; 22:693–710.

87. Davis JM, Abbasi S, Spitzer AR, Johnson L. Role of theophylline in pathogenesis of necrotizing enterocolitis. J Pediatr 1986; 109:344–347.

88. Grosfeld JL, Dalsing MC, Hull M, Weber TR. Neonatal apnea, xanthines, and necrotizing enterocolitis. J Pediatr Surg 1983; 18:80–84.

89. Zanardo V, Trevisanuto D, Cagdas S, Grella P, Cantarutti F. Prenatal theophylline and necrotizing enterocolitis in premature newborn infants. Pediatr Med Chir 1997; 19:153–156.

90. Milner ME, de la Monte SM, Moore GW, Hutchins GM. Risk factors for developing and dying from necrotizing enterocolitis. J Pediatr Gastroenterol Nutr 1986; 5:359–364.

91. Santulli TV, Schullinger JN, Heird WC, et al. Acute necrotizing enterocolitis in infancy: a review of 64 cases. Pediatrics 1975; 55:376–387.

92. Frantz ID III, L'heureux P, Engel RR, Hunt CE. Necrotizing enterocolitis. J Pediatr 1975; 86:259–263.

93. Buch NA, Ahmad SM, Ali SW, Hassan HM. An epidemiological study of neonatal necrotizing enterocolitis. Saudi Med J 2001; 22:231–237.

94. Tam AL, Camberos A, Applebaum H. Surgical decision making in necrotizing enterocolitis and focal intestinal perforation: predictive value of radiologic findings. J Pediatr Surg 2002; 37:1688–1691.

95. Fasoli L, Turi RA, Spitz L, Kiely EM, Drake D, Pierro A. Necrotizing enterocolitis: extent of disease and surgical treatment. J Pediatr Surg 1999; 34:1096–1099.

96. Ade-Ajayi N, Kiely E, Drake D, Wheeler R, Spitz L. Resection and primary anastomosis in necrotizing enterocolitis. J R Soc Med 1996; 89:385–388.

97. O'Connor A, Sawin RS. High morbidity of enterostomy and its closure in premature infants with necrotizing enterocolitis. Arch Surg 1998; 133:875–880.

98. Griffiths DM, Forbes DA, Pemberton PJ, Penn IA. Primary anastomosis for necrotising enterocolitis: a 12-year experience. J Pediatr Surg 1989; 24:515–518.

99. Kliegman RM, Fanaroff AA. Necrotizing enterocolitis. N Engl J Med 1984; 310:1093–1103.

100. Ladd AP, Rescorla FJ, West KW, Scherer LR III, Engum SA, Grosfeld JL. Long-term follow-up after bowel resection for necrotizing enterocolitis: factors affecting outcome. J Pediatr Surg 1998; 33:967–972.

101. Stanford A, Upperman JS, Boyle P, Schall L, Ojimba JI, Ford HR. Long-term follow-up of patients with necrotizing enterocolitis. J Pediatr Surg 2002; 37:1048–1050.

102. Weber TR, Lewis JE. The role of second-look laparotomy in necrotizing enterocolitis. J Pediatr Surg 1986; 21:323–325.

103. Sugarman ID, Kiely EM. Is there a role for high jejunostomy in the management of severe necrotising enterocolitis? Pediatr Surg Int 2001; 17:122–124.

104. Luzzatto C, Previtera C, Boscolo R, Katende M, Orzali A, Guglielmi M. Necrotizing enterocolitis: late surgical results after enterostomy without resection. Eur J Pediatr Surg 1996; 6:92–94.

105. Vaughan WG, Grosfeld JL, West K, Scherer LR III, Villamizar E, Rescorla FJ. Avoidance of stomas and delayed anastomosis for bowel necrosis: the 'clip and drop-back' technique. J Pediatr Surg 1996; 31:542–545.

106. Demestre X, Ginovart G, Figueras-Aloy J, et al. Peritoneal drainage as primary management in necrotizing enterocolitis: a prospective study. J Pediatr Surg 2002; 37:1534–1539.

107. Ahmed T, Ein S, Moore A. The role of peritoneal drains in treatment of perforated necrotizing enterocolitis: recommendations from recent experience. J Pediatr Surg 1998; 33:1468–1470.

108. Cass DL, Brandt ML, Patel DL, Nuchtern JG, Minifee PK, Wesson DE. Peritoneal drainage as definitive treatment for neonates with isolated intestinal perforation. J Pediatr Surg 2000; 35:1531–1536.

109. Rovin JD, Rodgers BM, Burns RC, McGahren ED. The role of peritoneal drainage for intestinal perforation in infants with and without necrotizing enterocolitis. J Pediatr Surg 1999; 34:143–147.

110. Noble HG, Driessnack M. Bedside peritoneal drainage in very low birth weight infants. Am J Surg 2001; 181:416–419.

111. Cheu HW, Sukarochana K, Lloyd DA. Peritoneal drainage for necrotizing enterocolitis. J Pediatr Surg 1988; 23:557–561.

112. Wang YH, Su BH, Wu SF, et al. Clinical analysis of necrotizing enterocolitis with intestinal perforation in premature infants. Acta Paediatr Taiwan 2002; 43:199–203.

113. Camberos A, Patel K, Applebaum H. Laparotomy in very small premature infants with necrotizing enterocolitis or focal intestinal perforation: postoperative outcome. J Pediatr Surg 2002; 37:1692–1695.

114. Moss RL, Dimmitt RA, Henry MC, Geraghty N, Efron B. A meta-analysis of peritoneal drainage versus laparotomy for perforated necrotizing enterocolitis. J Pediatr Surg 2001; 36:1210–1213.

115. Nadler EP, Upperman JS, Ford HR. Controversies in the management of necrotizing enterocolitis. Surg Infect (Larchmt) 2001; 2:113–119.

116. Masumoto K, Suita S, Taguchi T. The occurrence of unusual smooth muscle bundles expressing alpha-smooth muscle actin in human intestinal atresia. J Pediatr Surg 2003; 38:161–166.

117. Roberts HE, Cragan JD, Cono J, Khoury MJ, Weatherly MR, Moore CA. Increased frequency of cystic fibrosis among infants with jejunoileal atresia. Am J Med Genet 1998; 78:446–449.

118. Snyder CL, Miller KA, Sharp RJ, et al. Management of intestinal atresia in patients with gastroschisis. J Pediatr Surg 2001; 36:1542–1545.

119. Werler MM, Sheehan JE, Mitchell AA. Maternal medication use and risks of gastroschisis and small intestinal atresia. Am J Epidemiol 2002; 155:26–31.

120. Danismend EN, Frank JD, Brown S. Morbidity and mortality in small bowel atresia. Jejuno-ileal atresia. Z Kinderchir 1987; 42:17–18.

121. Kullendorff CM. Atresia of the small bowel. Ann Chir Gynaecol 1983; 72:192–195.

122. Touloukian RJ. Diagnosis and treatment of jejunoileal atresia. World J Surg 1993; 17:310–317.

123. Rescorla FJ, Grosfeld JL. Intestinal atresia and stenosis: analysis of survival in 120 cases. Surgery 1985; 98:668–676.

124. Waldhausen JH, Sawin RS. Improved long-term outcome for patients with jejunoileal apple-peel atresia. J Pediatr Surg 1997; 32:1307–1309.

125. Festen S, Brevoord JC, Goldhoorn GA, et al. Excellent long-term outcome for survivors of apple peel atresia. J Pediatr Surg 2002; 37:61–65.

126. Tam PK, Nicholls G. Implications of antenatal diagnosis of small-intestinal atresia in the 1990s. Pediatr Surg Int 1999; 15:486–487.

127. Louw JH. Resection and end-to-end anastomosis in the management of atresia and stenosis of the small bowel. Surgery 1967; 62:940–950.

128. Nixon HH. Intestinal obstruction in the newborn. Arch Dis Child 1955; 13–22.

129. Takahashi A, Tomomasa T, Suzuki N, et al. The relationship between disturbed transit and dilated bowel, and manometric findings of dilated bowel in patients with duodenal atresia and stenosis. J Pediatr Surg 1997; 32:1157–1160.

130. Sheth NP, Chainani M. Deflating proximal enterostomy for jejunoileal atresia. Pediatr Surg Int 1998; 13:455–456.

131. Turnock RR, Brereton RJ, Spitz L, Kiely EM. Primary anastomosis in apple-peel bowel syndrome. J Pediatr Surg 1991; 26:718–720.

132. de Lorimier AA, Harrison MR. Intestinal plication in the treatment of atresia. J Pediatr Surg 1983; 18:734–737.

133. Weber TR, Vane DW, Grosfeld JL. Tapering enteroplasty in infants with bowel atresia and short gut. Arch Surg 1982; 117:684–688.

134. Takahashi A, Tomomasa T, Suzuki N, et al. Gastrointestinal manometry findings in a case with dilated small bowel and disturbed transit treated successfully with bowel plication. Neurogastroenterol Motil 1995; 7:97–100.

135. Takahashi A, Suzuki N, Ikeda H, et al. Results of bowel plication in addition to primary anastomosis in patients with jejunal atresia. J Pediatr Surg 2001; 36:1752–1756.

136. De Lorimier AA. The letter to the editor. J Pediatr Surg 1998; 33:950.

137. Alexander F, Babak D, Goske M. Use of intraluminal stents in multiple intestinal atresia. J Pediatr Surg 2002; 37:E34.

138. Elhalaby EA. Tube enterostomy in the management of intestinal atresia. Saudi Med J 2000; 21:769–770.

139. Hatch EI Jr, Schaller RT Jr. Surgical management of multiple intestinal atresias. Am J Surg 1986; 151:550–552.

140. Soutter AD, Askew AA. Transumbilical laparotomy in infants: a novel approach for a wide variety of surgical disease. J Pediatr Surg 2003; 38:950–952.

141. Rothenberg SS. Laparoscopic duodenoduodenostomy for duodenal obstruction in infants and children. J Pediatr Surg 2002; 37:1088–1089.

142. Bax NM, Ure BM, van der Zee DC, van Tuijl I. Laparoscopic duodenoduodenostomy for duodenal atresia. Surg Endosc 2001; 15:217.

143. Fujimoto T, Hata J, Yokoyama S, Mitomi T. A study of the extracellular matrix protein as the migration pathway of neural crest cells in the gut: analysis in human embryos with special reference to the pathogenesis of Hirschsprung's disease. J Pediatr Surg 1989; 24:550.

144. Rosenfield NS, Ablow RC, Markowitz RI, et al. Hirschsprung disease: accuracy of the barium enema examination. Radiology 1984; 150:393–400.

145. Alizai NK, Batcup G, Dixon MF, Stringer MD. Rectal biopsy for Hirschsprung's disease: what is the optimum method? Pediatr Surg Int 1998; 13:121–124.

146. Park WH, Choi SO, Kwon KY, Chang ES. Acetylcholinesterase histochemistry of rectal suction biopsies in the diagnosis of Hirschsprung's disease. J Korean Med Sci 1992; 7:353–359.

147. So HB, Becker JM, Schwartz DL, Kutin ND. Eighteen years' experience with neonatal Hirschsprung's disease treated by endorectal pull-through without colostomy. J Pediatr Surg 1998; 33:673–675.

148. Cilley RE, Statter MB, Hirschl RB, Coran AG. Definitive treatment of Hirschsprung's disease in the newborn with a one-stage procedure. Surgery 1994; 115:551–556.

149. Wilcox DT, Bruce J, Bowen J, Bianchi A. One-stage neonatal pull-through to treat Hirschsprung's disease. J Pediatr Surg 1997; 32:243–245.

150. Mir E, Karaca I, Gunsar C, Sencan A, Fescekoglu O. Primary Duhamel–Martin operations in neonates and infants. Pediatr Int 2001; 43:405–408.

151. van der Zee DC, Bax KN. One-stage Duhamel–Martin procedure for Hirschsprung's disease: a 5-year follow-up study. J Pediatr Surg 2000; 35:1434–1436.

152. Teitelbaum DH, Cilley RE, Sherman NJ, et al. A decade of experience with the primary pull-through for Hirschsprung disease in the newborn period: a multicenter analysis of outcomes. Ann Surg 2000; 232:372–380.

153. Georgeson KE. Laparoscopic-assisted pull-through for Hirschsprung's disease. Semin Pediatr Surg 2002; 11:205–210.

154. Georgeson KE, Cohen RD, Hebra A, et al. Primary laparoscopic-assisted endorectal colon pull-through for Hirschsprung's disease: a new gold standard. Ann Surg 1999; 229:678–682.

155. Rothenberg SS, Chang JH. Laparoscopic pull-through procedures using the harmonic scalpel in infants and children with Hirschsprung's disease. J Pediatr Surg 1997; 32:894–896.

156. Gao Y, Li G, Zhang X, et al. Primary transanal rectosigmoidectomy for Hirschsprung's disease: preliminary results in the initial 33 cases. J Pediatr Surg 2001; 36:1816–1819.

157. Albanese CT, Jennings RW, Smith B, Bratton B, Harrison MR. Perineal one-stage pull-through for Hirschsprung's disease. J Pediatr Surg 1999; 34:377–380.

158. Shankar KR, Losty PD, Lamont GL, et al. Transanal endorectal coloanal surgery for Hirschsprung's disease: experience in two centers. J Pediatr Surg 2000; 35:1209–1213.

159. Teeraratkul S. Transanal one-stage endorectal pull-through for Hirschsprung's disease in infants and children. J Pediatr Surg 2003; 38:184–187.

160. Van Leeuwen K, Geiger JD, Barnett JL, Coran AG, Teitelbaum DH. Stooling and manometric findings after primary pull-throughs in Hirschsprung's disease: perineal versus abdominal approaches. J Pediatr Surg 2002; 37:1321–1325.

161. Carcassonne M, Guys JM, Morrison-Lacombe G, Kreitmann B. Management of Hirschsprung's disease: curative surgery before 3 months of age. J Pediatr Surg 1989; 24:1032–1034.

162. Ikeda K, Goto S. Total colonic aganglionosis with or without small bowel involvement: an analysis of 137 patients. J Pediatr Surg 1986; 21:319–322.

163. Bickler SW, Harrison MW, Campbell TJ, Campbell JR. Long-segment Hirschsprung's disease. Arch Surg 1992; 127:1047–1050.

164. Ikawa H, Masuyama H, Hirabayashi T, Endo M, Yokoyama J. More than 10 years' follow-up to total colonic aganglionosis—severe iron deficiency anemia and growth retardation. J Pediatr Surg 1997; 32:25–27.

165. Coran AG, Teitelbaum DH. Recent advances in the management of Hirschsprung's disease. Am J Surg 2000; 180:382–387.

166. Endo M, Watanabe K, Fuchimoto Y, Ikawa H, Yokoyama J. Long-term results of surgical treatment in infants with total colonic aganglionosis. J Pediatr Surg 1994; 29:1310–1314.

167. Fouquet V, De Lagausie P, Faure C, et al. Do prognostic factors exist for total colonic aganglionosis with ileal involvement? J Pediatr Surg 2002; 37:71–75.

168. Rescorla FJ, Morrison AM, Engles D, West KW, Grosfeld JL. Hirschsprung's disease. Evaluation of mortality and long-term function in 260 cases. Arch Surg 1992; 127:934–941.

169. Levy M, Reynolds M. Morbidity associated with total colon Hirschsprung's disease. J Pediatr Surg 1992; 27:364–366.

170. Sarioglu A, Tanyel FC, Buyukpamukcu N, Hicsonmez A. Clinical risk factors of Hirschsprung-associated enterocolitis. I. Preoperative enterocolitis. Turk J Pediatr 1997; 39:81–89.

171. Sarioglu A, Tanyel FC, Buyukpamukcu N, Hicsonmez A. Clinical risk factors of hirschsprung-associated enterocolitis. II. Postoperative enterocolitis. Turk J Pediatr 1997; 39(1):91–98.

172. Elhalaby EA, Coran AG, Blane CE, Hirschl RB, Teitelbaum DH. Enterocolitis associated with Hirschsprung's disease: a clinical-radiological characterization based on 168 patients. J Pediatr Surg 1995; 30:76–83.

173. Blane CE, Elhalaby E, Coran AG. Enterocolitis following endorectal pull-through procedure in children with Hirschsprung's disease. Pediatr Radiol 1994; 24:164–166.

174. Yoo SY, Jung SH, Eom M, Kim IH, Han A. Delayed maturation of interstitial cells of Cajal in meconium obstruction. J Pediatr Surg 2002; 37:1758–1761.

175. Neal MR, Seibert JJ, Vanderzalm T, Wagner CW. Neonatal ultrasonography to distinguish between meconium ileus and ileal atresia. J Ultrasound Med 1997; 16:263–266.

176. Burke MS, Ragi JM, Karamanoukian HL, et al. New strategies in nonoperative management of meconium ileus. J Pediatr Surg 2002; 37:760–764.

177. Rescorla FJ, Grosfeld JL. Contemporary management of meconium ileus. World J Surg 1993; 17:318–325.

178. Harberg FJ, Senekjian EK, Pokorny WJ. Treatment of uncomplicated meconium ileus via T-tube ileostomy. J Pediatr Surg 1981; 16:61–63.

179. Steiner Z, Mogilner J, Siplovich L, Eldar S. T-tubes in the management of meconium ileus. Pediatr Surg Int 1997; 12:140–141.

180. Nguyen LT, Youssef S, Guttman FM, Laberge JM, Albert D, Doody D. Meconium ileus: is a stoma necessary? J Pediatr Surg 1986; 21:766–768.

181. Mak GZ, Harberg FJ, Hiatt P, Deaton A, Calhoon R, Brandt ML. T-tube ileostomy for meconium ileus: four decades of experience. J Pediatr Surg 2000; 35:349–352.

182. Myers NA. The early history of oesophageal atresia and tracheoesophageal fistula. In: Beasley SW, Myers NA, Auldist AW, eds. Oesophageal Atresia. London: Chapman and Hall Medical, 1991:1–16.

183. Merei JM, Hutson JM. Embryogenesis of tracheo esophageal anomalies: a review. Pediatr Surg Int 2002; 18:319–326.

184. Crisera CA, Connelly PR, Marmureanu AR, et al. Esophageal atresia with tracheoesophageal fistula: suggested mechanism in faulty organogenesis. J Pediatr Surg 1999; 34:204–208.

185. Spilde TL, Bhatia AM, Marosky JK, et al. Complete discontinuity of the distal fistula tract from the developing gut: direct histologic evidence for the mechanism of tracheoesophageal fistula formation. Anat Rec 2002; 267:220–224.

186. Ioannides AS, Henderson DJ, Spitz L, et al. Role of sonic hedgehog in the development of the trachea and oesophagus. J Pediatr Surg 2003; 38(1):29–36.

187. Crisera CA, Maldonado TS, Longaker, MT, et al. Defective fibroblast growth factor signaling allows for nonbranching growth of the respiratory-derived fistula tract in esophageal atresia with tracheoesophageal fistula. J Pediatr Surg 2000; 35:1421–1425.

188. Spilde TL, Bhatia AM, Ostlie D, et al. A role for sonic hedgehog signaling in the pathogenesis of human tracheoesophageal fistula. J Pediatr Surg 2003; 38:465–468.

189. Langer JC, Hussain H, Khan A, et al. Prenatal diagnosis of esophageal atresia using sonography and magnetic resonance imaging. J Pediatr Surg 2001; 36:804–807.

190. Rothenberg SS. Thorascopic repair of tracheoesophageal fistula in newborns. J Pediatr Surg 2002; 37:869–872.

191. Little DC, Rescorla JL, Grosfeld KW, et al. Long-term analysis of children with esophageal atresia and tracheoesophageal fistula. J Pediatr Surg 2003; 38:852–856.

192. Romeo C, Bonanno N, Baldari S, et al. Gastric motility disorders in patients operated on for esophageal atresia and tracheoesophageal fistula: long-term evaluation. J Pediatr Surg 2000; 35(5):740–744.

193. Filston HC, Shorter NA. Esophageal atresia and tracheoesophageal malformations. In: Ashcraft KW, Murphy JP, Sharp RJ, eds. Pediatric Surgery. 3rd ed. Philadelphia: WB Saunders, 2000.

194. Torfs CP, Curry CJ, Bateson TF, et al. A population-based study of congenital diaphragmatic hernia. Teratolog 1992; 46: 555–565.

195. Katz AL, Wiswell TE, Baumgart S. Contemporary controversies in the management of congenital diaphragmatic hernia. Clin Perinatol 1998; 25:219–248.

196. deLorimer AA, Tierney DF, Parker HR. Hypoplastic lungs in fetal lambs with surgically produced congenital diaphragmatic hernia. Surgery 1967; 62:12–17.

197. Keijzer R, Liu J, Deimling J, et al. Dual-hit hypothesis explains pulmonary hypoplasia in the Nitrofen model of congenital diaphragmatic hernia. Am J Pathol 2000; 156:1299–1306.

198. Guilbert TW, Gebb SA, Shannon JM. Lung hypoplasia in the nitrofen model of diaphragmatic hernia occurs early in development. Am J Physiol Lung Cell Mol Physiol 2000; 279: 1159–1171.

199. Kluth D, Tenbrinck R, von Ekesparre, et al. The natural history of congenital diaphragmatic hernia and pulmonary hypoplasia in the embryo. J Pediatr Surg 1993; 28:456–463.

200. Iritani I. Experimental study on embryogenesis of congenital diaphragmatic hernia. Anat Embryol 1984; 169:133–139.

201. Acosta JM, Thebaud B, Castillo C, et al. Novel mechanisms in murine nitrofen-induced pulmonary hypoplasia: FGF-10 rescue in culture. Am J Physiol Lung Cell Mol Physiol 2001; 281:250–257.

202. Unger S, Copland I, Tibboel D, et al. Down-regulation of sonic hedgehog expression in pulmonary hypoplasia is associated with congenital diaphragmatic hernia. Am J Pathol 2003; 162:547–555.

203. Hirschl R. Innovative therapies in the management of newborns with congenital diaphragmatic hernia. Semin Pediatr Surg 1996; 5:256–265.

204. Reyes C, Chang LK, Waffarn F, et al. Delayed repair of congenital diaphragmatic hernia with early high frequency oscillatory ventilation during preoperative stabilization. J Pediatr Surg 1998; 33:1010–1016.

205. Boloker J, Bateman DA, Wung JT, et al. Congenital diaphragmatic hernia in 120 infants treated consecutively with permissive hypercapnea/spontaneous respiration/elective repair. J Pediatr Surg 2002; 37:357–366.

206. Lally KP. Congenital diaphragmatic hernia. Curr Opin Pediatr 2002; 14:486–490.

207. Hedrick MH, Estes JM, Sullivan KM, et al. Plug the lung until it grows (PLUG): a new method to treat congenital diaphragmatic hernia in utero. J Pediatr Surg 1994; 29:612–617.

208. Flake AW, Crombleholme TM, Johnson MP, et al. Treatment of severe congenital diaphragmatic hernia by fetal tracheal occlusion: clinical experience with fifteen cases. Am J Obstet Gynecol 2000; 183:1059–1066.

209. Kamiyama M, Kawahara H, Okuyama H, et al. Gastroesophageal reflux after repair of congenital diaphragmatic hernia. J Pediatr Surg 2002; 37:1681–1684.

210. Skandalakis JE, Gray SW, Ricketts R, et al. The small intestines. In: Skandalakis JE, Gray SW, eds. Embryology for Surgeons. Baltimore: Williams & Wilkins, 1994:184–189.

211. Clark LA, Oldham KT. Malrotation. In: Ashcraft KW, Murphy JP, Sharp RJ, eds. Pediatric Surgery. 3rd ed. Philadelphia: WB Saunders, 2000.

212. Mehall JR, Chandler JC, Mehall RL, et al. Management of typical and atypical intestinal malrotation. J Pediatr Surg 2002; 37:1169–1172.

213. Prasil P, Flageole H, Shaw KS, et al. Should malrotation in children be treated differently according to age? J Pediatr Surg 2000; 35:756–758.

214. Ladd WE, Gross RE. Intestinal obstruction resulting from malrotation of the intestines and colon. In: Abdominal Surgery of Infancy and Childhood. Philadelphia: WB Saunders, 1941.

215. Bass KD, Rothenberg SS, Chang JHT. Laparoscopic Ladd's procedure in infants with malrotation. J Pediatr Surg 1998; 33:279–281.

60

Physiologic Considerations in the Elderly Surgical Patient

Ronnie Ann Rosenthal and Melissa F. Perkal

INTRODUCTION

Physicians and surgeons have long understood that the physiological and pathological processes characteristic of the neonatal period are considerably different from those of the mature adult. The same is true of physiological and pathological characteristics at the other extreme of life. Although internists have recognized the need to provide special "geriatric" care for more than four decades, the adjustment of surgical practice to meet the specific needs of the elderly has only recently begun in a programmatic way. The "graying" of the population has created the need to provide surgical care to an ever-increasing number of older patients, and the technological explosion has provided the means to do so safely.

In the next 25 years, the portion of the population over the age of 65 is expected to grow from the present 12.4% to nearly 20%, or over 70 million people. Persons over the age of 85 comprise the most rapidly growing segment of this population. Their number is expected to increase fivefold, to over 20 million, by 2050 (Fig. 1) (1). As the number of elderly persons continues to grow, so does the average life expectancy at all ages. At present, life expectancy for a male at age 65 is 16.6 years and at age 85 is 5.7 years. For a female, life expectancy at 65 and 85 years of age is 19.5 years and 6.9 years, respectively (2).

The rise in the number of surgical procedures performed on older patients is, in part, a reflection of this aging population. In 1980, 19% of all operations performed in nonfederally funded, short stay hospitals were on patients over 65 years of age. By 2002, this portion reached 36%, and if obstetrical procedures are excluded, this portion was 43% (3). In federally funded hospitals, this proportion is even higher. For example, in 2002, in the General Surgical Service at the Veterans Affairs Medical Center in West Haven, Connecticut, 83% of patients having major abdominal operations were over the age of 60, and 53% were over the age of 70.

This increase is not, however, only a reflection of the increased number of older people, but also of the growing awareness that older patients can truly benefit from such surgical intervention. Although age was previously a contraindication to operations such as pancreaticoduodenectomy, major hepatic resection, major cardiac revascularization, and transplantation, these and other major procedures are now performed routinely on older patients with results that are comparable to those in younger patients.

The indication for surgical treatment in the elderly, therefore, is increasingly determined by the need to provide maximal disease management rather than the desire to avoid surgical risk. It is important, however, to remember that the elderly surgical patient is frequently not physiologically equivalent to the younger patient and that comorbid illnesses can impact enormously on the surgical outcome. Understanding the physiological and pathological differences and adjusting care accordingly is essential for successful management.

PHYSIOLOGY AND PATHOLOGY OF AGING

The processes of maturation, aging, and senescence describe the life cycle of most living organisms, including man. Aging and senescence are commonly used interchangeably to refer to the myriad molecular and cellular events that eventually lead to the demise of the organism. These terms are not necessarily synonymous, although in clinical medicine the aging process is believed to incorporate predetermined or programmed cellular events that inevitably contribute to a limitation of longevity. The development of some diseases in the elderly patient may be directly linked to cellular events related to senescence, whereas the clinical presentation of others may be altered by aging-related changes in the physiological milieu. Cristafalo et al. (4) have identified five attributes that characterize the human aging process, which are as follows:

- An increase in mortality with increasing age (after maturation)
- A change in the biochemical composition of the body

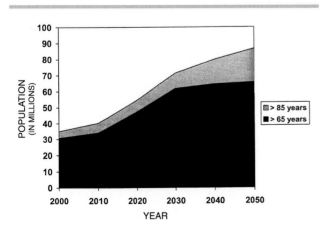

Figure 1 Projected population growth of persons over the age of 65 in the United States. *Source*: From Ref. 1.

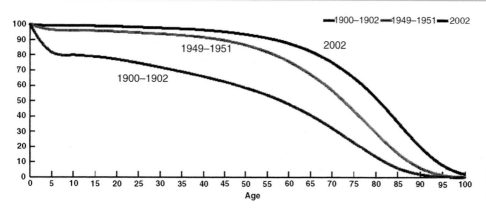

Figure 2 Life expectancy in the United States, 1900 to 1988. *Source:* From Ref. 2.

- A decline in physiological function
- A decreased ability to adapt to the environment
- An increased susceptibility to disease

Although the elucidation of molecular and cellular events is necessary for a complete understanding of the process of aging and senescence, an awareness of the clinical manifestations of the characteristics listed above is essential for the provision of appropriate care to the elderly patient.

Increasing Mortality with Age

The risk of death increases exponentially with increasing age, as described initially in 1825 by Gompertz (5). The relationship between age and survival is frequently shown as a Gompertzian function. Figure 2 shows the average or median survival of a population (the age at which 50% of the population is alive) (2). In the past century, there has been a rectangularization of the survival curve with a larger and larger percentage of the population living into old age. Although the median survival of man has more than doubled since the time of Hippocrates, the maximum lifespan potential (MLSP) has remained essentially constant at 100 to 115 years. The dramatic shift in median survival has been attributed to an elimination of the causes of early mortality and an improvement in sanitation and nutrition. Although these changes have paralleled the expansion of medical knowledge, no modern medical breakthrough has impacted greatly on median survival or altered MLSP. Recently, the National Institute on Aging (NIA) has begun a new effort to increase life expectancy and longevity by challenging investigators to make novel proposals with this goal (6). Under the auspices of the NIA's Interventions Testing Program, several compounds are presently being tested for their effects on prolonging life (7).

The above observations suggest that survival in all species may be limited in a predetermined way, and experimental observations support this concept (Fig. 3). Human fibroblasts maintained in culture undergo a predictable number of proliferative cycles, or doublings, before dying. This number is many times greater than the number of doublings for mouse fibroblasts maintained in identical culture (8).

In intact animals, the only intervention that consistently increases median survival and MLSP is caloric restriction (CR). This effect was first described by McCay in 1935 (9). In 1985, Yu et al. (10) showed that rats fed a diet containing

only 60% of the calories consumed by ad libitum fed littermates had a 50% higher median survival and MLSP than the animals receiving the full caloric load (Fig. 4). Over the past two decades, there has been a great increase in interest in the molecular explanation for the benefit of CR. Many theories have been proposed but two have gained widespread recognition. The first attributes the benefit to a decrease in oxidative damage caused by a decrease in intracellular accumulation of reactive oxygen species. The second credits the improvement in glucose and insulin metabolism associated with CR (11). Recently, there is growing opinion that the effects of CR are mediated through the stress response genes. The Hormesis Hypothesis, as it is called, suggests that a low intensity stressor, such as CRs, stimulates a survival response

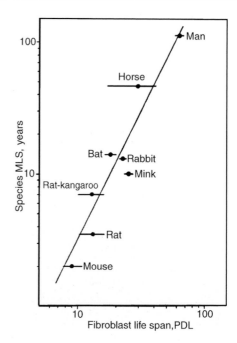

Figure 3 Correlation between PDL and MLS potential. Fibroblasts from longer-lived species undergo more cell divisions before senescence than cells derived from shorter-lived species. *Abbreviations*: MLS, maximal life span; PDL, population-doubling capacity. *Source:* From Ref. 8.

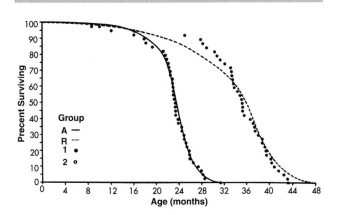

Figure 4 Survival curve for ad libitum fed (*solid circles*) and calorically restricted (*open circles*) rats. Restriction of calories to 60% of ad libitum–fed levels results in a dramatic increase in life span and maximum life-span potential. *Source*: From Ref. 10.

characterized by metabolic changes and augmented host defenses (12). This theory provides a unifying framework for many of the observations made about oxidative damage and glycemic modulation. Although CR has been shown to increase MLSP in experimental animals, longitudinal studies in humans show a small survival advantage for the elderly who are slightly "overweight" (body composition below) (13).

Whether or not human life-span potential is actually increasing, the elderly now represent the fastest growing segment of our population. The number of persons reaching their 100th birthday has increased so greatly that their names can no longer be read on the morning television programs. The number reaching their 110th birthday, however, is still quite small.

Changes in Body Composition

Aging is associated with specific biochemical, anatomical, and functional changes in virtually all body tissues and organs. Age-related effects have been documented at the chromosomal level, at the protein-processing level, and at the level of catabolism. Changes in molecular structure may be expressed in a tissue-specific manner, however, and organ systems must be evaluated individually to assess how age-related changes in composition are manifested in any single patient.

Compositional changes contribute to changes in organ function, such as the deposition of lipofuscin or "age pigment" in Purkinje cells, which results in conduction disturbances and altered cardiac contractility (14). Increased cross-linking of matrix molecules such as collagen (15) or the accumulation of increased amounts of protein due to impaired protein catabolism (16) can also alter the function of specific organs. An explanation for the increased occurrence of cross-linking of nucleic and matrix molecules is the age-related increase in oxidative damage to proteins due to excess free-radical formation (17). Impaired metabolism of reactive oxygen species may cause extensive damage to proteins, which in turn provides a favorable site for glucose moieties to bind to amino acids. This glycation reaction may promote the cross-linking of proteins such as osteocalcin and the lens protein crystalin, which may result in altered bone density or cataract formation (4).

Alterations in musculoskeletal tissues account for the physiognomic changes associated with aging, including shortened stature, impaired ambulation, and decreased chest wall excursion (Fig. 5) (18). These changes impact greatly on the postoperative recovery of elderly patients by increasing susceptibility to complications such as atelectasis, pneumonia, and pulmonary embolism. However, because tissue composition is not uniformly affected in all elderly patients, it is inappropriate to institute compensatory measures, such as prolonged endotracheal intubation, based only upon older age.

Nutritional effects account for some of the most important changes in body composition in the elderly (19). A significant prevalence of undernutrition has been documented in noninstitutionalized, free-living elderly, and reduced protein intake is common even among affluent

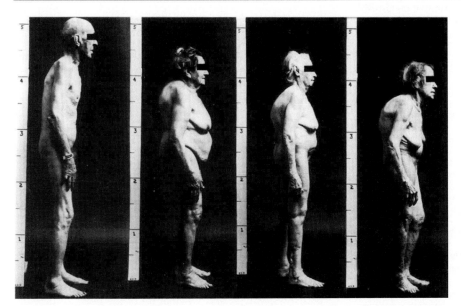

Figure 5 Four randomly selected patients from the ambulatory section of a nursing home, illustrating short stature, osteoporotic kyphosis, and relatively long extremities. Ages from left to right: 82, 78, 79, and 94 years. *Source*: From Ref. 18.

older persons (19–21). These dietary changes are multifactorial (Table 1), but are thought to contribute to the significant loss of lean body mass (muscle) in elderly subjects. This loss translates into reduced strength and mobility, as well as a decline in creatinine excretion. The shift from lean body mass to increase adipose tissue may also be mediated in part through an age-related decline in pituitary growth hormone (GH) activity (22).

Within the aging muscle, the synthesis of contractile proteins declines, as does the number of actual muscle fibers. Declining metabolic activity of the muscles combined with alterations in the neuromuscular junctions results in less efficient muscular activity and easy fatigability (23).

In addition to impairing the strength and mobility of the elderly patient, the decrease in muscle mass results in a smaller pool of amino acids available for the synthesis of other body proteins. Protein intake, therefore, must be maintained at levels sufficient to prevent further muscle mass losses. Decreased levels of exercise further exacerbate the loss of muscle mass, and together with a relative increase in percent body fat, contributes to progressive insulin resistance and a lower basal metabolic rate (24,25). Reduced calcium and vitamin D intake contributes to osteoporosis and loss of bone mass, which is further compounded by reduced levels of 25-hydroxyvitamin D due to reduced exposure of the skin to sunshine.

The shift in body mass from muscle to adipose tissue is complicated by the use of inaccurate methods to assess obesity in older persons (26), and by the metabolic consequences of increased adipose tissue. The standard comparisons of height to weight is an unreliable method to measure obesity in the elderly, due to both the shift in body mass from muscle to fat and the changes in skeletal configuration. Because weight generally increases linearly with the square of body height, the computation of a body mass index (BMI = wt/ht^2), using metric units of measurement, partially corrects weight for height and affords a better estimate of obesity. The computation of BMI must be corrected for age, however, to normalize indices of obesity in the elderly. The establishment of "normal" ranges of BMI for the elderly still ignores the effects of the increased "fatness" on metabolism and mortality. A comprehensive analysis of 4.2 million insurance policy holders indicates that the lowest mortality risks are associated with a progressive rise in BMI with age (27). The BMI associated with the lowest mortality increases from 21.4 in the 20- to 29-year-old group, to 22.9 in the 40- to 49-year-old group, and to 26.6 in the 60- to 69-year-old group. This roughly corresponds to an increase

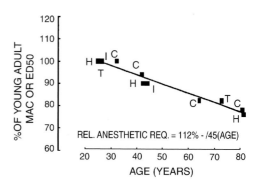

Figure 6 The decrease in relative anesthetic requirement with age in unsedated humans. *Abbreviations*: C, cyclopropane; H, halothane; I, isoflurane; T, thiopental. *Source*: From Ref. 30.

of about 10 pounds per decade in the weight of the best survivors. Recent data from the National Health and Nutrition Examination Survey (NHANES I, II, III) confirmed that mildly increased BMI (25 to < 30) in persons over the age of 70 is not associated with increased risk of death, whereas underweight (BMI < 8.5) and obesity (BMI > 30) are (15).

In addition to a progressive loss of lean body mass, and a corresponding increase in adiposity, aging is also associated with a decrease in total body water. Red cell mass is usually maintained in healthy individuals, but circulating plasma volume is reduced, particularly in debilitated patients (28). This decreased volume of distribution can result in higher than expected concentrations of administered drugs, and a correspondingly exaggerated drug effect. For example, the initial volume of distribution of thiopental in 20 to 40 year old subjects is 15 to 30 L, although in 60 to 90 year olds, it is 3 to 7 L (29). This fact dictates a reduction in dosing levels of many anesthetic drugs (Fig. 6) (30).

The increase in relative body fat also has significant pharmacological implications for surgical management, due to an increased distribution compartment for lipid-soluble drugs. The increase in the reservoir of lipid-soluble agents can result in a lower than expected plasma concentration of the agents initially, with a longer drug effect due to protracted clearance (30). These changes in body composition, together with changes in the functions of organs responsible for the clearance of drugs, mandate more careful anesthetic management and closer postoperative surveillance of elderly surgical patients.

Decline in Physiologic Function

With increasing age, there is a clear decline in physiologic function, although the rate and significance of the decline may vary considerably among individuals and among organ systems. In the resting state, these changes may have minimal consequences, but when physiological reserves are needed to respond to a stress such as surgery, overall performance may deteriorate.

Cardiovascular Function

Morphological changes in the myocardium, conducting pathways, valves, and vasculature of the heart accompany advancing age, although it is often difficult to separate the

Table 1 Findings in the Medical History Suggesting Increased Risk for Nutrient Deficiency

Recent weight loss
Restricted dietary intake (limited variety and food avoidances)
Psychosocial situation (depression, cognitive impairment, isolation, and economic difficulties)
Problems with eating, chewing, and swallowing
Previous surgery
Increased losses resulting from gastrointestinal disorders such as malabsorption and diarrhea
Systemic disease interfering with appetite or eating (chronic lung, liver, heart, and renal disease, abdominal angina, and cancer)
Excessive alcohol use
Medications that interfere with appetite and/or nutrient metabolism

Source: From Ref. 21.

changes associated with aging from those caused by disease. The functional implications of many of these changes are also variable and frequently not well defined (Table 2). The overall weight of the heart increases slightly in females but not in males, whereas the thickness of the ventricular septum increases significantly regardless of gender (31). There is also an increase in the fat content of the epicardium overlying the right ventricle. The number of myocytes declines whereas the size of the cells and the content of lipofuscin, the degenerative pigment, increases. The deposition of amyloid protein increases significantly with age, and some form of the protein can be found in the hearts of nearly half of the persons over the age of 70 (32). Collagen and elastin content also increases and fibrotic areas may appear throughout the myocardium. Whereas any one of these features alone may be of limited functional significance, the sum of these changes is a decline in ventricular compliance (33).

In the conducting system, the most pronounced change is the replacement of nearly 90% of the autonomic cells in the sinus node by fat and connective tissue (34). There is also a less impressive increase in fibrosis in the intranodal tracts and partial loss of proximal bundle fascicles between the left bundle and the bundle of His. These changes may contribute to the high incidence of sick sinus syndrome, atrial arrhythmias, and bundle branch blocks.

Valvular anatomy is also altered with aging. Sclerosis and calcification of the aortic valve is most common, but is usually of little functional importance (35). Calcification and sclerosis occurs less frequently in the mitral valve, but because of the juxtaposition of the valve to the atrioventricluar (AV) node and conducting bundles, calcification at this location may be responsible for AV nodal and bundle branch blocks. Progressive dilation of all four valvular annuli has also been described (36). It is thought that this dilation may be responsible for the multivalvular regurgitation frequently demonstrated in healthy older people.

Lastly, morphological changes can be seen in both the coronary and peripheral vessels. The endothelial cells lining the vessels change size and shape and flow may become more turbulent. The subendothelial and medial layers thicken, and calcification in these layers increases independent of atherosclerosis. As a result, the vessels become progressively more rigid and less distensible (37). These changes in the peripheral vasculature probably contribute to an increase in systolic blood pressure, an increased resistance to ventricular emptying, and a compensatory loss of myocytes with thickening of the ventricular wall (38). These degenerative changes in the coronary vessels may appear as calcifications on radiographs and, therefore, may be mistaken for the calcifications caused by atherosclerotic disease.

The functional implications of aging on the heart have been difficult to accurately assess because alterations in body composition, metabolic rate, general states of fitness, and underlying disease all influence cardiac performance (37). It is now generally accepted that *systolic* function, both at rest and in response to exercise, does not change with age. Cardiac output and ejection fraction at rest are maintained in spite of the increased afterload imposed by the stiffening of the outflow tract (39). In younger persons, cardiac output during periods of increased demand is maintained by increasing heart rate. With aging, the heart becomes less responsive to catecholamines, possibly secondary to changes in receptor function, and thereby loses the ability to augment cardiac output by increasing rate (37). Maintenance of cardiac output, therefore, becomes more dependent on ventricular filling (preload). Because of this dependence on preload, even minor hypovolemia may result in severe compromise in cardiac performance.

Diastolic function, which depends on myocardial relaxation rather than contraction, is more significantly affected by aging. In 50% of patients over the age of 80 with heart failure, systolic function is preserved whereas diastolic function is impaired (40). Because relaxation requires greater energy expenditure and, therefore, more oxygen consumption than does contraction, it is more susceptible to declining oxygen availability. With age, there is a progressive decrease in the partial pressure of arterial oxygen. As a consequence, relaxation is prolonged and even mild additional hypoxia from stress can result in significant diastolic dysfunction (41). This prolongation of relaxation, combined with the decreased ventricular compliance that results from progressive fibrosis, leads to decreased ventricular filling and higher diastolic pressures. This in turn can result in pulmonary vascular congestion and signs of heart failure.

As a result of impaired early diastolic filling, maintenance of adequate preload becomes more dependent on the contribution of the atrium. Loss of this atrial contraction or even minor hypovolemia can, therefore, result in significant impairment of cardiac function (41).

Alterations at the cellular level have also been implicated in the diastolic dysfunction that accompanies aging. A decline in the rate of calcium sequestration by the sacroplasmic reticulum following myocardial excitation and an increase in net calcium influx across the sacroplasmic reticulum (42) have both been suggested as possible etiologic factors.

Distinguishing systolic from diastolic dysfunction may be difficult. Systolic failure is usually gradual in onset and progressive, whereas diastolic failure is abrupt and the decline is rapid. Some distinguishing features are listed in Table 3 (43). The treatment is also different. Although digitalis and diuretics are indicated in systolic failure, the use of these agents in diastolic dysfunction may exacerbate the derangement. Diastolic abnormalities are treated with agents that improve preload and ventricular relaxation, such as calcium channel blockers, angiotensin-converting enzyme inhibitors, and beta-adrenergic antagonists (Table 4) (43,44).

Table 2 Age-Related Changes in the Heart and Great Vessels

Morphologic changes	Functional significance
↓ Number of myocytes	↓ Ventricular compliance
↑ Interstitial collagen content	↑ Diastolic pressure
↑ Amyloid deposition	↑ Diastolic relaxation time
↑ Ventricular septal thickness	↑ End diastolic volume
↑ Myocardial fibrosis	
↓ Elasticity	
↓ Atrial pacemakers	Bundle of His damage
Replacement of autonomic tissue	↑ Bundle branch blocks
Fibrosis of the cardiac skeleton	AV conduction abnormalities
Calcification at base of aortic valve	↑ Atrial arrhythmias
↑ Stiffness of the great vessels and outflow tract	↑ Afterload on the LV
	Compensatory LVH
↓ Reactivity of baroreceptors	↑ Systolic blood pressure

Abbreviations: LVH, left ventricular hypertrophy; AV, Atrioventricular.

Table 3 Clinical Differentiation of Diastolic Vs. Systolic Dysfunction in Patients with Heart Failure

	Systolic dysfunction	Diastolic dysfunction
Past history	Hypertension	Hypertension
	Myocardial infarction	Renal disease
	Diabetes	Diabetes
	Chronic valvular insufficiency disorders	Aortic stenosis
Presentation	Younger than 65 yrs	65 yrs or older
	Progressive shortness of breath	Acute pulmonary edema
Physical examination	Displaced PMI	Sustained PMI
	S$_3$ gallop	S$_4$ gallop
Radiographic findings	Pulmonary congestion	Pulmonary congestion
	Cardiomegaly	Normal sized heart
Electrocardiogram	Q waves	LVH
Echocardiogram	Decreased LVEF	Normal or increased LVEF

Abbreviations: LVEF, left ventricular ejection fraction; LVH, left ventricular hypertrophy; PMI, point of maximal impact.
Source: From Ref. 43.

It is also important to remember that the manifestation of cardiac diseases in the elderly may be nonspecific and atypical. Whereas chest pain is still the most common symptom of myocardial infarction, as many as 40% of older patients will present in a nonclassical manner with symptoms such as shortness of breath, syncope, acute confusion, or stroke (45).

Cardiac complications are the most common cause of death in the postoperative period. Identification of patients at risk for postoperative cardiac events is the basis for most preoperative evaluation strategies (Table 1).

Respiratory Function

The normal decline in respiratory function that accompanies aging can be attributed to changes in the chest wall and the lung (Table 5) (46). There is a decline in chest wall compliance secondary to changes in structure caused by kyphosis and exaggerated by vertebral collapse. There is decreased

Table 5 Age-Related Changes in the Chest Wall and Lung

Morphologic change	Functional significance
Thorax	
Calcification of bronchial and costal cartilage	↑ Resistance to deformation of chest wall
↑ Costovertebral stiffness	↑ Use of diaphragm in ventilation
↑ Rigidity of chest wall	↑ Tidal volume
↑ Anteroposterior diameter (kyphosis)	Response to exercise hyperpnea
Wasting of respiratory muscles	↓ Maximal voluntary ventilation
Lung	
Enlarged alveolar ducts	↓ Surface area for gas exchange
↓ Supporting duct frame work, enlarged alveoli	↑ Physiologic dead space
Thinning, separation of alveolar membrane	↓ Lung elastic recoil VC, RV/TLC
↑ Mucous gland	↓ Ventilatory flow rate
↑ Number, thickness of elastic fibers (?)	↓ Ventilation distribution
↑ Tissue extensibility (alveolar wall)	↑ Resistance to flow in small airways
↓ Pulmonary capillary network	↓ Ventilation: blood flow equality
↑ Fibrosis of pulmonary capillary intima	

Abbreviations: RV, residual volume; TLC, total lung capacity; VC, vital capacity.
Source: From Ref. 46.

mobility of the ribs caused by calcification of the costal cartilage and contractures of the intercostal muscles (12). There is also a progressive decrease in the strength of the respiratory muscles (47), which leads to as much as a 50% decline in the maximum inspiratory and expiratory force generated, and easy fatigability.

In the lung, the major change with age is the loss of elastic recoil in the alveoli. The elastic properties of the lung are responsible for maintaining the patency of the small airways. Loss of elasticity leads to increased alveolar compliance with collapse of these airways and subsequent uneven alveolar ventilation and air trapping (48). Uneven alveolar ventilation leads to ventilation–perfusion

Table 4 Pharmacologic Management of Heart Failure Secondary to Diastolic Dysfunction

Therapeutic agents	Goals of therapy	Considerations
Diuretics	Decrease in blood volume Decrease in ventricular filling pressure	Abrupt reduction in volume may produce hypotension and decreased CO; close monitoring for hypotension and renal dysfunction necessary; no effect on regression of LVH
ACE inhibitors	Decrease in afterload Regression of LVH Regression of myocardial interstitial fibrosis Enhanced ventricular relaxation	Agents with most marked effect on regression of LVH; acute unloading effects may produce hypotension and decreased CO; close monitoring of BP and renal function necessary
Calcium channel blockers	Decrease in afterload Regression of LVH Relief of myocardial ischemia Slow heart rate[a] Enhanced ventricular relaxation	Acute unloading effects may produce hypotension and decreased CO; anti-ischemic effects are beneficial in patients with CAD; may be detrimental when both systolic and diastolic dysfunction present and beneficial in slowing heart rate in patients with atrial fibrillation[a]; combination with β-blockers may cause severe bradycardia[a]
β-Blockers	Decrease in afterload Regression of LVH Relief of myocardial ischemia Slow heart rate Enhance ventricular relaxation	Limited effect on LVH regression; anti-ischemic effect beneficial in patients with CAD; beneficial in slowing heart rate in patients with atrial fibrillation

[a]Verapamil and diltiazem.
Abbreviations: ACE, angiotensin-converting enzyme; BP, blood pressure; CAD, coronary artery disease; CO, cardiac output; LVH, left ventricular hypertrophy.
Source: From Ref. 43.

mismatches, which in turn cause a decline in arterial oxygen tension of approximately 0.3% or 0.42 mmHg/yr. Although there is a decline in the partial pressure of oxygen, the partial pressure of CO_2 does not change, in spite of an increase in the dead space or wasted ventilation. This may be due, in part, to the decline in the production of CO_2 that accompanies the falling basal metabolic rates. Air trapping is also responsible for an increase in the residual volume (RV) or the volume remaining after maximal expiration.

The loss of support of the small airways also leads to compression during forced expiration, which limits dynamic lung volumes and flow rates. Forced vital capacity (VC) decreases by 14 to 30 cc/yr and one second forced expiratory volume decreases by 23 to 32 cc/yr (in males) (48). The overall effect of loss of elastic inward recoil is balanced somewhat by the decline in chest wall outward force. Total lung capacity (TLC), therefore, remains unchanged, and there is only a mild increase in resting lung volume or functional residual capacity. Because TLC remains unchanged, the increase in RV results in a decrease in VC (Fig. 7) (46).

Changes in the control of ventilatory responses with age are not yet fully clarified. Older data in men describe a fall in response to hypoxia and hypercapnia by 50% and 40%, respectively (49). Recent studies in healthy women show no change in hypoxic response with age (50).

In addition to these intrinsic changes, pulmonary function is affected by alterations in the ability of the respiratory system to protect against environmental injury and infection. There is a progressive decrease in T-cell function (see below) and a decline in mucociliary clearance. The loss of cough reflex secondary to neurologic disorders may predispose one to aspiration (51). The increased frequency and severity of pneumonia in older persons has been attributed to these factors and to an increased incidence of oropharyngeal colonization with gram negative organisms. This colonization correlates closely with comorbidity and with the ability of older patients to perform activities of daily living (ADL). This fact lends support to the idea that functional capacity is a crucial factor in assessing the risk of pneumonia in older patients (52).

Renal Function

Morphologic and functional changes also occur in the kidney and lower urinary tract with aging (Table 6). Between the ages of 25 and 85, there is a progressive decrease in kidney size, length, and volume. The majority of the tissue loss is in the cortex where approximately 40% of the nephrons become sclerotic and the remaining functional units hypertrophy in a compensatory manner. Sclerosis of the glomeruli is accompanied by atrophy of the afferent and efferent arterioles, and by a decrease in renal tubular cell number. Renal blood flow also falls by approximately 50%. This decline is thought to be secondary to changes in the vessels supplying the kidneys or to increased renal vascular resistance (53).

The functional result of these changes is a fall in glomerular filtration rate (GFR) by approximately 45% at the age of 80. This fall in GFR is reflected in a decline in creatinine clearance of 0.75 mL/min/yr in healthy elderly men. Serum creatinine, however, remains unchanged, because there is a concomitant decrease in lean body mass and, thus, a decrease in creatinine production. Estimates of creatinine clearance in the healthy aged can be made from the serum creatinine by using the formula derived by Cockcroft and Gault (54): [(140 − age in years) × (weight in kg)] / [72 × (serum creatinine in mg/dL)].

Caution must be exercised when applying this formula to critically ill patients or those on medications that directly affect renal function.

Renal tubular function also declines with advancing age. The ability to conserve sodium and excrete hydrogen ion falls, resulting in a diminished capacity to regulate fluid and acid–base balance (55). Dehydration becomes a particular problem, because losses of sodium and water from nonrenal causes are not compensated for by the usual mechanisms: increased renal sodium retention, increased urinary concentration, and increased thirst. The inability to retain sodium is thought to be due to a decline in the activity of the renin–angiotensin system (56). The increasing inability to concentrate the urine, which has been well documented (57), is related to changes in antidiuretic hormone (ADH). Measurements of ADH indicate that with advancing age there is a normal or exaggerated ADH response to a variety of stimuli. The defect in concentrating ability, therefore, is probably secondary to a decline in end organ responsiveness to ADH rather than a change in hormone

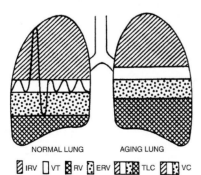

Figure 7 Changes in lung volumes with aging. Note the decrease in VC and increase in RV. *Abbreviations*: RV, residual volume; VC, vital capacity; IRV, inspiratory reserve volume; VT, tidal volume; ERV, expiratory reserve volume; TLC, total lung capacity. *Source*: From Ref. 46.

Table 6 Age-Related Changes in the Kidney and Lower Urinary Tract

Morphologic changes	Functional significance
↓ Kidney size, length, volume	↓ GFR
↑ Sclerosis of nephrons	↓ Creatinine clearance
↑ Sclerosis of glomeruli	
Atrophy of afferent/efferent arterioles	
↓ Renal blood flow	
↓ Renal tubular cell number	↓ Ability to conserve sodium
↓ Renal tubular function	↓ Ability to excrete hydrogen
↓ Renin–angiotensin system	↓ Ability to concentrate urine
↓ Responsiveness to ADH	↓ Ability to excrete free water
↑ Collagen content of bladder	↓ Bladder distensibility
↑ Detrusor activity	Impaired emptying
↑ Prostatic hypertrophy	↑ Incontinence
↓ Estrogen responsiveness	↑ Urinary tract infections

Abbreviations: GFR, glomerular filtration rate; ADH, antidiuretic hormone.

production. The marked decline in the subjective feeling of thirst is also well documented (58), but not well explained. Alterations of osmoreceptor function in the hypothalamus may be responsible for the failure to recognize thirst in spite of significant elevations in serum osmolality (59).

In the perioperative period, the decline in renal function combined with the changes in cardiovascular compensatory mechanisms leaves older patients at increased risk from both hypovolemia and fluid overload: Postural instability and syncope results when cardiovascular reflexes and tubular function cannot compensate for even minor volume depletion (42), whereas congestive heart failure and pulmonary edema result when excess fluid cannot be excreted rapidly enough, due to the inability to augment cardiac output, improve renal perfusion, and increase GFR.

Alterations in renal function also have great impact on the types and doses of drugs used in older patients. Although drugs are handled by the kidney in several different ways, most changes in renal drug processing parallel the decline in GFR. Therefore, creatinine clearance can be used to determine the appropriate clearance of most agents processed by the kidney (60).

Changes also occur in the lower urinary tract with aging. In the bladder, increased collagen content leads to limited distensiblity and impaired emptying (61). Overactivity of the detrusor secondary to neurological disorders or idiopathic causes has also been identified (62). In women, decreased circulating levels of estrogen and decreased tissue responsiveness to this hormone cause changes in the urethral sphincter, which predispose the person to urinary incontinence. In males, prostatic hypertrophy impairs bladder emptying. Together, these factors lead to urinary incontinence in approximately 10% to 15% of elderly persons living in the community and 50% of those in nursing homes (63).

There is also an increased prevalence of asymptomatic bacteriuria with age, which varies from 10% to 50% depending on gender, level of activity, underlying disorders, and place of residence. Urinary tract infections alone are responsible for 30% to 50% of all cases of bacteremia in older patients (64). Alterations in the local environment and declining host defenses are thought to be responsible. Because of the lack of symptoms in elderly patients with bacteriuria, preoperative urinalysis becomes increasingly important.

Hepatobiliary Function

Morphological changes in the liver with age include a decrease in overall weight and size, and a decrease in the number of hepatocytes. There is, however, a compensatory increase in cell size and increase in binucleated cells with a proliferation of bile ducts. Functionally, hepatic blood flow falls by approximately 1% per year to about 40% of earlier values, after the age of 60 (65).

Although the synthetic capacity, as measured by the standard test of liver function, remains unchanged (66), the metabolism of and sensitivity to certain kinds of drugs is altered. Drugs requiring microsomal oxidation (Phase I reactions) prior to conjugation (Phase II reactions) may be metabolized more slowly whereas those requiring only conjugation may be cleared at a normal rate (67). Drugs that act directly on hepatocytes, such as coumadin, may produce the desired therapeutic effects at lower doses in the elderly due to an increased sensitivity of the cells to these agents (68).

The most significant correlate of altered hepatobiliary function in the aged is the increased incidence of gallstones and gallstone-related complications. Gallstone prevalence rises steadily with age, although there is variability in the absolute percentages, depending on the population studied (Table 7) (69–71). Stones have been demonstrated in as many as 80% of nursing home residents over the age of 90 (72). Biliary tract disease is the single most common indication for abdominal surgery in the elderly population (Table 8) (3).

Although pigment gallstones are found with more frequency in older people (73), cholesterol stones have also been shown to increase with advancing age (74). The formation of all types of gallstone first requires a change in the bile itself that promotes stone formation. This lithogenic bile is necessary but not sufficient for stone formation. Factors that promote nucleation and allow stone growth (stasis) are also necessary. Included in these factors is the glycoprotein mucin, which serves as a nidus for stone formation and forms a gel layer lining the gallbladder mucosa, which provides the environment for stone growth. The formation of this mucin gel precedes the development of both types of stones and is closely related to gallbladder stasis. The increased development of gallstones in the elderly is thought to result from both changes in the composition of bile and impaired biliary motility.

Alterations in the composition of bile with advancing age include an increase in the activity of 5-hydroxy-3-methylglutaryl-coenzyme A (the rate-limiting enzyme in the synthesis of cholesterol), and a decrease in the activity of 7α-hydroxylase (the rate-limiting enzyme in the synthesis of bile salts from cholesterol) (75). This results in supersaturation of the bile with cholesterol and a decrease in the primary bile salt pool (76). The ratio of secondary to primary bile salts also increases. It is postulated that these secondary bile salts promote cholesterol gallstone formation by enhancing cholesterol synthesis, increasing protein content of the bile, decreasing nucleation time, and increasing

Table 7 Prevalence of Gallbladder Disease (%)

Age	Pima Indians (70) (cholecystography)		New Haven, Connecticut (71) (necropsy)		Age	Rome (72) (ultrasound)	
	Male	Female	Male	Female		Male	Female
15–24	0	13	7	4	20–29	0	2
25–34	4	73	2	5	30–39	1	4
35–44	11	71	9	10	40–49	4	6
45–54	32	76	13	16	50–59	11	12
55–64	66	62	18	20	60–69	10	23
> 65	68	90	22	28			

Table 8 Distribution of Abdominal Operations Per Year in the United States (2002)

	Total	Age > 65 yr
Cholecystectomy	436	151 (35%)
Lysis of adhesions	342	93 (27%)
Appendectomy (planned)	329	25 (8%)
Partial excision of large intestines	263	145 (55%)

Source: Data from Ref. 3.

the production of specific phospolipids that are thought to effect the production of mucin (77). It has also been suggested that the increase in secondary bile salts in the aged may promote a recycling of bilirubin, which in turn leads to the unconjugated bilirubin supersaturation necessary for pigment stone formation.

Alterations in gallbladder motility and bile duct motility are thought to be central to the development of cholesterol stones and brown pigment stones, respectively. The role of motility in black pigment formation, however, is less clear (77). Biliary motility is a complex interaction of hormonal and neural factors; however, the major stimulus of gallbladder emptying is cholecystokinin (CCK). The sensitivity of the gallbladder wall to CCK has been shown to decrease with increasing age in animal models (78). Exogenous administration of CCK to animals fed a lithogenic diet inhibits the age-dependent development of cholesterol gallstones (79). In humans, gallbladder sensitivity to CCK is also decreased. However, there is a compensatory increase in the production of CCK in response to stimuli, which results in normal gallbladder contraction (80). The production of the hormone pancreatic polypeptide, which inhibits gallbladder contraction and promotes relaxation, has also been shown to increase with increasing age in humans (81,82). The significance of this observation with regard to gallstone formation, however, is unknown. Further studies to elucidate changes in biliary motility with age are necessary.

Regardless of the pathogenesis, gallstones are associated with complications in 40% to 60% of older patients requiring treatment for the disease, as compared to less than 20% of younger patients (83). In a study of over 20,000 open cholecystectomies in the elderly, nearly two-thirds of patients required emergency operation (84). The increased rate of complicated disease seen in older patients may be directly attributable to the increased severity of the disease or to increased prevalence of comorbid illnesses like atherosclerosis and diabetes mellitus. It is more likely, however, a result of delays in diagnosis and treatment, caused by the frequent absence of typical biliary tract symptoms. Biliary colic, or episodic right upper quadrant pain radiating to the back, precedes the development of a complication only half as often in older than younger patients (85). Even in the presence of acute cholecystitis, one-quarter of older patients may have no abdominal tenderness, one-third will have no elevation in temperature or white blood cell count, and as many as one-half will have no peritoneal signs in the right upper quadrant (86). Unfortunately, mortality in the emergent setting is at least three times the elective mortality (83). Until predictors of impending complications other than symptoms are identified, improving the outcome of biliary tract disease in the elderly will be difficult. Until that time, increased awareness of the atypical presentation of gallstone-related illness in this age group is essential.

Hematopoietic Function

Long-term culture studies of bone marrow reveal that the maintenance of in vitro hematopoiesis varies inversely with the age of the donor (87). Additional studies corroborate the observation that the ability of progenitor spleen–colonizing stem cells to replicate is an age-dependent process (88,89), probably analogous to the species-dependent limits on cell replication. The replicative capacity of spleen-colonizing stem cells far exceeds the life span of the host, however, making it unlikely that exhaustion of erythroid precursor proliferation accounts for the diminished hematopoietic reserve seen in the elderly. In addition, marrow taken from young donors and transplanted into elderly recipients proliferates at a rate that is indicative of the recipient, not the donor (90).

Erythropoiesis is dependent upon the stimulation of erythroid progenitor replication by erythropoietin. Under basal conditions, the rate of erythroid turnover and erythroid kinetics are essentially normal in healthy elderly subjects. Under the condition of increased demand, as in the response to hemorrhage, however, the elderly patient has a delayed or absent erythroid response. Diminished erythropoiesis in the elderly is, therefore, due to a combination of inherent and environmental factors that alter the erythroid response to increased demand and result in a loss of functional reserve. The reasons for altered red cell responses to stress are not well defined, but insufficient levels of erythropoietin, and/or other growth factors, or decreased sensitivity to these factors may contribute. Inflammatory cytokines have also been implicated as the mediators of this declining sensitivity (91). Neutrophils form the first line of defense by their role in phagocytosis and bacterial killing. The bactericidal action of neutrophil superoxides and lysosomal enzymes is dependent upon the neutrophil response to a series of stimuli. When young and old neutrophils are compared in their basal and stimulated responses, basal rates of enzyme release are similar whereas the response to a challenge is measurably impaired in the old neutrophils. The diminished response may be associated with an age-related but reversible alteration in the lipid composition of neutrophil plasma membranes (92).

Clinically, the neutrophil response to bacterial invasion in elderly patients is generally intact if drugs, metabolic stress, or concurrent disease do not supervene. However, nutritional deficiency is an important variable, because the bactericidal function of neutrophils is significantly impaired by relatively short-term malnutrition of the host. However, protein-calorie repletion by the intravenous route carries its own risk of infectious problems, so the selection of treatment strategies that minimize the risk of ileus followed by an early enteral feeding is the best support for the aged leukocyte system.

Metabolic and Endocrine Function

The regulation of intermediary metabolism and the neurocrine–paracrine–endocrine mediation of cellular events are complex processes with multiple potential points of failure. The age-related loss of functional reserve of endocrine responsiveness or the changes in nutrient metabolism seen commonly in elderly patients have multiple causes. Age-related alterations in hormone levels are inconsistent, with some being quite elevated and others nearly absent. For example, plasma levels of CCK are elevated in elderly patients, although levels of gastrin are reduced. Gallbladder CCK receptor function is depressed in elderly subjects, however, as is parietal cell gastrin receptor function (83,93).

Therefore, diminished cholecystokinesis in the elderly is probably a result of receptor loss or dysfunction, but hypochlorhydria appears to be a consequence of primary hormone insufficiency. Altered endocrine function may result from changes at several points in the pathway—alterations in hormone (or receptor) gene expression, in protein processing within the cell of origin (including protein assembly, storage, or vesicle trafficking), in hormone release due to stimulus–secretion–coupling abnormalities, in hormone distribution due to circulatory dysfunction or vascular occlusion, and in target cell responsiveness (due to impaired receptor binding, faulty ligand internalization, or diminished target cell postreceptor activation). Studies of endocrine dysfunction in the elderly are further confounded by the use of reference measurements originally made in hospitalized patients.

The hypothalamic-pituitary-adrenal axis is the classical neuroendocrine feedback loop. Subtle and varied age-related changes have been described in the release of corticotropin-releasing hormone (CRH), adrenocorticotropic hormone (ACTH), and glucocorticoids, but the loop appears to remain essentially intact despite advanced age. Glucocorticoid inhibition of CRH and ACTH release has been documented to be impaired (94), which suggests that the central neuroendocrine response to stress is actually prolonged in elderly surgical patients.

The release of GH from the anterior pituitary declines progressively with increasing age, and is associated with lower levels of insulin-like growth factor-I (IGF-I). GH stimulates IGF-I production by the liver, the replacement of which in aging animals has been shown to reverse age-related defects in gene expression and immune function, and to prolong life expectancy (95,96). Protein catabolism has been shown to be reversed in critically injured patients by GH replacement therapy, and the role of GH in the treatment of impaired wound healing in the elderly is currently under study.

The adrenal glands undergo gradual changes with aging, which include fibrosis or nodular hyperplasia. Glucocorticoid or mineralocorticoid excess is unusual, but can result from a functional adrenal adenoma or adrenocortical carcinoma. Deficiency of mineralocorticoid or glucocorticoid is more common, but is usually apparent in the setting of increased demand. Loss of adrenal reserve may result from hemorrhage, infection, infiltrative or metastatic disease, or autoimmune destruction. Unexplained hemodynamic instability or frank shock in an elderly patient should be treated with a trial of glucocorticoids, in addition to other necessary agents.

Thyroid diseases are common in elderly patients, and are often insidious in their presentation. Fibrosis, decreased follicle size, and atrophy are frequently seen, and hypothyroidism occurs in up to 4% of the elderly population (97). Nonspecific symptoms, such as constipation, lethargy, and dry skin, are frequent and may be confused with constitutional complaints attributed to "aging." Hyperthyroidism is fairly common among older patients as well, and some studies suggest it may be more prevalent in the elderly than in younger patients (98). Thyroid enlargement, commonly observed in younger hyperthyroid patients, may be absent in elderly. Older hyperthyroid patients also lack the exophthalmos seen in younger patients, and nodular goiter, rather than Graves' disease, is the most frequent cause of thyroid hyperfunction. The presenting symptoms are also disturbingly misleading—weight loss, tremor, muscle weakness, anorexia, and arrhythmias may easily be mistaken for signs of "aging." Masked and apathetic hyperthyroidism, terms originally used to describe advanced cardiac and toxic forms of hyperthyroidism, are now used to describe the typical presentation of the disease in the elderly.

Thyroid nodules and degenerative cysts occur with increased frequency in the elderly. Sonographic imaging is helpful to identify those cystic lesions that require only aspiration. Solid lesions, however, need to be evaluated with thyroid function studies and fine needle aspiration (FNA), because of the substantial risk of malignancy. Of the 20% to 25% of euthyroid patients with "suspicious" FNA cytology of a discreet nodule, a final pathologic diagnosis of malignancy will be observed in 11% to as many as 71% of cases (99), with the majority of these being papillary or follicular carcinoma.

Hyperparathyroidism is more prevalent in the elderly as well, and is frequently unsuspected at diagnosis. Automated blood chemistry–screening accounts for most newly diagnosed cases, and in the elderly, the sporadic or nonfamilial forms of the disease is most common. With persistence of the disease, nephrocalcinosis, bone demineralization, mental status changes, and constitutional symptoms may develop, but many patients remain seemingly asymptomatic despite elevated calcium levels. This has resulted in controversy over whether or not to advocate parathyroidectomy in elderly patients with few or no symptoms. A National Institute of Health (NIH) consensus conference held in 1990 recommended that only patients with overt signs and symptoms of known target organ complications be managed surgically (100). At a more recent NIH workshop in 2002, a panel reconsidered therapy for asymptomatic primary hyperparathyroidism (101). The threshold for parathyroidectomy was reduced to include patients with a serum calcium greater than 1 mg/dL above the upper limits of normal. This definition still leaves uncertain whether "weakness" and "depression" indicate symptomatic disease, although roughly 40% of patients with hyperparathyroidism have one or both complaints. Furthermore, in a recent case–control study, only 4.6% of hyperparathyroid patients were found to be truly asymptomatic, and the majority of patients felt better overall, after surgery (102). Because there is no medical treatment of hyperparathyroidism, there is no means of predicting when or if severe complications of the disease, such as nephrocalcinosis or bone disease, will develop. Because the morbidity and mortality risk of surgery is low even in older patients, parathyroidectomy remains the treatment of choice unless other comorbid conditions preclude surgery (103) (see "Preoperative Evaluation, Risk Assessment, and Outcome").

Diabetes and changes in glucoregulatory hormones constitute a common set of concerns in elderly surgical patients. Hyperglycemia after carbohydrate ingestion or glucose administration is so common in the elderly that age-adjusted nomograms are used in standardized glucose tolerance testing. Glucose homeostasis is the net result of the interactions of a series of interrelated systems or processes: (i) gastric emptying of nutrients, (ii) enteric nutrient absorption, (iii) insulin release by elevated circulating glucose levels, (iv) the potentiating effect of enteric hormones, called incretins, which augment the insulin response, (v) the distribution of insulin to visceral and peripheral tissues, (vi) insulin actions including receptor binding, glucose transport, and inhibition of glucose production, and (vii) metabolism of glucose by insulin-dependent and insulin-independent tissues. Abnormalities in one or more of these processes may lead to impaired glucose tolerance or frank diabetes, and it should be apparent that multiple etiologies of abnormal glucose metabolism are possible.

The most common abnormality in glucose metabolism with aging is an increased insulin resistance. Even in healthy elderly elderly volunteers, enteral glucose stimulates an exaggerated insulin response accompanied by higher glucose levels than those found in younger controls (Fig. 8) (104). The higher degree of body fat in the elderly may contribute to this insulin resistance. Hyperglycemia is common in elderly patients who receive intravenous alimentation, and insulin therapy is commonly, albeit transiently, required in many sick elderly patients.

A variety of abnormalities are apparent in gastroentero-pancreatic function in older patients, and may contribute to surgical disease in the elderly. Altered esophageal motility and sphincter function results in an increased incidence of reflux and aspiration (105). Hypochlorhydria and diminished gastric emptying are common (106), but there is a paradoxical increase in the incidence of peptic ulcer disease in the elderly (107,108). This may be secondary to an age-related decrease in duodenal bicarbonate secretion (109), and a breakdown in mucosal defense mechanisms. Small bowel absorption of fat and carbohydrates is basically unaltered in healthy aging (110), and the enteric hormonal response to nutrients is essentially intact. Serum levels of some hormones actually rise with aging, including CCK and pancreatic polypeptide, probably in response to declining end organ sensitivity (81). Absorption of calcium is significantly impaired in aging secondary to decreased renal production of 1,25-hydroxycholecalciferol, as well as to a decrease in the amount and/or sensitivity of intestinal mucosal calcium-binding proteins (110). Mucosal changes are seen in the aging colon, where progressive loss of muscularis propria function and increased thickness of the colon wall contribute to the age-related incidence of diverticular disease.

Exocrine pancreatic secretion appears to change minimally with advancing age, although duct ectasia and dilatation of acini are seen (111). Lipase deficiency may contribute to altered fat absorption, but secretory function of the gland remains intact (112). The incidence of nonalcoholic pancreatitis increases in the elderly, due to the increased incidence of gallstones and the increased incidence of acute idiopathic pancreatitis. This entity is disproportionately present in the elderly, and carries a mortality risk of 25% or more (113). The age-related increase in the death risk due to pancreatitis may result from a higher likelihood of coexisting diseases, but is also a reflection of an altered presentation as well as an altered response to the disease process in the older patient.

Decreased Ability to Adapt to Changes in the Environment

Altered Response to Stress

Alterations in the neuroendocrine response(s) to stress in the elderly may account for some aspects of the "diminished reserve," which characterizes many aging effects on organ systems. Catecholamine responses to a variety of stressors are altered in aging, although it has been difficult to achieve consensus on age-related effects on the actual levels of the catecholamines. Considerable evidence demonstrates a decline in the beta-adrenergic regulation of arterial and venous dilatation and myocardial contractility (114,115). These effects are thought to be related to altered beta-adrenergic receptor function, rather than changes in catechol levels, per se (116,117). Adrenocortical responses to stress are retained in most studies, but the anterior pituitary response to surgical stress is greatly diminished in the elderly, and is virtually eliminated when spinal analgesia is used (118). It remains unknown whether the loss of this neuroendocrine response contributes to the risk of hemodynamic instability in elderly patients undergoing operation.

Surgical stress is usually accompanied by catabolism and protein loss. The administration of appropriate nutritional support is, therefore, an important part of the care of the critically ill patient. Elderly patients are particularly vulnerable in the postoperative period, because subtle preoperative malnutrition, usually secondary to poor nutrient intake and concomitant disease, is so common in this age group. In addition, compensatory protein synthesis is impaired in older persons secondary to the shrinking amino acid reservoir that results from the replacement of lean muscle mass with fat (119). However, elderly patients also have a significant intolerance for protein administration despite standard calculation of their needs (120). The inaccuracy in standard formulae probably arises from the relatively lower lean body mass, and calculation of the basal energy expenditure (BEE) should be modified to compensate for the age-related changes. The Harris–Benedict equation, which does incorporate an age factor, accurately predicts BEE when a correction factor of 1.75 is used for trauma, or 1.5 for general surgery patients.

Altered Response to Pain and Temperature

Neurosensory responses to stress are also altered in elderly patients, and this is particularly evident in the perception of pain and in the maintenance of body temperature. Although the data are somewhat conflicting, elderly patients appear to have a higher threshold for pain perception (121), which complicates the diagnosis of abdominal surgical disease. Peptic ulcer disease, for example, may be associated with diminished or even absent pain in as many as a third of elderly patients (122). Moreover, when analgesics are given, a lowered dose is frequently required (see section "Changes in Body Composition"), because the unwanted effect of respiratory depression is not reduced (123). Pulse-oximetry is always an appropriate monitoring aide when narcotic analgesic agents are used in older patients.

Diminished sensation of cold and an impaired sensitivity to temperature changes are causes of altered thermoregulation in the elderly (124). Altered autonomic

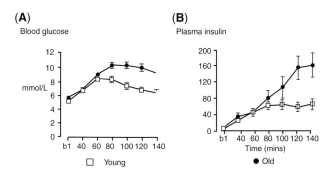

Figure 8 Serum glucose and insulin response to an enteric glucose load in old and young healthy subjects. *Source*: From Ref. 104.

vasoconstrictor responses to cold may contribute to a basal core temperature as low as 35°C in older individuals. Decreased thermogenesis secondary to reduced lean body mass with concomitant decreased basal metabolic rate, and a variety of coexisting endocrine and metabolic conditions including hypothyroidism and hypoglycemia, may also increase the risk of hypothermia. In the operating room, the use of body warmers, head covers, and warmed irrigation fluids are helpful to avoid the risk of hypothermia in elderly patients.

The most significant immediate complications of severe hypothermia (below 32°C) are arrhythmias and cardiorespiratory arrest. The electrocardiogram may show a characteristic "J" wave or Osborn wave following the QRS complex, which disappears when the hypothermia is reversed (125). Hypothermia has also been implicated as a contributing factor to postoperative wound infections (126).

Just as hypothermia represents a failure to compensate for ambient low temperatures in the elderly, hyperthermia may reflect an inability to increase evaporative heat loss in the setting of high external temperature. The inability to generate a fever in response to a serious infection or injury is another manifestation of altered thermoregulation in the older patient (127). Whereas younger individuals can mount a fever in response to relatively minor infections or inflammatory processes, the elderly patient may lack a febrile response to even suppurative peritonitis (128). When fever does occur in an elderly patient, it usually implies a significant pathologic process and should never be ignored.

Altered Wound Healing

The response to a wound is also a form of reaction to the environment, and represents an attempt to preserve or restore physical homeostasis. This response involves the complex interaction of systemic and local immune processes as well as tissue repair processes, and both sets of events can be impaired in elderly patients (129). In addition, impaired wound healing is associated with nutritional deficiencies and other disease states that cause tissue hypoxia, all of which occur with increasing frequency in older persons. Unfortunately, because normal wound healing requires such a complex constellation of coordinated events, actual data confirming the changes associated with increased aging, per se, are few. In one study of experimental wounding in healthy volunteers, epithelialization was delayed in older patients compared to younger patients, but collagen content of the wounds appeared equal. The accumulation of noncollagenous proteins, however, was decreased in the older group (130). In another study, the rate of healing of ischemic wounds in old animals was impaired by 40% to 65% compared to that of younger animals (131). More recent studies suggest that impaired wound healing in the elderly is associated with an exaggerated inflammatory response and excess matrix degradation. Matrix production is also reduced secondary to altered cytokine-mediated fibroblast function (132).

When immune responsiveness is enhanced in elderly subjects, as with the oral administration of arginine, cellular and chemical parameters of wound healing are also enhanced (133). Other strategies to enhance wound healing in the elderly are presently under investigation. These include the restoration of protein–calorie balance, and the induction of endogenous growth factor synthesis, such as IGF-I, by GH administration.

Increased Vulnerability to Disease
Alterations in the Immune System

Immune competence, like other physiologic parameters, declines with advancing age. This immunosenescence is characterized by an increased susceptibility to infections, an increase in autoantibodies and monoclonal immunoglobulins (Igs), and an increase in tumorogenesis. Also, like other physiological systems, this decline may not be apparent in the nonchallenged state. For example, there is no decline in neutrophil count with age, but the ability of the bone marrow to increase neutrophil production in response to infection may be impaired (134). Elderly patients with major infections frequently have normal WBC counts, but the differential count will show a profound shift to the left, with a large proportion of immature forms. Although the study of immunosenescence in humans is complicated by the increasing prevalence of other diseases, the inability to effectively sample all of the elements of the immune system, and the inability to separate environmental effects from biological effects, several specific changes have been defined.

The most consistent of the changes in the immune system with age is the involution of the thymus gland and the decline in the production of thymic polypeptide factors such as thymosin a-1 (135). This and other thymic hormones control the differentiation and proliferation of thymocytes into mature T-lymphocytes. T-cell proliferation (136) and IL-2 production (137) in response to stimulation have been shown to decrease with increasing age, and diminished T-cell responsiveness to a variety of antigens has been demonstrated in studies using skin tests (138).

B-cell defects have not been as clearly established, although it is thought that the functional deficits are related to altered T-cell regulation (134) rather than to intrinsic B-cell changes. The mix of Igs, however, does change— IgM levels decrease whereas IgG and IgA levels increase slightly. There is also a significant rise in the prevalence of monoclonal Igs to more than 10% in the population of people over the age of 80 (139). There is also an increase in the prevalence of autoantibodies, but this does not appear to correlate with overt clinical disease.

Changes in the immune system with aging are similar to those seen in chronic inflammation and cancer. In addition to the reduced mitogenic responses of T-cells, there is an increase in the levels of "acute phase" proteins. It is hypothesized that persistently elevated levels of inflammatory cytokines may be responsible for downregulation of IL-2 production by chronically stimulated T-cells (134).

The clinical manifestations of these changes are difficult to ascertain, because the increased susceptibility to many infectious agents is more likely a result of comorbid disease than of physiologic decline. There is no good evidence to support the contention that immunosenescence alone is responsible for the observation that older patients are more likely to contract an infectious illness and less able to eradicate it quickly. However, the decline in physiologic reserve of other organ systems combined with comorbid illnesses may make recovery prolonged and more difficult.

Oncogenesis

There is a clear increase in most common cancers in people over the age of 65 and two-thirds of all cancer deaths occur in this age group. The increased incidence of cancer in the elderly is related to several biological factors including longer exposure to environmental carcinogens, increased susceptibility of cells to carcinogens, decreased immune surveillance of abnormal cells, and abnormalities in the rate of occurrence or repair of acquired DNA damage. Alterations in the expression or amplification of oncogenes or tumor suppressor genes may play a role in oncogenesis as well as in the aging process itself. The biological basis for both oncogenesis and aging may be more closely related than was previously realized (140).

Aging is characterized by a general decrease in cellular proliferative capacity, as discussed earlier. Some age-related illnesses, including prostatic hypertrophy and early atherosclerosis, may represent disease processes characterized by hyperproliferation of certain cells types. This altered control of cell-specific proliferation may be genetically programmed or acquired, but contributes to the limits of life span for that species. Although neoplasia frequently occurs in actively dividing cells, it also occurs in nonreplicating tissues. This suggests that factors that determine replicating capacity (and life span) may be directly and indirectly linked to those processes that regulate oncogenesis. Experimental evidence for this proposal is still incomplete, but interesting evidence for a reciprocal relationship between cellular aging and oncogenesis is found in animal studies of CR. In this model of maximal life-span prolongation in mammalian species, the extension of average life span is accompanied by a decrease in the occurrence of neoplasia (141).

The control of proliferation at the molecular level is the subject of great interest in both aging and oncology circles. The end of each chromosome is capped by a telomere, a nucleoprotein structure with tandem repeating six nucleotide sequences. This structure protects the chromosomal DNA from degradation and fusion, and has multiple functions in cell division and nuclear spatial organization (142). With each cell division, the telomere is shortened until a critical length is reached at which point proliferation ceases and the cell enters replicative senescence. It is postulated that in tissue, changes in gene expression in senescent cells may cause alterations in adjacent cells, which effect overall homeostasis and facilitate the processes of aging and tumor development (143). Physiological evidence of this, however, is lacking. The enzyme telomerase, not normally found in most somatic cells, can restore telomere length and allow for continuing replication. Although telomerase expression has been identified in the great majority of tumor cells tested, it does not cause malignant transformation, but rather permits proliferation (142).

As the gene pool represented by the older population continues to enlarge, the increased occurrence of late programmed events may result in a greater than expected incidence of cellular alterations (malignancy) linked to the end to the predetermined replicative cycle. This may explain the disproportionate increase in malignant diseases in older persons.

In addition, there are several specific mechanisms whereby the aging process may contribute to malignant transformation. First, it is possible that aging or the passage of time simply allows the accumulation of a required sequence of cellular events to transform cells. Second, there may be increased susceptibility in aging to exposure to carcinogens (144). Third, it has been shown that DNA damage once incurred is repaired less efficiently or less completely in aged cells. This may explain why increased karyotypic abnormalities are seen in both normal elderly subjects and in patients with malignancies. Fourth, activation or amplification of oncogenes may be greater in the older subject. An increased amplification of protogenes has been documented in aging

fibroblasts (145), and c-myc transcript levels are increased in aging mouse livers (146). Alternatively, cancer suppressor genes may be inactivated, because p53 has been shown to be altered in both tumorogenesis and in senescence (147). Fifth, although a loss of immune surveillance has been implicated in some tumors, it remains uncertain whether this is a common aging effect that facilitates tumorogenesis.

Finally, in addition to specific effects of cellular aging on oncogenesis, other aspects of the aged host may alter the natural history of the tumor or the response to specific therapy. Although there is no evidence that cancers in older people respond differently to treatment than those in younger people (144), the presence of significant comorbid illness in the aged may require that treatment protocols be adjusted to avoid severe side effects and complications. Unfortunately, data defining appropriate drug regimens and dosing schedules for elderly patients with most types of cancer are lacking because, until recently, elderly patients have been excluded from most clinical trails of cancer treatments.

PREOPERATIVE EVALUATION, RISK ASSESSMENT, AND OUTCOME

In keeping with previous discussions of risk assessment, we will refer to risk primarily as the chance of postoperative mortality and morbidity. Risk in the elderly, however, should also be assessed in terms of restoration of preoperative functional status and quality of life, because survival is not necessarily the only important issue for patients in this age group. Preoperative assessment of risk in the elderly must provide an accurate assessment of the extent of physiological decline and the presence of other coexisting disease processes. This does not necessarily require an extensive evaluation of each separate system. An assessment of functional status, nutritional status, cognitive function, and level of psychosocial support is frequently all that is necessary to evaluate risk and formulate a postoperative recovery plan.

Although the physiological changes that accompany aging are myriad, the impact of these changes on the outcome of uncomplicated elective surgery in otherwise healthy, functional older patients is minimal. As a result of these physiological alterations, however, the response to the surgical disease in the elderly is frequently "atypical." The lack of the classical signs and symptoms of disease often leads to delays and errors in diagnosis, which result in the increased need for "acute" surgical intervention. In one series of patients over the age of 70, emergency operation carried a 10-fold higher mortality rate than the elective rate of 1.9% (148). Almost regardless of the type of procedure, emergency surgery is associated with at least a threefold increase in mortality and morbidity. It is also associated with a higher rate of long-term hospital stay (>30 days), greater need for postoperative intensive care, and larger decline in functional status with consequent increase in the need for nursing home placement (149).

Assessment of Comorbid Illnesses

Although physiologic decline may impair the ability of the elderly patient to compensate appropriately for the additional stress of complicated or emergency surgery, it is the presence of comorbid illnesses, or pathological processes other than the primary surgical disease, that is the most important determinant of surgical outcome. Comorbidity has been implicated both in the development of acute disease and in increased surgical mortality and morbidity. For example, Boyd et al. studied the impact of comorbidity on the mortality from colon surgery in 357 patients over the age of 50 (150). The preoperative incidence of additional pathologic conditions other than the primary surgical disease rose steadily with age, such that by age 80, only 5% of patients had no comorbid illnesses (Table 9). In patients over the age of 70, the mortality rate rose, in association with the number of comorbid conditions, from 1.5% with zero to one conditions to 16% with two or more. A similar increase in mortality was observed in patients younger than 70 years of age, and age as an isolated factor was seen to have no effect on mortality. In a more recent Veterans Affairs study, which included 26,648 patients over the age of 80 (5% of total subjects), both age and comorbidity were found to be independent predictors of postoperative mortality, but 10 other patient characteristics were better predictors than age. These included American Society of Anesthesiologists classification, low albumin, emergency surgery, impaired functional status, elevated blood urea nitrogen, disseminated cancer, do not resuscitate order, history of weight loss, elevated liver enzymes, and complexity of the operation (151).

Unfortunately, as is the case with the surgical disease itself, the manifestations of these comorbid illnesses in the elderly are frequently less specific and less "typical" than they are in younger patients. Silent myocardial infarction, apathetic hyperthyroidism, moderate cognitive impairment, and malnutrition are among the many disorders that may not be apparent from initial history and physical examination. The search for comorbid illness must, therefore, be diligent. In one study of hospitalized patients over 70 years of age, 60% of moderate to severe cognitive deficits and 42% of nutritional deficits had been previously unrecognized by the primary caregiver (152).

The identification of cardiac comorbidity is most important in the elderly surgical patient, because cardiac events are the leading cause of perioperative complications and death. For this reason, preoperative evaluation of "cardiac risk" has been extensively studied. The American College of Cardiology and the American Heart Association Task Force on Practice Guidelines has recently published an in depth set of guidelines for perioperative cardiovascular evaluation, which addresses all the major concerns (153). Stratification of risk based on clinical factors and operative factors is discussed. More detailed applications of these strategies are discussed elsewhere in the text, and for elderly patients with known cardiac disease, rigorous workup may be necessary. For most other elderly patients, however, assessments of functional status and exercise tolerance are accurate predictors of outcome (see section "Assessment of General Health and Functional Status").

Table 9 Prevalence of Preoperative Pathologic Conditions (%)

Condition	Age (yr)				
	50–59	60–69	70–79	>80	Total
Cardiovascular	36	52	57	85	53
Pulmonary	8	17	20	17	16
Renal	5	8	24	15	13
Hepatic	7	10	16	20	12
Nutritional	2	7	10	22	8
Other	13	18	21	20	18

Source: From Ref. 150.

Assessment of General Health and Functional Status

For decades, anesthesiologists have successfully predicted postoperative mortality in patients of all ages using the Dripp's American Society of Anesthesiology Physical Status Scale. This scale assigns patients to one of five categories, depending on extent of underlying systemic disease. Using this scale Djokovic and Hedley-White studied mortality in 500 consecutive surgical patients aged more than 80 years (154). No patient in this study was classified as Class 1, because an age of 80 or more is an exclusion criterion for this category. Mortality rate correlated well with the severity of illness, increasing from less than 1% in Class 2 patients (mild systemic disease) to 25% in Class 4 patients (incapacitating systemic disease). For each and every class, the figures are similar to those seen in younger patients. These data support the concept that severity of illness and comorbidity rather than age alone are the significant factors in postoperative mortality.

Standard measures of functional status have also proven to be predictive of postoperative outcome. The ability to perform the ADL or the simple tasks of life like feeding, continence, transferring, toileting, dressing, and bathing has been correlated with operative mortality and morbidity. In one study, patients identified as inactive (defined as unable to leave their homes on of their own efforts at least twice a week) were shown to have a higher incidence of all major surgical complications (155). In another study of noncardiac surgical cases, mortality in patients with severely limited activity (defined as bedridden or only able to transfer from bed to chair) was 9.7 times higher than in active patients. Of the risk factors studied, inactivity was found to be the single strongest predictor of death (156).

Even for patients with less obvious limitations, functional capacity or exercise tolerance is the single most important predictor of cardiac complications following noncardiac surgery. In a study comparing Dripps Criteria and Goldman Clinical Criteria (noninvasive ventricular functional assessment and exercise tolerance), Gerson et al. (157) demonstrated that the inability to raise the heart rate to 99 beats/min while doing two minutes of supine bicycle exercise was the most sensitive predictor of postoperative cardiac complications and death.

The physiologic basis for this finding has been further clarified by a study in which patients performed supine ergometry while being connected by mouthpiece to a metabolic cart (158). The authors identified an anaerobic threshold, defined as the level of oxygen consumption above which circulatory supply could not meet metabolic demand, and correlated this threshold with surgical outcome. For those patients able to reach an anaerobic threshold of 11 mL/kg/min or more, the mortality was 0.8%, compared to 18% for those unable to reach this threshold. Even in patients with preoperative ischemia identified at the time of exercise testing, this threshold level was highly predictive of postoperative mortality (Table 10).

Should all preoperative elderly patients, therefore, be subjected to this type of exercise testing? Clearly this is neither practical nor necessary. The metabolic requirements for many routine activities have already been determined and are quantitated as metabolic equivalents (METs). One MET, 3.5 mL/kg/min, is basal oxygen consumption or that amount of oxygen consumed by a 70 kg, 40-year-old man at rest. Estimated energy requirements for various activities are shown in Table 11. By asking appropriate questions

Table 10 Anaerobic Threshold and Postoperative Mortality

AT (mL/min/kg)	No. of pts.	No. of CVS deaths	% Mortality
All patients			
< 11	55	10	18[*]
> 11	132	1	0.8
Patients with preoperative ischemia			
< 11	19	8	42[**]
> 11	25	1	4

[*]$p < 0.001$.
[**]$p < 0.01$.
Abbreviations: AT, anaerobic threshold, CVS, cardiovascular system.
Source: From Ref. 158.

about the level of activity, or by using a standardized self-assessment tool such as the Duke's Activity Status Index (159), the functional status can be determined. The inability to function above 4 METs has been associated with increased perioperative cardiac events and long-term risk (153).

Diminished preoperative functional capacity may be the result of chronic anemia. The prevalence of anemia rises steadily after the age of 65 and more sharply after the age of 80. World Health Organization defines anemia as the hemoglobin (Hgb) levels less than 13 in men, and less than 12 in women (91). Anemia in older people, whether of known etiology (80%) or undefined, is a strong predictors of both disability in the community and in the hospital (160). Studies of elderly disabled women show women with Hgb levels of 13–14 have the best results on mobility test, whereas those with Hgb < 12 have the worst (161). In a study of patients with hip fracture repair, mobility, as measured in the distance walked, rose steadily with rising Hgb (Fig. 9) (162).

Other nonspecific indices have recently been shown to predict poor outcome and mortality in elderly patients with a wide variety of medical and surgical illnesses. Among these, low levels of serum albumin have emerged as an independent and sensitive predictor of increased length of stay, increased rates of readmission, unfavorable disposition, and increased all cause mortality (163). Whether this finding is related to poor nutritional status or unidentified complex chronic illness has not been clarified. In a large study of surgical patients, low preoperative serum albumin was shown also to be an independent and sensitive predictor of both operative mortality and morbidity (164).

Preoperative cognitive impairment has been shown to have a similar, although far less well defined, negative

impact on many surgical outcomes. It has been suggested that the increased operative mortality seen in this group of patients is related, in part, to delays in diagnosis (165). In addition, preoperative cognitive dysfunction is a major cause of postoperative delirium. Postoperative delirium has significant impact on all other surgical outcomes including mortality, major morbidity, length of stay, and discharge to long-term care or rehabilitation facilities (166). Delirium in the ICU is also associated with higher mortality and prolonged length of stay (167).

Persistent cognitive dysfunction can occur in the postoperative period, even in the patients without preexisting deficits. This dysfunction has been shown to persist for as long as three months after operation in a significant percent of elderly patients (168). Following cardiac bypass surgery, early cognitive deficits are common and persist at six months (169).

Overall Outcome

Over the past 30 years, there has been a clear decline in the overall surgical mortality in older age groups (170), even for the highest risk operations like aneurysmorraphy and major cancer resections. Overall, long-term survival does not appear to be adversely affected by the need for surgical intervention, even in patients over the age of 90 (Fig. 10) (171).

However, because of comorbidity and declining physiologic reserves, older patients are less able to tolerate postoperative complications. In the VA study mentioned earlier, mortality in patients over the age of 80 increased from 3.7% in patients without complications to 26% in patients with one or more complications (151).

Data regarding the functional outcome and return to the same (or better) preoperative status are available primarily for procedures that directly address improving these outcomes, such as total joint replacement and aortic valve replacement. For other procedures, the data are less clear. In the SUPPORT study (Study to Understand Prognoses and Preferences for Treatment), designed to develop a model to predict outcome in seriously ill medical and surgical patients, prior ability to perform the ADL was the most important predictor of functional outcome (172).

In a more recent study of functional recovery after major elective open abdominal operations, better recovery and short time to recovery of ADLs and instrumental ADL was nearly always predicted by a better preoperative physical performance status, as measured by three simple tests of strength and mobility (173).

Minimal access techniques, which have been shown to limit postoperative pain and promote a more rapid return

Table 11 Estimated Energy Requirements for Various Activities

1 MET	Can you take care of yourself?	4 METs	Climb a flight of stairs or walk up hill?
	Eat, dress, or use the toilet?		Walk on level ground at 4 mph or 6.4 km/h?
	Walk indoors around the house?		Run a short distance?
			Do heavy work around the house like scrubbing floors or lifting or moving heavy furniture?
	Walk a block or two on level gound at 2–3 mph or 3.2–4.8 km/h?		Participate in moderate recreational activities like golf, bowling, dancing, doubles tennis, or throwing a baseball or football?
4 METs	Do light work around the house like dusting or washing dishes?	10 METs	Participate in strenuous sports like swimming, single tennis, football, basketball, or skiing?

Abbreviation: MET, metabolic equivalent.
Source: From Ref. 153.

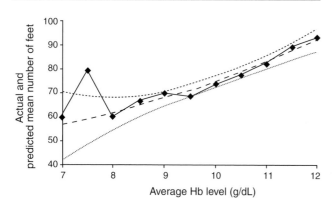

Figure 9 Functional recovery after hip fracture. The distance walked at discharge increases with increasing hemoglobin concentration. *Source*: From Ref. 162.

to normal function in younger patients, may also improve functional outcome in older patients. However, the advanced nature of the pathology frequently found in the aged often complicates or even precludes the laparoscopic approach. Studies do show that when laparoscopic techniques are possible, mortality and morbidity are comparable to open procedures (174).

Further clarification of the factors that may have an impact on the outcomes of death, nursing home placement, and total hospital days in patients with medical or surgical illnesses can be found in a study of 12 conditions common in the geriatric population (175). These "geriatric-targeting criteria" include socioeconomic problems, vision impairment, hearing impairment, appetite loss, weight loss, incontinence, confusion, depression, dementia, falls, and prolonged bed rest. In this prospective study of 507 acutely ill male veterans, over 65 years of age, only confusion was associated with all three negative outcomes. Weight loss was the strongest predictor of death, although appetite loss, depression, falls, and socioeconomic problems were also significantly associated. Polypharmacy and prolonged bed

rest predicted nursing home placement, and falls and prolonged bed rest were associated with increased total hospital days.

The elderly are also more susceptible to the sequela of the surgical intervention that may not be directly related to the operative procedure itself. Bed rest, for example, is associated with a variety of physiological changes that can have a great impact on an elderly patient's ability to recover from the surgical insult. In addition to the well-known sequela such as pressure ulcers, deep venous thrombosis, and muscle wasting, inactivity can quickly lead to deconditioning, which by itself can be considered an illness different from the original surgical disease. The deconditioned patient will demonstrate changes in multiple organ systems: depression and lethargy; anorexia and dehydration; neuromuscular instability, decreased bone density, muscular weakness, and incoordination; altered bladder and bowel function with retention and constipation; and urinary and fecal incontinence. Once these changes occur, the road back to independent functioning is all uphill. It is estimated that in severely deconditioned patients, the time to recovery can be three times the length of the period of inactivity (176).

In a study of hospitalized elderly medical patients, initial admission to a special care unit, which emphasized a multidisciplinary approach to assessment and treatment, was found to have a positive effect on the outcomes of maintenance of independence and discharge to home (177). Similar studies of surgical patients are not yet available. It is likely, however, that careful attention to the assessment and treatment of elderly surgical patients in a multidisciplinary manner that emphasizes early recognition of surgical disease and comorbidity and addresses deficits appropriately will have equally beneficial results.

SUMMARY

In the next 50 years, the portion of the population older than 65 years is expected to grow from the present 12.4% to 20% or more, encompassing nearly 80 million people. This being the case, it is incumbent on the surgeon to have a comprehensive understanding of the physiologic changes that occur with aging and how these could potentially impact on the outcome from a surgical procedure. Several important changes occur in body composition, including a reduction in lean body mass and the expansion of the extracellular compartment. Recognizing these body compositional changes ensures the appropriate use of drugs and fluids. Aging is also associated with specific changes in cellular function affecting cardiac, pulmonary, and renal responses to stress, which could impact adversely on perioperative management. Recognition of these changes enables appropriate risk assessment preoperatively. Altered responses to pain and temperature control and wound healing are likewise commonly encountered in elderly patients and can influence both preoperative diagnosis of surgical disease and postoperative complications. Accordingly, knowledge of this information in the older patient pays rich dividends in ensuring appropriate risk assessment preoperatively, precise management intraoperatively, and a smooth postoperative course. Although postoperative recovery and rehabilitation may sometimes be prolonged in elderly patients, returning these individuals to a functioning state after being subjected to surgical illness is an achievable goal.

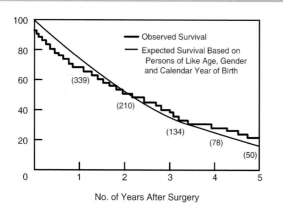

Figure 10 Postoperative survival in patients aged 90 years and older. *Source*: From Ref. 171.

REFERENCES

1. U.S. Census Bureau. U.S. Interim Projections by Age, Sex, Race and Hispanic Origin, 2004. http://www.census.gov/ipc/www/usinterimproj/. Internet release date: March 18, 2004.
2. Arias E. United states life tables, 2002. National Vital Statistics Reports. Vol. 53, Number 6, November 2004.
3. DeFrances CJ, Hall MJ. 2002 National hospital discharge survey. CDC Advanced Data from Vital and Health Statistics. Number 342, May 2004.
4. Cristafalo VJ, Gerhard GS, Pignolo RJ. Molecular biology of aging. In: Zenilman ME, Roslyn JJ, eds. Surgery in the Elderly Patient. Surg Clin North Am 1994; 74:1.
5. Gompertz B. On the nature of the function expressive of the law of human mortality and on a new mode of determining life contingencies. Philos Trans R Soc Lond 1825; 115:513.
6. Warner HR, Ingram D, Miller RA, et al. Program for testing biological interventions to promote healthy aging. Mech Ageing Dev 2000; 115:199–207.
7. Beckman M. Placing bets, National Institute on Aging Committee chooses three compounds for the definitive longevity testing. Sci Aging Knowledge Environ 2004:14.
8. Rhome D. Evidence for a relationship between longevity of mammalian species and life spans of normal fibroblasts in vitro and erythrocytes in vivo. Proc Natl Acad Sci USA 1981; 78:5009.
9. McCay, Cromwell M, Maynard L. The effect of retarded growth upon the length of life and upon ultimate size. J Nutr 1935; 10:63.
10. Yu BP, Masoro EJ, McMahon CA. Nutritional influences in aging of Fischer 344 rats. I. Physical, metabolic and longevity characteristics. J Gerontol 1985; 40:664.
11. Masoro EJ. Caloric restriction and aging: an update. Exp Gerontol 2000; 35:299.
12. Sinclair DA. Toward a unified theory of caloric restriction and longevity regulation. Mech Aging Dev 2005; 126:987–1002.
13. Flegal KM, Graubard BI, Williamson DF, Gail MH. Excess death associated with underweight, over weight and obesity. JAMA 2005; 293:1861–1867.
14. Goldman R. Decline in organ function with aging. In: Rossman I, ed. Clinical Geriatrics. 2nd ed. Philadelphia: Lippincott, 1979.
15. Reiser KM, Hennessey SM, Last JA. Analysis of age-associated changes in collagen cross linking in the skin and lung in monkeys and rats. Biochem Biophys Acta 1987; 926:339.
16. Bjorksten J. Cross linkage and the aging process. In: Rothstein M, ed. Theoretical Aspects of Aging. New York: Academic Press, 1974.
17. Harman D. Aging: A Theory Based on Free Radical and Radiation Chemistry. J Gerontol 1956; 11:298.
18. Rossman I. Anatomy of aging. In: Rossman I, ed. Clinical Geriatrics. 2nd ed. Philadelphia: Lippincott, 1979.
19. Elahi VK, Elahi D, Andres R, Tobin JD, Butler MG, Norris AH. A longitudinal study of nutritional intake in man. J Gerontol 1983; 38:162.
20. Vin SC, Love AGH. Nutritional status of institutionalized and non-institutionalized aged in Belfast, Northern Ireland. Am J Clin Nutr 1979; 32:1934.
21. Rosenberg IH. Nutrition and aging. In Hazzard WR, ed. Principles of Geriatric Medicine and Gerontology, 3rd ed; New York: McGraw-Hill, 1994. Reprinted with permission of The McGraw-Hill Companies.
22. Rudman, et al. Effect of human growth hormone in men over 60 years old. N Engl J Med 1990; 323:1.
23. Trmiras P. Aging of the skeleton, joints and muscles. In: Timiras PS, ed. Physiological Basis of Aging and Geriatrics. Boca Raton: CRC Press, Inc., 1994.
24. Tzankoff SP, Norris AH. Effect of muscle mass decrease on age-related BMR changes. J Appl Physiol 1977; 43:1001.
25. Shock NW. Energy metabolism, caloric intake, and physical activity in the aging. In: Carlson LA, ed. Nutrition in Old Age, Symposia of the Swedish Nutrition Foundation. Uppsala: Almquist and Wiksell, 1972.
26. Shimokata H, et al. Studies on the distribution of body fat: I. Effects of age, sex, and obesity. J Gerontol 1989; 44:M66.
27. Andres R. Mortality and obesity: the rationale for age-specific height-weight tables. In: Hazzard WR, Bierman EL, Blass JP, Ettinger WH Jr, Halter JB, eds. Principles of Geriatric Medicine and Gerontology. 3rd ed. New York: McGraw-Hill, 1994.
28. McLeskey CH. Anesthesia for the elderly patient. In: Barash PG, Cullen BF, Stoelting RK, eds. Clinical Anesthesia. 2nd ed. Philadelphia: JB Lippincott, 1992.
29. Homer TD, Stanski DR. The effect of increasing age on the disposition and anesthetic requirement. Anesthesiology 1985; 62:114.
30. Buxbaum JL, Schwartz AJ. Perianesthetic consideration for the elderly patient. In: Zenilman ME, Roslyn JJ, eds. Surgery in the Elderly Patient. Vol. I. Surg Clin North Am 1994; 74:41–58.
31. Kitzman DW, Edwards WD. Minireview: age-related changes in the anatomy of the normal human heart. J Gerontol 1990; 45:M33.
32. Lakatta EG, et al. Human aging: changes in structure and function. J Am Coll Cardiol 1987; 10:42A.
33. Nixon JV, et al. Ventricular performance in human hearts aged 61–73 years. Am J Cardiol 1991; 56: 932.
34. Davies MJ. Pathology of the conducting system. In: Caird FL, Dalle JLC, Kennedy RD, eds. Cardiology in Old Age. New York: Plenum Press, 1976.
35. Sahasakul Y, et al. Age-related changes in aortic and mitral valve thickness: implications for two-dimensional echocardiography based on an autopsy study of 200 normal human hearts. Am J Cardiol 1988; 62:424.
36. Kitzman, et al. Age-related changes in normal human hearts during the first ten decades. Part II (Maturity): A quantitative anatomic study of 765 specimens from subjects 20–99 years old. Mayo Clin Proc 1988; 63:137.
37. Lakatta EG. Cardiovascular regulatory mechanisms in advanced age. Physiol Rev 1993; 73:413.
38. Yin FCP. The aging vasculature and its effect on the heart. In: Weisfeldt ML, ed. The Aging Heart: Its Function and Response to Stress. Aging. 12. Vol. 12. New York: Raven Press, 1980.
39. Lewis JF, Maron BJ. Cardiovascular consequences of the aging process. In: Lowenthal DT, ed. Geriatric Cardiology. Cardiovascular Clinics. Vol. 22. Philadelphia: FA Davis Co, 1992.
40. Lachi RJ, et al. Left ventricular function in hospitalized geriatric patients. J Am Geriatr Soc 1982; 30:700.
41. Manning WJ, et al. Reversal of changes in left ventricular diastolic filling associated with normal aging using diltiazem. Am J Cardiol 1991; 67:894.
42. Wei JY. Age and the cardiovascular system. N Engl J Med 1992; 327:1735.
43. Tresch DD, McGough MF. Heart failure with normal systolic function: a common disorder in older people. J Am Geriatr Soc 1995; 43:1035.
44. Wei JY. Use of calcium entry blockers in elderly patients: special considerations. Circulation 1989; 80(suppl IV):171.
45. Wenger NK. Cardiovascular disease. In: Cassel CK, Riesenberg DE, Sorensen LB, Walsh JR, eds. Geriatric Medicine. 2nd. New York: Springer-Verlag, 1990.
46. Timiras PS. Aging of the respiration, erythrocytes, and the hematopoietic system. In: Timiras PS, ed. Physiological Basics of Aging and Geriatrics. Boca Raton: CRC Press, 1988.
47. Pfitzenmeyer P, et al. Lung function in advanced age: study of ambulatory subjects aged over 75 years. Gerontology 1993; 39:267.
48. Tockman MS. Aging of the respiratory system. In: Katlic MR, ed. Geriatric Surgery. Baltimore: Urban & Schwarzenberg, 1990.
49. Kronenberg RS, Drage CW. Attenuation of the ventilatory and heart rate responses to hypoxia and hypercapnia in with aging in men. J Clin Invest 1973; 52:1812.
50. Pokorski M, Walski M, Dymecka A, Marczak. The aging carotid body. J Physiol Pharm 2004; 55(suppl 3):107–113.
51. Marik PE. Aspiration pneumonitis and aspiration pneumonia. N Engl J Med 2001; 344:665–671.

52. Bartlett JG. Pneumonia. In: Andres R, Bierman EX, Hazzard WR, eds. Principles of Geriatric Medicine. 1st. New York: McGraw-Hill, 1985.

53. Lindeman RD. Overview: renal physiology and pathophysiology of aging. Am J Kidney Dis 1990; 16:275.

54. Cockroft DW, Gault MH. Prediction of creatinine clearance from serum creatinine. Nephron 1976; 16:31.

55. Macias Nunez JF, et al. Physiology and disorders of water balance and electrolytes in the elderly. In: Macias Nunez JF, Cameron JS, eds. Renal function and Disease in the Elderly. Stoneham, MA: Butterworth, 1987.

56. Tsundo K, et al. Effect of aging on the renin-angiotensin-aldosterone system in normal subjects: simultaneous measurement of active and inactive renin, renin substrate and aldosterone in plasma. J Clin Endrocrinol Metab 1986; 62:384.

57. Rowe JW, et al. The influence of age on urinary concentrating ability in man. Nephron 1976; 17:270.

58. Phillips PA, et al. Reduced thirst after water deprivation in healthy elderly men. N Engl J Med 1984; 12:753.

59. Mukherjee AP, Coni NK, Davidson W. Osmoreceptor function among the elderly. Gernotol Clin 1973; 15:227.

60. Lindeman RD. Changes in renal function with aging: implications for treatment. Drugs & Aging 1992; 2:423.

61. Susset JG, et al. Collagen in 155 human bladders. Invest Urol 1978; 16:204.

62. Brocklehurst JC, Dilane JB. Studies of the female bladder in old age: I. Cystometricograms in non-incontinent women. Gerontol Clin 1968; 10:242.

63. Mohide EA. Prevalence and scope of urinary incontinence. Clin Geriatr Med 1986; 2:639.

64. Esposito AL, et al. Community acquired bacteremia in the elderly: analysis of one hundred consecutive episodes. J Am Geriatr Soc 1980; 28:315.

65. Mooney H, et al. Alterations in the liver with aging. Clin Gastroenterol 1985; 14:757.

66. Kampmann JP, Sinding J, Moller-Jorgenson L. Effect of age on liver function. Geriatrics 1975; 30:91.

67. Schmucker DL. Aging and drug disposition: an update. Pharmacol Rev 1985; 37:133.

68. Shepherd MM, et al. Age as a determinant of sensitivity to warfarin. Br J Clin Pharmacol 1977; 4:315.

69. Sampliner RE, et al. Gallbladder disease in Pima Indians. Demonstration of prevalence and early onset by cholecystography. N Engl J Med 1979; 283:1358.

70. Simonivis NJ, Wells CK, Feinstein AR. In-vivo and post-mortem gallstones: support for the validity of the "epidemiologic necropsy" screening technique. Am J Epidemiol 1991; 133:922.

71. The Rome Group for the Epidemiology and Prevention of Cholelithiasis (GREPCO). The epidemiology of gallstone disease in Rome, Italy, Part 1. Prevalence in men. Hepatology 1988; 8:904.

72. Ratner J, et al. The prevalence of gallstone disease in very old institutionalized persons. JAMA 1991; 265:902.

73. Trotman BW, Sotoway RD. Pigment vs cholesterol cholelithiasis: clinical epidemiological aspects. Dig Dis 1975; 20:735.

74. Bateson MC. Gallbladder disease and cholecystectomy are independently variable. Lancet 1984; 2:621.

75. Bowen JC, et al. Gallstone disease: pathophysiology, epidemiology, natural history, and treatment options. Med Clin North Am 1992; 76:1143.

76. Einarsson K, et al. Influence of age on secretion of cholesterol and synthesis of bile acids by the liver. N Engl J Med 1985; 313:277.

77. Carey MC. Pathogenesis of gallstones. Am J Surg 1993; 165:410.

78. Khalil T, et al. Decreased gallbladder responsiveness to CCK-8 in aged rabbits. Gastroenterology 1984; 86:1134.

79. Poston GJ, et al. Effect of age and sensitivity to cholecystokinin on gallstone formation in the guinea pig. Gastroenterology 1990; 98:993.

80. Khalil T, et al. Effects of aging on gallbladder contraction and release of cholecystokinin-33 in humans. Surgery 1985; 98:423.

81. Berger D, et al. Effects of age on fasting plasma levels pf pancreatic polypeptide in man. J Clin Endocrinol Metab 1978; 47:1183.

82. Brunicardi FC, et al. Regulation of pancreatic polypeptide secretion in the isolated perfused human pancreas. Am J Surg 1988; 155:63.

83. Rosenthal RA, Andersen DK. Surgery in the elderly: observations on the pathophysiology and treatment of cholelithiasis. Exp Gerontol 1993; 28:459.

84. Escarce JJ, et al. Outcomes of open cholecystectomy in the elderly: a longitudinal analysis of 21,00 cases in the prelaparoscopic era. Surgery 1995; 117:156.

85. Wenckhert A, Robertson B. The natural history of gallstone disease. Gastroenterology 1966; 50:376.

86. Morrow DJ, Thompson J, Wislon SE. Acute cholescystitis in the elderly. A surgical emergency. Arch Surg 1978; 113:1149.

87. Lipschitz DA, et al. The use of long term marrow culture as a model for the aging process. Age 1983; 6:122.

88. Reincke U, et al. Proliferative capacity of murine hematopoietic stem cells in vitro. Science 1982; 215:1619.

89. Albright JA, Makinodan T. Decline in the growth potential of spleen-colonizing bone marrow stem cells of long lived aging mice. J Exp Med 1976; 144:1204.

90. Lipschitz DA. Aging of the hematopoietic system. In: Hazzard WR, Bierman EL, Blass JP, Ettinger WH Jr, Halter JB. Principles of Geriatric Medicine and Gerontology. 3rd ed. New York: McGraw Hill, 1994.

91. Balducci L. Epidemiology of anemia in the elderly: information on diagnostic evaluation. J Am Geriatr Soc 2003; 51(suppl):S2-S9.

92. Lipschitz DA, et al. Evidence that microenvironmental factors account for the age-related decline in neutrophil function. Blood 1987; 70:1131.

93. Evers BM, Townsend CM, Thompson JC. Organ physiology of aging. In: Zenilman ME, Roslyn JJ, eds. Surgery in the Elderly Patient. Vol. I. Surg Clin North Am 1994; 74:23–39.

94. Simpkins JW, Millard WJ. Influence of age or neurotransmitter function. Endocrinol Metab Clin North Am 1987; 16:893.

95. Khansari DN, Gustad TV. Effect of long term, low dose growth hormone therapy on immune function and life expectancy of mice. Mech Aging Dev 1991; 57:87.

96. Forster JA, et al. Effect of age and IGF-I administration on elastin gene expression in rat aorta. J Gerontol 1990; 45: B113.

97. Burrows V, Shenkman L. Thyroid function in the elderly. Am J Med Sci 1982; 283:8.

98. Ronnov V, Kirkegaard C. Hyperthyroidism—A disease of old age? Br Med J 1973; 1:41.

99. Norton JA, Levin B, Jensen RT. Cancer of the endocrine system. In: DeVita VT Jr, Hellman S, Rosenberg SA, eds. Cancer: Principles and Practice of Oncology. 4th ed. Philadelphia: JB Lippincott, 1993.

100. Potts JT, Ackerman IP, Barker CF, et al. Diagnosis and management of asymptomatic primary hyperparathyroidism: consensus development conference statement. Ann Intern Med 1991; 114:593.

101. Bilezikian JP, Potts JT, Fuleihan GH. Summary statement from a workshop on asymptomatic primary hyperparathyroidism: a perspective for the 21st century. J Clin End & Metab 2002; 87(12):5353–5361.

102. Chan AK, Duh QY, Katz MH, Siperstein AE, Clark OH. Clinical manifestations of primary hyperparathyroidism before and after parathyroidectomy. Ann Surg 1995; 222:402.

103. Chen H, Parkerson S, Udelsman R. Parathyroidectomy in the elderly: Do the benefits outweigh the risks? World J Surg 1998; 22:533–536.

104. Macintosh CG, Horowitz M, Verhagen MA, et al. Effect of small intestinal nutrient infusion on appetite, gastrointestinal

hormone release, and gastric myoelectrical activity in young and older men. Am J Gastroenterol 2001; 96:997–1007.

105. Soergel K, Zboralske F, Amberg J. Presbyesophagus: esophageal motility in nonagenarian. J Clin Invest 1964; 43:1472.

106. Khalil T, Poston GJ, Thompson JC. Effects of aging on gastrointestinal hormones. In: Prinsley DM, Shustead HH, eds. Progress in Clinical and Biological Research, Nutrition, and Aging. Vol. 326. New York: Alan R. Liss, 1990.

107. Bonnevie O. The incidence of duodenal ulcer in Copenhagen County. Scand J Gastroenterol 1975; 10:385.

108. Kurata JH, Honda GD, Frankl H. The incidence of duodenal and gastric ulcers in a large health maintenance organization. Am J Public Health 1985; 75:625.

109. Kim SW, Parekh K, Townsend CM, et al. Effect of aging on duodenal bicarbonate secretion. Ann Surg 1990; 212:332.

110. Russel RM, Koruda MJ. The aging process as a modifier of metabolism. Am J Clin Nutr 2000; 72:529s–532s.

111. Kreel L, Sandlin B. Changes in pancreatic morphology associated with aging. Gut 1973; 14:962.

112. McEvoy A. Investigation of intestinal malabsorption in the elderly. In: Evans J, Caird F, eds. Advanced Geriatric Medicine. London: Pittman, 1982.

113. Browder W, Patterson MD, Thompson JL, Walters DN. Acute pancreatitis of unknown etiology in the elderly. Ann Surg 1993; 217:469.

114. Pan HY, et al. Decline in beta adrenergic receptor-mediated vascular relaxation with aging in man. J Pharmacol Exp Ther 1986; 239:802.

115. Lakatta EG. Altered autonomic modulation of cardiovascular function with adult aging: perspectives from studies ranging from man to cell. In: Stone HL, Weglicki WB, eds. Pathobiology of Cardiovascular Injury. Boston: Nojhoff, 1985.

116. Vestal RE, et al. Reduced beta-adrenoreceptor sensitivity in the elderly. Clin Pharmacol Ther 1979; 26:181.

117. Feldman RD, Limbird LE, Nadeau J, Robertson D, Wood JJ. Alteration in leukocyte β-receptor affinity with aging: a potential explanation for altered β-adrenergic sensitivity in the elderly. N Engl J Med 1984; 310:815.

118. Arnetz BB. Endocrine reactions during standardized surgical stress: the effects of age and methods of anesthesia. Age Aging 1985; 14:96.

119. Rolandelli RH, Ulrich JR. Nutritional support of the frail elderly surgical patient. Surg Clin North Am 1994; 74:79.

120. Clevenger FW, Rodriguez DJ, Demarest GB, Osler TM, Olson SE, Fry DE. Protein and energy tolerance by stressed geriatric patients. J Surg Res 1992; 52:135.

121. Gibson SJ, Helme RD. Age-related differences in pain perception and report. Clin Geriatr Med 2001; 17:433–456.

122. Clinch D, Banerjee AK, Ostick G. Absence of abdominal pain in elderly patients with peptic ulcer. Age Aging 1984; 13:120.

123. Moore AK, et al. Differences in epidural morphine requirements between elderly and young patients after abdominal surgery. Anesth Analg 1990; 70:316.

124. Collins KJ, Exton-Smith AN. Thermal homeostasis in old age. J Am Geriatr Soc 1983; 31:519.

125. Wongsurwat N, et al. Thermoregulatory failure in the elderly. J Am Geriatr Soc 1990; 38:899.

126. Kurz A, Sessler DI, Lenhardt R. Perioperative normaothermia to reduced the incidence of surgical wound infection and shorten hospitalization: study of wound infection and temperature group. N Engl J Med 1996; 334:1209–1215.

127. Frankenfiled D, Cooney RN, Smith JS, Rowe WA. Age-related differences in the metabolic response to injury. Trauma 2000; 48:49–62.

128. Norman DC, et al. Fever and aging. J Am Geriatr Soc 1985; 33:859.

129. Mikinodan T, Kay MMB. Age influences the immune system. In: Kunkel HG, Dixon FJ, eds. Advances in Immunology. New York: Academic Press, 1980.

130. Holt DR, et al. Effects of age on wound healing in healthy human beings. Surgery 1992; 112:293.

131. Quirina A, Viidik A. The influence of age on the healing of normal and ischemic incisional skin wounds. Mech Ageing Dev 1991; 58:221–232.

132. Ashcroft GS, Mills SJ, Ashworth JJ. Ageing and wound healing. Biogerontology 2002; 3:337–345.

133. Kirk SJ, et al. Arginine stimulates wound healing and immune function in elderly human beings. Surgery 1993; 114:155.

134. Currie MS. Immunosenescence. Comprehensive Ther 1992; 18:26.

135. Lewis VM, et al. Age, thymic involution and circulating thymic hormone activity. J Clin Endocrinol Metab 1978; 47:145.

136. Hefton JM, et al. Immunologic studies of aging. V. Impaired proliferation of PHA responsive human lymphocytes in culture. J Immunol 1980; 125:1007.

137. Ershler WB, et al. IL-2 and aging: decrease IL-2 production in healthy older people does not correlate with reduced helper cell numbers or antibody response to influenza vaccine and is not corrected in vitro by thymosinal. Immunopharmacology 1985; 10:11.

138. Roberts-Thomson JC, et al. Aging, immune response and mortality. Lancet 1974; 2:368.

139. Crawford J, Eye MK, Cohen HJ. Evaluation of monoclonal gammopathies in the well elderly. Am J Med 1987; 82:39.

140. Cohen HJ. Biology of aging as related to cancer. Cancer 1994; 74:2092.

141. Weindruch R, Walford RL. The retardation of aging and disease by dietary restriction. Springfield, II: Chas. C. Thomas, 1988.

142. Urquidi V, Tarin D, Goodison S. Role of telomerase in senescence and oncogenesis. Ann Rev Med 2000; 51:65–79.

143. Shay JW, Wright WE. Senescence and immortalization: role of telomeres and telomerase. Carcinogenesis 2005; 26:867–874.

144. Ershler WB, Longo DL. Aging and cancer. Issues of basic and clinical science. J Natl Cancer Inst 1997; 89:1489–1497.

145. Srivastava A, et al. C-Ha-ras-1 protooncogenes amplification and over expression during the limited replicative lifespan of normal fibroblasts. J Biocommun 1985; 260:6404.

146. Matocha MF, et al. Selective elevation of c-myc transcript leels in the liver of the aging Fischer-344 rat. Biochem Biophys Res Commun 1987; 147:1.

147. Shay JW, Pereora DM, Wright WE. A role for both RB and p53 in the regulation of human cellular senescence. Exp Cell Res 1991; 196:33.

148. Keller SM, et al. Emergency and elective surgery in patients over age 70 years. Am Surg 1987; 53:636.

149. Zenilman ME. Considerations in surgery in the elderly. In: Andersen DK, ed. Master Series in Surgery. 2. Advances in Surgery in the Elderly. New York: World Medical Press, 1993.

150. Boyd BJ, et al. Operative risk factors pf colon resection in the elderly. Ann Surg 1980; 192:743.

151. Hamel MB, Henderson WG, Khuri SF, Daley J. Surgical outcomes for patients age 80 and older: morbidity and mortality from noncardiac surgery. J Am Geriatr Soc 2005; 53: 424–429.

152. Pinholt EM, et al. Functional assessment of the elderly. A comparison of standard instruments with clinical judgement. Arch Intern Med 1987; 147:484.

153. Eagle KA, et al. ACC/AHA Task Force Report. Guidelines for perioperative evaluation for noncardiac surgery. Circulation 1996; 93:1279.

154. Djokovic JL, Hedley-White J. Prediction of outcome of surgery and anesthesia in patients over 80. JAMA 1979; 242:2301.

155. Seymour DG, Pringle R. Post-operative complications in the elderly surgical patient. Gerontology 1983; 29:262.

156. Browner WS, Mangano DT. In hospital and long-term mortality in male veterans following noncardiac surgery: the study of perioperative ischemia research group. JAMA 1992; 268:228.

157. Gerson MC, et al. Cardiac prognosis in noncardiac geriatric surgery. Ann Intern Med 1985; 103:832.

158. Older P, et al. Preoperative evaluation of cardiac function and ischemia in elderly patients by cardiopulmonary exercise testing. Chest 1993; 103:701.

159. Hlatky MA, et al. A brief self-administered questionnaire to determine functional capacity (the Duke's Activity Status Index). Am J Cardiol 1989; 64:651.

160. Lipschitz D. Medical and functional consequences of anemia in the elderly. J Am Geriatr Soc 2003; 51(S):S10-S13.

161. Chaves P, Ashar T, Guralnik JM, et al. Looking at the relationship between hemoglobin concentration and previous mobility difficulty in older women. Should criteria used to define anemia in older people be changed? J Am Geriatr Soc 2002; 50:1257–1264.

162. Lawrence VA, Silverstein JH, Cornell JE, et al. Higher Hb level is associated with better early functional recovery after hip fracture repair. Transfusion 2003; 43:1717.

163. Corti M, et al. Serum albumin level and physical disability as predictors of mortality in older persons. JAMA 1994; 272:1036.

164. Gibbs J, Cull W, Henderson W, et al. Preoperative serum albumin level as a predictor of operative mortality and morbidity. Arch Surg 1999; 134:36–42.

165. Berstein GM, Offenbartl SK. Adverse surgical outcomes among patients with cognitive impairments. Am Surg 1991; 57:682.

166. Marcantonio ER, et al. A clinical prediction rule for delirium after elective noncardiac surgery. JAMA 1994; 271(2):134.

167. Ely EW, Shintani A, Bernadrd G, et al. Delirium in the ICU is associated with higher mortality and prolonged length of stay. J Am Geriatr Soc 2002; 50(suppl):S166.

168. Moller JT, et al. Long-term postoperative cognitive dysfunction in the elderly: ISPOCDl study. Lancet 1998; 351(9106): 857.

169. Newman MF, Kirchner JL, Philips-Bute B, et al. For the Neurological Research Group and the Cardiothoracic Anesthesiology Research Endeavors Investigators. Longitudinal assessment of neurocognitive function after coronary-artery bypass surgery. N Engl J Med 2001; 344; 395.

170. Thomas DR, Ritchie DS. Preoperative assessment of older adults. J Am Geriatr Soc 1995; 43:211–215.

171. Hosking MP, et al. Outcomes of surgery in patients 90 years of age and older. JAMA 1989; 261:1909.

172. Wu AW, et al. Predicting future functional status for seriously ill hospitalized adults. The SUPPORT prognostic model. Ann Intern Med 1995; 122:342.

173. Lawrence VA, Hazuda HP, Cornell JE, et al. Functional Independence after major abdominal surgery in the elderly. J Am Coll Surg 2004; 199:762–772.

174. Effron DT, Bender JS. Laparoscopic surgery in older adults. J Am Geriatr Soc 2001; 49:658–663.

175. Satish S, et al. Geriatric targeting criteria as predictors of survival and health care utilization. J Am Geriatr Soc 1996; 44:914.

176. Rader MC, Vaughen JL. Management of the frail and deconditioned patient. Southern Med J 1994; 87:61.

177. Landefeld CS, et al. A randomized trial of care in a hospital medical unit especially designed to improve the functional outcome of acutely ill older patients. N Engl J Med 1995; 332:1338.

61

Surgery for Morbid Obesity

Eric J. DeMaria, Ramzi Alami, and Robert E. Brolin

INTRODUCTION

At the present time, it is estimated that more than 40% of the population of the United States is clinically overweight (1). A 1999 report in JAMA indicated that the prevalence of obesity in the 18- to 29-year-old group had increased from 12.0% in 1991 to 18.9% in 1999 (2). It is not surprising, therefore, that most centers across the United States now offer some form of surgical therapy for morbid obesity.

Obesity is currently reported in terms of body mass index (BMI), which is expressed as body weight in kilograms divided by the height in meters squared. Obesity is defined as a BMI of 30 kg/m² or greater. Morbid obesity is defined as a BMI of 40 kg/m² or greater or a BMI of 35 kg/m² with associated comorbidities. Since the recognition by the 1985 National Institutes of Health (NIH) Consensus Development Panel that obesity is a disease that adversely affects health and longevity (3), there has been a growing interest in the pathology and treatment of morbid obesity. This culminated in the 1991 NIH Consensus Development Conference that set forth guidelines for the surgical treatment of clinically severe obesity (4).

The definition of "morbid" obesity evolved in conjunction with the introduction of surgery as a viable treatment alternative for the massive overweight. Minimum weight limits for morbid obesity were initially established in the range of 100 pounds or 100% above ideal body weight. After the NIH Consensus Development Conference, morbid obesity was redefined as a minimum BMI of 40 kg/m⁴. Obesity of this magnitude is surprisingly common in the United States. One estimate suggests that between 6 and 10 million Americans are more than 100 pounds overweight. Even two decades ago in 1980, Abraham and Johnson (5) estimated that 7.2% of American women and 5% of American men were morbidly obese.

The concept of superobesity has gradually evolved to describe a group of patients whose weight far exceeds the minimum weight criteria required for surgical treatment (6,7). Several definitions have been used to describe this magnitude of overweight including more than 225% of ideal body weight, a weight greater than 200 pounds overweight or a BMI greater than 50 kg/m². Individuals in this extreme category frequently do not live longer than 45 years unless substantial weight loss is achieved.

Apart from the excessive weight, morbid obesity carries a constellation of other life threatening syndromes including hypertension, diabetes mellitus, hyperlipidemia, cardiovascular atherosclerosis, cardiomyopathy, and sleep apnea. Morbid obesity has also been clearly linked with several other conditions including degenerative arthritis, cholelithiasis, pseudotumor cerebri, varicose veins, venous stasis ulcers, gastroesophageal reflux, urinary incontinence, dysmenorrhea, infertility, and all types of hernias. Morbidly obese individuals also face social prejudice and discrimination often resulting in depression or low self-esteem. The initial approach to the morbidly obese individual focuses on nonsurgical therapy. Although it is widely accepted that most of the patients that fit the morbidly obese profile will fail this approach, it is recommended that attempts at dietary changes as well as lifestyle changes be made before consideration for surgery. Once patients have failed nonsurgical management, the 1991 panel recommended that gastric restrictive or bypass procedures be considered for patients that meet the criteria (4). Over the years, the surgical approach to morbid obesity has undergone several changes with many of the initial procedures being abandoned in favor of other operations and with the application of new technologies as they evolve. Over the last decade, the biggest change has been the adaptation of laparoscopic techniques to bariatric surgery.

ETIOLOGY AND PATHOPHYSIOLOGY

An excess of calorie intake in comparison with reduced energy expenditure results in gradual expansion of the body's primary energy storage depot, which is fat. In normal weight humans, the percentage of body weight as fat varies from 15% to 25%. The majority of excess fat is usually found in subcutaneous tissues. However, in men the intra-abdominal storage depot is occasionally larger than the subcutaneous depot. As the magnitude of obesity increases, the weight of the lean body mass, particularly bone and skeletal muscle, is also increased. A greater lean body mass is probably necessary to provide adequate structural support for the obese.

During the past two decades, it has been learned that the distribution of body fat is of greater importance in terms of health risk than the weight of the fat mass per se. The risks of cardiovascular complications are significantly greater in patients with a preponderance of abdominal fat (so-called central or android obesity) as opposed to individuals with a gluteal preponderance [so-called peripheral or gynoid obesity (8)]. The gluteal fat distribution pattern is more prevalent in women. However, there is considerable heterogeneity of body fat distribution patterns in both sexes. There is also considerable variability in the size of fat cells from specific depots in both men and women. Women typically have larger fat cells in the gluteal region, whereas men tend to have their largest fat cells in the mesentery and omentum (9). The fat distribution pattern is commonly expressed in terms of waist-to-hip ratio (WHR) measurements, although other anthropomorphic measurements such as sagittal diameter or neck-to-thigh ratio may be more predicitive of cardiovascular risk.

The precise mechanisms that explain the relationship between increased abdominal fatness and morbidity are not well understood. Furthermore, the biochemical and genetic mechanisms that result in deposition of excess fat in abdominal or gluteal depots are also incompletely explained. The primary mechanism for weight fluctuation in adults is change in fat cell size. However, fat cells may continue to increase in number throughout early adult life, particularly in individuals who are substantially overweight. Once formed, fat cells do not undergo involution. The failure of fat cells to undergo involution provides one explanation for the failure of postoperative morbidly obese patients to reach ideal weight even with a remarkably low level of daily calorie intake.

There is convincing evidence that the development of obesity has a strong genetic component. Children of normal weight parents have only a 10% chance of becoming obese, whereas the children of obese parents have an 80% to 90% probability of developing obesity in early adulthood. There is also a strong correlation between the weight of adopted children and that of their biologic parents (10). Studies comparing the degree of fatness in monozygotic versus dizygotic twins have shown a considerably stronger correlation in the monozygotic group (11). Other studies have shown a close correlation of basal metabolic rate, body fat distribution pattern, and energy expenditure among family members.

There is also a growing body of evidence that obese patients have lower levels of thermogenesis, which is a major component of the body's means of energy expenditure. Several studies comparing thermogenesis in obese and lean subjects have shown that the obese have substantially lower levels of thermogenesis in comparison with the lean subjects. Conversely, the resting metabolic rate of obese patients is remarkably similar to that of normal weight patients.

Although it is generally conceded that environmental factors also contribute to the development of obesity, there is little hard scientific data that confirm this relationship. Morbid obesity is predominantly an American disease, suggesting that the American diet and culture play an important role in its development. In the United States, morbid obesity is generally recognized as a disease of lower socioeconomic groups. Lack of good nutrition education and diets with high-fat content are two frequently cited causes for the preponderance of severe obesity in lower class people in the United States. Recent studies in animals and man have suggested that a disproportionately high intake of fat in the diet contributes to development of obesity. It has been estimated that the percentage of dietary fat consumed by Americans has increased by 10% in the past 50 years. Because dietary fat is converted to body fat with nearly 25% greater efficiency than carbohydrate, weight gain is promoted by a high-fat diet. A greater consumption of fast foods, which are notoriously high in fat, is also cited as a major factor contributing to the increased prevalence of obesity in the United States.

Physical exercise is an extremely important means of energy expenditure and weight control. Because physical activity in morbidly obese patients is severely limited by their weight, they are notoriously sedentary. Poor diet habits and a sedentary lifestyle coupled with an inherently reduced capability of energy expenditure make morbid obesity a disease that is highly resistant to nonsurgical treatment.

RISKS AND COMPLICATIONS OF SEVERE OBESITY

The relationship of body weight to mortality and other medical illnesses is shown in Figure 1. The prevalence of

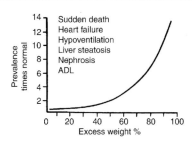

Figure 1 The estimated relative risk of medical illnesses and complications in relation to percentage above desirable weight. *Source*: From Ref. 12.

complications related to severe obesity increases sharply at a level corresponding to approximately 60% above desirable weight (12,13). At that level there is a twofold increase in morbidity and mortality. However, the slope of the "risk curve" rises almost exponentially above the 60% overweight level, so that the complication rate corresponding to 100% above ideal weight is in the range of 13 to 14 times normal. Unfortunately, there is a paucity of life table statistics for adults who are more than 100 pounds overweight. These data are particularly lacking among women who are the most common subjects of obesity operations. The 1980 study of Drenick et al. (14) of mortality in 200 morbidly obese men, which is shown in Figure 2, is the only clinical series in which all the patients were heavy enough to qualify for surgical treatment. The most striking finding in the study was the 12-fold increase in mortality in the youngest age group. The most common causes of death among the overweight men in Drenick's study were myocardial infarction and stroke.

A list of medical problems and other illnesses that have been associated with severe obesity is shown in Table 1.

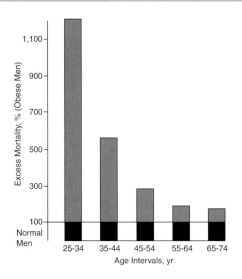

Figure 2 Comparison of excess mortality in men with morbid obesity (*light shaded bars*) vs. normal weight men (*black boxes*) by age interval. *Source*: From Ref. 15.

Table 1 Diseases Associated with Severe Obesity

Comorbidity	Incidence (%)[a]
Hypertension	20–55
Cholelithiasis	25–45
Degenerative osteoarthritis	20–35
Hyperlipidemia	15–25
Diabetes mellitus	10–25
Asthmatic bronchitis	10–15
Coronary artery disease	5–15
Heart failure (right ventricular and/or left ventricular)	5–15
Stasis ulcers/venous insufficiency	5–15
Gastroesophageal reflux	5–15
Stress overflow urinary incontinence	5–15
Obesity hypoventilation/sleep apnea syndrome	5–12
Pseudomotor cerebri	1–2
Sexual hormone imbalance/infertility	–[b]
Malignancy (uterine, colon, gallbladder)	–[b]
Pulmonary embolism/thrombophlebitis	–[b]
Necrotizing subcutaneous infections	–[b]
Mental depression	–[b]

[a]There is considerable variability in the reported incidence of nearly all the diseases that have been associated with morbid obesity.
[b]Statistical data relative to the incidence of these conditions in patients ≥100 pounds overweight are absent.

Many of these conditions can be controlled or eliminated with substantial weight loss. It is generally acknowledged that there is an inverse relationship between the magnitude of overweight and the age of onset of many of these comorbid conditions. Problems such as sleep apnea and cardiovascular disease are frequent causes of premature death in the morbidly obese. Congestive heart failure is generally a consequence of left ventricular or biventricular hypertrophy caused by a combination of increased demand for blood flow through the excess adipose tissue and increases in both systemic and pulmonary artery blood pressure. The obesity hypoventilation syndrome is caused by the increased weight placed on the chest wall and diaphragm, which results in restricted breathing. Systemic hypoxemia and hypercarbia gradually ensue. Gradual desensitization of the central chemoreceptors to carbon dioxide may result in daytime somnolence. The obstructive sleep apnea syndrome is caused by fat deposition in the hypopharynx, which results in constriction of the upper airway. During sleep, the narrowed upper airway produces loud snoring and can become completely obstructed, resulting in episodic apnea and cardiac arrhythmias. Sudden wakening is caused by hypoxic stimulation of the desensitized chemoreceptors. Prolonged hypoxia also can result in cardiac arrest, which is the usual cause of death in these patients.

Necrotizing subcutaneous infections can be life threatening in morbidly obese patients. These infections are usually polymicrobial, and typically develop in the perineum or the underside of a large abdominal paniculus. Diabetes frequently is an associated factor. The infections are extremely difficult to treat because the affected tissue has an inherently poor blood supply. Extensive soft tissue debridement is frequently necessary.

Diabetes, hypertension, and atherosclerosis typically occur in patients with an "abdominal" fat distribution pattern, which is characterized by a WHR of 0.9 or greater (8). Diabetes associated with severe obesity almost invariably begins in adulthood and is typically resistant to insulin due a marked downregulation of insulin receptors. Oral hypoglycemic agents are also usually ineffective in controlling serum glucose levels. Coronary artery disease is usually found in patients with either diabetes or hyperlipidema. Approximately 20% of morbidly obese patients have elevated serum levels of total cholesterol and triglycerides (15). However, angina in these patients is relatively uncommon, probably because they are only capable of low levels of physical exertion.

Other conditions such as degenerative arthritis, venous stasis, and urinary incontinence frequently result in serious long-term disability in the morbidly obese. Many orthopedic surgeons consider morbid obesity to be a contraindication for both prosthetic joint replacement and lower back operations, because of the likelihood of a poor result. Urologists and gynecologists are reluctant to attempt surgical correction of urinary continence problems for the same reason. This attitude creates a "catch-22" for the morbidly obese, in that the immobility resulting from both degenerative arthritis and massive overweight also contributes to their difficulty in losing weight.

There are a number of other diseases that are increasingly prevalent in severely obese patients, including gastroesophageal reflux, sex hormone imbalance, pseudotumor cerebri, and several types of malignancy. Morbidly obese women of childbearing age are known to have a high incidence of infertility and other menstrual and hormonal problems. Grace et al. (16) and Deitel (17) have independently reported preoperative abnormalities in sex hormone–binding globulin (SHBG) in infertile morbidly obese women who were attempting pregnancy. An epidemiologic study conducted by the American Cancer Society has shown an increased risk for colon cancer in men ≥40% overweight and an increased incidence of uterine cervix and gallbladder neoplasms in women ≥40% overweight.

Many of the morbidly obese suffer from low self-esteem and mental depression. The social stigma associated with severe obesity is apparent in a number of areas. Discrimination in obtaining employment is common particularly when the job requires some degree of public exposure. Fat people are often the objects of ridicule and unkind jokes. Their social activity is restricted by the inability to buy clothes at conventional clothing stores or to sit in airplane and theater seats. The most severely obese often have problems maintaining an acceptable level of personal hygiene. Morbid obesity is commonly associated with problematic marriages. Often obesity in one spouse is a "trade off" for a serious problem such as alcohol or drug addiction in the other. Many of the most severely obese become reclusive and housebound as a consequence of both the inability to ambulate and the embarrassment over their weight.

TREATMENT OF SEVERE OBESITY

Morbid obesity has been notoriously refractory to virtually every method of nonoperative treatment. The failure rate of diet and behavior modification treatment at two years in the morbidly obese approaches 100% (18). Likewise, the results of jaw wiring in this group of patients have been disappointing. Many morbidly obese patients gain substantial amounts of weight after unsuccessful attempts at dieting. The so-called yo-yo theory of dieting, namely transient weight loss followed by greater weight gain, is gaining popularity among many health professionals who provide nonsurgical treatment for obesity. The gist of this theory is that chronic dieters experience a diminished capability to lose regained weight after each successive weight fluctuation. However, the primary premise and justification for surgical treatment of morbid obesity has been the compelling evidence that severe obesity is associated with a shortened life span and a variety of other serious medical problems.

Early Obesity Operations

Kremen et al. (19) introduced the concept of surgery for morbid obesity in 1954, when they reported that resection of a large percentage of the small intestine resulted in massive weight loss. Kremen's concept of malabsorption-induced weight loss was later applied in the form of jejunoileal (intestinal) bypass as treatment for morbid obesity (20–22). Weight loss following jejunoileal bypass results entirely from malabsorption of ingested food. After experimenting with various lengths of jejunum and ileum, it was determined that the best weight loss occurred in patients with a functional intestinal length of approximately 18 in. Scott et al. (22) and Salmon (21) independently described a modification of jejunoileal bypass (Fig. 3) in which 12 in. of the proximal jejunum was anastomosed end-to-end to 6 in. of distal ileum.

During the 1960s and 1970s, thousands of intestinal bypasses were performed for treatment of morbid obesity. However, as more of these operations were done, reports of serious late sequelae, including hepatic failure, urinary calculi, arthritis, and vitamin deficiencies appeared in the literature (24,25). In 1975, Passaro et al. (26) described the bypass enteritis syndrome, an entity characterized by intermittent episodes of abdominal pain, bloating, and diarrhea, which occasionally was mistaken for peritonitis or intestinal obstruction. Many patients with bypass enteritis went on to develop arthralgias, skin rashes, and cachexia. Drenick et al. (27) later incriminated bacterial overgrowth of the distal bypassed bowel as a cause for the syndrome.

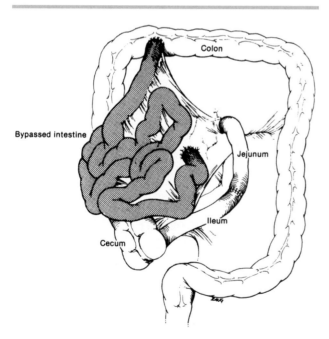

Figure 3 Jejunoileal bypass in which a 12-in. segment of jejunum is anastomosed end-to-end to 6 in. of the terminal ileum. The remainder of the small bowel (*dark shaded area*) is totally excluded from digestive continuity. The distal end of the excluded bowel is anastomosed to the transverse colon. *Source*: From Ref. 24.

The first public repudiation of jejunoileal bypass was delivered by Ravitch and Brolin (28) in 1979. During the next several years, many other prominent surgeons abandoned intestinal bypass as treatment for severe obesity (29,30). Today, jejunoileal bypass is no longer recommended for treatment of morbid obesity.

The concept of gastric restriction as treatment for morbid obesity was introduced by Mason and Ito (31) in 1967. At that time, Mason's operations received little support from the surgical community both because they were technically difficult to perform and because weight loss was less consistent than with jejunoileal bypass. Moreover, the early gastric restrictive operations were associated with a high incidence of postoperative complications. Complication rates with gastric bypass decreased after Alden (32) introduced the concept of stapling the stomach in continuity rather than dividing it. In addition, use of the Roux-en-Y technique eliminated problems with bile reflux esophagitis that were common after loop gastric bypass.

In 1979 Pace et al. (33) introduced stapled gastric partitioning, touting its technical ease in performance and low incidence of operative complications relative to gastric bypass. However, an unacceptably high incidence of early staple-line breakdown subsequently led to a proliferation of modifications using this approach. Many of these stapling techniques were performed in an uncontrolled manner. However, during the 1980s two gastric restrictive operations, vertical banded gastroplasty (VBG) and Roux-en-Y gastric bypass (RYGB), have become recognized as procedures that have produced satisfactory weight loss in patients at 5 to 10 years postoperatively.

Current Open Operations

As obesity surgery gained more acceptance and its role in the treatment of morbid obesity became better recognized and defined, the gastric restrictive procedures became the most popular method of surgical treatment. All the current gastric operations are designed to restrict oral intake. The less than 50 mL capacity upper gastric pouch and the calibrated less than 12 mm diameter outlet effectively limit the quantity of solid food that can be consumed at one time. Conversely, intake of liquids is not limited by these operations.

There are three basic categories of gastric restrictive operations: (i) gastroplasty in which the stomach is partitioned close to the gastroesophageal junction, creating a small upper gastric pouch with a small calibrated outlet leading from the upper pouch to the remainder of the digestive tract; (ii) gastric banding in which a calibrated piece of prosthetic material is wrapped around the upper portion of the stomach; and (iii) gastric bypass in which the upper stomach is closed off, thereby excluding more than 95% of the stomach, all of the duodenum, and 10 to 15 cm of proximal jejunum, from digestive continuity.

Gastroplasty

There is no malabsorption associated with gastroplasty operations. Weight loss results exclusively from reduced calorie intake. Current techniques have evolved in favor of stapling in a vertical direction along the lesser curvature of the stomach, which has facilitated reinforcement of the outlet with prosthetic materials to prevent progressive stomal dilation. Horizontal gastroplasty techniques have now been largely abandoned because of an unacceptably high incidence of staple-line disruption and stomal dilation.

The two most popular techniques of gastroplasty are VBG and vertical silicone elastomer (Silastic) ring gastroplasty (SRG), which are shown in Figs. 4 and 5. The stoma located at the distal end of a vertically oriented staple-line is reinforced with prosthetic material to prevent gradual dilation. VBG was first described in detail by Mason (34) in 1982. SRG was first described by Laws (35) in 1981 and has since been refined by others (36,37). The incidence of transmural erosion of the Silastic ring has been greatly reduced by not covering it with the surrounding stomach as Laws had originally described.

Morbidity and mortality rates with both VBG and SRG have been low. Mason et al. (38) have reported an overall morbidity rate of under 10% and a mortality rate of 0.25% in a series of more than 1200 VBGs. In 1987, Willbanks (37) reported a 3% complication rate with no deaths in a series of 305 SRG patients.

Gastric Banding

Gastric banding is a technique that has enjoyed popularity in Europe, but has not received much attention in the United States. The majority of techniques of gastric banding employ a premeasured strip of prosthetic material to restrict oral intake (Fig. 6). The circumference of the band is generally in the range of 5 cm, similar to the measurement used in VBG. Most techniques of gastric banding lack precision in measuring the volume of stomach above the band. With some techniques, the band is sutured to both itself and the stomach to prevent "slipping." Kuzmak (39) introduced the concept of an inflatable silicone band in which the diameter of the band can be adjusted by infusion of saline through a subcutaneous reservoir. Kuzmak's reported that weight loss results and complication rates are better than those observed after other banding techniques in which strips of polypropylene or Teflon are used.

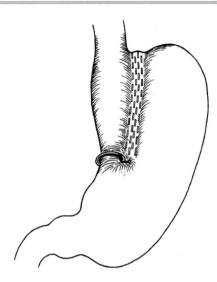

Figure 5 Vertical Silastic ring gastroplasty in which the 15 to 20 mL capacity upper gastric pouch empties through a 5 cm circumference Silastic ring. The ring is secured at the distal end of the vertical staple-line using a heavy suture of either nylon or polypropylene. *Source*: From Ref. 24.

Complication rates with the European techniques of gastric banding have been relatively high with morbidity and mortality rates in the range of 30% and 3%, respectively. Stenosis and/or erosion of the band have been reported in 10% to 30% of cases. Stenosis and erosion can result in leaks and stomal obstruction, which frequently require reoperation. Kuzmak has not reported erosion of his inflatable silicone band. However, problems with the subcutaneous reservoir are common.

Gastric Bypass

Gastric bypass combines gastric restriction with a small amount of malabsorption. However, malabsorption of protein, carbohydrate, and fat has not been reported after

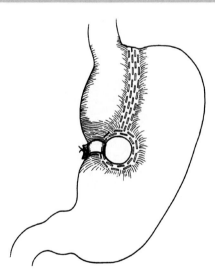

Figure 4 Vertical-banded gastroplasty in which the upper gastric pouch, measured at 15 to 20 mL capacity, empties into the remainder of the stomach through a calibrated stoma. The stoma is reinforced with a strip of polypropylene (Marlex) mesh measuring 5 cm in circumference resulting in a 1.6 cm internal diameter stoma. The mesh is placed around the stoma through a "window" created by firing a circular stapling instrument alongside a No. 32 French diameter bougie. The mesh is sutured to itself rather than the stomach, a modification that has reduced the incidence of outlet stricture and leaks. *Source*: From Ref. 24.

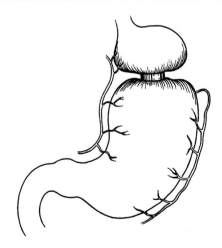

Figure 6 Gastric banding in which the upper portion of the stomach is encircled by a calibrated prosthetic band. The volume of the stomach above the band is crudely estimated by most surgeons who perform this operation. *Source*: From Ref. 24.

conventional gastric bypass. The anatomic parameters required for successful weight loss with gastric bypass were defined by Mason et al. (40) in 1975 and include a small ≤50 mL capacity upper gastric pouch and a ≤1.2 cm diameter gastrojejunostomy stoma. The RYGB, shown in Figure 7, is currently the preferred method of almost every surgeon who performs gastric bypass. Further, a number of surgeons are now transecting the upper stomach rather than stapling it in continuity.

The postoperative complication rates and weight loss observed with current modifications of RYGB improved substantially during the 1980s. In 1984, Flickinger et al. (42) reported a 10% complication rate and two deaths (1%) in a series of 210 consecutive RYGB patients. Sugerman et al. (43) reported a 5% morbidity rate and no mortality in their series of 182 patients who had RYGB. Yale (44) reported two deaths (0.8%) and a 10% incidence of major early postoperative complications in a series of 251 gastric bypass operations.

Gastric bypass occasionally produces symptoms of the "dumping syndrome," which include nausea, bloating, diarrhea, and colic. Dumping is thought to be due to rapid emptying of the small gastric pouch directly into the small bowel. Symptoms of "late" dumping such as light-headedness, palpitations, and sweating also occur in a smaller percentage of patients. These vasomotor symptoms are the consequence of rebound hypoglycemia and typically occur one to two hours after ingestion of a carbohydrate-laden meal. After gastric bypass, the incidence of dumping is variable with some patients reporting no symptoms, others having symptoms associated with eating specific foods such as milk products or sweets, and a few patients who report troublesome symptoms after almost every meal.

Biliopancreatic Bypass

Biliopancreatic bypass (BPB), also known as distal gastric bypass, is an operation that combines a modest amount of gastric restriction with a substantial amount of malabsorption. The concept of BPB was introduced by Scopinaro in the late 1970s. An early modification of this procedure is shown in Figure 8.

The technique includes performance of a subtotal gastrectomy leaving an approximately 250 to 500 mL capacity gastric remnant, which is anastomosed to the proximal ileum. All the jejunum is excluded from digestive continuity and is anastomosed end to side to a "common channel" of ileum at a point between 50 and 100 cm proximal to the ileocecal junction. Because this degree of malabsorption predisposes to cholelithiasis, cholecystectomy is also an integral part of the operation. Scopinaro et al. (45) have modified his original operation several times to further reduce gastric capacity to ≤200 mL in superobese patients (the so-called very little stomach modification) and has lengthened the "common channel" in less obese patients to reduce the incidence of malabsorption-related sequelae. Sugerman et al. (46) suggested that there is no need to perform gastrectomy as part of BPB, and recommended stapling the stomach in continuity.

The incidence of early postoperative complications after BPB has been in the range of 10% to 15% with a 1% mortality rate (45,47). However, the incidence of metabolic complications within the first postoperative year has been high, including a 30% incidence of anemia, an 8% to 10% incidence of marginal ulcers, and a 20% incidence of hospitalization for treatment of protein-calorie malnutrition (45). As malabsorption is the primary source of both weight loss and weight maintenance, diarrhea and foul-smelling stools are common in patients after BPB has been performed.

An operation that was initially described for the management of duodenogastric reflux has been adapted for the

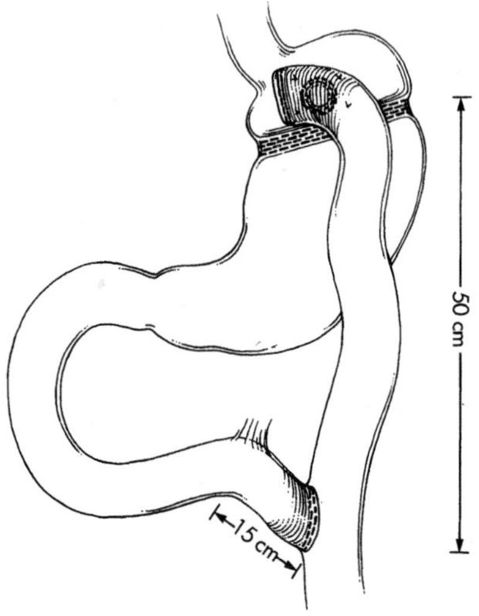

Figure 7   Roux-en-Y gastric bypass in which the TA 90B stapler (U.S. Surgical Corp., Norwalk, Connecticut, U.S.) is fired across the cardia of the stomach creating a 25±5 mL upper pouch. The jejunum is divided approximately 15 cm distal to the ligament of Treitz with the distal end anastomosed to the upper stomach using a circular stapler to create a 1.1 cm diameter anastomosis. The proximal end of jejunum is then anastomosed 50 cm below the gastrojejunostomy. *Source:* From Ref. 42.

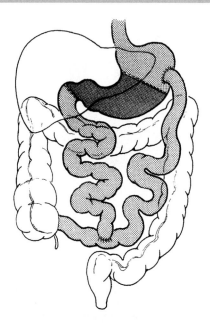

Figure 8   Biliopancreatic bypass in which the small bowel below the ligament of Treitz is bisected with the distal end of transected bowel anastomosed to the upper stomach and the proximal end anastomosed end to side to the "common channel" of distal ileum 50 cm proximal to the ileocecal junction. The distal stomach (*shaded in black*) is either resected (Scopinaro technique) or stapled in continuity. *Source:* From Ref. 24.

treatment of morbid obesity by Marceau et al. (48) This modification shown in Figure 9 combines a "parietal" gastrectomy with biliopancreatic diversion. Because the functional portion of the duodenum is diverted from digestive continuity, this procedure has been dubbed the "duodenal switch." The primary goal of this modification is reduction in the incidence of the serious metabolic sequelae that are associated with BPB. The so-called "parietal" gastrectomy preserves the pylorus and the vagal innervation along the lesser curvature, which in theory would facilitate both gastric emptying and vitamin B12 absorption. Elimination of the gastroenteric anastomosis might be expected to reduce the incidence of marginal ulcers. As one-third of the stomach is left intact, restriction of oral intake does not play a prominent role in postoperative weight loss.

Of the open procedures listed above, gastric bypass gained the most popularity in the United States. It was favored mostly because of the maintained weight loss that patients achieved long term. A study by Sugerman et al. (49) comparing gastric bypass with VBG showed significantly superior results from bypass surgery. The results revealed an average of 37% weight loss among the banding population compared to 64% among the bypass population at three years (49). Furthermore, a study from the Mayo Clinic looking at long-term results of VBG showed only a 26% success rate at 10 years follow-up (50). It is not surprising, therefore, that in a survey of the membership of the

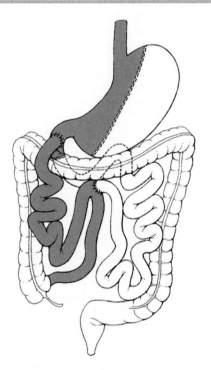

Figure 9 In a duodenal switch, two-thirds of the stomach is excised along the greater curvature using linear staplers. The duodenum is dissected from the head of the pancreas for a distance of 5 cm beyond the pylorus and stapled in continuity at that point. The ileum is then transected at a point 250 cm proximal to the ileocecal junction. The distal end of the transected ileum is anastomosed to the proximal duodenum using two layers of sutures. The remainder of the duodenum and proximal small bowel (*unshaded portion*) is diverted from the digestive stream. The distal end of the bypassed segment is reanastomosed to the ileum 100 cm proximal to the ileocecal junction to create the common channel.

Table 2 Common Surgeries for Morbid Obesity

Operation	Frequency performed (% of total)
RYGB	70
Biliopancreatic diversion	12
VBG	7
Gastric banding	5
Silastic ring gastroplasty	4
Laparoscopic bariatric surgery	3

Abbreviations: VBG, vertical banded gastroplasty; RYGB, Roux-en-Y gastric bypass.
Source: Courtesy of American Society of Bariatric Surgery, 1999.

American Society of Bariatric Surgery in 1999, 70% chose RYGB, while only 7% performed VBG (Table 2).

Laparoscopic Operations

The application of laparoscopic techniques to bariatric surgery is, by far, the most important advancement over the last decade. Laparoscopic approaches to bariatric surgery emerged in the early to mid-nineties. Because of the inherent technical difficulties of the procedures, especially gastric bypass, they did not gain widespread acceptance until the latter part of the decade. In fact, most centers where laparoscopic procedures are now common place went through a transition period using such bridging procedures as hand-assisted laparoscopic gastric bypass. Mirroring the results of the open techniques, lap gastric bypass, and lap gastric banding have emerged as the two most popular operations.

Interestingly, lap gastric banding is the preferred operation among most European centers, whereas lap gastric bypass has emerged as the operation of choice in the United States. Regardless of the choice of operation, laparoscopic surgery lends itself ideally to the morbidly obese population. In terms of technical difficulty, there is a long learning curve, especially for gastric bypass. Schauer et al. reported the learning curve as being 100 cases (51). Once the learning curve is overcome, the results from laparoscopic gastric bypass have so far been shown to be equivalent to those obtained with the open technique, which is the established gold standard. Moreover, with the minimally invasive approach, some of the short- and long-term complications associated with RYGB, most notably wound infections and incisional hernias, are diminished.

Laparoscopic Gastric Banding

Much like the open procedure, laparoscopic gastric banding is a purely restrictive procedure that involves the creation of a gastric pouch using an inflatable band with an adjustable subcutaneous reservoir buried in the abdominal wall. The reservoir is accessed and inflated with saline. Adjustments in the reservoir lead to tightening or releasing of the band, allowing adjustment of the luminal diameter of the band to decrease side effects or enhance weight loss. Again, this procedure is ideally suited for the minimally invasive approach in that it is technically easy and circumvents the complications associated with the open technique. In addition, one of its features is that it is totally reversible. This is currently the favored procedure in Europe and Australia where published series have shown comparable results to open banding (52–55). In the United States, the experience is much more limited with the Food and Drug Administration (FDA) approving the LAP-BAND in June 2001. The initial FDA-approved trials could not reproduce the data from studies elsewhere in the world (56). However, in a review by Ren et al. (57) of 500 LAP-BAND cases not included in the FDA trials, the percent excessive weight loss at nine months was 35.6% and at 12 months it was 41.6%. The study also had similar complication rates to those cited in the world literature (57). The general consensus is that laparoscopic gastric banding is a safe and effective procedure, though it fails at achieving the weight loss seen with gastric bypass.

Laparoscopic Gastric Bypass

As opposed to lap gastric banding, there is a lot of data from the United States on laparoscopic bypass. This is the procedure that has gained the widest acceptance in the circles of U.S. bariatric surgery. The operation itself is an adaptation of the open RYGB with minor modifications. The initial results from lap gastric bypass have shown a steep learning curve with higher complication rates. However, with time, the complication rates have been reduced to those seen in open gastric bypass. This is clearly demonstrated in several studies, an example of which was published by Demaria et al. of their first 281 consecutive laparoscopic gastric bypasses (58). In that series, the overall mortality was 0, with a leak rate of 5.1%. However, the leak rate for the last 164 patients and after modification of the gastrojejunostomy technique was only 1.8% (comparable to open RYGBP).

The results of laparoscopic gastric bypass have been very promising. The average excess weight loss is around 65% to 80% for most large series, which is comparable to the open technique. Improvement in comorbidities is most notable among type 2 diabetics, with resolution in about 85% of the patients. Anastomotic leak rate is around 2%, which again compares well to open gastric bypass. The reported mortality rate is around 0.2%. The most commonly reported complications were bowel obstruction and stomal stenosis in 3.1% and 4.7%, respectively. Wound complications of open gastric bypass, including wound infection and hernias, have been virtually eliminated by the laparoscopic technique (59). Conversion to open gastric bypass occurs in about 1.5%. Hospital stay is in the range of two to three days.

The operation is performed through five ports, and is essentially the same as the open procedure except that the stomach is usually divided and the jejunal limb is brought up in a retrocolic, retrogastric fashion. The gastrojejunostomy can be done with either a circular stapling device or can be performed in two layers, with an inner linear staple layer and an outer suture layer. The jejunojejunostomy is a stapled anastomosis.

PATIENT MANAGEMENT
Preoperative Patient Selection

All candidates for obesity operations should be interviewed in an outpatient setting prior to operation. During that interview, the surgeon should provide prospective patients with a clear understanding of the risks and goals of the operation as well as explain the mechanism by which the procedure produces weight loss. At the same time, the surgeon should obtain a complete medical history and make a preliminary assessment of a patient's operative risk. Psychologic stability should also be evaluated, particularly in terms of the patient's willingness to adjust to the permanent postoperative side effects of gastric restriction and malabsorption. At the conclusion of the interview, the patient should have obtained sufficient information to give informed consent.

Standard criteria used in selecting patients for obesity operations are shown in Table 3. Minimum weight limits for

Table 3   Criteria for Patient Selection

1. Weight
    a. 100 pounds or 100% above desirable weight
    b. BMI $\geq$ 40 kg/m^2
    c. BMI $\geq$ 35 kg/m^2 with coexisting medical problems
2. Failure of nonsurgical methods of weight reduction
3. Absence of endocrine disorders that can cause massive obesity
4. Psychologic stability
    a. Basic understanding of how surgery causes weight loss
    b. Realization that surgery itself cannot guarantee a good result
    c. Absence of alcohol and drug abuse

Abbreviation: BMI, body mass index.

surgical treatment of severe obesity were traditionally established in the range of 100 pounds or 100% above desirable weight as defined by standard life insurance tables. The 1991 NIH Consensus Development Panel (4) on gastrointestinal surgery for severe obesity suggested using the BMI rather than absolute body weight in evaluation of potential surgical candidates. The panel recommended that surgical treatment be considered for any patient with a BMI of 40 kg/m^2, who had failed serious attempts at nonsurgical treatment (4). The panel also recommended that surgery be considered for patients with a BMI of 35 kg/m^2, who have serious coexisting medical problems such as diabetes, hypertension, hyperlipidemia, or sleep apnea (4).

There are relatively few endocrine disorders that cause massive obesity. Although hypothyroidism is associated with both a decreased metabolic rate and obesity, it is virtually never the sole cause of morbid obesity. Hence, hypothyroidism is not a contraindication for obesity surgery. Conversely, Cushing's disease may occasionally cause massive obesity. Because successful treatment of Cushing's disease likely results in substantial weight loss, patients with untreated Cushing's disease should not undergo operations designed for treatment of morbid obesity. Adult-onset diabetes mellitus (AODM) is almost invariably associated with obesity. However, unlike Cushing's disease, AODM is effectively treated by weight reduction. Hence, AODM is considered an indication for obesity surgery.

Although patients with morbid obesity have been shown to have similar psychologic profiles to their normal weight counterparts, the psychologic stability of surgical candidates should be considered prior to operation. Although standardized psychologic tests and separate screening interviews with psychologists or psychiatrists have not proven useful in predicting postoperative outcome of obesity operations, a formal psychologic evaluation of patients with a documented history of mental illness is recommended. Patients should also be carefully queried regarding abuse of addictive drugs and alcohol prior to operation. All patients who undergo surgical treatment of obesity should be admonished that sustained long-term weight loss is not guaranteed merely by having an operation. This understanding is particularly important for patients who have gastric restrictive operations, which can be defeated by consuming large quantities of high-calorie liquids and soft junk foods.

Preoperative and Postoperative Care

Routine preadmission tests include a complete blood count, chem-21 screen, urinalysis, blood typing, chest X ray, electrocardiogram, and ultrasound of the gallbladder. An active peptic ulcer represents an absolute contraindication for bariatric surgery. It used to be routine to perform an upper gastrointestinal study to rule out ulcers. The current standard however is to screen for *Helicobacter pylori* and irradicate it if present. Because the incidence of cholelithiasis is 15% to 25% in morbidly obese patients, preoperative or intraopertaive screening for gallstones is recommended in all patients who have not had cholecystectomy. Ultrasonography is the most popular method of evaluation. Intraoperative ultrasonography is considered to be more sensitive than transabdominal examination in the morbidly obese. We recommend concomitant cholecystectomy for all patients with cholelithiasis. The association of obesity with sleep apnea also requires some attention. A room air arterial blood gas is therefore obtained in the clinic from all patients who are at high risk for having concomitant sleep apnea.

Patients who are scheduled to have gastric bypass or BPB operations should also have serum iron, iron-binding capacity, vitamin B12, and folate levels determined prior to operation. Baseline serum levels of fat-soluble vitamins should be obtained in patients prior to BPB. All patients who are scheduled to have revision of a failed bariatric procedure should have blood cross-matched for possible transfusion. Blood transfusion is necessary in nearly 50% of patients who undergo revision of failed gastric restrictive operations.

Preoperative preparation of patients for bariatric operations varies according to the underlying health of individual patients. Many young patients with no associated illnesses can be admitted to the hospital on the day of operation. Conversely, patients with severe sleep apnea syndrome or congestive heart failure require hospitalization for two or three days prior to operation to optimize their cardiopulmonary condition. Insertion of a Swan-Ganz catheter on the day prior to operation is advisable in many of these patients. All patients should be given intravenous prophylactic antibiotics in the perioperative period.

Morbidly obese patients tolerate general anesthesia remarkably well. However, endotracheal intubation may be difficult, particularly in patients who weigh more than 400 pounds. Awake intubation using intravenous sedation and topical pharyngeal anesthesia is often the safest way to establish an airway in the heaviest patients. Although an arterial line is not required during most bariatric operations, it is useful in some patients both for intraoperative blood pressure monitoring and for drawing blood for blood gases both during and following the operation.

A Foley catheter and nasogastric tube are inserted in all patients after induction of anesthesia. The Foley catheter is generally removed on the first postoperative day in all patients who spend their first night in the hospital. The nasogastric tube is helpful in identifying the gastroesophageal junction intraoperatively and is now routinely removed during the end of the case except in rare situations.

Less than 10% of patients require admission to the intensive care unit postoperatively. However, all patients with sleep apnea, congestive heart failure, and severe asthmatic bronchitis should spend one or two nights in the intensive care unit for close monitoring of their cardiopulmonary status. Many of these patients require overnight intubation. Incentive spirometry is used routinely for several days after extubation. Clinically significant atelectasis is remarkably uncommon in these patients postoperatively.

Obesity has traditionally been considered as a risk factor for postoperative pulmonary embolism. Hence, a variety of methods of prophylaxis have been employed toward prevention of this feared complication. These include subcutaneous low-dose heparin, pneumatic compression of the legs, elastic stockings or bandages, intravenous low-molecular weight dextran, and use of the Trendelenburg position intraoperatively. None of these methods have been proven to decrease the incidence of postoperative venous thromboembolism in bariatric surgical patients. Early postoperative ambulation is strongly encouraged and almost certainly contributes toward the low incidence of postoperative venous thromboembolism that has been reported in these patients. Patients are assisted in getting out of bed on the night of their operation and are walked on the first postoperative day. It is interesting to note that many of these patients move remarkably well.

Incisional pain is moderately severe during the first 48 to 72 hours postoperatively. This is obviously less severe with laparoscopic procedures. Nonetheless, patients are routinely maintained on narcotics via a patient-controlled analgesia pump in the first 24 hours. Oral narcotics are usually begun on the second or third postoperative day after intravenous fluids have been stopped. All pills and tablets are crushed and administered as a slurry with a liquid beverage. Patients are instructed not to swallow whole pills during the first four weeks postoperatively.

Ice chips and sips of water are given orally on postop day 1. Intravenous fluids are usually discontinued after clear liquids are tolerated without difficulty. A low calorie (maximum 1000 cal) pureed consistency diet is given on the next day and is continued until the time of discharge. Patients are usually discharged on the third postoperative day. Hospitalization for more than seven days is unusual in the absence of major complications. A limited upper gastrointestinal tract contrast study previously was routinely performed shortly before discharge, to examine the integrity of the staple-line and outlet stoma. This is only performed in cases with a high index of suspicion for a leak, or those who manifest signs and symptoms of a leak.

Postoperative Dietary Management and Follow-Up

Postoperative dietary counseling is essential in the long-term success of gastric restrictive operations. Patients are instructed to follow a modified liquid diet for four weeks after discharge. The modified liquid diet consists of liquids, pureed foods, and several soft solid foods such as mashed potatoes and cottage cheese. A liquid or chewable multivitamin supplement is taken during this phase of the diet. The purpose of the modified liquid diet is twofold: (i) to allow time for patients to adjust to their tremendously restricted stomach capacity by consuming foods that are relatively easy to chew and swallow and (ii) to minimize the likelihood of vomiting in the early postoperative period. Repeated episodes of vomiting in the early postoperative period have been associated with staple-line disruption and leaks. Patients are given a soft solid diet at the four-week visit and then gradually progress to a normal diet. Patients can resume swallowing whole pills and tablets after solid food is well tolerated.

Postoperative follow-up is extremely important in bariatric surgical patients. All patients should have easy access to the operating surgeon and a clinical nutritionist. During the first year visits are scheduled at four weeks postoperatively and then at three-month intervals thereafter. Two follow-up visits are scheduled at six-month intervals during the second year. After the second year, all bariatric surgical patients should be followed indefinitely by annual physician office visits. However, some patients may require more frequent follow-up. Weight and blood pressure should be recorded at each visit along with the laboratory studies, which are needed to check for postoperative metabolic sequelae and to follow up preoperative medical problems such as diabetes or hyperlipidemia.

Patients who have malabsorptive operations require periodic blood tests postoperatively to check for possible metabolic and nutritional deficiencies. These patients should take a daily multivitamin supplement with minerals for the rest of their lives. Menstruating women who have had gastric bypass or BPB should also take a prophylactic iron supplement postoperatively. After BPB, many patients require additional protein and other nutritional supplements.

RESULTS OF SURGICAL TREATMENT
Weight Loss
Early weight loss results with both VBG and SRG have been generally acceptable. Mason et al. (38) reported a mean loss of 62% of excess weight in a series of 226 patients followed for a mean five years after VBG. MacLean et al. (7) reported a mean 60% excess weight loss in 57 patients followed for five years after VBG. However, a substantial number of their patients required surgical revision for either complications or inadequate weight loss during the five-year study period. Willbanks (37) reported a mean 61% excess weight loss in his series of 305-SRG patients who were followed for a minimum of two years. Weight loss maintenance after VBG and SRG has been somewhat problematic, in that many patients regain at least 15% to 20% of their lost weight between three and five years postoperatively.

Open gastric banding has given way to laparoscopic gastric banding. Most large series are reported from Europe and reveal a 40% to 60% mean EWL over three to five years (52–55). The U.S. experience with LAP-BAND is much more limited and has not consistently reproduced the results seen in the larger European trials (56).

Weight loss results with RYGB have been generally superior to those observed after other gastric restrictive operations. Studies over the last two decades regarding open gastric bypass have consistently shown a better maintained weight loss with most large series showing an average of 49% to 80% EWL over 5 to 15 years (60–66).

Weight loss results with BPB have been almost uniformly good. Scopinaro et al. (45) reported a mean loss of 75% of the preoperative weight in a series of 916 patients followed for a mean five years with excellent weight maintenance after stabilization. Sugerman et al. (46) reported a mean 71% excess weight loss at one year in their series of 25 superobese patients. Early weight loss results with the "duodenal switch" have been comparable to those reported after BPB.

Over the years, there have been several prospective comparisons of bariatric procedures that have shown significant differences between operations both in terms of weight loss outcome and in terms of the incidence of postoperative complications. Pories et al. (66), Naslund et al. (67), and Lechner and Callender (68) independently performed prospective randomized comparisons of horizontal gastroplasty with gastric bypass and reported significantly better weight loss after gastric bypass and no difference in the early complication rate between the two procedures. Sugerman et al. (69) prospectively compared VBG with RYGB and again found that gastric bypass resulted in significantly greater weight loss. Surgeons from Adelaide, Australia prospectively compared gastrogastrostomy, vertical gastroplasty, and RYGB in 310 patients (70). At five

years postoperatively, weight loss after gastric bypass was significantly greater than with either gastroplasty or gastrogastrostomy. The early postoperative complication rates were similar among the three procedures. These prospective studies clearly show that gastric bypass is a better weight loss–producing operation than any modification of gastroplasty.

Sugerman et al. (46) prospectively compared conventional RYGB with Scopinaro's BPB in a group of superobese patients and found that weight loss was significantly better at one year after BPB. However, because the incidence of serious complications was considerably higher after BPB, Sugerman et al. concluded that BPB was too risky to be recommended as a primary procedure for treatment of morbid obesity (46).

Successful weight loss in superobese patients has generally been problematic after conventional gastroplasty and gastric bypass procedures. Two reports have described modifications of conventional operations with the goal of improving long-term weight loss (6,71). One study employed a "long-limb" modification of RYGB in which the Roux limb length was measured at 150 cm. The long-limb modification was prospectively compared with a standard technique of gastric bypass and resulted in significantly greater weight loss versus the conventional method after 12 months postoperatively (6). Another investigator proposed a two-stage approach consisting of a jejunocolic bypass at the outset, which was subsequently converted to a VBG after weight stabilization (71). This two-stage method resulted in excellent weight loss in a group of eight superobese patients. It appears that some degree of intestinal malabsorption is necessary to achieve satisfactory weight loss in these extremely heavy patients.

The results from laparoscopic RYGBP have been just as good as those obtained from open gastric bypass. The largest series so far by Higa et al. (72) reports an excess weight loss of 70% at 12 months. These figures are reproduced in all the large series so far published (58,59,73,74). These results are shown in Table 4.

Amelioration of Comorbidities
Amelioration of obesity-related medical problems is a primary goal of all bariatric operations. Improvement or resolution of morbid obesity-associated diabetes, including a significant decrease in insulin resistance after weight reduction surgery, has been reported by many investigators (63,75–77). Pories et al. (63,76) have extensively studied postoperative changes in glucose metabolism in morbidly obese patients with diabetes. In 1995, they reported that 121 of 146 (82.9%) patients with overt type 2 diabetes became euglycemic after RYGB (63). Moreover, 98.7% (150 of 152 patients) with glucose impairment maintained normal levels of blood glucose, glycosylated hemoglobin, and insulin (63).

Weight reduction surgery also has salutary effects on obesity-related hypertension and cardiovascular dysfunction.

Table 4 Weight Loss Results Using Laparoscopic Gastric Bypass

Author	N	BMI (mean)	Follow-up (months)	Excess weight loss (%)
Demaria (59)	281	48	12	70
Higa (73)	1040	46	12	70
Schauer (74)	275	48	30	77
Wittgrove (75)	500	NI	60	73

Abbreviation: BMI, body mass index.

Alpert et al. (78) used echocardiography to measure a number of parameters of ventricular function in 62 morbidly obese patients and found that surgically induced weight loss was associated with significant improvement of left ventricular ejection fraction and lesser, but measurable improvements in mean blood pressure, cardiac chamber size, and ventricular wall thickness.

Sugerman et al. (77) queried their database of 1025 patients between 1981 and 2000. They showed a 69% resolution of hypertension at one year and 66% at five to seven years. The response of hypertension to weight loss following gastric restrictive operations was also reported by two other groups of investigators (79,80). Each group defined hypertension as a blood pressure reading ≥160/90 and noted improvement or resolution of hypertension in approximately 70% of patients at four years postoperatively. However, there were conflicting results regarding the relationship between blood pressure reduction and weight loss, with one group showing a correlation between blood pressure improvement and the amount of weight loss (79) and the other reporting a significant correlation between improved blood pressure and proximity to ideal weight after weight stabilization (80).

The beneficial effects of weight reduction surgery on obesity-related hyperlipidemia have been documented by a number of investigators. Gleysteen et al. (81), Rucker et al. (82), Nanji and Freeman (83), and Gonen et al. (84) independently reported significant decreases in both total cholesterol and triglyceride levels after gastric restrictive operations for morbid obesity. They also showed a favorable increase in the high-density lipoprotein/low-density lipoprotein ratio after gastric bypass, suggesting that the risk of atherosclerosis may be decreased by weight loss in this group of patients. Gleysteen et al. (81) have shown that these lipid reductions persist for as long as weight loss is satisfactorily maintained. Conversely, patients who regain a substantial portion of their lost weight tend to have concomitant regression of the salutary changes in lipid profile.

The obesity hypoventilation syndrome probably poses the greatest immediate risk to life of any of the obesity-related medical illnesses. Following gastric restrictive operations, Sugerman et al. (85) and Charuzi et al. (86) have independently reported complete resolution of sleep apnea symptoms and significant improvements in both arterial blood gases and polysonmographic studies. Sugerman et al. (85) also reported significant reductions in mean pulmonary artery pressures in patients with obesity hypoventilation syndrome between three and nine months after RYGB. Many patients in these reports were incapacitated by their condition preoperatively, but after losing weight were able to lead normal and productive lives.

Weight loss has a salutary effect on sex hormone balance and fertility in women. After gastroplasty-induced weight loss, Grace et al. (16) and Deitel (17) independently reported significant improvement in SHBG levels and a significantly decreased incidence of irregular menses. Both androgen levels and hirsutism decreased with substantial weight loss. A number of previously infertile women became pregnant and delivered normal babies, following surgically induced weight loss. Printen and Scott (87) reported similar results after gastric bypass. Although these women are able to eat only small amounts, adequate nutritional status can be maintained for both the mother and the developing fetus. Pregnancy is not recommended during the first postoperative year in which the great majority of weight loss occurs

Postoperative Complications

In experienced hands, bariatric operations can be performed with anticipation of a perioperative morbidity rate of under 10% and a mortality rate of approximately 1%. The advent of laparoscopic techniques was at first faced with a higher incidence of complications due to the learning curve, especially with gastric bypass. With time and experience, the laparoscopic approach has proven superior as it is associated with fewer wound-associated complications (58,59,72–74).

Early Complications

The most serious early complications are gastrointestinal tract anastomotic leak and pulmonary embolism. Fortunately, the incidence of these two serious problems is reported in the range of 1% to 2% in most large series of bariatric operations (41,43,44,88–90). The incidence of pulmonary embolism does not seem to be altered by the routine use of intermittent decompression stockings or subcutaneous heparin. However, nearly all bariatric surgeons use some method of deep venous thrombosis prophylaxis in the perioperative period. Early postoperative ambulation is always emphasized and is surprisingly well tolerated by most patients.

Gastrointestinal tract leaks can be difficult to recognize after gastric restrictive procedures, because fever and abdominal tenderness are frequently absent during the first 48 hours after a leak has occurred. Persistent tachycardia and progressive tachypnea are the most common early signs. Hence, it is not unusual to initially suspect pulmonary embolism in a patient with a gastric leak. However, a ventilation-perfusion scan is generally interpreted as "low probability" for pulmonary embolism. An isolated left-sided pleural effusion is a common finding on the plain chest radiograph. Most surgeons initially attempt to identify leaks using radiographic gastrointestinal tract contrast studies. However, a normal result from contrast study by no means excludes the diagnosis, because leaks from the gastric staple-line are usually not identified by upper gastrointestinal tract contrast studies. Because failure to recognize a leak can result in death, exploratory laparotomy should be empirically performed in patients with progressive tachypnea and tachycardia in whom pulmonary embolism has been ruled out. This approach has been modified in the laparoscopic population in whom a drain is routinely placed posterior to the anastomosis, with one-third of these patients not requiring any further intervention, one-third undergoing laparoscopic drainage and one-third undergoing laparotomy (58).

Although severe obesity is reported to be associated with a high incidence of postoperative wound problems, in experienced hands, the incidence of major wound infection after gastric restrictive operations is reported in the range of 1% to 3% (41,43,44). The potential for wound dehiscence after bariatric operations is increased because of the great tension placed on the wound closure by massive overweight. Hence, the abdominal fascia should be closed with heavy absorbable or nonabsorbable suture. Again, this has not been a problem with the laparoscopic techniques.

Late Complications

Previous studies have documented a high incidence of gallstone formation following rapid weight loss in obese patients. The incidence of symptomatic gallbladder disease reported after gastric restrictive operations varies from 3% to greater than 30% (91). Hence, removing the gallbladder "prophylactically" at the time of gastric restrictive surgery is a controversial issue among bariatric surgeons. Several surgeons who have recommended prophylactic cholecystectomy report histologic evidence of gallbladder pathology in nearly 90% of cases. Other surgeons believe that the incidence of symptomatic cholecystitis after gastric restrictive operations is not high enough to justify routine removal of the gallbladder in patients who do not have gallstones. Scopinaro et al. (45) have recommended cholecystectomy as an integral part of BPB, because more than 50% of the patients in his early experience developed symptomatic gallstones. The risks of adding cholecystectomy to an elective gastric restrictive procedure are negligible.

A multicenter, randomized, double-blind, prospective trial evaluated three oral doses of ursodiol (Actigall) versus placebo during the first six months after RYGB (92). Of 233 patients who had postoperative ultrasonography, gallstones formed in 32% of the placebo group versus 4% of the higher-dose treatment groups. The investigators concluded that ursodiol at doses of 600 and 1200 mg/day was effective in preventing cholelithiasis during the rapid weight-loss phase after gastric bypass.

Although vomiting is a common side effect of most gastric restrictive operations, severe, intractable vomiting is quite rare. Most cases of severe vomiting have followed banded gastric restrictive operations and are usually caused by stenosis of the outlet stoma. Patients with vomiting who cannot tolerate liquids should be hospitalized and given intravenous fluids. In most cases, the stomal edema that results from protracted vomiting resolves without further intervention. Patients who cannot tolerate liquids after several days of nothing by mouth and intravenous fluids should undergo upper endoscopy and stomal dilation using balloon-tipped catheters. Stomal dilation is almost always successful in patients after RYGB, but is more problematic in patients with prosthetic stomal reinforcement.

Many patients report great difficulty with eating meat and fresh fruit and vegetables after banded gastric restrictive operations. Hence, these patients often consume large quantities of soft high-calorie foods such as cookies, chips, and ice cream.

Incisional hernia is a common late complication after gastric restrictive operations, with an incidence ranging from 10% to 15%, in most large series of open RYGB. Again, this is a rarely encountered complication after laparoscopic RYGB. The incidence of marginal ulcer in patients after RYGB and BPB ranges from 3% to 10%. These ulcers typically develop on the jejunal side of the gastroenterostomy and are caused by excessive production of gastric acid. Serum gastrin levels are normal or subnormal. This potentially serious complication has been associated with breakdown of the gastric staple-line after RYGB (89). Marginal ulcers that are not associated with disruption of the stapled gastric partition almost always respond to H2 blocking drugs or pump inhibitors. Conversely, ulcers that occur in patients with staple-line breakdown are often intractable to medications and require operative treatment.

Patients who have either RYGB or BPB are at risk for developing metabolic sequelae as a consequence of malabsorption. Table 5 shows the incidence of metabolic complications typically associated with gastric bypass (15,90,93). Because iron absorption occurs primarily in the duodenum, malabsorption of ingested iron is the primary cause of iron deficiency after gastric bypass. Smith et al. (94) demonstrated that vitamin B12 deficiency after gastric bypass is the result of failure to cleave food-bound vitamin B12 in the upper gastric pouch. Conversely, crystalline vitamin B12 is absorbed normally in the distal ileum. The cause of folate deficiency after gastric bypass is not known. Deficiencies in each of these micronutrients can result in anemia. Because these deficiencies are relatively common, daily prophylactic multivitamin/mineral supplements are recommended for all patients. However, the efficacy of multivitamin supplements alone in prevention of these deficiencies has not been clearly established.

In our experience, a daily multivitamin supplement does not consistently prevent development of iron deficiency and anemia in women who have had gastric bypass. Fortunately, the majority of vitamin and mineral deficiencies after gastric bypass are mild and easily corrected with oral supplements of the deficient micronutrients. Injection therapy is rarely required in patients who are willing to take oral supplements. Hospitalization for treatment of these deficiencies is extremely uncommon.

Due to the fact that fat malabsorption is a primary component of both the BPB and the duodenal switch, patients who have these procedures are prone to develop deficiencies in fat-soluble vitamins. Sugerman et al. (46) reported a 50% incidence of serious complications, metabolic sequelae, and two deaths during the first year after BPB in a series of 25 superobese patients. More than half of Sugerman's patients had deficiencies in fat-soluble vitamins after BPB. Calcium deficiency and hypoproteinemia have been noted in 10% to 20% of patients after BPB (47). Moreover, approximately 3% of the lighter patients ($<220\%$ overweight) in Scopinaro's series (45) became "underweight" with gross manifestations of malnutrition. Marceau et al. (48) reported a comparative study of the duodenal switch versus conventional BPB, which disclosed significant reductions in the incidence of hypocalcemia, hypoalbuninenemia, anemia, and malodorous flatus in patients who had the duodenal switch.

Revision Operations

Occasionally, bariatric operations require revision for either inadequate weight loss or late complications. The incidence of major postoperative complications following revision of bariatric procedures is high, with reports ranging from 15% to 60%. The mortality rate reported after revision operations ranges from 5% to 30%. Undoing an original bariatric operation without conversion to another weight reduction procedure is invariably associated with prompt regaining of the lost weight. The indication for revision (unsatisfactory weight loss or complications) generally dictates the planned approach.

Table 5 Metabolic Deficiencies after Gastric Bypass[a]

Report/year	Iron	Vitamin B_{12}	Folate	Anemia	Follow-up
Halverson (1981) (91)	20%/17 mo	26%/20 mo	9%/13 mo	18%/–	20 mo
Amaral (1985) (94)	49%/15.6 mo	70%/13 mo	18%/–	35%/20 mo	33.2 mo
Brolin et al. (1990) (16)	33%/13.4 mo	37%/12.8 mo	16%/10.7 mo	22%/12 mo	24.2 mo

[a]The mean incidence and time of deficiency recognition reported in each series are listed in columns 2 through 5 with the mean follow-up shown at far right.

Patients who undergo revision operations for complications frequently have lost a sufficient amount of weight after their initial procedure. These patients should generally be offered a gastric restrictive rather than a malabsorptive procedure. Patients who require takedown of an intestinal bypass for metabolic complications and are no longer overweight are best suited by conversion to a banded gastroplasty for weight maintenance. Conversely, patients who remain substantially overweight after intestinal bypass are best converted to RYGB with the hope of providing further weight loss.

Gastroplasty patients with stornal stenosis and an intact staple-line may initially undergo stomal dilation via upper endoscopy. Unfortunately, because less than 50% of patients with stomal stenosis have permanent relief with dilation, operative revision is frequently required. Revision should include removal of the reinforcing band and conversion to RYGB.

Patients with staple-line disruption after gastroplasty or RYGB need only to have the stomach restapled. After observing a high incidence of subsequent disruption in patients who had restapling in continuity, MacLean et al. (89) recommended transection of the stomach between staple-lines in patients who require reoperation for staple-line breakdown. Patients with unsatisfactory weight loss after gastroplasty are best converted to PYGB or, in some cases, BPB.

Patients with anatomically intact operations and unsatisfactory weight loss after gastric bypass have almost certainly "outeaten" the operation. These patients may be converted to a BPB with anticipation of further weight loss. Unfortunately, patients with intact gastric restrictive operations who are converted to BPB frequently suffer severe metabolic complications. At present, many surgeons believe that BPB should only be used in revision of patients with unsatisfactory weight loss after an anatomically intact banded gastroplasty or gastric bypass (95,96). There are also a small number of morbidly obese patients who outeat any bariatric operation or die trying. Whenever a patient has failed a second technically sound and intact operation, surgeons should approach the prospect of a further revision with considerable caution and skepticism. Rejection of such patients for another operation is frequently a prudent decision.

Quality of Life Changes

Nearly all morbidly obese patients with satisfactory postoperative weight loss experience substantial improvement in their overall lifestyle. Health status is generally markedly improved as characterized by increased exercise tolerance and improvement or resolution of obesity-related comorbidities. Patients' abilities to interact with others in social situations are also enhanced. They are delighted to be able to buy clothes at major department stores, sit comfortably in an airplane seat, or even climb a flight of stairs.

Employment opportunities also increase. Approximately 75% of patients who were receiving public assistance prior to gastric restrictive surgery were able to find full-time jobs at two years postoperatively. Other patients have received promotions in the same workplace, which seemed unattainable prior to losing weight. Weight loss can suddenly make a patient attractive to the opposite sex. However, increased self-esteem and sexual awareness probably results in divorce as often as marriage. Generally, divorce can be viewed as a positive step for these patients, because they are usually leaving a pathologic marriage in which they were "trapped" by their severe obesity.

SUMMARY

As stated at the beginning of this chapter, it is estimated that more than 40% of the U.S. population is clinically overweight. Many of these individuals are clearly obese, and of this subset a substantial number are morbidly obese. Despite attempts at dietary changes as well as lifestyle modifications, the ability to successfully lose weight and keep it lost once morbid obesity has occurred is virtually impossible. Thus, surgery has evolved as an effective treatment option. In the early history of surgical intervention for morbid obesity, jejunoileal bypass was the most popular operation. Although effective in eliciting weight loss, problems with severe malabsorption and metabolic complications quickly demonstrated that it was more harmful than beneficial. At the same time that jejunoileal bypass was falling into disfavor, a variety of gastric restrictive or bypass procedures were demonstrating their ability to initiate weight loss and keep this loss maintained with an acceptable complication rate, most of which were easily managed. As operative strategies have been refined and new technological approaches have evolved, it is now possible to manage morbid obesity using laparoscopic techniques. The minimal complication rates associated with these new procedures have made surgical management of morbid obesity the treatment of choice.

REFERENCES

1. Popkin BM, Udry JR. Adolescent obesity increases significantly in second and third generation US immigrants: The National Longitudinal Study of Adolescent Health. J Nutr 1998; 128:701.
2. Mokdad AH, Serdula MK, Deitz WH, et al. The spread of the obesity epidemic in the United States 1991–1998. JAMA 1999; 282:1519.
3. National Institutes of Health Consensus Development Panel. Health implications of obesity. Ann Intern Med 1985; 103:1073.
4. National Institutes of Health Consensus Development Panel. Gastrointestinal surgery for severe obesity. Am J Clin Nutr 1992; 55(suppl):615.
5. Abraham S, Johnson CL. Prevalence of severe obesity in adults in the United States. Am J Clin Nutr 1980; 33:364.
6. Brolin RE, et al. Long-limb gastric bypass in the super-obese: a prospective randomized study. Ann Surg 1992; 215:387.
7. MacLean LD, Rhode BM, Forse RA. Late results of vertical banded gastroplasty for morbid and super obesity. Surgery 1990; 107:20.
8. Larsson B, et al. Abdominal adipose tissue distribution, obesity and risk of cardiovascular disease and death, 13 year follow up of participants in the study of men born in 1913. Br Med J 1984; 288:1401.
9. Fried SK, Krai JG. Sex differences in regional distribution of fat cell size and lipoprotein lipase activity in morbidly obese patients. Int J Obes 1987; 11:129.
10. Stunkard AJ, et al. An adoption study of human obesity. N Engl J Med 1986; 314:193.
11. Stunkard AJ, Foch TT, Zdenek H. A twin study of human obesity. JAMA 1986; 256:51.
12. Kral JG. Morbid obesity and health risks. Ann Intern Med 1985; 103:1043.
13. Van Itallie TB. Health implications of over-weight and obesity in the United States. Ann Intern Med 1985; 103:983.
14. Drenick EJ, et al. Excessive mortality and causes of death in morbidly obese men. JAMA 1980; 243:443.
15. Brolin RE, et al. Serum lipids after gastric bypass surgery for morbid obesity. Int J Obes 1990; 14:939.
16. Grace DM, Nisker JA, Hammond GL. Changes in menstrual cycle pattern and sex hormone binding after gastroplasty. Abstract presented at the Second Annual Meeting of the American Society for Bariatric Surgery, Iowa City, June 13, 1985.

17. Deitel M. Gynecologic-obstetrics changes after massive weight loss. Abstract presented at the Third Annual Meeting of the American Society for Bariatric Surgery, Iowa City, June 19, 1986.

18. Anderson T, et al. Randomized trial of diet and gastroplasty compared with diet alone in morbid obesity. N Engl J Med 1984; 310:352.

19. Kremen AJ, Linner JH, Nelson CH. An experimental evaluation of nutritional importance of the proximal and distal small intestine. Ann Surg 1954; 140:439.

20. Payne JH, DeWind LT. Surgical treatment of obesity. Am J Surg 1969; 118:141.

21. Salmon PA. The results of small intestinal bypass operations for the treatment of obesity. Surg Gynecol Obstet 1971; 132:965.

22. Scott HW Jr, et al. Results of jejunoileal bypass in two hundred patients with morbid obesity. Surg Gynecol Obstet 1977; 145:661.

23. Brolin RE. In: Levine BA, et al., eds. Current Practice of Surgery. Vol. 3. New York: Churchill Livingstone, 1993.

24. Halverson JD, et al. Jejunoileal bypass. Late metabolic sequelae and weight gain. Am J Surg 1980; 140:347.

25. Starkloff GB, et al. Metabolic intestinal surgery: its complications and management. Arch Surg 1975; 110:652.

26. Passaro E Jr, Drenick EJ, Wilson SE. Bypass enteritis. Am J Surg 1976:131.

27. Drenick EJ, et al. Bypass enteropathy. JAMA 1976; 236:269.

28. Ravitch MM, Brolin RE. The price of weight loss by jejunoileal shunt. Ann Surg 1979; 190:382.

29. Griffen WO Jr, Bivens BA, Bell RM. The decline and fall of the jejunoileal bypass. Surg Gynecol Obstet 1983; 157:301.

30. Hocking MP, et al. Late hepatic histopathology after jejunoileal bypass for morbid obesity. Am J Surg 1981; 141:159.

31. Mason EE, Ito C. Gastric bypass in obesity. Surg Clin North Am 1967; 43:1345.

32. Alden JE. Gastric and jejunoileal bypass: a comparison in the treatment of morbid obesity. Arch Surg 1977; 112:799.

33. Pace WG, et al. Gastric partitioning for morbid obesity. Ann Surg 1979; 190:392.

34. Mason EE. Vertical banded gastroplasty for obesity. Arch Surg 1982; 117:701.

35. Laws HL. Standardized gastroplasty orifice. Am J Surg 1981; 141:393.

36. Eckhout GV, Willbanks OL, Moore JT. Vertical ring gastroplasty for morbid obesity: five year experience with 1463 patients. Am J Surg 1986; 152:713.

37. Willbanks OL. Long-term results of silicone elastomer ring vertical gastroplasty for the treatment of morbid obesity. Surgery 1987:606.

38. Mason EE, et al. Vertical banded gastroplasty (VBG) for treatment of obesity: an eight year review. Abstract presented at the 75th Clinical Congress of the American College of Surgeons, Atlanta, October 17, 1989.

39. Kuzmak LL. Gastric banding. In: Dietel M, ed. Surgery for the Morbidly Obese Patient. Philadelphia: Lea & Febiger, 1989:225.

40. Mason EE, et al. Optimizing results of gastric bypass. Ann Surg 1975; 182:405.

41. Brolin RE, et al. The dilemma of outcome assessment after operations for morbid obesity. Surgery 1989; 105:337.

42. Flickinger EG, et al. The Greenville gastric bypass: progress report at 3 years. Ann Surg 1984; 157:93.

43. Sugerman HJ, et al. Weight loss with vertical banded gastroplasty and Roux-en-Y gastric bypass for morbid obesity with selective versus random assignment. Am J Surg 1989; 157:93.

44. Yale CE. Gastric surgery for morbid obesity: complications and long term weight control. Arch Surg 1989; 124:941.

45. Scopinaro N, et al. Evolution of biliopancreatic bypass. Clin Nutr 1985; 5(suppl):137.

46. Sugerman HJ, et al. Conversion of failed standard to distal gastric bypass for superobesity. J Gastrointest Surg 1997; 1:167.

47. Scopinaro N, et al. Biliopancreatic diversion for obesity. Probl Gen Surg 1992; 9:362.

48. Marceau P, et al. Biliopancreatic diversion with a new type of gastrectomy. Obes Surg 1993; 3:29.

49. Sugerman HJ, Starley JV, Birkenhauer R. A randomized prospective trial on gastric bypass vs vertical banded gastroplasty for morbid obesity and their effects on sweets vs non sweets eaters. Ann Surg 1987; 205:613.

50. Balsiger BM, Poggio JL, Mai J, et al. Ten and more years after vertical banded gastroplasty as primary operation for morbid obesity. J Gastrointest Surg 2000; 4:598.

51. Schauer P, Ikramuddin S, Hamad G, Goursh W. The learning curve for laparoscopic roux en y gastric bypass is 100 cases. Surg Endosc 2003; 17:212.

52. Fielding GA, Rhodes M, Nathanson LK. Laparoscopic gastric banding for morbid obesity: surgical outcomes in 335 cases. Surg Endosc 1999; 13:550.

53. Belachew M, Legrand M, Vincent V, et al. Laparoscopic adjustable gastric banding. World J Surg 1998; 22:995.

54. Dargent J. Laparoscopic adjustable gastric banding: lessons from the first 500 patients in a single institution. Obes Surg 1999; 9:446.

55. O'Brien PE, Brown WA, Smith A, et al. Prospective study of a laparoscopically placed adjustable gastric band in the treatment of morbid obesity. Br J Surg 1999; 86:113.

56. Rubenstein RB. Laparoscopic adjustable gastric banding at a U.S. center with up to 3-year follow-up. Obes Surg 2002; 12: 380–384.

57. Ren CJ, Horgan S, Ponce J. US experience with the LAP-BAND system. Am J Surg 2002; 184:46S.

58. Demaria EJ, Sugerman HJ, Kellum JM, Meador JG, Wolfe LG. Results of 281 consecutive total laparoscopic Roux-en-Y gastric bypasses to treat morbid obesity. Ann Surg 2002; 235:640.

59. Pondos YD, Jiminez JC, Wilson SE, Stevens CM, Nguyen NT. Complications after laparoscopic gastric bypass: a review of 3464 cases. Arch Surg 2003; 138:957.

60. Linner JH. Comparative effectiveness of gastric bypass and gastroplasty. Arch Surg 1982; 117:695.

61. Sugerman HJ, Londrey GL, Kellum JM, et al. Weight loss with vertical banded gastroplasty and Roux -en-Y gastric bypass for morbid obesity with selective vs. random assignment. Am J Surg 1989; 157:93.

62. Brolin RE, Kenler HA, Gorman JH, et al. Long limb gastric bypass in the superobese: a prospective randomized trial; Ann Surg 1991; 215:387.

63. Pories WJ, Swanson MS, Mac Donald KG, et al. Who would have thought it? An operation proves to be the most effective therapy for adult-onset diabetes mellitus. Ann Surg 1995; 222:339.

64. Capella JF, Capella RF. The weight reduction operation of choice: vertical banded gastroplasty or gastric bypass. Am J Surg 1996; 171:74.

65. Fobi MAL, Lee H, Holness R, et al. Gastric bypass operation for obesity. World J Surg 1998; 22:925.

66. Pories WJ, et al. The effectiveness of gastric bypass over gastric partition in morbid obesity. Ann Surg 1982; 196:389.

67. Naslund I, et al. A prospective randomized comparison of gastric bypass and gastroplasty: complications and early results. Acta Chir Scand 1986; 152:681.

68. Lechner GW, Callender K. Subtotal gastric exclusion and gastric partitioning: a randomized prospective comparison of one hundred patients. Surgery 1981; 90:637.

69. Sugerman HJ, Starkey JV, Birkenhauer R. A randomized prospective trial of gastric bypass vs. vertical banded gastroplasty for morbid obesity and their effect on sweets vs. nonsweets eaters. Ann Surg 1987; 205:613.

70. Hall JC, et al. Gastric surgery for morbid obesity. The Adelaide Study. Ann Surg 1990; 211:419.

71. Grant JR. Duke procedure for super-obesity: preliminary report with 3.5 year follow-up. Surgery 1994; 115:718.

72. Higa KD, Boone KB, Ho T. Complications of the laparoscopic Roux-en-Y gastric bypass: 1,040 patients—what have we learned? Obes Surg 2000; 10:509.

73. Schauer PR, Ikramuddin S, Gourash W, Ramanthan R, Luketich J. Outcomes after laparoscopic Roux-en-Y gastric bypass for morbid obesity. Ann Surg 2000; 232:515.

74. Wittgrove AC, Clark GW. Laparoscopic gastric bypass: a five year prospective study of 500 patients followed from 3 to 60 months. Obes Surg 1999; 9:123.

75. Herbst CA, et al. Gastric bariatric operation in insulin-treated adults. Surgery 1984; 95:209.

76. Pories WJ, et al. The control of diabetes mellitus (NIDDM) in the morbidly obese with the Greenville gastric bypass. Ann Surg 1987; 206:316.

77. Sugerman HJ, Wolfe LG, Sica DA, Clore JN. Diabetes and hypertension in severe obesity and effects of gastric bypass-induced weight loss. Ann Surg 2003; 237:751.

78. Alpert MA, Terry BE, Kelly DL. Effect of weight loss on cardiac chamber size, wall thickness and left ventricular function in morbid obesity. Am J Cardiol 1985; 56:783.

79. Foley EF, et al. Impact of gastric restrictive surgery on hypertension in the morbidly obese. Am J Surg 1992; 163:294.

80. Carson JL, et al. The effect of gastric bypass surgery on hypertension in morbidly obese patients. Arch Intern Med 1994; 154:193.

81. Gleysteen JJ, Barboriak JJ, Sasse EA. Sustained coronary-risk factor reduction after gastric bypass for morbid obesity. Am J Clin Nutr 1990; 51:774.

82. Rucker RD, et al. Lipid effects of obesity operations. J Surg Res 1981; 30:229.

83. Nanji AA, Freeman JB. Rate of weight loss after vertical banded gastroplasty in morbid obesity.Relationship to serum lipids and uric acid. Int Surg 1985; 70:323.

84. Gonen B, Halverson JD, Schonfeld G. Lipoprotein levels in morbidly obese patients with massive surgically induced weight loss. Metabolism 1983; 32:492.

85. Sugerman HJ, et al. Hemodynamic dysfunction in obesity-hypoventilation syndrome and the effects of treatment with surgically induced weight loss. Ann Surg 1988; 207:604.

86. Charuzi I, et al. The effect of surgical weight reduction on sleep quality in obesity-related sleep apnea syndrome. Surgery 1985; 97:535.

87. Printen KJ, Scott DS. Pregnancy following gastric bypass for the treatment of morbid obesity. Am Surg 1982; 48:363.

88. Benotti PN, et al. Gastric restrictive operations for morbid obesity. Am J Surg 1989; 157:150.

89. MacLean LD, et al. Results of the surgical treatment of obesity. Am J Surg 1993; 65:155.

90. Halverson JD, et al. Gastric bypass for morbid obesity: a medical-surgical assessment. Ann Surg 1981; 194:152.

91. Amaral JF, Thompson WR. Gallbladder disease in the morbidly obese. Am J Surg 1985; 149:551.

92. Sugerman HJ, et al. Prophylactic ursodiol acid prevents gallstone formation following gastric bypass induced rapid weight loss: a multicenter, placebo controlled, randomized, double-blind, prospective trial. Am J Surg 1994; 169:91.

93. Amaral JF, et al. Prospective hematologic evaluation of gastric exclusion surgery for morbid obesity. Ann Surg 1985; 201:186.

94. Smith CD, et al. Gastric acid secretion and vitamin B-12 absorption after vertical Roux-en-Y gastric bypass for morbid obesity. Ann Surg 1993; 218:91.

95. Linner JH. Comparative effectiveness of gastric bypass and gastroplasty. Arch Surg 1982; 117:695.

96. Flanigan L. Does initial pouch volume influence weight loss results in the Roux-en-Y gastric bypass procedure? Abstract presented at the 6th Annual Meeting of the American Society for Bariatric Surgery, Nashville, 1989.